Clinical Diabetes Mellitus
A Problem-Oriented Approach

THIRD EDITION

Clinical Diabetes Mellitus
A Problem-Oriented Approach

THIRD EDITION

John K. Davidson, M.D., Ph.D.

Professor of Medicine Emeritus
Emory University School of Medicine
Founding Director, Diabetes Unit
Grady Memorial Hospital
Atlanta, Georgia

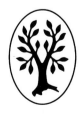

2000
Thieme
New York • Stuttgart

Thieme New York
333 Seventh Avenue
New York, NY 10001

Editor: Andrea Seils
Editorial Director: Ave McCracken
Editorial Assistant: Michelle Carini
Developmental Manager: Kathleen P. Lyons
Director, Production and Manufacturing: Anne Vinnicombe
Production Editor: Janice G. Stangel
Marketing Director: Phyllis Gold
Sales Manager: Ross Lumpkin
Chief Financial Officer: Seth S. Fishman
President: Brian D. Scanlan
Cover Designer: Tony Scarlatos
Compositor: Prepare
Printer: Canale

Library of Congress Cataloging-in-Publication Data

Clinical diabetes mellitus: a problem oriented approach / [edited by] John K.
Davidson. — 3rd ed.
    p.   cm.
  Includes bibliographical references and index.
  ISBN 0-86577-840-X
  1. Diabetes. I. Davidson, John K.
  [DNLM: 1. Diabetes Mellitus. WK 810 C64081 1999]
  RC660 .C459 1999
  616.4'62 21—dc21

                                                      99-042914

Important note: Medical knowledge is ever-changing. As new research and clinical experience broaden our
knowledge, changes in treatment and drug therapy may be required. The authors and editors of the material
herein have consulted sources believed to be reliable in their efforts to provide information that is complete and
in accord with the standards accepted at the time of publication. However, in view of the possibility of human
error by the authors, editors, or publisher of the work herein, or changes in medical knowledge, neither the
authors, editors, publisher, nor any other party who has been involved in the preparation of this work, warrants
that the information contained herein is in every respect accurate or complete, and they are not responsible for
any errors or omissions or for the results obtained from use of such information. Readers are encouraged to
confirm the information contained herein with other sources. For example, readers are advised to check the
product information sheet included in the package of each drug they plan to administer to be certain that the
information contained in this publication is accurate and that changes have not been made in the recommended
dose or in the contraindications for administration. This recommendation is of particular importance in
connection with new or infrequent used drugs.

Some of the product names, patents, and registered designs referred to in this book are in fact registered
trademarks or proprietary names even though specific reference to this fact is not always made in the text.
Therefore, the appearance of a name without designation as proprietary is not to be construed as a
representation by the publisher that it is in the public domain.

Printed in Italy

5 4 3 2 1

TNY ISBN 0-86577-840-X
GTV ISBN 3-13-117681-4

Dedication

The third edition of *Clinical Diabetes Mellitus: A Problem-Oriented Approach* is dedicated with profound gratitude to the inspired research, teaching, and leadership of Charley Best, co-discoverer of insulin with Fred Banting in August, 1921.

I had the pleasure of working with Dr. Best as a Ph.D. student (1960–1965) and as an assistant and associate professor of physiology (1965–1968). Charley and his colleagues taught me how to do research, how to teach, and how to provide excellent clinical care to those who have diabetes mellitus.

During our eight years in Toronto, Dr. and Mrs. Best and Bebe, I, and our children spent much time together. We celebrated two of Dr. Best's birthdays in our home and visited their home in Schooner Cove, Maine.

Charley became famous just as he was entering medical school at the University of Toronto. In 1925 he graduated as the Gold Medalist, and in 1929 on the recommendation of J.J.R. MacLeod he became Chairman of the Department of Physiology. He remained active until 1968, conversing with faculty and students about their research while drinking coffee with them in the morning and tea with them in the afternoon.

Charley died in 1978 "after a distinguished career, known, loved, and revered by millions of diabetics all over the world" (quote from Dr. Barbara Hazlett, Chapter 1). And as we remember, Barbara, "known, loved, and revered" who he befriended and trained to become academic diabetologists.

Contents

A.M. Albisser, Ph.D.
Professor of Medicine
BCMC Better Control Medical Computers, Inc.
Director of Disease Management
Miami Beach, Florida

James H. J. Anderson, M.D.
Clinical Associate Professor
Indiana University School of Medicine
Medical Advisor
Diabetes Care and Endocrinology
Eli Lilly Research Laboratories
Eli Lilly and Company
Indianapolis, Indiana

Kathryn Arnold
Infectious Disease Epidemiologist
Georgia Division of Public Health
Department of Human Resources
Atlanta, Georgia

Judy Ashworth, M.D.
Guest Investigator
Sansum Medical Research Foundation
Santa Barbara, California

Jean-Philippe Assal, M.D.
Professor of Medicine
Chief, Diabetes Treatment and Teaching Unit
Hopital Cantonal Universitaire, and
Director, WHO Collaborating Centre
Geneva, Switzerland

David J. Ballard, M.D., Ph.D., F.A.C.P.
Professor of Medicine
Emory University
Atlanta, Georgia

Brian Beauchamp
Account Executive
Mitchell Martin, Inc.
New York, New York

David S.H. Bell, M.B.
Professor of Medicine
Department of Medicine
The University of Alabama at Birmingham
Birmingham, Alabama

Michael Berger, M.D., Ph.D.
Professor of Medicine
Department of Metabolic Diseases and Nutrition
(WHO Collaborating Center for Diabetes)
Heinrich-Heine University Düsseldorf
Düsseldorf, Germany

William G. Blackard, M.D.*
Professor of Medicine
Chairman, Division of Endocrinology
Virginia Commonwealth University
Medical College of Virginia
Richmond, Virginia

Peter C. Butler, M.D.
Professor of Medicine
Department of Endocrinology
University of Southern California
Los Angeles, California

Ronald E. Chance, B.S., M.S., Ph.D.
Eli Lilly Research Laboratories
Eli Lilly and Company
Indianapolis, Indiana

Steven D. Chessler, M.D., Ph.D.
Senior Fellow
Department of Medicine
Division of Metabolism,
Endocrinology and Nutrition
University of Washington,
R.H. Williams Laboratory
Seattle, Washington

John N. Clore, M.D.
Professor of Medicine
Division of Endocrinology
Department of Internal Medicine
Medical College of Virginia/Virginia
Commonwealth University
Richmond, Virginia

William C. Coleman, D.P.M.
Podiatry Section Head
Department of Orthopedics
Ochsner Clinic
New Orleans, Louisiana

* Deceased

John A. Colwell, M.D., Ph.D.
Professor of Medicine
Department of Medicine
Medical University of South Carolina
Charleston V.A. Medical Center
Charleston, South Carolina

Gerald R. Cooper, M.D., Ph.D.
Medical Officer
Division of Laboratory Science
National Center for Environmental Health,
  Centers for Disease Control and
  Prevention (CDC)
Atlanta, Georgia

Catherine C. Cowie, Ph.D.
Director, Type 1 Diabetes Clinical
  Trials Program
National Institute of Diabetes,
  Endocrinology, and Metabolic Diseases
National Institutes of Health, NIDDK
Bethesda, Maryland

Barbara S. Daniels, M.D.
Associate Professor of Medicine
Department of Medicine
University of Minnesota
Minneapolis, Minnesota

John K. Davidson, M.D., Ph.D.
Emeritus Professor of Medicine
Emory University School of Medicine, and
Founding Director, Diabetes Unit
Grady Memorial Hospital
Atlanta, Georgia

Mario Di Girolamo, M.D.
Professor of Medicine
Professor of Physiology
Emory School of Medicine
Grady Memorial Hospital
Emory University Hospital (CRC)
Atlanta, Georgia

Richard C. Eastman, M.D.
Director, Division of Diabetes,
  Endocrinology, and Metabolic Diseases
National Institute of Diabetes,
  Endocrinology, and Metabolic Diseases
National Institutes of Health, NIDDK
Bethesda, Maryland

S.C. En Chao, MASc
Systems Director
BCMC Better Control Medical
  Computers, Inc.
Miami Beach, Florida

Michael M. Engelgau, M.D., M.S.
Chief, Epidemiology and Statistics Branch
Division of Diabetes Translation
National Center for Chronic Disease
  Prevention and Health Promotion
Centers for Disease Control and Prevention
Atlanta, Georgia

Judith Fradkin, M.D.
Deputy Director, Endocrinologist
National Institute of Diabetes,
  Endocrinology, and Metabolic Diseases
National Institutes of Health, NIDDK
Bethesda, Maryland

Michael E. Fritz, D.D.S, M.S., Ph.D.
Charles Howard Candler Professor
  of Dental Medicine
Department of Surgery
Emory University
Atlanta, Georgia

Steven G. Gabbe, M.D
Chairman
Department of Obstetrics and Gynecology
University of Washington
Seattle, Washington

Sanford A. Garfield, Ph.D.
Senior Advisor for Biometry and
  Behavioral Research
National Institute of Diabetes,
  Endocrinology, and Metabolic Diseases
National Institutes of Health, NIDDK
Bethesda, Maryland

Leonard C. Glass, M.D.
Resident, Department of Medicine
University of Texas Health Science Center
  at San Antonio, Texas
San Antonio, Texas

Frederick C. Goetz, M.D.
Professor (Emeritus)
Department of Medicine
University of Minnesota
Minneapolis, Minnesota

Dorothy Gohdes, M.D.
Director
Indian Health Service Diabetes Program
Albuquerque, New Mexico

John H. Graham, IV, B.A.
Chief Executive Officer
American Diabetes Association
Alexandria, Virginia

Sara G. Grossi, D.D.S, M.S.
Associate Professor, Oral Biology
State University of New York
Buffalo, New York

Angelika Gruessner, Ph.D.
Research Associate
Department of Surgery
University of Minnesota
Minneapolis, Minnesota

Rainer W.G. Gruessner, M.D., Ph.D.
Professor of Surgery
Department of Surgery
University of Minnesota
Minneapolis, Minnesota

George Grunberger, M.D., F.A.C.P.
Henry L. Brasza Professor and Director
Center for Molecular Medicine and Genetics
Professor, Department of Internal Medicine
Director, Diabetes Program
Wayne State University School of Medicine/
  Detroit Medical Center
Detroit, Michigan

Thomas M. Guest, M.D.
Fellow in Cardiology
Division of Cardiology, Emory University
Atlanta, Georgia

W. Dallas Hall, M.D., M.R.C.P.
Emeritus Professor of Medicine
Department of Medicine
Emory University School of Medicine
Atlanta, Georgia

William D. Hammonds, M.D.
Associate Professor of Anesthesiology
Department of Anesthesiology—Center for Pain
  Medicine
Emory University School of Medicine
Atlanta, Georgia

Joan T. Harmon, Ph.D.
Senior Advisor for Diabetes
National Institute of Diabetes, Endocrinology,
  and Metabolic Diseases
National Institutes of Health, NIDDK
Bethesda, Maryland

Maureen I. Harris, Ph.D.
Director, Diabetes Epidemiology Program
National Institute of Diabetes, Endocrinology,
  and Metabolic Diseases
National Institutes of Health, NIDDK
Bethesda, Maryland

Michael D. Harris, M.D.
Clinical Associate Professor of Medicine
Department of Endocrinology
UCLA School of Medicine/
  Cedars-Sinai Medical Center
Beverly Hills, California

Ronald I. Harris, M.D.
Clinical Programs Director
Penn. State Geisinger Health Systems
Wilkes-Barre, Pennsylvania

Barbara E. Hazlett, M.D., F.R.C.P.(C)
Retired
Elora, Ontario, Canada

William H. Herman, M.D., M.P.H.
Associate Professor of Medicine and Epidemiology
Department of Internal Medicine
  University of Michigan
Ann Arbor, Michigan

Edwin Hobgood, B.S., D.P.M.
Assistant Professor of Medicine
Department of Endocrinology
Emory University School of Medicine
Podiatrist, Diabetes Unit (Retired)
Grady Memorial Hospital
Atlanta, Georgia

Nancy M. Holekamp, M.D.
Clinical Assistant Professor
Department of Ophthalmology and Visual Sciences
Washington University School of Medicine
St. Louis, Missouri

William D. James, M.D.
Professor of Dermatology
Department of Dermatology
University of Pennsylvania
Philadelphia, Pennsylvania

Jak Jervell, Ph.D.
Professor of Medicine
Department of Medicine
Oslo University
Oslo, Norway

Viktor Jörgens, M.D.
Executive Director
European Association for Study of Diabetes
Düsseldorf, Germany

Lois Jovanovic, M.D.
Director and Chief Scientific Officer
Sansum Medical Research Institute
Clinical Professor of Medicine, USC.
Santa Barbara, California

Hilary King, M.D.
Medical Officer Responsible for Diabetes
World Health Organization
Geneva, Switzerland

Mark B. Landon, M.D.
Associate Professor and Vice-Chairman
Department of Obstetrics and Gynecology
The Ohio State College of Medicine
Columbus, Ohio

Ake Lernmark, D.Sc.
Robert H. Williams Professor
Department of Medicine
University of Washington
Seattle, Washington

Marvin E. Levin, M.D.
Professor of Clinical Medicine
Department of Internal Medicine
Washington University School of Medicine
St. Louis, Missouri

Errol Marliss, M.D., F.R.C.P.(C)
Professor of Medicine
McGill Nutrition Center
Royal Victoria Hospital
Montreal, Quebec, Canada

Ruchi Mathur, M.D.
Clinical Instructor
Department of Endocrinology and Metabolism
Cedars-Sinai Medical Center
Los Angeles, California

John E. McGowan, Jr., M.D.
Professor of Pathology and Laboratory
  Medicine
Emory University School of Medicine, and
Director, Clinical Microbiology
Grady Memorial Hospital
Atlanta, Georgia

Malachi J. McKenna, M.D., M.R.C.P.I.
Robert and Jane Gurwin Research
Diabetologist, Division of Endocrinology and
  Metabolism
Henry Ford Hospital
Detroit, Michigan

John A. McKnight, M.D., F.R.C.P.
Consultant Physician/Honorary Senior Lecturer
Diabetes Centre
Western Central Hospital
United Kingdom

Donald E. McMillian, A.E., M.D.
Professor Emeritus of Internal Medicine
University of South Florida
Tampa, Florida

Curtis L. Meinert, Ph.D.
Professor of Epidemiology and Biostatistics
The Johns Hopkins University
School of Hygiene and Public Health
Baltimore, Maryland

Travis A. Meredith, M.D.
Clinical Professor of Ophthalmology
Washington University School of Medicine
St. Louis, Missouri

Boyd E. Metzger , M.D.
Professor of Medicine
Department of Medicine
Division of Endocrinology
Northwestern University
Chicago, Illinois

John Mills, Ph.D.
Professor of Biochemistry Emeritus
Department of Biochemistry
Emory University School of Medicine
Atlanta, Georgia

Richard E. Mullins, B.S., Ph.D.
Associate Professor
Department of Pathology and
  Laboratory Medicine
Emory University Hospital
Atlanta, Georgia

Dara Murphy, M.P.H.
Chief, Program Development Branch
Division of Diabetes Translation
National Center for Chronic Disease Prevention
  and Health Promotion Centers for Disease
  Control and Prevention
Atlanta, Georgia

Gary L. Myers, Ph.D.
Chief, Special Activities Branch
Division of Laboratory Sciences
National Center for Environmental Health,
  Centers for Disease Control and Prevention
Atlanta, Georgia

Steven Offenbacher, D.D.S., Ph.D., M.M.Sc.
Professor
Department of Periodontics
School of Dentistry
University of North Carolina at Chapel Hill
Chapel Hill, North Carolina

Donald R. Parker, Ph.D., DABCC, P.A.C.D.
Director
Clinical Trials/Clinical Research
Bayer Corporation
Elkhart, Indiana

I.D. Parson, M.A.Sc., Ph.D.
Production Director
BCMC Better Control Medical Computers, Inc.
Miami Beach, Florida

Charles M. Peterson, M.D.
Clinical Professor
University of Southern California, and
Director of Research
Sansum Medical Research Foundation
Santa Barbara, California

Michael Poon, M.D.
Assistant Professor of Medicine
Department of Medicine/Cardiovascular Institute
Mount Sinai School of Medicine
New York, New York

Thaddeus E. Prout, M.D., F.A.C.P.
Associate Professor Emeritus
Department of Medicine
The Johns Hopkins Hospital
Baltimore, Maryland

Lisa P. Purdy, M.D., C.M., M.P.H.
Assistant Professor of Medicine
Department of Medicine
Division of Endocrinology and Metabolism
University of Rochester
Rochester, New York

Marvin L. Rallison, B.S., M.D., F.A.C.E.
Professor of Pediatrics
Chief, Division of Pediatric Endocrinology
University of Utah Health Sciences Center
Salt Lake City, Utah

Elliot J. Rayfield, M.D.
Clinical Professor of Medicine
Department of Medicine
Division of Endocrinology and Medicine
Mount Sinai School of Medicine
New York, New York

Janice M.T. Redmond, M.B., B.Ch., M.R.C.P.I.
Fellow in Clinical Neurophysiology Research
Department of Neurology
Henry Ford Hospital
Detroit, Michigan

Bernd Richter, M.D.
Research Associate, Clinical Pharmacology
Department of Metabolic Diseases and Nutrition
(WHO Collaborating Center for Diabetes)
Heinrich-Heine University Düsseldorf
Germany

Carol Rodgers, Ph.D.
Associate Professor of Exercise Metabolism
 and Physiology
Faculty of Physical Health and Education
University of Toronto
Toronto, Ontario, Canada

Jesse Roth , M.D.
President and Chief Executive Officer
Professor, The Picower Graduate School of
Molecular Medicine
Director, Laboratory of Diabetes and Aging
Picower Institute for Medical Research
Manhasset, New York

S. Sakkal, M.D.
Metabolic Care Center
Greenville, Pennsylvania

Atef A. Salam, M.D.
Professor of Surgery
Department of Vascular Surgery
Emory University Hospital
Atlanta, Georgia

Eric J. Sampson, Ph.D.
Director, Division of Laboratory Sciences
National Centers for Disease Control
 and Prevention
Atlanta, Georgia

Dawn W. Satterfield, RN, M.S.N., A.N.P., C.D.E
Centers for Disease Control
Division of Diabetes Translation
Health Education Consultant, and
Former Professional Course Coordinator
Grady Memorial Hospital, Diabetes Unit
Atlanta, Georgia

Robert Schwartz, M.D.
Professor of Pediatrics and Medical Sciences
Brown University, and
Pediatrician (Senior), Rhode Island Hospital
Providence, Rhode Island

Joe V. Selby, M.D., M.P.H.
Director, Division of Research
Kaiser Permanente Medical Care Program
Oakland, California

Jin-Xiong She, Ph.D.
Associate Professor
Department of Pathology
University of Florida
Gainesville, Florida

Shobana Sood, M.D.
Assistant Professor of Dermatology
Department of Dermatology
University of Pennsylvania
Philadelphia, Pennsylvania

Russell Swiegowski, M.P.H.
Chief, Health Systems Section
Division of Diabetes Translation
Centers for Disease Control and Prevention
Atlanta, Georgia

Jean-Pierre Sorensen, M.D.
International Marketing Director
Customer Relations/ Market Development
Novo Nordisk A/S
Bagsvaerd, Denmark

Laurence S. Sperling, M.D.
Assistant Professor of Medicine
Medical Director of Preventive Cardiology
Emory University School of Medicine
Atlanta, Georgia

George Steiner, BA, M.D.
Professor of Medicine and Physiology
Department of Medicine
Toronto General Hospital/
  University of Toronto
Toronto, Ontario, Canada

David E.R. Sutherland, M.D., Ph.D.
Professor
Department of Surgery
University of Minnesota Hospital
Minneapolis, Minnesota

Bix E. Swain, M.S.
Consultant, Division of Research
Kaiser Permanente Medical Care Program
Oakland, California

Frank Vinicor, M.D., M.P.H.
Director, Division of Diabetes Translation
Centers for Disease Control and Prevention
Atlanta, Georgia

Aaron I. Vinik, M.D., Ph.D., F.C.P., F.A.C.P
Professor of Internal Medicine, Anatomy, and
  Neurobiology
Director, The Strelitz Diabetes Research Institutes
Eastern Virginia Medical School
Norfolk, Virginia

Mladen Vranic, M.D., D.Sc., F.R.C.P.(C), F.R.S.C.
Professor of Physiology and Medicine
Department of Physiology
University of Toronto
Toronto, Ontario, Canada

John Ward, M.D.
Professor of Medicine
University of Sheffield
United Kingdom

Joseph Webb, M.D.
Assistant Professor of Anesthesiology
Department of Anesthesiology
Emory University School of Medicine
Atlanta, Georgia

William S. Weintraub, M.D.
Professor of Medicine
Department of Cardiology
Emory University
Atlanta, Georgia

Charles A. Wells, Ph.D.
Senior Advisor for Diabetes Prevention
National Institute of Diabetes,
  Endocrinology, and Metabolic Diseases
National Institutes of Health, NIDDK
Bethesda, Maryland

Fred W. Whitehouse, M.D.
Division Head, Emeritus
Division of Endocrinology and Metabolism
Henry Ford Hospital
Detroit, Michigan

C.H. Wilson, Jr., M.D.*
Professor of Medicine
Founder of the Division of Rheumatology
Emory University School of Medicine
Atlanta, Georgia

W. Hayes Wilson, M.D.
Chief of Rheumatology
Piedmont Medical Clinic
Piedmont Hospital
Atlanta, Georgi

* Deceased

Preface to the Third Edition

Since the second edition of this book was published in 1991, a number of changes have occurred in the field of diabetes mellitus.

In 1997 *new diagnostic criteria* were introduced by an American Diabetes Association Expert Committee. It defined non-gestational diabetes mellitus as *impaired fasting plasma glucose* ≥ 126 mg/dl or 7.0 mmol/l or random plasma glucose ≥ 200 mg/dl or 11.1 mmol/l plus symptoms. The committee discouraged the use of the glucose tolerance test. This recommendation has been severely criticized by the European Diabetes Epidemiology Study Group. No changes for the diagnosis of gestational diabetes were recommended. Typing was changed: IDDM is now type 1, NIDDM is now type 2, GDM remains GDM. Each type has its subtypes.

Methods of monitoring metabolic control by the patient have improved with the availability of better monitors, data-management systems, finger-sticking devices, and glycohemoglobin measurements. Beginning in 1999, Medicare will pay for prescribed monitoring supplies and patient education by a team of diabetes professionals (MD, RN, RD, DPM, etc.).

In many diabetes centers in the USA and Europe, evaluation, education, and follow-up by a diabetes team are firmly entrenched. Efforts to bridge science with clinical care by widespread data collection and analysis are underway in Europe. Implementation of the recommendations of the St. Vincent Declaration (1989) has already led to a reduction of some of the chronic complications (i.e., lower extremity amputations). Similar efforts to reduce the incidence and prevalence of complications in the USA and world-wide have been initiated by the CDC, NIH, WHO, IDF, and ADA.

Intensive reduced caloric intake (minus 500 to 1000 calories) below that needed to maintain body weight in overweight NIDDMs continues as the preferred initial method of treatment. If hyperglycemia persists, insulin therapy is needed. During 20 years of follow-up in the UKPDS Study of NIDDM, stepped oral agent therapy progressing to insulin therapy failed to attain adequate plasma glucose control.

In the Diabetes Control and Complications Trial (DCCT) in IDDMs, the intensive control group attained better control (mean PG 155 mg/dl, HbA1c 7.2%) than the conventional control group (mean PG 232 mg/dl, HbA1c 9.1%). In the intensive control group, the development and progression of retinopathy, albuminuria, and neuropathy were prevented or delayed. In the intensive control group severe hypoglycemia (coma) occurred more than three times as frequently, and significantly more excess weight was gained.

The DCCT Study has stimulated efforts to improve metabolic control in those with IDDM, and to prevent and control NIDDM and to prevent and delay the development of its complications. New tools are in hand: new human insulins and rapid-acting insulin analogues (LISPRO) and better continuous subcutaneous insulin infusion (CSII) devices. Yet we are still unable to attain and continuously maintain normoglycemia in IDDMs.

NIDDM and obesity have attained epidemic status in the USA and other developed countries in the last two decades, with 10.3 million Americans having diagnosed diabetes (over 95% NIDDMs) and 5.4 million more having undiagnosed NIDDM. For assessment and treatment of overweight and obesity and NIDDM, see Chapters 2 and 16.

One hundred and four contributors joined me in the preparation of the third edition. Each devoted many hours to preparation of his or her sections of the book, and I am most grateful for those efforts. Each chapter and appendix was critiqued by one or more reviewers. I thank each of them for sharing their expertise with the users of the book. An attempt was made to minimize repetition and avoid omission of significant data. Factual errors and failure to record universally accepted significant facts are the responsibility of the editor.

I express my sincere thanks to Dr. Steven Darsey for his help in using a computer to prepare manuscripts.

Thieme Medical Publishers, Inc., has been very supportive during the preparation and production of the third edition. I extend special thanks to Janice Stangel, Production Editor, Anne Vinnicombe, Director of Production and Manufacturing, Thomas Soper and Jennie Kim, Editorial Assistants, and Andrea Siles, Aquisitions Editor.

John K. Davidson, M.D., Ph.D.
Atlanta, Georgia—November 1999

Preface to the Second Edition

Since the first edition of this book was published in 1986, some significant changes have occurred in our understanding of the nature and treatment of diabetes mellitus. Both non-insulin-dependent diabetes mellitus (NIDDM) and insulin-dependent diabetes mellitus (IDDM) have emerged as distinct clinical entities. It is now clear that the most successful method of treatment for the overweight NIDDM is reduced caloric intake with weight loss to ideal body weight. The National Institutes of Health Consensus Conference and the European NIDDM Policy Group have recommended that aggressive diet therapy be implemented as the cornerstone of therapy for those with NIDDM.

Human insulin (rDNA) therapy has been successful, and immunologic resistance, allergy, and lipoatrophy are much less common today than they were 5 years ago. Self-monitoring of blood glucose (SMBG) and measurement of glycated hemoglobin have increased the knowledge of metabolic control levels for patients and the professionals who work with them.

There have been disappointments along the way. It has not been possible to develop a reliable closed-loop portable continuous subcutaneous insulin infusion device that will maintain long-term normoglycemia. The aldose reductase inhibitor drugs, which promised much for the treatment of diabetic neuropathy, have been relatively ineffective and have had some serious (including fatal) side effects.

Considerable progress has been made in the treatment of three of the chronic complications: (1) cataract removal and replacement with a corrective plastic lens for distant vision, laser and vitrectomy therapy with preservation of useful vision; (2) slowing of development of end-stage renal disease by low protein diet and hypertension control with later (if needed) dialysis and transplantation (kidney or kidney plus pancreas); and (3) more successful treatment of atherosclerosis of the carotid, coronary, and leg arteries utilizing bypass surgery and angioplastic procedures.

The NIH Diabetes Data Group criteria for diagnosis of diabetes mellitus and its classification into sub-groups have been generally accepted. I express my sincere thanks to Dr. Maureen Harris, Director of the Diabetes Data Group, NIH, for critiquing Chapter 11, "Screening for Diabetes."

Ninety-two contributors joined me in the preparation of this edition. Each has devoted many hours to the preparation of his or her portions of the book, and for that I am most grateful. Each chapter and appendix was read by at least one other professional, most were read by several. An attempt was made to minimize repetition and omissions. Errors in the citing or recording of universally accepted facts are the responsibility of the editor.

I owe a great deal of gratitude to Shirley Langella, my secretary-administrative assistant for the last 12 years, who not only prepared the revised and new manuscript texts, tables, and exhibits, but also coordinated my research, teaching, and practice schedule as the book contents were being developed.

Many of the figures were drawn by Lee Burns and Dwight Williams, and glossies and color slides were prepared by Eddie Jackson, all of the Department of Medical Illustration, Emory University School of Medicine. The A.W. Calhoun Medical Library of Emory University was the source of most of the journals and books cited in the lists of references.

The publisher, Thieme Medical Publishers, Inc., has been very supportive during the preparation and production of the second edition. I extend special thanks to Hilary Evans, Editor-in-Chief, Kim Wright, Editorial Assistant, Elyse Dubin, Manager of Production and Manufacturing, and Laura Giesman, Production Editor. Betty Hamilton, the copy editor, has been extremely helpful in locating and correcting many typographical and other errors and has relieved me of what was a very stressful chore when the first edition was being prepared.

John K. Davidson, M.D., Ph.D.
Atlanta, Georgia

Preface to the First Edition

The frequently quoted aphorism, "Know diabetes and you know all of medicine" is an exaggeration. Yet it is true that the disease and its complications embrace or relate closely to many other diseases and to many therapeutic modalities and procedures that have been developed during the last 40 years.

Diabetes mellitus has been my primary area of practice and research during this period (1945–1985). In 1978 the decision to write this book was made, and work began in earnest in 1981. About 75 professional colleagues, many of whom are friends of long standing, were invited to write chapters that reflect their expertise. The participation of these individuals has given the book an international flavor, because contributors from the United States have been joined by those from Canada and several European countries.

The problem-oriented format and many of the changes now occurring in the delivery of health care are described in the Introduction and in several of the appendices. The problem-oriented medical record seems to be the most efficient way to deal with the rapidly proliferating facts that continue to expand the knowledge base of epidemiologic, clinical, and basic researchers and practitioners.

With increasing frequency medical practitioners are forming alliances with other professionals who provide education and service for people with diabetes. This approach in turn improves the quality of health care and its cost-effectiveness, and for these reasons this book has highlighted *team care* as an essential component of the delivery of optimal contemporary care.

An attempt has been made to consolidate and index contemporary knowledge of diabetes so that it will be quickly available to the practicing physician and to other health care professionals. The contents have been arranged to facilitate the physician's search for information needed to assess the nature of a patient's problems and their optimal treatment.

In diabetes, there has long been disagreement and controversy over the definition of terms and diagnostic criteria, as well as over the safety and effectiveness of

recommended therapeutic modalities. Not all readers will agree with the definitions and recommendations used in this book (*see* Table 1 in the Introduction). My feeling is that most genuine controversies result from inadequate knowledge. The field of diabetes mellitus is awash with controversies that need to be resolved by carefully designed and executed epidemiologic, clinical, and basic research. After the needed research is completed, most of the controversies almost certainly will recede into the fog of history. Universal agreement will gradually emerge in the use of standardized terms and diagnostic criteria, and on the relative safety and effectiveness of various therapeutic modalities.

In addition to the 75 who contributed to the book, I owe a special debt of gratitude to Peter Bennett who critiqued Chapter 9, "Diagnosis of Diabetes," and to John Galloway and Ron Chance who critiqued and provided additional material for Chapter 16, "Insulin Therapy."

Each chapter was read by at least one other professional; most were read by several. An attempt was made to minimize repetition and omissions. Errors in the citing or recording of universally accepted facts are the responsibility of the Editor.

Without the dedicated work of Tom Sellers, my editorial associate for the last three years, the book would not have been completed. He coordinated with good humor and thoroughness the literature searches, the writing and revising of the text contents, the correspondence with contributors and publisher, and other more mundane activities. I owe a very special debt of gratitude to Tom as well as to Shirley Langella and Betty White who prepared many versions of the manuscript text, tables, and exhibits.

Many of the figures were drawn by Lee Burns of the Emory University School of Medicine, Department of Medical Illustration. James Johnson, Administrative Assistant of the Diabetes Unit of Grady Memorial Hospital, was responsible for the coordination of my research, teaching, and practice schedule as the book contents were being developed. Bonita Bryan of the

A.W. Calhoun Medical Library of Emory University provided invaluable assistance in searching the literature and checking references.

Our publisher, Thieme Inc., has worked with us patiently during production. We extend special thanks to Jill Rudansky, Vice President/Publisher, James Costello, Managing Editor, Alan Fischer, Production Editor, and Joseph Pomerantz, Copy Editor.

John K. Davidson, M.D., Ph.D.
Atlanta, Georgia
August 1985

Introduction

The discovery of insulin 78 years ago and its successful clinical use in 1922 have become benchmarks in the history if medicine.[1] By 1923, it was possible to treat those who were dying of diabetic ketoacidosis (DKA); and to keep them alive for many decades thereafter. Worldwide in 1998, it is estimated that at least 25 million individuals are alive because insulin therapy is available.[2] It should be noted, however, that even though DKA is preventable, over 100,000 cases each year are still hospitalized in the USA alone.[3]

Because of the incidence, prevalence, and costs of the chronic complications of diabetes mellitus, during the last two decades attention has shifted strongly to efforts directed to *primary prevention* (type 2 and type 1 diabetes mellitus) and after diagnosis to *secondary prevention* (of acute and chronic complications) and *tertiary prevention* [prevention or delay of complications leading to morbidity (such as lower extremity amputations, blindness, renal failure, and severe neuropathy), and mortality].

In the last 25 years, there also has been explosive growth of diabetes patient education and follow-up programs.[4-7] In 1998, there were more than 8,000 certified diabetes educators (CDEs), many of whom are RNs and RDs. In addition to teaching individual patients about diet and exercise therapy, CDEs with physician supervision have been very effective in helping patients control their blood (or plasma) glucose and glycosylated hemoglobin (HbA1c) levels. With home self-monitoring of blood glucose (SMBG), individuals can learn to appropriately adjust insulin dose, exercise, and diet.[8] It is estimated that in 1998 over five million individuals own and use blood glucose meters. Recently Medicare announced that it would pay for diabetes education, meters, and monitoring supplies.

In 1997, the American Diabetes Association Expert Committee changed the criteria for diagnosis and typing of diabetes mellitus.[9] Thus non-gestational diabetes was defined as having fasting plasma glucose $\geq$ 126 mg/dl (7.0 mmol/l) $\times$ 2 and impaired fasting plasma glucose $\geq$ 110 mg/dl and < 125 mg/dl (6.0 - 7.0 mmol/l) $\times$ 2. Random plasma glucose > 200 mg/dl (11.1 mmol/l) plus symptoms was defined as diabetes demanding immediate treatment. Use of the glucose tolerance test was discouraged. The European Diabetes Epidemiology Study Group (EASD) has suggested that the recommendations of the ADA Expert Committee are *very unwise* and that the consequences of abandoning the GTT 2-hour glucose level to screen for diabetes needs to be evaluated in many population subgroups.[10] See Chapter 12. Criteria for diagnosis of gestational diabetes mellitus (GDM) remained unchanged.[9] Typing of diabetes was changed: *insulin-dependent diabetes mellitus* (IDDM) became type 1, *non-insulin-dependent diabetes mellitus* (NIDDM) became type 2, GDM remained the same. Each type was divided into subtypes.

Therapy of type 1 consists of insulin plus an appropriate diet to promote normal growth in individuals under 20 years of age (see Chapter 15). Therapy of type 2 diabetes in those who are overweight consists of a reduced energy intake to produce sufficient weight loss to attain normoglycemia.[11-16] If hyperglycemia persists, insulin therapy may be essential. See Chapters 16 and 18.

Two studies (UGDP[17] and UKPDS[18,19]) have generated worries concerning the lack of safety and effectiveness of oral agent (sulfonylureas, metformin, etc.) therapy. Most oral agents are more expensive than insulin therapy. See Chapters 20 and 54.

The diabetes control and complications trial (DCCT)[20-23] evaluated the effect of intensive versus conventional treatment of insulin-dependent diabetes mellitus on the development and progression of long-term complications. Conventional control (mean plasma glucose 232 mg/dl, mean HbA1c 9.1%) versus intensive control (mean plasma glucose about 155 mg/dl, mean HbA1c 7.2%) resulted in intensive control outcomes over a mean follow-up period of about 6.5 years of significant prevention or delay in progression of retinopathy, albuminuria, and neuropathy. *Many individuals are not candidates for intensive insulin therapy* (those less than 7 years of age, many with chronic complications, hypoglycemic unawareness, etc).[24] Family, professional, and financial resources must be available if intensive therapy is to succeed. Even in ideal candidates, severe hypoglycemia is more than three times as common as with conventional therapy, and excess weight gain occurs more frequently.[22]

It has been documented that plasma glucose levels are unsatisfactory in many individuals being treated for diabetes.[25] For example, in three university diabetes clinics, mean fasting plasma glucose levels were 199, 217, and 224 mg/dl. Mean fasting plasma glucose level in the DCCT conventional study group was 232 mg/dl (12.5 mmol/l). Thus if ideal or even adequate control of plasma glucose levels are to be attained and maintained in the general population (see table Intro-1), more successful methods of administering insulin are needed to attain normoglycemia and maintain it without hypoglycemia.

In NIDDMs more attention needs to be directed to the reduction of excess body weight and the treatment of comorbid factors: hypertension, obesity, hyperlipidemia, and smoking.

The intent of the third edition of *Clinical Diabetes Mellitus: A Problem-Oriented Approach* is the same as that of the second edition: to provide easy access to contemporary knowledge of clinical diabetes mellitus for all members of the health care team. Thousands of users of the second edition have informed the editor that this objective was achieved. The contents of the third edition are divided into seven sections containing 55 chapters (four new) and 12 appendices (one new). Each has been completely rewritten or extensively revised. Of the 66 chapters and appendices, more than three-fourths are in the problem-oriented format. This format was not appropriate for 14 chapters and appendices. Exhibit Intro-1 outlines the POMR approach.

The Problem-Oriented Medical Record (POMR)

In 1918, Codman[26] hypothesized that complete, carefully maintained hospital records would improve efficiency, but his suggestion was not accepted by his peers. The problem-oriented approach to medical record keeping and to the planning of initial and follow-up evaluation, education, and therapy was introduced in 1968 by Weed.[27,28] It has been shown to be of outstanding value in clinical care, teaching, and research by Hurst and his colleagues.[29,30] In 1998 it is accepted as the most efficient method for the systematic collection of a defined data base using a problem-oriented diabetes mellitus dictionary. It simplifies record-keeping and the complete follow-up of individuals and groups with a chronic disease or diseases over a long period of time. See Exibits Intro-2 and Intro-3, Appendices VII and VIII. The POMR is computer-compatible and facilitates the collection, storage, retrieval, analysis, and assessment of data for both individuals and groups. It can increase the accuracy of diagnoses, differential diagnoses, decision-tree analyses related to processes of care and statistical probabilities of outcomes. The POMR facilitates the monitoring of the safety and effectiveness of alternative therapeutic modalities.

Major US organizations interested in diabetes mellitus have set up websites which are listed in Exhibit Intro-4.

The Team Approach to Patient Evaluation, Education, and Follow-up

In the last 25 years, physicians have joined forces with nurses, dietitians, podiatrists, social workers, and others to improve the care of those with diabetes. This has been designated the *team approach*[4-7] and it has become increasingly popular in developed countries. It was a critical component of the DCCT study.[20-24] This book takes the view that the *team approach* is an essential element in the provision of optimal contemporary diabetes care.

EXHIBIT INTRO–1   Outline of Book Chapter Format

Historical Perspective
How did our knowledge get from there (none) to here (present)?
Epidemiology
What do we know about the prevalence (number of cases in a defined population), incidence (number of new cases in a defined period of time, normally 1 year, in a defined population), etiology, and natural history of diabetes mellitus and of its complications (yearly increase or decrease in a defined population), in various population groups classified by age, sex, race, duration of diagnosed diabetes, and geographic distribution? What do we know about correlating diabetes with excess body weight, genetic background, etc.?
Pathophysiology
What is our present knowledge of the whole body, organ, tissue, cell, biochemical, immunologic, and other abnormalities of diabetes mellitus and its acute and chronic complications?
The Problem-Oriented Medical Record
See Exhibits 2 and 3.
Patient Adherence (or Lack of Adherence) to Therapy
What factors exert an influence and how can they be modified?
Audits of Data
Identify and correct deficiencies. Appropriately revise therapeutic strategy. How can we improve what we have been doing (in terms of mortality, morbidity, costs)?
Author's Summary of Research
Perspectives on current and future research that may increase knowledge and that may lead to better therapeutic modalities oriented toward prevention, improved metabolic control, and/or cure of diabetes mellitus.

TABLE INTRO–1 Some Diagnostic Terms and Criteria Used in CDM:POA (3)

Term	Criteria
I. Diagnosis DM (after 1997)	**Non-gestational**
Research in progress to evaluate new criteria	DM = FPG ≥126 mg/dl × 2 or GTT (2hr) >200 mg/dl × 2 or RPG >200 mg/dl + symptoms
	IGM = IFG = 110-125 mg/dl
	$IGTT$ = 2 hr ≥140 and <200 mg/dl
See Chapters 40, 41	*Normoglycemia* = FPG <110 mg/dl GTT 2 hr <140 mg/dl
	Gestational
	GDM if GTT (100 gm) 2 levels above upper normal limits:
	FIOS, 1 hr/90, 2 hr 165, 3 hr 145 mg/dl
Diagnosis DM (before 1997)	
See Chapter 12	
II. Screening for DM	**Non-gestational**
See Chapter 11	Note upper normal limits above of FPG, RPG, and GTT; random urine glucose ≤25 mg/dl
See Chapters 40,41	**Gestational**
	If PG 1 hr after 50 gm glucose load >140 mg/dl, do 100 gm glucose GTT as above
III. Typing DM (after 1997)	Type 1 preferred to IDDM (Insulin-Dependent Diabetes Mellitus)
Subtypes being characterized by genetic and other research methods	Type 2 preferred to NIDDM (Non-Insulin Dependent Diabetes Mellitus)
	Gestational Diabetes Mellitus (GDM)
See Chapters 2, 3, 4, 5, 8, 9, 10	
IV. Acute Complications	
See Chapter 24	
DKA	Metabolic acidosis: hyperglycemia, ketonemia
Mild	CO_2 21–28 mEq/l, pH >7.30
Moderate	CO_2 11–20 mEq/l, pH 7.10–7.30
Severe	CO_2 ≤10 mEq/l, pH <7.10
HHS	>350 mOsm/kg serum
DKA + HHS	Any level of metabolic acidosis plus serum osmolality >350 mOsm/kg
V. Chronic Complications	
Macrovascular	Premature arterial disease
See Chapters 28, 29, 30, 34, 38, 39	
Microvascular	Premature capillary disease
See Chapter 26	
Kidney	Nephropathy
See Chapter 27	
Nervous system	Neuropathy
Peripheral	
See Chapters 35, 37	
Autonomic	
See Chapter 36	
VI. Hypoglycemia	
Exogenous	PG <60 mg/dl on insulin, sulfonylurea, other drugs, toxins
See Chapters 18 and 20	
Endogenous	
Fasting	PG <50 mg/dl
Reactive	PG <40 mg/dl with parallel symptoms at NADIR during 6 hr GTT
See Chapter 12	

VII. Desirable levels*† of Plasma Glucose and HbA1c Control

	Fasting	*mg/dl (mm)*	*1 hr PPPG mg/dl (mm)*	*HbA1c*
For mild DM				
Ideal		<110 (6.0)	<110 (6.0)	≤5%
Adequate		<130 (7.2)	<170 (9.4)	≤6%
Inadequate		>130 (7.2)	>170 (9.4)	>7%
For severe diabetes				
Ideal		≤110 (6.0)	≤110 (6.0)	≤5%
Adequate		≤170 (9.4)	≤170 (9.4)	≤7%
Inadequate		>170 (9.4)	>170 (9.4)	>8%
		2 hr after 100 gm CHO meal		
Normal (+ 2SD)		94 (119) mg/dl	105 (152) mg/dl	4–5%
See Chapters 12 and 18				

† Inferred by Molnar and DCCT† studies references 52 and 24.

EXHIBIT INTRO–2   The Strategy of Collecting a Defined Data Base and of Contructing a Problem-Oriented Medical Record (POMR) for Those with Diabetes Mellitus

1. **Problem Statement**
   A statement of the problem as defined in a Problem Dictionary
   A. *Subjective*: symptoms, personal and family history, review of systems
   B. *Objective*: physical and/or laboratory abnormalities that may be present
   C. *Assessment*: criteria for establishing the presence or absence of the problem (the diagnosis). What is the sensitivity, specificity, and predictive value of present accepted diagnostic criteria? What other problems (disease processes) should be considered in the differential diagnosis, and how should they be diagnosed or excluded?
   D. *Plan*:
      • *Therapy*: What is the selected therapy versus the alternative therapies that might have been selected? What are the benefits, risks, and costs of each?
      • *Education*: Patient and family, qualifications of professional teachers, standards of programs, available teaching aides
      • *Consultation and Cooperation with Other Professionals*: the team concept of primary care: physician (family practitioner, internist, pediatrician, etc.), dietitian, nurse, podiatrist, social worker, and others. Consult physicians (diabetologists, endocrinologists, ophthalmologists, nephrologists, cardiologists, urologists, cardiovascular surgeons, etc.)
      • *Follow-up*: MD(s) only or team: Are continuity and continuing access assured?

   • *Outcomes*: (Automatically follow process[es]) (mortality, morbidity, individual, group). Two elements contribute: (1) natural history of the disease as it would evolve if it were untreated (standard mortality and morbidity indices); (2) change in mortality and morbidity indices as a result of therapy or therapies that are used. If a study is to be without bias, (1) it should have an appropriately selected control group; (2) it should be prospective (rather than retrospective); (3) patients should be randomly assigned to the treatment (drug [procedure] or placebo [mock procedure]) group; (4) the study should be double blind (neither investigator nor patient know whether patient is on drug or placebo); and (5) a plan for the proper design for appropriate statistical analysis of the results should be built into the study design before it is started.

   A drug or any other intervention therapy has the potential to be safe or unsafe, therapeutically effective or ineffective, and cost-effective or ineffective. Ideally, outcomes in a control group (the natural history in the untreated group) should be compared to the outcomes in the treated group (drug or procedure) to determined safety and/or effectiveness, including morbidity (adverse drug and procedure reactions), mortality (increased or decreased length of life).

2. **Audit**
   Evaluation of outcomes and correction of deficiencies in processes of care.

EXHIBIT INTRO–3   The Procedures for Collecting a Defined Data Base and for Assessing a Complete Problem-Oriented Medical Record (POMR) for Those with Diabetes Mellitus

1. **Problem Statement**—A statement of the problem as defined in a Problem Dictionary.
2. **Defined Data Base—(see Appendix VI)**
   A. Subjective (History) —43 elements (1–43)
   B. Objective
      (1) Physical, 22 elements (44-65)
      (2) ECG, one element (66)
      (3) Dietetic evaluation, education, and plan, seven elements (67-73)
      (4) Laboratory evaluation, eight elements (81–88)
      (5) Podiatry evaluation, education, and plan, seven elements (74-80)
3. **Assessment of Data Base**—List each problem on the complete problem list, and assess it at its highest level of reso-

   lution that available data permit. Plan appropriate additional data collection to provide eventually the highest possible level of problem resolution.
4. **Plan for Patient Education and Therapy**—See patient checklist
   A. Initial: See Appendix VI and VIIa
   B. Follow-up
      (1) See Appendices VIIb, VIIc, VIId, VIIe
      (2) Complications: Diagnosis, evaluation, and therapy
5. **Audit**
   See Appendix VIIf and VIIg for adult forms for (1) diabetic ketoacidosis (DKA) and the hyperglycemic hyperosmolar state (HHS) and (2) lower extremity amputations.

The St. Vincent Initiative

The St. Vincent Declaration for care and research in diabetes was formulated in 1989 in St. Vincent, Italy, at a meeting attended by people with diabetes, health care professionals, government representatives, and industry.[31] Its impact on the quality of diabetes care already has been significant in many European countries.[32] The St. Vincent Group plans a 10th anniversary meeting for 1999. See Appendix XI.

EXHIBIT INTRO–4   Major USA Organizations Interested in Diabetes Mellitus and their Web Sites

American Association of Diabetes Educators (AADE):
    http://www.diabetesnet.com/aade.html
American Diabetes Association (ADA):
    http://www.diabetes.org
Centers for Disease Control and Prevention (CDCP):
    http://www.cdc.gov/diabetes
Department of Veterans Affairs (DVA):
    http://www.va.gov/health/diabetes
Health Resources and Services Administration (HRSA):
    http://www.hrsa.dhhs.gov
Indian Health Service (IHS):
    http://www.ihs.gov/IHSMAIN.html

Juvenile Diabetes Foundation International (JDFI):
    http://www.jdfcure.com
National Diabetes Educational Program (NDEP):
    Internet page under construction
National Institute of Diabetes and Digestive and Kidney Diseases (NIDDK) and National Institutes of Health (NIH):
    http://www.niddk.nih.gov
U.S. Department of Health and Human Services (US DHHS) and Office of Minority Health (OMH):
    http://www.omrhc.gov
American Dietetic Association:
    http://www.eatright.org

The Genesis and Trajectory of the American Health Care System

In 1974 Freymann described the genesis and trajectory of the American Health Care System.[33] He contended that the attitudes of physicians and the organization and operation of hospitals were still turned largely toward the past. He felt that the education of health professionals was just beginning to free itself of 19th-century traditions which shackled it to the *crisis-oriented approach* of that era. He advocated a *preventive approach to chronic diseases with early diagnosis and optimal treatment* in ambulatory care facilities to decrease the impact of crisis-induced hospitalizations.

Until less than 200 years ago, medical practice was dominated by folkways and religious beliefs that had evolved over thousands of years.[34] The decisive step that permitted a systematic response to disease, usually an infectious disease epidemic, occurred in the 19th century when the forerunners of modern hospitals and medical schools were organized in Europe. One result was that during an 1883 epidemic in Egypt, Robert Koch discovered the cholera bacillus. By 1893 a vaccine to combat the desease had been developed. Since that time the infectious nature of many other diseases has been established. Vaccines to prevent many of them, and antibiotics and chemotherapeutic agents to cure others, have been developed. One disease (small pox) has been eradicated, and public health programs with the aim of eradicating others are in progress.

A number of European physicians, including Bouchardat, Naunyn, and VonNoorden, had a special interest in diabetes treatment (primarily dietary) before the turn of the 20th century. In the same year (1893) that the cholera vaccine was used to control an epidemic, Elliot Joslin in Boston saw his first diabetes patient.[35] Yet the hormone (insulin) that could have controlled that patient's blood glucose did not become available until 29 years later. By that time, the almost inevitably fatal outcome of diabetic coma was well known.

In recent years, great emphasis has been placed on primary, secondary, and tertiary prevention and eventual cure of diabetes mellitus and its complications.

Disease and Procedure Coding (ICD-9-CM), Diagnosis-Related Groups (DRGs), and Prospective Payment Systems (PPS)

Coding for diabetes mellitus and diabetes-related disease categories is shown in Appendix IXa, for diabetes drug-related adverse reactions in IXb, and for procedures frequently carried out for diabetes and its complications in Appendix IXc.[36] ICD-9-CM categories are used in assigning hospitalized patients to diagnosis-related groups (DRGs), which in turn play an important role in the calculation of prospective payments (PPS) to hospitals by Medicare, Medicaid, and other third party payers (Appendix X). It has been suggested that ICD-9-CM may be replaced by ICD-10-CM in the year 2000.

Changes in Health Care Delivery and its Financing in the 1990s

The estimated one trillion dollar health care industry in the USA has undergone radical restructuring during the decade of the 1990s. Actions of federal and state governments, of corporate America, and of third-party payers have had a dramatic effect on the way health care is delivered and financed.[37-40]

Traditional *fee-for-service* medical care has been replaced by alternative methods of payment in which Medicare, Medicaid, HMOs, PPOs, and others establish hospital and physician payment (or denial of payment) schedules and *almost always without hospital or physician agreement.*

Hospitalization is eliminated or severely restricted by required *preadmission certification for an approved diagnosis or procedure* and *limitations of length of stay by utilization review*. HMOs, to avoid spending money whenever possible, have established the *gate-keeper physician concept*. This requires their covered patients to select *one physician to provide and supervise all of their medical care* and *rewards the gatekeeper with money* for severely limiting referral for specialist and/or hospital care. Such rules clearly limit patient free-choice and access to the highest quality care. To the previously noted constraints have been added by HMOs very long delays and denial of payment of claims. Relman recently described this mix of apparently insoluble problems as the *decline and fall of managed care*.[37]

Hospitalization accounts for more than half of the health care costs in the USA, and for 85% of the health care costs related to diabetes and its complications. Thus many in-hospital health care activities have been moved to ambulatory care areas in the 1990s. With well-organized, comprehensive, and frequent follow-up of those with diabetes mellitus in an ambulatory care unit, many complications can be prevented or minimized and hospitalizations can be decreased by more than 50%. This approach will not only provide higher quality care, it will save money.[41,42]

Changes in Medical Education and its Financing in the 1990s

During the 1990s, there have been not only drastic changes in the practice of medicine and its financing, there also have been drastic changes in the education of specialists (diabetologists, endocrinologists, etc.) and the financing of that education.[43-45,47] The training of specialists has been decreased, where as that of primary care physicians (generalists) has been increased. As the mass of medical knowledge has increased almost exponentially in the last 50 years, the ability of a physician to learn more than a small fraction of the total medical knowledge base has demanded that the highest quality of care must be provided by specialists working in concert with generalists and with *patients having free access to both*.[43-45,47]

Training of residents in academic medical centers has remained intensive, and scrutiny of resident's working hours in New York has increased.[48,49] An unexpected death in a New York City teaching hospital in 1984 provoked a grand jury investigation. The grand jury was highly critical of *inadequate supervision* of interns and residents *by faculty physicians* and of the *long work hours* by residents (greater than 95 hours per week by 20% of residents).[49] In a May 1998 press release,[48] the New York State Department of Health reported that physicians training in New York hospitals were working hours that *far exceed the limits* set earlier by the State to protect

patients. Since then, the department has levied $30,000 in fines against two New York City hospitals, and additional actions are expected.

During the 1990s medical students have been subjected to the rising costs and mounting debts incident to acquiring a medical degree. In 1997, average yearly tuition and fees for private medical schools was $24,930. The average debt for a 4-year medical education was $80,462.[50-51] After that, the student has to start the arduous task of repayment on a resident's salary. Of course this problem influences life-style and type-of-practice decisions.

Definition of Terms Used in Clinical Diabetes Mellitus: A Problem-Oriented Approach (Third Edition)

Terms and criteria used in the third edition of *Clinical Diabetes Mellitus: A Problem-Oriented Approach* are listed in Table Intro-1. These relate to diagnosis, screening, and typing of diabetes mellitus, acute and chronic complications of diabetes, hypoglycemia, and desirable levels of plasma glucose control. It has been 20 years since West requested that diabetes definitions, classifications, and reporting become epidemiologically standardized.[46] Since that time, progress has been made in improving communication, but there is still serious disagreement concerning criteria for diagnosis as proposed by the ADA Expert Committee (see Chapters 11 and 12). For instance, the European Diabetes Epidemiology Study Group[54] feels that using fasting plasma glucose levels will fail to diagnose early at least 30% of those with NIDDM. The problems are yet to be resolved by research that is underway. Research is also underway concerning the genetics and other characteristics of type 1 and type 2 diabetes mellitus, and knowledge is increasing rapidly. See Chapters 2, 3, 4, 5, 8, 9, and 10. There is essential agreement on subtypes of acutely decompensated diabetes mellitus (diabetic ketoacidosis and the hyperglycemic hyperosmolar state). See Chapter 24. Much research is underway to understand and characterize the chronic complications of diabetes. These include the macrovascular (Chapters 28, 29, 30, 34, 38, and 39), microvascular (Chapter 26), kidney (Chapter 27), and peripheral and cranial (Chapters 35 and 37) and autonomic (Chapter 36) nervous system problems presented by diabetes mellitus. There is now essential agreement on the various types of hypoglycemia and their causes, although some remain idiopathic. See Chapters 12, 18, and 20.

Tools to attain and maintain continuously desirable levels of plasma (or blood) glucose control and hemoglobin A1c control as advocated by Molnar, et al. in

1974[52] and the DCCT in 1993[24] are desirable but not yet available. When they become available, plasma glucose and HbA1c control in the general diabetic population should improve significantly.

As new knowledge continues to accumulate from clinical and basic research and from epidemiologic studies, we can anticipate that definitions will become more precise and will be more generally used. As Dr. Michael Berger pointed out in the 27th Claude Bernard Lecture of the EASD[53], it is essential that we continue to build the bridge between science and patient care in the field of diabetes mellitus.

References

1. Campbell WR, Macleod JJR: Insulin. Medicine 3:195–308. 1924.

2. West KM: Epidemiology of Diabetes and Its Vascular Lesions. New York: Elsevier, 1978.

3. Fishbein H, Palumbo PJ: Acute metabolic complications in diabetes in: Diabetes in America, second edition, NIH Diabetes Data Group, NIH Publication No. 95–1468, pp 283–291, 1995.

4. Berkowitz KJ, Anderson LA, Panayioto RM, Ziemer DC, Gallina DL: Mini-residency on diabetes care for health care providers: Enhanced knowledge and attitudes with unexpected challenges to assessing behavior change. The Diabetes Educator: 24:143–150, 1998.

5. Assal JP, Mulhauser I, Pernet A, et al.: Patient education as the basis for diabetes care in clinical practice and research. Diabetologia 28:602–613, 1985.

6. Davidson JK: What does the doctor do when allied health professionals take over? The view of a medical convert. In: Larkins R, Zimmet P, Chisholm D (eds): Diabetes 1988, Elsevier, Amsterdam, 1989, pp 955–958.

7. Day JL, Johnson P, Raymond G, Walker R: The feasibility of a potentially "ideal" system of integrated diabetes care and education based on a day centre. Diabetic Med 5:70–75, 1988.

8. Goldstein DE, Little RR, Lorenz RA, Malone JI, Nathan D, Peterson CM: Tests of glycemia in diabetes (technical review). Diabetes Care 18:896–909, 1995.

9. American Diabetes Association: Report of the Expert Committee on the diagnosis and classification of diabetes mellitus. Diabetes Care 21(suppl.1):S5–S19, 1998.

10. European Epidemiology Study Group: Epidemiological considerations related to the new diagnostic criteria for diabetes mellitus. Diabetologia 41: EASD News Section 51–52, 1998. (Nov.)

11. Davidson JK, Lebovitz H: Diet therapy is the cornerstone of treatment for non-insulin-dependent diabetes. In: Debates in Medicine. Chicago: Mosby-Yearbook, 1991.

12. Davidson JK: Plasma glucose lowering effect of caloric restriction in obesity-induced insulin-treated diabetes mellitus. (Abstr.) Diabetes 26:355, 1977.

13. National Institutes of Health. Consensus development conference on diet and exercise in non-insulin-dependent diabetes mellitus. Diabetes Care 10:639–644, 1987.

14. European NIDDM Policy Group: Management of non-insulin-dependent diabetes mellitus in Europe. A consensus view. Diabetic Med 5:275–281, 1988.

15. Davidson JK, Delcher HK, Englund A: Spin-off cost/benefits of expanded nutritional care. J Am Diet Assoc 75:250–257, 1979.

16. Davidson JK, Vander Zwaag R, Cox CL, et al.: The Memphis and Atlanta continuing care programs for diabetes. II. Comparative analyses of demographic characteristics, treatment methods, and outcomes over a 9–10 year follow-up period. Diabetes Care 7:25–31, 1984.

17. University Group Diabetes Program VIII. Evaluation of insulin therapy: Final report. Diabetes 31(suppl. 5-Part 2):1–81, 1982.

18. NKPDS No. 33: Intensive blood-glucose control with sulfonylureas or insulin compared with conventional treatment and risk of complications in patients with type 2 diabetes. Lancet 352:837–853, 1998.

19. NKPDS No. 34: Effect of intensive blood-glucose control with metformin and complications in overweight patients with type 2 diabetes. Lancet: 352:854–865, 1998.

20. The Diabetes Control and Complications Trial Research Group: The absence of a glycemic threshold for the development of long-term complications: the perspective of the Diabetes Control and Complications Trial. Diabetes 45:1289–1298, 1996.

21. The Diabetes Control and Complications Trial Research Group: The effect of intensive treatment of diabetes on the development and progression of long-term complications in insulin-dependent diabetes mellitus. N Engl J Med 329:977–986, 1993.

22. The Diabetes Control and Complications Trial Research Group: Lifetime benefits and costs of intensive therapy as practiced in the Diabetes Control and Complications Trial. JAMA 276:1409–1415, 1996.

23. The Diabetes Control and Complications Trial Research Group: The relationship of glycemic exposure (HbA1c) to the risk of development and progression of retinopathy in the Diabetes Control and Complications Trial. Diabetes 44:968–983, 1995.

24. American Diabetes Association: Implications of the Diabetes Control and Complications Trial. Diabetes Care 21(suppl. 1):S88–S90, 1998.

25. Harris MI: Screening for undiagnosed non-insulin-dependent diabetes mellitus. In (eds): Alberti KGMM, Mazze RS: Frontiers of diabetes research: current trends in non-insulin-dependent diabetes mellitus. Amsterdam: Excerpta Medica, International Congress Series 859, 1989, pp. 119-131.

26. Codman EA: A study in hospital efficiency. Boston: Thomas Todd Co, Printers, 1918.

27. Weed LL: Medical records that guide and teach. N Engl J Med 278:593–599, 652–657, 1968.

28. Weed LL: Medical Records, Medical Education, and Patient Care: The Problem-Oriented Record as a Basic Tool. Cleveland: Case Western Reserve University Press, 1969.

29. Hurst JW, Walker HK: The problem-oriented system. New York. Medcom, 1972.

30. Walker HK, Hurst JW, Woody MF: Applying the problem-oriented system. New York: Medcom, 1973.

31. Specialist UK Workgroup Reports: Saint Vincent and improving diabetes care. Diabetic Med: 13(suppl. 4): S1–S128, 1996.

32. Home P, Keen H: Making progress with diabetes care: Story from the United Kingdom. IDF Bulletin 43:8–12, 1998.

33. Freymann JG: The American health care system: ITS genesis and trajectory. New York: Medcom, 1974.

34. McNeill WH: Plagues and peoples. Garden City, NY: Doubleday Anchor Books, 1976.

35. Joslin Clinic educates diabetics in how to live with the disease: Scope Weekly Aug. 20, 1958, p. 7.

36. AMA ICD–9–CM, 1999. American Medical Association Order Dept. 100 Enterprise Place, P.O. Box 7046, Dover, DE 19903–7046. Phone 800–621–8335, Fax 312–464–5600.

37. Relman A: The decline and fall of managed care. Hospitals and health networks. July 5, 1998: pp. 70, 72.

38. Smothers: Delays and denials on HMO claims said to hurt doctors. Sept. 3, 1998: A 27.

39. Doctor discontent. New Engl J Med 339:1543–1545, 1998.

40. Brett AS: New guidelines for coding physician's services. A step backward. New Engl J Med 339:1705–1708, 1998.

41. Carter Center of Emory University: Closing the gap: The problems of diabetes mellitus in the United States. Diabetes Care 8:391–406, 1985.

42. American College of Physicians: Position on access to health care. ACP Observer 10(4):7–9, 1990.

43. Jonas S: The case for change in medical education in the United States. Lancet 1:452–454, 1984.

44. Huth EJ: The humanities, science, and the medical curriculum. Ann Intern Med 101:864–865, 1984.

45. Panel on the General Professional Education of the Physician and College Preparation for Medicine. Physicians for the twenty-first century. J Med Educ 59:1–208, 1984.

46. West KM: Standardization of definition, classification, and reporting diabetes-related epidemiologic studies. Diabetes Care 2:65–76, 1979.

47. Tosteson DC: New pathways for medical education. Jour Am Med Assoc 265:1022–1023, 1991.

48. Office of Public Affairs Health Department Releases Residency Review Report (press release). Albany, NY: Dept. of Health, May 18, 1998.

49. DeBuono BA, Osten WM: The medical resident workload: The case of New York State. JAMA 280:1882–1883, 1998.

50. Naradzay JF: Into the deep well: The evolution of medical school loan debt. JAMA 280:1881–1883, 1998.

51. Stockwell A: The Guerrilla Guide to Mastering Student Loan Debt. Harper-Perennial, NY, NY. 1997.

52. Molnar GD, Taylor WF, Langworthy A: On measuring the adequacy of diabetes regulation: Comparison of continuously monitored blood glucose patterns with values at selected time points. Diabetologia 10:139-143, 1974.

53. Berger M: The 27th Claude Bernard Lecture: To bridge science and patient care in diabetes. Diabetologia 39:749–757, 1996.

54. The European Diabetes Epidemiology Group (EDEG): Epidemiological considerations related to the new diagnostic criteria for diabetes mellitus. Diabetologia 41: EASD News Section pp. 51–52, 1998.

Section I.
The Nature of Diabetes Mellitus

1

Historical Perspective: The Discovery of Insulin

Barbara E. Hazlett

The disease diabetes, whose name is derived from the Greek word meaning "siphon," was named by Aretaeus of Cappadocia (AD 81–138), but it was probably described much earlier in the Egyptian papyrus Ebers of 1500 BC. The cardinal symptoms of the disease, polyuria, polydipsia, polyphagia, and weight loss, were later described in detail by Celsus (30 BC-AD 50) and in Chinese writings of AD 200–600. The ancients noticed that ants were attracted by a "sweetness of the urine" and that carbuncles frequently plagued victims of this disease. Paracelsus (AD 1493–1541) thought the white deposit left by the urine of diabetics was salt and advised salt loading as proper treatment.

Thomas Willis (1621–1675) tasted the urine of diabetics and found it "wondrous sweet, as if imbued with honey," and a century later, William Dobson realized that the serum of diabetics was also sweet. Cullen (1710–1790) added the word "mellitus," meaning honey, to the name diabetes. Quantitative sugar determinations were later done on the urine, and by 1910, sugar determinations were possible on the blood. By 1920, only 0.1 mL of blood was needed for these tests.

In 1788, Cawley reported destruction of the pancreas in a diabetic patient, and 100 years later (1889), Joseph von Mering and Oskar Minkowski in Strasbourg produced diabetes in a dog by removing its pancreas. They observed that merely ligating the pancreatic duct did not cause diabetes.

In 1869, a medical student named Paul Langerhans described systems of cells in the pancreas which he thought were lymph glands. G.E Laguesse later named these cells the "islets of Langerhans." In 1901, Eugene Opie of Johns Hopkins University, Baltimore, associated diabetes with an alteration in the islets of Langerhans and proposed that they were the source of an internal secretion. At the turn of the century, other "ductless" glands were being described, and for their chemical messengers Starling coined the word "hormone."

In the 1850s a French physician, Piorry, advised increasing sugar and starch in the diet of diabetic patients to make up for urinary loss. Bouchardat, also French, advised against this, noting improvement in diabetic patients when he subjected them to fast days and increased exercise.

Bernard Naunyn (1848–1914) had a clinic for diabetics in Strasbourg. He also recommended carbohydrate-restricted diets and fast days, even locking patients in their rooms to achieve this. He introduced the term "acidosis" for decompensated diabetes and advised treating acidosis with bicarbonate.

Claude Bernard about this time began to describe intermediary metabolism and ascribed the problems of diabetes to overproduction of sugar by the liver.

In the United States, another advocate of undernutrition as a therapeutic measure was Frederick Allen. He published a massive work in 1919 entitled *The Total Dietary Regulation of Diabetes Mellitus*. He did subtotal pancreatectomies on animals and produced an illness not unlike many cases of human diabetes.

Once diabetes was ascribed to a form of pancreatic insufficiency, attempts to make extracts of the pancreas were legion. Minkowski observed a temporary fall in urine sugar of dogs, but his extract had harmful side effects.

Laguesse suggested using fetal or fish pancreas to make extracts. In fish the islets are separate from the exocrine portion of the gland, simplifying the extraction.

In 1902, two Scottish researchers (John Rennie and Thomas Fraser) tried an oral pancreatic extract on four patients with negative results.

A German scientist, Georg Ludwig Zuelzer, believed that the purpose of the pancreatic secretion was to neutralize adrenalin. On June 21, 1906, he injected 8 mL of his extract subcutaneously into a patient in diabetic coma and the patient's condition improved. He called his extract "acomatol." Zuelzer needed financial support to continue his work and accepted help from the Schering Pharmaceutical Company. In 1907 he tried again, but his extract produced serious reactions with convulsions in five patients. Glycosuria was notably reduced. Another German, J. Forschbach, tested samples of Zuelzer's extract and found them too toxic for use. Schering withdrew its support, but Hoffmann-La Roche offered their support in 1911, and in 1912 Zuelzer applied for a U.S. patent. In his newly subsidized laboratory, he made another batch of pancreatic extract which again caused convulsions in patients. World War I intervened. It is noteworthy that had Zuelzer been able to measure blood sugar, he might have found that the convulsions caused by his extracts were hypoglycemic in nature.

In 1906, in the United States, Lydia Dewitt began to work on pancreatic extracts prepared by ligating the ducts prior to extraction of the glands. She did no animal or human testing.

E.L Scott, a medical student at the University of Chicago in 1911, began a project for his master's thesis, believing that the secretions of the exocrine glands digested the internal secretion of the pancreas before it could be extracted. When Dewitt's method failed, he used alcohol as a solvent to make his extract. It lowered the blood sugar level in four dogs, but his thesis adviser discouraged him from continuing the work.

In 1913 Frederick Allen pronounced that all pancreatic extracts to that date had been failures.

John James Rikard (J.J.R.) Macleod had come to Case Western Reserve University in Cleveland from Scotland as Professor of Physiology in 1903 at the age of 27. He was invited to the University of Toronto in 1918. His treatise on carbohydrate metabolism was already familiar to most investigators in this field.

In 1915, in the United States, Israel Kleiner in association with SJ. Meltzer at the Rockefeller Institute injected a pancreatic emulsion in association with glucose into animals, and observed the disappearance of glucose from the blood. The war interrupted Kleiner's work temporarily but he resumed it in 1919. He injected an emulsion of ground-up fresh pancreas suspended in salted distilled water IV into depancreatized dogs and measured their blood sugar levels. In 16 experiments, the animals' blood sugars fell significantly. In 1919, Kleiner left the Rockefeller Institute and did not return to this work.

In Romania, Nicolas Paulesco, Professor of Physiology in Bucharest, began to experiment on pancreatic extracts in 1916. Because of the postwar turmoil, his research was delayed until 1919. He also measured blood sugar levels and noticed a spectacular drop in sugar when his extract, which he call "pancreine," was given IV. He published material in French on the results of his work; his articles appeared between April and June of 1921.

A series of events that set the stage for the discovery of insulin then occurred.[1] On November 14, 1891, Frederick Grant Banting had been born in Alliston, Ontario, Canada, the youngest of five children of Methodist farming parents. He entered the Faculty of

Arts at the University of Toronto in 1911 but dropped out of arts and entered medical school the following year with his cousin, Fred Hipwell. They were in the class of 1917, and both meant to become medical missionaries. The war changed that; the entire class of 1917 enlisted after an accelerated graduation in 1916. Fred Banting was in England in 1917 as a battalion medical officer. In France he sustained an arm wound at Cambrai, winning the Military Cross for courage under fire. While convalescing in England, he studied for the examinations of the Royal College of Surgeons. He returned to Christie Street Military Hospital in Toronto in 1919. By September of that year he was fully recovered and began a surgical residency at the Hospital for Sick Children with an interest in orthopedics.

He was not offered a staff appointment in surgery in Toronto, but his friend, Edith Roach, was teaching school near London, Ontario, so Banting settled there. In July 1920 he bought a house that he used for an office. He got a part-time job at $2 an hour as a demonstrator in surgery and anatomy to subsidize his income. He assisted the professor of physiology whose interest was in neurology. Banting's own medical practice was very slow. In his spare time he tinkered with his car and began to paint in oils.

On October 30, 1920, Banting was preparing a seminar on carbohydrate metabolism. He was quite interested in an article in the November 1920 issue of the journal *Surgery, Gynecology and Obstetrics* which had just arrived. It was entitled "Relation of the Islets of Langerhans to Diabetes with Reference to Cases of Pancreatic Lithiasis," and the author was Moses Barron. Barron reported that a stone blocking the main pancreatic duct had resulted in atrophy of the acinar cells, leaving the islet cells intact. Banting wrote in his notebook "Diabetus—Ligate pancreatic ducts of dog. Keep dogs alive till acini degenerate leaving Islets. Try to isolate the internal secretions of these to relieve glycosurea." (Banting's original spelling has been retained.)

The next day he mentioned his idea to Prof. F.R. Miller who suggested that Banting go to Toronto and see Prof. J.J.R Macleod, by then well known for his expertise in carbohydrate metabolism. It was known that the University of Toronto, unlike many smaller schools, could afford laboratories, animals, and animal operating rooms. Banting made an appointment to see Macleod, who listened to the idea but was not impressed by Banting's obvious inexperience and unfamiliarity with the literature. However, Macleod knew of E.L. Scott's work and agreed to give Banting laboratory space and dogs if Banting was willing to take time off to do the work. He told Banting that "even negative results would be of great physiologic value."

Banting thought it over and wrote to Macleod that he would come to Toronto for May, June, and July 1921. However, he did not put all his hopes on the

Toronto experiment. He also made an application to join an oil exploration expedition to the Northwest Territories. Fortunately, the expedition decided not to take a physician.

On April 26, 1921, Banting took the train to Toronto. He went to see Professor Macleod and they planned the work. By coincidence, James Bertram Collip also was in Macleod's office that day, planning a sabbatical in Toronto the next year. Professor Collip, from the University of Alberta, already had acquired some expertise in glandular secretions and the making of tissue extracts. Professor Macleod also had two fourth-year students in Honors Physiology and Biochemistry who had shared the silver medal and were working as student assistants for the summer. Charley Best (Charles Herbert Best) and Clark Noble (E.C. Noble) planned to do their master's degrees the following year and were looking for thesis material. Macleod offered the job as Banting's helper to the students, sweetening the offer by telling them that they would see some surgery. The two young men decided to split the summer, one working in May and June and the other in July and August.

Charley Best won the toss of a coin for the earlier start, which was preferable because the weather would not be as warm. Best was 22, the son of a Canadian-born general practitioner in Maine and was a returned artillery sergeant from World War I. Best knew the techniques of qualitative and quantitative urine and blood sugar and nitrogen determinations. He wrote his last examination on May 16,1921, following which he and Banting cleaned their laboratory space thoroughly. On May 17, Macleod joined them, instructing and assisting in their first pancreatectomy on a dog. They decided to use Hedon's two-stage procedure, leaving a remnant of pancreas under the abdominal wall to be removed 1 week later. They also prepared duct-ligated dogs. All their early dogs died, most of infection, others due to bleeding and anesthesia. Macleod left for a summer in Scotland after the two young men had been working for 1 month, leaving them suggestions for their summer's work.

By the end of June, they had had little success. Since he was familar with the experimental procedures, Best decided to stay on despite the summer heat, dirt, and stench, and Noble concurred. Best and Banting had to help look after their own dogs and frequently had to run up and down two flights of stairs between their bench space in a former storeroom and the animal quarters on the roof of the Medical Building.

Finally, on Saturday, July 30, 1921, they made an extract from the shrivelled pancreas of the original duct-ligated dog (animal no. 391). They sliced up the pancreas in a cold mortar, suspended it in ice-cold Ringer's solution kept in freezing brine, then macerated the pancreas with sand and filtered it through cheese cloth and blotting paper. They warmed the filtrate and injected it IV, a procedure in which they had become very proficient, into a white terrier (animal no. 410). The preinjection blood sugar was 0.20 g%. In 1 hr, the blood sugar level had fallen to 0.12 g%. Success spurred them on, and they worked on dog after dog. They called their first extract "isletin." Banting wrote Macleod on August 8, 1921, telling him of their success and saying that he and Charley would like to continue to work together but needed financial assistance and better operating facilities.

In fact, Banting was penniless. He lived in a $2 a week boarding house and ate in the laboratory or with friends. He sold his instruments and house in London to finance the work. Banting and Best, 29 and 22 years old, respectively, worked day and night, singing war songs to keep awake, at first using duct-ligated dog pancreas to make isletin and then extracting it with acid. On August 17, they achieved an equally good result from extract made with fresh whole pancreas, but for some reason they did not realize the significance of this. The fact that they could use fresh pancreas belied Banting's whole hypothesis. In fact, they wasted time trying to increase the yield of extract from duct ligated pancreas by giving secretin. They had considerable difficulty with their experiments and not nearly all their extracts were effective.

On September 21, 1921, Macleod returned to Toronto.

Banting demanded a salary, living quarters, more assistants in the animal quarters, and improved operating room facilities. It is said that he threatened to go elsewhere if his demands were not met. Professor of Pharmacology Velyien Henderson offered Banting a job as a special lecturer in pharmacology at the then-magnificent salary of $250 a month. In October 1921, Banting suggested to Macleod that Collip, also 29, by then back in Toronto and working in the field of pathologic chemistry, be invited to help purify their extract. They also talked to Dr. J.D. Fitzgerald, the director of the Connaught Anti-toxin Laboratories, hoping for some assistance. Macleod encouraged the two to work alone until they had a clear solution.

In October 1921, for the first time, Banting and Best reviewed the literature while waiting for the pancreas to atrophy in dogs in which they had ligated the ducts. As previously mentioned, Paulesco also had worked on pancreatic extracts; his results had been published in French, a language which neither Banting nor Best could read well. Thus, they misunderstood Paulesco's writings. By some misadventure, they also missed the writings of Zuelzer and E.L. Scott.

Macleod asked the two young men to give a preliminary report of their work at the Physiological Journal Club on November 14, 1921. Macleod, in his introduction, devastated Banting by saying things that Banting had intended to say. Banting's paranoia became more evident at this time. A longevity experiment in a dog was suggested in the discussion after the meeting. In December, the researchers' first longevity experiment ended because the dog died in convulsions. On December 6, they started the famous dog Marjorie (no. 33), depancreatized on November 18, on a longevity experiment.

They obtained fetal calf pancreas from an abattoir as had been suggested earlier by Laguesse. The extract lowered a dog's blood sugar from 0.30 to 0.20 g% in 45 min. Another 10 mL lowered the blood sugar level from 0.17 to 0.08 g% in 1 hr and the dog's urine became sugar-free.

Banting and Best began to use a Berkefeld filter to sterilize their extracts. Banting himself took 1.5 mL of extract subcutaneously without any untoward side effects. They did not measure blood sugar levels when they experimented on themselves. In December 1921 Banting and Best sent their first paper on "The Internal Secretion of the Pancreas" to the *Journal of Laboratory and Clinical Medicine,* listing only themselves as authors. The paper was accepted for publication in the February 3, 1922 issue. It is interesting that in their submission, Banting and Best claimed 75 good results although their records suggest that only 42 of 75 dogs had a good result.

Macleod invited Banting and Best to present their work at a meeting of the American Physiological Society in New Haven, Connecticut on December 30, 1921. A Canadian studying at Johns Hopkins University wrote to Elliott Joslin in Boston and to George Clowes, the research director of Eli Lilly and Company in Indianapolis, telling them what was to be on the program.

On December 8, 1921, Banting and Best used fresh adult beef pancreas extracted with alcohol and evaporated at cold temperature, as suggested by Macleod, to concentrate their extract. They then redissolved the dry residue in saline solution. On December 11, 6 cc of this extract lowered the blood sugar of dog no. 35 from 0.35 to 0.116 g% in 4 hr.

J.B. Collip was now anxious to participate in the experiments. Rumor has it that his first extracts did not work because the sweetbreads he ordered the laboratory assistant to obtain were thymus, not pancreas. After this, Collip used whole beef pancreas and followed Macleod's suggestion to test the potency of the extract on rabbits instead of dogs. Collip became interested in the effect of the extract on liver glycogen and on ketone body formation. On December 21, 1921, his first extract was effective in a diabetic Airedale.

By mid-December, Banting and Best had modified their method to make an alcohol extract of fresh beef or dog pancreas which they dialyzed through a semipermeable membrane, then washed with toluene.

On December 15, they addressed physicians at the Toronto General Hospital on their progress. It is certain that Dr. Duncan Graham, the professor of medicine, and Dr. Walter Campbell were among those present, and both were interested.

On December 20, Banting and Best tried their extract on a classmate of Banting's, Joe Gilchrist, who had become diabetic in 1917 and was going downhill on the semistarvation Allen treatment. They used extract that was potent in a dog, but when they gave it to Gilchrist by mouth it had no effect.

On December 30, they went to New Haven, and a nervous Banting presented his paper. Kleiner and Scott were in the audience. Macleod, as chairman of the session, protected Banting by answering most of the questions himself. The experts who were present took cautious interest. Clowes offered the facilities of Eli Lilly and Company if Macleod would consider collaboration.

On December 2, 1921, a 12-year-old boy, Leonard Thompson, [2] was admitted to the Toronto General Hospital to the service of Dr. W.R. Campbell. Diabetic for $2\frac{1}{2}$ years, he had been on the Allen starvation treatment and was reaching the terminal stages of the disease. His father carried him into Duncan Graham's office, and Graham turned him over to Campbell's care.

Banting pressured Macleod to arrange a clinical trail with Dr. Graham. He and Best were enthusiastic because the longevity experiment on the dog Marjorie was very successful. Marjorie had been alive for many weeks. Banting was also afraid that Collip would prepare a more purified extract than his and Best's, and would present it for a clinical trial before they had had a chance.

Best made a batch of extract from beef pancreas, washed it twice with toluene, then sterilized it by passing it through the Berkefeld filter. They tried it on a dog, then gave each other injections. It was a thick brown muck, Dr. Campbell said later. They took it over to Ward H in the hospital where Leonard Thompson lay. The boy and his father had agreed to the experiment. Dr. Campbell asked the intern on the ward, Dr. Edward Jeffrey, to give the boy the first injection. They settled on half the dose that would be used on a dog of similar weight. Dr. Jeffrey gave the boy 15 cc, 7.5 cc into each buttock. Banting and Best waited in the hall and were refused a specimen of urine from the boy. Eventually they walked back to their laboratory. Leonard Thompson's blood sugar level did not fall dramatically, only from 0.440 to 0.320 g%. Seven days later an abscess was noted at one injection site. Such was the embarrassment caused by premature testing.

Collip worked on, trying one thing after another, and finally on January 16, 1922 he made a breakthrough. He discovered that at 90% concentration of alcohol, the active principle precipitated. On January 23, Leonard Thompson was given Dr. Collip's serum, and a significant fall in blood sugar resulted. After the boy had received injections of the extract for several days his condition visibly improved (see Fig. 18–3).

Collip is said to have refused to tell Banting and Best how his improvements were made and even threatened to take out a patent in his own name. A fight ensued. Dr. Fitzgerald of the Anti-toxin Laboratories became the arbitrator. On January 25, Fitzgerald agreed to offer his facilities to Banting, Best, Collip, and Macleod in an effort to obtain an extract. They all agreed to reveal any and all modificiations to one another.

Word had leaked to the *Toronto Star* daily newspaper, and letters began to arrive from diabetics and their physicians. Macleod was interviewed, and according to Banting he used the pronoun "we" too frequently. Banting began to tell his friends that Macleod was stealing both the applause and the work. Others tried to mollify Banting, and Macleod agreed henceforth to publish alphabetically, meaning that his name would come last.

Banting and Best killed the dog Marjorie on January 27, 1922 after she had lived 70 days. A careful post mortem was done by the chief pathologist of the Toronto General Hospital, Dr. W.L. Robinson. A 3 mm nodule of pancreas was found, but no islet cells were seen under a microscope.

In the next month, Dr. Campbell and Dr. A.A. Fletcher treated six patients, all with good results. In February 1922, the discoverers presented their work to the Toronto Academy of Medicine, and later that month their article appeared in the *Journal of Laboratory and Clinical Medicine*. In March a clinical article appeared in the *Canadian Medical Association Journal* entitled "Pancreatic Extracts in the Treatment of Diabetes Mellitus" by Banting, Best, Collip, Campbell, and Fletcher. There was no doubt now that their extract had unquestionable value. The *Toronto Star* agreed, calling it "epochmaking" and "one of the greatest achievements in modern medicine."

Banting was unhappy in his love life and bitter about Macleod's taking credit for his discoveries. The discoverers were invited to present their work to the Association of American Physicians in Washington, D.C. On May 3, 1922, Campbell went to the American meeting, but Banting and Best stayed in Toronto, not having the money to make the trip. The paper that was delivered carried the following names: Banting, Best, Collip, Campbell, Fletcher, Macleod, and finally E.C. Noble. It was accepted with a standing ovation.

Macleod named the extract "insulin" from the Latin word meaning "island."

Production of insulin in quantity was undertaken by the Connaught Anti-toxin Laboratories. Initially, the results were disastrous. Nothing worked when production of large quantities was attempted. Diabetics were dying in the spring of 1922 from lack of insulin. By mid-May, probably because of a small adjustment in pH, the producers gained the ability to make insulin in quantity and Dr. Peter Moloney, a chemist, joined the team.

Fearing they might lose the credit, they took out patent applications in the name of the lay members of the group, Best and Collip, assigning the rights to insulin to the University of Toronto.

Banting was denied a clinical appointment at the Toronto General Hospital because he had no experience in treating diabetics, so he opened a private office granting him the right to admit his private patients to the hospital. He also headed a new diabetes clinic at Christie Street Military Hospital. Connaught Laboratories distributed one third of its insulin to Banting for his private patients, one third to the clinic at Christie Street, and one third to Toronto General and the Hospital for Sick Children. Macleod began to refer to Banting as "my clinical associate."

Joe Gilchrist received his second dose of insulin this time subcutaneously on May 15, 1922 and thereafter made himself a human guinea pig, allowing each batch to be tested on himself after animal testing and before it went to patients.

On May 21, 1922, Jim Havens, the son of the vice-president of Eastman Kodak in Rochester, New York, became the first U.S. citizen to receive insulin. His physician, Dr. John Williams, came to Toronto begging for insulin for the dying boy. Banting went to Rochester to assist in the boy's treatment.

Eli Lilly and Company was a family firm which had been in business for 46 years. The first of its kind, it had established a research facility and hired an English research chemist, George Clowes, to direct it. Macleod knew Clowes and admired him as a scientist. Lilly agreed to pool all knowledge and supply insulin free for clinical trials for 1 year. The following year, the firm would supply insulin at cost and pay royalties for all insulin sold. An Insulin Committee to decide policies was established in Toronto and headed by Colonel Albert Gooderham, chairman of the board of the Connaught Laboratories. Best and Collip went to Indianapolis to assist Lilly in their first attempts to make insulin, following which Collip returned to the University of Alberta.

Lilly was not in fact the first in the United States to make insulin. Banting had corresponded with a Dr. W.B. Sansum in Santa Barbara, California, and had supplied him with directions to make the extract. Sansum made his insulin with sheep pancreas, but his attempts at large-scale production failed. Dr. Rollin T. Woodyatt of Chicago was also prepared to make his own insulin.

In the summer of 1922, Macleod went to New Brunswick to investigate the possibility of using fish insulin, since fish islets are separate from the acinar cells. Clark Noble was also sent to New Brunswick some time later to do a feasibility study on fish insulin.

The governors of the University of Toronto now realized that Banting had no university status and that their hospital, Toronto General, was not getting insulin to test. Banting received several offers to go elsewhere but turned them down, and in August, the university agreed that Graham, Campbell, Fletcher, and Banting would begin clinical trials at the Toronto General Hospital in a newly established diabetes clinic. Banting was to be paid $6,000 a year.

Unfortunately, supplies of insulin were scarce, and by the time Havens, Gilchrist, and a few at Christie Street were supplied, there was little for anyone else. Banting received a letter from the mother of 14-year-old Elizabeth Hughes, the diabetic daughter of the U.S. Secretary of State, Charles Evans Hughes. Banting discouraged treatment with insulin at that time because Jim Havens was complaining of painful injections, the volume of the shots sometimes being 8 mL.

In July, a Dr. W. Palmer brought a lady with a gangrenous foot to Banting. With insulin she became the first diabetic patient to survive an amputation.

George Walden, a biochemist at Lilly, worked full-time on insulin. He modified the recipe, finding that the filtrate had even more potency than the precipitate previously used. Lilly called its product Iletin. For a time, Lilly supplied insulin for Toronto. Eli Lilly himself liked Banting and backed him to the hilt.

Another chemist, David Scott, was added to the Toronto team. He and Banting visited Indianapolis to learn the new methodology. They saw the expensive vacuum stills that Lilly was using for its successful production. When Banting returned to Toronto, he asked the university for money to purchase such a vacuum still, but was refused. He wrote to Dr. Geyelin of New York City, who immediately asked the father of a diabetic boy for the money. Geyelin was put on a distribution list for insulin.

Eli Lilly began to supply physicians across the United States. Joslin received his first supply on August 6, 1922. Frederick Allen got his first batch 2 days later. By the end of August, both Lilly and Connaught were producing good insulin.

Elizabeth Hughes, the 14-year-old who weighed 52 pounds, came to Toronto with her nurse in August of 1922 and lived close to Banting's office. With insulin and the 2,700 calorie diet which he prescribed, she gained $2\frac{1}{2}$ pounds per week. (Banting was not rigid in his diet prescription, as were the people who had treated diabetes by starvation.) Elizabeth wrote remarkable letters to her mother, describing her time in Toronto. She later married, had children, and lived until 1981, when she died of a myocardial infarct.

By September 1922, Lilly was supplying insulin for the United States, and Connaught made insulin for testing in four cities in eastern Canada, while Collip made insulin in Edmonton, Alberta.

In October 1922, Leonard Thompson, weighing 55 pounds, was again admitted to the Toronto General in

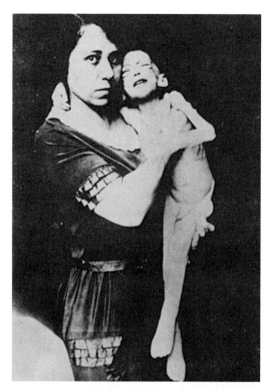

Figure I–I. *Before insulin*: "J.L." Age 3 years, weight 15 pounds. December 15, 1922. (*Source*: Bliss M: The Discovery of Insulin. Toronto: McClelland and Stewart, 1982. Photograph courtesy of Elli Lilly and Co., Ltd. With permission.)

diabetic ketoacidosis. His life was saved by insulin, which he received continuously thereafter.

Late in November 1922, leading clinicians came to Toronto for a workshop on insulin treatment. All related anecdotes of their early experiences with the "miracle" substance. By February of 1923, 250 physicians, 60 clinics, and 1,000 patients in the United States and Canada were being supplied with insulin. In those days there was a 25% difference in potency from batch to batch which had to be resolved. In the United States, a boy named Randall Sprague was started on insulin on September 21, 1922 when he was 16. He had an anaphylactic reaction to Iletin, but 6 days later he was able to tolerate a new batch well. Sprague later became president of the American Diabetes Association.

In February of 1923, Nicolas Paulesco wrote to Banting, enclosing one of his articles, but his letter was in French. Banting once more could not understand it and did not answer.

The introduction of insulin to Europe was slow. A Spanish physician who had done postgraduate work at Harvard and Yale in 1921–1922 tried to make insulin in Spain. Jonathan Meakins, a Canadian, wrote to Banting from Edinburgh in June 1923 because he had a colleague who was diabetic. Meakins did nothing further about it, however, until January 1924. The British Medical Research Council was skeptical about accepting patent rights to insulin and sent Henry Dale, the council's Director of Pharmacology and Biochemistry, to Indianapolis and Toronto. Dale was enthusiastic but recommended a period of testing before large-scale production was begun. By mid-June 1924, insulin from Burroughs Wellcome, Allen & Hanbury, British Drug Houses (BDH), and Eli Lilly and Company were all available in Britian.

Professor August Krogh, a 1920 Nobel laureate, visited Toronto in November 1922. Upon his return to Denmark, he and H.C. Hagedorn established the non-profit Nordisk Insulin Laboratory, using pork pancreas from Danish bacon factories.

In Germany, large-scale production was begun in 1924–1925, although van Noorden and Naunyn believed that the insulin story was "an American exaggeration." Oskar Minkowski read Macleod's article in the *British Medical Journal* of November 22, 1922. France was the last to join in insulin production.

Lilly, with the most financial support, supplied insulin for Canada and Britain until midway through 1923. In the United States, it was sold at cost, but in Britain insulin was sold at a profit. Lilly's George Walden made another advance in insulin production, discovering that from a pH of 4.0 to 6.5 a potent, stable material formed during salt precipitation. This isoelectric precipitation method replaced the previous method in October 1922. At about the same time, Drs. Doisy, Somogyi, and P. Shaffer at Washington University in St. Louis discovered the same isoelectric precipitation method for the manufacture of insulin. Both groups claimed the discovery, and it is still felt in Washington University that this institution should have received more recognition in the insulin story.

Treatment at this time cost up to $1 per day, equivalent to $15 at today's costs. Lilly was anxious to patent Walden's method, calling the product Iletin.

Collip and Best's application for a U.S. patent was turned down because of two previous U.S. patents including that of Zuelzer in 1912. Letters from clinicians and influential patients were sought, and Lilly amended its patent applications to remove all conflict with Toronto. Banting, Best, and Collip assigned their patent rights, once granted, to the Board of Governors of the University of Toronto for $1.

In September 1923, Lilly allowed that insulin would be the generic name rather than Iletin and agreed to enter a patent pool available to all manufacturers.

In mid-September of 1923, 25,000 U.S. diabetics were taking insulin prescribed by 7,000 physicians.

Determination of the basic unit and international standardization of insulin was decided by the League of Nations (1923–1926). The results of the mouse convulsion test and the production of hypoglycemia in rabbits were the bioassays accepted (See Exhibit 18–1).

The press, meanwhile, raved over this "victory over diabetes." Only the antivivisectionists were outraged. Several references in the press gave Macleod credit for masterminding the discovery. The antagonism between Banting and Macleod flared anew. Banting accused Macleod of stealing his work. Macleod issued a carefully worded statement, saying that the idea for duct ligation (and only that idea) was Banting's. Macleod's position became so uncomfortable that he eventually left Toronto.

Col. Albert Gooderham, as chairman of the Insulin Committee, tried to resolve the situation by asking the three—Banting, Best, and Macleod—each to write his version of the story. Macleod described it as "a collaborative investigation among diverse groups, successful in giving to medical science a practically completed piece of work in a few months' time." Banting's account stressed the obstacles and was vindictive towards Macleod. Best wrote a fair account, giving credit to Macleod for suggesting alcohol extraction and immediate chilling and to Collip for determining the highest concentration of alcohol in which the active principle was soluble.

No reconciliation took place and a comprehensive document was not written. The three accounts were deposited in the archives of the University of Toronto and were sealed until after the death of the last participant (C.H. Best) in 1978.

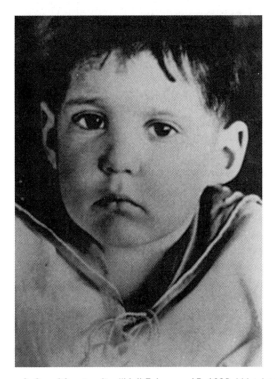

Figure 1–2.   After insulin: "J.L." February 15, 1923. Weight 29 pounds. (*Source:* Bliss M: The Discovery of Insulin. Toronto: McClelland and Stewart, 1982. Photograph courtesy of Elli Lilly and Co., Ltd. With permission.)

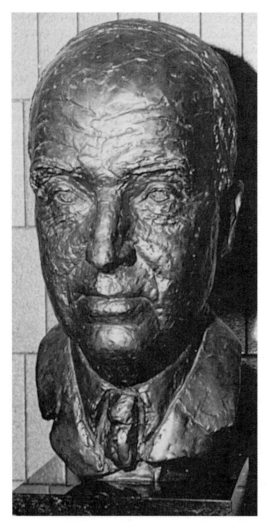

Figure 1–3. Charles Herbert Best, 1899–1978. Bust stands in the foyer of the Medical Sciences Builing, University of Toronto.

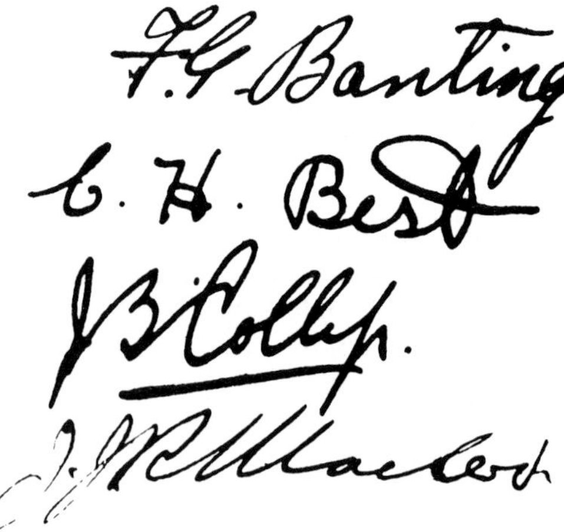

Figure 1–4. Signatures of Banting, Best, Coolip, and Macleod (*Source*: The Discovery of Insulin. Toronto: McClelland and Stewart, 1982. With permission.)

The early papers were criticized; weaknesses and flaws were pointed out, and the discoverers were accused of manipulating the numbers and ignoring the fact that whole pancreatic extract was more effective than the duct-ligated pancreas. In fact, the body of work was called a "wrongly conceived, wrongly conducted, and wrongly interpreted series of experiments."

Banting[3] did have the initial idea, and he and Best began the process that led to the successful outcome, but Collip and Macleod played important roles in the discovery of insulin. There was no doubt that the group had produced a nontoxic preparation that lowered the blood sugar and reduced the cardinal symptoms of diabetes in human beings.

Zuelzer had an extract that was more effective than theirs, but it was too toxic for use.

The presentation of work to the Association of American Physicians by the Toronto group—Banting, Best, Collip, Campbell, Fletcher, Macleod, and Noble—

on May 3, 1922 was perhaps the most important landmark in the early events surrounding the discovery.

Banting was hailed in both the United States and Canada as the discoverer. A Chair of Medical Research was endowed by the Canadian Government to be held by Banting for $10,000 a year. The government also gave him an annuity of $7,500 a year for life. Friends of Best and Collip sought more recognition for them, but the government declined. Macleod was awarded the highly esteemed Cameron Prize by the University of Edinburgh.

Banting and Macleod were nominated singly and together for the 1923 Nobel Prize in Physiology and Medicine for a discovery conferring the greatest benefit on mankind. A joint prize was awarded to them on October 25, 1923. Banting was about to refuse the award because of having to share it with Macleod, but his mind was changed by Col. Gooderham with a reminder of the meaning of the award to Canada and its people. No Canadian had previously won a Nobel Prize. Gooderham offered to pay Banting's expenses to Stockholm to accept the award.

Banting decided almost immediately to share his prize with Best, and Macleod wired Collip the next day, asking if he would share his half of the award. (The *Toronto Star* reporter on the Nobel Prize story was Ernest Hemingway.) Zuelzer and Paulesco protested to the Nobel Committee but were ignored.

J.J.R. Macleod returned to Scotland in 1928 as Regis Professor at the University of Aberdeen. He died with severe arthritis in 1935 at the age of 59. Banting never forgave Macleod and refused to attend the farewell dinner given for him in Toronto.

C.H. Best graduated in medicine as gold medalist in 1925 and later succeeded Macleod as Professor of Physiology at the University of Toronto (he was Macleod's

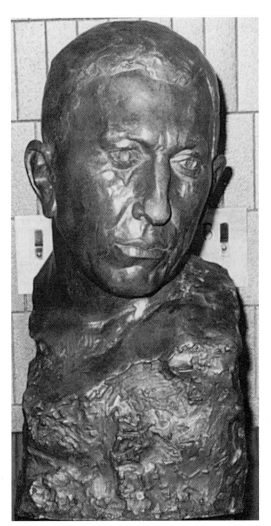

Figure 1–5. Frederick Grant Banting, 1891–1941. Bust stands in the foyer of the Medical Sciences Building, University of Toronto.

choice to fill the position). He was 29. He later married Margaret Mahon. He had done postgraduate work in physiology in London with his friend Sir Henry Dale. He died in 1978 after a distinguished career, known, loved, and revered by millions of diabetics all over the world. Margaret Best lived until 1998.

Banting occupied the Banting and Best Chair, which later became the Banting and Best Department of Medical Research. He was knighted by King George V in 1934, becoming Sir Frederick Banting, KBE. He began to paint seriously and became friends with some of the Canadian "Group of Seven." He traveled throughout Canada, painting mostly on plywood in oils. His paintings hang in many galleries and are a reminder of this remarkable man—simple, bullheaded, and tremendously talented.

Banting's first marriage in 1924 to Marion Robertson ended in divorce in 1932. He married Henrietta Ball, one of his technicians, in 1939. Their marriage ended in 1941 with his tragic death in a plane crash in Newfoundland. Banting had again become friends with Collip in the 1930s and spent his last night with Collip in Montreal. Collip died in 1967.

Zuelzer immigrated to the United States, where he died in 1952. Frederick Allen died at 88 in 1964. Walter Ruggles Campbell died at 90 in 1980.

Leonard Thompson died on April 20, 1935, when he was 27 years old. He succumbed to staphylococcal pneumonia, complicated by diabetes. Jim Havens died of cancer at the age of 59. Elizabeth Hughes Gossett died April 25, 1981. after 58 years on insulin.

The University of Toronto has established the endowed Charles H. Best Lectureship and Award which is to be presented every two years in perpetuity.[4] Dr. Donald Steiner was the first lecturer in 1995. He spoke on his discovery of proinsulin, and subsequent research on it and related peptides. Dr. Martin Rodbell, Nobel Laureate in medicine and physiology, was the second lecturer, 1997. He spoke of his discovery of G - proteins, and their relationships to insulin action and cellular signal transduction.

The celebration of the 75th anniversary of the Discovery of Insulin took place in Toronto October 4–6, 1996. Over 500 scientists from more that 35 countries attended, as did the sons of Banting (Mr. William Banting) and Best (Dr. Henry Best), and the daughter of Collip (Dr. Barbara Wyatt).[5]

References

1. Bliss M: The Discovery of Insulin. Toronto: McClelland and Stewart, 1982.
2. Burrow GN, Hazlett BE, Phillips MF: "A case of diabetes mellitus." N Engl J Med 306:340–343,1982.
3. Bliss M: Banting—A Biography. Toronto: McClelland and Stewart, 1984.
4. The University of Toronto Bulletin 51 :5, 16 (Oct. 14, 1997).
5. The Toronto Star: Oct. 7, 1996, A2 and A6

2

Non-Insulin-Dependent (Type 2) Diabetes Mellitus and Obesity

John K. Davidson and Mario DiGirolamo

Historical Perspective

What has been designated since 1979 as non-insulin-dependent diabetes mellitus (NIDDM or type 2 diabetes mellitus)[1,2] was described three thousand years ago by Hindu physicians who noted that the disease was associated with gluttony and obesity.[3] Bouchardat found more than a century ago that his overweight patients with diabetes became aglucosuric coincidental to the shortage of food and the weight loss that occurred during the siege of Paris (Franco-Prussian War).[4] His observations prompted him to prescribe a reduced caloric intake and exercise to promote weight loss. Prior to the clinical use of insulin in 1922, diet and exercise therapy were the only effective treatments available to abolish or diminish glucosuria.

During both world wars (1914–1918, 1939–1945), in countries where supplies were inadequate to meet the needs, food was rationed. In England and Wales, there was a parallel decrease in sugar (and calorie) consumption and in diabetes mortality indices (Fig. 2–1).[5]

Less than 2 years after the introduction of insulin therapy, Campbell and Macleod (1924)[6] warned against the use of insulin in the treatment of overweight individuals who were not in diabetic ketoacidosis: "the so-called 'luxury use' of insulin was a matter of some concern during the earlier period of treatment with the drug, while supplies were still relatively scarce. At that time it was considered justifiable to place a limit on the amount of insulin obtainable by any patient in order that others "should not suffer". The large supply of insulin now available [*editor's note: i.e., available in 1924*] has brought about its use by many physicians who are more or less unfamiliar with the clinical course of diabetes, and who are using it unnecessarily (luxury use). The use of insulin and precariously high-calorie diets to fatten a diabetic unduly, or to satisfy a gluttonous appetite, or to avoid the necessity of dieting, reveals a lack of intelligent foresight on the part of the physician as well as a lack of resourcefulness in the treatment of his patients. For the patient himself, there is an increased danger of hypoglycemia, of hyperglycemia and glucosuria, and of degenerative phenomena associated with diabetes."[6] These comments are as true in 1998[7] as they were in 1924.

Himsworth (1936)[8] reported that patients who were "insensitive" to the plasma-glucose-lowering effects of insulin therapy had eaten more calories and were more

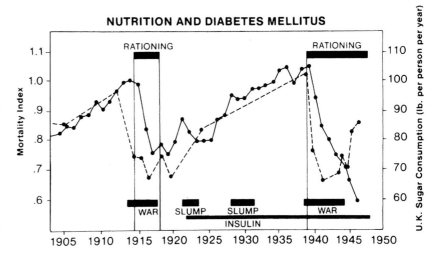

Figure 2–1 Diabetes mortality indices for England and Wales (1938 was used as the base year). With food rationing during both world wars, there was a dramatic drop in the diabetes mortality index. There was a parallel drop in the amount of sugar consumed (dashed line) during the wars. [*Source:* Drash A: Influence of the level of nutrition on diabetes mellitus; world-wide dietary and ethnic factors in evaluation of the disease. *In* Gardner LI, Amacher P (eds): Endocrine Aspects of Malnutrition. Santa Ynez, CA: Kroc Foundation, 1973, pp. 257–287. With permission.]

likely to be overweight, even obese, than were those who were "sensitive" to the plasma-glucose-lowering effects of insulin therapy.

During the last 40 years (see Chapter 16, Historical Perspective section), investigators have noted that: (1) many overweight individuals with diabetes were hyperinsulinemic or normoinsulinemic,[9,10] (Fig. 2–2); (2) that cellular insulin receptor numbers were down-regulated by hyperinsulinemia and that coincidentally insulin-responsive tissues became "resistant" to the metabolic effects of both endogenous and exogenous insulin[11]; (3) that weight gain in nondiabetic normal

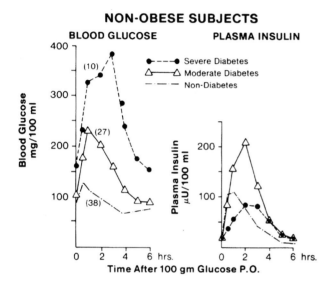

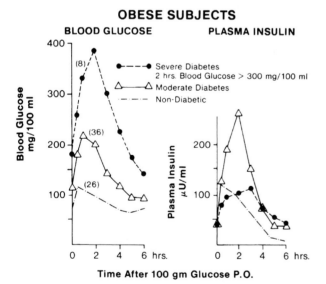

Figure 2–2 Comparison of blood glucose and plasma insulin levels in nonobese and obese subjects without diabetes and with moderate and severe diabetes. In moderate diabetes plasma insulin levels are increased, but in severe diabetes plasma insulin levels in the first phase of insulin secretion in response to the glucose load are decreased. (*Source:* Yalow RS, Glick SM, Roth J, et al.: Plasma insulin and growth hormone levels in obesity and diabetes. Ann NY Acad Sci 131:357–373, 1965. With permission.)

weight individuals increased tissue "resistance" to insulin; (4) that decreased caloric intake and/or increased caloric expenditure with weight loss decreased tissue "resistance" to insulin[12,13]; and (5) that hyperglycemia in those with NIDDM frequently decreased or disappeared (normal glucose tolerance test) during restricted caloric intake and weight loss even in those who had been treated with insulin.[14–17]

Yet NIDDM remains an enigma,[18] and controversy continues concerning the role of insulin resistance in its etiology. As in the *chicken-egg debate*, the questions are: (1) Is the resistance *the cause* of NIDDM, or (2) is it the *consequence* of NIDDM?[19,21,54] The insulin receptor is the best characterized component of the insulin-signaling pathway in insulin-sensitive cells (see Chapters 8 and 9). Yet it is only one of several components in a complex regulatory pathway, and attempts to define insulin resistance at the molecular level have been hampered by an imperfect understanding of insulin action.[22–26] Although certain rare forms of severe insulin resistance (lipoatrophic diabetes, Robson-Mendenhall syndrome, leprechaunism, extreme insulin resistance type A, and others) are associated with inherited defects in insulin receptor function,[18,27] there is little evidence for heritable defects in receptor function in NIDDM in which insulin-binding affinity is normal and receptor number is modulated *only* as a reversible consequence of hyperinsulinemia.[27]

In a few Pima Indians whose receptors have been sequenced in a search for mutations, the receptor sequence has been normal.[28,29] Thus receptor mutations, though they may occur in a very small subset of cases of NIDDM, appear to be only one of several factors contributing to the etiology of the disease.[18] See Chapters 8, 9, and 5.

In the early 1990s two important discoveries revealed the beginning and end of a cascade of reactions that link the interaction of insulin and its receptor and the stimulation of the uptake of glucose into mammalian cells. First was the discovery that the occupied insulin receptor is a tyrosine kinase leading to both tyrosine autophosphorylation of the receptor beta-subunit and of cellular substrates; second was the discovery that glucose transporters reside mainly in intracellular membrane vesicles in the absence of insulin and that insulin stimulation leads to an increase in the recruitment of these transporters to the plasma membrane. This translocation accounts for the increased rates of glucose transport into the stimulated cells. Recently PI3-kinase has been characterized as a mediator of insulin signaling to glucose transport. Additional questions yet to be answered center around the specificity of PI3-kinase effects on glucose transporter translocation: do specific IRS molecules, PI3-kinases, phosphatidyl-inositol binding proteins, serine/threonine kinases and/or G proteins produce the required specificity?[30]

West (1978)[17] summarized his classic international epidemiologic studies on the relationship between nutritional status and diabetes prevalence rates by concluding that excess adiposity secondary to excess caloric intake (caloric overload in the body's adipose tissue depots), rather than any specific component of the diet (i.e., sugars, carbohydrate, fat, protein, and so forth) accounted for the vast majority of cases of diabetes in the world. The nature of the *obesity-NIDDM connection* will be explored in much greater detail later in this chapter.

The University Group Diabetes Program Study (UGDP, 1982) reported no measurable influence(s) of insulin treatment on mortality or morbidity outcomes in those with NIDDM (see Chapters 18, 20, 54, and 55). Another study in two diabetes clinics (Memphis and Atlanta)[15,16] that used different treatment strategies in the decade of the 1970s showed that the standard mortality ratios in the two clinics were almost identical. Age accounted for 73% and duration of diabetes accounted for 15% of the deaths. The effects of other risk factors (hypertension, obesity, hyperlipidemia, smoking) on mortality and morbidity rates of those with NIDDM are unknown.[15,16] Whether or not removal of those risk factors (including return of normoglycemia due to therapeutically induced weight loss) can reduce contemporary mortality and/or morbidity rates for NIDDM is also unknown.[14,15]

Epidemiology

The prevalence of diagnosed diabetes has increased sixfold in the last 40 years in the USA. The centers for disease control reported the prevalence of diabetes in the United States in late 1997 to be 15.7 million (5,9% of the population, 10.3 million diagnosed, 5.4 million undiagnosed).[20] 798,000 new cases are diagnosed each year.

It is estimated that 90-95% of those with diabetes have type 2 (NIDDM) and 5-10% have type 1 (IDDM). There are at least 123,000 children and teen-agers with type 1 diabetes in the USA.

A new category designated *Impaired Fasting Plasma Glucose (IFPG)* was introduced by the American Diabetes Association in 1997 (fasting plasma glucose 110-125 mg/dl). It is estimated that 13.4 million Americans (7% of the population) fall into that category.

The complications of diabetes account for most of its morbidity and mortality. 65% of individuals with diabetes have *high blood pressure*. *Heart disease* and *stroke* death rates in diabetics are 2-4 times higher than in non-diabetics. *Diabetic retinopathy* causes from 12,000 to 24,000 new cases of blindness per year, with diabetes being the leading cause of new cases of blindness in adults 20 to 70 years of age. 27,851 diabetics developed *end-stage renal disease* in 1995, and during that same

year 98,872 Americans with diabetes underwent dialysis or kidney transplantation. Diabetes now accounts for about 40% of new cases of renal failure.[20] About two-thirds of those with diabetes have *nerve problems*, with *lower extremity neuropathy* being a major contributor to *lower extremity amputation.* From 1993 to 1995 each year in the USA, 67,000 lower extremity amputations were performed in individuals who had diabetes. *Periodontal disease* is present in 30% of type 1 diabetics over 18 years of age. *For infant and mother* diabetes causes many *major complications of pregnancy.*[20]

The total costs of diabetes in the USA in 1992 was $92 billion ($45 billion direct medical costs, $47 billion indirect costs due to disability, work loss, and premature mortality).[20]

The studies of West[17] (Figs. 2–3 and 2–4) had shown an increased prevalence of diabetes that was strongly correlated with an increased percent of mean group weight in different countries. Diabetes prevalence increased from 2% in East Pakistan (mean group weight = 75% of mean standard weight) to 6.9% in Uruguay (mean group weight = 123% of mean standard weight) to 25% in the North Carolina Cherokee Indians, whose mean group weight was even greater.

The age-adjusted incidence rates for diabetes in Pima Indians by body mass index showed a marked increase in incidence of new cases of diabetes per thousand person-years as body mass index increased from less than 20 (1 per 1,000 person-years) to 40 or higher (60 per 1,000 person-years).[35] Prevalence of new cases was greater in children of mothers-only-diabetic than in mothers-and-fathers-diabetic than in fathers-only-diabetic than in mothers-and-fathers-nondiabetic.[35] As the body mass index increased from

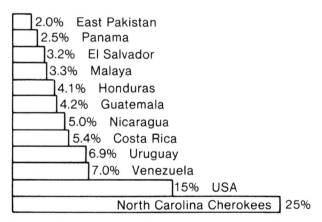

Figure 2–3 Prevalence of abnormal glucose tolerance (2-hr venous plasma glucose concentration greater than 170 mg/dL after a 75 g glucose load at time zero). In all population samples the mean age was about 50 years, and all subjects were more than 29 years of age. (*Source:* West KM: Epidemiology of Diabetes and Its Vascular Lesions. New York: Elsevier, 1978. With permission.)

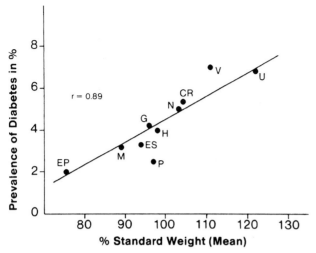

Figure 2–4   Relationship of average fatness (expressed as percent of mean standard weight) and prevalence of diabetes in ten countries [East Pakistan, Malaya, El Salvador, Guatemala, Panama, Honduras, Nicaragua, Costa Rica, Venezuela, and Uruguay, as designated by their initials: e.g., EP (East Pakistan)]. All individuals were more than 29 years of age. (*Source:* West KM: Epidemiology of Diabetes and Its Vascular Lesions. New York: Elsevier, 1978. With permission.)

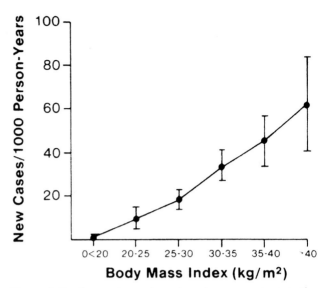

Figure 2–5   Age- and sex-adjusted incidence rates (with 95% confidence intervals) for diabetes in Pima Indians, by body mass index. [*Source:* Knowler WC, Bennett PH, Pettitt DJ, et al.: Obesity and diabetes in Pima Indians: the effects of parental diabetes on the relationship of obesity and the incidence of diabetes. *In* Melish JS, Hanna J, Baba S (eds): Genetic environmental Interaction in Diabetes Mellitus. Amsterdam: Excerpta Medica, 1982, pp. 95–100. With permission.]

less than 20 to greater than 40, the prevalence of new cases of diabetes increased almost fourfold even in those whose mothers and fathers were nondiabetic. This finding again highlights the remarkable correlation between overweight and NIDDM. As Fig. 2–6 illustrates, the prevalence of obesity in the United States increases with increasing age up to age 50 years. The prevalence of obesity in females is more than twice the prevalence in males, with prevalence being greater in African American females than in Caucasian females and greater in Caucasian males than in African American males.[36]

Studies have shown that African Americans have a 50% higher rate of NIDDM than do Caucasians in the United States. Although African American to Cau-

casian rate ratios for diabetes were identical at desirable body weight, African American to Caucasian rate ratios increased to 1.6 at body weight 125% of desirable and to 1.8 at body weight 150% of desirable. These findings suggest that interventions directed at reducing excess weight or maintaining normal weight may be the most important actions needed to ameliorate the racial disparity in diabetes.[37]

Studies of age-standardized prevalence of diabetes in the Pacific region (1975–1980) in those more than 20 years of age by 1980 World Health Organization criteria varies from 0.8 to 30.3% (Table 2–1).[38] Prevalence is highest in "westernized" Micronesians (Nauru), high in Fiji Indians, and lowest in rural Melanesians. There appear to be ethnic differences in susceptibility to

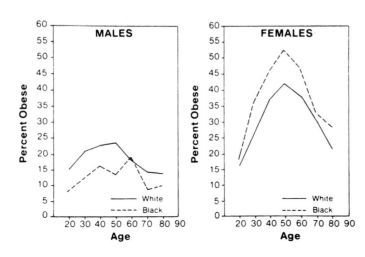

Figure 2–6   Prevalence of obesity (>120% of ideal body weight) by age, sex, and race in combined samples of ten states in the nutrition survey of 1968–1970 by the Department of Health, Education and Welfare. (*Source:* Department of HEW Ten-State Nutrition Survey 1968–1970. Publication 72-8131 (HSM), Vol. 3, p. 44, West KM: Epidemiology of Diabetes and Its Vascular Lesions. New York: Elsevier, 1978. With permission.)

TABLE 2–1 Age-Standardized Diabetes Prevalence—Pacific Region (1975–1980)[a]

Geo-Ethnic Group	No. Individuals Studied[b]	Diabetes Prevalence[c] (%)
Micronesians		
Nauru	456	30.3
Polynesians		
Tuvalu	397	3.9
Western Samoa		
R	745	2.7
U	744	7.0
Melanesians		
Loyalty	535	2.0
New Caledonia	172	1.5
Fiji		
R	477	1.8
U	861	6.9
Papua (R)	105	0.8
New Guinea (U)	184	15.4
Indians		
Fiji		
R	452	13.3
U	848	14.8

[a] Age standardized to Western Samoa Census (1976).

[b] More than 20 years.

[c] See WHO Criteria, 1980.

Abbreviations: R, rural; U, urban.

[*Source:* Zimmet P, Kirk JR, Serjeantson S, et al.: Diabetes in Pacific populations—genetic and environmental interactions. *In* Melish JS, Hanna J, Baba S (eds): Genetic Environmental Interaction in Diabetes Mellitus, Amsterdam: Excerpta Medica, 1982, pp. 9–17. With permission.]

develop NIDDM, but additional studies will be needed to confirm this hypothesis.[39,40]

Data analyses (cited before) have shown the remarkably close correlations between prevalence and duration of obesity (or overweight) and prevalence and incidence of NIDDM in different parts of the world and in different ethnic groups. Weight differences appear to be related primarily to differences in energy intake, with excess intake (intake calories > caloric expenditures) leading to overweight or obesity and to hyperglycemia. Although the prevalence of NIDDM is more common in some families and in some ethnic groups than in others, the significance of the genetic contribution to the overall prevalence and incidence of NIDDM in different ethnic groups is yet to be determined.[40] See Chapter 5.

Pathophysiology

When energy intake exceeds energy use, the excess calories are stored in adipose (or fat) tissue as triglycerides (Tables 2–2 and 2–3, Figs. 2–4, 2–5, and 2–6). As triglycerides accumulate, fat cells hypertrophy (increase in size) and may increase in number (hyperplasia) (Figs. 2–7, 2–8, and 2–9).[31]

Table 2–2 illustrates the approximate caloric content of energy depots in hypothetical lean, desirable weight, overweight males of medium frame and 1.73 meters in height. Table 2–3 shows the 1998 classification of

TABLE 2–2 Approximate Calorie Content of Energy Depots in Hypothetical Lean, Desirable Weight, Overweight, and Obese Males of Medium Frame and 68 In. (1.73 M) in Height

	Lean Example Below (2% Body Fat)	Desirable Male: 9–18% Female: 18–28% Example Below (10% Body Fat)	Overweight Example Below = 30% Body Fat	Obese Example Below = 50% Body Fat
Body weight				
Pounds	142.1	154	184.8	277.2
Kg	64.6	70	84	126
% IBW (Hamwi)	91.5	100	120	180
Body mass index (kg/m^2)	21.6	23.4	28.1	42.1
Body specific gravity[a]	1.10	1.085	1.04	1.00
Body water (L)	45.9	46	46.1	46.6
% of body weight	71	66	49	37

	Energy Stores[b]							
	g	cal	g	cal	g	cal	g	cal
Carbohydrate	300	1,200	300	1,200	300	1,200	300	1,200
Glucose	70	280	70	280	70	280	70	280
Glycogen	230	920	230	920	230	920	230	920
Liver	75	300	75	300	75	300	75	300
Muscle	155	620	155	620	155	620	155	620
Protein	7,300	29,200	7,300	29,200	7,300	29,200	7,300	29,200
Fat	1,400	10,700	7,000	53,500	25,200	192,800	63,000	482,000

[a] Specific gravity of skeleton = 1.56 (15% of body weight), of adipose tissue = 0.90, of other tissues = 1.06.

[b] Based on dry weight of the tissues and allowing 4 cal/g for carbohydrate and protein, and 9 cal/g for fat (triglyceride). It has been assumed that adipose tissue contains 15% water.

TABLE 2–3 Classification of Overweight

Classification	% of Ideal Body Weight	BMI (kg/m²)
Underweight	<90	<18.5
Normal Range	90–109	18.5–24.9
Overweight	≥110	25.0 or higher
Pre-obese	110–119	25.0–29.9
Obese class I	120–149	30.0–34.9
Obese class II	150–199	35.0–39.9
Obese class III	≥200	40 or higher

The classification according to BMI is based on data from the International Obesity Task Force. World Health Organization. Obesity: Preventing and managing the global epidemic (World Health Organization, Geneva, 1998). The two classifications may be close but they have not been matched as yet.

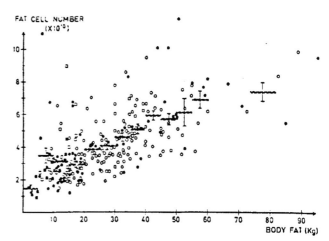

Figure 2–7 Dependence of body fat on fat cell number in young men (filled squares) (*Sjöström, Smith, Krotkiewski and Björntorp* 1972, *Björntorp, Berchtold and Tibblin* 1971), young women (open squares) (*Sjöström et al.* 1972), middle-aged men (filled circles) (*Björntorp et al.* 1971) and women (open circles) (*Björntorp et al.* 1971) and obese men (filled circles) and women (open circles). Group means ± SEM denoted for each body fat class of 5 kg up to 60 kg. Body fat above 60 kg treated as one group.

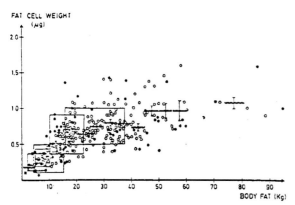

Figure 2–8 Dependence of body fat on fat cell weight in the same materials as in Fig. 1. Rectangles denote mean ± one standard deviation of values for medical students (body fat 2-9 kg) (*Sjöström et al.* 1972), young athletes (body fat 5-10 kg) (*Björntorp et al.* 1972b), middle-aged athletes (body fat 3-15 kg) (*Björntorp et al.* 1972b), randomly selected middle-aged men (body fat 10-22 kg) (*Björntorp et al.* 1971) and men with endogenous hypertriglyceridemia (body fat 16-38 kg) (*Björntorp, Gustafson and Persson* 1971).

overweight (as % ideal body weight) as compared to Body Mass Index (BMI) of the world health organization obesity task force.[32] The body mass index table is shown in Table 2–4.[32] Excess amounts of body adipose tissue correlate with increased mortality rates (Fig. 2–10).[42]

Obesity in the westernized world has reached epidemic proportions,[33,34] and the prevalence of non-insulin dependent diabetes has increased in a parallel fashion.[33,34]

It has been known for over 60 years that about two thirds of the body weight of "normal" adults is related to its water content, with the remaining one third being accounted for by the dry weight of the skeleton, skin, muscles, tissues and other organs, and adipose tissue.[43]

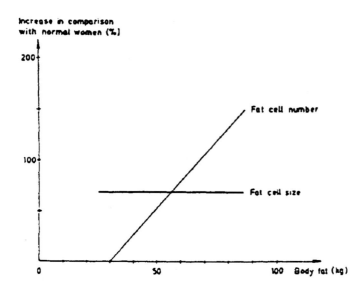

Figure 2–9 Dependence of adipose tissue increase on fat cell size and fat cell number increase in obese patients in comparison with randomly selected women (from *Björntorp and Sjöström* 1971).

TABLE 2–4 Body Mass Index Table

BMI	19	20	21	22	23	24	25	26	27	28	29	30	31	32	33	34	35
Height (inches)							**Body Weight (pounds)**										
58	91	96	100	105	110	115	119	124	129	134	138	143	148	153	158	162	167
59	94	99	104	109	114	119	124	128	133	138	143	148	153	158	163	168	173
60	97	102	107	112	118	123	128	133	138	143	148	153	158	163	168	174	179
61	100	106	111	116	122	127	132	137	143	148	153	158	164	169	174	180	185
62	104	109	115	120	126	131	136	142	147	153	158	164	169	175	180	186	191
63	107	113	118	124	130	135	141	146	152	158	163	169	175	180	186	191	197
64	110	116	122	128	134	140	145	151	157	163	169	174	180	186	192	197	204
65	114	120	126	132	138	144	150	156	162	168	174	180	186	192	198	204	210
66	118	124	130	136	142	148	155	161	167	173	179	186	192	198	204	210	216
67	121	127	134	140	146	153	159	166	172	178	185	191	198	204	211	217	223
68	125	131	138	144	151	158	164	171	177	184	190	197	203	210	216	223	230
69	128	135	142	149	155	162	169	176	182	189	196	203	209	216	223	230	236
70	132	139	146	153	160	167	174	181	188	195	202	209	216	222	229	236	243
71	136	143	150	157	165	172	179	186	193	200	208	215	222	229	236	243	250
72	140	147	154	162	169	177	184	191	199	206	213	221	228	235	242	250	258
73	144	151	159	166	174	182	189	197	204	212	219	227	235	242	250	257	265
74	148	155	163	171	179	186	194	202	210	218	225	233	241	249	256	264	272
75	152	160	168	176	184	192	200	208	216	224	232	240	248	256	264	272	279
76	156	164	172	180	189	197	205	213	221	230	238	246	254	263	271	279	287

BMI	36	37	38	39	40	41	42	43	44	45	46	47	48	49	50	51	52	53	54
58	172	177	181	186	191	196	201	205	210	215	220	224	229	234	239	244	248	253	258
59	178	183	188	193	198	203	208	212	217	222	227	232	237	242	247	252	257	262	267
60	184	189	194	199	204	209	215	220	225	230	235	240	245	250	255	261	266	271	276
61	190	195	201	206	211	217	222	227	232	238	243	248	254	259	264	269	275	280	285
62	196	202	207	213	218	224	229	235	240	246	251	256	262	267	273	278	284	289	295
63	203	208	214	220	225	231	237	242	248	254	259	265	270	278	282	287	293	299	304
64	209	215	221	227	232	238	244	250	256	262	267	273	279	285	291	296	302	308	314
65	216	222	228	234	240	246	252	258	264	270	276	282	288	294	300	306	312	318	324
66	223	229	235	241	247	253	260	266	272	278	284	291	297	303	309	315	322	328	334
67	230	236	242	249	255	261	268	274	280	287	293	299	306	312	319	325	331	338	344
68	236	243	249	256	262	269	276	282	289	295	302	308	315	322	328	335	341	348	354
69	243	250	257	263	270	277	284	291	297	304	311	318	324	331	338	345	351	358	365
70	250	257	264	271	278	285	292	299	306	313	320	327	334	341	348	355	362	369	376
71	257	265	272	279	286	293	301	308	315	322	329	338	343	351	358	365	372	379	386
72	265	272	279	287	294	302	309	316	324	331	338	346	353	361	368	375	383	390	397
73	272	280	288	295	302	310	318	325	333	340	348	355	363	371	378	386	393	401	408
74	280	287	295	303	311	319	326	334	342	350	358	365	373	381	389	396	404	412	420
75	287	295	303	311	319	327	335	343	351	359	367	375	383	391	399	407	415	423	431
76	295	304	312	320	328	336	344	353	361	369	377	385	394	402	410	418	426	435	443

The Practical Guide to the Identification, Evaluation, and Treatment of Overweight and Obesity in Adults with Permission from ref. 33.

The skeleton contains about 22% water and adipose tissue contains about 15%. Other tissues contain 72 to 83% water. The specific gravity of the skeleton (1.56), other tissues (1.06), and fat (0.90) are known. The total body density (or specific gravity) can be determined by underwater weighing. When body specific gravity is known, the percentage of body water and percentage of body fat, which are inversely correlated, can be calculated (Figs. 2–11 and 2–12).[44]

Although there is much controversy about what should be regarded as a "normal" or desirable weight and a "normal" or desirable amount of body adipose tissue (see Chapter 16 on diet therapy for NIDDM), insurance company statistics indicate that the mortality ratio is lowest for those with a body mass index from 19 to 25, and rises progressively for those with a body mass index greater than 25 (Fig. 2–10).[42] The progressive increase in the mortality ratio with increasing

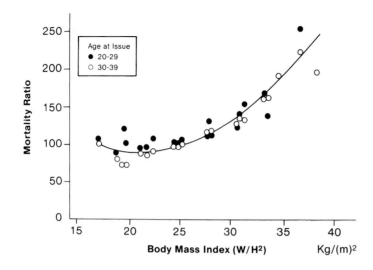

Figure 2–10 Relation of body mass index to mortality. Adapted from data in the Build and Blood Pressure Study of 1959. As body mass index rises, the excess mortality increases. (*Source:* Bray GA: Definition, measurement, and classification of syndromes of obesity. Int J Obesity 2:99–112, 1978. With permission.)

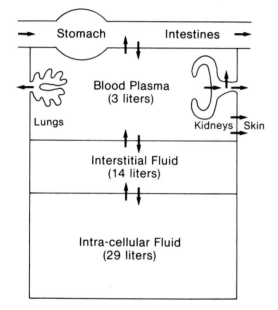

Figure 2–11 Diagrammatic illustration of the three fluid compartments (modified from Gamble). Figures in parentheses have been inserted to show volume of water in each compartment of a subject weighing 154 pounds (70 kg), whose total water content is assumed to be 46 L (2/3 of body weight). [*Source:* Gregersen ML: Total body water and the fluid compartments. *In* Bard P (ed): Medical Physiology, Ed. 11. St. Louis: C.V. Mosby, 1961, pp. 301–316. With permission.]

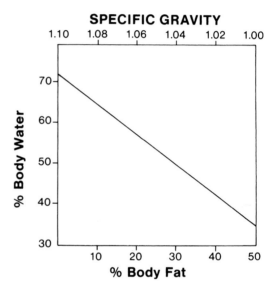

Figure 2–12 Schema showing relationship of body specific gravity to percent body water and percent body fat. [*Source:* Gregersen MI: Total body water and the fluid compartments. *In* Bard P (ed): Medical Physiology, Ed. 11. St. Louis: C.V. Mosby, 1961, pp. 301–316. With permission.]

body mass was more obvious for those age 30 to 39 years than for those age 20 to 29 years at time of issue of insurance. It is clear that the prevalence of obesity and NIDDM increases with increasing age and increasing body mass (see Figs. 2–5 and 2–6).

The relationships between body weight, percent ideal body weight (HAMWI), body mass index (BMI), body specific gravity, body water content, and energy stores (carbohydrate, protein, fat) in lean, "desirable weight," "overweight," and "obese" individuals are shown in Table 2–2. Table 2–3 shows the 1998 comparison of % of ideal body weight broken

down into underweight, normal weight, and overweight (pre-obese, and obese classes I, II, and III) according to the world health organization international obesity task force.[32] The desirable percentage of body fat in males is 9-18%, and in females is 18-32%. Body fat in excess of 22% in the male or 28% in the female has been found to be associated with increased health risks.[33]

Extensive studies of the effects of obesity in animals and humans (including the development of NIDDM and its complications) have been carried out in the last 40 years.

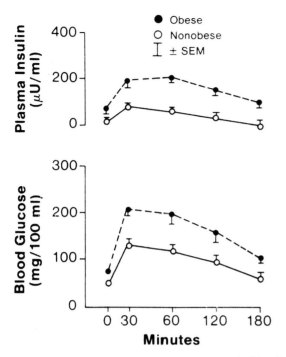

Figure 2–13 Influence of spontaneous obesity on the blood glucose and plasma insulin response to an oral glucose load. The values represent the mean blood glucose and plasma insulin levels of ten obese and ten nonobese patients during oral glucose tolerance tests. [*Source*: Salans LB, Cushman SW: Relationship of adiposity and diet to the abnormalities of carbohydrate metabolism in obesity. *In* Katzen HL, Mahler J (eds): Advances in Modern Nutrition, Vol. 2. Diabetes, Obesity, and Vascular Disease. New York: John Wiley & Sons, 1978, pp. 267–302. With permission.]

Obese individuals are "resistant" to their endogenous insulin during a glucose tolerance test, and the glucose level is significantly higher despite the fact that endogenous insulin levels are significantly higher (both fasting and after a glucose load) (Fig. 2–13).[45] During infusion of exogenous insulin (Fig. 2–14), the glucose

uptake by forearm muscle is significantly greater in nonobese nondiabetics than in obese nondiabetics.[46]

Sims[13] has shown that humans who are fed hypercaloric diets (more calories than needed to maintain ideal body weight) gain weight and increase their plasma glucose and insulin levels. These changes revert to normal after a decreased caloric intake and weight loss (less calories than needed to maintain body weight).

The relationship of obesity to the development of NIDDM is unquestioned, both from animal and human studies.[5,17,49,50] It is also clear that prevention of obesity, or correction of obesity even to a modest degree, can reduce or delay the manifestations of carbohydrate intolerance in individuals with an inherited predisposition to diabetes.

There are, however, several considerations that must be kept in mind in order to understand the complex interaction between obesity and obesity-related development of NIDDM.

Not all obese subjects are diabetic. Actually, only a small proportion of obese subjects is diabetic. This may be due to lack of genetic propensity for diabetes, the limited duration of obesity, the size of the adipose mass, degree of pancreatic secretory capacity, or other factors, such as diet and exercise.

However, most, if not all, obese subjects with normal carbohydrate tolerance are hyperinsulinemic, both in the basal state and during a glucose challenge. And most, if not all, obese subjects are insulin-resistant, as measured by the state-of-the-art euglycemic clamp method[51] or the minimal model of insulin sensitivity of Bergman.[52]

From the data available, the following sequence of events has been postulated by several groups of investigators.[53,54] When a lean individual gains weight and body fat, by an excess of caloric intake over caloric expenditure, a state of insulin resistance develops that is accompanied by elevated levels of circulating insulin

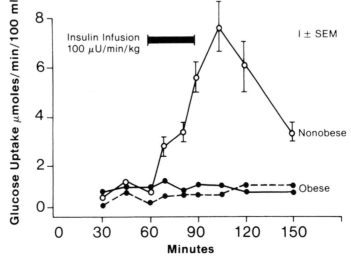

Figure 2–14 Comparison of basal and insulin-stimulated arterial deep-venous glucose concentration differences across forearm muscle in two obese and five nonobese individuals studied during periods of weight maintenance. [*Source:* Horton ES, Danforth E, Sims, EAH, et al.: *In* Burland WL, Samuel PD, Yudkin J (eds): Obesity. London: Churchill Livingstone, 1974, p. 217. With permission.]

and increased pancreatic secretion of insulin. The mechanisms of *insulin resistance*[54] are not clear and may vary from tissue to tissue. In some tissues, such as adipose, the resistance to insulin appears to be mostly postreceptor in nature, reflecting a limited capacity for the adipose cell to convert glucose to fatty acids and other metabolic products. Adipocyte binding of insulin in obesity has been reported to be normal, decreased, or even increased.[55] In other tissues, such as muscle, the resistance to insulin appears to be both at the receptor level with demonstrated reduction in insulin binding and at the postreceptor level, resulting in reduced oxidative and nonoxidative utilization of glucose.[56] Similarly, the mechanism of hyperinsulinemia is still unexplained, and the specific message reaching the pancreas to increase insulin production in obesity as in other conditions of insulin resistance is unknown.

In the early stages of obesity, the insulin resistance is partially compensated for by the hyperinsulinemia, which is effective in promoting glucose utilization, restraining hepatic glucose production, and inhibiting catabolic events such as lipolysis and proteolysis by a "shift to the right" of the dose response. In this early stage of obesity, fasting and postchallenge glucose levels may remain within normal limits and the free fatty acid (FFA) levels may be normal.[53,54] Later, however, the increased demands on the pancreatic secretion of insulin produced by greater degrees of obesity and prolonged duration of obesity leads to an inability of the pancreas to keep up with the demands of insulin resistance and the insulin secretory rate progressively declines and becomes insufficient to maintain glucose and fatty acid homeostasis. Some have referred to this failure of the beta cells as *Starling's law of the pancreas*. When this stage is reached, the zenith of the circulating hyperinsulinemia is quickly followed by progressively lower insulin levels and progressively rising levels of blood glucose and FFAs. Experimental data have clearly demonstrated[54] that a rise in FFAs can lead to an increase in hepatic gluconeogenesis, and thus promotes hyperglycemia. Reduction of obesity may be more effective in the early stages of hyperglycemia when pancreatic insulin secretion is not exhausted and reduction of insulin resistance by weight loss may lead to improvement of glycemia[12–16,53].

In patients who become diabetic after having become obese, it is not clear in many cases whether the obesity is a necessary concomitant of the inherited genetic abnormality that ultimately culminates in NIDDM or whether obesity is an independent aggravating factor. In the human, genetic propensity for diabetes is frequently associated with genetic propensity for obesity and epidemiologic studies have shown a high concordance rate, in identical twins, of middle to late adult-onset NIDDM.[57] Thus, in certain individuals, development of obesity could represent the result of a genetic predisposition expressed initially in progressive obesity and later as diabetes. Recent developments in application of molecular biology tools may clarify this point, once the genes for obesity and diabetes become known. A focus of investigation is also the possibility that genetic abnormalities may reside in the secretory capacity of the beta cells of the pancreatic islets, thus explaining the early appearance of NIDDM in some predisposed individuals (see Chapters 3, 5, 6, and 10).

In other individuals, however, without obvious genetic predisposition, obesity promoted by excessive caloric intake over caloric expenditure could lead to carbohydrate intolerance by similar mechanisms.

Animal Models of Obesity and Diabetes

The complex relationship between obesity and diabetes has led to the search for animal models and experimentalists have identified models of "spontaneous" diabetes associated with various degrees of obesity in numerous animal species, including rodents, carnivora, and ruminants.[49,50,58,59] Although some of these[49,50,58,59] reports are sporadic, several models have been sufficiently established to be used consistently in investigations of the various parameters contributing to diabetes. An extensive review of animal models of diabetes is provided in a monograph by E. Shafrir and the late A.E. Renold.[50]

Table 2–5 lists some of the most common rodent models of the obesity/diabetes syndrome. It should be noted: (1) That in some models the obesity is not present or is minimally present, and this may be associated with greater degrees of ketosis; and (2) that a variety of different presentations and metabolic manifestations are observed in these animal models of obesity/hyperglycemia. Among the better known obesity/diabetes models in which obesity is accompanied by insulin resistance, hyperinsulinemia and hyperglycemia are the obese ob/ob mice, New Zealand obese (NZO) mice and the Zucker "fatty rat." In these models, however, the hyperglycemia can at times be modest.

In the obese Zucker rats, enlarged adipocytes present a diminished binding of insulin and a markedly reduced intracellular capacity to metabolize glucose.[56] The soleus muscle in the obese Zucker rat, besides showing decreased insulin receptor numbers, is defective in its basal glucose utilization and capacity for glycogen synthesis; the dose-response curve for hexose transport and glucose phosphorylation is shifted to the right.[56]

Among the primate models, the diabetes occurring in black Celebes apes (*Macaca nigra*)[58] and the diabetes occurring in overfed and obese rhesus monkeys[59] provide useful animal models.

TABLE 2–5 Features of Inappropriate Hyperglycemia and Obesity in Rodents

Name	Inheritance	Obesity	Adipocyte Hyperplasia	Increased Serum IRI	Islet Changes	Ketosis
Diabetes (*db*)	Auto. rec.	+	−	Trans	++	++
Spiny mice	Polygenic (?)	+	ND	++	++	+
Sand rats	Polygenic (?)	+	ND	Trans	+	+
Obese (*ob*)	Auto. rec.	++	+	++	++	−
PBB/Ld	Polygenic (?)	++	+	+	−	−
Yellow	Auto. dom.	++	−	+	+	−
NZO	Polygenic	++	+	+	+	−
KK mice	Polygenic	+	ND	+	+	−
$C_2H1 \times 1$	Hybrids (F_1)	+	ND	+	+	−
Zucker rat	Auto. rec.	++	+	++	−	−
Chinese hamster	Polygenic	−	ND	Trans	+	++
S. African hamster	Polygenic	−	ND	ND	+	+

Abbreviations: Auto = autosomal; dom. = dominent; IRI = immunoreactive insulin; ND = no data available; rec. = recessive; Trans = transient. [*Source:* Adapted from Hunt CE, Lindsey JR, Walker SW: Animal models of diabetes and obesity, including the PBB/Ld mouse. Fed Proc 35:1206–1217, 1976. With permission.]

Regional Adiposity and Risk of Diabetes

Another important aspect of the relationship between obesity and diabetes results from observations of the last 2 decades indicating that a regional pattern of adiposity, the upper body segment obesity (UBSO), is more readily associated with health risk factors, including diabetes, than the obesity distributed in the lower body segment (LBSO)[60,61] (Figs. 2–15 and 2–16).

The UBSO includes individuals, mostly but not exclusively males, with accumulated fat in the abdominal region, both subcutaneously and in the visceral intra-abdominal area. This pattern has been nicknamed "apple" to be contrasted to the LBSO with accumulation of fat in the buttocks and hips, nicknamed "pear" (Fig. 2–17).

The UBSO has been found to have a greater association with carbohydrate intolerance than the LBSO.[62] Furthermore, a recent study has indicated that within subjects with UBSO, individuals with predominantly visceral fat distribution had greater insulin elevation and greater carbohydrate intolerance than individuals with predominantly abdominal subcutaneous fat distribution[63] (Table 2–6; Fig. 2–18).

The mechanisms of this association are unclear. The suggestion has been advanced that abdominal fat in obese subjects may release more FFAs than adipose tissue in other locations.[64] A greater level of FFAs may interfere with peripheral glucose utilization, according to the Randle hypothesis.[65] Furthermore, abdominal fat may, by virtue of its proximity to the liver and portal venous effluent, carry more FFA to the liver with resulting reduction in insulin clearance and consequent hyperinsulinemia.[64] Although preliminary support for this hypothesis has been found, several questions remain before these observations can be converted into acceptable conclusions (see Table 2–6).

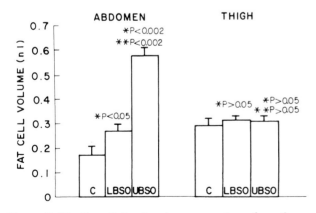

Figure 2–15 Fat cell sizes in subcutaneous tissue from the abdominal and thigh regions. Values are the mean ± SE. P denotes statistical significance. *, compared 16 upper body segment obese (UBSO) and nine lower body segment obese (LBSO) to nine control (C) subjects. **, compares UBSO versus LBSO. [*Source:* Kissebah AH, Vydekungum N, Murray R, et al.: Relation of body fat distribution to metabolic complications of obesity. J Clin Endocrinol Metab 54:254–260, 1982. With permission.]

Adipose Tissue Cellularity and Metabolic Functions in Lean and Obese

Since obesity is frequently a forerunner of NIDDM, investigators have attempted to elucidate the components of the adipose mass in normal lean men and

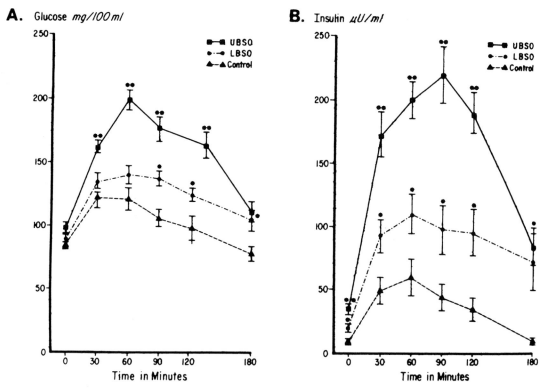

Figure 2–16   Glucose and insulin levels in relation to body fat distribution. Control subjects were not obese. *Abbreviations:* LBSO: lower body segment obese; UBSO: upper body segment obese. [*Source:* Kissebah AH, Vydelingum N, Murray R. et al.: Relation of body fat distribution to metabolic complications of obesity. J Clin Endocrinol Metab 54:254–260, 1982. With permission.]

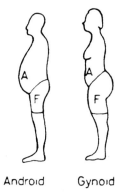

Figure 2–17   Different types of body fat distribution. *Abbreviations:* A (abdominal) obesity = upper body segment obesity (UBSO); F (femoral) obesity = lower body segment obesity (LBSO).

women, and then followed the changes taking place in the enlarging adipose mass of obesity, in the hope of identifying some pathophysiologic component linking obesity to NIDDM.

The morphology, cellularity, and chief functions of adipose tissue are briefly discussed with the main focus being on changes produced by progressive degrees of obesity.

Adipose tissue is a specialized tissue with unique features:

1. It is ubiquitous in the body with diffuse representation around organs such as the heart, kidney, and pancreas, as well as showing distinct accumulation in depots such as mesenteric, omental, and retroperitoneal.

2. The fat mass can be markedly reduced or increased from its normal levels in lean subjects (9 to 18% of body weighs in men, 18 to 28% in women), depending on nutritional and endocrine status. Deviation from normality can be seen with fat mass as low as 3 to 5% body weight in cachetic or athletic individuals, and as high as 70 to 80% in massively obese subjects.

3. The water content of adipose tissue is low (about 5 to 15% of wet weight) compared with that of most lean organs (about 70 to 72%).

4. The main constituent of adipose tissue is the adipocyte, which stores triglyceride lipids with a high caloric density. For example, 1 kg of fat contains approximately 7,700 kcal (mostly triglyceride) whereas 1 kg of muscle contains approximately 1,200 kcal (mostly glycogen and protein).

The number of fat cells present in the body of an adult lean man is around 30 to 40 billion; of an adult lean woman, 40 to 50 billion.[66] In infancy and adolescence, the number of adipocytes grows from a

TABLE 2–6 Metabolic Features of Obese Subjects with Increase in Visceral or Subcutaneous Fat[a]

	Visceral Fat/Subcutaneous Fat					
	All		Men		Women	
	≥0.4	<0.4	≥0.4	<0.4	≥0.4	<0.4
Number	18	28	8	7	10	21
Age (yr)	55 ± 18	34 ± 16	46 ± 20	20 ± 6	61 ± 12	39 ± 15
Onset of obesity (yr)	34 ± 17	17 ± 13	27 ± 18	5 ± 2	39 ± 15[b]	21 ± 12
Duration of obesity (yr)	21 ± 13	17 ± 8	19 ± 14	15 ± 6	22 ± 13	18 ± 9
Body mass index (kg/m^2)	32 ± 4	35 ± 6	31 ± 48	39 ± 5	34 ± 3	34 ± 6
Fasting serum glucose (mg/dL)	130 ± 46[c]	93 ± 17	139 ± 60[b]	87 ± 10	123 ± 33[b]	95 ± 18
Glucose area (mg min/dL) $\times 10^{-2}$	409 ± 155[d]	247 ± 78	432 ± 180[b]	238 ± 35	390 ± 140[b]	250 ± 89
Fasting plasma insulin (μU/mL)	15 ± 7	16 ± 8	12 ± 5	20 ± 9	17 ± 8	14 ± 7
Insulin area (μU · min/ml) $\times 10^{-2}$	116 ± 76	139 ± 83	77 ± 44[b]	170 ± 95	148 ± 84	129 ± 78
Total cholesterol (mg/dL)	256 ± 38	216 ± 29	268 ± 42[b]	214 ± 31	246 ± 33[b]	217 ± 30
Triglycerides (mg/dL)	226 ± 107[b]	145 ± 50	276 ± 129	170 ± 50	186 ± 69	136 ± 48
HDL-cholesterol (mg/dL)	46 ± 11	48 ± 16	42 ± 9	49 ± 26	50 ± 12	48 ± 12

[a] Values are means ± s.d.
[b] $p < 0.05$.
[c] $p < 0.01$.
[d] $p < 0.001$.

[*Source:* Matsuzawa Y, Fujioka S, Tokunage K, Tarui S: A novel classification: visceral fat obesity and subcutaneous fat obesity. *In* Berry, Blondheim, Eliahou, Shafrir (eds): Proceedings of the 5th International Congress on Obesity, Jerusalem. London: John Libbey, 1986, pp. 92–96. With permission.]

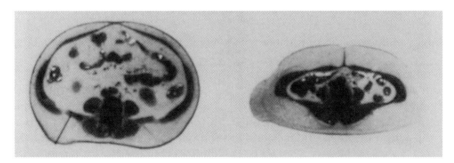

Figure 2–18 Computed tomography scans at level of the umbilicus of two typical obese types: case 1, intra-abdominal visceral; case 2, subcutaneous.

"preadipocyte pool" in response to nutritional and hormonal stimuli. At puberty, greater accumulation of adipocytes is seen in women in areas such as breasts, hips, and buttocks. In contrast to earlier notions indicating that adipocyte number becomes fixed at maturity,[67] it is now recognized that adipocyte number can be increased at any stage of life, including maturity, by excessive nutritional intake, which initially leads to lipid accumulation and cell enlargement and secondarily "triggers recruitment" of cells from the adipocyte precursor pool.[68] Numerous studies have shown that an acquired adipocyte number cannot be reduced by weight loss. Only the fat cell size can be modified[67] when weight loss occurs.

A corollary of this is that, in adolescent obesity, a judicious use of restricted diet can slow down the accretion of new cells and possibly prevent an increased fat cell number when maturity is reached. In obesity developing after maturity (age 20 to 25 years), fat accumulation results in increased size and number of fat cells; weight loss by caloric deprivation can reduce only the cell size, not the cell number.

The main conventional functions of the adipocytes are: (1) lipid synthesis and storage; and (2) triglyceride breakdown with release of glycerol and FFAs. Lipid accumulation in the fat cells takes place when the fatty acids synthesized de novo in situ or taken up from the circulation are esterified with alpha-glycerophosphate derived from glucose or other substrates (lactate, pyruvate); the resulting triglyceride is stored in the fat cell. The FFA moiety of the triglyceride derives from several sources: uptake of circulating FFA in the FFA-albumin complex; FFA liberated from circulating triglyceride-rich lipoproteins (chylomicra, very low density lipoprotein) by the action of an enzyme, lipoprotein lipase produced in fat cells and secreted to be strategically located on the endothelial surface; FFA derived from the constant hydrolysis of triglycerides; and FFA synthesized de novo from glucose.[69] See Chapter 7.

Glucose uptake and metabolism are very active in fat cells. Specialized glucose transporters carry glucose inside the cell and the resulting major metabolic products are: carbon dioxide, glycogen, triglyceride, lactate, and pyruvate. Work in the last few years has shown that glucose conversion to lactate by adipocytes is an important process of previously unrecognized magnitude: 50 to 75% of total glucose metabolized is converted to lactate in adipocytes from mature and obese animals and humans.[70,71]

The implications for the body's metabolic economy of the conversion of glucose to lactate by the adipocyte have not yet been fully elucidated. Evidence suggests that the conversion plays a significant role in providing substrate for hepatic gluconeogenesis during fasting, and that hepatic glycogen synthesis by this *indirect pathway*[72] during feeding after a fast requires extrahepatic (such as adipocyte) conversion of glucose to lactate.

Triglyceride breakdown and subsequent mobilization of glycerol and fatty acids is facilitated by an intracellular lipase enzyme (hormone-sensitive lipase) which initially converts triglycerides to diglycerides. This is followed by the action of diglyceridases and monoglyceridases.[73]

The hormonal stimulation of the adipocyte metabolic processes is exquisitely regulated by lipogenic hormones (mostly insulin) and lipolytic hormones (several catecholamines, peptide hormones, among others, with considerable species specificity). Insulin regulates glucose transport by facilitating translocation of glucose transporters from an intracellular microsomal location to the plasma membrane and prompting glucose metabolism by enzyme activation and protein synthesis.[74] Insulin also possesses an important antilipolytic action.[73] Lipolytic hormones activate the hormone-sensitive lipase through activation of the adenylate system and elevation of intracellular cyclic adenosine monophosphate.

Morphologic and Metabolic Consequences of Obesity and Diabetes

Obesity is characterized by increased body weight and body mass index (>30 kg/m^2 in men and women), greater accumulation of body fat ($>22\%$ of body weight in men, $>32\%$ in women), larger fat cells, and later more numerous fat cells[66] (see Tables 2–2 and 2–3).

The metabolic functions of adipocytes are altered in enlarged adipocytes from obese animals and humans; reduced fatty acid synthesis and glucose oxidation are observed in association with a moderate rise in glucose conversion to glyceride-glycerol (enhanced triglyceride reesterification) and a marked rise in glucose conversion to lactate. Total glucose metabolism is not markedly altered. Basal lipolysis increases in obesity[75] and lipoprotein lipase activity increases in relation to adipocyte size. The hormonal stimulation of adipocytes is altered in obesity with markedly reduced responsiveness to insulin in its glucose-transport promoting effect and generally reduced responsiveness to lipolytic stimuli.[73]

The alterations in cells from diabetic animals and humans are similar to those of obesity, with even more suppression of de novo fatty acid synthesis and nearly absent response to insulin.[76] These cellular events in the enlarging adipose mass of obese individuals are seen in concomitance with the deranged carbohydrate metabolism and insulin resistance. Since enlargement of the fat mass is the most obvious abnormality in obesity, attempts have been made to relate, so far with limited success, the adipose changes to the overall metabolic changes.

Older studies[77] had indicated that adipose tissue takes up 1 to 2% of circulating glucose. These calculations were modified once the magnitude of glucose conversion to lactate became known.[78] It is now believed that adipose tissue from a lean individual takes up 10 to 20% of circulating glucose, and that of an obese individual, up to 30%, or more in individual cases. Even though these studies have revised upward the utilization by adipose tissue of circulating carbohydrate, it is unlikely that carbohydrate intolerance of obesity-related NIDDM derives from significantly reduced glucose utilization by adipose tissue.

Two types of metabolic alterations in adipose tissue functions have been linked to the metabolic alterations seen in obesity/diabetes syndromes. FFA elevation, resulting from enhanced lipolysis in obesity, could contribute to reduced peripheral (mostly muscle) glucose utilization, according to Newsholme and Randle,[65] and to hyperinsulinemia in view of the reported effects of FFA on hepatic insulin clearance.[64] It must be recognized, however, that elevation of FFA in obesity is not present in the early stages of obesity and may be a relatively late event related to the loss of the restraining effect of insulin on lipolysis once insulin levels are reduced by the "exhausted" pancreatic insulin secretion.

Recent studies by Lovejoy et al.[79] and others[80,81] have identified another possible link between enlarged adipose mass and the typical metabolic alterations of obesity. Obese subjects have been found to have significantly raised circulating levels of lactate.[79,80] These elevated levels of lactate may derive from increased lactate production by enlarged and more numerous adipocytes in obesity or from other tissues.[79,81]

In a recent study with lean and obese subjects with normal carbohydrate tolerance, Lovejoy et al.[79] have found a positive and significant correlation between body mass index and basal and integrated glucose levels. This has led to the following postulated series of events: obesity leads to greater baseline lactate production from glucose and higher circulating levels of lactate. This may result in enhanced hepatic glucose production. The raised circulating levels of glucose may be due to elevated hepatic glucose output or to reduction in peripheral utilization of glucose. Insulin levels rise in parallel with elevated glucose levels and as a result of insulin resistance. Furthermore, elevated levels of lactate have been found to suppress glucose utilization (by a glucose-sparing effect) overall[82] and in several tissues such as lung and muscle.[83–85] Thus, lactate elevation secondary to obesity could contribute to the early metabolic derangements of obesity-NIDDM and combine with elevated FFA as a later expression of pathophysiologic mechanisms.

More recently, the triglyceride content of tissues, such as skeletal muscle, liver and pancreas have been found to be elevated in animals that have insulin resistance and hyperinsulinemia. The precise link of tissue hypertriglyceridemia with deficient insulin secretion and effectiveness is not clear, but it has been postulated that elevated FFA, as a derivative of triglyceride, may have both inhibitory effects on insulin secretion by the pancreas and also on glucose utilization by peripheral tissues, such as skeletal muscle.

More work needs to be done, in human and animal models, to test these working hypotheses. The clinical observation that reversal of obesity prior to, or in the early stages of, carbohydrate intolerance reverts many of the pathophysiologic abnormalities (and reduces lactate levels) toward normal underscores both the *definite metabolic link between enlarged fat mass and diabetes and the importance of obesity prevention and/or correction in the control of NIDDM and its many complications.* See Chapter 7.

Extensive studies have been done in an attempt to understand how the body adjusts its food intake so as to regulate its energy stores.[86–88] These studies have been subdivided into four categories: (1) the brain as the controller of food intake, (2) the role of spontaneous eating (meal patterns) as the controller of food intake, (3) satiety: its components and its sequence as a controller of food intake, and (4) depot fat as a controller of food intake through feedback hormone and substrate loops to assure that adipose tissue energy stores (triglycerides) are not depleted.[86]

A major development in the understanding of food intake regulation and the relationship between body fat stores and the hypothalamus has been the discovery of leptin, the product of the ob gene in rodents and humans.[89] Ob/ob mice are deficient in leptin and become obese. Leptin is produced by the fat cells and is released into the circulation. Since leptin is produced in proportion to body fat mass, an obese animal or human produces larger amounts of circulating leptin. Thus, leptin could be a potential signal to the brain about the size of the adipose tissue lipid storage. In mice, mutations of the Ob gene results in lack of circulating leptin, food intake increases and obesity develops. Administration of leptin either intracerebrally or intraperitoneally to rodents produces reduction in food intake, body weight and body fat.

In db/db mice that become obese, the amounts of circulating leptin is increased, but these animals have an hypothalamic defect which prevents the effect of leptin on limiting food intake and the animals become obese.

When studies were done in the human, it has been found that circulating leptin is higher in women than in men[89] and that obese subjects have higher serum leptin concentrations than normal-weight controls. A significant correlation is found between percentage body fat and leptin levels.

When obese subjects were given food restriction for 8-12 weeks, a 10 percent decrease in body weight was associated with a reduction of 53% in serum leptin. These findings have reinforced the concept that adipocytes inform the brain, through leptin production, release and serum levels, about the size of the fat storage. However, the increased serum leptin in the human is not accompanied by reduction of food intake, and it has been postulated that "leptin resistance" may be present and that the human hypothalamus in the obese subjects may become less sensitive to leptin, thus reducing the effect of leptin on central mechanisms regulating food intake and energy expenditure.

More studies are necessary to fully understand the physiological and pathophysiological implications of the leptin-generating system and the response of the brain in lean, obese and diabetic subjects.

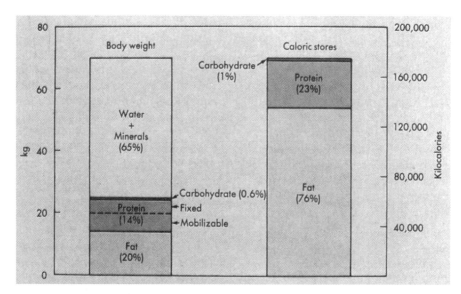

Figure 2–19   The composition of an average 70 kg human is shown in terms of weight (left) and caloric stores (right). Note the trivial proportion of carbohydrate stores in relation to fat stores. (*Source:* Berne, Levy: Physiology. St. Louis: C.V. Mosby, 1988. With permission.)

The desirable or optimal adipose mass in lean men and women has been noted previously. Figure 2–19 shows the body composition and the calorie stores of a 70 kg human. Note that the major component of body weight is water and minerals (65%), whereas the major component of caloric storage is fat. A body fat content of 20% of the body weight contains approximately 76% of total calories and 140,000 kcal. Protein storage makes approximately 23% of total caloric stores and carbohydrate barely 1%.

An optimal caloric storage can be defined as the amount of calories necessary to maintain body functions during the usual alterations in fasting and feeding, and to survive prolonged starvation when the caloric intake is reduced in part or in total by war, famine, starvation, or other causes.

Protein storage is partly structural and partly metabolic. Approximately one third to one half of the protein calories are available for metabolic use during starvation. Once the "structural" proteins are utilized, major metabolic functions (locomotion, heart action, enzymatic activities, and so on) may be affected negatively.

Too little body fat (i.e., <5% of body weight) may provide insufficient reserve for states of increased caloric demands (such as stress and starvation). Too much body fat (i.e., >30 to 40% of body weight), even though it may provide an advantage during times of reduced food availability, is usually accompanied by metabolic and cardiovascular alterations such as hyperlipidemia, insulin resistance, carbohydrate intolerance, hypertension, and other cardiovascular abnormalities.

How does the body regulate its energy stores? The answer lies in a complex interaction between regulation of energy intake and energy expenditure (Table 2–7).

TABLE 2–7   Energy Balance[a]

$$E_{in} = E_{out}\left(E_B + E_{tef} + E_{u+s} + E_{pa} \pm E_{sto}\right)$$

Where E_{in} = gross energy intake
  E_{out} = caloric expenditure
  E_B = basal metabolic rate (approximately 60%)
  E_{tef} = thermic effect of food (approximately 5 to 10%)
  E_{u+s} = Energy loss in urine and stool (approximately 10%)
  E_{pa} = Physical activity expenditure (approximately 10 to 20%)
  E_{sto} = Energy stored in fat and muscle (usually 0 at equilibrium)

[a] See text for explanation.

E_{in} (energy intake) represents calories ingested. In normal individuals, caloric intake depends on total caloric expenditure and is regulated by a variety of humoral, hormonal, and neurosensory components. Hunger is generated by a state of relative caloric deficiency (perceived by peripheral tissues and hypothalamic regions of the brain).

In the early 1990s, leptin was discovered. In ob/ob mice, its absence and failure to function as the "satiety factor" to suppress appetite after optimal feeding leads to massive obesity. Leptin is produced by adipocytes in many animals and humans. It is now being researched extensively as a product produced by adipocytes to signal the hypothalmus and related brain structures in their role of controlling food intake to maintain fat tissue mass at an optimal level.[89,90] Virtually all obese humans have increased levels of immunoreactive leptin in the blood that correlate positively with degree of adiposity and that decline with sustained significant weight loss.[91]

Food intake follows the hunger stimulus. Satiety is generated by ingested calories through short-term satiety signals produced in the gastrointestinal tract. Factors that *increase food intake* are divided into *central* [norepinephrine-α receptor, neuropeptide y (NPY), melanin-concentrating hormone (MCH), galanin, growth hormone-releasing hormone (GHRH), opioid peptides] and *peripheral* (hypoglycemia). Factors that *decrease food intake* are divided into *neurotransmitters* (norepinephrine-β receptor, dopamine, serotonin), *hypothalamic peptides* [cortotropin-releasing factor (CRF), urocortin, glucagon-like peptide 1 (GLP-1), cholecystokinin (CCK)], and *peripheral factors* (leptin-long term signal, CCK-meal-related signal, and the insulin-effect observed after its central administration).[92]

The normal mechanisms of hunger and satiety can be altered by voluntary reduction in caloric intake leading to anorexia and cachexia on one side, and obesity on the other.

Basal metabolic rate (BMR) is by far the largest component of energy expenditure. BMR is raised by fever, a cold ambient environment, and stress, is elevated in obese subjects, and is reduced by caloric deprivation.

The thermic effect of food is the energy expenditure linked to food ingestion, absorption, and storage. It is highest for protein sources (approximately 10% of calories ingested), intermediate for carbohydrate sources (approximately 4 to 6%), and lowest for fat sources (2 to 4%). Obligatory losses in energy loss in urine and stool may be proportional to total caloric intake and dietary composition. In uncontrolled diabetes, up to 300 g glucose (1,200 kcal) per day may be excreted in the urine.

The caloric expenditure of physical activity varies with type and degree of activity, and with conditioning and may vary from 3 to 5% of total energy expenditure in a sedentary individual to 40 to 50% in a heavy construction worker or marathon runner. See Chapter 17.

Energy storage is minimal in individuals in energy balance. Energy storage in muscle and skeleton may be enhanced during growth and development; energy storage in fat tissue is enhanced during pregnancy, overeating, and in any condition in which caloric intake exceeds energy expenditure.

Recent studies have suggested that dietary composition, over and beyond caloric intake, can influence accumulation of energy storage in fat. In animals, equicaloric diets high in fat content produce greater accumulation of body fat with limited or no change in body weight.

In the human, a diet high in fat content (i.e., 45 to 50% of total calories) appears to lead to body fat accumulation greater than if an isocaloric diet high in carbohydrate and/or protein had been ingested.

This observation is of paramount importance in the understanding of obesity, and its related complications. Partly for these reasons, the American Diabetes Association, American Dietetic Association, and American Heart Association have recommended to the general population a prudent diet made up of 30% or less fat, 15 to 20% protein, and 50 to 55% carbohydrate (mostly nonrefined starches).

The reasons why a diet high in fat leads to greater caloric storage in adipose tissue are not clear: (1) On one side, a lesser thermic effect of food may reduce the thermogenic caloric expenditure; (2) conversion of dietary protein and carbohydrate to stored lipid is energetically more costly than conversion of dietary fat; (3) it has been suggested that the body responds to dietary carbohydrate intake with a more regulated caloric expenditure than dietary fat; and (4) other unknown factors may contribute, such as ethnic preference and genetic predisposition.

Further elucidation of some of the regulating mechanisms may help physicians, patients, and the general population to maintain caloric storage at its "optimal" or "ideal" level for essential body functions and necessary reserves for times of increased caloric demands or decreased caloric supply.

What emerges from an examination of the body-weight behavior of various mammals, including man, is that the defense against the depletion of energy stores is much more rigorous than is the defense against a surfeit of stores (as is also the case with hypoglycemia and hyperglycemia). It is evident that body energy stores are regulated with far less precision than are the blood pH and the body temperature,[86,87] and that substantial changes in the size of the adipose depot can occur without evident immediate harm, although long-term harm (NIDDM, hypertension, hyperlipidemia, and so on) may occur.

A great deal of research has been done on the psychiatric, psychologic, and environmental determinants of behavior.[88] Yet there is little convincing evidence that in the majority of obese individuals behavior modification therapy alone, or self-help weight control groups, or hypnotherapy change eating habits and result in permanent weight loss over the long term (see Chapter 16 on diet therapy for NIDDM).

The central importance of the therapeutic alliance between professionals and patients in stimulating motivation and adherence to programs designed to promote loss of excess weight by those with NIDDM has been reviewed and reemphasized.[93] It is now clear, as the 1986 National Institutes of Health Concensus Conference on Treatment of NIDDM with Diet and Exercise emphasized,[94] that the only proven effective method for treatment of those who have NIDDM and are overweight is a reduced caloric intake, exercise if appropriate, and weight loss. Medication should be reserved for those who fail to respond to weight loss from aggressively prescribed and intensively monitored reduced caloric intake and exercise. A similar view has been expressed by the European NIDDM Policy Group[95] and others.[96] (See Chapter 20).

It has been proposed that a new social policy perspective directed at the prevention of, and at the more effective treatment of obesity, needs to be developed and implemented.[97]

The goals and mechanisms of such a policy would aim at achieving primary prevention by weight management for life, and by secondary prevention of the consequences of overweight.[97] The program would require education of the public and of professionals about good nutritional practices for children and adults. Portion sizes in school lunch rooms and in the public cafeterias and in homes should be varied by age, sex, and activity. Food intake should be adjusted to attain and maintain normal growth and ideal body weight for life. Food production, distribution, and advertising would require appropriate adjustment in order to encourage fitness and optimal intake and expenditure of energy.[97] Should such a program be implemented, and should it succeed, it is reasonable to predict that the incidence and prevalence of NIDDM would decline dramatically in the United States.

Problem Statement

Noninsulin-dependent diabetes mellitus (NIDDM or type 2 diabetes mellitus).

Subjective and Objective

See Exhibit 2–1.

Assessment

See Exhibit 2–1, and Table 2–8. The primary objective is to determine whether the nonpregnant patient has NIDDM or IDDM. If the patient is above ideal body weight and has no history of diabetic ketoacidosis, a serum C-peptide measurement can be helpful[98,99] (Table 2–8). If there is still doubt, the therapeutic test of a 1 week total fast may resolve the problem. If during the fast the plasma glucose falls to normal or near-

---

EXHIBIT 2–1   Data Base for Non-Insulin-Dependent Diabetes Mellitus

1. *Subjective:* Patient's weight history (maximum, at age 20, at time of diagnosis of diabetes), family weight history, previous attempts to lose weight, previously prescribed diets, food intake habits, patient's concept of normal weight, preferred body image, history of treatment for diabetes (diet, exercise, sulfonylurea, insulin), plasma glucose and lipid levels and relation to weight loss or gain, medications and relation to weight loss or gain.

2. *Objective:* Measure weight (pounds or kilograms), height (inches or centimeters), estimate frame size [wrist circumference, finger size, caliper-measured elbow breadth (Tables 16–10 and 16–11)]. Measure the *smallest circumference of the abdomen or waist* (inches or centimeters) to the *largest circumference of the hips* and calculate the *waist to hip ratio* (WHR). The normal ratio for females is <0.8, and for males is <0.9. A WHR substantially in excess of normal (by ≥0.2) reflects upper body segment obesity (UBSO) or an *"apple"* distribution, whereas a WHR substantially less than normal (by ≤0.2) reflects lower body segment obesity (LBSO) or a *"pear"* distribution. With experience, the clinician can become proficient in estimating the approximate amount of fat in adipose tissue depots (abdomen, upper arms, for example) by palpation. Skinfold thickness measurements are useful. *In research studies*, the adipose mass and lean body mass may be measured by a method or methods that are selected to meet the research objectives and that consider the limitations of each method and includes an understanding of practical matters (cost, ease of operation, technical skills required, and subject cooperation). The *available methods* include: measurement of *total body water* (deuterium, oxygen-18, tritium), *body potassium*-40, *muscle metabolites* (urinary creatinine excretion, total plasma creatinine, endogenous urinary 3-methylhistidine excretion), *densitometry* (immersion, plethysmography), anthropometry (bone mass, skinfold thickness, arm and wrist circumference), *neutron activation, photon absorptiometry, electrical conductivity and impedance, computed tomography, ultrasound, infrared interactance, and magnetic resonance imaging.*[101]

3. *Assessment:* Calculate patient's ideal (desirable) body weight (pounds or kilograms), percentage of ideal body weight (actual divided by ideal), and excess body weight (actual minus ideal). Calculate body mass index (BMI) as kg/m^2. Measure serum C-peptide (in NIDDM, >0.3 nM fasting and >0.6 nM 1 hour after 240 ml Sustacal or 1 mg glucagon; in IDDM, <0.3 nM fasting and <0.6 nM after 240 mL Sustacal or 1 mg glucagon).[98,99] Differentiate NIDDM from IDDM as noted in Table 2-8. NIDDMs are usually overweight, have no history of ketoacidosis, have normal or high serum C-peptide and insulin levels, and return to normoglycemia or near-normoglycemia during a 1-week total fast. IDDMs are usually underweight or normal weight, frequently are in ketoacidosis or have a history of ketoacidosis, have low serum C-peptide and insulin levels, and do not become normoglycemic during a 1-week total fast (see Chapter 16).

4. *Plan:* See Chapters 15 and 16 for discussion of how to prescribe and implement effective diet and exercise therapy.

TABLE 2–8   Some Suggestions for Differentiating NIDDM from IDDM[98,99]

	NIDDM	IDDM
Age	>40 YR	<40 YR
Weight	>100% IBW	<100% IBW
Ketoacidosis	UNCOMMON	COMMON
Urine ketones	USUALLY < 1 mmol	USUALLY > 1 mmol
Serum C-peptide		
Fasting	>0.3 nM	<0.3 nM
One hr after stimulation with 1 mg glucagon or 140 ml Sustacal	>0.6 nM	<0.6 nM
Fasting plasma glucose after 1 week total fast	Fasting plasma glucose returns to normal or near-normal (<8.3 mmol or <150 mg/dL)	Fasting plasma glucose remains significantly elevated (>8.3 mmol or >150 mg/dL)

normal and carbon dioxide content does not fall below 15 mEq/L, the patient has NIDDM (see Chapter 16).

Plan

Initial: If the patient has NIDDM and is overweight, a low calorie diet (including an initial 1 week total fast if appropriate) and exercise therapy (if not contraindicated) should be prescribed (see Chapters 16, 17, and 18) and maintained until ideal bodyweight and normoglycemia are attained.

Follow-up: About 3% of NIDDMs progress to IDDM each year. See Chapter 12. An example of an individual with what was initially diagnosed as NIDDM, but which progressed unexpectedly after about 1 year of follow-up to IDDM, is noted in Exhibit 2–2.

Recently Berger and colleagues[100] have recommended that when there is a need to initiate pharmacologic therapy for type 2 diabetes mellitus (NIDDM), it is safer and probably more effective to start with insulin therapy alone. See Chapters 20 and 54.

Adherence and Audit

See Chapter 16.

Research Considerations

It is well known that individuals with high normal glucose tolerance tests or impaired glucose tolerance (IGT) are at increased risk of progressing to NIDDM, and that NIDDMs are at increased risk of progressing to IDDM. See Chapters 11 and 12.

Yet, although there is a multitude of possible reasons for a decline in the pancreatic beta cell's ability to produce sufficient amounts of insulin to prevent this progression, the reasons responsible are not yet known.

The possibilities under consideration include: (1) a decreased genetic potential for beta cell division and growth;[102,103] (2) increased susceptibility of *stressed* beta cells to damage or destruction by viral infections or autoimmune processes;[102,103] (3) "exhaustion" or premature death of stressed beta cells that are maximally synthesizing and exporting protein (including insulin) as a result of sustained hyperglycemia ("glucose toxicity");[102–104] or (4) that amylin, which is cosecreted with insulin and is deposited in beta cell granules that contain insulin, may be involved in the post-translational processing of insulin, and that a defect in this process may be responsible for an accumulation of excess amylin in the beta cells of patients with NIDDM.[105–109] Several groups of investigators are trying to determine the pathophysiologic consequences of amylin production, metabolism, and deposition.

Obesity as a risk factor for development of NIDDM is being researched on a broad front,[110] especially as it relates to being an independent risk factor for cardiovascular disease.[111,112] The significance of upper-body and visceral obesity (as identified by waist-girth measurements) is widely recognized.[113–115] The value of very low calorie diets in the prevention and treatment of overweight are widely recognized in 1998.[116,117] Yet many physicians and patients prefer drug treatment[118–120] and some elect to have dangerous, permanently disabling surgery.[121] Beginning in 1992, long-term use of fenfluramine, dexfenfluramine, and combined phentermine and fenfluramine (with FDA approval) were used until regurgitant valvular lesions and deaths started appearing in hundreds of users.[118–120] Two new drugs for long-term use have appeared recently: (sibutramine,[122] FDA-approved in August, 1998, and orlistat,[33] now being FDA-evaluated). Use of either of these drugs should be approached with caution since long-term safety has not been shown for either.

See Chapters 3 and 16 (section on Research Considerations).

EXHIBIT 2–2   Example of a Case of NIDDM That Progressed to IDDM

A case report of diabetes mellitus in a 55-year-old obese female who presented as NIDDM (insulin-treated) which remitted to normoglycemia with discontinuation of insulin therapy, reduced caloric intake, and weight loss, and whose diagnosis 10 months later had become B-cell-antibody-positive IDDM.

Problems (4/29/83)
- NIDDM, insulin treated
- Local allergy to purified pork insulin
- Allergic rhinitis
- Obesity
- Hypertension (11 years), treated with reserpine and hydrochlorothiazide
- Hypothyroidism, treated with synthyroid 0.2 mg/day, no change after thyroidectomy for "tumor" of isthmus

Subjective

Weight age 25 years = 125 pounds; 2/83, 187 pounds (85.0 kg); weight loss 17 pounds (7.7 kg) to 170 pounds (77.3 kg) by 4/15/83, polyuria, polydipsia, polyphagia, blurring of vision, numbness and tingling of hands, vaginal itching. Diabetes diagnosed 4/15/83 and 35 U beef-pork insulin therapy started with local wheal-and-flare reaction which persisted when insulin therapy was changed to purified pork. Her weight increased 14 pounds (6.4 kg), to 184 pounds or 83.6 kg in 2 weeks. She was seen in consultation 2 weeks later (4/29/83) with the problems noted above. Brother, IDDM for 20 years, died of myocardial infarction at age 50 years.

Objective

Height 64 in. (163 cm), 184 pounds (83.6 kg), medium frame ideal body weight (IBW) (Hamwi) = 120 pounds (54.5 kg), 64 pounds (29.1 kg) above IBW, body mass index (BMI) = 32.4. Indurated wheal-and flare reactions at insulin (pure pork) injection sites both anterior thighs.

Assessment

Noninsulin-dependent diabetes mellitus being treated with insulin, local allergy to purified pork insulin, obesity (153% of IBW).

Plan

Initial

Patient hospitalized in ambulatory care unit 4/29/83, discharged 5/8/83. Insulin therapy discontinued abruptly, total fast for 1 week. Weight decreased 15 pounds (6.8 kg), from 184 pounds (83.6 kg) to 169 pounds (76.8 kg), plasma glucose (PG) decreased from 99 to 66 mg/dL, blood pressure (BP) decreased from 150/90 (on reserpine and hydroflumethiazide) to 114/80 on no medication. Five hundred calorie lactovegetarian diet (skim milk, vegetables, fruits) started 2 days prior to hospital discharge.

Follow up

Remission of NIDDM, Then Development of IDDM

Dates 5/27/83–3/28/84: Weight decreased from 165 to 156 lb. Random PG ranged from 64 to 140 mg/dL, BP from 110–180/70–102 on 4 mg trichlormethiazide + 20 mEq potassium/day.

Dates 4/1–4/27/84: Recurrence of polyuria, polyphagia, polydipsia, vaginal itching, constipation, 8 lb weight loss; PG 330, trace urine ketones, weight 152 lb.

Dates 5/4–6/27/84: Self-monitoring blood glucose at home consistently 180 to 300 mg/dL, symptoms continued; on 6/28 readmitted to ambulatory care unit for reevaluation (6/28–7/3/84). On 4th day fast, weight decreased from 152 to 142 lb, but PG remained in range from 294 to 304 mg/dL. Computed tomography scan revealed no evidence of pancreatic lesion, serum C-peptide (normal 0.7 to 3.3 ng/mL) fasting: 0.5 ng/mL; Sustacal stimulated, 0.8 ng/mL. Serum cytoplasmic islet cell antibodies (courtesy Dr. George Eisenbarth, Joslin Clinic Research Laboratory) were strongly positive. On 7/3/84, 20 U rDNA neutral protamine Hagedorn (NPH) human insulin therapy every a.m. started.

Date 7/13/84: Weight 148, PG 116 mg/dL. Continue 20 U NPH insulin.

Date 8/10/84: Weight 161, PG 67. Prebreakfast and prelunch hypoglycemia. (? honeymoon). Insulin reduced to 10 U.

Date 11/2/84: Weight 165, PG 185, BP 190/115, 10 U NPH insulin every a.m. Referred for follow-up to primary care MD. By 2/17/89: Weight 194 lb, PG 138 mg/dL, BP 180/110, on 30 U NPH insulin a.m.; 20 U NPH + 6 U regular every p.m. (total insulin dose, 56 U/day).

Dates 2/17/89–7/6/90: Weight decreased to 160 lb on 500 calorie lactovegetarian diet, insulin decreased to total dose 30 U/day; PG 172 mg/dL, BP 140/90 on captopril 50 mg twice daily.

References

1. National Diabetes Data Group: Classification and diagnosis of diabetes mellitus and other categories of glucose intolerance. Diabetes 28:1029–1057, 1979.

2. Expert Committee on Diabetes Mellitus: Technical Report Series 646. Geneva: World Health Organization, 1980.

3. Papaspyros NS: The History of Diabetes Mellitus, Ed. 2. Stuttgart: Georg Thieme Verlag, 1964.

4. Bouchardat A: De la Glycosurie ou Diabete Sucre, Vol. 2. Paris Germer-Bailliere, 1875.

5. Drash A: Influence of the level of nutrition on diabetes mellitus; world-wide dietary and ethnic factors in evaluation of the disease. *In* Gardner LI, Amacher P (eds): Endocrine Aspects of Malnutrition. Santa Ynez, CA: Kroc Foundation, 1973, pp. 257–287.

6. Campbell WR, Macleod JJR: Insulin. Medicine 3:195–308, 1924.

7. Kromann H, Borch E, Gale EA: Unnecessary insulin treatment for diabetes. Br Med J 183:1386–1388, 1981.

8. Himsworth HP: Diabetes mellitus: its differentiation into insulin-sensitive and insulin-insensitive types. Lancet 117–120, 1936.

9. Karam JH, Grodsky GM, Forsham PH: Excessive insulin response to glucose in obese subjects as measured by immunochemical assay. Diabetes 12:197–204, 1963.

10. Yalow RS, Glick SM, Roth J, et al.: Plasma insulin and growth hormone levels in obesity and diabetes. Ann NY Acad Sci 131:357–373, 1965.

11. Rifkin H (ed): The American Diabetes Association Clinical Education Program: The Physician's Guide to Type II Diabetes (NIDDM), Diagnosis and Treatment. New York: American Diabetes Association, 1984.

12. Roth J, Kahn CR, Lesniak MA, et al.: Receptors for insulin, NSILA-5, and growth hormone: applications to disease states in man. Recent Prog Horm Res 31:95–139, 1976.

13. Sims EAH: Endocrine and metabolic effects of experimental obesity in man. Recent Prog Horm Res 29:457–496, 1973.

14. Davidson JK: Plasma glucose lowering effect of caloric restriction in obesity-induced insulin treated diabetes mellitus. Diabetes 26 (Suppl 1):355 (abstr), 1977.

15. Davidson JK, Vander Zwaag R, Cox CL, Runyan JW et al.: The Memphis and Atlanta continuing care programs for diabetes. II. Comparative analyses of demographic characteristics, treatment methods, and outcomes over a 9–10 year followup period. Diabetes Care 7:25–31, 1984.

16. Vander Zwaag R, Runyan JW, Davidson JK, et al.: A cohort study of mortality in two clinic populations of patients with diabetes mellitus. Diabetes Care 6:341–346, 1983.

17. West KM: Epidemiology of Diabetes and Its Vascular Lesions. New York: Elsevier, 1978.

18. Editorial: NIDDM enigma. Lancet 335:1187–1188, 1990.

19. DeFronzo RA: The triumvirate: B cell, muscle, liver. A collusion responsible for NIDDM. Diabetes 37:667–687, 1988.

20. Diabetes surveillance 1997. Geiss L, (Ed.) Centers for Disease Control and Preventions Division of Diabetes Translation ms K10, Atlanta, GA.

21. Taylor R: Aetiology of non-insulin dependent diabetes. Br Med Bull 45:73–91, 1989.

22. Czech MP: The nature and regulation of the insulin receptor: structure and function. Annu Rev Physiol 47:357–381, 1985.

23. Goldfine ID: The insulin receptor: molecular biology and transmembrane signaling. Endocr Rev 8:235–255, 1987.

24. Zick Y: The insulin receptor: structure and function. Crit Rev Biochem Mol Biol 24:217–269,1989.

25. Rosen OM: After insulin binds. Science 237:1452–1458, 1987.

26. Honsley MD, Siddle K: Molecular basis of insulin receptor function. Br Med Bull 45:264–284, 1989.

27. Flier JS: Insulin receptors and insulin resistance. Annu Rev Med 34:145–160, 1983.

28. Moller DE, Yokota A, Flier JS: Normal insulin receptor cDNA sequence in Pima Indians with NIDDM. Diabetes 38:1496–1500, 1989.

29. Gama A, Patterson AP, Kadowaki T, et al: The amino acid sequence of the insulin receptor is normal in an insulin resistant Pima Indian. J Clin Endocrinol Metab 70: 1155–1161, 1990.

30. Holman GD, Kasuga M: From receptor to transporter: insulin signalling to glucose transport. Diabetologia 40: 991–1003, 1997.

31. Björntorp P: Size, number and function of adipose tissue cells in human obesity. Horm and metabolic res (SUPPL) 1974, pp. 77–83.

32. World health organization. Obesity. Preventing and managing the global epidemic of obesity. Report of the WHO consultation on obesity. Geneva, 3-5 June 1997.

33. Practical guide to the identification, evaluation, and treatment of overweight and obesity in adults. National heart, lung, and blood institute of the national institutes of health, and the North American Association for the study of obesity. Pre print Sept. 1998.

34. Kulzmarski RJ, Flegal KM, Campbell SM, Johnson CL: Increasing prevalence of overweight among US adults. The National Health and Nutrition Examination Surveys, 1960 to 1991. JAMA 272: 205–211, 1994.

35. Knowler WC, Bennett PH, Pettitt DJ, et al.: Obesity and diabetes in Pima Indians: the effects of parental diabetes on the relationship of obesity and the incidence of diabetes. *In* Melish JS, Hanna J, Baba S (eds): Genetic Environmental Interaction in Diabetes Mellitus. Amsterdam: Excerpta Medica, 1982, pp. 95–100.

36. Department of HEW: Ten State Nutrition Survey 1968–1970. Publication 72-8131 (HSM), Vol. 3, p. 44.

37. Cowie CC, Harris MI, Silverman RE, Johnson EW: Are blacks at greater risk of diabetes after considering other diabetic risk factors? (Abstr 293) Diabetes 39 (Suppl 1): 74A, 1990.

38. Zimmet P, Kirk JR, Serjeantson S, et al.: Diabetes in Pacific populations—genetic and environmental interactions. *In* Melish JS, Hanna J, Baba S (eds): Genetic Environmental Interaction in Diabetes Mellitus. Amsterdam: Excerpta Medica, 1982, pp. 9–17.

39. King H, Zimmet P, Pargeter K et al.: Ethnic differences in susceptibility to non-insulin-dependent diabetes: a comparative study of two urbanized Micronesian populations. Diabetes 33:1002–1007, 1984.

40. Dowse GK, Zimmet PZ: The prevalence and incidence of non-insulin-dependent diabetes mellitus. *In* Alberti KGMM, Masse RS (eds): Current Trends in Non-Insulin-Dependent Diabetes Mellitus, Excerpta Medica International Congress Series 859, New York, 1989, pp. 57–60.

41. Stern JS, Johnson PR: Size and number of adipocytes and their implications. *In* Katzen HM, Mahler RJ (eds): Advances in Modern Nutrition, Vol.2, Diabetes, Obesity, and Vascular Disease. New York: John Wiley & Sons, 1978, pp. 303–340.

42. Bray GA: Definition, measurement, and classification of syndromes of obesity, Int J Obesity 2:99–112, 1978.

43. Skelton, H: The storage of water by various tissues of the body. Arch Intern Med 49:140–152, 1927.

44. Gregersen MI: Total body water and the fluid compartments. *In* Bard P (ed): Medical Physiology, Ed. 11. St. Louis: C.V. Mosby, 1961, pp. 301–316.

45. Salans LB, Cushman SW: Relationship of adiposity and diet to the abnormalities of carbohydrate metabolism in obesity. *In* Katzen HL, Mahler RJ (eds): Advances in Modern Nutrition; Vol. 2. Diabetes, Obesity, and Vascular Disease. New York: John Wiley & Sons, 1978, pp. 267–302.

46. Horton ES, Danforth E, Sims EAH, et al.: *In* Burland WL, Samuel PD, Yudkin J (eds): Obesity. London: Churchill Livingstone, 1974, p. 217.

47. Kahn CR: Insulin resistance, insulin insensitivity, and insulin unresponsiveness: a necessary distinction. Metabolism 27 (Suppl 2):1893–1902, 1978.

48. Olefsky JM: Insulin resistance and insulin action: an in vitro and in vivo perspective. Diabetes 30:148–162, 1981.

49. Hunt CE, Lindsey JR, Walker SW: Animal models of diabetes and obesity, including the PBB/Ld mouse. Fed Proc 35:1206–1217, 1976.

50. Shafrir E, Renold AE: Frontiers in Diabetes Research: Lessons from Animal Diabetes II. London: John Libbey, 1988.

51. DeFronzo RA, Tobin JD, Andres R: Glucose clamp technique: a method for quantifying insulin secretion and resistance. Am J Physiol 237:E214–223, 1979.

52. Bergman RN: Toward physiological understanding of glucose tolerance. Minimal-model approach. Diabetes 38:1512–1527, 1989.

53. Golay A, Felber J-P, Jequier E, et al.: Metabolic basis of obesity and non-insulin-dependent diabetes mellitus. Diabetes Metab Rev 4:727–747, 1988.

54. Reaven GM: Role of insulin resistance in human disease. Diabetes 37:1595–1607, 1988.

55. Lonnroth P, DiGirolamo M, Krotkiewski M, at al: Insulin binding and responsiveness in fat cells from patients with reduced glucose tolerance and Type II diabetes. Diabetes 32:748–754, 1983.

56. Czech MP, Richardson DK, Becher SG, et al.: Insulin response in skeletal muscle and fat cells of the genetically obese Zucker rat. Metabolism 27 (Suppl 2): 1967–1981, 1978.

57. Friedman JM, Fialkow PJ: The genetics of diabetes mellitus. Prog Med Genet 4:199–232, 1980.

58. Howard CF Jr: Longitudinal studies on the development of diabetes in individual Macaca nigra. Diabetologia 29:301–306, 1986.

59. Hansen BC, Bodkin NL: Heterogeneity of insulin responses: phases leading to type 2 (non-insulin dependent) diabetes mellitus in the rhesus monkey. Diabetologia 29:713–719, 1986.

60. Kissebah AH, Vydelingum N, Murray R, et al.: Relation of body fat distribution to metabolic complications of obesity. J Clin Endocrinol Metab 54:254–260, 1982.

61. Krotkiewski M, Sjostrom L, Bjorntorp P, Smith U: Regional adipose tissue cellularity in relation to metabolism in young and middle-aged women. Metabolism 24:703–710, 1975.

62. Krotkiewski M, Bjorntorp P, Sjostrom L, Smith U: Impact of obesity on metabolism in men and women: importance of adipose tissue distribution. J Clin Invest 72:1150–1162, 1983.

63. Matsuzawa Y, Fujioka S, Tokunage K, Tarui S: A novel classification: visceral fat obesity and subcutaneous fat obesity. *In* Berry, Blondheim, Eliahou, Shafrir (eds): London: John Libbey: 1986, pp. 92–96.

64. Peiris AN, Mueller RA, Smith GA, Struve MF, Kissebah AH: Splanchnic insulin metabolism in obesity: influence of body fat distribution. J Clin Invest 78:1648–1657, 1986.

65. Newsholme EA, Randle PJ: Regulation of glucose uptake by muscle. 7 effects of fatty acids, ketone bodies and pyruvate, and of alloxan-diabetes, starvation, hypophysectomy and adrenalectomy on the concentrations of hexose phosphates, nucleotides and inorganic phosphate in perfused rat heart. Biochem J 93:641–651, 1964.

66. Hirsch J, Batchelor B: Adipose tissue cellularity in human obesity. Clin Endocrinol Metab 5:299–311, 1976.

67. Hirsch J, Han PW: Cellularity of rat adipose tissue: effects of growth, starvation and obesity. J Lipid Res 10:77–89, 1969.

68. Faust IM, Johnson PR, Stern JS, Hirsch J: Diet-induced adipocyte number increase in adult rats: a new model of obesity. Am J Physiol 4:E279–E286, 1978.

69. DiGirolamo M, Fried SK: In vitro metabolism of adipocytes. *In* Housmann GJ, Martin RJ (eds): Biology of the Adopocyte: Research Approaches. New York: Van Nostrand Reinhold 1987, pp. 120–147.

70. Crandall DL, Fried SK, Francendese AA, Nickel M, DiGirolamo M: Lactate release from isolated rat adipocytes: influence of cell size, glucose concentration, insulin and epinephrine. Horm Metab Res 15:326–329, 1983.

71. Kashiwagi A, Verso MA, Andrews J, Vasquez B, Reaven G, Foley JE: In vitro insulin resistance of human adipocytes isolated from subjects with non-insulin-dependent diabetes mellitus. J Clin Invest 72:1246–1254, 1983.

72. Foster DW: Banting Lecture 1984. From glycogen to ketones—and back. Diabetes 33:1188–1199, 1984.

73. DiGirolamo M: Effeas of age and nutrition on adipose tissue growth, metabolism, and responsiveness to hormones. *In* Hensen B (ed): Controversies in Obesity, Endocrine and Metabolism Series, Vol 5. New York, Praeger, 1984, pp. 91–121.

74. Wardzala LJ, Cushman SW, Salans LB: Mechanism of insulin action on glucose transport in the isolated rat adipose cell. J Biol Chem 253:8002–8005, 1978.

75. DiGirolamo M: Fat cell size, metabolic capacities and hormonal responsiveness of adipose tissue in spontaneous obesity in the rat. Isr J Med Sci 8:807, 1972.

76. Newby FD, Bayo F, Thacker SV, Sykes M, DiGirolamo M: Effects of streptozocin-induced diabetes on glucose metabolism and lactate release by isolated fat cells from young lean and older moderately obese rats. Diabetes 38:237–243, 1989.

77. Bjorntorp P, Sjostrom L: Carbohydrate storage in man: speculations and some quantitative considerations. Metabolism 27 (Suppl 2):1853–1865, 1978.

78. Marin P, Rebuffe-Scrive M, Smith U, Bjorntorp P: Glucose uptake in human adipose tissue. Metabolism 36:1154–1160, 1987.

79. Lovejoy J, Mellen B, DiGirolamo M: Lactate generation following glucose ingestion: Relation to obesity, carbohydrate tolerance and insulin sensitivity. Int J Obesity 1990. In press.

80. Doar JWH, Cramp DG: The effects of obesity and maturity-onset diabetes on L(+) lactic acid metabolism. Clin Sci 39:271–279, 1970.

81. Vendsborg PB, Bach-Mortensen N: Fat cell size and blood lactate in humans. Scand J Clin Lab Invest 27:317–320, 1977.

82. Issekutz B Jr, Miller HI, Paul P, Rodahl K: Effect of lactic acid on free fatty acids and glucose oxidation in dogs. Am J Physiol 209:1137–1144, 1965.

83. Fisher AB, Dodia C: Lactate and regulation of lung glycolytic rate. Am J Physiol 246:E426–E429, 1984.

84. Pearce FJ, Connett RJ: Effect of lactate and palmitate on substrate utilization of isolated rat soleus. Am J Physiol 238:C149–C159, 1980.

85. Stanley WC, Gertz EW, Wisneski JA, Morris DL, Neese RA, Brooks GA: Systemic lactate kinetics vary during graded exercise in men. Am J Physiol 249:E595–E602, 1985.

86. Van Itallie TR, Gale, SK, Kissileff HR: Control of food intake in the regulation of depot fat: an overview. *In* Katzen HL, Mahler RJ (eds): Advances in Modern Nutrition, Vol. 2. Diabetes, Obesity, and Vascular Disease. New York: John Wiley & Sons, 1978, pp. 427–492.

87. Cioffi LA, James WPT, Van Itallie TB (eds): The Body Weight Regulatory System: Normal and Disturbed Mechanisms. New York: Raven Press, 1981.

88. Stunkard AJ, Stellar E (eds): Eating and Its Disorders, Association for Research in Nervous and Mental Disease Vol 62. New York: Raven Press, 1984.

89. Caro JF, Siriha MK, Kolaczynski JW, Zhary PL, Considine RV: Leptin: The Tale of an obesity gene. Diabetes 45:1455–1462, 1996.

90. Campfield L, Smith F, Guisez Y, et al.: Recombinant mouse ob protein: evidence for a peripheral signal linking adiposity and central neural networks. Science 269:546–548, 1995.

91. Considine RV, Sinha M, Heiman M, et al.: Serum immunoreactive Leptin concentrations in normal weight and obese humans. N Engl J Med 334: 292–295, 1995.

92. Flier JS, Foster DW: Eating disorders: *In* Williams text book of endocrinology, ninth edition, p. 1067 (Table 22–2), WB Saunders, Philadelphia, 1998.

93. Sims EAH, Sims D: Motivation, adherence, and the therapeutic alliance. Diabetes Spectrum 2:18–27, 49–51, 1989.

94. National Institutes of Health. Concensus development conference on diet and exercise in non-insulin-dependent diabetes mellitus. Diabetes Care 10:639–644, 1987.

95. European NIDDM Policy Group: Management of non-insulin–dependent diabetes mellitus in Europe: A concensus view. Diabetic Med 5:275–281, 1988.

96. Davidson JK, Lebovitz HE: Diet is the therapy of choice in adult non-insulin-dependent diabetes mellitus. *In* Barnes HV (ed): Debates in Medicine. Chicago: Mosby Year Book Medical Publishers, 1991.

97. Fullarton JR: Obesity: A new social policy perspective. Int J Obes 2:267–285, 1978.

98. Welborn TA, Garcia-Webb P, Bouser AM: Basal C-peptide in the discrimination of type I from type II diabetes. Diabetes Care 4:616–619, 1981.

99. Hother-Nielsen O, Faber O, Sorensen NS, Beck-Nielsen H: Classification of newly diagnosed patients as insulin-requiring or as non-insulin-requiring based on clinical and biochemical variables. Diabetes Care 11:531–537, 1988.

100. Berger M, Jurgen SU, Muhlhauser I: Rationale for the use of insulin therapy alone as the pharmacological treatment of type 2 diabetes. Diabetes Care 22(Suppl. 3): C71–C75, 1999.

101. Lukaski HC: Methods for the assessment of human body composition: traditional and new. Am J Clin Nutr 46:537–556, 1987.

102. Logothetopoulos J, Bell G: Histological and autoradiographic studies of the islets of mice injected with insulin antibody. Diabetes 15:205–211, 1966.

103. Brosky G, Logothetopoulos J: Streptozotocin diabetes in the mouse and guinea pig. Diabetes 18:606–611, 1969.

104. Karam JH: Vulnerability of the pancreatic beta cell to hyperglycemia in non-insulin-dependent diabetes. *In* Melish JS, Hanna J, Baba S (eds): Genetic Environmental Interaction in Diabetes Mellitus. Amsterdam: Excerpta Medica, 1982, pp. 192–197.

105. Ehrlich JC, Ratner IM: Amyloidosis of the islets of Langerhans: a restudy of islet amylin in diabetic and nondiabetic individuals. Am J Pathol 38:49–59, 1961.

106. Westermark P, Wernstedt C, O'Brien TD, Hayden DW, Johnson KH: Islet amyloid in type 2 human diabetes mellitus and adult diabetic cats contains a novel putative polypeptide hormone. Am J Pathol 127:414–417, 1987.

107. Cooper GJS, Leighton B, Dimitriadis GD, Parry-Billings M, Kowalchuk JM, Howland K, Rodbard JB, Willis AC, Reid KBM: Amylin found in amyloid deposits in human type 2 diabetes mellitus may be a hormone chat regulates glycogen metabolism in skeletal muscle. Proc Natl Acad Sci USA 85:7763–7766, 1988.

108. Porte D, Kahn SE: Hyperproteininsulinemia and amyloid in NIDDM: clues to etiology of islet B-cell dysfunction? Diabetes 38:1333–1336, 1989.

109. Butler PC, Chou J, Carter WB, Wang Y-N, Bu B-H, Chang D, Chang J-K, Rizza RA: Effects of meal ingestion on plasma amylin concentration in NIDDM and nondiabetic humans. Diabetes 39:752–756, 1990.

110. Perry H, Wannamethee SG, Walker MK, Thomson AG, Whincup PH, Shaper AG: Prospective study of risk factors for development of non-insulin dependent diabetes in middle-aged British men. BMJ 310:560–564, 1995.

111. Hubert HB, Feinleib M, McNamara PM, Castelli WP. Obesity as an independent risk factor for cardiovascular

disease: a 26-year follow-up of participants in the Framingham Heart Study. Circulation. 1983;67:968–977.

112. Young T, Palta M, Dempsey J, Skatrud J, Weber S, Badr S. The occurrence of sleep-disordered breathing among middle-aged adults. N Engl J Med. 1993;328:1230–1235.

113. Dowling HJ, Pi-Sunyer FX. Race-dependent health risks of upper body obesity. Diabetes. 1993;42:537–543.

114. Chan JM, Rimm EB, Colditz GA, Stampfer MJ, Willett WC. Obesity, fat distribution, and weight gain as risk factors for clinical diabetes in men. Diabetes Care. 1994;17:961–969.

115. Lemieux S, Prud'homme D, Bouchard C, Tremblay A, Despres J. A single threshold value of waist girth identifies normal-weight and overweight subjects with excess visceral adipose tissue. Am J Clin Nutr. 1996;64:685–693.

116. Very low-calorie diets. National Task Force on the Prevention and Treatment of Obesity, National Institutes of Health. JAMA. 1993;270:967–974.

117. Wadden TA. The treatment of obesity. *In* Stunkard AJ, Wadden TA, eds. Obesity: Theory and Therapy. New York: Raven Press; 1993:197–217.

118. Connolly HM, Crary JL, McGoon MD, et al. Valvular heart disease associated with Fenfluramine-Phentermine. N Engl J Med. 1997;337:581–588.

119. Centers for Disease Control. Cardiac valvulopathy associated with exposure to Fetfluramine or Dexfenfluramine: U.S. Department of Health and Human Services interim public health recommendation, November 1997. MMWR Morb Mortal Wkly Rep. 1997;46:1061–1065.

120. Long-term pharmacotherapy in the management of obesity. National Task Force on the Prevention and Treatment of Obesity. JAMA. 1996;276:1907–1915.

121. Gastrointestinal surgery for severe obesity. National Institutes of Health Consensus Development Conference Statement. Am J Clin Nutr. 1992;55:615S–619S.

122. Bray GA, Ryan DH, Gordon D, Heidingsfelder S, Cerise F, Wilson K. A double-blind randomized placebo-controlled trial of sibutramine. Obes Res. 1996;4:263–270.

3

Type 1 (Insulin-Dependent) Diabetes Mellitus

Steven D. Chessler and Åke Lernmark

Historical Perspective

Diabetes Before 1921

Diabetes mellitus has affected human beings since ancient times (Exhibit 3–1).[1] Two early Hindu physicians, Sushruta and Charaka (1000 B.C.), described syndromes interpreted to represent two forms of diabetes: one associated with emaciation, dehydration, polyuria, and lassitude, and the other with stout build, gluttony, obesity, and sleepiness. The diabetes syndrome was a fatal disease, it caused humans to "urinate honey" leading to a rapid death. There was no remedy for diabetes until 1921 when insulin was discovered. Aretaeus of Cappadocia (AD 81–138) documented:

Diabetes is a wonderful affection, not very frequent among men, being a melting down of the flesh and limbs into urine. Its cause is of a cold and humid nature, as is dropsy. The course is the common one, namely, the kidneys and bladder for the patients never stop making water, but the flow is incessant, as if from the opening of aqueducts. The nature of the disease, then, is chronic, and it takes a long period to form, but the patient is short-lived, if the constitution of the disease be completely established; for the melting is rapid, the death is rapid.

Moreover, life is disgusting and painful, thirst is unquenchable; excessive drinking, which is disproportionate to the large volume of urine, for more urine is passed; one cannot stop them either from drinking, their mouths become parched and their bodies dry, the viscera seem as if scorched up; they are affected with nausea, restlessness, and a burning thirst; and in no distant term they die.

Hence, the terms diabetes, meaning "to run through a siphon" and mellitus, meaning "honey sweet" were introduced. However, the anatomical localization and the metabolic alteration causing diabetes remained a mystery. Galaeus (A.D. 131–201) thought that diabetes was caused by a kidney disease while Dobson (1776) argued that the sugar present in the blood increased before glucosuria was apparent. In the 18th century Morgagni (1761) wrote that diabetes was a fatal disease, the location of which was impossible to establish, and Claude Bernard (1859) could not but conclude that the liver was an organ of internal secretion and that its increased secretion of sugar explained diabetes.

Experiments in animals would eventually prove the relationship between diabetes and the pancreas. Brunner (1683) performed partial pancreatectomies in dogs, which resulted in polydipsia and polyuria; however, the relationship to diabetes was not noted. This relationship was first clearly demonstrated by von Mering and Minkowski (1889),[2] and Hedon (1893) completed the postulate of an internal secretion by demonstrating

EXHIBIT 3–1 Some Historic Perspectives of Diabetes

1000 BC	Sushruta and Charaka, Hindu physicians	Recognized two forms of diabetes
AD 100	Aretaeus of Cappadocia	Designation and clinical symptoms of diabetes
1683	Brunner	Polydipsia and polyuria after pancreatectomy in dogs
1869	Langerhans	Described pancreatic islets
1889	Minkowski, Hedon	Physiologic demonstration of the endocrine pancreas
1893	Laguesse	Islets of Langerhans recognized as possible source of an internal secretion
1907	Lane	A and B cells
1909	De Mayer	Insuline (or insulin): a factor from the pancreas
1910	Weichelsbaum	Pathologic changes of the islets in diabetes
1921	Banting and Best	Extraction of insulin
1950	Harris	Juvenile- and maturity-onset diabetes have different modes of inheritance

that pancreas transplantation to pancreatectomized dogs prevented the development of diabetes. The origin of a pancreatic factor that controlled glucose homeostasis remained to be determined. Following the discovery of the pancreatic islets by Langerhans in 1869, Laguesse (1893) suggested that the pancreatic islets were a possible source of an internal secretion. A likely connection to diabetes was evidenced by Dieckhoff's observations in 1894 that the pancreas of diabetic patients had a greatly diminished number of pancreatic islets.[3]

Technical advancements, particularly in techniques of microscopy and histology, allowed Lane (1907) and Bensley (1911) to describe the pancreatic α and β cells, and De Mayer (1909) proposed insulin as the factor from the pancreatic islets that controlled blood sugar. A search for insulin was undertaken by many workers but was greatly hindered by the extensive proteolytic activity in pancreatic extracts and the specific requirements to solubilize insulin. It was not until 1921 that Banting and Best successfully prepared pancreatic extracts containing sufficient amounts of biologically active insulin (see Chapters 1 and 18).

Diabetes After 1921

The discovery of insulin had a dramatic effect on the therapy of diabetes: it was now possible to keep patients alive. Treatment during the period preceding the discovery of insulin was characterized by a starvation diet or undernutrition, with the patients allowed to receive very few calories each day. Before 1922 the life expectancy of a child or young adult with diabetes was 1 year from diagnosis. By 1924, the life expectancy had risen to 7 to 8 years, and it improved rapidly with increased knowledge of insulin action and better training of physicians and nurses. Insulin had a marked social impact; it was long thought to be the cure for diabetes. However, 78 years of insulin therapy have proved the hormone only maintains survival in a chronic disorder associated with a 200 to 300% excess mortality.[4]

The etiology and pathogenesis of diabetes remained unexplained. In the disease affecting the young, several investigators in the early years of this century described that the pancreatic islets were altered by fibrosis, hyalinosis, atrophy, and infiltration by inflammatory cells. The complexity of the islet organ precluded systematic and quantitative studies, and it was not until later that careful studies by Gepts[5] focused interest on the islets as the primary target tissue in diabetes. The previous recognition of the β cells as the source of insulin[6] and the α cells of glucagon[7] permitted further investigations of the role of these two blood glucose-controlling hormones in the development of diabetes. Later additions to the complexity of the endocrine pancreas are the δ cells producing somatostatin and the PP cells which secrete pancreatic polypeptide (PP).

Epidemiology

The epidemiology of type 1 (insulin-dependent) diabetes mellitus has not been clearly delineated, primarily due to the fact that diagnostic criteria of diabetes have drifted throughout the years (See Chapters 11 and 12). Retrospective analyses are likely to be biased, and stringent prospective analyses are necessary to define prevalence and incidence as well as sex and seasonal variations.

Prevalence

The prevalence rate (i.e., the frequency of type 1 diabetes at a particular time in a particular group) has been repeatedly estimated by different methods in several parts of the United States and in other countries. The diagnosis of insulin dependency is less ambiguous in children and young adults, and prevalence data from such individuals are shown in Table 3–1. However, the true prevalence is difficult to establish due to the necessity of distinguishing type 1 diabetes from other disorders of glucose metabolism, such as the so-called maturity-onset diabetes of the young (MODY).

The prevalence of diabetes mellitus increases with age, due primarily to an increasing frequency of non-insulin-dependent diabetes with age. The prevalence of diabetes mellitus among Caucasians in general ranges from 0.05% in the very young to 3 to 4% in individuals older than 60 to 70 years of age.[8,9] The prevalence among African-Americans is 0 to 1.8%. The proportion of individuals with *undetected diabetes mellitus is thought to be high*, especially among the elderly, and prevalence rates up to 10 to 15% have been estimated. The prevalence rate of type 1 diabetes among individuals younger than 20 years of age (Table 3–1) is

TABLE 3–1 Prevalence of Diabetes Mellitus in Individuals Below the Age of 20 Years in the General Population

Country	Year of Study or Publication	Prevalence Rate (%)
United States	1978	0.1
Wisconsin	1980	0.2
Minnesota	1979	0.15
Canada		
Montreal	1975	0.04
Great Britain	1968	0.2
France	1977	0.03
Denmark	1980	0.14
Sweden	1985	0.15
Finland	1982	0.20

about 0.1 to 0.2% in most countries, with most studies in the United States indicating a prevalence around 0.17% (meaning ~123,000 individuals age 19 or younger have type 1 diabetes in the United States). This makes type 1 diabetes one of the most common chronic diseases of childhood. In Europe, for unclear reasons, there seems to be a secular trend toward increased prevalence of type 1 diabetes.[9]

Because diabetes is not a reportable disease, accurate statistical information is not always available. Initiatives taken by physicians to establish Diabetes Registries of incident cases have improved the epidemiological understanding of diabetes.[9] Still, attempts to define the prevalence of type 1 diabetes are complicated by increasing evidence that the disease occurs at all ages. It has been estimated that a population (Caucasians of Northern Europe or Northern European extraction) of 10^7 give birth to about 10^5 children each year. Among these children, 10^3 will develop type 1 diabetes during their lifetime: 40% of them before 14 years of age, 30% between 15 and 34 years and the remaining 30% when older than 35 years of age. In the United States, approximately 7.4% of patients between 30 and 74 years of age diagnosed with diabetes mellitus have type 1 diabetes, or 0.3% of all adults in this age group.[8]

Incidence

The *incidence rate* is the frequency of new cases of type 1 diabetes that occur in a population during a defined period. The rate is usually expressed as the annual number of newly diagnosed cases per 100,000 individuals. Incidence studies have been carried out in a number of countries,[8,9] but the populations observed have been primarily Caucasian. The reliability of data from most countries has suffered from the absence of clearly defined degrees of ascertainment and of demographic as well as geographic delineation of the group subject to investigation.[9] In an attempt to improve epidemiological data, the World Health Organization began the Multinational Project for Childhood Diabetes (DiaMond) in 1990 to track the incidence of type 1 diabetes in various areas worldwide.[10] Reliable incidence data is crucial because, for example, data indicating geographical variation (see below) or epidemic-like trends could provide important insights into the etiology of the disease or potential preventative measures. Currently, there are about 168 type 1 diabetes registries throughout the world monitoring about 7% of the global population.[10] The diagnosis of type 1 diabetes is more readily established in children, and the standardized criteria for inclusion as a case in a DiaMond-associated registry includes the necessity of insulin therapy before age 15.[10]

In the United States, incidence varies between approximately 10 and 20 new patients per 100,000 (<15

years old), depending on region. Incidence also varies depending on race and ethnicity; for example, the incidence in non-Hispanic Caucasian children and African-American children in Allegheny County, Pennsylvania was 18.1 and 10.2 per 100,000, respectively, typical of the lower incidence of type 1 diabetes in African-American children throughout the country. About 40% of the up-to twofold regional differences in incidence in the United States are accounted for by local differences in race and ethnicity.[8,11]

Geographic Distribution

The incidence of type 1 diabetes varies even more dramatically around the world (Table 3–2), and the geographic variability of type 1 diabetes incidence is one of the greatest of any noncommunicable disease. The highest reported rate in children is in Finland (35.3 per 100,000 per year). Mexico has the lowest rate in North America (0.6 per 100,000) and one of the lowest in the world; the region of highest incidence in North America is Prince Edward Island (23.9 per 100,000). In the past, there has been the suggestion that there is a gradient of increasing incidence as distance from the equator increases or average daily temperature decreases, but this no longer seems to be the case. For example, in Europe, which has the greatest intracontinental variability, type 1 diabetes incidence is high in the north, especially in the Scandinavian countries, but a southern region, Sardinia in Italy, has the second highest rate (30.2 per 100,000). With improving worldwide data on incidence, though, it is becoming clear that type 1 diabetes is more common in the northern hemisphere than the southern, where annual incidence does not surpass 15 per 100,000.[12] The variation in incidence around the world remains to be explained. Both genetic factors perhaps primarily associated with different human lymphocyte antigen (HLA-DR) or DQ specificities of the major histocompatibility complex on chromosome 6—as well as environmental factors, including infectious agents and diet, will need to be considered. It will also be important to determine why the incidence of type 1 diabetes seems to be increasing steadily in Europe while, in the United States, there have been transient increases suggestive of epidemics.

Variation with Age and Sex

Until recently, type 1 diabetes was thought to occur almost exclusively in children and adolescents. Autoimmunity to islet antigens, though, can be detected in essentially all age groups and in many patients classified with type 2 diabetes, often making difficult classification of the disease in individuals past school-age. For example, there is increasing evidence

TABLE 3–2   Incidence of Insulin-Dependent Diabetes Mellitus in Various countries (Under Age 15; per 100,000 per Year).

Country, Region	Total Incidence	Male: Female Ratio	Study Period
Finland	35.3	1.2	1987–1989
Sweden	24.4	1.1	1978–1987
Canada			
Prince Edward Island	23.9	1.3	1978–1986
Montreal	9.8	1.0	1971–1985
United States			
North Dakota	18.9	1.3	1980–1986
Rochester, NY	17.1	0.9	1965–1979
San Diego, CA	9.4	1.1	1978–1981
United Kingdom	13.5	1.0	1988
France	7.8	1.0	1989–1990
Brazil			
Sao Paulo	7.6	0.6	1987–1991
Sudan			
Khartoum	6.4	?	1987–1990
Israel	4.5	1.0	1975–1980
Japan			
Hokkaido	1.7	0.6	1974–1986
Korea	0.6	0.8	1985–1986

Data from Karvonen et al.[12]

that many patients initially diagnosed with type 2 diabetes have autoimmunity to islet cell antigens and progress to insulin-dependence as a result of β-cell depletion.[13,14] Clinical classification of diabetes mellitus will likely evolve to reflect a growing understanding of the underlying etiological and pathogenic mechanisms. Still, type 1 diabetes is primarily a disease associated with youthful onset: it estimated that the annual incidence in the United States (per 100,000) is 18.2 for individuals less than 19 years old versus 9.2 for those older.[8]

Though the prevalence of type 1 diabetes is approximately equal in males and females, the incidence rate varies between the sexes at different ages (Fig. 3–1). Type 1 diabetes is rare in newborn children. The incidence rate increases with increasing age, reaching a peak for males and females between 11 and 14 years. Also, an additional peak at the ages of 4 to 6 years (Great Britain) or 7 to 8 years (Denmark) has been observed.[9] The peak incidence among female type 1 diabetes patients occurs earlier than in males. There is an excess of males in the age group of 0 to 4 years and over 10 years of age. The minor incidence peak observed at the ages of 4 to 6 years has been interpreted as being associated with the children entering preschool or school programs. The major peak at the ages of 11 to 14 years is thought to be linked with puberty and the maximal velocity of pubertal growth. The difference between females and males, in this respect, would then be explained by the earlier appearance of pubertal changes in females. It is also commonly reported that there is a marked decline in

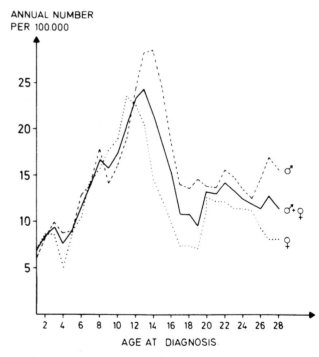

ANNUAL NUMBER
PER 100.000

AGE AT DIAGNOSIS

Figure 3–1.   Incidence of insulin-dependent diabetes mellitus in relation to the age at clinical diagnosis. (*Source:* Christau B, Akerblom H, Joner G, et al.: Incidence of insulin-dependent diabetes mellitus (0–29 years at onset) in Denmark. Acta Med Scand Suppl 24:54–60, 1979. With permission.)

incidence after puberty.[15] The incidence rate seems to remain relatively stable thereafter, although a slight increase may occur among individuals in older age groups (55 to 65 years old).[16] The variation in incidence rate with the patient's age has not been explained. Boys in the prepubertal ages were found to be taller at the clinical onset of type 1 diabetes, and newly diagnosed type 1 diabetes children of both sexes showed an advanced skeletal maturity.[17] It is therefore speculated that the age variation in the occurrence of new type 1 diabetes patients is related to unknown changes in metabolism, hormone levels, or both before type 1 diabetes is clinically detected. The problem of the age-related onset of type 1 diabetes remains an enigma, and any hypothesis formulated to explain the etiology and pathogenesis of type 1 diabetes needs to take the age-related phenomenon into account.

Etiology

Type 1 diabetes is caused by destruction of the pancreatic islet β cells, resulting in deficient insulin production and eventual dependence on insulin-replacement therapy for survival. Almost always, β-cell destruction is mediated by the patient's immune system and is therefore referred to as an autoimmune *process* when it precedes the clinical onset and an autoimmune *disease* at the time of diagnosis and classification. Type 1 diabetes is characterized by an islet-specific inflammatory process, called insulitis (other, far less frequent, causes of islet cell depletion—such as from pancreatic insufficiency caused by pancreatitis, hemochromatosis, or pancreatectomy—will not be discussed here). A single factor that triggers the autoimmune process has not been discovered. Rather, a variety of data suggests that the *origin of the disease is multifactorial*. Inheritance plays a role, as an increased risk of the disease has been linked, with varying degrees of certainty, to approximately 10 genetic loci, most notably to certain of the genes (HLA genes) that help control the immune response.[18–20] However, environmental factors clearly are also important, as concordance of the disease in identical twins is less than 50% (see Chapter 5). Epidemiological data and experiments in animals have revealed a variety of possible, nongenetic etiological factors (Table 3–3). Infections, most notably mumps, coxsackie, rheo, or congenital rubella, are frequently reported to precede the clinical onset of type 1 diabetes (see Chapter 4). Gestational infections[21,22] or ingestion of cow's milk in the first months of life,[23] for example, has been linked to an increased risk of type 1 diabetes, and in utero factors seem to be important as well: the offspring of a mother with the disease is at a lower risk of developing type 1 diabetes than the offspring of an affected father.[24]

Certain chemicals, such as streptozotocin and alloxan, are β-cell toxins and cause diabetes in susceptible animals by directly depleting β cells or by damaging the cells in such a way that an autoimmune

TABLE 3–3　Possible Etiological Factors in IDDM

Viruses
　Coxsackie (including maternal infections)
　Mumps
　Rubella (congenital rubella)
Chemical
　Alloxan (mostly rodents)
　Streptozocin (mostly rodents; diabetes rarely seen in
　　streptozocin-treated patients with endocrine tumors)
　Pyriminil (Vacor; rodenticide, diabetogenic in man)
Pharmaceuticals
　Pentamidine
　L-Aspariginase
Nutritional factors
　Intake of cows milk during infancy
　Breast-feeding (may have independent protective effect)
　Diets containing hydrolyzed, versus intact, protein
　　(primarily animal experiments)
In utero environment
　Maternal enterovirus infections
　Presence of type 1 diabetes in mother (protective)
　Increased age of mother

response is initiated. In humans, the ability of streptozotocin and alloxan to induce diabetes is unclear. Streptozotocin is used in the treatment of certain gastrointestinal tumors, including insulinomas and glucagonomas; however, type 1 diabetes rarely develops in these patients. This could be due either to the dose being too small or to resistance of the human β cell to the diabetogenic action of this drug.[25] A number of compounds structurally related to streptozotocin and alloxan have also been implicated as possible pathogenic factors in type 1 diabetes. These include uric acid and its structurally related metabolites, which are related to alloxan, and some nitrosamines, which are related to streptozotocin. Pyriminil (Vacor), a rodenticide, was found to be highly diabetogenic in humans.[26] Individuals developing diabetes after ingestion of Pyriminil were positive for islet cell surface antibodies, indicating that islet antibodies (see below) may develop after a primary lesion has been inflicted on the β cells.

Several lines of evidence suggest that certain viral infections can result in type 1 diabetes. First, there seems to be seasonal variation in the incidence of the disease, with, in general, fewer cases being diagnosed in summer. Second, in some regions there have been periods of increased incidence of the disease that have coincided with viral epidemics: for example, a transient increase in new cases of type 1 diabetes diagnosed in Birmingham, Alabama in 1983 coincided with a similar spike in cases of coxsackie virus infection.[27] In experimental animals, there are several viruses, including encephalmomyocarditis virus, rubella virus, cytomegalovirus, and reovirus that are capable of inducing type 1 diabetes.[28]

Some of these viruses may cause diabetes primarily by β-cell destruction, while others have been shown to induce autoimmunity including a strong polyclonal autoantibody response. Virus-induced autoimmunity, if it indeed does play a role, could be caused by the production of antibodies that—in addition to recognizing viral antigens—cross-react with β-cell proteins. A region of sequence similarity between a Coxsackie virus protein and the cytoplasmic β-cell protein GAD65 may be responsible for the apparent link between the virus and type 1 diabetes in this manner.[29,30] It also has been observed that combined treatment with a subdiabetogenic dose of streptozotocin followed by the inoculation of a variety of diabetogenic viruses rendered certain strains of mice diabetic despite their normally being resistant to the virus alone.[28] This observation may be significant to type 1 diabetes in humans, because it is possible that repeated injuries to the pancreatic β cells over several years may, in the presence of concomitant autoimmunity, eventually precipitate β-cell deficiency.

Pathophysiology of the Endocrine Pancreas

Morphological Abnormalities

Studies of the postmortem morphology of the pancreatic islets in type 1 diabetes patients demonstrate a marked reduction in the endocrine pancreas (Table 3–4). The total mass of the islets is clearly reduced in a type 1 diabetes pancreas,[31] and the pancreas is often smaller, particularly the lobe poor in PP cells. This may be due to atrophy or reduced growth of the pancreas after the onset of type 1 diabetes, because the pancreas is often normal-sized at the time of diagnosis. It has not been possible to study thoroughly the pancreas of newly diagnosed type 1 diabetes patients. In general, the islets are small and appear pseudoatrophic. The endocrine cells are primarily α, δ, and PP cells (Table 3–4) and these cells may be scattered throughout the exocrine parenchyma. The lack of β cells is a major feature of the diabetic endocrine pancreas (Table 3–4). Islets with β cells showing signs of hyperactivity have also been detected in the pancreas of newly diagnosed type 1 diabetes patients, and β cells may also be detected in the close vicinity of duct cells, suggesting neoformation of cells. However, one of the characteristics of a pancreas of a newly diagnosed type 1 diabetes child is the presence of inflammatory cells adjacent to islets or cords of newly formed β cells.[5,32]

The presence of inflammatory cells in the diabetic pancreas had been demonstrated by the turn of this century. The term insulitis was introduced in 1947 by von Meyenburg[33] and the phenomenon was clearly established by the careful studies of Gepts,[5] who found

TABLE 3–4 The Endocrine Pancreas in Normal and Insulin-Dependet Diabetes Mellitus Individual's[a]

Cell Type	Total Mass of Endocrine Cells in Pancreas (mg)	
	Control Subjects	IDDM Subjects
B + A + D + PP	1,395	413
B	850	0
A	230	150
D	125	97
PP	190	166

[a] For details, see Rahier J, Goebbels RM, Henquin JC: Cellular composition of the human diabetic pancreas. Diabetologia 24:336–371, 1983.

insulitis in 16 of 23 individuals with type 1 diabetes who died within 6 months of the diagnosis. Because the mass of the β cells is already markedly reduced at the time of diagnosis, the presence of inflammatory cells in large numbers is perhaps not to be expected. It is speculated that the antigen that attracts the inflammatory cells in fact is a β-cell-specific determinant. It is therefore an important task to determine which cell type(s) in the immune system might be populating the pancreatic islets at the time of diagnosis of type 1 diabetes, especially during the period preceding the actual clinical onset of the disease. One interpretation of the histopathological appearance is that the islets of Langerhans at the time of clinical onset are end-stage islets with signs of chronic inflammation. These islets have already lost their β cells; therefore, no inflammatory cells will be present either. In a few patients with newly diagnosed type 1 diabetes, there was evidence that nearly all cells thought to be involved in an inflammatory response were present in the insulitis.[34] The role of the different immune cells in the process leading to the disappearance of β cells from the endocrine pancreas remains to be determined. The appearance of a chronic inflammatory reaction at the time of diagnosis again suggests that the pathophysiology of β-cell loss might start long before the actual clinical onset of type 1 diabetes.[35] It has not yet been possible to define the sequence of events that trigger the migration or attraction of inflammatory cells to the pancreatic islets.

It is possible that surface modification of the pancreatic β cells suffices for certain clones of T lymphocytes to become activated. Cell surface antigens which may trigger an immune reaction may develop in virus-infected cells, and it is interesting that insulitis has been observed in virus-infected nondiabetic children.[36]

Functional Abnormalities

The histopathological changes in the endocrine pancreas in type 1 diabetes of short duration correspond to a drastic decrease in the ability to release insulin

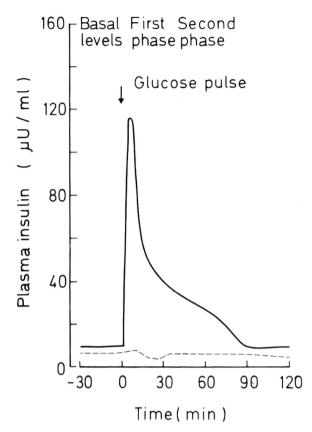

Figure 3–2. Schematic representation of insulin release in response to an IV injection of D-glucose. The dotted line is the response in a patient with insulin-dependent diabetes.

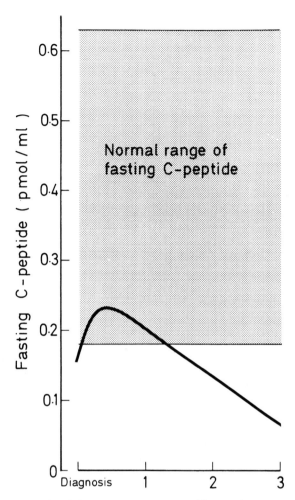

Figure 3–3. Schematic representation of fasting plasma C-peptide immunoreactivity range in healthy individuals. The solid line is the average fasting C-peptide level for insulin-dependent diabetic patients in relation to duration of the disease in years.

(Fig. 3–2). Highly sensitive and specific radioimmunoassays for the proinsulin C-peptide[37] permit studies of residual β-cell function despite a patient being treated with insulin. The use of the C-peptide radioimmunoassay is based on the observation that insulin and C-peptide are released in equimolar amounts from the cells. Fasting C-peptide is reduced, often to a level below the normal range (Fig. 3–3). The initial insulin treatment appears to increase the level of fasting C-peptide during the first 3 to 6 months after diagnosis After that, C-peptide levels continuously decrease, reaching values below the detection limit of the assay (about 0.05 pmol/ml) after 3 to 4 years of type 1 diabetes.[38–40] The extent to which fasting or stimulated levels of C-peptide reflect the residual mass of pancreatic β cells remains to be clarified. It is clear that, within hours, removal of exogenous insulin hampers the ability of a type 1 diabetic patient to control blood sugar. However, it is not clear whether the residual amount of C-peptide and its fluctuation following dietary control or intensified insulin therapy reflect changes in the number of residual β cells or in the function of those remaining β cells.

To be able to estimate the residual mass of insulin-producing cells, it is important to understand not only the development of an insulin-dependent state but also the efficacy of therapy. It should be kept in mind that pancreatectomy in humans and experimental animals indicates that as much as 70 to 80% of the pancreas can be removed before difficulties arise in the control of fasting blood glucose.

Although the total pancreatic insulin content in experimental animals appears to correlate well with the total β-cell mass, it cannot be excluded that a diminished β-cell mass alters the rate of insulin biosynthesis and secretion in remaining β cells. It has been hypothesized that an increased and sustained demand on remaining cells exhausts these cells leading to their death and to a diminished β-cell mass. However, at present, there are no experimental data to support this hypothesis.

Immunological Abnormalities

Numerous autoimmune diseases are associated with genetic markers in the major histocompatibility complex (MHC) on the short arm of chromosome 6.[18,41]

The MHC, a unique part of the human genome, contains genes encoding many of the proteins necessary for the normal functioning of the immune system. Many of these genes are polymorphic, with numerous different alleles creating great diversity among individuals. The HLA class I and class II molecules are polymorphic cell-surface proteins encoded within the MHC. The HLA cell surface proteins are important in the immune response and also as highly reactive molecules involved in transplant rejection. Type 1 diabetes was initially associated with the class I HLA-B8 and B15 specificities,[42,43] two alleles of the class I B gene (there are also A and C genes that encode class I molecules). Subsequently, the class II molecules, which are expressed by the specialized antigen-presenting cells of the immune system (e.g., macrophages and B lymphoctyes) were discovered, and a tighter linkage was made to the class II HLA-DR3 and DR4 specificities, which are disproportionately co-inherited with HLA-B8 and B15.[44] More than 90% of Caucasian type 1 diabetes patients younger than 30 years of age at onset carry HLA-DR3 and/or DR4.[45] Subsequent molecular cloning and sequence analysis revealed that linkage with the DR locus may be secondary to another primary genetic factor for diabetes risk, as will be explained next.

In addition to the DR locus, class II molecules are encoded by genes at loci called DQ and DP.[18] Detailed genetic analyses in families[46] and in case-control[47–49] studies have shown that DQ confer a higher risk for type 1 diabetes than DR. Among Caucasians it is DQ8 (the haplotype is called DQA1*0301-B1*0302 in WHO nomenclature) and DQ2 (DQA1*0501-B1*0201), which confer the highest susceptibility to Type 1 diabetes. The DQ genes are necessary but not sufficient for type 1 diabetes, and the particular genes may vary depending on the race and ethnic group studied. The analysis of the linkage between genes within the MHC (HLA region) and type 1 diabetes is complicated by the phenomenon of "linkage disequilibrium," meaning that genes are separated by crossing over during meiosis at a rate lower than expected based on their distance apart on the chromosome. Also, different combinations of HLA types confer different degrees of risk: for example, inheriting DQ2-DR3 from one parent and DQ8-DR4 from the other results in a greater risk for type 1 diabetes than homozygosity for either.[50] While it is clear, then, that a gene or genes in the HLA region are important in determining susceptibility to type 1 diabetes and that these genes encode components of class II proteins, their precise identities and the extent of their contribution to the development of type 1 diabetes remain to be determined.[50] Other genetic elements in the MHC complex may also contribute to the development of type 1 diabetes, as the HLA region contains genes encoding a variety of proteins that play diverse roles in immunity, including tumor necrosis factor (TNF), heat-shock proteins, and complement factors C2 and C4 (see Chapter 5).

In addition to the locus in the HLA region (referred to as *type 1 diabetes1*), approximately 10 other genetic loci have been linked to Type 1 diabetes with varying degrees of certainty.[20] Another contributing genetic factor (*type 1 diabetes2*) maps to a region of repeated DNA sequence (known as a VNTR marker, for variable number of tandem repeats) just upstream of the insulin gene.[51] The other loci are less well defined, and the mode of inheritance of the disease is still not clear. More than 80% of new type 1 diabetic patients have no family history of the disease, but the lifetime risk of the disease is increased in family members of those affected. Siblings of patients have an approximately 7–8% risk and children have a 5% risk, which is substantially higher than the less than 0.2% prevalence of type 1 diabetes in the population less than 20 years old. Prevalence in the parents of type 1 diabetes patients is about 3% and it is higher for fathers than mothers. In families with several affected members, the occurrence of type 1 diabetes is about 15% if the parent or sibling shares both HLA markers with the proband (HLA identical), and 1% or less if HLA nonidentical.[52] Overall, it is emphasized that HLA types that confer susceptibility to the disease seem to be necessary, but not sufficient, for the development of type 1 diabetes while environmental factors and other genes likely play an important role.[18,20] The threefold reduced risk of type 1 diabetes in the offspring of mothers with the disease as compared to the offspring of affected fathers may be due to the development, in utero, of tolerance to the predisposing HLA type.

The hypothesis that some HLA class II molecules, such as HLA-DQ, are able to bind a peptide from an autoantigen ("diabetogenic peptide") to render the trimolecular complex (class II protein with bound peptide) diabetogenic is attractive.[53] HLA class II molecules with bound peptide promote cell–cell interactions between T-helper lymphocytes and antigen-presenting cells (APC), such as macrophages and dendritic cells. Immunogens taken up by phagocytosis are processed intracellularly by APC into peptides. These are bound to class II molecules within small prelysosomal vesicles before being presented on the surface of the APC bound to class II proteins. T-helper cells, in turn, can recognize the antigen-class II protein complex if they have the appropriate T-cell receptor for that particular trimolecular complex. The antigen-specific T-helper cells are stimulated by the interaction with the antigen-HLA-class II protein complexes to produce cytokines, which then stimulate the development of cytotoxic T and B lymphocytes that produce antibodies to the immunogen. The class II specificities linked to type 1 diabetes may be important because they bind and present diabetogenic antigens, possibly including islet cell proteins. Normally, T lymphocytes that bear receptors recognizing self (as opposed to foreign) antigens are killed in the thymus during late fetal and early prenatal life. One possibility, then, is that individuals who are at risk of developing diabetes fail to delete self-reactive T lymphocytes.

Cellular Immunopathophysiology

In type 1 diabetes one or more constituents of the islet β cells are treated by the immune system as foreign, and, as a result, the β cells are attacked in much the same way that an invasive pathogen would be. The reason that otherwise normal proteins become aberrantly recognized by the immune system is unknown. APC in humans are macrophages, dendritic cells or B lymphocytes, which all are capable of transporting the antigenic peptides to their cell surface complexed to HLA class II molecules.[54] It is not known whether APC activity is altered in type 1 diabetes patients or in individuals susceptible to this disease. Studies with immunoglobulin G (IgG)-sensitized autologous erythrocytes have shown that normal individuals with a DR3 HLA haplotype have an abnormally prolonged Fc-receptor-mediated mononuclear phagocyte system. It should be noted, however, that phagocytosis is also greatly reduced in polymorphonuclear leukocytes in type 1 diabetic patients due to poor metabolic control.[55] In contrast, leukocyte chemotaxis was decreased not only in type 1 diabetic patients but also among their first-degree relatives. The mitogenic transformation of normal lymphocytes was, on the other hand, markedly reduced in cells cultured in serum from poorly controlled diabetes. However, when repeating the experiments with serum from the same diabetic patients after improving their diabetes control, the lymphocyte transformation was normal. There are several examples of similar observations in which the insulin-deficient diabetic state markedly influenced cellular function or distribution of immunologically competent cells.[55] The importance of studying diabetic patients in good metabolic control cannot be too highly stressed.

Tests for leukocyte migration inhibition or blast formation have indicated that type 1 diabetes patients may be sensitized to pancreatic antigens.[56] T-cell proliferation to islet cell autoantigens, in particular to the glutamic acid decarboxylase (GAD) autoantigen is increased among new onset patients as well as first-degree relatives.[57,58] There is also indication of GAD-specific cytotoxic T cells in new onset type 1 diabetic patients.[59] The precise role of cell-mediated immunity in the development of type 1 diabetes is yet to be determined in humans, though, in some rodent models of the disease, type 1 diabetes can be transferred from a diabetic to a diabetes-prone animal by infusing the latter with T lymphocytes from the former.[60,61] The most readily apparent manifestation of a cell-mediated immune mechanism in the disease is insulitis, the characteristic islet lesion that precedes the clinical onset of symptoms. Insulitis, as discussed earlier, consists of what appears to be an inflammatory infiltrate involving the pancreatic islets but sparing the rest of the gland. CD4 (cytotoxic/suppressor) as well as CD4 (helper) positive T lymphocytes are present in the inflamed islets, with a preponderance of the former. Most or all of the other circulating cell types that mediate immune function, such as B lymphocytes, macrophages, and natural killer (NK) cells, are present also, though in what proportion is unclear. Also unclear is how this inflammatory process mediates β-cell death. The elaboration of cytokines, such as interleukin-1, members of the interferon family and tumor necrosis factor by the inflammatory cells almost certainly plays a role, perhaps by killing the β cells directly or by injuring them in a way that allows otherwise intracellular proteins to become accessible to the immune system. As an increasing number of β-cell proteins become targeted, an enhanced immune attack perhaps develops, a phenomenon called antigen spreading. Antigen spreading may be relevant to T lymphocytes, but not to autoantibodies reactive with islet autoantigens.[62] Cytokines have also been linked to increased expression of MHC class I molecules by β cells and to an increased expression of class II molecules on islet nonendocrine cells.[63] The increased abundance of class I molecules on the β-cell surface could facilitate recognition and lysis of the β cells by CD8 cytotoxic lymphocytes, while expression of class II molecules could enable recognition of β-cell antigens, such as GAD65, by T-helper (CD4) cells. In addition to cytokine-mediated and CD8 T-cell-mediated toxicity, other mechanisms have been hypothesized to lead to β-cell destruction, such as damage by the free radicals produced by activated inflammatory cells. Antibody-mediated cytotoxicity may be especially important since islet cell surface antibodies are frequent in type 1 diabetes patients.

T lymphocytes participate in controlling the immune response in a positive (T-helper cells) and negative (T-suppressor or T-regulatory cells) manner. Several autoimmune disorders have been found to have an imbalance between T-helper and suppressor cells. This imbalance might be reflected in the peripheral blood, and the development of monoclonal antibodies detecting cell surface proteins has made the enumeration of circulating T-lymphocyte subsets feasible. Results so far have been conflicting, however, because decreased, normal and slightly elevated suppressor cell numbers have been found in patients with type 1 diabetes. The monoclonal antibody tests revealed a moderate reduction of total T lymphocytes at the expense of the T-helper subset or no alterations except an increase in the proportion of class II antigen-positive T lymphocytes.[64] As observed in other disorders of autoimmune character, a decrease in OKT8 (CD8 positive suppressor or cytotoxic T cells) positive cells or increased ratios of OKT4 (CD4 positive helper or inducer)/OKT8 positive cells was found in many type 1 diabetes patients. It remains to be determined whether these alterations are inherited or related to the pathogenesis of β-cell destruction. When newly diagnosed type 1 diabetes patients were assessed for the number of immunoglobulin-secreting cells in peripheral blood, several patients with type 1 diabetes of short duration had an elevated spontaneous secretion of immunoglobulin. These type 1 diabetes patients were found to have not only higher fasting C-peptide levels, but also higher average titers of islet cell cytoplasmic antibodies compared with patients with normal levels of spontaneous in vitro antibody secretion.[65] It is therefore possible that the clinical onset of type 1 diabetes is associated with a polyclonal B-lymphocyte activation and that this immunoregulatory malfunction is associated with the simultaneous presence of residual β cells and islet cell antibodies. An approach to determining the relevance of the just mentioned cellular immune functions to the pathogenesis of β-cell destruction is the use of β-cell-specific antigens.[62,66] In a system with isolated pancreatic islets from guinea pigs, it was observed that patients with newly diagnosed type 1 diabetes had diminished activities of islet cell antigen-specific suppressor cells.[66] In a system with human islets, newly diagnosed patients had an increased T-helper cell activity to multiple antigens.[62] In a patient with high residual C-peptide production, it is therefore possible that a decreased suppressor-cell activity would lead to the formation of islet cell antibodies. Similar antigen-specific tests in HLA-DR/DQ-matched type 1 diabetes and control individuals should allow a proper test of the hypothesis that a specific immunoregulation abnormality, that involved β-cell antigens, is associated with the development of type 1 diabetes.

Humoral Immunopathophysiology

Humoral antibodies reacting with an autologous tissue preparation is taken as evidence for the presence of autoantibodies. A large number of autoantibodies associated with different disorders have been documented. The autoantibody response may be organ-specific, such as in myasthenia gravis, or broad, such as in systemic lupus erythematosus. Autoantibodies reacting with the affected tissue are highly prevalent in organ-specific endocrine diseases. Several assay systems have been

used to show that the sera from patients with type 1 diabetes have antibodies that react with pancreatic islet cells.[67,68] These antibodies are called islet cell antibodies (ICA) and, when allowed to bind to sections of frozen human pancreas and then detected using indirect immunofluorescence, are found to bind specifically to the islet endocrine cells. The ICA are a mixture of antibodies specific for various islet cell antigens. Though much progress has been made in determining the identity of islet antigens (Exhibit 3–2), this is an area of active investigation and the list of proteins bound by ICA may continue to grow. The antibodies detected using immunofluorescence are primarily directed to cytoplasmic antigens, raising the important and unanswered question of how they initially become accessible to the immune system. Because they seem to be present in all of the islet endocrine cells, they may represent components involved in the formation or secretion of islet cell hormones. The identification of GAD65, IA-2, and insulin as the major autoantigens in type 1 diabetes does not fully explain the cytoplasmic immunofluoresence reaction in all the islet endocrine cells.

The ICA are detected in 0.1 to 1% of the general population and in 15 to 30% of type 1 diabetes patients.[68,69] However, at the time of clinical onset, 70 to 80% of patients younger than 30 years of age are ICA-positive. The prevalence decreases with increasing duration of type 1 diabetes, being roughly 20 to 30% after 2 years. Determination of ICA titers indicated that the patients who have antibodies persisting for 2 years had higher titers at the time of diagnosis. The indirect immunofluorescence assay for ICA has been standardized and ICA levels are expressed in JDFI units.[70,71] In newly diagnosed patients, high levels of ICA are the mark of a more rapid loss of endogenous β-cell function.[38,39] The levels of ICA in newly diagnosed children are unaffected by both age at onset and sex and do not

EXHIBIT 3–2   Islet Cell Autoantibodies in Type I IDDM

Antigen:	Tissue distribution	% Type 1 Diabetes Patients Positive
Insulin	Beta cells	40–70
GAD65	Neuroendocrine	50–80
GAD67	Neuroendocrine	10–20
IA-2 (ICA512)	Neuroendocrine	50–80

Other candidate antigens
  Pancreatic sialoglyconconjugate
  Carboxypeptidase H
  Pancreatic sulfatide
  Beta-cell glucose transporter
  Heat-shock protein 65
  38-kd, 52-kd, and 150-kd proteins

For details see Schranz and Lernmark.[122]

show seasonal variation. ICA are also at least 10 to 20 times more frequent among healthy children (3%) compared with the prevalence of the disease (0.15 to 0.2%).[72] In the general population, ICA are therefore a poor positive predictive marker for type 1 diabetes. In first-degree relatives, on the other hand, the positive predictive value for type 1 diabetes may be as high as 100% among a subgoup of relatives with high levels of islet cell antibodies.[73] In many studies of first-degree relatives, ICA were found between 2–8 years before the clinical onset.[74,75] Previous analyses indicated that ICA were observed for several years in patients initially treated with oral hypoglycemic agents and later with insulin and in subjects in whom the onset of diabetes was preceded by viral infection. However, any assessment of the risk for an individual of developing diabetes will depend on the ability accurately to determine the presence of antibodies in a prospective analysis. This is particularly important, because ICA may appear temporarily in healthy individuals, children with recent viral infections, as well as in newly diagnosed patients.[76,77]

Antibodies in type 1 diabetes sera bind to human pancreatic islet cells, preferentially to β cells if the patients are diagnosed before the age of 30 years. The observation that antibodies are capable of binding to living β cells is important because it allows testing of the possibility that surface-bound antibodies either mediate immune effector mechanisms or directly affect the function of the β cells. The former phenomena may include complement-mediated cytotoxicity or antibody-dependent cellular cytotoxicity. Either mechanism would possibly contribute to killing pancreatic β cells provided the in vitro phenomenon is also occurring in vivo. The evidence obtained with both monolayer cultures of pancreatic islet cells from newborn rats and cloned rat islet tumor cells is that the cytotoxic ICA correlate well with the presence of islet cell surface antibodies but not with islet cell cytoplasmic antibodies.[68] In fact, it was found that some patients have both types of antibodies whereas others have either cytoplasmic or cell-surface antibodies.

Autoantibodies against unique β-cell antigens may explain the specific loss of the insulin-producing cells in type 1 diabetes. Autoantibodies against insulin and proinsulin have been reported in 30–50% of patients with new-onset type 1 diabetes as well as in selected first-degree relatives studied retrospectively after developing type 1 diabetes.[78] The levels of insulin autoantibodies tend to be higher in individuals who develop diabetes at a younger age or who have a more rapid progression toward clinical disease. Along with insulin, GAD65, an isoform of the γ-aminobutyric acid (GABA)-synthesizing enzyme, is one of the best-characterized islet cell autoantigens.[79–82] Though, unlike insulin, GAD65 is not unique to islets or β cells, in islets, the protein is expressed primarily or solely in the β cells. GAD65 is also synthesized in the brain, where it is associated with *the autoimmune disease stiff-man syndrome*, a disorder characterized by muscle rigidity and painful spasms.[80] Interestingly, there is a *markedly increased incidence of diabetes in patients with this syndrome*, suggesting that antibodies to GAD65, rather than being simply a byproduct of β-cell destruction, may play a role in the pathogenesis of type 1 diabetes.[83] Whether they are a cause of the disease or a marker of the disease process, though, antibodies to GAD65 are proving to be among the most useful islet cell autoantibodies for predicting progression to type 1 diabetes, as they are both one of the most sensitive and most specific islet cell autoantibodies for detecting the disease. Up to 80% of newly diagnosed individuals but less than 2% of controls have autoreactivity to GAD65. Furthermore, probably because it is a marker or cause of ongoing β-cell destruction, autoreactivity to GAD65 is a predictor of eventual insulin-dependent diabetes when detected in patients with type 2 diabetes[13] or pregnancy-associated diabetes.[84] GAD65 has also been found to be an antigen for cell-mediated autoimmunity in type 1 diabetes, as T cells from some patients seem to be specifically targeted to this protein.[57,85] *Assays for GAD65 antibodies—probably in conjunction with assays for antibodies to IA-2, another specific marker, and insulin—may soon come into more widespread clinical use for detecting pre-symptomatic β-cell damage.*[86,87]

GAD65 antibody levels at the time of diagnosis do not seem to predict the residual β-cell function 12 to 30 months later, though IA-2 (ICA512) autoreactivity has more recently been shown to sometimes be linked to a more rapid progression of the disease.[86,88] Also, the antigenic stimulation that precipitates the formation of islet cell autoantibodies remains an enigma, and the early formation of immunoglobulin M (IgM) and its isotypic shift to IgG are yet to be detected. Also, more fundamentally, the importance of antibody-mediated autoimmunity relative to cell-mediated mechanisms, of which insulitis is the most obvious manifestation, is yet to be determined.

Problem Statement I: Diagnosis of type 1 (Insulin-Dependent) Diabetes

Classification of diabetes mellitus has been problematic because the disease is heterogeneous in its etiology as well as in its clinical manifestations, and it can be difficult to determine the underlying pathogenesis from the clinical presentation. The classification scheme recommended in 1979 by the National Diabetes Data Group[89] and by the WHO[90] eliminated the prior category of juvenile onset diabetes and substituted insulin-dependent diabetes mellitus (IDDM), reflecting the necessity of insulin treatment in these patients. As understanding of the various etiologies of the disease increases, though, it is becoming increasingly desirable for the classifications to reflect the underlying disease process rather than the therapeutic intervention. Because of this, in 1997 an expert committee convened by the American Diabetes Association proposed that the classification IDDM be eliminated and type 1 be used to denote diabetes mellitus caused by either autoimmune or idiopathic β-cell destruction and typically resulting in ketosis if not treated.[91] Other causes of diminished β-cell function, such as from toxins or diffuse pancreatic disease, are not included in this category. *The committee also decreased the fasting plasma glucose necessary to diagnose diabetes from 140 mg/dL to 126 mg/dL to better reflect the threshold glycemic level* at which the risk of diabetes-related complications markedly increases.[91]

Type 1 diabetes typically manifests in youth, though, as discussed earlier, patients with type 1 diabetes can present at all ages. The elevated blood glucose causes polyuria and polydipsia from the osmotic diuretic effect of glucose. Continued hyperglycemia and glucosuria results in hunger, fatigue, and weight loss. The symptoms often have an abrupt onset in children and a more insidious onset with increasing age. Girls often have monilial vaginitis. Patients may present initially with the classic ketoacidosis of diabetes including air hunger with rapid, deep (Kussmaul) respirations, metabolic acidosis, acetone (fruity) odor on the breath, dehydration, hyperglycemia, glucosuria, ketonemia, and ketonuria (see Chapter 24).

β-Cell Function

The major defect in type 1 diabetes is the deficiency in insulin production. Following an injection of glucose, the β cells in healthy individuals are capable of releasing 10 to 20 times the basal rate of insulin (see Fig. 3–2). However, in type 1 diabetes patients there is often a total lack of any response to glucose.

Because the diagnosis of an insulin-dependent state requires immediate administration of insulin and because a substantial portion of endogenous insulin is quickly taken up by the liver, residual β-cell function is most commonly assessed by measuring levels of C-peptide, a processing byproduct of the insulin precursor molecule. All patients treated with insulin also develop insulin antibodies that interfere in the immunoassays used to detect serum or plasma insulin. The C-peptide is a 31-amino acid fragment cleaved from proinsulin and released by the β cells in equimolar amounts to insulin. Its half-life is approximately 30 min, versus about 3 min for insulin. At the time of diagnosis, C-peptide levels are often undetectable. Strict metabolic control with exogenous insulin (β-cell rest) and clinical remission (honeymoon period) early in the

course of the disease are often associated with increased levels of fasting and of meal- or glucagon-stimulated C-peptide (Fig. 3–3). It is unclear why early, aggressive insulin therapy can slow β-cell depletion; one possibility is that improved glycemic control decreases expression by the β cell of autoantigens such as GAD65. In any case, with increased duration of type 1 diabetes, there is a continuous decrease in fasting C-peptide levels (Fig. 3–3).

The range of C-peptide values in type 1 diabetes patients is considerable, reflecting variability in the rate of loss of endogenous insulin production.[40] C-peptide levels near the normal range have been found to be associated with improved diabetes control. However, other factors are also important for metabolic control, as the absence of C-peptide or very low levels are found in stable and unstable type 1 diabetes patients. Several methods are used—primarily in an investigative context—to assess β-cell reserve by stimulating insulin, and thus C-peptide, production; these include injection of glucagon, injection of insulin secetatogues such as glucose or L-arginine or ingestion of a meal.

Islet Cell Antibodies

Up to 80–90% of patients newly diagnosed with type 1 diabetes have either ICA, insulin autoantibodies (IAA), or antibodies to GAD65 or IA-2 (ICA512) (see Exhibit 3–2 and Table 3–5). The usefulness of the assays for these antibodies has improved due to increased standardization, the result of a series of international workshops.[71,92,93] The use of reference sera and quantitative analysis are two techniques that have improved the sensitivity (positivity in disease), specificity (negativity in health), and the positive predictive value for type 1 diabetes of antibody testing.[73]

The role in the care of patients with type 1 diabetes of immunofluorescence assays for detection of ICA or of specific assays for defined ICA is still being determined, and they are not yet in widespread clinical use. Due to their sensitivity for type 1 diabetes, they will likely be valuable aids in classifying newly detected hyperglycemic patients, helping to differentiate type 1 from type 2. Their role in predicting the clinical course of type 1 diabetes is still under investigation, though there is evidence that ICA antibodies predict a more rapid decline in insulin synthetic capacity.[38,39] Because they are markers of ongoing autoimmune β-cell depletion, in patients with type 2[13,14] or gestational diabetes mellitus,[84] these antibody assays potentially will be useful as predictors of eventual progression to insulin-requiring diabetes. Finally, if therapies become available to slow or prevent the onset of type 1 diabetes, these assays may help determine which patients are at risk, as they are present prior to the clinical onset of the disease.[87] For screening, the currently available anti-

TABLE 3–5 Prevalence of Islet Cell Antibodies at the Time of Diagnosis

Antibody	Tissue Preparation	Assay	Prevalence (%)
Insulin autoantibodies	Insulin	Radiobinding assay	40–70
GAD65 antibodies	Recombinant GAD65	Radiobinding assay	50–80
IA-2 (ICA512)	Recombinant IA-2	Radiobinding assay	50–80
IA-2β	Recombinant IA-2β	Radiobinding assay	30–40
Islet cell cytoplasmic	Sections of frozen human tissue	Indirect immunofluorescence	60–80
Islet cell surface	Living pancreatic islet cells	Indirect immunofluorescence	60–80
		Protein A	35–50
Cytotoxic	Living pancreatic islet cells	^{51}Cr-release	50–70
		Dye exclusions	

body assays will have to be combined with other predictive methods; even when testing for dual GAD65 and insulin autoantibody positivity, which has the best specificity (99.7% in the Swedish population tested), the positive predictive value is only 25%, with a sensitivity of only 41% (as expected, the sensitivity of antibody testing decreases when more than one test is required to be positive).[94]

Tissue Type

Tissue typing by serological or cellular techniques has shown that type 1 diabetes is associated with certain HLA-DR and DQ genes.[18,95] At first type 1 diabetes was found to be associated with HLA-B8 and B15. Later the serologically defined HLA-DR specificities showed that the latter associations were secondary to the increases in HLA-DR3 and DR4, respectively (Table 3–6). Molecular cloning techniques and the definition of HLA genotypes suggest that the HLA-DR association in turn is secondary to the increases in HLA-DQ2 (DQ A1*0501-B1*0201) and DQ8 (DQ A1*0301-B1*0302), respectively. This phenomenon is explained by the pronounced linkage disequilibrium among various loci within the HLA region. Thus, certain alleles tend to appear together in the same person more often than expected from the individual frequencies of the alleles. HLA-B8, DR3, and DQ2 as well as HLA-B15, DR4, and DQ8 are in linkage disequilibrium. The relative risk value (Table 3–6) indicates the strength of the association between a given HLA specificity and the disease. It reveals the increased frequency with which the disease occurs in a group of individuals that has a specificity compared with a group that lacks it.

Currently typing for HLA-DQ genotypes show an increased frequency of HLA-DQ2, DQ8, or both in the diseased population.[96] In some studies nearly all patients have been found to be either DQ2 or 8 positive. The interpretation of such results should be cautious because most investigations are not carried out in representative incident cases of patients. More importantly, the controls are usually not representative of the

TABLE 3–6 HLA-DR Specificities Associated with IDDM Among Nonrelated Individuals

HLA-DR Genotype	Control Subjects (%)	IDDM (%)	Relative Risk
3/4	6	51	14.3
3/X	24	20	0.8
4/X	28	27	1.0
X/X	42	3	0.1
3 and/or 4	58	98	1.4

general population. It has been suggested that a particular amino acid, position 57 in the HLA-DQ-β chain, confers resistance or susceptibility to type 1 diabetes.[97] The amino acid Asp in position 57 would represent a resistance allele. Transracial comparison has not supported this hypothesis.[18,98] DNA sequencing of the HLA-DQ locus in type 1 diabetes patients and controls has revealed several sequences in the DQ-locus that are identical between patients, however, these sequences are also found among 10–20% of the controls, that is, in the general population. These individuals would carry the risk of developing type 1 diabetes but it should be kept in mind that in high-risk populations the prevalence rate is only 0.3–0.4%. Again, the HLA susceptibility sequences are necessary but not sufficient for the development of type 1 diabetes. Genotyping in individuals at risk such as ICA-positive healthy individuals monozygotic twins or first-degree relatives would currently only confirm the risk and only marginally improve the positive predictive value for type 1 diabetes.[94] *It will be necessary to develop methods that measure ongoing β-cell destruction to predict accurately the clinical onset of type 1 diabetes.*

HLA-DR typing has shown that more than 90% of young type 1 diabetes patients are positive for HLA-DR 3 and/or 4 (Table 3–6), however, it is notable that nearly 60% of Caucasian control subjects also have these specificities. The risk of developing type 1 diabetes among roughly half the population would be about eight times that among the other half. HLA typing of sporadic patients therefore provides little diagnostic value since less than 0.5% of the HLA-DR3 and/or 4 positive population have type 1 diabetes.[94]

Other Endocrine Abnormalities

IDDM is associated with an increased incidence of other autoimmune disorders such as Graves thyrotoxicosis, thyroiditis, and Addison's disease. The disease-associated autoantibodies listed in Table 3–7 are found with increased prevalence in type 1 diabetes patients, consistent with aberrant functioning of the immune system in these patients.

Problem Statement II: Early Detection of type 1 Diabetes

The large majority of type 1 diabetes patients are detected as sporadic cases as opposed to familial ones.[24] A highly effective screening assay for a representative disease marker would be required to detect individuals at risk of developing type 1 diabetes. Early detection would serve two purposes. One would be to forestall ketoacidosis and thereby, perhaps, prevent an accelerated loss of β cells. The other would be to introduce preventive measures, once they become available. At present the individuals with the greatest risk of developing diabetes represent family members. However, it should be noted in this respect that even among monozygotic twins the rate of concordance, that is, of both twins developing diabetes, is only 50% or less. However, the risk increases among HLA-DR3 or 4-positive twins. It seems also that, if type 1 diabetes develops in a sibship, the second sib is most frequently diagnosed 1 to 2 years after the first. Is it possible that HLA-typing, determination of ICA and β-cell function have value in predicting a later onset of type 1 diabetes?

HLA genotypes, which consist of two haplotypes, one inherited from the father, the other from the mother, are determined by HLA-typing of complete families. The probability of any pair of siblings, HLA-identical (both haplotypes in common), haploidentical (one haplotype in common), or nonidentical (neither haplotype in common) to develop type 1 diabetes is 25, 50, and 25%, respectively. However, in several studies of families with two or more children with type 1 diabetes, the expected random distribution was disturbed. Thus, it has been possible to calculate that an HLA-identical sibling has a 90-fold increased risk, a haplo identical 40-times, and an HLA non-identical sibling virtually no risk of developing type 1 diabetes.[18] HLA-typing of families may therefore provide guidance to the early detection of new type 1 diabetes patients. Prospective studies of first-degree relatives, although they represent only 7–10% of new-onset patients, have established that the clinical onset is preceded by a prodromal phase of islet autoimmunity. ICA, IAA,

GAD65, and IA-2 antibodies alone or in combination have been detected up to 8 years before the clinical onset.[75,86,88] The sensitivity and predictive value of ICA for the future onset of type 1 diabetes was calculated in a 10-year prospective study of 719 first-degree relatives.[99] Type 1 diabetes developed in 16 (2%) individuals, 14 had ICA, two did not. However, as many as 40 (6%) had ICA, hence only one third of these relatives developed type 1 diabetes. In all five relatives with the highest level (80 JDFI units) of ICA type 1 diabetes developed within a follow-up of 7 years. The predictive value to develop type 1 diabetes within 10 years ranged from 100% (80 JDFI units) to 40% (threshold 4 JDFI units).[73] The presence of ICA may therefore reflect either a previous insult to the β cells or a general immunoregulatory defect in genetically predisposed individuals. This notion is supported by observations that ICA may occur temporarily in the general population,[76] among first-degree relatives or in children after mumps infection.[77] Studies of the ability of the β cells to release insulin in ICA-positive nondiabetic individuals are inconclusive. As expected, in those individuals studied retrospectively because they developed type 1 diabetes, there is a continuous decline in the ability to release insulin in response to glucose.[100] An impaired β-cell function is found in many ICA-positive or HLA identical first-degree relatives or twins. Because the likelihood of subsequent type 1 diabetes decreases with greater duration of discordance, it is possible that the diabetogenic process in these individuals has remitted.[101,102] Another risk group for type 1 diabetes is that of patients who are initially diagnosed as having non-IDDM (type 2 diabetes), but later fail to respond to oral hypoglycemic agents.[13,14] In fact, *as many as 10% of new-onset type 2 diabetes patients may have ICA.* The conversion rate from type 1 diabetes to type 2 diabetes in such patients is high[13,103]. The sensitivity, specificity, and predictive value for insulin treatment among ICA-positive patients have been estimated to be 72, 96, and 84%, respectively. A low plasma C-peptide value at the clinical diagnosis was an additional risk factor for later insulin treatment. It remains to be determined whether this is a form of a mild onset type 1 diabetes or type 2 diabetes as a risk factor for type 1 diabetes. However, rather than providing direct evidence for reliable markers to detect a disease process that eventually precipitates type 1 diabetes, these observations underline our need to clearly define the genetic predisposition to type 1 diabetes to be able to understand its etiology and pathogenesis.[46]

Prevention of an Immune Response Against the Pancreatic β Cell

Differences in clinical and pathological features suggest heterogeneity in the acquirement of type 1 diabetes. However, as it appears from the previous description of pathophysiological phenomena, type 1 diabetes may represent a failure in some immune mechanisms that leads to a specific destruction of pancreatic β cells.

We define an autoimmune response as being directed against self-antigen(s): several lines of evidence indicate that B-lymphocyte clones capable of producing autoantibodies exist in normal individuals but are kept under stringent control. Autoreactive T lymphocytes are thought to be effectively deleted in the thymus during the development and maturation of the human immune system. The removal of autoreactive T-helper lymphocytes is an effective means by which autoreactive B lymphocytes, which develop in the bone marrow, are prevented from being activated. The process by which the thymus deletes T lymphocytes is yet to be fully clarified but expression of self-antigens may be important to the deletion of autoreactive T lymphocytes.[104] However, the fact that B lymphocytes able to produce autoantibodies are not deleted makes it possible for such cells to be activated. Autoreactive B-lymphocyte clones against thyroglobulin can, for instance, be detected in most individuals. Polyclonal activation may be associated with the development of type 1 diabetes, because already new-onset type 1 diabetes patients tend to have a multitude of autoantibodies (Table 3–7).

Another example is autoreactive B-lymphocyte clones participating in the idiotypic network by producing idiotype antibodies. Immunization with a receptor ligand such as insulin may produce antibodies capable of binding to the insulin combining site of the receptor. This is normally a transient phenomenon, but perturbation of the idiotype network might result in a prolonged production of such antibodies.[105] The cause of type 1 diabetes as well as other autoimmune diseases may be multifactorial, however, and possible primary insults by infectious agents or chemicals on the immune system or on the pancreatic β cell need to be distinguished from secondary phenomena. Several immunosuppressive drugs have been tested on new-onset type 1 diabetes patients with limited success.[106] Treatment with plasmapheresis, azathioprine, prednisone and numerous other immune suppressive drugs has had little if any effects. Open as well as randomized double-blind placebo-controlled trials with cyclosporine have shown improved β-cell function and an increased rate of remission during the first year of type 1 diabetes. These effects were, however, dependent on the duration of symptoms and that the drug treatment was initiated soon after the clinical diagnosis.[107] Cyclosporine was found to be unsafe because kidney biopsies showed histopathological alterations.

Knowledge of the detailed mechanisms of β-cell destruction may eventually provide means of specific prevention without undesirable side effects. An approach currently under investigation, for example, is the treatment of individuals identified as being at risk with insulin injections prior to the appearance of any clinical manifestations of the disease.[108] There is evidence in animal models of type 1 diabetes that exogenous insulin, probably by suppressing the expression of β-cell autoantigens, can delay or prevent the onset of clinical diabetes.[109,110] Such prophylactic therapies are especially promising because it will probably be more effective and more feasible to slow or stop the progression of islet cell destruction than to restore or attempt to reproduce the elegant glycemic control afforded by functional islets.

Changes in Antigen Structure, Concentration, or Presentation

Structural modulation of antigen either by viral infections or by chemicals might trigger an immune response against the altered self-antigen. Although in some experimental systems altered self-antigen does not seem to be a prerequisite, abnormalities in the antigen structure may help to initiate an autoimmune response. Changes in antigen concentrations on the cell surface or in circulation might also disturb the balance

TABLE 3–7 Autoantibodies Found at an Increased Prevalence Among Type I Diabetes Patients

Target Antigen	Antibody	Antigen
Organ-specific		
Thyroid	Thyroid microsomal	Thyroid peroxidase
	Thyroglobulin	Thyroglobulin
Stomach	Gastric-parietal cell	H^+,K^+-ATPase
	Intrinsic factor	
Adrenals	Adrenal cell	21-hydroxylase
Pituitary	Pituitary cell	unknown
Nonorgan-specific		
Peripheral lymphocytes	Lymphocytotoxic	unknown
Nucleic acids	Single-stranded DNA	
	Double-stranded DNA	
Cell constituents	Tubulin	

between T-helper and T-suppressor cells to evoke an immune response.

One of the possibilities suggested for the mechanisms of self-tolerance is that self-molecules do not normally associate with class II antigens (HLA-DR, -DQ, and -DP in humans). An immune response resulting in T-lymphocyte help to B lymphocytes or cytotoxic T lymphocytes requires that protein antigens be recognized in connection with class II antigens on the surface of an antigen-presenting cell (APC). Pancreatic β cells normally express class I antigens, but it has not been possible to establish that these endocrine cells themselves express class II antigens and become functional as an APC. Class II expression is not sufficient because co-stimulatory molecules are also necessary. Other cells able to engulf, process, and present antigens such as macrophages or dendritic cells (APC) will be necessary for proper antigen presentation to T-helper cells. In this case the approach to prevention would be to stall the T-helper recognition of self-antigen.

The presentation of antigen is dependent on the secretion of interleukin-1 (IL-1), TNF, and gamma interferon from the APC. These growth factors are necessary for the proliferation and differentiation of the T-helper lymphocyte to initiate an immune response. These cytokines, however, affect many cell types including the target β cells in the islets of Langerhans.[111] In vitro experiments suggest, for example, that IL-1 at low concentrations stimulates the β-cell function, while high concentrations are inhibitory and sometimes cytotoxic.[112] Effector molecules such as cytokines may therefore be of pathogenetic importance. Injection of IL-1 to BB rats or NOD mice that spontaneously develop type 1 diabetes have shown protection from type 1 diabetes at a low dose and an earlier age of onset at pharmacological dosages.[113]

The successful prevention of spontaneous islet autoimmunity by treating NOD mice with recombinant GAD65 further emphasizes the importance of autoantigens in the development of autoimmune diseases.[114,115] Prevention of an autoimmune response against the pancreatic β cells may therefore be achieved by the administration of autoantigens that are found in close association with type 1 diabetes. Hence, unresponsiveness to self may be generated by elimination of T-helper cells specific for self-antigens.

Defect in T-Suppressor Cell Function

A general defect in T-suppressor cells could account for the clustering of autoimmune disorders seen in some individuals. A depletion of circulating T-suppressor cells was found in multiple sclerosis; however, similar analyses in type 1 diabetes patients are conflicting. T-suppressor lymphocytes express the CD8 lymphocyte marker and are thought to be programmed in the thymus to suppress autoreactive T lymphocytes of the helper phenotype (CD4). This mechanism is antigen-driven. It is of interest therefore that the immunoresponse in type 1 diabetes patients against their own islet β cells seems to be antigen-dependent. In segmental pancreas transplantation without immunosuppression between healthy and diabetic co-twins being type 1 diabetes discordant for about 20 years, the β-cell function ceased within 6 weeks after transplantation.[116] Histologic analysis of the grafts showed the presence of a lymphocytic infiltration and, in some of the twins, ICA reappeared in the circulation. The autoimmune reaction against the β cells was therefore reestablished after transplantation most likely due to an activation of memory T lymphocytes. Such T lymphocytes are thought to be generated only in antigen-dependent processes. T-suppressor cells are unable to suppress this form of acquired immunity. Evidence of recurrence of disease has also been observed in patients receiving isolated pancreatic islets demonstrating an increase in GAD65 antibody levels at the time of functional loss of the islet graft.[117]

Abnormal T-Cell Help

Helper T cells generated against antigens of infectious agents that show structural similarity to self-antigens (molecular mimicry) could provide the help necessary for activation of existing autoreactive B-lymphocyte clones. Antibodies against the thyroid-stimulating hormone receptor in Graves disease cross-react with antigenic determinants of the Gram-negative *bacillus Yersinia enterocolitica* and a high frequency of *Y. enterocolitica* infection is also found in these patients.[118] The rapid progress in molecular cloning of cellular viral and bacterial proteins have made it possible to search for homologous amino acid sequences between cell proteins and antigens in infectious agents.[119] Shared epitopes may be identified. For example, the acetylcholine receptor in myasthenia gravis shows sequence homology to one of the antigens in polio virus. GAD65 in type 1 diabetes shows sequence homology to an antigen in Coxsackie virus.[29,57] Coxsackie virus is implicated as a risk factor for the disease in offspring to pregnant mothers,[21,22] as well as in association with epidemics.[27] This information may be useful in future strategies to develop antigen-specific immunosuppressive therapies.

Polyclonal B-Lymphocyte Activation

Lipoproteins, lipopolysaccharides, and other mitogenic agents including some viruses and parasites act as polyclonal β-cell activators. The spectrum of monoclonal antibodies that can be isolated from type 1 diabetes patients is compatible with a polyclonal activation.[120] *Reovirus* induces a polyendocrine autoimmune disease in mice and autoantibodies are generated against a range of antigenic determinants in different organs.[121] Assuming that a similar virus induces an autoimmune diabetes in humans vaccination against the appropriate virus would then prevent type 1 diabetes. The possible role of virus immunity aquired by infection or following vaccination for prevention or initiation of type 1 diabetes and other autoimmune diseases is controversial.

Research Considerations

Several important questions need to be answered to understand the etiology and pathogenesis of type 1 diabetes. First, the HLA genes that confer risk or protection for type 1 diabetes need to be fully defined and their ability to present β-cell antigens to initiate or maintain an autoimmune response established. This information will be important to help identify healthy individuals in the background population who are at risk of developing type 1 diabetes. This information will also be important for investigations aimed at identifying other diabetogenic genes and to determine mechanisms of risk and protection. Second, the autoantigen or autoantigens that direct the immune system to the islet β cells need to be defined. Currently, GAD65 is a major candidate because up to 80% of new-onset type 1 diabetes patients have antibodies against this protein. GAD65 antibodies have been detected many years before the clinical onset of type 1 diabetes and, within islets, this protein is β-cell specific. The understanding of the islet autoantigen is central to an understanding of the autoimmune process. It should be possible to detect the initial appearance of GAD65 antibodies as IgM and IgG in the healthy population using quantitative assays. The role of insulin as an autoantigen in primarily children also needs to be understood. Is the autoantigen preproinsulin or proinsulin rather than insulin? The IA-2 and IA-2β autoantigens also need to be investigated beyond their utility as markers for islet autoimmunity. Why are the IA-2 antibodies appearing closer to the onset of hyperglycemia? Third, the formation of the inflammatory lesion in the islets of Langerhans needs to be defined. What is the role of APC and the subsequent production of cytokines in establishing the insulitis and in affecting the islet β cells? What is the relative importance of humoral compared to cellular immunity? It is clear that one cannot function without the other, but how do they interact to maintain islet autoimmunity? The examples presented are but a few, given to indicate possible avenues for future studies of means by which to prevent the onset of type 1 diabetes in humans. The large number of additional examples that can be generated rather reflect our lack of knowledge and a need for further research on the etiology and pathogenesis of type 1 diabetes.

Acknowledgment

The research in the authors' laboratory was supported by the National Institutes of Health (grant Nos. DK26190, DK42654, DK53384, DK53004, and AI42380), by the Diabetes Endocrinology Research Center (DK17047) and the Juvenile Diabetes Foundation International including a Research Followship to S.D.C.

References

1. Papaspyros NS: The History of Diabetes Mellitus, 2nd ed. Stuttgart, 1964.

2. von Mering J, Minkowski O: Diabetes Mellitus nach Pankreasextirpation. Arch Exp Pathol Pharmakol 26:371–387, 1889.

3. Dieckhoff C: Beiträge zur pathologischen anatomie des Pankreas, mit besonderer Berücksichtigung der Diabetes Frage (Diss). Rostock:Number of 1894, Pages.

4. Borch-Johnsen K, Kreiner S, Deckert T: Mortality of Type 1 (insulin-dependent) diabetes mellitus in Denmark: A study of relative mortality in 2930 Danish Type 1 diabetic patients diagnosed from 1933 to 1972. 29:767–772, 1986.

5. Gepts W: Pathologic anatomy of the pancreas in juvenile diabetes mellitus. Diabetes 14:619–633, 1965.

6. Dunn JS, McLetchie SH: Necrosis of the islets of Langerhans produced experimentally. Lancet 1:484–487, 1943.

7. Baum J, Simmons BE, Unger RH: Localization of glucagon in the B-cells in the pancreatic islets by immunofluorescence. Diabetes 11:371–374, 1962.

8. DPT-1 Study Group: Diabetes in America, 2nd ed. Bethesda: National Institutes of Health, 1995.

9. Green A, Gale EA, Patterson CC: Incidence of childhood-onset insulin-dependent diabetes mellitus: the EURODIAB ACE Study. Lancet 339:905–909, 1992.

10. Diamond: Childhood Diabetes, Epidemics and Epidemiology: An approach for controlling diabetes. Am. J. Epidem. 135:803–816, 1992.

11. Diabetes Epidemiology Research International Group. Secular trends in incidence of childhood IDDM in 10 countries. Diabetes 39: 858–864, 1990.

12. Karvonen M, Tuomiletho J, Libman I, et al.: A review of the recent epidemiological data on incidence of type 1 (insulin-dependent) diabetes mellitus worldwide. Diabetologia 36:883–892, 1993.

13. Hagopian WA, Karlsen AE, Gottsater A, et al.: Quantitative assay using recombinant human islet glutamic acid decarboxylase (GAD-64) showed 64K autoantibody positivity at onset predicts diabetes type. J Clin Invest 91:368–374, 1993.

14. Tuomi T, Groop LC, Zimmet PZ, et al.: Antibodies to glutamic acid decarboxylase reveal latent autoimmune diabetes mellitus in adults with a non-insulin-dependent onset of disease. Diabetes 42:359–362, 1993.

15. Nyström L, Dahlquist G, Östman J, et al.: Risk of developing insulin-dependent diabetes mellitus (IDDM) before 35 years of age: Indications of climatological determinants for age at onset. Int J Epidemiol 21:352–358, 1992.

16. Christau B, Kromann H, Christy M: Incidence of insulin-dependent diabetes mellitus (0–29 years at onset) in Denmark. Acta Med Scand 624:54–60, 1979.

17. Edelsten AD, Hughes IA, Oakes S: Height and skeletal maturity in children with newly diagnosed juvenile-onset diabetes. Arch Dis Child 56:40–44, 1981.

18. Wassmuth R, Lernmark Å: The genetics of susceptibility to diabetes. Clin Immunol Immunopathol 53:358–399, 1989.

19. Todd JA, Farrall M: Panning for gold: Genome-wide scanning for linkage in type 1 diabetes. Hum Molec Genetics 5:1443–1448, 1996.

20. Field LL, Tobias R: Unraveling complex trait: The genetics of insulin-dependent diabetes mellitus. Clin Invest Med 20:41–47, 1997.

21. Dahlquist G, Ivarsson S, Lindberg B et al.: Maternal enteroviral infection during pregnancy as a risk factor for childhood IDDM. Diabetes 44:408–413, 1995.

22. Hyöty H, Hiltunen M, Knip M et al.: A prospective study of the role of coxsackie B and other enterovirus infections in the pathogenesis of IDDM. Childhood Diabetes in Finland (DiMe) Study. Diabetes 44:652–657, 1995.

23. Åkerblom HK, Savilahti E, Saukkonen TT et al.: The case for elimination of cow's milk in early infancy in the prevention of type 1 diabetes. Diabetes Metab Rev 9:456–462, 1994.

24. Dahlquist G, Blom L, Tuvemo T, et al.: The Swedish Childhood Diabetes Study—Results from a nine year case register and one year case-referent study indicating that type 1 (insulin-dependent) diabetes mellitus is associated with both type 2 (non-insulin-dependent) diabetes mellitus and autoimmune disorders. Diabetologia 32:2–6, 1989.

25. Wilson GL, Leiter EH: Streptozotocin interactions with pancreatic beta cells and the induction of insulin-dependent diabetes. Curr Top Microbiol Immunol. 27:54, 1990.

26. Karam JH, Lewitt PA, Young CW, et al.: Insulinopenic diabetes after rodenticide (Vactor) ingestion. A unique model of acquired diabetes in man. Diabetes 29:971–978, 1980.

27. Wagenkneckt LE, Roseman JM, Herman WH: Increased incidence of insulin-dependent diabetes mellitus following an epidemic of coxsackie virus B5. Am J Epidemiol 132:1024–1031, 1991.

28. Yoon JW: Role of viruses in the pathogenesis of IDDM. Ann Med 23:437–45, 1991.

29. Kaufman DJ, Erlander MG, Clare-Salzler M, et al.: Autoimmunity to two forms of glutamate decarboxylase in Insulin-dependent diabetes mellitus. J Clin Invest 89:283–292, 1992.

30. Gerling I, Chatterjee NK, Nejman C: Coxsackie virus B4-induced development of antibodies to 64,000 Mr islet autoantigen and hyperglycemia in mice. Autoimmunity 6:49–56, 1991.

31. Rahier J: The Diabetic Pancreas: A pathologist's view. In Lefebvre P, Pipeleers D (eds): The Pathology of the Endocrine Pancreas. Berlin/Heidelberg: Springer-Verlag, 1988, pp. 17–40.

32. Lernmark Å, Klöppel G, Stenger D, et al.: Heterogeneity of human islet pathology in newly diagnosed childhood insulin-dependent diabetes mellitus. Macrophage infiltrations and expression of HLA-DQ and glutamic acid decarboxylase. Virchows Archiv 425:631–640, 1995.

33. von Meyenburg H: Über "Insulitis" bei Diabetes. Schweitz Med Wochenschr 21:554–561, 1940.

34. Bottazzo GF, Dean BM, McNally JM, et al.: *In situ* characterization of autoimmune phenomena and expression of HLA molecules in the pancreas in diabetic insulitis. N Engl J Med 313:353–360, 1985.

35. Foulis AK, McGill M, Farquharson A: Insulitis in Type 1 (insulin-dependent) diabetes mellitus in man—Macrophages, lymphocytes, and interferon-λ containing cells. J Pathol 165:97–103, 1991.

36. Jenson AB, Rosenberg HS, Notkins AL: Pancreatic islet-cell damage in children with fatal viral infections. Lancet ii:354–358, 1980.

37. Rubenstein AH, Kuzuya H, Horwitz DL: Clinical significance of circulating C-peptide in diabetes mellitus and hypoglycemic disorders. Arch Intern Med 137:625–632, 1977.

38. Wallensteen M, Dahlquist G, Persson B, et al.: Factors influencing the magnitude, duration, and rate of fall of B-cell function in type 1 (insulin-dependent) diabetes children followed for two years from their clinical diagnosis. Diabetologia 31:664–669, 1988.

39. Marner B, Agner T, Binder C, et al.: Increased reduction in fasting C-peptide is associated with islet cell antibodies in type I (insulin-dependent) diabetic patients. Diabetologia 28:875–880, 1985.

40. Agner T, Damm P, Binder C: Remission in IDDM: prospective study of basal C-peptide and insulin dose in 268 consecutive patients. Diabetes Care 10:164–169, 1987.

41. Nepom BS: The role of the major histocompatibility complex in autoimmunity. Clin Immunol Immunopathol 67:S50–S55, 1993.

42. Nerup J, Platz P, Anderssen OO: HL-A antigens and diabetes mellitus. Lancet 2:864–866, 1974.

43. Singal DP, Blajchman MA: Histocompatibility (HL-A) antigens, lymphocytotoxic antibodies and tissue antibodies in patients with diabetes mellitus. Diabetes 22:429–432, 1973.

44. Platz P, Jakobsen BK, Morling M, et al.: HLA-D and DR-antigens in genetic analysis of insulin-dependent diabetes mellitus. Diabetologia 21:108–115, 1981.

45. Wolf E, Spencer KM, Cudworth AG: The genetic susceptibility to type 1 (insulin-dependent) diabetes: Analysis of the HLA-DR association. Diabetologia 24:224–230, 1983.

46. Davies JL, Kawaguchi Y, Bennett ST, et al.: A genome-wide search for human type 1 diabetes susceptibility genes. Nature 371:130–136, 1994.

47. Sanjeevi CB, Lybrand TP, DeWeese C, et al.: Polymorphic amino acid variations in HLA-DQ are associated with

systematic physical property changes and occurrence of IDDM. Diabetes 44:125–131, 1995.

48. Owerbach D, Lernmark Å, Platz P, et al.: HLA-D region β-chain DNA endonuclease fragments differ between HLA-DR identical healthy and insulin-dependent diabetic individuals. Nature 303:815–817, 1983.

49. Todd JA, Bell JI, McDevitt HO: HLA DQ β gene contributes to susceptibility and resistance to insulin-dependent diabetes mellitus. Nature 329:599–604, 1987.

50. Thorsby E, Rønningen KS: Particular HLA-DQ molecules play a dominant role in determining susceptibility or resistance to Type 1 (insulin-dependent) diabetes mellitus. Diabetologia 36:371–377, 1993.

51. Bell GI, Aorita S, Koran JH: A polymorphic locus near the human insulin gene is associated with insulin-dependent diabetes mellitus. Diabetes 33:176–183, 1984.

52. Tillil H, Köbberling K: Age-corrected empirical genetic risk estimates for first-degree relatives of IDDM patients. Diabetes 36:93–99, 1987.

53. Nepom GT: A unified hypothesis for the complex genetics of HLA associations. Diabetes 39:1153–1157, 1990.

54. Teyton L, O'Sullivan D, Dickson PW, et al.: Invariant chain distinguishes between the exogenous and endogenous antigen presentation pathways. Nature 348:39–44, 1990.

55. Scott J, Nerup J, Lernmark Å: Immunologic factors in diabetes mellitus. In Rose WF (ed): Clinical Immunology Update. New York: Elsevier, 1985, pp. 53–85.

56. Scott FW, Monegeau R, Kardish M, et al.: Diet can prevent diabetes in the BB rat. Diabetes 34:1059–1062, 1985.

57. Atkinson MA, Bowman MA, Campbell L, et al.: Cellular immunity to a determinant common to glutamate decarboxylase and coxsackie virus in insulin-dependent diabetes. J Clin Invest 94:2125–2129, 1994.

58. Honeyman MC, Stone N, de A-H, et al.: High T cell responses to the glutamic acid decarboxylase (GAD) isoform 67 reflect a hyperimmune state that precedes the onset of insulin-dependent diabetes. J Autoimmun 10:165–173, 1997.

59. Panina-Bordignon P, Lang R, van Endert PM, et al.: Cytotoxic T cells specific for glutamic acid decarboxylase in autoimmune diabetes. J Exp Med 181:1923–1927, 1995.

60. Crisá L, Mordes JP, Rossini AA: Autoimmune diabetes mellitus in the BB rat. Diabetes Metab Rev 8:9–37, 1992.

61. Wicker LS, Miller BJ, Mullen Y: Transfer of autoimmune diabetes mellitus with splenocytes from Nonobese Diabetic (NOD) Mice 35:855–860, 1986.

62. Brooks-Worrell BM, Starkebaum GA, Greenbaum C, et al.: Peripheral blood mononuclear cells of insulin-dependent diabetic patients respond to multiple islet cell proteins. J Immunol 157:5668–5674, 1996.

63. Pipeleers D, Ling Z: Pancreatic beta cells in insulin-dependent diabetes. Diabetes Metab Rev 8:209–227, 1992.

64. Peakman M, Vergani D: The T lymphocyte in type 1 diabetes. In Marshall SM, Home PD (ed): The Diabetes Annual/8. Amsterdam: Elsevier, 1994, 53–73.

65. Papadopoulos G, Petersen J, Andersen V: Spontaneous in vitro immunoglobulin secretion at the diagnosis of insulin-dependent diabetes. Acta Endocrinol 105:521–527, 1984.

66. Fairchild RS, Kyner JL, Abdou NI: Specific immunoregulation abnormality in insulin-dependent diabetes mellitus. J Lab Clin Med 99:175–186, 1982.

67. Bottazzo GF, Florin-Christensen A, Doniach D: Islet cell antibodies in diabetes mellitus with autoimmune polyendocrine deficiencies. Lancet 2:1279–1283, 1974.

68. Lernmark Å: Islet cell antibodies-theoretical and practical implications. Diabetic Med 4:285–292, 1987.

69. Greenbaum CJ, Brooks-Worrell BM, Palmer JP, et al.: Autoimmunity and prediction of insulin dependent diabetes mellitus. Diabetes Ann 8:21–52, 1994.

70. Bonifacio E, Lernmark Å, Dawkins RL: Serum exchange and use of dilutions have improved precision of measurement of islet cell antibodies. J Immunol Methods 106:83–88, 1988.

71. Greenbaum CJ, Palmer JP, Nagataki S, et al.: Improved specificity of ICA assays in Fourth International Immunology of Diabetes Serum Exchange Workshop. Diabetes 41:1570–1574, 1992.

72. Landin-Olsson M, Palmer JP, Lernmark Å, et al.: Predictive value of islet cell and insulin autoantibodies for type 1 (insulin-dependent) diabetes mellitus in a population-based study of newly-diagnosed diabetic and matched control children. Diabetologia 35:1068–1073, 1992.

73. Bonifacio E, Bingley PJ, Shattock M, et al.: Quantification of islet cell antibodies and prediction of insulin dependent diabetes. Lancet 335:147–149, 1990.

74. Gorsuch AN, Spencer KM, Lister J, et al.: Evidence for a long prediabetic period in Type 1 (insulin-dependent) diabetes mellitus. Lancet ii:1363–1365, 1981.

75. Bingley PJ: Interactions of age, islet cell antibodies, insulin autoantibodies, and first-phase insulin response in predicting risk of progression to IDDM in ICA(+) relatives: The ICARUS data set. Diabetes 45:1720–1728, 1996.

76. Landin-Olsson M, Karlsson A, Dahlquist G, et al.: Islet cell and other organ-specific autoantibodies in all children developing type 1 (insulin-independent) diabetes mellitus in Sweden during one year and in matched controls. Diabetologia 32:387–395, 1989.

77. Helmke K, Otten A, Willems WR, et al.: Islet cell antibodies and the development of diabetes mellitus in relation to mumps infection and mumps vaccination. Diabetologia 29:30–33, 1986.

78. Palmer JP, Asplin CM, Clemons P, et al.: Insulin antibodies in insulin-dependent diabetics before insulin treatment. Science 222:1337–1339, 1983.

79. Baekkeskov S, Nielsen JH, Marner B, et al.: Autoantibodies in newly diagnosed diabetic children immunoprecipitate human pancreatic islet cell proteins. Nature 298:167–169, 1982.

80. Baekkeskov S, Aanstoot HJ, Christgau S, et al.: Identification of the 64K autoantigen in insulin-dependent diabetes as the GABA-synthesizing enzyme glutamic acid decarboxylase. Nature 347:151–156, 1990.

81. Karlsen AE, Hagopian WA, Grubin CE, et al.: Cloning and primary structure of a human islet isoform of glutamic acid decarboxylase from chromosome 10. Proc Natl Acad Sci US 88:8337–8341, 1991.

82. Grubin CE, Daniels T, Toivola B, et al.: A novel radioligand binding assay to determine diagnostic accuracy of isoform-specific glutamic acid decarboxylase antibodies in childhood IDDM. Diabetologia 37:344–350, 1994.

83. Solimena M, Folli F, Aparisi R, et al.: Autoantibodies to GABA-ergic neurons and pancreatic beta cells in stiff-man syndrome. N Engl J Med 322:1555–1560, 1990.

84. Petersen JS, Dyrberg T, Damm P, et al.: GAD65 autoantibodies in women with gestational or insulin dependent diabetes mellitus diagnosed during pregnancy. Diabetologia 39:1329–1333, 1996.

85. Worsaae A, Hejnaes K, Moody A, et al.: T cell proliferative responses to glutamic acid decarboxylase-65 in IDDM are negatively associated with HLA-DR3/4. J Autoimmun 22:183–189, 1995.

86. Verge CF, Gianani R, Kawasaki E, et al.: Prediction of type I diabetes in first-degree relatives using a combination of insulin, GAD, and ICA512bdc/IA-2 autoantibodies. Diabetes 45:926–933, 1996.

87. Bingley PJ, Bonifacio E, Williams AJK, et al.: Prediction of IDDM in the general population: Strategies based on combinations of autoantibody markers. Diabetes 46:1701–1710, 1997.

88. Kulmala P, Savola K, Petersen JS, et al.: Prediction of insulin-dependent diabetes mellitus in siblings of children with diabetes—A population-based study. J of Clin Inves 101:327–336, 1998.

89. The National Diabetes Data Group. National Institute of Health (NIH). Classification and diagnosis of diabetes mellitus and other categories of glucose tolerance. Diabetes 1039–1057, 1979.

90. WHO. Study Group Diabetes mellitus. WHO Technical Report Series. 1985: 727.

91. Gavin JR, Alberti KGMM, Davidson MB, et al.: Report of the Expert Committee on the Diagnosis and Classification of Diabetes Mellitus. Diabetes Care 20:1183–1197, 1997.

92. Greenbaum CJ, Palmer JP, Kuglin B, et al.: Insulin autoantibodies measured by radioimmunoassay methodology are more related to insulin-dependent diabetes mellitus than those measured by enzyme-linked immunosorbent assay: Results of the Fourth International Workshop on the Standardization of Insulin Autoantibody measurement. J Clin Endcrinol Metab 74:1040–1044, 1992.

93. Schmidli RS, Colman PG, Bonifacio E: Disease sensitivity and specificity of 52 assays for glutamic acid decarboxylase antibodies. The Second International Glutamic Acid Decarboxylase Workshop. Diabetes 44:636–640, 1995.

94. Hagopian WA, Sanjeevi CB, Kockum I, et al.: Glutamate decarboxylase-, insulin- and islet cell-antibodies and HLA typing to detect diabetes in a general population-based study of Swedish children. J Clin Invest 95:1505–1511, 1995.

95. Nepom GT: Immunogenetics and IDDM. Diabetes Rev 1:93–103, 1993.

96. Sanjeevi CB, Kockum I, Lernmark Å: The role of major histocompatibility complex in insulin-dependent diabetes mellitus. Curr Sci 2:3–11, 1995.

97. Todd JA, Acha-Orbea H, Bell JL, et al.: A molecular basis for MHC class II-associated autoimmunity. Science 240:1003–1009, 1988.

98. Yamagata K, Nakajima H, Hanafusa T, et al.: Aspartic acid in position 57 of DQβ chain does not protect against type 1 (insulin-dependent) diabetes mellitus in Japanese subjects. Diabetologia 32:762–764, 1989.

99. Riley WJ, Maclaren NK, Krischer J, et al.: A prospective study of the development of diabetes in relatives of patients with insulin-dependent diabetes. N Engl J Med 323:1167–1172, 1990.

100. Srikanta S, Ricker AT, McCulloch DK, et al.: Autoimmunity to insulin, beta cell dysfunction, and development of insulin-dependent diabetes mellitus. Diabetes 35:139–142, 1986.

101. McCulloch DK, Klaff LJ, Kahn SE, et al.: Nonprogression of subclinical β-cell dysfunction among first degree relatives of IDDM patients: 5-yr follow-up of the Seattle family study. Diabetes 39:549–556, 1990.

102. Bärmeier H, McCulloch DK, Neifing JL, et al.: Risk for developing type 1 (insulin-dependent) diabetes mellitus and the presence of islet 64K antibodies. Diabetologia 34:727–733, 1991.

103. Gottsäter A, Landin-Olsson M, Lernmark Å, et al.: Glutamate decarboxylase antibody levels predict rate of beta-cell decline in adult onset diabetes. Diabetes Res Clin Pract 27:133–140, 1995.

104. Pugliese A, Zeller M, Fernandez J A, et al.: The insulin gene transcribed in the human thymus and transcription level correlate with allelic variation at the INS VNTR-IDDM2 susceptibility locus for type 1 diabetes. Nature Genet 15:293–297, 1997.

105. Cleveland WL, Wassermann HH, Sarangarajan R, et al.: Monoclonal antibodies to the acetylcholine receptor by a normally functioning auto-anti-idiotypic mechanism. Nature 305:56–57, 1983.

106. Skyler JS, Marks JB: Immune intervention in type 1 diabetes mellitus. Diabetes Rev 1:15–42, 1993.

107. The Canadian-European Randomized Control Trial Group: Cyclosporin-induced remission of IDDM after early intervention: Association of 1 yr of cyclosporin treatment with enhanced insulin secretion. Diabetes 37:1574–1582, 1988.

108. Group D-S: The Diabetes Prevention Trial-type 1 diabetes (DPT-1): Implementation of screening and staging of relatives. Transplant Proc 27:3377, 1995.

109. Gotfredsen CF, Buschard K, Frandsen EK: Reduction of diabetes incidence of BB Wistar rats by early prophylactic insulin treatment of diabetes-prone animals. Diabetologia 28:933–935, 1985.

110. Atkinson MA, Maclaren NK, Luchetta R: Insulitis and diabetes in NOD mice reduced by prophylactic insulin therapy. Diabetes 39:933–937, 1990.

111. McDaniel ML, Hughes JH, Wolf BA, et al.: Descriptive and mechanistic considerations of interleukin 1 and insulin secretion. Diabetes 37:1311–1315, 1988.

112. Eizirik DL, Welsh N, Hellerstrom C: Predominance of stimulatory effects of interleukin-1 beta on isolated human pancreatic islets. J Clin Endocrinol Metab 76:399–403, 1993.

113. Vertrees S, Wilson CA, Ubungen R, et al.: Interleukin-1β regulation of islet and thyroid autoimmunity in the BB rat. J. Autoimmun 4:717–732, 1991.

114. Kaufman DL, Clare-Salzler M, Tian J, et al.: Spontaneous loss of T-cell tolerance to glutamic acid decarboxylase in murine insulin-dependent diabetes. Nature 366:69–72, 1993.

115. Tisch R, Yang XD, Liblau RS, et al.: Administering glutamic acid decarboxylase to NOD mice prevents diabetes. J Autoimmun 7:845–850, 1994.

116. Sutherland DER, Sibley RK, Xu X-Z, et al.: Twin-to twin pancreas transplantation: Reversal and reenactment of the pathogenesis of type I diabetes. Trans Assoc Am Physicians 97:80–87, 1984.

117. Jaeger C, Hering BJ, Dyrberg T, et al.: Islet cell antibodies and glutamic acid decarboxylase antibodies in patients with insulin-dependent diabetes mellitus undergoing kidney and islet-after-kidney transplantation. Transplantation 62:424–426, 1996.

118. Weiss M, Ingbar SH, Winblad S, et al.: Demonstration of a saturable binding site for thyrotropin in Yersinia enterocolitica. Science 219:1331–1333, 1983.

119. Dyrberg T, Michelson B, Oldstone M: Virus and host cell antigen sharing in myasthenia gravis and autoimmune diabetes. *In* Lernmark Å, Dyrberg T, Terenius L, Hökfelt B (ed): Molecular Mimicry in Health and Disease. Amsterdam: Excerpta Medica, 1988 pp. 245–254.

120. Satoh J, Prabhakar BS, Haspel MV, et al.: Human monoclonal autoantibodies that react with multiple endocrine organs. NEJM 309:73–76, 1983.

121. Haspel MV, Onodera T, Prabhakar BS, et al.: Multiple organ-reactive monoclonal autoantibodies. Nature 304:73–76, 1983.

122. Schranz D, Lernmark Å: Immunology in diabetes: An update. Diabetes Metab Rev in press.

4

Viral Infection and Other Factors

Elliot J. Rayfield and Michael Poon

Historical Perspective

Since 1864, when the Norwegian physician J. Stang reported that diabetes developed in one of his patients soon after mumps infection, a succession of case reports have appeared in the medical literature in which diabetes has been noted to follow a viral infection. The hypothesis that viruses are one cause of insulin-dependent diabetes mellitus (IDDM) is based on (1) its abrupt onset, (2) its seasonal incidence, (3) studies of pancreatic pathological states—the presence of inflammatory cells in the islets (insulitis) and destruction of B cells, (4) many case reports showing a temporal relationship between the onset of viral infections (e.g., mumps, rubella, Coxsackievirus B group) and the subsequent development of diabetes, (5) epidemiological studies in which elevated specific viral antibody titers (Coxsackievirus B group) are correlated with an increased frequency of IDDM, and (6) animal models of virus-induced diabetes.[1,2]

The best evidence that viruses have a causative role in diabetes has come from animal studies with encephalomyocarditis (EMC) virus. Some evidence exists to support a role for viruses in the etiology of noninsulin-dependent diabetes mellitus (NIDDM).[3] In addition to viruses, the genetic background of the host and autoimmunity, toxins, drugs, and endocrine-metabolic factors may also be involved in the pathogenesis of diabetes. New information has emerged regarding the genetic predisposition for IDDM. It is well accepted that there is an increased frequency of DR3 and DR4 serotypes of the major human lymphocyte antigen (HLA) types in IDDM.[1] However, sequence analysis of HLA-DQ alleles has revealed to date eight allelic variants at the DQ α alleles locus and 13 at the DQ β locus.[4] Thus, polymorphism within the DQ alleles (which reside next to the DR alleles) can be correlated with the known susceptibility to major HLA types in IDDM.

Horn et al.[4] have also searched for homology between segments of the HLA-DQ proteins and human viruses that are potentially diabetogenic. These viruses have developed mechanisms to evade their host's immune defenses and some of these mechanisms may be related to mimicry with portions of molecules that are part of the human major histocompatibility complex. For example, the E1 envelope protein of rubella virus has been sequenced and contains at position 261 a segment of five amino acids (GPPAA) identical to a segment encoded by the IDDM-associated DQ β 3.2 allele.[4] Several review articles of general interest concerning viral–autoimmune interrelationships have been published in the past several years.[5–7] Environmental factors may also play a critical role in the induction, acceleration, and modification of the progression of diabetes.[2,6] Exhibit 4–1 summarizes several chemical agents that can induce diabetes.

EXHIBIT 4–1 Chemical Agents that can induce Diabetes Mellitus

Irreversible	Reversible
Alloxan	6-Aminoicotinamide
Streptozotocin	Azide
Diphenylthiocarbazine	Cyanide
Oxine-9-hydroxyquinolone	Cyproheptadine
Pyriminil	Dehydroascorbic acid
Pentamidine isethionate	Fluoride
	Iodoacetate
	Malonate
	Thiazides
	2-Deoxyglucose
	Mannoheptulose
	Interferon α

(*Source:* Adapted from Mordes JP, Rossini AA: Animal models of diabetes. Am J Med 70:353–360, 1981. With permission.)

Mechanisms of Virus-Induced Cell Disease

Four general mechanisms exist by which virus infection can lead to cell disease irrespective of the tissue involved.[2] The first mechanism involves a highly lytic virus, such as EMC, which initially must attach to virus-specific receptors on the cell membrane. On entry into the cell, virus replication is initiated, with focal areas of cytoplasmic degeneration within several hours. Soon, necrosis of the B cells occurs with concomitant infiltration of mononuclear cells that phagocytize cellular debris. If 90% of the B-cell mass is lysed, fasting hyperglycemia will develop. A second way a virus can lead to cellular dysfunction is by causing a persistent infection. Lymphocytic choriomeningitis, rubella, and cytomegalovirus (CMV) are protoypes of this phenomenon. In a persistent infection, the viral genome persists for a prolonged period of time, frequently the lifetime of the host, irrespective of the presence of the disease symptoms. It has been shown that cells chronically infected with rubella virus have a decreased life span that could be applicable to pancreatic B cells.[8] Chronic islet cell inflammation is thought to play a major role in the destruction of islet cells in mice infected with a diabetogenic strain (E2) of Coxsackievirus B4 (CVB4).[9] A persistent infection could account for the frequently long lag time between the occurrence of the congenital rubella syndrome at birth and the development of clinical diabetes mellitus 5 to 20 years later. A latent infection is another mechanism by which a virus such as simian virus 40 (SV-40) can induce cellular disease. The virus first gains entry into the target cell by membrane receptors. In a latent infection, the virus's nucleic acid becomes integrated into the host genome; virus gene products can be detected, but infectious virus particles are not produced. Thus, a viral infection could have the capacity to result in the altered synthesis of or the release of insulin from the B cells by this means. In addition to a persistent infection explaining a 5- to 20-year lag time between a viral infection and frank diabetes, one can postulate three infections with diabetogenic lytic viruses, each of which destroys 30% of the B-cell mass. It would not be until the third infection that hyperglycemia would be detectable. The fourth mechanism by which a viral infection can result in diabetes is by triggering an autoimmune process. Rubella and *Reovirus* Type 1 are examples of this mechanism. Rubella virus is surrounded by a lipoprotein coat that originates from the host cell membrane when the virus buds through. Therefore rubella virus could insert, expose, or alter antigens in the plasma membrane of the host cell during infection.[2]

Virus-Induced Diabetes in Animals

Encephalomyocarditis Virus

EMC virus, one of the smallest ribonucleic acid (RNA) viruses, belongs to the picornavirus family. When this virus infects the susceptible cells, RNA and protein synthesis of the host are inhibited within 3 to 5 hr after infection. Following EMC virus infection, pancreatic B cells exhibit degranulation and coagulation necrosis, other endocrine cells appear normal, and acinar necrosis rarely occurs.[10,11] When mice are infected with the M-variant of EMC virus, certain inbred strains such as SJL/J, SWR/J, and DBA/2 develop diabetes, whereas other strains such as C57BL/6J, CBA/J, and ARK/J do not develop diabetes. Susceptibility to EMC virus-induced diabetes is inherited as an autosomal recessive trait. The genetic factors that determine susceptibility operate at the level of the B cells with respect to permissiveness to infection with EMC virus. Genetic studies suggest that B-cell susceptibility to EMC virus infection is under the control of a single locus that influences two or more alleles.

Initial studies with EMC virus-induced diabetes used the M-variant. However, recent studies have shown that the M-variant is made up of at least two populations of viruses: one diabetogenic and tropic for insulin-producing B cells and the other nondiabetogenic with no tropism for insulin-producing B cells.[12] These two populations of the M stock pool have been isolated (plaque purified) into two stable variants: the D-variant is diabetogenic and the B-variant is nondiabetogenic.[12]

After inoculation of the D-variant of EMC virus into male SJL/J mice, hyperglycemia develops in over 90% of the animals in 3 days. In contrast, mice inoculated with the B-variant do not become hyperglycemic. Tissue culture experiments demonstrate that the B-variant induces considerably more interferon than the D-variant. In vivo studies show that interferon appears earlier and in greater amounts in the circulation of animals infected with the B-variant in contrast to the D-variant. The data point to a role for the interferon system in EMC virus-induced murine diabetes. Another study has shown that the repeated administration of interferon or an interferon inducer reduces the development of diabetes in mice infected with D-variant of EMC virus.[13] More recent studies provide evidence that immunization with the B-variant completely prevents the development of diabetes in mice subsequently challenged with the D-variant. It is thus conceivable that in nature antigenically similar but nondiabetogenic variants suppress the more serious outcome of coexisting diabetogenic variants. Furthermore, these data show, at least in mice, virus-induced diabetes can be prevented by a live attenuated virus.

Using an athymic nude mice model, Yoon et al.[14] infected the nude mice with EMC-D virus and showed a nearly identical diabetogenic response as compared with heterozygous littermates. In addition, passive transfer of lymphocytes from mice made diabetic with EMC-D virus into normal mice failed to produce diabetes. The results of these studies argued for the direct destruction of B cells by the virus and against the immune response as a major contributor to the pathogenesis of EMC-D-induced diabetes.

The isolation of the D-variant of EMC virus permitted experiments to be performed in which the long-term complications of virus-induced diabetes could be examined.[15] Mice inoculated with the D-variant of EMC virus develop severe hyperglycemia lasting 6 months along with some of the long-term complications of diabetes, including reduced life span, glomerulosclerosis, and ocular changes.[15] The renal complications documented include thickening of the mesangium, the peripheral basement membrane, and Bowman's capsule, nodular and diffuse glomerular basement, which was thickened as much as fourfold compared with control mice.[15] These changes have not been well documented in the diabetes induced by alloxan or streptozotocin in which there was varying degrees of mesangial thickening of the peripheral glomerular basement membranes. Ocular changes included lesions similar to human corneal erosions, a decrease in the number of pericytes in retinal vessels, and a thickening of the basement membrane of the retinal capillaries.[15] Bae et al.,[16] from the Yoon laboratory, have determined the complete nucleotide sequences of EMC-D and EMC-B and found that EMC-D (7829 bases) differs from EMC-B (7825 bases) by only 14 nucleotides. The differences include two deletions of five nucleotides, one base insertion, and eight point mutations. Among these differences, some of the five-point mutations found in the VP1 gene are likely to influence the attachment of the virus to pancreatic B cells because the major portion of the VP1 gene product is exposed on the surface of the virus particles. Recently, the VP1 protein has been successfully cloned and expressed in *Escherichia coli* by Jun et al. Five- to 6-week-old male SJL/J mice were immunized intraperitoneally with purified VP1 protein and then challenged with highly diabetogenic EMC-D virus. All of the VP1-immunized mice did not develop diabetes and showed intact pancreatic islet architecture. In comparison, most of the infected control mice showed severe β-cell necrosis and lymphocytic infiltration of their pancreatic islets.[17] Most recently, Jun et al.[18] has identified a single point mutation at nucleotide position 3155 or 3156 of the recombinant EMC viral genome, located on the major capsid protein VP1, which causes an amino acid change and results in the gain or loss of viral diabetogenicity.

Coxsackievirus B4

Early studies showed that CVB4 could attack the acinar cells of the pancreas, but spare the islets of Langerhans. However, when CVB4 is passaged 14 times in β-cell cultures prepared from SJL/J mice, the tropism changes so that the virus can now destroy pancreatic B cells in certain inbred strains of mice.[19] Histologic examination of the pancreas reveals destruction of β cells, and immunofluorescent techniques using fluorescence-labeled anti-CVB4 antibody show viral antigens within the β cells in the islets of Langerhans.[19]

Chatterjee and colleagues[20] have characterized a diabetogenic strain (E4) of CVB4 isolated from a human source. This strain contains two types of particles: virions and membrane-bound virions (MBV). MBVs are lighter and significantly less infectious than virions. In contrast, MBVs are more diabetogenic than virions. More recently, Hou et al.[21] from the Chatterjee laboratory, have identified a threefold increase expression of a 64K islet autoantigen in islets of mice infected with a diabetogenic strain of CVB4 at 72-hr postinfection.[21] This autoantigen was identified as the enzyme glutamic acid decarboxylase.[21] Glutamic acid decarboxylase antibodies are an early marker of type 1 diabetes.[22] Recent population-based studies conducted in Finland and Sweden demonstrated that children of mothers whose sera were postive for Coxsackie B virus antibodies by capture radioimmunoassay carried an increased risk for developing childhood onset IDDM suggesting the possible virus-induced antoimmunity or persistent infection as a cause of progressive β-cell destruction.[23,24]

Rubella

Menser et al.[25] have shown that experimental congenital rubella infection in white rabbits (Castle Hill Laboratory strain, University of Sydney) results in B-cell degranulation with necrosis. Hyperglycemia was not present in these animals. Mento and Rayfield[26] reported in preliminary form that rubella virus vaccine strain (RA 27/3: Merck, Sharp, and Dohme, lot 0647D)-induced hyperglycemia in a hamster model.

We reported on an animal model for rubella virus-induced diabetes using golden Syrian hamsters. Seven- to 10-day-old male LVG strain golden Syrian hamsters were inoculated with a diabetogenic (P5) variant of the vaccine strain (RA27/3) of rubella virus or sham inoculated with diluent and followed longitudinally. All hamsters developed hyperglycemia and hypoinsulinemia that was sustained during the 15-week period.

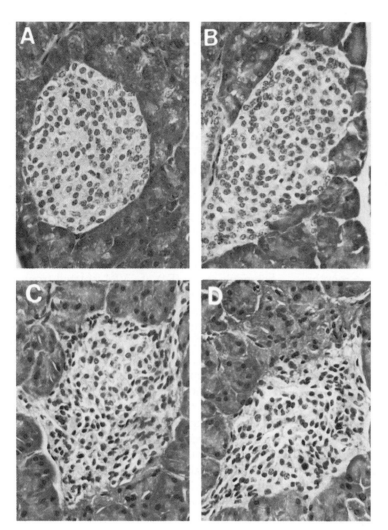

Figure 4–1. Histopathological findings from four hamsters infected with P5 rubella virus. A and B: Islets exhibiting first signs of inflammation with few mononuclear cells infiltrating parenchyma of endocrine tissue (14 days). There are occasional endocrine cells with pyknotic nuclei. In both islets illustrated, and in most of the other islets examined, there is disruption of the connective tissue capsule delimiting the islet. Islet in B is more severely affected. Exocrine tissue is histologically unaffected by viral infection. C and D: Islets showing marked inflammatory responses in ~50% of islets (21 days). Numerous mononuclear cells have infiltrated the islets. In these islets, there is complete disruption of normal architecture and marked loss of parenchymal cells. Occasional mitotic figures were seen in infiltrated islets. Exocrine pancreas remains histologically normal. (Hematoxylin and eosin stains ×300)

Histopathological studies revealed a marked mononuclear infiltration of 34.5% of islet cells from infected hamsters 21 days following rubella virus inoculation (Fig. 4–1). Rubella virus was isolated from the pancreas of all 10 hamsters tested. Cytoplasmic islet cell antibodies were documented in 8 of 20 sera obtained 21 to 32 days following infection. These data suggest that autoimmunity is a major mechanism accounting for the diabetes that develops in these hamsters. Rubella virus [similar to Venezuelan encephalitis (VE) virus] is a member of the togavirus family of enveloped viruses that are surrounded by a lipoprotein coat formed when the maturing virus buds through the host cell membrane. Thus, the virus has the potential to insert, alter, or expose antigens in the plasma membrane of the host cell during intracellular infection. An alternative possibility is that the autoimmunity might result from lysis or activation of subpopulations of lymphocytes (helper or suppressor T cells) that regulate the immune response of the host.

Reovirus

Onodera et al. have shown that when 5-to 7-day-old SJ (male and female) mice are inoculated with *Reovirus* type I (*Reo*-1), infection occurs in the pancreas and pituitary leading to mild hyperglycemia or impaired glucose tolerance and growth retardation. Autoantibodies were found that reacted with antigens in the pancreatic islets, the anterior pituitary, and gastric mucosa, as well as antibodies to insulin and growth hormone.[25] The impaired glucose tolerance and retarded growth induced by *Reo*-1 could be prevented by treatment with antilymphocyte serum, antithymocyte serum, or cyclophosphamide. In the *Reovirus* model, although some lysis of islet cells occurs, the autoimmune component appears to predominate. In contrast to *Reo*-1, *Reovirus* type 3 (*reo*-3) was reported to cause transient diabetes by destruction of beta cells without an autoimmune mechanism.[27] Because in human IDDM, islet cell cytoplasmic antibodies or surface antibodies are found in patients' serum in addition to an increased incidence of autoimmunity of other endocrine glands, *Reo*-1 virus-induced diabetes in mice may have clinical relevance in understanding the pathogenesis of the human disease.

Venezuelan Encephalitis Virus

VE belongs to a group of viruses (togaviruses) that are enveloped and in which viral proteins become incorporated into membranes of host tissues during viral replication. Golden Syrian hamsters inoculated with the virulent Trinidad strain of VE virus were shown to have mature virions and viral antigens in B cells by electron microscopy and immunofluorescence.[27] Viral growth occurred in the pancreas with both the Trinidad strain and the vaccine (TC-83) strain of VE virus. Following inoculation with TC-83 VE, hamsters developed glucose intolerance of 24 days' duration and markedly diminished plasma insulin levels that lasted at least 90 days following infection.

TC-83 VE virus was shown to inhibit glucose-stimulated insulin release in three genetic variants of C57BL/Ks mice (db/db, db/+, and +/+).[28] Furthermore, the Trinidad strain of VE virus resulted in impaired glucose tolerance and hypoinsulinemia in one group of young rhesus monkeys (2 to 3 years old) but not in a slightly older group of monkeys (3 to 4 years old). Interestingly the monkeys in the first experiment were febrile and exhibited coughing and rhinorrhea, in contrast to the second experiment in which monkeys had no respiratory symptoms and only three were febrile. In vitro studies were next carried out in perifused islets from control animals and 24-day post-VE virus-infected hamsters.[29] These experiments were done to assess insulin secretion accurately without the influence of neural and hormonal factors that are present in vivo. In the presence of 20 mM glucose, VE-infected islets exhibited a 45% diminution in insulin release in comparison with control islets, which was similar to in vivo findings. This decrease in glucose-stimulated insulin release persisted for 8 months following VE inoculation in the perifusion system in hamsters, which were not hyperglycemic in vivo. The phosphodiesterase inhibitor theophylline and cyclic adenosine monophosphate (cAMP) analogs (dibutyryl cAMP and 8-bromo cAMP) were able to normalize insulin release in the presence of 20 mM glucose.[29] These observations suggested that the virus-induced defect in insulin release was possibly at or close to the B-cell membrane, but that events distal to the cAMP system of the B cell are intact. Morphological and morphometric evaluation of VE-infected islet cells (21 days following virus inoculation) showed no changes in islet volume density, B-cell density, and B-cell granulation.[29]

Further studies have more directly pointed to an abnormality in the cAMP system in VE-infected islet cells by measuring islet cAMP content in response to various secretagogues.[29] Thus, in the presence of 10 mM glucagon plus 1 mM isobutylmethylxanthine or 20 mM glucose plus 1 mM RO 20-1724, cAMP generation is significantly decreased in VE-infected in contrast to control islet cells when measured over a 20-min period. Isobutylmethylxanthine and RO 20-1724 are added to the system to retard the degradation of cAMP.[29] The precise mechanism by which VE virus impairs glucose-stimulated insulin secretion remains to be determined. The model is interesting in that it suggests that environmental factors may act in subtle ways to alter cellular biochemistry and, thus, impair insulin secretion.

Association of Viral Infection in Humans with Insulin-Dependent Diabetes Mellitus

In Vitro Studies

The possibility that viruses might cause some cases of IDDM by infecting and destroying pancreatic B cells has received considerable attention. However, it is difficult to demonstrate in vivo that viruses replicate in human B cells and produce diabetes in humans. As a practical approach, an in vitro system has been developed to determine if viruses are capable of infecting and destroying human B cells in culture. Because the cells in these cultures were not pure B cells, a double-label immunofluorescent antibody technique was used to show unequivocally that it was the B cells, and not contaminating non-B cells, that became infected. Antibody to virus was labeled with fluorescein isothicyanate and antibody to insulin was labeled with tetramethyl rhodamine isothiocyanate. By this method, it was clearly shown that several common human viruses, including mumps, Coxsackievirus B3 (CVB3), CVB4, and reo-3, could infect human B cells.[30] Also, it was shown that the infection markedly decreased the insulin content of B cells as measured by decreased insulin content of B cells as measured by radioimmunoassay. Thus, at least under in vitro conditions, human B cells are susceptible to viral infection.

However, there is no way to prove that these viruses actually infect and destroy human pancreatic B cells and cause diabetes in the in vivo situation. It is known that some viruses will grow in cultured cells derived from animals that are resistant to infection.

In vivo studies

Isolation of virus. As mentioned in the previous section, in vitro susceptibility of B cells may not be a true reflection of in vivo susceptibility. A more direct approach is to isolate virus from the pancreas of children dying form acute-onset IDDM. In 1979, such a case was reported by Yoon and colleagues.[31] A healthy 10-year-old boy was admitted to the hospital in diabetic ketoacidosis within 3 days after the onset of a flu-like illness. Despite intensive therapy, the child died of cerebral edema 7 days later. At autopsy, lymphocytic infiltration of the islets of Langerhans was noted, which was similar to that of mice that developed diabetes after infection with EMC or Coxsackievirus. A piece of the boy's pancreas was homogenized and then inoculated into a number of different cell lines. Several days later, cytopathological changes were observed in tissue culture and a variant of CVB4 was isolated.[31] Studies on the patient's serum revealed a rise in neutralizing antibody titer to this isolate from less than 4 on the second hospital day to 32 on the day of death. Neither the earlier nor later serum neutralized the diabetogenic variant of EMC virus that was being studied in the laboratory. In addition, when sections of the child's brain were stained with fluorescein-labeled anti-CVB4 antibody, a few cells were found to contain viral antigens. These findings supported the idea that the virus actually came from the child and was not a laboratory contaminant.

However, the possibility still remained that the infection with CVB4 was completely unrelated to the cause of the patient's diabetes. The animal models proved to be of great value. When several inbred strains of mice were inoculated with the human isolate, SJL/J male mice developed diabetes, while CBA/J, 57BL/6J, and BALB/c mice did not develop diabetes.[31] Moreover, examination of the pancreas from diabetic mice revealed extensive infiltration of inflammatory cells, destruction of B cells, and viral antigens in the islets of Langerhans. Based on the patient's clinical picture, the virus isolation studies, and the induction of diabetes in mice, the evidence supported the conclusion that the patient's diabetes was virus-induced.

The notion that viruses can trigger diabetes in humans has been strengthened by two additional case reports. The first is that of a 16-month-old child who developed a Coxsackievirus B5 (CVB5) infection and a few days later was diagnosed as having diabetes.[32] This virus was isolated from the feces of the child and produced impaired glucose tolerance tests when inoculated into mice. The second case was a 5-year-old girl who had myocarditis and diabetes 2 to 3 weeks after having open heart surgery. At necropsy, her islet cells showed a lymphocytic infiltrate and B cell necrosis. By immunofluorescence examination, CVB4 antigens were sectioned from five of eight neonates who died of Coxsackievirus B infections that showed insulitis and B-cell damage observed at autopsy. Although the cited cases do not prove that a virus caused them, they do provide further in vivo support for the idea that under certain circumstances, some viruses are capable of infecting B cells.

The frequency of diabetogenic variants of Coxsackieviruses in the human population is not known. However, it is evident that diabetes is not a common consequence of CVB4 infection because anti-CVB4 antibody is present in about half the population, and less than 1% of the population develops IDDM. It is also known that CVB4 is not the only cause of diabetes, because approximately half the children with IDDM do not have anti-CVB4 antibody. It is possible that B-cell tropic viruses are far more common than previously suspected, producing a spectrum of disease from a subclinical infection with minimal B-cell damage and no overt diabetes to the unusual case with severe B-cell damage and clinically apparent diabetes. In some patients, diabetes may follow multiple infections with different viruses or a virus infection may trigger an autoimmune process that leads to diabetes several years later. Thus, IDDM appears to be several diseases with different causes. Viruses would be only one of the causes, and more than one virus or virus group may be involved.

Epidemiological Studies and Case Reports

In 1969, Gamble et al.[33] reported that IDDM of recent onset (within 3 months) had a higher neutralizing antibody titer to Coxsackievirus than did either normal subjects or IDDM of a duration longer than 3 months.[33] However, other epidemiological studies have not confirmed this finding. In 1974, Templeton and colleagues[39] reported a case documenting the acute onset of IDDM in children in association with a Coxsackievirus B2. More recently, it has been reported that the frequency of CVB4 viral antibody in Asia was significantly higher in IDDM patients (80%) than in the control population (15%). A cross-sectional study performed in Finland in 1988 among 273 children and adolescents with newly diagnosed IDDM supported the hypothesis that autoimmune mechanisms may play a more active role in young children, whereas environmental factors may be of greater importance in older children contracting the disease.[33] In this study, Coxsackie B4 virus-specific immunoglobulin A autobodies were more common in the complement fixing (CF) islet cell antibody negative than in the CF islet cell-positive groups of children with the new onset of IDDM. The CF islet cell-negative group represented the older children. The role of Coxsackieviruses of the B group in the pathogenesis of human diabetes awaits further epidemiological studies.

Mumps Virus. The initial case report of an association of mumps infection with diabetes mellitus in the 19th century by Harris[1] has since been followed by numerous others. Mumps virus has been the virus most frequently reported in association with diabetes mellitus with symptoms of diabetes developing from a few days to several months following parotitis or parotitis with pancreatitis. Several cases of mumps pancreatitis examined pathologically during autopsy have shown acute inflammation with edema, mononuclear cell infiltration, and degeneration of epithelioid cells, but this may not be the rule. An epidemiologic study performed by Sultz and coworkers[1] in Erie County, New York, found a mean lag time of 3.8 years between mumps infection for vaccination and development of symptomatic diabetes. In contrast, a study from South India showed no correlation between antibody titers to mumps virus in a group of recent-onset IDDM patients compared with nondiabetic control subjects. Subsequently, Gamble[33] reported that diabetes starting in childhood may result in a small proportion of cases from recent mumps infection.

Rubella Virus. To date, more than 80 documented cases of diabetes mellitus have been reported in patients with the congenital rubella syndrome. The oldest studied series has been performed by Menser and associates[25] in Australia. They have shown that there is a greater than 20% incidence of either clinical diabetes or impaired glucose tolerance in patients with the congenital rubella syndrome (CRS). In this same group of patients, HLA-B8 was present in 50% of the diabetics in contrast to 24% of a control population. This HLA type is known to be increased in IDDM. A 50-year follow-up of the Menser series has recently been reported without any significant changes in the prevalence of diabetes.[35] Monif and co-workers[36] also reported persistent rubella virus infections of the pancreas of infants with the congenital rubella syndrome. However, in some pathological studies of infants dying with the congenital rubella syndrome, lesions in the islets of Langerhans have not been found.[37] More recently, Patterson and colleagues[38] reported that there is an association between insulitis and recent-onset diabetes with CRS.

One of the earliest clues that the endocrine abnormalities in CRS might have an autoimmune basis was the observation in 1984 of an increased prevalence of islet cell surface antibodies (ICSA) in 21% of the entire CRS population in the New York study as well as 50 to 80% of patients with altered carbohydrate metabolism.[39,40] In addition, antithyroid microsomal or antithyroid globulin autoantibodies, or both, were found in 26% of patients with CRS.[39,40] Adrenal antibodies were not found in any of the 66 CRS patients studies. Thirteen percent of the patients with CRS and IDDM exhibited insulin autoantibodies in comparison with less than 1% of the control population and 49% of new-onset IDDM.[37] The patients with both CRS and IDDM also tended to be ICSA positive, but no clear association with the DR3 or DR4 haplotype has been found. Although most patients with CRS and IDDM

have decreased circulating insulin levels, 18.4% of CRS patients have hyperinsulinemia. Of the 17 patients who were hyperinsulinemic at the time of the first study, three have become hypoinsulinemic; all are DR3 and DR4 and have ICSA.[41] T4/T8 (helper/suppressor) lymphocyte studies performed in 17 patients with CRS revealed that the ratios were low normal, with 9 of 17 CRS patients having below normal ratios.[41] Only one of these patients was insulin dependent.

The precise mechanisms resulting in the endocrine abnormalities as well as congenital defects in CRS is not completely known. Possibilities include: (1) persistence of virus in tissues resulting in a reduced growth rate and shortened life span of the cells, (2) autoimmune responses, (3) genetic factors, and (4) vascular damage by the viral infection with further stenosis or occlusion of the vessels later. This model is particularly important because the autoimmune features of the diabetes accompanying CRS are similar to those of IDDM without CRS.

Cytomegalovirus and Others. In 1947, Cappell and McFarlane reported that CMV can cause pancreatic lesions in humans. Furthermore, diabetes mellitus has been associated temporally with viral infections from cytomegalovirus, measles, polio, influenza, tick-borne encephalitis, and infectious hepatitis.[12] However, a recent prospective study examined 76 Swedish CMV-infected infants from a cohort of 16,474 newborns screened by virus isolation in urine. Only 1 out 76 CMV-infected infants developed type 1 diabetes, during the study period extending from 1977 through 1993, which was not statistically different from the uninfected controls who were born and followed during the same period ($p = 0.14$).[42] Using DNA amplification and in situ hybridization techniques, two separate groups of investigators from Japan and Sweden could not detect CMV or Epstein–Barr virus DNA and RNA in sections of pancreas tissues from patients with recent onset IDDM of less than 7 months in duration.[42] The results do not conclusively exclude CMV as a virus pathogen for IDDM. In patients with chronic cirrhosis and hepatitis C, but not hepatitis B virus infection, there is an increased incidence of diabetes in contrast to hepatitis C-negative cirrhotic controls.[44,45]

Toxins and Chemicals Associated with Diabetes Mellitus

These are summarized in Exhibit 4–1.[3] Alloxan and streptozotocin have been the most extensively studied agents. The mechanisms of alloxan-induced diabetes is through an initial interaction with the B-cell membrane. Glucose and to a lesser extent fructose and mannose can prevent or reduce the ensuing hyperglycemia if these sugars are administered before alloxan. This protection is stereo-specific, with a greater effect by the α-anomers.

Streptozotocin-induced diabetes also required B-cell membrane binding as its first step in the ensuing cell damage. It is thought that the glucose moiety of streptozotocin enhances its uptake into the B cell, allowing for concentration of the cytotoxic nitrosourea component of the molecule. Within the B cell, streptozotocin decreases levels of nicotine adenine dinucleotide by decreasing its synthesis and increasing its breakdown. When given as multiple small doses (each of which is subdiabetogenic), streptozotocin produces a diabetes-like syndrome in mice associated with mononuclear cell infiltrates and type C virus particles in the pancreatic islets. Depending on the dose of streptozotocin administered to the rat, one can produce an animal model resembling NIDDM or severe IDDM with ketoacidosis. This dose dependency may hold true for toxins in their ability to damage human B cells in nature.

Pentamidine isethionate is used for the treatment of *Pneumocystis carinii* pneumonia.[46] This agent has been reported to cause hypoglycemia, sometimes followed by IDDM.[47] The time course of the metabolic response with pentamidine is that of a direct β-cell toxin. N-3-pyridylmethyl N'-nitrophenyl urea (pyriminil) is also known as the rodenticide, Vacor. When pyriminil has been taken accidentally or deliberately as a suicidal gesture, IDDM with severe neuropathy ensues.[48]

Recently, case reports of patients with hepatitis developed adult onset diabetes while receiving interferon α suggesting the possible autoimmune mechanism of the development of diabetes in response to interferon treatment.[49,50]

Research Considerations

Evidence of environmental factors participating in the pathogenesis of diabetes mellitus continues to grow.

The mechanisms operative in the development of viral diabetes include cell lysis, a persistent infection, a latent infection, and autoimmunity.

The data accrued from animal models are much more solid than those obtained from human studies.

EMC virus-induced diabetes in mice remains the most extensively studied animal model, although the model does not cause human disease. A new model of rubella virus-induced diabetes in the hamster has been shown to share the autoimmune features observed in patients with IDDM who also have the congenital rubella syndrome. Other viruses that cause diabetes-like syndromes in animals include the Coxsackieviruses and *Reovirus*. Although mumps virus, CVB4, and CMV may be associated with human diabetes, the most convincing data come from clinical studies of children and young adults with CRS.

The toxins alloxan and streptozotocin have been extensively studied in animal models. Pentamidine and pyriminil can produce unequivocal diabetes in man, but are not agents to which humans are ordinarily exposed.

Genetics data have recently pointed to DQB alleles as playing a role in conferring susceptibility to or protection from IDDM.

The question is no longer whether viruses can trigger diabetes mellitus, but rather how often they do and under what circumstances. The answer to this conundrum will require further studies utilizing advanced techniques of immunology and molecular biology.

Acknowledgments

The authors thank Ariel Kohane for his excellent technical assistance and a grant from Mansfred and Anne Lehmann Research Foundation.

References

1. Rayfield EJ, Seto Y: Viruses and the pathogenesis of diabetes mellitus. Diabetes 27:1126–1140, 1978.

2. Rayfield EJ, Ishimura K: Environmental factors and insulin-dependent diabetes mellitus. Diabetes Metab Rev 3:925–957, 1987.

3. Rayfield EJ, Mento SJ: Viruses may be etiologic agents for non-insulin-dependent (type II) diabetes. Rev Infect Dis 5:341–345, 1983.

4. Horn GT, Bugawan TL, Long CM, et al.: Allelic sequence variation of the HLA-DQ loci: Relationship to serology and to insulin-dependent diabetes susceptibility. Proc Natl Acad Sci USA 85:6012–6026, 1988.

5. von Herrath MG, Oldstone MB: Virus-induced autoimmune disease. Curr Opin Immunol 8:878–885, 1996.

6. Leslie RD, Elliott RB: Early environmental events as a cause of IDDM. Evidence and implications. Diabetes 43:843–850, 1994.

7. Boitard C, Larger E, Timsit J, et al.: IDDM: An islet or an immune disease? Diabetologia 37(Suppl 2):S90–S98, 1994.

8. Rayfield EJ, Kelly KJ, Yoon JW: Rubella virus-induced diabetes in the hamster. Diabetes 35:1278–1281, 1986.

9. See DM, Tilles JG: Pathogenesis of virus-induced diabetes in mice. J Infect Dis 171:1131–1138, 1995.

10. Craighead JE: The role of viruses in the pathogenesis of pancreatic disease and diabetes mellitus. Prog Med Virol 19:161–214, 1975.

11. Craighead JE, Huber SA, Sriram S: Animal models of picornavirus-induced autoimmune disease: Their possible relevance to human disease. Lab Invest 63:432–446, 1990.

12. Yoon JW, McClintock PR, Onodera T, et al.: Virus-induced diabetes mellitus. XVIII. Inhibition by a nondiabetogenic variant of encephalomyocarditis virus. J Exp Med 152:878–892, 1980.

13. Giron DJ, Agostini HJ, Thomas DC: Effect of interferons and poly(I):poly(C) on the pathogenesis of the diabetogenic variant of encephalomyocarditis virus in different mouse strains. J Interferon Res 8:745–753, 1988.

14. Yoon JW, McClintock PR, Bachurski CJ, et al.: Virus-induced diabetes mellitus. No evidence for immune mechanisms in the destruction of beta-cells by the D-variant of encephalomyocarditis virus. Diabetes 34:922–925, 1985.

15. Yoon JW, Rodrigues MM, Currier C, et al.: Long-term complications of virus-induced diabetes mellitus in mice. Nature 296:566–569, 1982.

16. Bae YS, Eun HM, Yoon JW: Molecular identification of diabetogenic viral gene. Diabetes 38:316–320, 1989.

17. Jun HS, Yoon SW, Kang Y, et al.: Cloning and expression of the VP1 major capsid protein of diabetogenic encephalomyocarditis (EMC) virus and prevention of EMC virus-induced diabetes by immunization with the recombinant VP1 protein. J Gen Virol 76:2557–2566, 1995.

18. Jun HS, Kang Y, Notkins AL, Yoon JW: Gain or loss of diabetogenicity resulting from a single point mutation in recombinant encephalomyocarditis virus. J Virol 71:9782–9785, 1997.

19. Yoon JW, Onodera T, Notkins AL: Virus-induced diabetes mellitus. XV. Beta cell damage and insulin-dependent hyperglycemia in mice infected with coxsackie virus B4. J Exp Med 148:1068–1080, 1978.

20. Chatterjee NK, Nejman C, Gerling I: Purification and characterization of a strain of coxsackievirus B4 of human origin that induces diabetes in mice. J Med Virol 26:57–69, 1988.

21. Hou J, Sheikh S, Martin DL, et al.: Coxsackievirus B4 alters pancreatic glutamate decarboxylase expression in mice soon after infection. J Autoimmun 6:529–542, 1993.

22. Pietropaolo M, Peakman M, Pietropaolo SL, et al.: Combined analysis of GAD65 and ICA512(IA-2) autoantibodies in organ and non-organ-specific autoimmune diseases confers high specificity for insulin-dependent diabetes mellitus [In Process Citation]. J Autoimmun 11:1–10, 1998.

23. Hyoty H, Hiltunnen M, Knip M, et al.: A prospective study of the role of coxsackie B and other enterovirus infections in the pathogenesis of IDDM. Childhood Diabetes in Finland (DiMe) Study Group. Diabetes 44:652–657, 1995.

24. Dahlquist G, Frisk G, Ivarsson SA, et al.: Indications that maternal coxsackie B virus infection during pregnancy is a risk factor for childhood-onset IDDM. Diabetologia 38:1371–1373, 1995.

25. Menser MA, Forrest JM, Bransby RD: Rubella infection and diabetes mellitus. Lancet 1:57–60, 1978.

26. Mento SJ, Rayfield EJ: Comparison of the diabetic effects of a vaccine and a street strain of rubella virus in hamsters. Diabetes 31:45, 1982.

27. Yoon JW, Selvaggio S, Onodera T, et al.: Infection of cultured human pancreatic B cells with reovirus type 3. Diabetologia 20:462–467, 1981.

28. Rayfield EJ, Seto Y, Goldberg SL, et al.: Venezuelan encephalitis virus-induced alterations in carbohydrate metabolism in genetically diabetic mice. Diabetes 28:799–803, 1979.

29. Rayfield EJ, Seto Y, Walsh S, et al.: Virus-induced alterations in insulin release in hamster islets of Langerhans. J Clin Invest 68:1172–1181, 1981.

30. Yoon JW, Onodera T, Jenson AB, et al.: Virus-induced diabetes mellitus. XI. Replication of coxsackie B3 virus in human pancreatic beta cell cultures. Diabetes 27:778–781, 1978.

31. Yoon JW, Austin M, Onodera T, et al.: Isolation of a virus from the pancreas of a child with diabetic ketoacidosis. N Engl J Med 300:1173–1179, 1979.

32. Champsaur HF, Bottazzo GF, Bertrams J, et al.: Virologic, immunologic, and genetic factors in insulin-dependent diabetes mellitus. J Pediatr 100:15–20, 1982.

33. Gamble DR, Kinsley ML, FitzGerald MG, et al.: Viral antibodies in diabetes mellitus. Br Med J 3:627–630, 1969.

34. Templeton AA, Kerr MG, Cole RA, et al.: Laparoscopic sterilization with silastic-band technique. Br Med J 1:1007–1008, 1977.

35. McIntosh ED, Menser MA: A fifty-year follow-up of congenital rubella. Lancet 340:414–415, 1992.

36. Monif GRG, Avery BG, Korones SB, et al.: Postmortem isolation of the rubella virus from the organs of three children with rubella syndrome defects. Lancet. 1:723–727, 1965.

37. Singer DB, Rudolph AJ, Rosenberg HS, et al.: Pathology of the congenital rubella syndrome. J Pediatr 71:665–675, 1967.

38. Patterson K, Chandra RS, Jenson AB: Congenital rubella, insulitis, and diabetes mellitus in an infant [letter]. Lancet 1:1048–1049, 1981.

39. Ginsberg-Fellner F, Witt ME, Fedun B, et al.: Diabetes mellitus and autoimmunity in patients with the congenital rubella syndrome. Rev Infect Dis 7(Suppl 1):S170–176, 1985.

40. Ginsberg-Fellner F, Witt ME, Yagihashi S, et al.: Congenital rubella syndrome as a model for type 1 (insulin-dependent) diabetes mellitus: Increased prevalence of islet cell surface antibodies. Diabetologia 27(Suppl):87–89, 1984.

41. Yoon JW, Morishima T, McClintock PR, et al.: Virus-induced diabetes mellitus: Mengovirus infects pancreatic beta cells in strains of mice resistant to the diabetogenic effect of encephalomyocarditis virus. J Virol 50:684–690, 1984.

42. Ivarsson SA, Lindberg B, Nilsson KO, et al.: The prevalence of type 1 diabetes mellitus at follow-up of Swedish infants congenitally infected with cytomegalovirus. Diabetes Med 10:521–523, 1993.

43. Itoh N, Hanafusa T, Yamagata K, et al.: No detectable cytomegalovirus and Epstein–Barr virus genomes in the

pancreas of recent-onset IDDM patients. Diabetologia 38:667–671, 1995.

44. Allison ME, Wreghitt T, Palmer CR, et al.: Evidence for a link between hepatitis C virus infection and diabetes mellitus in a cirrhotic population [see comments]. J Hepatol 21:1135–1139, 1994.

45. Fraser GM, Harman I, Meller N, et al.: Diabetes mellitus is associated with chronic hepatitis C but not chronic hepatitis B infection [see comments]. Isr J Med Sci 32: 526–530, 1996.

46. Lillehei JP, Funke JL, Drage CW, et al.: Pneumocystis carinii pneumonia. Needle-biopsy diagnosis and successful treatment. JAMA 206:596–600, 1968.

47. Bouchard P, Sai P, Reach G, et al.: Diabetes mellitus following pentamidine-induced hypoglycemia in humans. Diabetes 31:40–45, 1982.

48. Prosser PR, Karam JH: Diabetes mellitus following rodenticide ingestion in man. JAMA 239:1148–1150, 1978.

49. Fabris P, Betterle C, Floreani A, et al.: Development of type 1 diabetes mellitus during interferon alfa therapy for chronic HCV hepatitis [letter] [see comments]. Lancet 340:548, 1992.

50. Koivisto VA, Pelkonen R, Cantell K: Effect of interferon on glucose tolerance and insulin sensitivity. Diabetes 38:641–647, 1989.

5

Genetic Factors in Diabetes Mellitus

Jin-Xiong She

Diabetes mellitus is a heterogeneous group of diseases in which homeostasis of blood glucose is disrupted. These diseases have been grouped into two major *subtypes* based on insulin-dependency: insulin-dependent diabetes mellitus (IDDM, type 1 or juvenile diabetes) and noninsulin-dependent diabetes mellitus (NIDDM, type 2 or adulthood diabetes). Within each major type, the clinical phenotypes are also heterogeneous. For example, about 2% of the NIDDM patients have an early age of onset and the disease is referred to as maturity-onset diabetes of the young (MODY). A subtype of diabetes that is neither type 1 nor type 2 has also been described in African-Americans and is known as atypical diabetes mellitus (ADM) or type 1.5 diabetes. ADM patients present with an initial phase of insulin requirement and later become noninsulin-dependent. Other less common types of diabetes such as J-type (Jamaican) diabetes and gestational diabetes have also described but will not be discussed here.

Heritability and Mode of Inheritance of Diabetes Mellitus

Most, if not all, forms of diabetes have a genetic basis. Some are clearly genetic disorders determined by a defect in a single gene since they show Mendelian segregation ratios and mode of inheritance. MODY and ADM belong to this category and are dominantly inherited.[1-3] However, the most common forms of diabetes (IDDM and late onset NIDDM) do not fit any Mendelian pattern. Therefore, the disease could be determined by any combination of genetic and environmental factors, ranging from 100% genes to 100% environment. These diseases are known as multifactorial or complex diseases and include the majority of the common diseases such as diabetes, hypertension, cancer, and many others. Several epidemiological methods have been developed to demonstrate the

influence of genes in multifactorial diseases. Familial aggregation and twin studies are commonly used in diabetes research.

Familial Aggregation

Genetic contribution implies that there must be familial aggregation (clustering of multiple cases in families) because relatives share genes to a greater extent than do unrelated people in the general population. Table 5–1 lists the recurrence risk in relatives of diabetic patients. The risk to develop IDDM in first-degree relatives of IDDM patients is approximately 5–6%, which is significantly higher than the general population prevalence (0.4%). This increased risk in relatives compared to the population prevalence suggests a familial aggregation. The degree of familial aggregation of a disease (λ_s) can be estimated from the ratio of the risk for siblings of patients and the population prevalence.[4] The λ_s for IDDM is about 15 (6%/0.4%). The risk of developing NIDDM in relatives of NIDDM patients and the population prevalence of the disease vary greatly in different populations. Consequently, the λ_s value for NIDDM also varies in different populations (3–10 in most studies). Significant familial aggregation may indicate either shared genetic or environmental (nongenetic) factors. These factors can be best delineated using twin studies.

TABLE 5–1 Familial Aggregation of Diabetes Mellitus

Relatives	IDDM	NIDDM
MZ twins	50%	90–100%
DZ twins	5–10%	20–40%
Siblings	6%	20–40%
Children	5%	20–40%
Parents	5%	20–40%
Population prevalence	0.4%	5–10%
λ_s	15	3–10

Twin Studies

Monozygotic (MZ; or identical) twins are identical for all their germline genes, while dizygotic (DZ; or fraternal) twins are only as similar genetically as ordinary siblings (25% identical). The concordance rate [# concordant/(# concordant + # discordant)] is used to measure the degree of similarity for the disease between twin pairs. Twins are concordant for a disease if they are both affected, discordant if only one is. Because both MZ and DZ twins usually share similar environmental factors, a genetic contribution is indicated by a significantly higher concordance rate in MZ twins than in DZ twins (or siblings). The higher the concordance rate, the stronger the genetic contribution to the disease. The MZ concordance for complex disease is rarely 100%, suggesting the involvement of environmental as well as genetic components in these diseases. The concordance rate for NIDDM is virtually 100% for MZ twins and 20–40% for DZ twins,[5] suggesting a strong contribution by genes to NIDDM. It should be noted that this high concordance rate does not necessarily exclude environmental contribution to NIDDM. It rather indicates the importance of genetic factors in the specific environment in which the studied twins live. Indeed, environmental contribution to NIDDM is suggested by the severalfold variation of disease incidence in migrant populations. In contrast to NIDDM, the concordance rate for IDDM is only 30–50% ($\approx$50% in most studies) for MZ twins and 10% for DZ twins,[5] suggesting that environmental factors also play an important role in IDDM.

The concordance rates in twin studies should be interpreted with caution because they may vary according to a number of factors. The age of the twins studied may greatly affect concordance rate. If the twins are young, the unaffected twin may become affected later in life resulting in an underestimation of concordance rates. Second, concordance rate may depend on the genetic liability to the disease in the twin population studied. Both factors may be consequential in the case of IDDM because of the younger age of onset and the possibility that in some IDDM patients the disease may have a stronger environmental influence. Overall, the higher the genetic liability in twins, the more concordant the twin pairs.

Genetic Mapping Methods

Several genetic mapping methods have been developed to search for genes involved in human diseases. The choice of methods depends on the mode of inheritance of the disease, the number of genes involved and the availability of patient materials. The methods widely used in genetic studies of diabetes include parametric (lod score) linkage analysis, affected sibpair analysis, and association (linkage disequilibrium) analysis.

Linkage Analysis

Linkage analysis maps genes by their proximities to marker loci on the same chromosome. According to Mendel's law of independent segregation (assortment), transmission of genes from one generation to the next should occur at random. This law does not hold when genes are physically close on the same chromosome. Linkage is the tendency of genes of close proximity to segregate together. The closer the genes are to each other, the more frequently they will be transmitted together because the chance for crossing over (recombination) in meioses is proportional to genetic distance between genes. The rate of recombination is used to define the genetic distance between genes (1% recombination = 1 centi-Morgan; cM). Unlinked genes (50 cM or more apart) segregate independently.

Genetic polymorphisms (variations at appreciable frequencies in the population) are essential to linkage analysis. Polymorphic markers that were widely used in the past include red cell antigens, human leucocyte antigens (HLA), isoenzymes, serum proteins, and restriction fragment-length polymorphism (RFLP). Recently, simple sequence length polymorphism (SSLP), also known as microsatellite, di-, tri-, or tetra-nucleotide repeats, have become the most useful genetic markers for linkage analyses. SSLPs are simple nucleotide repeats such as (CA)n flanked on both sides by unique DNA sequences.[6,7] The number of repeat units varies in different individuals and can be determined by the use of the polymerase chain reaction (PCR) and unique primers at the flanking sides. SSLPs are extremely polymorphic and abundant in the human genome. They can be easily and cheaply assayed in large numbers of samples using semi-automated procedures.

Localization of disease genes requires a large number of markers randomly distributed throughout the entire human genome, which is about 3000 cM or 3×10^9 bases. A total of 150–200 markers spaced at approximately 20 cM would provide an adequate coverage in most linkage studies. The segregation of these genetic markers in pedigrees with multiple affected individuals are studied and the location of the disease gene (linkage) is indicated by marker(s) that co-segregate with the disease phenotype. Linkage is usually measured by the logarithm of odds (lod), a ratio of the maximum likelihood probability that the disease gene is linked to a marker versus the probability that the gene is not linked to that marker. Conventionally, a lod score of >3 (e.g., the disease gene and the marker is 1000:1 more likely than not linked) is required to declare linkage.

The lod score linkage analysis is the most powerful method to map disease genes. However, the application of this technique requires the availability of large pedigrees with multiple affected individuals. Such pedigrees are usually only available for monogenic diseases, or multigenic diseases with a major gene. Knowledge of the mode of inheritance, the prevalence of disease and other parameters such as marker gene frequencies in the study population is also essential for successful linkage studies. As discussed below, this method has been extremely efficient in mapping three genes responsible for MODY, but has not been useful in the studies of IDDM or late onset NIDDM.

Affected Sibpair Analysis

Affected sibpair (ASP) analysis is the simplest form of affected relative pair (allele-sharing) methods, which test whether the inheritance pattern of chromosomal regions in affected relatives is consistent with random Mendelian segregation. Linkage is indicated by increased sharing of identical alleles at marker loci, that is, identity-by-descent (IBD) as compared to random expectation. In affected sibpair analyses, allele-sharing is measured in families with two or more affected siblings and normal parents. A sibpair can share 2, 1, or 0 copies of any locus with a 25, 50, and 25% distribution expected under random segregation. When IBD data are separately scored for the paternal and maternal chromosomes, a sibpair shares either 1 or 0 allele with a 50–50% distribution under random expectation. In either case, affected sibpairs are expected to share more alleles than randomly expected at a marker locus that is linked to the disease gene. The excess of allele-sharing can be measured with a simple Chi-square χ^2 test, although more complicated and powerful statistical methods have been developed. ASP analyses have played an important role in the studies of IDDM, NIDDM, and many other complex diseases.

Association Studies

Association refers to a concurrence greater than that predicted by chance between a specific allele of a gene and a disease (such as diabetes) that may or may not have an obvious genetic basis. When a gene is associated with a disease trait, that gene is often considered as a cause or contributing factor to the trait. In this case, the same association would be expected to occur in all populations.

Association can also occur when a gene does not cause the trait, but is in linkage disequilibrium with the actual disease gene. Linkage disequilibrium refers to the phenomenon that specific alleles at two different loci are found together more often than expected by chance. When two loci (A and B) are unlinked (on dif-

ferent chromosomes or far apart on the same chromosome), all combinations of alleles (for example, A1B1, A1B2, A2B1, and A2B2 for two alleles at each locus) are found in the population at a frequency based on the allelic frequency of the alleles. The genes are said to be in equilibrium. With linkage disequilibrium, a particular combination, such as A1B2, would be present in the population at a higher (or lower) frequency than expected from the allelic frequencies, implying that these two alleles segregate in a nonrandom manner. Linkage disequilibrium usually only occurs between tightly linked genes (usually <0.3 cM or 300 kb of DNA). The closer the genes are, the more generations it takes to randomize the combinations of alleles through recombination. Linkage disequilibrium may also occur between loosely linked or unlinked genes due to such factors as random chance, natural selection, or recent admixture between two differentiated populations.

Case/control studies compare the frequencies of an allele or genotype at a locus in a patient group and a control group. The two groups must be matched for ethnicity and most often geographical origins due to large variations in gene frequencies among different populations. A genotype or allele is considered to be positively associated or predisposing (susceptible) when its frequency is significantly higher in patients than in normal controls. It is said to be negatively associated or protective when it occurs at a significantly lower frequency in patients than in controls. The strength of association is usually measured by the relative risk (RR): $RR = [a(b + d)/b(a + c)]$, where a and b are the numbers of patients and controls with a given genotype, c and d are the corresponding numbers without the genotype. The odds ratio (OR), $OR = ad/cb$, is often used as an approximation to the RR and is referred to as approximate relative risk or simply RR. The greater the RR, the more frequently the genotype is found among patients and the less frequently it is found among controls. A predisposing effect is indicated by a RR that is $\gg 1$, a protective effect (negative association) is indicated by a RR $\ll 1$, while a neutral effect is indicated by a RR that is not significantly different from 1.

The results from case/control studies must be interpreted with caution. The most serious concern is that association may be due to mismatches in ethnicity or geographical regions between the control and patient groups (e.g., spurious association or population stratification). A second concern is association due to random chance. This is particularly serious when the association is weak and/or when a large number of association tests are performed. Therefore, highly significant evidence is required before an association could be declared. To avoid such artefacts, the probability value is usually corrected by multiplying the p value by the number of alleles tested (Bonferoni correction). It is important to keep in mind that replication of association in multiple studies (especially in different populations, ethnic groups and/or different laboratories) is extremely useful to confirm real association.

Family-based (intrafamilial) association is a study design that can avoid the confounding effect of spurious association. Families with one or more affected children can be analyzed in family-based association studies. The transmission/disequilibrium test (TDT)[8] has been widely used in many studies due to its simplicity in principle and practice. TDT considers parents who are heterozygous for an allele associated with disease and evaluates how often that allele is transmitted or not transmitted to affected offspring. Significant deviation of transmission from the randomly expected 50% is considered as indication for association between the disease and the tested gene.

The Genetics of MODY

MODY, representing 2% of all NIDDM cases, is transmitted as an autosomal dominant trait. Due to its early age of onset (frequently before 25 years of age), multigenerational pedigrees have been identified. These large pedigrees are extremely useful for linkage analysis because MODY is genetically heterogeneous. Until the early 1990s, linkage studies of MODY concentrated on the use of candidate genes without much success. In 1991, the first linkage for MODY was described with a polymorphic marker associated with the adenosine deaminase (ADA) gene on chromosome 20 (Table 5–2) in a large well-characterized pedigree (the R–W pedigree, which includes more than 360 members spanning 6 generations and 74 members with diabetes including those with MODY).[1] This linkage was later confirmed in the same pedigree by use of other polymorphic markers.[9,10] Analyses of key recombinants in the R–W pedigree localized the MODY gene (designated as MODY1) to a 13-cM interval. However, analyses of a large collection of French MODY families did not reveal linkage with the MODY1 locus.[2] Linkage was then tested with two other key candidate genes: glucokinase (GCK) and glucose transporter 2 (GLUT2). Significant linkage with GCK on chromosome 7p (designated as MODY2) was revealed in several families. Mutation analyses in patients from families linked to MODY2 revealed a large number of mutations that cause β cells to secrete less insulin in response to glucose, leading to hyperglycemia. This locus accounts for about 50% of all French MODY cases and MODY1 has not been identified in France.[11] Thus, other MODY loci must exist and account for the remaining 50% of MODY cases. To identify the other MODY genes, a genome-wide search using microsatellite markers evenly spaced in the entire human genome was undertaken. A third MODY locus (MODY3) was localized to the long arm of chromosome 12 in 6 of the 12 French families that are not linked to MODY1 or MODY2.[11]

Localization of MODY1 and MODY3 to a chromosomal region represents the first step toward the identification of the defective genes. However, the regions that may contain the disease genes are very large [7 million bases (Mb) of DNA for MODY1[12] and 3 Mb for MODY3].[13] Each of these regions may contain 30–70 genes, one of which is MODY1 or MODY3. It is a daunting task to identify the disease gene from such a large number of candidates, most of which are yet to be identified from genomic sequences. The investigators had to search for mutations in patients from all genes in the critical regions one by one and correlate the mutations with the disease status to find the defective gene. Sequence analyses of 10 candidate genes in the MODY3 region identified a mutation in the hepatocyte nuclear factor-1α (HNF-1α) gene that resulted in a frameshift and synthesis of a truncated mutant protein.[13] This mutation was found in all affected members but none of the unaffected members of the families or other normal controls, convincingly suggesting that the HNF-1α gene is MODY3. The demonstration of HNF-1α gene as

TABLE 5–2   List of MODY and NIDDM Genes

Symbols	Genes	Location	Evidence	Functions
MODY1	HNF-4α	20q12–q13	Linkage	Hormone receptor
MODY2	GCK	7p13–p15	Linkage	β-cell glucose sensor
MODY3	HNF-1α	12q22–qter	Linkage	Transcription factor
NIDDM1	Unknown	2q34–q37	Linkage (sibpair)	Unknown
NIDDM2	= MODY3 ?	12q22–qter	Linkage (sibpair)	Unknown
—	= MODY1 ?	20q12–q13	Linkage (sibpair)	Unknown
—	GCG-R	17q25	Association	Insulin release
—	SUR	11p15	Association	Insulin release
—	tRNA	mtDNA	Rare mutations	Energy production
—	GCK	7p13–p15	Rare mutations	β-cell glucose sensor
—	INS	11p15	Rare mutations	Glucose homeostasis
—	INS-R	19p13	Rare mutations	Glucose homeostasis
—	IRS-1	2q36	Rare mutations	Glucose homeostasis

MODY3 prompted the same group of investigators to search for mutations in the *HNF-4α* gene, which is located in the *MODY1* region. In the R-W pedigree, which contains *MODY1*, a nonsense mutation in the *HNF-4α* gene was found.[14] *HNF-4α* is a member of the steroid/thyroid hormone receptor superfamily and is highly expressed in liver, kidney, and intestine.[15,16] It is also expressed in pancreatic islets and insulinoma cells.[17] *HNF-4α* is a key regulator of hepatic gene expression and is a major activator of *HNF-1α*, which in turn activates the expression of a large number of liver-specific genes, including those involved in glucose, cholesterol, and fatty acid metabolism. The role of *HNF-4α* and its downstream product *HNF-1α* in the regulation of gene expression in pancreatic beta cells is still unclear, although *HNF-1α* is known to be a weak transactivator of the insulin gene.[18] *MODY1–3* only explain about 75% of the French MODY cases and their contribution to MODY in other countries is now under investigation. It will not be surprising to see several other MODY genes identified in the near future.

The Genetics of NIDDM

The search for genes responsible for late onset NIDDM has many difficulties. First is the difficulty of identifying suitable study pedigrees. Large pedigrees are typically not available due primarily to the late age of onset. Sibpairs affected by NIDDM can be found, but parents are often not available for study. The second major problem is the unclear mode of inheritance of NIDDM. Segregation analyses suggest that NIDDM is likely to be polygenic, although one or more major genes could also be involved. However, the number of genes and relative contribution of each gene to the disease are unknown. The third major problem is etiological and genetic heterogeneity that evidently exists for most highly prevalent diseases. Both etiological and genetic heterogeneity could exist between populations or between families within a population. NIDDM is recognized to arise from a combination of insulin resistance and impaired β-cell function. Because the phenotypes in NIDDM patients are highly variable, uniform and well-defined criteria for identifying diabetes are absolutely essential for successful genetic studies. Genetic factors are likely to contribute to the development of insulin resistance and β-cell function, which involve many different pathways. Each of the genetic defects in any of the steps in the glucose regulation pathways, either alone or in concert with other defects, could result in NIDDM. In addition, obesity, a major determinant of insulin resistance, also contributes to the development of NIDDM. As obesity is genetically determined,[19] genetic factors involved in insulin sensitivity, β-cell function, as well as appetite control and other metabolic factors are also

likely to contribute to NIDDM. Each of these processes involves complex regulatory pathways that may be influenced by genetic factors. It is more likely than not that the genetic factors in NIDDM are heterogeneous in different families and populations. Even with all these difficulties, some impressive progress has been made on discovery of NIDDM genes in the last few years.

Association Studies of Candidate Genes

Most early genetic studies on NIDDM focused on the testing of specific candidate genes using case/control and more recently family-based association study designs. These studies have been reviewed by several authors.[5,20] Therefore, only the most recent studies will be discussed here.

Insulin (*INS*), Insulin receptor (*INSR*), Insulin Receptor Substrate-1 (*IRS-1*). A number of mutations in these genes have been identified in a small number of NIDDM patients. Weak association with these genes was found in some but not other studies.[5,20] Therefore, they are unlikely major NIDDM genes.

Genes that are Unlikely Involved in NIDDM. A number of genes have been extensively studied in NIDDM. Association with these genes was found in some studies but not confirmed in others. These genes include glucose transporters (*GLUT2* and *GLUT4*), Glycogen-synthase (*GSY*), lipoproteins, HLA genes, and Haptoglobin (*Hp*).

Glucokinase (*GCK*). Because mutations in *GCK* are responsible for many MODY cases, extensive studies were undertaken to search for mutations in the *GCK* gene in late onset NIDDM patients. Several mutations in *GCK* have been identified in a small number of late onset NIDDM patients, but the majority of Caucasians and Japanese NIDDM patients do not have mutated *GCK*.[21–23]

Association between *GCK* polymorphism and NIDDM has also been reported in some studies[24,25]; however, the association is usually weak and not confirmed in other studies.[26] In addition, no linkage was detected between *GCK* and late onset NIDDM.[21,23] These studies together suggest that GCK mutations may contribute to late onset NIDDM in a small number of patients, but it is unlikely a major NIDDM gene.

Glucagon Receptor (*GCG-R*). Glucagon plays an important role in controlling hepatic glucose production and is involved in the regulation of insulin secretion. Most NIDDM patients have elevated concentrations of glucagon in peripheral blood, despite their basal hyperglycemia as a result of increased hepatic glucose output by elevated glucagon.[27] Glucagon action is mediated through its binding to a specific receptor in the superfamily of G protein-coupled transmembrane receptors. Mutations in the *GCG-R* gene could thus contribute to NIDDM. The human *GCG-R* has been mapped to chromosome 17q. Hager and co-workers[28] scanned mutations in a French cohort of NIDDM patients and identified a Gly to Ser missense substitution in the *GCG-R* gene. This polymorphism was associated with NIDDM in a pooled French and Sardinian data set ($p = 0.0001$) and linkage evidence ($p = 0.01$) was also found in a small set of sibpair families. These results by themselves are not sufficient to confirm the role of *GCG-R* in NIDDM. Receptor binding studies using cultured cells expressing the Gly/Ser mutation showed that the mutation results in a threefold lower affinity receptor compared to the wild type receptor. The genetic and functional studies together provide convincing evidence for a role of glucagon receptor gene in NIDDM. However, only approximately 5% of French and 8% of Sardinian patients are heterozygous carriers of this mutation. Additional studies in other populations will be important to confirm these findings and assess the importance of the *GCG-R* mutations in NIDDM.

Sulfonylurea Receptor (*SUR*). Signals derived from the metabolism of glucose in pancreatic β cells lead to a sequence of events including closure of ATP-sensitive potassium channels (I_{KATP}), membrane depolarization, activation of voltage-gated Ca^{2+} channels, which results in increased intracellular Ca^{2+} and insulin exocytosis. Sulfonylurea directly inhibits β-cell I_{KATP} and leads to depolarization and insulin release. The β-cell K_{KATP} is a heteromultimeric structure composed of two subunits, one of which is the sulfonylurea receptor. Given the essential role of *SUR* in the regulation of insulin secretion, mutations in the *SUR* gene could play a role in NIDDM susceptibility. Linkage analysis using a microsatellite marker near the *SUR* gene failed to reveal significant linkage with NIDDM.[29] Mutation analyses in *SUR* coding sequence revealed eight mutations in Caucasians.[29] Two mutations were found to be associated with Caucasians from the United Kingdom and United States. One of the mutations was also found to be more common in NIDDM patients and morbid obesity than in controls in the French population.[30] Sibpair analyses in French NIDDM families did not reveal significant linkage, but one French obesity family gave suggestive evidence for linkage. Together, these studies suggest that *SUR* may be a contributor to NIDDM susceptibility.

Mitochondrial Genes. Mitochondrial oxidative phosphorylation is involved in peripheral glucose metabolism, as well as, in glucose stimulation of β-cell insulin secretion. Deletions/insertions[31] and point mutations[32,33] in mitochondrial DNA have been described in patients with diabetes as part of the complex encephalomyopathic syndromes. A particular point mutation in position 3243 of the mitochondrial DNA encoding tRNA Leu$^{(UUR)}$ has been found repeatedly in patients with

maternally inherited diabetes associated with deafness.[32,33] Preliminary studies suggest that the mitochondrial mutation is only found in <1% of Caucasian NIDDM patients. Diabetes due to this mitochondrial mutation may have a progressive nature. Insulin secretory capacity progressively decreases and eventually reaches an insulin-dependent state in most patients in Japan.[34] Surprisingly, the mutation is often observed in ICA (islet cell autoantibodies)-positive IDDM patients who were initially noninsulin-dependent (so-called slowly progressive IDDM).[34]

Genome-Wide Search for NIDDM Genes

To identify genes responsible for late onset NIDDM, several groups of investigators have carried out genome scans for NIDDM genes using affected sibpair analyses. Two of the studies successfully identified two major NIDDM genes, designated *NIDDM1* and *NIDDM2*. In the first study, the primary study group consisted of 408 Mexican-American individuals (330 affected sibpairs from 170 sibships) from a rural county in Texas, where the frequency of NIDDM is the highest among all counties in Texas.[35] This Mexican-American population has approximately 31% of its contemporary gene pool from Native-American ancestry. The increased incidence of diabetes in this population is consistent with the contribution of susceptibility alleles derived from admixture with Native-Americans.[36] This admixing may increase the power to detect NIDDM genes through linkage analysis. A genome scan using 490 markers in this sample set[37] identified two markers (*D2S125* and *D2S126*) on chromosome 2 that showed suggestive linkage (lod = 2.6, $p < 0.0005$) and 19 other markers with nominal evidence for linkage ($p < 0.05$). A second group of 110 Mexican-American affected sibpairs from the same county was analyzed for the markers suggested by the genome screen. In the combined data set, the marker D2S125 revealed linkage evidence that met the criteria for significant linkage in a genome-wide screen ($p < 10^{-6}$, lod = 4.1). This locus, designated *NIDDM1*, may explain 21–30% of the familial clustering of NIDDM in the study population.

The second genome wide screen was conducted using affected sibpair analysis of NIDDM families from Finland.[38] The Finnish population is particularly suitable for linkage analysis of many diseases because of its homogeneity and enrichment of certain disease genes due to founder effect. The genome scan was performed in 26 families (comprising 217 individuals) from an isolated population in western Finland. No significant evidence for linkage was found when these families were analyzed together, but strong evidence for linkage was found when families were classified according to mean insulin levels (revealed during oral glucose tolerance testing) in affected individuals. Families with the lowest insulin levels showed linkage ($p < 2 \times 10^{-5}$) to the marker *D12S1349* on chromosome 12. This disease locus has been designated *NIDDM2*. Interestingly, this region also contains the *MODY3* gene and it is possible that *NIDDM2* and *MODY3* represent different alleles of the same gene.[38]

Other affected sibpair studies have been reported for selected genomic regions and suggestive evidence for linkage was found for several regions.[39-41] However, these linkages have not been confirmed in additional data sets. *NIDDM1* and *NIDDM2* appear to be major susceptibility genes in the populations studied. It is not yet clear whether they are also implicated in NIDDM in other populations. The localization of these genes represents a major step forward for the identification of NIDDM genes, but a difficult task remains to identify the exact disease genes in the *NIDDM1* and *NIDDM2* intervals and to localize other NIDDM genes. The studies discussed above indicate that analyses in well-characterized isolated populations will continue to be a revealing approach to map NIDDM genes.

Studies on Intermediate Phenotypes

Phenotypic heterogeneity is one of the major confounding factors reducing the power of linkage studies. One good approach to analyze such heterogeneous phenotypes is to use "intermediate" phenotypes such as insulin resistance and obesity. Insulin resistance and hyperinsulinemia are familial traits that may precede and predict the onset of NIDDM. In some populations, the distribution of fasting insulin levels and measures of in vivo insulin action suggest the effects of a single gene.[42] A study in the Pima Indians of Arizona, the group with the highest incidence of NIDDM in the world, have suggested that a gene on chromosome 4q may influence insulin sensitivity.[43] Analyses of other

intermediate phenotypes of NIDDM may reveal other important genes.

The Genetics of IDDM

As indicated by the concordance rate in MZ twins, IDDM also has a significant genetic component. As a typical multifactorial (complex) disease, a number of genes appear to contribute to the development of IDDM. These genes are referred to as susceptibility genes because the gene carriers are only more susceptible to the disease than the noncarriers. None of the susceptibility genes is either necessary or sufficient for the development of disease. Individuals carrying a susceptibility allele may have a higher RR of disease, but some carriers may be unaffected, and some noncarriers may be affected. The lack of a perfect correspondence between genotype and phenotype complicates the task of genetic mapping. Despite these difficulties, a tremendous amount of progress has been made in the identification of IDDM susceptibility genes in the last three decades and particularly since the early 1990s (Table 5-3).

HLA Class II Genes (*IDDM1*)

The HLA is a large genetic complex located on chromosome 6p21. Several key features of the HLA are important to understand its function and importance in diseases such as diabetes. First, it is a multigene family containing many genes with similar structure and functions. Second, strong linkage disequilibrium occurs between genes in the region. The alleles at multiple loci have been maintained together in the population as stable haplotypes through evolutionary time spans. Third, most genes in the HLA complex are extremely polymorphic with a large number of alleles and most individuals are heterozygous (with two different alleles).

TABLE 5-3 List of IDDM Susceptibility Intervals

Loci	Region	Genes	Status	Mechanism
IDDM1	6p21	DR, DQ	Identified	Antigen presentation
IDDM2	11p15	INS-VNTR	Identified	Tolerance induction
IDDM4	11q13	?	Confirmed	Unknown
IDDM5	6q25	?	Confirmed	Unknown
IDDM8	6q27	?	Confirmed	Unknown
IDDM12	2q33	CTLA4 ?	Confirmed	Apoptosis ?
IDDM3	15q26	?	Suggestive	Unknown
IDDM6	18q	?	Suggestive	Unknown
IDDM7	2q33	?	Suggestive	Unknown
IDDM9	3q	?	Suggestive	Unknown
IDDM10	10q	?	Suggestive	Unknown
IDDM11	14q24–q31	?	Significant	Unknown
IDDM13	2q33	?	Significant	Unknown
IDDM15	6q21	?	Significant	Unknown

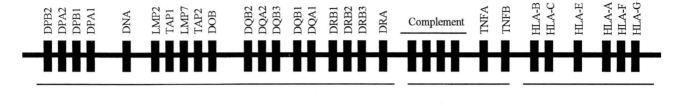

Figure 5–1. Genomic location of HLA genes on chromosome 6p.

The HLA genes are structurally and functionally divided into three subregions (Fig. 5–1). The products of class I genes are ubiquitously expressed on all nucleated human cells and are important in the presentation of viral antigens. Class I molecules (A, B, and C) are heterodimers of one class I chain and β2-microglobulin that is encoded outside of the HLA. Class II molecules are heterodimers comprising one α chain and one β chain, encoded by an α gene and a β gene within the HLA, respectively (Fig. 5–1). There are three major class II molecules (DR, DQ, and DP) that are expressed in humans. All class II genes with the exception of DRA (α gene for DR) are polymorphic. Therefore, the functional properties of DR molecules are solely determined by the polymorphic DRB genes, while the DQ and DP molecules are determined by both α and β genes. All DQ α and β chains encoded by alleles located on the same chromosome (haplotype) can form functional DQ dimers (known as *cis*-complementation). At least some functional molecules can be formed between one DQα chain encoded on one haplotype (chromosome) and one DQβ chain encoded on a different haplotype (e.g., *trans*-complementation). The following discussion is a brief summary extracted from an extensive review on HLA in IDDM.[44] Readers interested in more details should consult that review.

Association with DQ and DR. HLA class II genes are recognized as the most important genetic factors in IDDM. Because HLA was the first identified IDDM susceptibility region, it has been referred to as *IDDM1*. The role of the HLA region in IDDM was first suggested by associations with HLA class I alleles (B8 and B15). Subsequent studies indicate that virtually all genes in the HLA region are associated with IDDM in all studied populations. These findings are not surprising in light of the strong linkage disequilibrium between genes in the region. The question has been, since the early 1970s, which gene or genes are responsible for the association. One approach to address this question is to compare the relative strength of association with genes in the region. The real susceptibility locus should have the strongest association. Soon after the studies with class I molecules, stronger association was found with the *DRB1* locus. Subsequently, the *DQB1* gene was shown to be even more strongly associated with IDDM in many

Caucasian populations. Therefore, it was believed that the *DQB1* gene was the "true" disease locus. This belief was supported by a number of additional observations. First, the degree of susceptibility/protection of HLA is correlated with key amino acid positions of the *DQB1* gene. Specifically, position 57 is thought to play an important role in determining IDDM susceptibility.[45] All DQB1 alleles with an aspartic acid at DQβ residue 57 (*0301, *0303, *0401, *0402, *0503, *0601, *0603) confer neutral to protective effects, while the two *DQB1* alleles with an alanine (*0201 and *0302) confer strong susceptibility in all ethnic groups (Table 5–4). DQB1 *0604 and *0501 have a valine at this position and appear to confer disease predisposition. DQB1 *0502 has a serine at residue 57 and probably confers weak susceptibility. The second line of evidence for the DQ as the primary factor was from comparisons of susceptibility effects conferred by a same *DRB1* allele on haplotypes with different *DQB1* alleles. For example, DR4 (DRB1 *0400 in the new nomenclature) on the haplotypes with DQB1 *0302 is positively associated (RR = 6–28), but DR4 on the haplotypes with DQB1 *0301 is negatively associated (RR ≈ 0.3) in Caucasian populations, suggesting that *DQB1* alleles are important. The third line of evidence is provided by the observation that several heterozygous genotypes confer much stronger risk than the corresponding homozygous genotypes (e.g., synergistic effect). The first synergistic effect was observed for DR3/4 (DRB1 *0301/DRB1 *0400 in the new nomenclature) heterozygotes (RR ≈ 20), which confer much higher risk than DR4/4 (RR ≈ 15) or DR3/3 (RR ≈ 7) in most Caucasian populations. Synergistic effect was also observed for many other heterozygotes (DR3/9 in Chinese and Africans, DR8/9, DR9/13, DR4/8 and DR4/13 in Japanese).[44] These findings can be best explained by DQα/β heterodimers formed through *trans*-complementation.[44]

It is now accepted by all investigators that DQ molecules are a key susceptibility factor in IDDM. The remaining question is whether any other genes are also implicated. A few authors have argued and some continue to argue that the association with DR is due to linkage disequilibrium with *DQB1* and *DQA1* genes.[46–49] If indeed DQ is the only susceptibility factor in the HLA region, the association between DQ and IDDM must be consistent in all populations. This is,

TABLE 5–4 Susceptibility Effects of HLA-DR/DQ Molecules

Effect	DRB1	DQ α/β	DQA1	DQB1	DQB1 57
1. Highly susceptible	0405	0301/0201	0301	0201	Ala
	0402	0301/0302		0302	Ala
2. Susceptible	0401	0301/0604	?	0604	Val
	0301	0301/0501		0501	Val
		0301/0502		0502	Ser
3. Neutral to susceptible	0404	0301/0303	0501?	—	—
	01, 08	0501/0201			
	09	0501/0302			
4. Neutral to protective	07	Others	Others	0303	Asp
	12			0503	
	15			0601	
	16			0603	
5. Protective	11	Others	Others	0301	Asp
	13			0401	
	14			0402	
6. Highly protective	0403	All/0602	—	0602	Asp
	0406				
	0408				

however, not true at all. For example, DQB1 *0302 is not positively associated with IDDM in Asian populations even though it confers high risk in Caucasians and Africans. Some investigators attempted to explain these discrepancies by hypothesizing that the same DQ allele may confer susceptibility in one population but neutral or protective effects in another population.[46–48] This hypothesis is not supported by any experimental data and is not consistent with the functional properties of the HLA molecules.[44] The more likely explanation is that the *DRB1* gene, tightly linked to the *DQB1* and *DQA1* genes, is responsible for the discrepant associations of DQ alleles. To demonstrate the independent effect of the *DRB1* locus, one can simply compare the RR between haplotypes that have the same *DQA1* and *DQB1* alleles. For example, the relative risk conferred by the DRB1 *0405-DQA1 *0301-DQB1 *0302 haplotype (RR $\approx$ 34) is much higher than that for the 0406-0301-0302 haplotype with the same DQ genes (RR $\approx$ 0.2) in Chinese.[50] Similar results are also found in many other populations, suggesting that DR molecules contribute independently to IDDM susceptibility.

There are a large number of DR and DQ alleles in the human population. Their effect on IDDM susceptibility varies greatly and range from highly susceptible to strongly protective. Table 5–4 tentatively groups all DR and DQ alleles or molecules into six categories based on comparative association studies in many different ethnic groups and geographical populations.[44] In several instances, susceptible DR and DQ alleles are found on the same haplotypes. For example, the DRB1 *0301-DQA1 *0501-DQB1 *0201 and the DRB1 *0401-DQA1 *0301-DQB1 *0302 haplotypes in Caucasians encode susceptible DR and DQ molecules. The alleles on these

haplotypes are all positively associated with IDDM. On other haplotypes such as DRB1 *0403-DQA1 *0301-DQB1 *0302 contain protective *DRB1* alleles and susceptible DQ alleles. The effect of such haplotypes is determined by the balancing outcome of the DR and DQ molecules. Because DRB1 *0403 is a highly protective allele, the haplotype is overall weakly protective. The HLA-linked risk to IDDM is determined by the complex interactions of not only the molecules encoded on one haplotype but also all HLA molecules present in a given individual.[44] The molecules can enhance or counteract the effect of each other. Generally, a predisposing genotype contains several susceptible DR and DQ molecules. By contrast, the presence of one highly protective DR or DQ molecule is sufficient to overcome the effects of all susceptibility molecules in an individual. For example, the DR3/4 heterozygous subjects with DRB1 *0403 are protected against diabetes probably due to the dominant protection of DRB1 *0403 (Table 5–5). Several other alleles (DRB1 *0406, DRB1 *0408, and DQB1 *0602) also confer similar dominant protection. Therefore, DR and DQ genotypes must be considered to assess an individual's risk to develop IDDM.[44]

The Immunological Mechanisms. Even though DR/DQ molecules are undoubtedly involved in IDDM, the exact mechanism by which they contribute to the disease is still unclear. Most likely, HLA class II molecules influence IDDM susceptibility through presentation of diabetogenic antigens (peptides). Due to structural differences of HLA molecules, their binding affinity to β-cell antigens may be different. Nepom[51] first proposed that competition of antigens between HLA molecules in an individual may be the functional

TABLE 5–5   Risks Conferred by HLA DR/DQ Genotypes in Caucasians in Florida

Genotypes DRB1-DQB1/DRB1-DQB1	Frequency (%)			
	Controls	Patients	RR	AR
0301-0201/0401-0302	1.8	35.0	20	1/15
0401-0302/0401-0302	0.7	10.0	15	1/20
0301-0201/0301-0201	1.5	9.0	7	1/45
0100-0501/0401-0301*	0.6	2.0	5	1/60
0401-0302/0800-0201*	0.5	2.0	5	1/60
0401-0302/1300-0604*	0.7	3.0	5	1/60
0401-0302/0701-0201*	1.5	4.0	5	1/60
0100-0501/0401-0302*	2.0	3.0	5	1/60
0301-0201/X	16.0	12.0	0.7	1/450
X/X	50.7	20.0	0.5	1/600
0301-0201/0403-0302	5	0.0	0.2	<1/1,250
1500-0602/others	24.0	2.0	0.02	1/15,000

X: Alleles not listed in the table. RR = Relative risk. AR = Absolute risk, estimated using RR × population prevalence (assuming a population prevalence of 1/300 for IDDM).

* The frequency for these genotypes are low in both controls and patient groups. The RR given here is an approximation.

basis of differential susceptibility effects of HLA molecules. In the Nepom model, some HLA molecules confer susceptibility because they bind and present a specific peptide or peptides so as to induce pathogenic immune responses to pancreatic β-cell antigens; other HLA molecules that are capable of more tightly binding such peptides (peptide sink), but without initiating pathogenic autoimmune responses, may behave as protective molecules. Later, Sheehy[52] proposed a model that is almost the mirror image of the Nepom model and focuses on the failure of the immune system to maintain tolerance to pancreatic β-cell antigens. In this model, protective HLA heterodimers have high binding affinity for certain β-cell peptides required to establish or maintain tolerance to β-cell antigens, while predisposing heterodimers have low affinity for the tolerogenic peptides or bind in the wrong configuration for inducing T-cell tolerance. It is not yet clear which model is the more likely mechanism for the HLA effect in IDDM, and it will not be surprising to see that both mechanisms are involved. Finally, it is also possible that the effects of protective and susceptible HLA class II molecules may not only be at the level of peptide binding but also at the level of immune responses either resulting in inflammatory responses (Th1 type) or the less diabetogenic humoral responses (Th2 type).

HLA and the Incidence of IDDM.   The incidence of IDDM has a strong correlation with the frequency of high risk HLA.[44,53,54] The high frequency of high-risk HLA (DRB1 *0301, DRB1 *0401, the 0301/0302 and 0301/0201 DQ dimers) correlates with the high incidence of IDDM in Scandinavians, while the high frequency of DRB1 *0301 is consistent with the high disease incidence in Sardinians. The above molecules

have lower frequencies in most other Caucasians compared with Scandinavians, correlating with their moderate incidence of the disease. The absence of the DR3 haplotype also correlates with the low incidence of IDDM in Japan. In addition, DR-DQ linkage, disequilibrium is also an important factor responsible for the differences in diabetes incidence. Linkage disequilibrium between highly susceptible DR and protective DQ alleles, or vice versa reduces the HLA-linked risk and consequently the incidence of IDDM in Asians.[44]

Other Genes in the HLA Complex.   Although DR and DQ genes and their linkage disequilibrium can satisfactorily explain the majority of the observations on HLA associations, other genes within the HLA complex may also contribute to IDDM. The HLA-DP genes,[55] HLA class I genes,[56,57] and class I antigen processing genes (LMP7 and LMP2)[58] have been shown to contribute to the development or the age of onset. Additional studies are needed to uncover how these additional genetic factors contribute to IDDM susceptibility.

The Insulin Gene (*IDDM2*)

The insulin (*INS*) gene is also an obvious candidate gene for IDDM. A variable number of tandem repeats (VNTR) polymorphism at the 5′ end of *INS* (INS-VNTR) was reported in 1984 to be associated with IDDM in a case-control study.[59] The finding was not seriously considered for many years for two reasons. First, linkage with *INS* could not be demonstrated in IDDM families,[60] suggesting that the observed association could be spurious. Second, case-control studies in some populations failed to replicate the observed association. Interest in the *INS* region was renewed in 1991 when linkage evidence with the INS region was demonstrated in paternal meioses using the affected sibpair analysis and transmission/disequilibrium test.[61] Because linkage was found only in paternal meioses, maternal imprinting was suggested as the most likely explanation for the gender effect, which was then confirmed in most populations except the United Kingdom.[62] The region containing the disease locus (now designated as *IDDM2*) was narrowed to a region of 19kb of DNA by showing absence of association with a polymorphic marker in the 3' neighboring locus IGF2 and a marker at the 5' neighboring locus tyrosine hydroxylase (TH). The two polymorphic sites encompass 19kb of DNA sequences. Immediately after the 1991 report, additional polymorphic markers were identified within the 19kb genomic interval using sequencing analyses. These additional polymorphic markers were analyzed in diabetic patients and normal controls in several laboratories. The studies established an association curve (a plot of association strength against marker distance as shown in Fig. 5–2), which defined *IDDM2* within a genomic interval of 4.1kb of DNA sequences. This interval includes *INS* and the *INS*-VNTR.[63,64]

Within the 4.1kb of DNA, there are >10 polymorphisms, one or more of which might be the etiological mutation for *IDDM2*. Each of these mutations was analyzed in a large collection of diabetic families and was able to pinpoint the etiological mutation to the *INS*-VNTR.[65] In the same period of time, functional studies

also showed that the VNTR sequence can influence the expression of its down-stream reporter genes.[66] These studies together suggest that the *INS*-VNTR could be the etiological mutation for *IDDM2*. The conclusion was further supported by the correlation of expression levels of INS mRNA and the linked VNTR alleles in human thymus.[65,67,68] It was shown that the expression of insulin in the thymus is several times higher with the protective VNTR than the susceptible ones, suggesting that the development of immunological tolerance to insulin in the thymus (negative selection of insulin-specific T cells) plays an important role in IDDM. Consistent with the maternal effect of *IDDM2*, *INS* is maternally imprinted in the thymus in a subset of individuals, although imprinting has not been found in the pancreas.[62]

It should be noted that IDDM2 only confers a relative risk of 2–4 in most populations.[62,69,70] IDDM2, like all other non-HLA IDDM genes, only modifies an individual's susceptibility to IDDM. The susceptibility alleles of IDDM2 are perfectly functional and normal genes. Their frequency in the general population is very high (40–60% in Caucasians). Although significant association with *IDDM2* was not found in some populations, *IDDM2* is probably implicated in IDDM in all populations. The absence of significant association may be related to the frequencies of the insulin gene in those populations. For example, the susceptible allele of *IDDM2* is found in about 95% of Chinese normal controls and its frequency reaches nearly 100% in IDDM

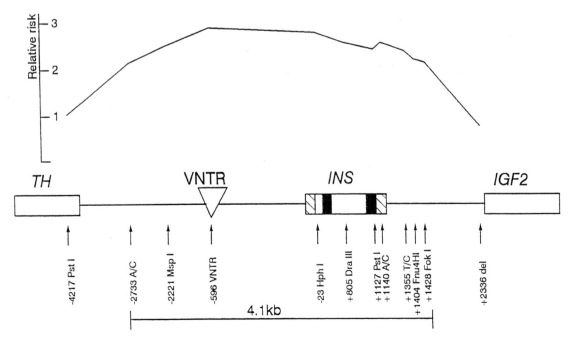

Figure 5–2. Genomic location of polymorphisms near the insulin gene and an association curve in IDDM.

patients. Therefore, a large data set is required to demonstrate significant association.

Other IDDM Susceptibility Genes

Both *IDDM1* and *IDDM2* were identified by association analyses of candidate genes. Less than 50% (most likely 20–40%) of the total familial aggregation of IDDM is explained by *IDDM1* and only about 5% by *IDDM2*. Therefore, there must be other IDDM susceptibility genes. It is a difficult task to identify the other genes because the number of genes implicated in IDDM may be large and genetic heterogeneity certainly exists. Parametric linkage analysis is not feasible due to genetic heterogeneity and lack of large pedigrees. Thus, several investigators set out in the early 1990s to map IDDM genes using the affected sibpair method. The common approach undertaken by these laboratories was to analyze a large number (200–400) of microsatellite markers throughout the entire human genome in 100–200 affected sibpair families. The first two genome-wide mapping studies revealed more than 20 linkage intervals that may contain IDDM susceptibility genes.[71,72] Similar studies were also reported by other investigators.[73–77] These results were exciting news but should be considered with caution because highly significant evidence ($p < 3 \times 10^{-5}$ or lod >3.6) and replication of the results in an additional data set ($p < 0.01$) are required to confirm a true linkage in genome-wide affected sibpair analyses.[78] Four of the intervals (*IDDM4* on chromosome 11q13, *IDDM5* on 6q25 and *IDDM8* on 6q27 and *IDDM12* on 2q33) have now been confirmed as real linkages (Table 5–3).

Support for *IDDM4* was obtained in several data sets.[71–74,76,79,80] *IDDM4* had a lod score of 1.3 in the U.K. data set[71] and a lod of 1.5 in a French data set.[72] In both studies, stronger statistical evidence was obtained after the data set was stratified based upon HLA sharing, or the HLA types of the affected sibpairs. This locus was then analyzed in a data set of 265 Caucasian families from the United States and Italy using several microsatellite markers in the 11q13 region.[79] This study revealed a lod score of 3.9 for *IDDM4* and provided, together with the two other reports, linkage evidence that met the criteria for confirmed linkage for complex disease genes.

Linkage evidence for *IDDM5* was obtained in two of the three data sets in the initial study.[71] Significant linkage evidence was obtained through fine-mapping analysis of a large Caucasian data set (lod = 4.5).[74,79] Together with the initial data (lod = 1.8), IDDM5 is thus confirmed. This locus has been localized within a region of 5cM between the markers *D6S476* and *D6S473* on 6q25. Linkage evidence for *IDDM8* has been obtained in several data sets [71,74] and the lod score in the combined data set was 3.6, which barely reached

the criterium for significant linkage. IDDM8 is localized to a 5 to 7-cm region on 6q27, about 40cM telomeric to *IDDM5*.

The final confirmed IDDM interval (designated *IDDM12*) maps to chromosome 2q33.[81,82] This region of the genome was examined because it contains two candidate genes (*CTLA4* and *CD28*), which play an important role in the regulation of T-cell activation. The initial evidence for linkage was found with a microsatellite marker within *CTLA4* in 48 Italian families (lod = 3.6).[81] A subsequent study in 338 affected sibpair families from United States, France, and Spain only revealed a lod score of 0.5.[82] The TDT was then used in both studies to evaluate association with the A/G polymorphism at position 49 of the *CTLA4* gene (CTLA4-A/G) in sibpair and simplex families. Association was detected in five different populations (Italian, Spanish, French, Mexican-American, and Korean).[81,82] The overall evidence for association is highly significant in the combined data set from these populations ($p = 10^{-9}$). The same trend of association is also found in the Caucasian-American data set. However, no association was found in a large data set of 284 U.K. families[81] or in the Chinese and Sardinian data sets.[81] When all data sets are included, the combined evidence for association is also highly significant ($p < 0.00005$), providing strong support for an IDDM susceptibility gene in the region surrounding *CTLA4*. In addition to the family-based studies, highly significant evidence for association was also reported in two independent case/control studies, one in the Belgian population ($p = 10^{-5}$)[81] and the other in the German population ($p = 10^{-5}$).[83] *CTLA4* has also been found to be associated with Graves disease, an autoimmune hypothyroidism, in several data sets,[81–84] further confirming the association between IDDM and *CTLA4*.

IDDM12 appears to be primarily in the Mediterranean-European populations (France, Spain, and Italy). The association with *CTLA4* in the Mexican American population may be due to genes from their Spanish ancestors. It is not yet clear why association was not detected in the United Kingdom and Sardinian data sets. Although different linkage disequilibrium patterns between the CTLA4-A/G and the *IDDM12* etiological mutation is a possible explanation, it is more likely that the *IDDM12* etiological mutation may have a low frequency in the U.K. population, thus reducing the chance to detect association. The weak association in the U.S. Caucasian data set is consistent with this hypothesis. Being an admixture of descendants from the United Kingdom with a low frequency of *IDDM12* and Mediterranean-European countries with a higher frequency of *IDDM12*, the strength of association in the U.S. Caucasians is expected to be intermediate. Ongoing studies in this author's laboratory have mapped *IDDM12* within a region of <100kb of DNA surrounding *CTLA4*. However, the exact gene for the disease locus has not been identified even though *CTLA4* is the most likely candidate gene.

More than 20 other intervals also showed some evidence for linkage with IDDM in one or more data sets. The evidence for three of these intervals was significant. *IDDM11* was mapped to 14q24.3-q31 using 254 sibpair families (lod = 4.0). This evidence meets the criteria for significant linkage. Analysis of >300 Caucasian families in this author's group revealed a lod score of only 1.0, suggesting that additional studies are required to confirm linkage with the locus. IDDM13 was mapped to 2q34 using 98 affected sibpairs from Australia and the United Kingdom (lod = 3.3).[75] This result was a surprise given the small number of sibpairs analyzed in the study. Linkage to this interval was not found in another U.K. data set.[71] Furthermore, this linkage cannot be confirmed by our own data. Therefore, *IDDM13* should not be considered as a confirmed linkage. Evidence for *IDDM15* on chromosome 6q21 was strong (p = 0.00003), but the interval is loosely linked with the HLA region. Additional studies are required to confirm this locus as well. Only weak evidence for linkage was obtained for all other intervals including the ones with designated names (*IDDM3, IDDM6, IDDM7, IDDM9, & IDDM10*). Although some of these intervals may contain IDDM susceptibility genes, many of the linkages may be falsely positive. These results are not unexpected because one would expect, by random chance, several linkages with weak lod scores in a genome scan.

Many valuable lessons for mapping complex disease genes are learned from the studies of IDDM. First, it has now become evident that genome-wide scan can be used to identify genes involved in common diseases, even though it remains a very difficult task. Second, a large number of sibpairs are required to obtain significant linkage and to confirm real disease genes. Allele-sharing by sibpairs may vary greatly in small data sets and consequently even significant linkage obtained from small data set may not be real. Third, linkage evidence may decrease very quickly as the distance from the disease gene increases. Therefore, a high density map of highly polymorphic markers would be helpful. Finally, genetic heterogeneity may significantly reduce the power of linkage analysis. The analysis of *IDDM12* provides an excellent illustration of the importance of a multi-ethnic approach when heterogeneity is present.

Localization and confirmation of the four novel IDDM intervals represent a step forward for identifying all IDDM genes. In addition to localization and confirmation of additional IDDM intervals, current research in IDDM focuses on the cloning of the confirmed genes using positional cloning techniques. This is an even bigger challenge because the genomic intervals containing the disease genes are generally large

(4–5 cM). Thousands of sibpair families will be required to further narrow the interval by affected sibpair statistics so that positional cloning techniques can be used to identify the disease gene. Fortunately, linkage disequilibrium mapping can be used to rapidly reduce the sizes of the genomic intervals. It is anticipated that some of these genes may soon be identified.

Clinical Applications

Diagnosis

The diagnosis of diabetes and its subtypes is not difficult in most circumstances; however, there are occasional cases where diagnosis is difficult at a given point of time. Genetic information may be helpful in determining the subtypes of diabetes. For example, the presence of IDDM-associated autoantibodies and high-risk HLA genes can provide valuable information for the diagnosis of IDDM because they are not present in the vast majority of NIDDM patients. Genetic information can be used to diagnose certain subtypes of diabetes even before the onset of clinical symptoms. Using mutations in the three MODY genes, approximately 75% of all MODY cases already can be identified. When additional MODY genes are found, the accurate diagnosis of MODY may approach 100% of the cases. The same may also be true for ADM when the ADM genes have been identified. However, it is not possible to use genetic information alone for the accurate diagnosis of IDDM and late onset NIDDM patients as most individuals with the susceptibility genes will not develop diabetes.

Prediction and Genetic Screening

One important application of genetic information for IDDM and late onset NIDDM is prediction of risk to develop diabetes. Genetic predisposition is a primary requirement for the development of type 1 and type 2 diabetes. The exact proportion of the population genetically at risk for diabetes is currently unknown. Risk prediction for IDDM has been extensively studied. Preliminary estimations suggest that 1–5% of individuals in most Caucasian populations may be genetically predisposed to IDDM. The specific risk for each individual in this group may also vary depending on the number and probably the combinations of susceptibility genes present in a given individual. Some of them may only have slightly higher risk than the population prevalence (0.4%), while others may have much higher risk. For example, the risk for DR3/4 heterozygous subjects is about 7% (Table 5–5). The risk for a small group of individuals may be as high as 50%, which is the concordance rate in MZ twins. The predicative power using currently known genetic markers (i.e., HLA) is much less than the theoretical maximum power. It is expected that the prediction power of genetic markers will significantly increase through the use of non-HLA IDDM genes.

In the mean time, family history is of great value for risk prediction. Risk assessment using genetic information and family history together has high specificity for IDDM prediction. The risk to develop IDDM in first-degree relatives of IDDM patients is approximately 6%, which is equivalent to the risk conferred by the high-risk HLA genotype DR3/4 (Table 5–5). In contrast, the risk is increased to 25–30% in first-degree relatives with the DR3/4 genotype. This increase is most likely due to the shared non-HLA IDDM genes between IDDM patient and their first degree relatives as well as, to some extent, shared environmental factors. Theoretically, when all IDDM genes are identified, the information gained through family history could be, at least partially, replaced by genetic testing of all IDDM genes.

Genetic markers combined with immunological and metabolic markers should provide the most efficient and economic tool for risk prediction of IDDM. Genetic testing is only required once in one's life time because genomic DNA (with a few exceptions) does not change over time. On the other hand, immunological and metabolic parameters are gradually changing. Annual or even more frequent monitoring is necessary from an early age and over a course of many years. Immunological and metabolic monitoring are important because they increase the specificity of disease prediction. Therefore, the screening strategy for IDDM in the general population should include population screening to identify the individuals genetically at high risk to develop IDDM and monitoring of the high-risk group using immunological and metabolic markers. Indeed, several such screening programs are now underway or under development.

The decision to undertake screening for a disease should be based on clearly defined criteria including the frequency and severity of the disease, availability of safe and cost-effective screening tests, availability of prevention or amelioration of the disease and/or its complications.[5] IDDM meets, at least partially, all three criteria. It is a common and severe disease afflicting millions of people in the world. A set of screening tests, although not perfect yet, are available. Tests using IDDM-associated autoantibodies could capture 80–90% of IDDM patients.[85–88] Genetic screening of the population followed by autoantibody testing in subjects with high risk genes should make the tests more affordable. Finally, preliminary studies in animal models and human trials suggest that IDDM may be preventable through antigen-driven therapies.[89–91]

Prevention and Therapy

Genetic information is valuable for prevention and therapy of diabetes in several aspects. First, gene therapy could be an efficient way to prevent or cure certain types of diabetes such as MODY and ADM, which are caused by a defect in a single gene in a given patient. This therapeutic avenue has not yet been explored. Second, genetic information is important to understand the pathogenesis of diabetes and thus provide novel prevention or intervention strategies. Finally, it is possible that the efficiency of prevention/therapy may depend on the genetic make up of the patients. If this proves to be true, genetic analysis will have to become a routine procedure of diabetes diagnosis, prevention, and care in the future.

References

1. Bell GI, Xiang K, et al.: The gene for non–insulin dependent diabetes mellitus (maturity–onset diabetes of the young subtype) is linked to DNA polymorphism on human chromosome 20q. Proc Natl Acad Sci USA 88:1484–1488, 1991.

2. Froguel P, Vaxillaire M, et al.: Close linkage of glucokinase locus on chromosome 7p to early- onset non–insulin–dependent diabetes mellitus. Nature 356:162–164, 1992.

3. Winter W, Maclaren N, et al.: Maturity onset diabetes of youth in Black Americans. N Engl J Med 316:285–291, 1987.

4. Risch N: Assessing the role of HLA–linked and unlinked determinants of disease. Am J Hum Genet 40:1–14, 1987.

5. Rotter JI, Vadheim CM, Rimoin DL: Diabetes mellitus. *In* King RA, Rotter JI, Motulsky AG (eds): Genetic Basis of Common Diseases. New York and Oxford: Oxford University Press, 1992, pp. 413–481.

6. Weber JL, May PE: Abundant class of human DNA polymorphisms which can be typed using the polymerase chain reaction. Am J Hum Genet 44:388–396, 1989.

7. Weber JL: Informativeness of human (dC–dA)n.(dG–dT)n polymorphisms. Genomics 7:524–530, 1990.

8. Spielman RS, Mcginnis RE, Ewens WJ: Transmission test for linkage disequilibrium: The insulin gene region and insulin–dependent diabetes mellitus (IDDM). Am J Hum Genet 52:506–512, 1993.

9. Bowden DW, Gravius TC, et al.: Identification of genetic markers flanking the locus for maturity-onset diabetes of the young on human chromosome 20. Diabetes 41:88–92, 1992.

10. Rothschild CB, Akots G, et al.: A genetic map of chromosome 20q12–q13.1: Multiple highly polymorphic microsatellite and RFLP markers linked to the maturity-onset diabetes of the young (MODY) locus. Am J Hum Genet 52:110–123, 1993.

11. Vaxillaire M, Boccio V, et al.: A gene for maturity onset diabetes of the young (MODY) maps to chromosome 12q. Nature Genet 9:418–423, 1995.

12. Stoffel M, Le Beau MM, et al.: A yeast artificial chromosome-based map of the region of chromosome 20 containing the diabetes susceptibility gene, MODY1, and a myeloid leukemia related gene. Proc Natl Acad Sci USA 93:3937–3941, 1996.

13. Yamagata K, Oda N, et al.: Mutations in the hepatocyte nuclear factor-1α gene in maturity-onset diabetes of the young (MODY3). Nature 384:455–458, 1996.

14. Yamagata K, Furuta H, et al.: Mutations in the hepatocyte nuclear factor-4α gene in maturity-onset diabetes of the young (MODY1). Nature 384:458–460, 1996.

15. Sladek FM, Zong WM, et al.: Liver-enriched transcription factor HNF-4 is a novel member of the steroid hormone receptor superfamily. Gene Dev 4:2352–2365, 1990.

16. Xanthopoulos KG, Prezioso SR, et al.: The different tissue transcription patterns of genes for HNF-1, C/EBP, HNF-3, and HNF-4, protein factors that govern liver–specific transcritpion. Proc Natl Acad Sci USA 88:3807–3811, 1991.

17. Miquerol L, Lopez S, et al.: Expression of the L-type pyruvate kinase gene and the hepatocyte nuclear factor 4 transcription factor in exocrine and endocrine pancreas. J Biol Chem 269:8944–8951, 1994.

18. Emens LA, Landers DW, Moss LG: Hepatocyte nuclear factor 1 alpha is expressed in a hamster insulinoma line and transactivates the rat insulin I gene. Proc Natl Acad Sci USA 89:7300–7304, 1992.

19. Stunkard AJ, Sorensen TIA, et al.: An adoption study of human obesity. N Engl J Med 314:193–198, 1986.

20. Kahn CR, Vicent D, Doria A: Genetics of non-insulin-dependent (type-II) diabetes mellitus. Annu Rev Med 47:509–531, 1996.

21. Froguel P, Zouali H, et al.: Familial hyperglycemia due to mutations in glucokinase. Definition of a subtype of diabetes mellitus. N Engl J Med 328:697–702, 1993.

22. Eto K, Sakura H, et al.: Sequence variations of the glucokinase gene in Japanese subjects with NIDDM. Diabetes 42:1133–1137, 1993.

23. Zouali H, Vaxillaire M, et al.: Linkage analysis and molecular scanning of glucokinase gene in NIDDM families. Diabetes 42:1238–1245, 1993.

24. Hinanta S, Nishi S, et al.: Mutations of glucokinase gene in Japanese subjects with NIDDM. Nippon-Rinsho 52:2702–2707, 1994.

25. Laakso M, Malkki M, et al.: Glucokinase gene variants in subjects with late-onset NIDDM and impaired glucose tolerance. Diabetes Care 18:398–400, 1995.

26. Shimokawa K, Sakura H, et al.: Analysis of the glucokinase gene promoter in Japanese subjects with non-insulin-dependent diabetes mellitus. J Clin Endocrinol Metab 79:883–886, 1994.

27. Baron AD, Schaeffer L, et al.: Role of hyperglucagonemia in maintenance of increased rates of hepatic glucose output in Type II diabetics. Diabetes 36:274–283, 1987.

28. Hager J, Hansen L, et al.: A missense mutation in the glucagon receptor gene is associated with non-insulin-dependent diabetes mellitus. Nature Genet 9:299–304, 1995.

29. Inoue H, Ferrer J, et al.: Sequence variants in the sulfonylurea receptor (SUR) gene are associated with NIDDM in caucasians. Diabetes 45:825–831, 1996.

30. Hani EH, Clement K, et al.: Genetic studies of the sulfonylurea receptor gene locus in NIDDM and in morbid obesity among French Caucasians. Diabetes 46:688–694, 1997.

31. Ballinger SW, Shoffner JM, et al.: Maternally transmitted diabetes and deafness associated with a 10.4 kb mitochondrial DNA deletion. Nature Genet 1:11–15, 1992.

32. Reardon W, Ross RJ, et al.: Diabetes mellitus associated with a pathogenic point mutation in mitochondrial DNA. Lancet 340:1376–1379, 1992.

33. Schulz JB, Klockgether T, et al.: Mitochondrial gene mutations and diabetes mellitus. Lancet 341:438–439, 1993.

34. Oka Y: NIDDM—genetic marker; glucose transporter, glucokinase, and mitochondria gene. Diabetes Res Clin Pract 24(Suppl):117–121, 1994.

35. Hanis CL, Chu HH, et al.: Mortality of Mexican Americans with NIDDM, retinopathy and other predictors in Starr county, Texas. Diabetes Care 16:82–89, 1993.

36. Hanis CL, Hewett-Emmett D, et al.: Origins of US Hispanics: Implication for diabetes. Diabetes Care 14:618–627, 1991.

37. Hanis CL, Boerwinkle E, et al.: A genome-wide search for human non-insulin-dependent (type2) diabetes genes reveals a major susceptibility locus on chromosome 2. Nature Genet 13:161–174, 1996.

38. Mahtani MM, Widen E, et al.: Mapping of a gene for type 2 diabetes associated with an insulin secretion defect by a genome scan in Finnish families. Nature Genet 14:90–94, 1996.

39. Ji L, Malecki M, et al.: New susceptibility locus for NIDDM is localized to human chromosome 20q. Diabetes 46:876–881, 1997.

40. Elbein SC, Bragg KL, et al.: Linkage studies of NIDDM with 23 chromosome 11 markers in a sample of whites of northern European descent. Diabetes 45:370–375, 1996.

41. Bowden DW, Sale M, et al.: Linkage of genetic markers on human chromosome 20 and 12 to NIDDM in Caucasian sib pairs with a history of diabetic nephropathy. Diabetes 46:882–886, 1997.

42. Schumacher MC, Hasstedt SJ, et al.: Major gene effect for insulin levels in familial NIDDM pedigrees. Diabetes 41:416–423, 1992.

43. Prochazka M, Lillioja S, et al.: Linkage of chromosomal markers on 4q with a putative gene determining maximal insulin action in Pima Indians. Diabetes 42:514–519, 1993.

44. She JX: Susceptibility to type I diabetes: HLA-DQ and DR revisited. Immunol Today 17:323–329, 1996.

45. Todd JA, Bell JI, McDevitt HO: HLA-DQ gene contributes to susceptibility and resistance to insulin-dependent diabetes mellitus. Nature 329:599–604, 1987.

46. Thorsby E, Ronningen KS: Role of HLA genes in predisposition to develop insulin-dependent diabetes mellitus. Ann Med 24:523–531, 1992.

47. Thorsby E, Ronningen KS: Particular HLA-DQ molecules play a dominant role in determining susceptibility or resistance to type 1 (insulin-dependent) diabetes mellitus. Diabetologia 36:371–377, 1993.

48. Thorsby E: HLA-associated disease susceptibility—which genes are primarily involved? Immunologist 3:51–58, 1995.

49. Sanjeevi CB, Hook P, et al.: DR4 subtypes and their molecular properties in a population-based study of Swedish childhood diabetes. Tissue Antigens 47:275–283, 1996.

50. Huang HS, Peng JT, et al.: HLA-encoded susceptibility to IDDM is determined by DR and DQ genes as well as their linkage disequilibrium in a Chinese population. Hum Immunol 44:210–219, 1995.

51. Nepom GT: A unified hypothesis for the complex genetics of HLA associations with IDDM. Diabetes 39:1153–1157, 1990.

52. Sheehy MJ: HLA and insulin-dependent diabetes, a protective perspective. Diabetes 41:123–129, 1992.

53. Dorman JS, LaPorte RE, et al.: Worldwide differences in the incidence of type I diabetes are associated with amino acid variation at position 57 of the HLA-DQ beta chain. Proc Natl Acad Sci USA 87:7370–7374, 1990.

54. Hu CY, Allen M, et al.: Association of insulin-dependent diabetes mellitus in Taiwan with HLA class II DQB1 and DRB1 alleles. Hum Immunol 38:105–114, 1993.

55. Erlich HA, Rotter JI, et al.: Independent association of HLA-DPB1 *0301 with insulin-dependent diabetes mellitus in Mexican-Americans. Diabetes 45:610–614, 1996.

56. Demaine AG, Hibberd ML, et al.: A new marker in the HLA class I region is associated with age at onset of IDDM. Diabetologia 38:623–628, 1995.

57. Fujisawa T, Igekami H, et al.: Class I is associated with age-at-onset of IDDM, while class II confer susceptibility to IDDM. Diabetologia 38:1493–1495, 1995.

58. Deng GY, Muir A, et al.: Association of LMP2 and LMP7 genes within the major histocompatibility complex with insulin-dependent diabetes mellitus: Population and family studies. Am J Hum Genet 56:528–534, 1995.

59. Bell GI, Horita S, Karam JH: A polymorphic locus near the human insulin gene is associated with insulin-dependent diabetes mellitus. Diabetes 33:176–183, 1984.

60. Cox NJ, Baker L, Spielman RS: Insulin-gene sharing in sib pairs with insulin-dependent diabetes mellitus: No evidence for linkage. Am J Hum Genet 42:167–172, 1988.

61. Julier C, Hyer RN, et al.: Insulin-IGF2 region on chromosome 11p encodes a gene implicated in HLA-DR4-dependent diabetes susceptibility. Nature 354:155–158, 1991.

62. Bui MM, Luo DF, et al.: Paternally transmitted IDDM2 influences diabetes susceptibility despite biallelic expression of the insulin gene in human pancreas. J Autoimmun 9:97–103, 1996.

63. Lucassen AM, Julier C, et al.: Susceptibility to insulin dependent diabetes mellitus maps to a 4.1 kb segment of DNA spanning the insulin gene and associated VNTR. Nature Genet 4:305–310, 1993.

64. She JX, Bui MM, et al.: Additive susceptibility to insulin-dependent diabetes conferred by HLA-DQB1 and insulin genes. Autoimmunity 18:195–203, 1994.

65. Bennett ST, Lucassen AM, et al.: Susceptibility to human type 1 diabetes at IDDM2 is determined by tandem repeat variation at the insulin gene minisatellite locus. Nature Genet 9:284–292, 1995.

66. Kennedy GC, German MS, Rutter WJ: The minisatellite in the diabetes susceptibility locus IDDM2 regulates insulin transcription. Nature Genet 9:293–297, 1995.

67. Pugliese A, Zeller M, et al.: The insulin gene is transcribed in the human thymus and transcription levels correlate with allelic variation at the INS VNTR-IDDM2 susceptibility locus for type 1 diabetes. Nature Genet 15:293–297, 1997.

68. Vafiadis P, Bennett ST, et al.: Insulin expression in human thymus is modulated by INS VNTR alleles at the IDDM2 locus. Nature Genet 15:289–292, 1997.

69. Bain SC, Prins JB, et al.: Insulin gene region-encoded susceptibility to type 1 diabetes is not restricted to HLA-DR4-positive individuals. Nature Genet 2:212–215, 1992.

70. Lucassen AM, Screaton GR, et al.: Regulation of insulin gene expression by the IDDM associated, insulin locus haplotype. Hum Molec Genet 4:501–506, 1995.

71. Davies JL, Yoshihiko K, et al.: A genome-wide search for human type 1 diabetes susceptibility genes. Nature 371:130–136, 1994.

72. Hashimoto L, Habita C, et al.: Genetic mapping of a susceptibility locus for insulin-dependent diabetes mellitus on chromosome 11q. Nature 371:161–164, 1994.

73. Field LL, Tobias R, Magnus T: A locus on chromosome 15q26 (IDDM3) produces susceptibility to insulin-dependent diabetes mellitus. Nature Genet 8:189–194, 1994.

74. Luo DF, Bui MM, et al.: Affected sibpair mapping of a novel susceptibility gene to insulin-dependent diabetes mellitus (IDDM8) on chromosome 6q25-q27. Am J Hum Genet 57:911–919, 1995.

75. Morahan G, Huang D, et al.: Markers on distal chromosome 2q linked to insulin-dependent diabetes mellitus. Science 272:1811–1813, 1996.

76. Delepine M, Pociot F, et al.: Evidence of a non-MHC susceptibility locus in type I diabetes linked to HLA on chromosome 6. Am J Hum Genet 60:174–187, 1997.

77. Field LL, Tobias R, et al.: Susceptibility to insulin-dependent diabetes mellitus maps to a locus (IDDM11) on human chromosome 14q24.3–q31. Genomics 33:1–8, 1996.

78. Lander ES, Schork NJ: Genetic dissection of complex traits. Science 265:2307–2048, 1994.

79. Luo DF, Buzzetti R, et al.: Confirmation of three susceptibility genes to insulin-dependent diabetes mellitus: IDDM4, IDDM5 and IDDM8. Hum Mol Genet 5:693–698, 1996.

80. Davies LD, Cucca F, et al.: Saturation multipoint linkage mapping of chromosome 6q in type 1 diabetes. Hum Mol Genet 5:1071–1074, 1996.

81. Nistico L, Buzzetti R, et al.: The CTLA4 gene region of chromosome 2q33 is linked to, and associated with, type 1 diabetes. Hum Mol Genet 5:1075–1080, 1996.

82. Marron MP, Raffel LJ, et al.: Insulin-dependent diabetes mellitus (IDDM) is associated with CTLA4 polymorphisms in multiple ethnic groups. Hum Mol Genet 8:1275–1282, 1997.

83. Donner H, Rau H, et al.: CTLA4 alanine-17 confers genetic susceptibility to Graves' disease and to type 1 diabetes mellitus. J Clin Endocrinol Metab 82:143–146, 1997.

84. Yanagawa T, Hidaka Y, et al.: CTLA4 gene polymorphism associated with Graves' disease in a caucasian population. J Clin Endocrinol Metab 80:41–45, 1995.

85. Schatz D, Krischer J, et al.: Islet cell antibodies predict insulin dependent diabetes in U.S. school age children as powerfully as in unaffected relatives. J Clin Invest 93:2403–2407, 1994.

86. Riley W, Maclaren N, et al.: A prospective study of the development of diabetes in relatives of patients with IDD. N Engl J Med 323:1167–1172, 1990.

87. Atkinson MA, Maclaren NK: Islet cell autoantigens in insulin-dependent diabetes. J Clin Invest 92:1608–1616, 1993.

88. Atkinson M, Maclaren N, et al.: 64,000 Mr autoantobodies as predictors of IDD. Lancet 335:1357–1360, 1990.

89. Ramiya VK, Shang X, et al.: Antigen based therapies to prevent diabetes in NOD mice. J Autoimmun 9:349–356, 1996.

90. Bowman MA, Leiter EH, Atkinson MA: Prevention of diabetes in the NOD mouse: Implications for therapeutic intervention in human disease. Immunol Today 15:115–120, 1994.

91. Eisenbarth GS, Verge CF, et al.: The design of trials for prevention of IDDM. Diabetes 42:941–947, 1993.

6

Insulin Deficiency

William G. Blackard* and John N. Clore

Most diabetics exhibit either an absolute or relative deficiency of insulin. The deficiency varies from an almost complete lack of insulin as seen in individuals with type 1 diabetes mellitus to relative insulin deficiency as seen in most individuals with type 2 diabetes mellitus. Approximately 80% of those with type 2 diabetes are obese and have variable degrees of insulin resistance related to their obesity. Although obese diabetic individuals may exhibit hyperinsulinism compared to nonobese subjects, the ability of type 2 diabetics to secrete insulin is clearly impaired compared to similarly obese, nondiabetic subjects.[1] Nevertheless, emphasis on insulin resistance and hyperinsulinism has tended to obscure the role of insulin deficiency in type 2 diabetes. The recognition that β-cell volume is reduced in type 2 diabetes suggests decreased insulin reserve and an impaired ability to compensate for insulin resistance from any cause, whether insulin resistance is brought about by hormonal antagonists (growth hormone), drugs (steroids), obesity, or immune abnormalities (anti-insulin receptor antibodies). Family history data and twin studies indicate that inherited factors are more important in type 2 than type 1 diabetes. Perhaps it is a genetically determined lack of β-cell reserve as a result of early islet senescence or failure of islets to regenerate which determines which obese persons develop diabetes.

Insulin Secretion in Diabetes

Type 1 diabetes is characterized by low basal levels as well as flat or negligible insulin responses to the commonly used secretagogues. Loss of insulin secretory capacity is often said to be abrupt but frequently the progression to severe insulin deficiency is more prolonged. High HbA1$_c$ values at the time of diagnosis indicate that even in those cases where onset was considered abrupt, the condition probably began at least weeks to months earlier. Studies in monozygotic twins initially discordant for type 1 diabetes have indicated that islet cell antibodies with presumed β-cell cytotoxicity may precede clinical diabetes by 5 to 8 years.[2]

After insulin treatment for acute onset type 1 diabetes, insulin secretory capacity chracteristically improves. This improvement in β-cell function is manifested by increased C-peptide peaks between 2 and 6 months after diagnosis.[3] Often in these patients, insulin secretion completely normalizes, resulting in a clinical remission called the "honeymoon period," lasting weeks to months. Significant endogenous insulin release may persist for 5 to 7 years after diagnosis. By 10 to 15 years, however, the prevalence of patients with type 1 diabetes with residual β-cell function decreases to about 15% and remains at that level.[4] Endogenous insulin secretion as measured by C-peptide levels correlates well with stability of control in patients with type 1 diabetes. Presumably, the ability to regulate insulin secretion even modestly helps prevent the extremes of hyperglycemia and hypoglycemia seen in those patients without this capacity.

In type 2 diabetes, basal and stimulated insulin levels may be normal, decreased, or even increased (Fig. 6–1). In mild diabetics with near-normal fasting plasma glucose (FPG), plasma insulin levels are higher than normal at 2 hr during a glucose tolerance test. With worsening glucose levels, insulin levels are reduced, particularly at early time points during the glucose tolerance test. Most studies in patients with type 2 diabetes have demonstrated an impaired early insulin response to a glucose challenge. The resulting hyperglycemia often results in hyperinsulinism, most apparent 2 to 4 hr after glucose ingestion. Many obese diabetic individuals have exceedingly elevated plasma insulin levels; yet these values are usually lower than those in similarly

---

*Deceased June, 1996.

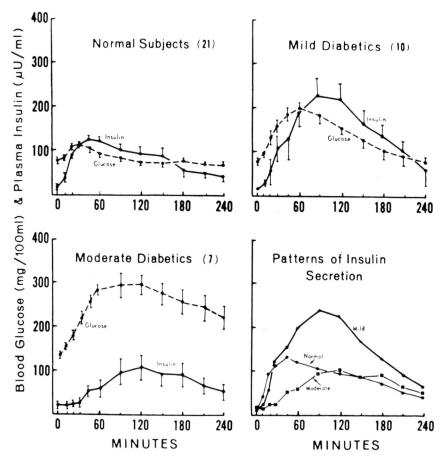

Figure 6–1. Plasma insulin levels in nonobese control and diabetic persons after oral glucose load. (*Source:* Selzer HS, Allen EW, Herron AL, et al: Insulin secretion in response to glycemic stimulus: Relation of delayed insulin release to carbohydrate intolerance in mild diabetes mellitus. J Clin Invest 46:323–335, 1967. With permission).

obese nondiabetic subjects.[1] Nonobese persons with type 2 diabetes also exhibit insulin resistance and in many cases increased insulin levels. However, as noted in the obese nondiabetic subjects, lean nondiabetic subjects matched for similar degrees of insulin resistance exhibit even greater basal and provoked insulin concentrations compared to diabetic individuals. Correction of insulin values for the glycemic stimulus shows that the insulin/glucose ratio is always decreased in diabetic subjects whether lean or obese.[5]

Limited longitudinal data on patients with type 2 diabetes exist. However, a spectrum of glucose-insulin profiles exists in type 2 diabetes, varying from mildly hyperglycemic, hyperinsulinemic patients to those with severe hyperglycemia and insulinopenia.[6] It is possible that the early diabetic with mild hyperglycemia and hyperinsulinemia becomes more severely hyperglycemic as the β-cell mass decreases and the ability of the β cell to respond to glucose fails. Conversely, the possibility that loss of β-cell function occurs as a result of hyperglycemia is consonant with the theory of glucose toxicity for which much evidence now exists.[7] Eventually, if the loss of β-cell mass and functional defect in insulin secretion is severe enough, the noninsulin-

dependent patients become severely insulinopenic and require insulin.

Islet Pathology in Diabetes

Islet cell and specifically β-cell mass is reduced in most diabetic patients.[8] The degree of reduction and the precise pathological picture depend on the type of diabetes and the duration of disease (Table 6–1). In cases of type 1 diabetes in which the pancreas has been examined shortly after onset of the disease, the islets are surrounded and invaded by round cells and inflammatory cells (Fig. 6–2). This appearance is called "insulitis" and resembles the pathological picture observed with autoimmune or viral destruction. This same picture is observed in autoimmune (BB rat, NOD mice) and viral-induced animal models of diabetes. The disappearance of β cells with relative sparing of α (glucagon secreting) and δ (somatostatin secreting) cells from involved islets suggests that the putative antigen for the autoimmune disturbance is derived from the β cell.

The pathological picture of insulitis is usually not observed a year or more after the onset of diabetes. Instead, a paucity of poorly granulated islets and even

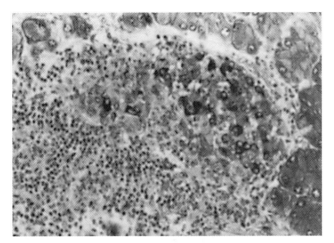

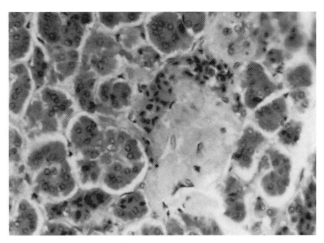

Figure 6–2. "Insulitis" in pancreas. Note intense round cell infiltration and loss of beta cells. Decreased aldehyde fuchsin staining indicates decreased insulin storage. (Photograph courtesy of A.A. Like.)

Figure 6–3. Section of pancreas from a patient with noninsulin dependent diabetes mellitus. Note islet hyalinization. (Photograph courtesy of Gordon Madge, MD.)

TABLE 6–1 Total Volumes of A, B, and D Cells, and Volume Ratio of B to A Cells[a]

Group	V_a (cm^3)	V_B (cm^3)	V_D (cm^3)	V_B/V_A
Nondiabetic	0.109 ± 0.28	0.636 ± 0.078	0.028 ± 0.008	7.2 ± 1.8
Diabetic				
Type 2	0.068 ± 0.013	0.388 ± 0.065	0.020 ± 0.009	6.3 ± 1.0
Type 1	0.026 ± 0.034	0.156 ± 0.114	0.007 ± 0.008	9.5 ± 6.7

islet cell replacement by fibrosis may be seen. Morphometry late after the onset of diabetes reveals reduced numbers of islet cells consisting mainly of α and δ cells. Insulin secretory cells are reduced to 10% of normal at onset and may persist at this low level for years. Beta cells appear singly throughout the pancreas or in regenerative islets composed mainly of hyperactive β cells. Alpha and δ cells also appear as single cells scattered throughout the endocrine pancreas.

In patients with type 2 diabetes, the loss of islets is not as severe as in those with type 1 diabetes. A reduction of islet cell mass to approximately 60% of normal is common (Table 6–1). A uniform loss of islet cell types has been reported using volumetric techniques, but some studies have shown a greater loss of β cells. In any case, the reduction in islet cell mass does not fully explain impaired insulin secretion because studies have suggested that 80% or more of the pancreas must be removed before hyperglycemia becomes manifest. However, the combination of reduced islet cell mass and a functional abnormality in insulin release to be described below probably accounts for the abnormal insulin release in this most common form of diabetes.

Hyalinization and fibrosis are also observed in the pancreas of diabetic patients (Fig. 6–3). These lesions are more charactersitic of the pancreas from older patients with type 2 diabetes and were first recognized in 1900. However, recent studies have identified the material forming these birefringent plaques as islet-specific amyloid.[9] Amyloid is present in over 70% of patients with type 2 diabetes in contrast to 10% of elderly nondiabetic persons (who parenthetically may be developing diabetes). A role for islet amyloid polypeptide (IAPP), also known as amylin, in progressive loss of β-cell mass and, perhaps function, has been proposed.

Physiology of Insulin Release and Potential Loci of Abnormalities in Insulin Release

Insulin deficiency may result from a reduced β-cell mass, aberrant biosynthesis, or a disturbance of the insulin release mechanism. Some insulin secretagogues stimulate synthesis and release, whereas others mainly affect release. In response to increased glucose phosphorylation within the β cell by glucokinase,[10] the insulin promoter is activated and gene transcription is initiated. Biosynthesis of insulin begins with translation of mRNA into preproinsulin.[11] The initial 24 amino acid segment of preproinsulin is thought to serve as a signal peptide for translocation of the nascent protein into the endoplasmic reticulum. Within

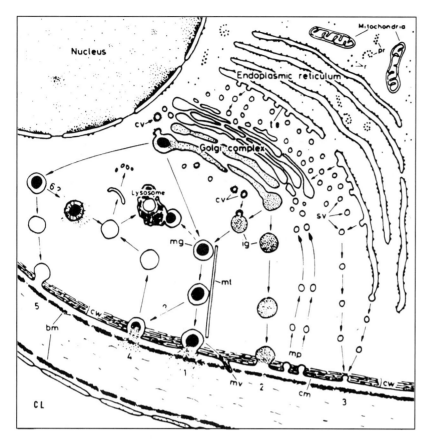

Figure 6–4. Schematic illustration of the morphological aspects of the secretory process in an insulin-producing cell. Insulin precursors are synthesized on the membrane-associated ribosomes of the endoplasmic reticulum (upper right) then transferred to the cisternae of the endoplasmic reticulum prior to transfer to the Golgi by way of microvesicular carriers. Packaging of insulin into granules occurs in the Golgi with cleavage of proinsulin to insulin in the granule. Possible release processes are also depicted. *Abbreviations:* bm = basement membrane; cm = cell membrane; cv = coated vesicles; cw = cell web; ig = immature granule; mg = mature granule; mp = micropinocytotic event; mt = microtubule; mv = microvillus; pr = polyribosomes; r = free ribosomes; sv = smooth vesicles. (Diagram courtesy Dr. A. Renold).

the lumen of the rough endoplasmic reticulum, the signal peptide is removed and the cleaved product, proinsulin (PI), undergoes folding and oxidation of its sulfhydral groups. The PI is then transferred by an energy-dependent process to the Golgi where granules destined for regulated secretion are formed. Finally, specific endopeptidases and carboxypetidases cleave the connecting peptide (C-peptide) from proinsulin to form insulin (see Fig. 6–4).

In response to stimulation of the β cell, granule products are released by a process of exocytosis in which granules are propelled to the plasma membrane, fuse with the plasma membrane, and the contents (insulin and C-peptide) are released in equimolar quantities. Some intact PI as well as intermediate cleavage products are also released. The proportion of insulin secreted as PI is small so that the relative proportion of immunoreactive insulin circulating in the plasma as PI rarely exceeds 15%. Recent studies using antibodies specific for insulin have indicated that this proportion is in large part the result of decreased clearance of PI; secretion of PI accounts for approximately 2–4% of total insulin release in vivo.

The complete sequence of events leading to exocytosis is not fully understood. However, nearly all recognized stimuli for insulin release have been associated with an increase in cytosolic calcium. It was previously speculated that the increase in cytosolic calcium might result from either enhancing calcium influx, inhibiting efflux, or translocating calcium from rough endoplas-

mic reticulum and mitochondria to the cytosol. However, in experiments in which calcium influx was inhibited, glucose failed to increase insulin secretion.[12] Thus, available data are consonent with the hypothesis that the increase in cytosolic calcium is mediated by enhanced influx. Activation of a muscarinic receptor on the β cell by acetylcholine with its consequent increase in phosphoinositide turnover and intracellular Ca^{++} appears to be involved in the cephalic phase of insulin secretion.[13] However, a rise in plasma glucose remains the predominant stimulus for insulin secretion. Following transport, phosphorylation and metabolism of glucose in the β-cell, the resultant increase in ATP (ATP/ADP ratio) results in inhibition of an ATP-sensitive potassium channel,[14] leading to depolarization of the membrane, activation of a voltage dependent Ca^{++} channel, and increased intracellular Ca^{++}.[12] This increase in cytosolic Ca^{++}, as well as changes in cell electrical activity manifested by bursts of action potentials, precede insulin secretion. Inhibitors (e.g., sulfonylureas) and activators (e.g., diazoxide) of the K+channel enhance or inhibit, respectively, insulin secretion via this mechanism. Increases in cAMP also promote glucose-stimulated insulin secretion by protein phosphorylation mediated through protein kinase A. However, the effect is glucose dependent; increases in cAMP in the absence of glucose are not associated with significant increases in insulin secretion. Activation of β-cell specific guanine nucleotide regulatory proteins by glucose or gastrointestinal hormones (e.g., glucagon-like peptide, GLP-1) increase cAMP and insulin secretion whereas prostaglandin E_2, epinephrine, and somatostatin inhibit adenyl cyclase, reducing cAMP and insulin secretion.[15] Additional sites of action for neurohumoral regulation of insulin secretion are under investigation.

The role of cytoskeletal microtubules in insulin secretion has been recognized as a result of experiments in vitro with agents that affect these cell elements. Vincristine, colchicine and deuterium oxide, which prevent the major constituent of microtubules (tubulin) from polymerizing and forming the channels necessary for granule transport to the cell surface, inhibit insulin release. On the other hand, cytochalasin B, which induces disruption and causes hypercontraction of microfilaments, has been demonstrated to stimulate insulin release. More recently, suppression of a microtubule-dependent ATPase (kinesin) involved in microtubular migration was also shown to inhibit insulin secretion in cultured mouse β cells.[16] Contractility of microtubules has not been demonstrated; however, a contractile property of microfilaments seems likely in view of their known content of actin. An attractive hypothesis, which is compatible with most of our present information, is as follows[17]: Glucose or some other secretagogue increases net calcium flux into the cytosol; the calcium binds to calmodulin (a calcium-dependent regulatory protein); in turn, calmodulin activates myosin light-chain kinase, which causes phosphorylation of myosin; this phosphorylation leads to its association with filamentous actin as actomycin; the contraction of the actomyosin may propel the granules through the microtubular channels; in addition, tubulin polymerization into microtubules may be enhanced by phosphorylation of tubulin or tubulin kinases activated by calmodulin.

The sequence just outlined supplies several attractive loci for defects in diabetes—a mutation in DNA with aberrant RNA synthesis producing an abnormal insulin, an abnormal PI that cannot be cleaved in the conventional manner, and an abnormality in the extrusion of granules. Evidence exists only for an abnormality in insulin biosynthesis. Although the clinical characteristics of diabetes caused by production of an abnormal insulin resemble those of diabetes due to any other cause, this abnormality may be suspected in persons with carbohydrate intolerance, hyperinsulinism, and normal sensitivity to exogenous insulin. The first case was detected by investigations in a patient showing a high concentration of immunoreactive insulin that exhibited poor biological activity (impaired binding to the insulin receptor). Sequencing of the insulin revealed a substitution of leucine for phenylalanine at amino acid 25 of the B-chain.[18] Other cases with similar B-chain mutations have been reported. The frequency of these mutations cannot be estimated at present, but a prevalence of abnormal insulins similar to that of abnormal hemoglobins would not be surprising. Many abnormal insulins might have normal biological activity, thus not resulting in the diabetic state (see Chapter 18).

Little evidence exists to indicate an abnormality in cleavage of PI to insulin as a cause of diabetes. Although patients with type 2 diabetes exhibit disproportionate proinsulin secretion, the increased release is considered secondary to increased demand on the residual stressed β cells rather than a primary abnormality.[19] In addition, in patients with familial hyperproinsulinemia, where a defect in conversion is known to occur, diabetes has rarely been observed. No abnormality in the exocytotic process has been demonstrated in diabetic persons although such a defect has been suggested for a diabetic animal model the spiny mouse. The failure of patients with type 2 diabetes to secrete insulin in response to glucose despite normal responses to other secretagogues suggests an abnormality in the release mechanism. However, the morphological counterpart of increased granules in β cells of persons with type 2 diabetes has not been reported in the limited pathological studies performed in humans.

Functional Impairment in β-Cell Insulin Secretion

In contrast to the virtual complete destruction of β cells in type 1 diabetes (certainly in C-peptide negative persons), type 2 diabetes is associated with relatively well-preserved albeit reduced numbers of β cells. The failure of β cells in persons with type 2 diabetes to secrete insulin maximally in the presence of hyperglycemia suggests a functional defect in insulin secretion in these patients. This functional defect has been characterized in a number of ways outlined in Exhibit 6–1 and discussed separately below.

The most consistently documented abnormality in insulin secretion in type 2 diabetes is an impaired early phase of insulin secretion. The insulin response to glucose occurs in two phases—an early phase that peaks

EXHIBIT 6–1 Functional Impairments in Insulin Secretion in Non-Insulin-Dependent Diabetes Mellitus

1. Impairment of early-phase insulin release with relative preservation of late-phase release
2. Impairment of insulin response to glucose with preservation of response to other secretagogues
3. Impaired potentiation of insulin release to nonglucose secretagogues by glucose
4. Increased adrenergic, serotonergic, prostaglandinergic tone inhibiting insulin release

at 2 min and lasts for approximately 5 to 7 min after an IV bolus of glucose, and a second phase beginning at 10 min and lasting until the hyperglycemic stimulus disappears. The nadir separating the two phases occurs at approximately 7 to 10 min and is more easily demonstrable in the portal vein than in a peripheral vein.[20] Even in the portal vein the nadir is partially obscured by recirculation of modest amounts of insulin in a closed loop system (Fig. 6–5). Several mechanisms have been proposed to explain the biphasic nature of insulin secretion. It was originally proposed that the first phase of insulin release was due to secretion of immediately releasable stores of insulin whereas the second phase was due to release of less-accessible insulin stores and in part to release of newly synthesized insulin. More recently it has been suggested that phasic insulin secretion might result from changes in sensitivity to cytoplasmic Ca^{2+}. In any case, patients with type 2 diabetes exhibit an impairment in the early phase of insulin release (often called acute insulin release; AIR), whereas the late phase is reasonably well preserved until the fasting plasma glucose exceeds 150 to 200 mg/dL.[21] That this abnormality is not due to hepatic destruction of insulin during the first phase release can be observed in the portal vein studies shown in Figure 6–5.[20]

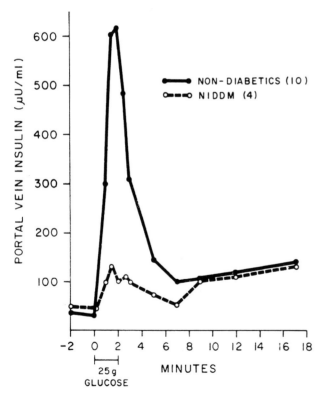

Figure 6–5. Portal vein insulin responses to IV glucose bolus in diabetic and nondiabetics. Note impairment of early phase release with preservation of late-phase secretion in diabetics. (*Source:* Blackard WG, Nelson NC: Portal vein insulin concentrations in diabetic subjects. Diabetes 20:286, 1971).

Those with type 2 diabetes also exhibit a selective impairment of insulin response to glucose but not to nonglucose stimuli. Despite a progressive loss of the early and then the later phase of insulin release to glucose as glucose intolerance becomes more severe (higher FPG), the insulin response to certain nonglucose stimuli may be well preserved in diabetic persons until the FPG exceeds 200 mg/dL (Fig. 6–6). The fact that the diabetic β cell will respond to these nonglucose stimuli (amino acids, isoproterenol, secretin, glucagon) and yet not respond to glucose has suggested a problem in signal recognition or in a putative glucoreceptor.

Patients with type 2 diabetes also exhibit impaired potentiation of nonglucose stimuli for insulin release by glucose. Porte and colleagues[22] have shown that glucose will potentiate the insulin response to nonglucose stimuli in normal and diabetic individuals (i.e., the higher the basal or steady-state glucose concentration, the greater the insulin response to nonglucose stimuli).[22] However, potentiation of insulin secretion at each glucose level is less in diabetic than in nondiabetic subjects (Fig. 6–7). These investigators have proposed that basal insulin levels are maintained relatively normal in mild and moderate diabetes as a result of a higher basal glucose level that potentiates the insulin response to nonglucose stimuli (metabolic and neural). In other words, basal insulin levels are maintained in the normal range at the expense of hyperglycemia. In this way, insulin is present for the suppression of hepatic glucose output and for peripheral glucose utilization in the mild diabetic. Only when this compensatory mechanism fails, as it does in more severe diabetes, is a fall in basal insulin concentration seen.

In many individuals with type 2 diabetes, the insulin secretory response to glucose can be restored by humoral and neural inhibitors. Alpha-adrenergic blockade with phentolamine was the first inhibitor shown to restore the AIR to normal in diabetic individuals. Similarly, inhibitors of prostaglandin synthesis have been shown to improve and even normalize first phase insulin release in patients with type 2 diabetes mellitus.

It is important to point out that these functional abnormalities in insulin secretion may not strictly characterize type 2 diabetes but may be more a reflection of the β cell under stress. The same qualitative abnormalities are observed in patients with type 2 diabetes as β-cell function begins to deteriorate.[23]

Postulated Etiologies of Insulin Deficiency

Loss of islet cell mass is more prominent in type 1 than in type 2 diabetes. Evidence exists for viral and autoimmune islet destruction (see Chapters 3 and 4). A popu-

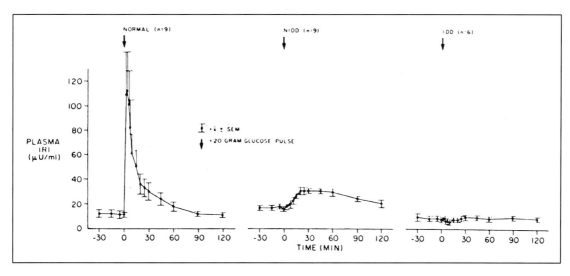

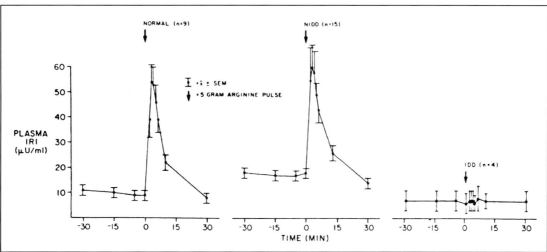

Figure 6–6. Plasma IRI response to glucose (upper panel) and the nonglucose stimulant arginine (lower panel) in normal and diabetic subjects. *Abbreviations:* NIDD = noninsulin dependent diabetes; IDD = insulin dependent diabetes; SEM = standard error of mean. (*Source:* Pfeiffer MA, Halter JB, Porte D Jr: Insulin secretion in diabetes mellitus. Am J Med 70:579, 1981. With permission).

lar scheme of pathogenesis suggests that viral infection[24] in a genetically susceptible person may lead to an autoimmune reaction that produces the pathologic changes seen in the pancreas of a patient with type 1 diabetes (Fig. 6–8). That an environmental factor is involved is supported by the low (~36%) concordance rate for type 1 diabetes mellitus in monozygotic twins[25] and the similarity of certain islet cell proteins with viral antigens. The observation that immunosuppressive therapy may prevent or ameliorate viral or chemical-induced diabetes in animals suggests that their effects may depend on producing an autoimmune reaction against the β cell. The pathological picture of "insulitis" and the experimental evidence implicating cytokines in the development of type 1 diabetes suggests that cell-mediated immunity is critical for islet cell destruction. However, although the detection of antibodies to numerous β-cell antigens (e.g., glutamic acid decarboxylase) has proven useful as a marker of type 1

diabetes, it is less clear if these autoantibodies are involved in antibody-mediated cytotoxicity.

In type 2 diabetes, where loss of islet cell mass is insufficient to explain insulin deficiency, several theories have been invoked to explain the functional impairment in insulin secretion. One of the most popular is that a defect in signal recognition for insulin release exists.[26] This defect could be either lack of a putative glucoreceptor (aprotein on the cell membrane capable of binding glucose) or disturbed islet metabolism responsible for triggering insulin release. There is now considerable support for the latter. Numerous studies indicate the requirement for glucose transport, phosphorylation, and metabolism for insulin release to occur. Of particular importance are the *islet specific glucose transporter GLUT-2 and/or glucokinase (GK)*, the rate limiting step in islet glucose metabolism. Levels of GLUT-2 are decreased in numerous animal models of type 2 diabetes[27] and there is increasing evidence

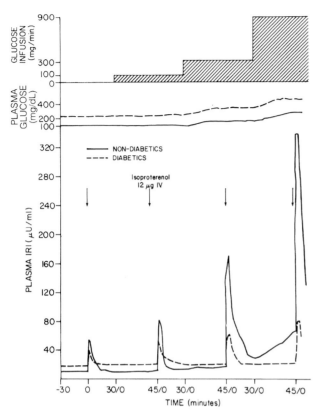

Figure 6–7. Potentiation of plasma IRI response to nonglucose stimulus (isoproterenol) by glucose in diabetics and nondiabetics. Note impaired potentiation by glucose in diabetics and also, "normal" IRI response to isoproterenol in diabetics at their preglucose infusion steady state. (*Source:* Halter JB, Graff RJ, Porte D Jr: Potentiation of insulin secretory responses by plasma glucose levels in man: Evidence that hyperglycemia in diabetes compensates for impaired glucose potentiation. J Clin Endocrinol Metab 48:946, 1979. With permission.)

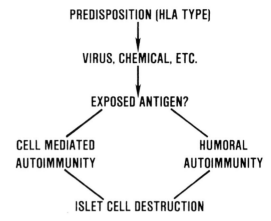

Figure 6–8. Postulated pathogenesis of insulin-dependent diabetes mellitus.

that the expression of GLUT-2 is regulated by the metabolic milieu. However, the contribution of diminished GLUT-2 to impaired insulin secretion in human diabetes is not known. No functional mutations in the GLUT-2 gene have been demonstrated in patients with type 2 diabetes and reduction in GLUT-2 in cultured cells does not appear to significantly reduce insulin secretion, perhaps because observed reductions in glucose transport in these models are not sufficient to impact the much lower rates of glucose phosphorylation in islets. The role of glucose phosphorylation in impaired insulin secretion in type 2 diabetes has been provided by studies in patients with maturity-onset diabetes of the young (MODY) and in transgenic animal models. With regard to the former, a mutation in a single allele of the GK gene (so-called MODY2) is characterized by a shift to the right in the insulin response to graded glucose infusion but relatively mild elevations in plasma glucose.[28] Similarly, when a knockout model of heterozygous GK deficiency (to mimic

MODY2) was developed in otherwise normal animals, only impaired glucose tolerance was observed. On the other hand, when heterozygous GK deficiency was paired with deficiency of insulin receptor substrate-1 (IRS-1) (to mimic peripheral insulin resistance), marked hyperglycemia developed.[29] As these studies suggest, a mutation in GK alone is unlikely to explain a significant proportion of classical type 2 diabetes mellitus. Indeed, it has been estimated that such mutations account for less than 1% of diabetes mellitus. However, the studies do support the notion that insulin resistance alone is insufficient to produce diabetes mellitus.

A second popular hypothesis for the functional impairment in insulin release espoused by some is that accentuation of certain neural or humoral factors known to depress β-cell secretion occurs. A probable partial listing of potential inhibitory factors includes catecholamines, serotonin, prostaglandins, and endorphins. The extensive network of autonomic nerve terminals in the pancreas as well as active prostaglandin synthesis occurring in the pancreas suggests that the modulating influence of these factors should not be underestimated. The fact that insulin secretion in diabetic patients can be improved with alpha-adrenergic blockade (phentolamine), the serotonin inhibitor (methylsergide), and inhibitors of prostaglandin synthesis (acetylsalicylic acid) indicates a possible role of these factors in type 2 diabetes.

A third popular hypothesis for impaired insulin release in type 2 diabetes mellitus is the exhaustion theory.[30] Exhaustion is not an ideal word to describe the progressive deterioration of the β-cell function in type 2 diabetes since ample cell content of insulin persists as determined by actual measurements and as indicated by the capacity of the β cells to respond to other stimuli. Nevertheless, it is a term that has been used to describe the progressive impairment in insulin secretion that occurs after years of insulin resistance, such as obesity-related diabetes. Although no precedent for overstimulation exists with other endocrine glands (adreno-corticotropic hormone-stimulated adrenal glands, etc.) the high prevalence of permanently impaired insulin release related to states of insulin resistance (steroid treatment, Cushings disease, acromegaly, etc.) suggests that this indeed is the case.

Several mechanisms have been proposed to explain this well-recognized clinical phenomen. The first mechanism is that hyperglycemia per se adversely affects β-cell function.[7] Experimental elevation of plasma glucose by glucose infusion results in a reproducible loss in insulin response to glucose ("glucose toxicity") and reduction in plasma glucose in diabetic animals restores insulin secretion.[31] Moreover, in studies performed in patients with type 2 diabetes mellitus in whom glucose levels were comparably reduced by diet, sulfonylurea or insulin administration, the insulin response to a glucose load was markedly increased.[32] Unfortunately, despite strong support for the role of hyperglycemia in acquired β-cell dysfunction, the intracellular processes responsible for this effect are not yet clear. Exhaustion could also represent senescence of the β-cell brought about prematurely by insulin resistance. Some studies have shown an impairment of insulin secretion in aging. A morphological correlation of this finding may be the increase in hyalinization of islets found in older individuals, an abnormality not found in young people and, more specifically, rarely found in those individuals with type 1 diabetes mellitus. As noted previously, the material forming these amyloid deposits has been identified as islet amyloid polypeptide or amylin. Amylin is co-secreted with insulin[33] so that conditions that demand increased insulin secretion (i.e., insulin resistant states) would be expected to demand increased amylin secretion as well. Thus, it is not surprising that amylin deposition in older persons with type 2 diabetes is three- to fourfold greater than in nondiabetic individuals of the same age. Progressive accumulation of amyloid deposits in monkeys that eventually developed type 2 diabetes has also been demonstrated.[34] However, insulin deficiency and type 2 diabetes develops in a minority of persons with insulin resistance and nondiabetic individuals with insulin resistance do not appear to have increased islet amyloid. A protective mecha-nism to prevent the deposition of amylin in β-cells of persons at lower risk for type 2 diabetes mellitus has been proposed to explain this paradox. A defect in this mechanism might then result in the structural and functional abnormalities found in patients with type 2 diabetes.

In addition to glucose intolerance and hyperglycemia, type 2 diabetes mellitus is also characterized by increased lipolysis and increased free fatty acids (FFA). While the effect of FFA to impair glucose disposal in peripheral tissues is well known, it has become apparent that FFA may play an important role in islet function as well. Acute exposure of nondiabetic islets to FFA is associated with an increase in insulin release. However, prolonged exposure to increased lipids leads to a loss of glucose-stimulated insulin release analogous to the effect of prolonged hyperglycemia.[35] Studies performed in obese prediabetic rats have shown a particular susceptibility to the FFA-induced impairment in glucose-stimulated insulin secretion. This susceptibility may be in part the result of increased triglyceride formation in islets[36] and enhanced nitric oxide formation.[37] Interestingly, inhibition of nitric oxide synthase in islets from prediabetic animals exposed to FFA restored insulin secretion and prevented the reduction in GLUT2 and β-cell mass and progression to hyperglycemia characteristic of this model of type 2 diabetes. Coupled with the considerable data linking increased lipolysis with peripheral insulin resistance and hyperglycemia, these studies suggest that the pathogenesis of β-cell dysfunction in type 2 may be tightly linked to abnormalities in lipid metabolism.

Insulin Deficiency Due to Other Causes

Insulin deficiency may occur as as result of other specific conditions (Exhibit 6–2). Surgical extirpation, pancreatitis, or hemochromatosis can cause diabetes. Evidence suggests that carbohydrate intolerance after partial pancreatectomy does not occur unless at least 80% of the pancreas has been removed. Similarly, diabetes can occur with major destruction of the pancreas

---

EXHIBIT 6–2   Insulin Deficiency Due to Other Causes

Destruction of pancreas	Drugs affecting insulin release
Surgical extirpation	Thiazides
Chronic pancreatitis	Phenytoin
Hemochromatosis	Pentamidine
Hormone-producing tumors inhibiting insulin release	Others
Pheochromocytoma	Antibodies producing insulin deficiency at cellular level
Somatostatinoma	Antibodies to insulin
Aldosteronoma	Antibodies to insulin receptor

in the form of chronic pancreatitis and hemochromatosis. The presence of microvascular complications of diabetes in these conditions suggests that these complications are related to the metabolic disturbance. Permanent carbohydrate intolerance less frequently occurs with acute pancreatitis. The transient glucose intolerance in these patients is best attributed to a combination of elevated glucagon and decreased plasma insulin levels.

Although quite a few endocrine disturbances are associated with diabetes, many are diabetogenic because the hormone in question is an insulin antagonist (growth hormone, cortisol, and glucagon). These conditions are discussed in Chapter 9). Two endocrine tumors, however, secrete hormones that act directly to inhibit β-cell secretion. These tumors are pheochromocytomas, which secrete catecholamines, and the rare somatostatinoma-secreting somatostatin. Another endocrine tumor, aldosteronoma, also impairs pancreatic insulin release, probably secondarily through its effect on lowering serum potassium.

Certain drugs have also been associated with impaired insulin release and diabetes. Thiazide diuretics inhibit insulin release as a result of drug-induced hypokalemia. The antiepileptic agent phenytoin can also impair pancreatic insulin release, but usually only when the drug is given in particularly high doses. Diazoxide inhibits insulin secretion by enhancing activity of the K^+ channel on the β cell (see above). The antiprotozoal agent pentamidine has also been associated with insulin deficiency and diabetes. This appears to be the result of β-cell lysis, with an initial phase of hypoglycemia followed by insulin-dependent diabetes mellitus, similar to that observed following streptozotocin treatment in animals. Retrospective analysis of patients with human immunodeficiency virus (HIV) infections treated with pentamidine suggest that hyperglycemia develops in up to 38% of patients and that the effect is related to cumulative dose.[38] The mechanism for the recent report of insulin deficiency and hyperglycemia in 84 HIV patients treated with protease inhibitors is not yet known.

Finally, carbohydrate intolerance can be produced by antibodies to insulin and to the insulin receptor. In the former case, the antibodies are usually the result of prior animal insulin injections. Antibodies to the insulin receptor occur rarely but are associated with severe insulin resistance rather than insulin deficiency.

References

1. Bagdade JD, Bierman EL, Porte D, Jr: The significance of basal insulin levels in the evaluation of the insulin response to glucose in diabetic and nondiabetic subjects. J Clin Invest 46:1549–1557, 1967.

2. Srikanta S. Ganda OP, Eisenbarth GS, et al.: Islet-cell antibodies and beta-cell function in monozygotic triplets and twins initially discordant for type I diabetes mellitus. N Engl J Med 308:322–325, 1983.

3. Block MB, Rosenfield RL, Mako ME, et al.: Sequential changes in beta-cell function in insulin-treated diabetic patients assessed by C-peptide immunoreactivity. N Engl J Med 288:1144–1148, 1973.

4. Madsbad S: Prevalence of residual B cell function and its metabolic consequences in type I (insulin-dependent) diabetes. Diabetologia 24:141–147, 1983.

5. Seltzer HS, Allen EW, Herron AL, et al.: Insulin secretion in response to glycemic stimulus: Relation of delayed internal release to carbohydrate intolerance in mild diabetes mellitus. J Clin Invest 46:323–335, 1967.

6. Fajans SS, Cloutier MC, Crowther RL: Clinical and etiologic heterogeneity of idiopathic diabetes mellitus. Diabetes 27:111–1125, 1978.

7. Leahy JL, Bonner-Weir S, Weir GC. β-cell dysfunction induced by chronic hyperglycemia: Current ideas on mechanisms of impaired glucose-induced insulin secretion. Diabetes Care 15:442–455, 1992.

8. Gepts W, Le Compte PM: The pancreatic islets in diabetes. Am J Med 70:105–115, 1981.

9. Clark A, Gooper GJS, Lewis CE, et al.: Islet amyloid formed from diabetes-associated peptide may be pathogenic in type-2 diabetes. Lancet 2:231–234, 1987.

10. German M. Glucose sensing in pancreatic beta cells: The key role of glucokinase and the glycolytic intermediates. Proc Nat Acad Sci USA 90:1781–1785, 1993.

11. Steiner DF, Kemmler W, Clark JL, et al.: The biosynthesis of insulin. In Steiner DE, Freinkel N (eds): Handbook of Physiology, Vol. 1. Baltimore: Williams & Wilkins, 1972, pp. 175–198.

12. Prentki M, Matchinsky FM: Ca^{2+}, cAMP and phospholipid-derived messengers in coupling mechanisms of insulin secretion. Physiol Rev 67:1185–1248, 1987.

13. Rasmussen H, Zawalich KC, Ganesan S, et al.: Physiology and pathophysiology of insulin secretion. Diabetes Care 13:655–666, 1990.

14. Ashcroft FM, Harrison DE, Ashcroft SJH. Glucose induces closure of single potassium channels in isolated rat pancreatic β-cells. Nature 312:446, 1984.

15. Robertson RP, Seaquist ER, Walseth TF. G proteins and modulation of insulin secretion. Diabetes 40:1–6, 1990.

16. Meng YX, Wilson GW, Avery MC, et al.: Suppression of the expression of a pancreatic beta cell form of the kinesin heavy chain by antisense oligonucleotides inhibits insulin secretion from primary cultures of mouse beta cells. Endocrinology 138:1979–1987, 1997.

17. Tomlinson S, Walker S, Brown BL: Calmodulin and insulin secretion. Diabetologia 11:1–5, 1982.

18. Given BD, Mako ME, Tager HS, et al.: Diabetes due to secretion of an abnormal insulin. N Engl J Med 302: 129–135, 1980.

19. Make ME, Starr JI, Rubenstein AH: Circulating proinsulin in patients with maturity onset diabetes. Am J Med 63:865–869, 1977.

20. Blackard WG, Nelson NC: Portal vein insulin concentrations in diabetic subjects. Diabetes 20:286–288, 1971.

21. Pfeiffer MA, Halter JB, Porte D, Jr: Insulin secretion in diabetes mellitus. Am J Med 70:579–588, 1981.

22. Halter JB, Graf RJ, Porte D, Jr: Potentiation of insulin secretory responses by plasma glucose levels in man: Evidence that hyperglycemia in diabetes compensates for impaired glucose potentiation. J Clin Endocrinol Metab 48:946–954, 1979.

23. Ganda OP, Srikanta S, Brink SJ, et al.: Differential sensitivity to B-cell secretagogues in "early" type I diabetes mellitus. Diabetes 33:516–521, 1984.

24. Cahill GF, Jr, McDevitt HO: Insulin-dependent diabetes mellitus: the initial lesion. N Engl J Med 304:1454–1465, 1981.

25. Olmos P, A'Hearn R, Heaton DA. et al.: The significance of concordance rate of Type I (insulin dependent) diabetes mellitus in identical twins. Diabetologia 31:747–750, 1988.

26. Ashcroft SJH: Glucoreceptor mechanisms and the control of insulin release and biosynthesis. Diabetologia 18:5–15, 1980.

27. Johnson JH, Ogawa A, Chen L, et al.: Underexpression of β cell high Km glucose transporters in non-insulin dependent diabetes mellitus. Science 250:546–549, 1990.

28. Byrne MM, Sturis J, Clemment K, et al.: Insulin secretory abnormalities in subjects with hyperglycemia due to glucokinase mutations. J Clin Invest 93:1120–1130, 1994.

29. Terauchi Y, Iwamoto K, Tamemoto H, et al.: Development of non-insulin dependent diabetes mellitus in the double knockout mice with disruption of insulin receptor substrate-1 and β cell glucokinase genes. J Clin Invest 99:861–866, 1997.

30. Weir GC: Non-insulin-dependent diabetes mellitus: Interplay between B cell inadequacy and insulin resistance. Am J Med 73:461–464, 1982.

31. Rossetti L, Shulman GI, Zawalich W, et al.: Effect of chronic hyperglycemia on in vivo insulin secretion in partially pancretectomized rats. J Clin Invest 80:1037–1044, 1987.

32. Kosaka K, Kuzuya T, Akanuma Y, Hagura R: Increase in insulin response after treatment of overt maturity-onset diabetes is independent of the mode of treatment. Diabetologia 18:23–28, 1980.

33. Blackard WG, Clore JN, Kellum JM: Amylin/insulin secretory ratios in morbidly obese man: Inverse relationship with glucose disappearance rate. J Clin Endocrinol Metab 78:1257–1260, 1994.

34. Howard CF. Longitudinal studies on the development of diabetes in individual Macaca nigra. Diabetologia 29: 301–306, 1986.

35. Zhou Y-P, Grill VE. Long term exposure of rat pancreatic islets to fatty acids inhibits glucose-induced insulin secretion and biosynthesis through a glucose fatty acid cycle. J Clin Invest 93:870–876, 1994.

36. Lee Y, Hirose H, Zhou Y-T, et al.: Increased lipogenic capacity of the islets of obese rats. Diabetes 46:408–413, 1997.

37. Shimabukuro M, Ohneda M, Lee Y, Unger RH: Role of nitric oxide in obesity-induced β cell disease. J Clin Invest 100:290–295, 1997.

38. Assan R, Perrone C, Assan D, et al.: Pentamidine-induced derangements of glucose homeostasis. Diabetes Care 18:47–55, 1995.

7

Substrate and Hormone Abnormalities in Diabetes Mellitus

John K. Davidson and John B. Mills

Historical Perspective

In 1979, the National Diabetes Data Group recommended that diabetes mellitus be divided into three types: type 1, or insulin-dependent diabetes mellitus (IDDM); type 2, or noninsulin-dependent diabetes mellitus (NIDDM); and gestational diabetes mellitus (GDM).[1,2] Each type is now divided into subtypes. The one *universal characteristic* shared by all types and subtypes of diabetes mellitus is glucose intolerance. Yet not only carbohydrate metabolism, but fat and protein metabolism are disturbed to varying degrees and at different stages in the natural history of IDDM, NIDDM, and GDM, as are hormone (particularly insulin) and enzyme control mechanisms.

The primary objective of this chapter is to review the biochemical aspects of metabolic homeostasis in normal individuals compared with abnormalities of metabolic homeostasis that occur in individuals with diabetes mellitus, and then to relate these abnormalities to the development of the complications of diabetes.

Metabolic Homeostasis in Normal Individuals

The digestion, absorption, storage, and metabolic transformations (of carbohydrate, protein, and fat) and their utilization for energy production, maintenance of body structure, and growth will be considered.[3]

Digestion and Absorption

Substrates are absorbed, usually after enzymatic breakdown, primarily from the small intestine (Fig. 7–1).

Carbohydrates

Starch, sucrose, and lactose are the principal carbohydrates in the human diet. Parotid and pancreatic secretions contain α-amylase, which converts starch to the disaccharides maltose and isomaltose. Brush border disaccharidases (maltase, lactase, sucrase) convert maltose and isomaltose to glucose, lactose to glucose and galactose, and sucrose to glucose and fructose. After digestion, the amount of each monosaccharide in the usual diet in the United Sates is about 80% glucose, about 10% fructose, and about 10% galactose. Glucose and galactose are absorbed by an energy-requiring, sodium-linked transport process and enter the portal circulation; fructose is absorbed by carrier-mediated facilitated diffusion and partially converted by the intestinal cells to glucose before entering the portal circulation.

Proteins

Proteins in the diet are hydrolyzed to amino acids by proteolytic enzymes (pepsin, trypsin, chymotrypsin, among others) in gastric and pancreatic juices and in the brush border of intestinal cells. Amino acids are absorbed by energy-requiring sodium-linked transport processes, at least five in number: (1) for neutral amino acids (such as alanine and valine), (2) for basic amino acids (such as lysine and arginine), (3) for acidic amino acids (such as aspartic and glutamic acids), (4) for glycine and imino acids (such as proline and hydroxyproline), and (5) for β amino acids (such as β alanine and taurine).

Twenty amino acids are required for protein synthesis in humans. Ten cannot be synthesized by the human body and are *essential* components of the diet (arginine, histidine, methionine, valine, isoleucine, threonine, phenylalanine , tryptophan, leucine, and lysine), whereas 10 can be synthesized by the human body and are classified as *nonessential* components of the diet (alanine, asparagine, glutamate, glycine, glutamine, proline, cysteine, serine, aspartate, and tyrosine).

The carbon chain of 18 amino acids can be converted by gluconeogenesis to *glucose* (alanine, asparagine, glutamate, glycine, glutamine, proline, cysteine, serine, aspartate, arginine, histidine, methionine, valine, isoleucine, phenylalanine, threonine, tryptophan, and

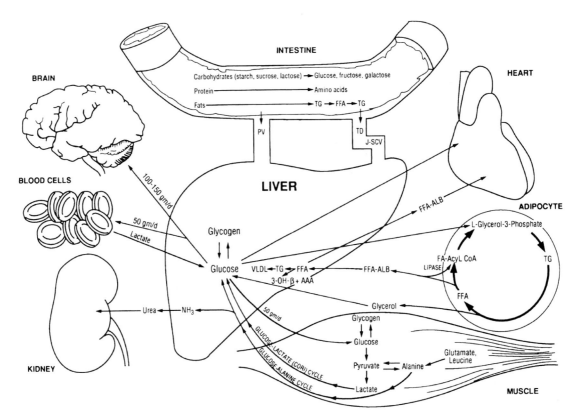

Figure 7–1. This figure illustrates the flow of substrates to and from the major organs involved their metabolic transformations and utilization. *Abbreviations:* PV, portal vein; TD, thoracic duct; J-SCV, jugular and subclavian veins; CO_2, carbon dioxide; NH_3, ammonia; FFA, free fatty acid; TG, triglyceride; FA Acyl Co A, fatty acid acyl CoA; Alb., albumin; β-OHB, beta-hydroxybutyric acid; AAA, acetoacetic acid.

tyrosine), whereas 7 amino acids can be converted to ketones [two (leucine and lysine) to *ketones only* and five (tyrosine, isoleucine, phenylalanine, threonine, tryptophan)] to *ketones and glucose.*

Amino acids from the portal vein are extracted by the liver, except for the branched chain amino acids valine, leucine, and isoleucine, which are extracted preferentially by skeletal muscle.

Fats

Triglycerides are hydrolyzed (by lipases) in the intestine to free fatty acids (FFA), monoglycerides, and glycerol. During absorption, they are resynthesized and coated with protein, and 88% are transported through the thoracic duct to the left jugular and subclavian veins.

Storage

Glucose

Glucose is stored in the liver as glycogen. Glycogen is broken down to glucose as needed to maintain normoglycemia and the amount of glucose needed for oxidation to supply energy (Fig. 7–1).

Amino Acids

Amino acids are not stored in appreciable quantity. Aside from the availability of the intracellular pool of amino acids, small amounts can be derived from circulating amino acids, blood proteins, and structural proteins. Normal protein synthesis depends upon a regular supply of amino acids derived from dietary protein. Surplus amino acids from the diet are soon converted to derivatives of the carbon skeletons and to urea or ammonia.

Fats

When triglyceride globules (chylomicrons) pass through the liver and adipose tissue, they are acted on by lipoprotein lipase present in endothelial cells to produce FFAs. These rapidly enter the liver and adipose cells and rapidly combine with glycerol-3-phosphate to reform the triglycerides for storage. Glucose can be converted to fatty acids and thence to triglycerides through a series of reactions during which acetyl coenzyme A (CoA) and malonyl-CoA residues combine sequentially until synthesis of the fatty acid chain is complete. Some amino acids in excess of need are also converted through acetyl-CoA to FFAs and triglycerides.

Major Metabolic Pathways and Changes During Anaerobic Glycolysis, Fasting, Feeding, and Exercise

Liver, muscle, adipose tissue, blood cells, and brain are the major organs involved in the metabolic transformations of carbohydrates (glucose), proteins (amino acids), and fats (fatty acids). The major metabolic pathways (Fig. 7–2) for glucose are: (1) the *Embden–Meyerhof–Parnas pathway* for glucose and glycogen *formation* (glucosis, gluconeogenesis) and *breakdown* (glycolysis); (2) *the pentose phosphate shunt* (phosphogluconate pathway); (3) the *glucuronic acid shunt* (pentose pathway); (4) *tricarboxylic acid cycle* (TCA or Krebs cycle), whereby acetyl CoA (from pyruvate) enters the TCA cycle to form citrate; and (5) the sorbitol pathway.[3–5] The intermediate acetyl CoA also lies on the pathway leading to fatty acid and triglyceride formation and to ketone (acetoacetate and β-hydroxybutyrate) production.

These pathways are integrated and balanced by substrate shuttles and hormone influences (insulin, glucagon, growth hormone, and catecholamines) to maintain plasma glucose in a narrow range by the normal physiological homeostatic mechanisms of: (1) glycolysis and gluconeogenesis; (2) the interaction of glucose and fructose; (3) changes in production, metabolic transformation, and utilization of glucose *during fasting, after feeding, and during and after exercise*.

Glucose is an obligatory substrate for the brain, and the liver provides 100 to 150 g/day of glucose to supply its energy needs. The liver also provides about 50 g/day to blood cells and 50 g/day to muscle. In turn, pyruvate and lactate (Cori cycle) and alanine (alanine cycle) return from muscle to liver, and glycerol and lactate return from adipose tissue to provide gluconeogenic substrates for the liver. Deaminated amino acids provide ammonia for production of urea, which is excreted by the kidney.

The normal circulating level of lactic acid is 0.4 to 1.4 mM (0.4 to 1.4 mEq/L). *Lactic acidosis* [lactic acid greater than 7 mM (>7 mEq/L)] may develop

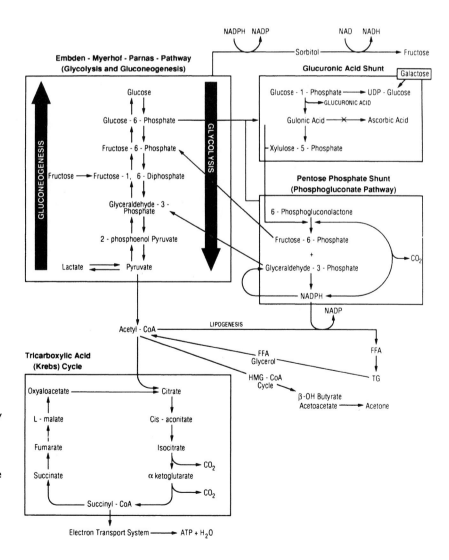

Figure 7–2. This figure illustrates the primary metabolic pathways for carbohydrate, protein, and lipid metabolism. *Abbreviations:* ATP-adenosine triphosphate; Acetyl CoA, acetylated form of coenzyme A; FFA, free fatty acids; TG, triglycerides; HMG-CoA, hydroxymethyl-glutaryl-CoA; NAD, nicotinamide-adenine dinucleotide; NADH, reduced form of nicotinamide-adenine dinucleotide; NADP, nicotinamide-adenine dinucleotide phosphate, NADPH, reduced form of nicotinamide-adenine dinucleotide phosphate; UDP, uridine diphosphate.

secondary to increased *anaerobic* glycolysis *(exercise, cardiogenic shock, hypovolemia, or severe infection)*. The *anti-gluconeogenic effect of ethanol*—a marked increase in the [NADH]/[NAD] ratio (reduced-nicotinamide-adenine dinucleotide to nicotinamide-adenine dinucleotide) incident to the metabolism of ethanol by the enzyme alcohol dehydrogenase with inhibition by NADH of conversion of lactate to pyruvate—may result in lactic acidosis (sometimes combined with ketoacidosis or hypoglycemia, or both). Shortly after excessive ethanol ingestion has ceased and little or no food has been eaten for 12 to 48 hr, excess fat utilization and insufficient gluconeogenesis may result in the development of *alcoholic ketoacidosis* or *alcoholic hypoglycemia.*

When food has not been ingested for 12 hr or more *(the fasted state)*, there is a small decrease in glucose and insulin and a rise in glucagon. Lipolysis, fatty acid oxidation, ketogenesis, and gluconeogenesis increase, and hepatic glucose production is maintained. Liver glycogen stores are depleted within 2 days, and within $2\frac{1}{2}$ days gluconeogenesis accounts for 97% of total hepatic glucose output.

When starvation is prolonged to more than 3 weeks, the rate of glucose utilization and gluconeogenesis are markedly reduced. There are reduced protein catabolism and alanine output by muscle. Ketones become important substrates for brain, and acetone formed by nonenzymatic decarboxylation of acetoacetic acid becomes a gluconeogenic precursor [in liver by conversion of acetone to pyruvaldehyde (methylglyoxal), in extrahepatic tissues by conversion of acetone to 1,2-propanediol].

In *the fed state*, plasma glucose increases; and glucose uptake by liver (glycogen and triglyceride synthesis), muscle (glycogen synthesis), and adipocytes (triglyceride synthesis) increases, keyed to a rise in serum insulin. Although investigators still disagree, it appears that after ingestion of oral glucose by humans, half as much or more is taken up by liver and the rest by peripheral tissues. Glycogen may be produced by one of two pathways (1) *direct* (from glucose), and (2) *indirect* (through pyruvate). Larger doses of glucose favor the direct pathway.

During *exercise*, there is a marked increase in glycogenolysis, glycolysis, gluconeogenesis, and lipolysis to supply energy. With brief exercise, muscle glycogen is the major substrate. When exercise lasts 1 to 2 hr, blood glucose accounts for 40% and FFAs for 60% of the utilized substrates. Glucose utilization by muscle increases up to 40 times the resting level, and glucose turnover may increase fourfold. During very prolonged exercise, fat utilization increases and glucose utilization decreases.

In spite of a decrease in splanchnic blood flow because of the marked increase in muscle blood flow, there is an increase in fractional extraction by the liver of the gluconeogenic precursors lactate and alanine. There is an increase in muscle output of alanine, lactate, and pyruvate and an increase in adipocyte output of glycerol, with a marked increase in hepatic uptake of these substrates for conversion to glucose.

About one third of the individuals who continue to exercise to the point of exhaustion will have a decrease in plasma glucose to less than 45 mg/dL ($<$ 2.5 mmol). During exercise, ingested glucose is absorbed and utilized by muscle.

During and after exercise, glycogen stores of resting muscle may be redistributed to exercising muscle. Presumably an increase in circulating catecholamines stimulates glycogenolysis and lactate production in resting muscle, liver gluconeogenesis increases, and the new glucose enters the muscle undergoing prolonged exercise. During the recovery phase after exercise is completed, the redistribution of glycogen stores from resting muscles to previously exercising muscles continues until a new resting steady state is reached.

Metabolic Pathways and Substrate Transformations

Glucose

Embden–Meyerhof–Parnas Pathway (Glycolysis, Gluconeogenesis). After glucose enters the cell, it is rapidly converted to glucose-6-phosphate. It may then enter the first initial pathway of glucose metabolism, the glycolytic or Embden–Meyerhof–Parnas pathway (liver, brain, muscle, adipose, and other tissues) with conversion to two molecules of pyruvate. Under aerobic conditions, pyruvate enters the mitochondria and is converted via the TCA (Krebs) cycle into carbon dioxide and water. Much of the energy derived from this process is conserved as adenosine triphosphate (ATP). Under energy-rich conditions, much of the glucose-6-phosphate is converted to glycogen, or pyruvate is converted via acetyl-CoA to fatty acids for energy storage (Figs. 7–1, 7–2, and 7–3).

Pentose Phosphate Shunt. A second initial pathway of glucose metabolism *(pentose phosphate shunt or the phosphogluconate pathway)* is present in liver, adrenal cortex, testis, red blood cells, and mammary gland. One of its major functions is to reduce the coenzyme nicotinamide-adenine dinucleotide phosphate (NADP to NADPH), an essential intermediate for the biosynthesis of fatty acids, steroids, and glutathione (to maintain normal structure of red blood cells). This pathway can synthesize and degrade nonhexose sugars (pentoses) that are used for nucleotide and nucleic acid synthesis. It can shorten the glucose chain by one carbon

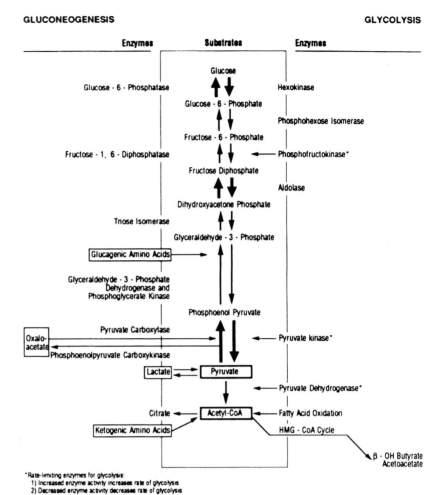

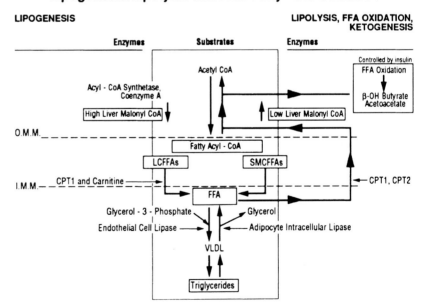

Lipogenesis/Lipolysis and Free Fatty Acid Oxidation

Figure 7–3. This figure illustrates the enzymes that control substrate flow during glycolysis, gluconeogenesis, lipogenesis, and lipolysis and free fatty acid oxidation and ketogenesis. The asterisks (*) represent points where two different enzymes control the flow so that it is directed toward gluconeogenesis or glycolysis so that the cycle does not become *futile* (no net flow in either direction). During lipogenesis, high liver malonyl CoA stimulates CPT1 with long chain FFA transport through the inner mitochondrial membrane and increased VLDL and TG synthesis and storage. Low malonyl CoA and suppressed CPT1 increases fatty acid oxidation and ketogenesis. Insulin secretion is sufficient to restrain ketogenesis during fasting, but it is not sufficient to restrain it during decompensated diabetes and diabetic ketoacidosis results. *Abbreviations:* HMG-CoA, hydroxymethyl glutarate; Acetyl CoA, acetylated form of coenzyme A; O.M.M., outer mitochondrial membrane; I.M.M., inner mitochondrial membrane; CPT1, carnitine palmitoyltransferase 1; CPT2, carnitine palmitoyltransferase 2; LCFFAs, long chain fatty acids; S,MCFFAs, short and medium chain free fatty acids; FFA, free fatty acids; VLDL, very low density lipoproteins.

(converting six glucose molecules to six molecules of ribulose-5-phosphate and six molecules of carbon dioxide). The six molecules of ribulose-5-phosphate can then be rearranged to form five molecules of glucose-6-phosphate, which can be recycled through the pentose phosphate shunt or metabolized through the glycolytic pathway.

Glucuronic Acid Shunt. A third initial pathway of glucose metabolism (glucuronic acid shunt) furnishes *glucuronic acid* for conjugation of bilirubin, adrenocortical hormones, and ingested drugs. Glucuronic acid is also converted to gulonic acid which, in turn, is converted to ascorbic acid. The enzyme that catalyzes this conversion is present in most plants and animals, but is absent in humans, primates, and guinea pigs. These animals must ingest preformed ascorbic acid to prevent scurvy.

Sorbitol Pathway. A fourth initial route of glucose metabolism (sorbitol pathway), a minor pathway when plasma glucose levels are normal, becomes a major pathway in the presence of diabetes mellitus and hyperglycemia (Fig. 7–4).

The Tricarboxylic Acid or Krebs Cycle. Under *aerobic conditions*, pyruvate is the end product of glycolysis in most cells. It is moved from the cytosol into mitochondria, where it is oxidatively decarboxylated with formation of acetyl CoA; then the carbon atoms of the acetyl CoA are oxidized in the TCA cycle to carbon dioxide. There is a close association in mitochondria between the *oxidative phosphorylation system* (to produce ATP) and the *electron transport system* (using the coenzymes NAD^+ and flavin-adenine dinucleotide (FAD) to produce hydrogen transfer by the enzymes isocitrate dehydrogenase, α-ketoglutarate dehydrogenase, malate dehydrogenase, and succinate dehydrogenase). The reduced coenzymes are then reoxidized through the electron transport system for oxidative phosphorylation and production of ATP. Thus, acetyl-CoA can form from pyruvate through the pyruvate dehydrogenase system, or through the β-oxidation pathway of fatty acids, and combine with oxaloacetate to enter the TCA as citrate. After one turn of the cycle, oxaloacetate is regenerated and is ready to accept another acetyl CoA.

The TCA cycle also has connections to amino acid metabolism. At the level of the pyruvate dehydrogenase reaction, pyruvate formed from transamination of alanine, and α-ketoglutarate formed from glutamate, and oxaloacetate formed from aspartate can enter the TCA cycle. Many other amino acids can convert their carbon chains to α-ketoglutarate, pyruvate, succinate, malate, fumarate, and acetyl CoA, and these in turn can enter the TCA cycle to be utilized for energy production.

Amino Acids

When more amino acids than are needed for protein synthesis are ingested, *glucogenic amino acids* are converted to glucose and glycogen. The metabolites of the glucogenic amino acids that enter the glycogenic (glucogenic) pathway are converted to pyruvate and perhaps to acetyl CoA. Acetyl CoA formed from glucogenic and ketogenic amino acids may be used for fatty acid synthesis or may be converted to energy in the TCA cycle.

Fats

When triglycerides are hydrolyzed, glycerol and fatty acids are formed. Glycerol can be used in the liver for glucose synthesis or metabolized to pyruvate and converted to acetyl CoA. At the outer mitochondrial membrane, *fatty acids* are converted by the enzyme acyl-CoA synthetase and the factor coenzyme A to fatty acyl-CoA.

Coenzyme A derivatives of long chain fatty acids (such as oleic acid) are unable to penetrate the inner mitochondrial membrane unless esterified with carnitine, a process catalyzed by the enzyme *carnitine palmitoyltransferase 1 (CPT1)*. Inside the mitochondrial membrane, the *long chain fatty acid is resynthesized* by the reverse process, which is catalyzed by *carnitine palmitoyltransferase 2 (CPT2)*.[6]

Medium chain fatty acids (such as octanoate) penetrate the inner mitochondrial membrane freely and have no need for esterification to carnitine.

The first specific step in fatty acid oxidation, which is catalyzed by the CPT enzyme system, is the primary regulator of fatty acid oxidation, which in excess leads to ketosis. The *controlling intermediate is malonyl CoA*, the primary substrate for long chain fatty acid synthesis. *Malonyl CoA* is derived from citrate and *inhibits CPT1 but not CPT2*. Thus CPT1 represents a pivotal site in the regulation of fatty acid metabolism.

In normal individuals, ingestion of carbohydrate (or of a mixed meal) results in elevated insulin and lowered glucagon levels, elevated liver malonyl CoA levels, brisk fatty acid synthesis and a block of fatty acid oxidation. Thus, in the *fed* state, the concentration of malonyl CoA can be viewed as the physiological mechanism for ensuring *unidirectional flow* of carbon from glucose and other pyruvate precursors into long chain fatty acids, triglycerides, and very low density lipoproteins by suppression of the activity of CPT1.

During *fasting* and in *uncontrolled diabetes*, insulin is lowered and glucagon elevated.[7-9] Malonyl-CoA synthesis falls, lipogenesis slows, CPT1 is activated, and

I. GLYCATION OF PROTEINS

Non-Enzymatic

Process:

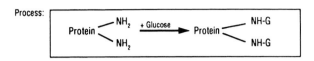

Enzymatic

Process:

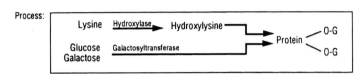

Proteins Affected: Hemoglobin, albumin, fibrinogen, low-density lipoproteins, basement membrane proteins, transferrin, α - 2 - macroglobulin, neural proteins, type IV collagen

Chronic Complications: Microangiopathy (retinopathy, nephropathy), macroangiopathy (capillary closure, accelerated atherogenesis) and neuropathy (see below).

II. SORBITOL SYNTHESIS AND ACCUMULATION

Process:

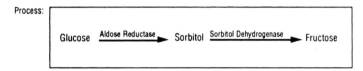

Effects: Glucose, sorbitol and fructose accumulate in the cell. Water uptake increases to satisfy Donnan Equilibrium, and increased osmolality disrupts the cell with leakage of myolnositol, amino acids, and ATP, which results in cell death.

Chronic Complications: Cataracts, neuropathy (peripheral, autonomic, cranial)

Figure 7–4. Proteins can be glycated as a result of nonenzymatic or enzymatic biochemical processes resulting from hyperglycemia (see Chapters 13 and 23). Hyperglycemia also results in excess sorbitol synthesis and accumulation in nerve and ocular lens cells, and contributes to blood vessel damage. Increased platelet agglutination and aggregation in uncontrolled diabetes mellitus contribute to the development of blood clots, capillary closure, and accelerated atherogenesis.

III. PLATELET AGGREGATION AND AGGLUTINATION

Process: Increased sensitivity of platelets from those with uncontrolled diabetes to a variety of aggregating agents (thromboxane, an arachidonic acid metabolite) and other non-thromboxane pathways. Platelet-plasma interactions (with Von Willebrand Factor, fibrinogen, immune complexes, glycated low-density lipoprotein) contribute.

Chronic Complications: Along with other risk factors, increased platelet aggregation and agglutination secondary to diabetes contribute to formation of blood clots, capillary closure, and accelerated atherogenesis.

tissue carnitine rises. The low insulin level increases adipocyte lipolysis by increased intracellular lipase activity. The increased amount of FFA substrate available to the liver results in a *fall in malonyl-CoA* levels and an increase in *FFA oxidation*, which is *the primary cause of all ketotic states.*

Rates of ketone utilization are not without limit (see Chapter 24), with the maximal disposal rate of 2.3 mmol/min/1.73 m² being attained at plasma levels of 10 to 12 mM, the highest levels attained during prolonged fasting in nondiabetics. The *insulin deficit* during *diabetic ketoacidosis* is responsible for even *higher levels of*

FFA oxidation and *ketone production*. Because there is no evidence of a ketone body removal defect in diabetes, it is now clear that *unrestrained (by insulin) ketone body overproduction* is the main factor leading to the uncontrolled hyperketonemia of diabetic ketoacidosis.[8,9]

Relationships Between Carbohydrate and Fat Metabolism

In normal fasting subjects, increased glucose production by the liver, plus a small increase by the kidneys, and decreased glucose oxidation by skeletal and cardiac muscles permit an adequate glucose supply to the brain even when liver glycogen is depleted.

Fat and carbohydrate metabolism converge in the *shared intermediate acetyl CoA* (Figs. 7–2 and 7–3). This, plus the effects of intermediates of one pathway on the enzymatic reactions in other pathways, result in several regulatory relationships between the *effects of augmented carbohydrate utilization on fat metabolism* and *the effects of augmented fat metabolism on carbohydrate utilization.*

After a meal containing carbohydrate, glucose utilization is increased, and FFA release is decreased because increased glycerol-3-phosphate is available for reesterification of FFAs. Also, the rise in plasma glucose stimulates insulin secretion, which suppresses the hormone-sensitive lipase in adipocytes. The rate-limiting enzyme for fat biosynthesis, *acetyl CoA carboxylase*, is induced by carbohydrate feeding. An increased availability of citrate (an activator of the enzyme) and a decrease in fatty acyl-CoA esters (inhibitors of the enzyme) plus utilization of glucose in the pentose phosphate shunt with increased production of NADPH, and increased plasma insulin levels, promote increased synthesis of fatty acids and triglycerides. Fatty acid oxidation and ketogenesis are reduced by the decreased levels of FFAs available and by the decreased activity of the enzyme carnitine acyltransferase.

The interaction between FFA and glucose metabolism is regulated by (1) *the glucose-fatty acid cycle* (interaction between adipocytes and muscle),[10] and (2) *stimulation of gluconeogenesis by FFA oxidation* (interaction between adipocytes and liver).

The *glucose-fatty acid cycle* was first described in heart muscle,[10] but more recently has been shown to be active in skeletal muscle.[11] When insulin is deficient, lipolysis is accelerated in muscle and adipose tissue. Muscle metabolizes FFA to form acetyl CoA and ATP, and these inhibit glycolysis by decreasing the activity of *phosphofructokinase, pyruvate kinase, and pyruvate dehydrogenase.* The last enzyme metabolizes pyruvate to acetyl CoA. The decrease in phosphofructokinase increases glucose-6-phosphate, which decreases glucose transport into the muscle cell. All of these effects are reversed by sufficient insulin and decreased lipolysis. Thus, glycolysis can proceed at a much greater rate.

In addition to the *inhibiting effects* of the *glucose-fatty acid cycle* on *muscle glucose metabolism, gluconeogenesis in liver* and *kidney* is *stimulated* by FFAs. A number of mechanisms to account for this stimulation have been proposed:[3] (1) oxidation of FFA by the liver results in increased ATP levels, and this high-energy phosphate bond donor provides the energy for gluconeogenesis; (2) the increase in ATP and concomitant decrease in adenosine monophosphate (AMP) results in increased activity of *fructose 1,6-diphosphatase* (which is one of the rate-limiting enzymes for gluconeogenesis); (3) FFA oxidation increases *pyruvate carboxylase* activity (another rate-limiting enzyme for gluconeogenesis); (4) increased acetyl CoA results in increased citrate formation, and thus increases the activity of *fructose-1,6-diphosphatase* [a rate-limiting enzyme for gluconeogenesis, see (2) above]; (5) the increased acetyl CoA decreases the activity of pyruvate dehydrogenase (an important enzyme that transforms pyruvate to acetyl CoA), and this makes a larger amount of pyruvate available to serve as a glucose precursor during gluconeogenesis; and (6) as previously noted, the intermediate *malonyl CoA* and the *CPT enzyme system* are pivotal regulators of FFA metabolism.[6]

The net effect of the glucose-fatty acid cycle in suppressing glucose utilization by muscle and the increase in gluconeogenesis by FFA utilization in liver and kidney increases glucose levels, which can terminate in significant hyperglycemia and eventually ketosis unless enough insulin (either endogenously produced or injected) is present to return the plasma glucose to normal levels.[12,13]

Utilization of Substrates for Energy Production, Maintenance of Body Structure, and Growth

Utilization of Substrates for Energy Production

Glycolysis is a pathway of special significance for production of ATP, the most widely used form of biologic energy. It is utilized by the human body for heat production, chemical and electrochemical processes, and to provide energy for muscular work and exercise.

When one molecule of glucose is transformed through glycolysis to two molecules of pyruvate, eight ATPs are formed. When the two molecules of pyruvate are transformed to six molecules of carbon dioxide and six molecules of water in the TCA cycle, 30 ATPs are formed. Thus, 38 ATPs are formed from one molecule of glucose.

In contrast, one molecule of fatty acid palmitic acid by β oxidation results in the formation of 129 ATPs. The remaining eight molecules of acetyl CoA are then oxidized in the TCA cycle.

Utilization of Substrates for Maintenance of Body Structure and Growth

Insulin is an anabolic hormone[14] that stimulates protein synthesis and limits protein breakdown; it also promotes wound healing. When nitrogen balance is negative (more excreted than ingested), protein degradation exceeds protein synthesis and the protein component of body structure is not maintained (muscle wasting, and so on). This is likely to occur in uncontrolled diabetes mellitus. Appropriate age- and sex-related body growth *before 20 years*, when growth is completed, requires a positive nitrogen balance and adequate protein synthesis. Carbohydrates and lipids participate to a less extent in maintenance of normal body structure and growth, again under the anabolic influence of insulin and of growth hormone. When uncontrolled diabetes is present, normal body growth does not occur, and in the adult there is a net loss of tissue protein.[15]

Hormone Control of Substrate Metabolism in Normal Individuals

During the *fed state*, increased secretion of insulin promotes *anabolism* of metabolites with storage in liver, muscle, and adipose tissue. During the *fasted state*, insulin secretion decreases and stored substrates (glycogen, triglycerides, and proteins) are mobilized in a *controlled catabolic fashion* (by increased secretion of glucagon, epinephrine, growth hormone, and cortisol) to maintain normoglycemia and to provide glucose and fatty acids for oxidation to produce energy.[7,16]

The normal human pancreas contains about 7 mg (200 U) of insulin. It is estimated that the normal amount secreted each day by the normal adult pancreas is in the range of 30 to 60 U (about 1 to 2 mg/day), and that the basal secretion rate is 0.5 to 1.0 U hr, with an additional secretion of about 5 to 10 U after feeding. The normal peripheral plasma insulin is 60 to 150 pM/mL (10 to 25 μU/mL); 0.5 to 1.5 hr after a meal, it rises to 180 to 600 pM/mL (30 to 100 μU/mL). *Hepatic glucose production* is half-maximally suppressed at 180 pM/mL (30 μU/mL), and is essentially totally suppressed at 600 pM/mL (100 μU/mL). *Peripheral glu-cose utilization* is half-maximal at 420 pM/mL (70 μU/mL), and maximal at 3,000 pM/mL (500 μU/mL). When *portal venous plasma insulin* levels reach 600 pM/mL (100 μU/mL), hepatic glucose output ceases because of the marked sensitivity of the liver to insulin.

Normal peripheral serum C-peptide levels are: fasting, 0.4 to 1.6 pM/mL (1.2 to 4.8 ng/mL); Sustacal- or glucagon-stimulated 0.4 to 12 pM/mL (1.2 to 36 ng/mL).

There is a prompt *first phase of insulin secretion* (within 10 min) in normals and a continuing *second phase* insulin secretion in response to a glucose load so that glucose tolerance remains normal (see Chapter 12).

As previously noted, during fasting insulin secretion continues at a rate sufficient to sustain normoglycemia during *stimulation of substrate release* by the contrainsulin hormones *glucagon, epinephrine, growth hormone, and cortisol.*

Failure of Metabolic Homeostasis in Diabetes Mellitus

At different times in the last half-century, attempts have been made to identify *single metabolic points* where insulin may act and account completely for the biochemical and pathophysiological problems presented by diabetes mellitus. *Hypotheses* have included: (1) inadequate transport of glucose into insulin-dependent tissues; (2) inadequate phosphorylation of glucose; (3) inability of glucose metabolism to generate adequate reducing power; (4) less than normally permeable basement membranes that prevent quick and adequate insulin secretion; (5) imbalance in insulin or glucagon secretion, and (6) an inadequate number or function of insulin receptors on insulin-sensitive cells.[5]

Although subsequent research has confirmed that there is a modicum of truth in several of these hypotheses, none explains more than a fraction of the metabolic abnormalities of diabetes. At the present time, hypotheses related to *insulin–receptor interaction, increased protein kinase activity,* and *"post-receptor"* actions of insulin are being considered.[16]

In NIDDM, *hepatic glucose production increases.*[12,13] Peripheral tissues take up glucose inefficiently because of down-regulated insulin receptors, inadequate insulin production and a *postreceptor defect* in cellular insulin action.

The pancreas of those with NIDDM at diagnosis contains about half the normal amount of insulin (100 U rather than 200 as in normals), although there may be great *variation between individuals* and at different times during the natural history of the disease. The nature of the islet cell problem in NIDDM is not understood (see

Chapter 6), but about 2% per year (despite weight loss to ideal body weight) of those diagnosed as NIDDM progress to insulin dependence and could for therapeutic purposes be reclassified as IDDMs.

The pancreas of those with IDDM usually contains less than 10% (less than 20 U) of the normal amount of insulin, and serum insulin levels are markedly reduced.

In addition to *primary changes* that occur in *carbohydrate, protein, and fat* metabolism related to inadequate insulin production by pancreatic beta cells, *secondary changes* (not dependent on insulin but dependent on the *hyperglycemia* of the diabetic state) occur (Fig. 7–4). These effects of hyperglycemia include: (1) non enzymatic *glucosylation* (previously designated *glycosylation*) of hemoglobin, albumin, lipoprotein, collagens, and basement membrane proteins;[17] (2) enzymatic glycoprotein synthesis; (3) increased functioning of the polyol (sorbitol) pathway with eye, nervous system, and kidney injury;[18] and (4) platelet aggregation and agglutination.[19] These secondary changes are thought now to account for much of the pathophysiology that underlies the development of the most important chronic complications of the disease.

Most diabetologists now accept the hypothesis that prolonged exposure to hyperglycemia is the primary causal factor for the complications. Although this statement must be immediately qualified by the caveat that genetic polymorphism, hypertension, hyperlipidemia, obesity, and smoking contribute significantly to the development and progression of vascular disease with its attendant morbidity and mortality in different individuals.

The pathophysiology and clinical manifestations of complications of diabetes reflect both *acute, insulin-reversible, and chronic, insulin-irreversible* problems.[17] *Insulin-reversible abnormalities include:* (1) increased polyol pathway; (2) increased protein kinase C activity in insulin-sensitive cells; (3) increased formation of early glycated products on proteins in plasma, matrix, and cells; and (4) increased hydrostatic pressure in the microcirculation. These insulin-reversible abnormalities (with persistent normoglycemia) are associated with increased vascular permeability, protein leakage, and extracellular matrix production. *Long-term hyperglycemia-induced insulin irreversible abnormalities* involve retinal and glomerular vessels, endoneurial microvessels, and coronary arteries, and include: (1) expanded extracellular matrix, (2) extravasated plasma protein deposits, and (3) cellular hypertrophy or hyperplasia. These problems cause progressive vessel narrowing and inadequate tissue perfusion.

The Diabetes Control and Complications Trial Research Group has concluded that IDDM intensive insulin therapy, with a view to maintaining glucose within normal limits at all times, is effective in preventing or delaying the onset of complications.[20]

An Overview of Contemporary Understanding of Substrate and Hormone Abnormalities in NIDDM, GDM, and IDDM

The primary changes in carbohydrate, fat, and protein metabolism that occur in diabetes have been noted earlier. They are: (1) hyperglycemia due to increased glucose production by the liver, (2) increased gluconeogenesis, (3) increased lipolysis, (4) preferential use of FFAs as an energy source, and (5) increased ketone production. Protein and fat catabolism accelerate, and this can lead to a negative nitrogen balance, hyperlipidemia, ketosis, and when far advanced, to diabetic ketoacidosis and death. All of these abnormalities will revert to normal with appropriate insulin therapy.

Resistance to insulin is a prominent feature of NIDDM.[21] Overweight increases insulin resistance, and more than 90% of those with NIDDM are overweight (see Chapter 2). Loss of excess adipose tissue by a short-term fast plus follow-up on a very low-calorie lactovegetarian diet (500 to 1000 cal) can return fasting and postprandial plasma glucose and lipid levels to normal in many individuals. This diet approach with weight loss, plus appropriate exercise when not contraindicated, is now accepted as the cornerstone of therapy for overweight NIDDMs.[22]

GDM may be viewed as NIDDM waiting to happen when the stress of weight gain of pregnancy, frequently superimposed on preexisting overweight, occurs. Glucose intolerance usually develops during the second trimester, and the metabolic abnormalities previously noted develop.

About 95% of those with GDM go into remission after delivery (normal glucose tolerance test), but about half of those followed up for 15 years develop symptomatic diabetes.

IDDM develops in the wake of pancreatic islet β-cell destruction secondary to a viral infection or an autoimmune process or both. Insulin content of the pancreas is only 5 to 10% of normal at diagnosis. Serum C-peptide levels may be undetectable in those with IDDM. The Diabetes Control and Complications Trial required for a diagnosis of IDDM a fasting C-peptide level <0.2 pM/mL (<0.6 ng/mL) and a 90-min Sustacal-stimulated level less than 0.5 pM/mL (<1.5 ng/mL); 0.33 pM (1 ng/mL) fasting and 0.5 pM (1.5 ng/mL) after glucagon stimulation have been suggested as the cut-points to distinguish NIDDM from IDDM.[15]

Frequently, especially when initially hyperglycemic, NIDDMs may have a fasting serum C-peptide as high or higher than 1.0 pM (>3.0 ng)/mL. Whenever the fasting level is more than 0.33 pM (1 ng/mL), the possibility that the patient may have NIDDM rather than IDDM should be considered. If such an individual is not in ketosis and is overweight, a trial of diet therapy with weight loss may be initiated.

In inadequately controlled diabetes mellitus and in other stressful states, glucagon, epinephrine, cortisol, and growth hormone levels increase, and the contrainsulin actions of each can reinforce the actions of the others.

In normals after feeding, an increase in plasma glucose and insulin secretion with a reciprocal decrease in glucagon secretion results in decreased glucose production by the liver and increased glucose utilization. In those with diabetes, a sufficient increase in insulin secretion is not possible, and hyperglycemia results. Inappropriately elevated glucagon levels occur in diabetes, and this promotes hepatic ketogenesis by increasing FFA oxidation through activation of the mitochondrial transport process.[6] During suppression of glucagon secretion by somatostatin, neither severe hyperglycemia or hyperketonemia develop in those with IDDM.

Epinephrine increases hepatic glucose production and lipolysis, impairs glucose uptake, and decreases insulin secretion.

Cortisol maintains key enzymes important to lipolysis, gluconeogenesis, and glycogen formation. Excess cortisol impairs the ability of insulin to stimulate glucose utilization and suppresses glucose production.

Growth hormone promotes growth by stimulating secretion of insulin-like growth factors I and II. It is also involved in maintaining metabolic homeostasis. When it is deficient, individuals are particularly sensitive to the hypoglycemic effects of insulin. Individuals who produce excess growth hormone (acromegaly) are insulin resistant. Excess growth hormone impairs the ability of insulin to stimulate glucose utilization and to suppress glucose production.

There are multiple defects in glucose counter regulation in those with long-standing diabetes. The plasma glucagon response to hypoglycemia is blunted, leaving those with diabetes dependent on epinephrine secretion. Those who have autonomic neuropathy fail to detect impending hypoglycemia (*hypoglycemic unawareness*) and also lose the metabolic effects of epinephrine. In some individuals, secretion of growth hormone or cortisol is impaired.

In insulin-treated patients, hyperglycemia may occur from: (1) waning of insulin action, (2) following hypoglycemia with an unopposed counter regulatory hormone response (Somogyi effect), or (3) the dawn phenomenon (early morning hyperglycemia), which occurs in IDDM and NIDDM.[7]

Conclusion

It is a common experience for otherwise knowledgeable clinicians to become frustrated because they do not understand all of the minutiae of biochemical and hormonal abnormalities of the different types of diabetes. It is reassuring, in reviewing the history of our understanding of the etiology, pathogenesis, and treatment of diabetes and its complications, to recognize that many favored hypotheses of the past have been discarded as being inadequate or incorrect, while others have been shown to be correct. Many hypotheses are now being tested, as most chapters in this book reveal. How many of them will be shown to be correct and clinically useful is yet to be determined. To prevent or delay the appearance and progression of the acute and chronic complications of diabetes, it is prudent to diagnose diabetes early, to classify it correctly, and to use appropriate therapy—diet and exercise and insulin, if needed, to attain and maintain normoglycemia and ideal body weight. Research, on a broad front, continues to explore the substrate and hormone defects and their etiology, pathogenesis, and consequences that characterize the disease.

References

1. National Institutes of Health Diabetes Data Group: Classification and diagnosis of diabetes mellitus and other categories of glucose intolerance. Diabetes 28: 1039–1057, 1979.
2. Harris MI: Screening for undiagnosed non-insulin-dependent diabetes. *In* Alberti KGMM, Mazze RM (eds): Frontiers in Diabetes Research: Current Trends in Non-insulin-Dependent Diabetes Mellitus. International Congress Series 859. Amsterdam: Excerpta Medica, 1989, pp. 119–131.
3. Feldman JM: Pathophysiology of diabetes mellitus. *In* Galloway JA, Potvin JH, Shuman CR (eds): Diabetes Mellitus. Indianapolis: Lilly Research Laboratories, 1988, pp. 17–44.
4. Felig P: Integrated physiology of carbohydrate metabolism. *In* Rifkin H, Porte D (eds): Diabetes Mellitus, Theory and Practice. Amsterdam: Elsevier, 1990, pp. 51–60.
5. Seifter S, England S: Carbohydrate metabolism. *In* Rifkin H, Porte D (eds): Diabetes Mellitus: Theory and Practice. Amsterdam: Elsevier, 1990, pp. 1–40.

6. McGarry JD, Foster DW: Ketogenesis. *In* Rifkin H, Porte D (eds): Diabetes Mellitus: Theory and Practice. Amsterdam: Elsevier, 1990, pp. 292–298.

7. Gerich JE: Hormonal control of homeostasis. *In* Galloway JA, Potvin JH, Shuman CR (eds): Diabetes Mellitus, Indianapolis: Lilly Research Laboratories, 1988, pp. 45–64.

8. Miles JM, Rizza RA, Haymond MW, Gerich JE: Effects of acute insulin deficiency on glucose and ketone body turnover in man: Evidence for the primacy of overproduction of glucose and ketone bodies in the genesis of diabetic ketoacidosis. Diabetes 29:926–930, 1980.

9. Fery F, Balasse EO: Ketone body production and disposal in diabetic ketosis: A comparison with fasting ketosis: Diabetes 34:326–332, 1985.

10. Randle PJ, Hales CN, Garland PB, Newsholme EA: The glucose-fatty acid cycle: Its role in insulin sensitivity and the metabolic disturbances of diabetes mellitus. Lancet 1:7285–7289, 1963.

11. Maizel EZ, Ruderman NB, Goodman MN, Lau D: Effect of acetoacetate on glucose metabolism in the soleus and extensor digitorium longus muscles of the rat. Biochem J 162:557–568, 1977.

12. DeFronzo RA, Ferrannini E: Regulation of hepatic glucose metabolism in humans. Diabetes Metab Rev 3:415–459, 1987.

13. Kahn SE, Porte D: Pathophysiology of type II (non-insulin-dependent) diabetes mellitus: Implications for treatment. *In* Rifkin H, Porte D (eds): Diabetes Mellitus: Theory and Practice. Amsterdam: Elsevier, 1990, pp. 436–456.

14. Galloway JA: Chemistry and clinical use of insulin. *In* Galloway JA, Potvin JH, Shuman CR (eds): Diabetes Mellitus, Indianapolis: Lilly Research Laboratories, 1988, pp. 105–138.

15. Nair KS, Schwenk WF: Protein metabolism in diabetes mellitus. *In* Marshall SM, Home PD, Rizza RA (eds): Diabetes Annual. Amsterdam: Elsevier, 1995, pp. 159–174.

16. Kitabchi AE, Duckworth WC, Stentz FB: Insulin synthesis; proinsulin and c-peptides. *In* Rifkin H, Porte D (eds): Diabetes Mellitus: Theory and Practice. Amsterdam: Elsevier, 1990, pp. 71–87.

17. Brownlee M: Advanced products of nonenzymatic glycosylation and the pathogenesis of diabetic complications. *In* Rifkin H, Porte D (eds): Diabetes Mellitus: Theory and Practice. Amsterdam: Elsevier, 1990, pp. 279–291.

18. Kinoshita JH, Datiles MB, Kador PF, Robison WG: Aldose reductase and diabetic eye complications. *In* Rifkin H, Porte D (eds): Diabetes Mellitus: Theory and Practice. Amsterdam: Elsevier, 1990, pp. 264–278.

19. Colwell JA: Antiplatelet drugs and the prevention of progression of macrovascular disease in diabetes mellitus. *In* Alberti KGMM, Mazze RM (eds): Frontiers in Diabetes Research: Current Trends in Non-Insulin-Dependent Diabetes Mellitus. International Congress Series 859. Amsterdam: Excerpta Medica, 1989, pp. 193–206.

20. The Diabetes Control and Complications Trial Research Group: The effect of intensive treatment of diabetes on the development and progression of long-term complications in insulin-dependent diabetes mellitus: N Engl J Med 329: 977–986, 1993.

21. Reaven GM: Insulin resistance abnormal free fatty acid metabolism, and fasting hyperglycemia in patients with non-insulin-dependent diabetes mellitus. *In* Alberti KGMM, Mazze RM (eds): Frontiers in Diabetes Research: Current Trends in Non-Insulin-Dependent Diabetes Mellitus. International Congress Series 859. Amsterdam: Excerpta Medica, 1989, pp. 167–176.

22. National Institutes of Health Consensus Development Conference Statement: On diet and exercise in non-insulin-dependent diabetes mellitus. Diabetes Care 10:639–644, 1987.

8

Insulin Interaction with Its Specific Receptor on Target Cells

George Grunberger and Jesse Roth

As a first approximation, all the cells of an organism are exposed to equal concentrations of the various hormones. Thus, a mechanism is needed to provide specificity for intercellular communication (Fig. 8–1). The target cell receptor ensures recognition of a particular hormone from among all other substances encountered by the cell. The two molecular entities, hormone and receptor, join together physically. In a way, they also provide a point for joining the informational resources of the secretory cell with the biochemical resources of the target cell. (Figuratively, the target cell can do everything but does not know when or how much, while the secretory cell knows what needs to be done but cannot do anything except tell the target cell what to do.)

The recognition of the hormone by the receptor is manifested by binding. The product of this union—a hormone-receptor complex—initiates activation of the biochemical processes leading eventually to the various metabolic events that we associate with insulin action. In the case of insulin, these include transport of glucose, amino acids, and ions; stimulation of synthesis (as well as inhibition of breakdown) of glycogen, fat, and protein; and glucose oxidation.

Clearly, both the hormone (or, more generally, the ligand) and the receptor are essential for hormone action, and a deficiency or absence of either leads to serious problems. However, an important scientific question is whether the information provided to the target cell by the hormone-receptor complex resides in the ligand, the receptor, or the complex (Exhibit 8–1). Examples of each of these possibilities have been encountered in various biological systems. For most hormones, neurotransmitters, and other mediators of intercellular communication, it is the receptor, rather than the ligand, that contains the full program for activation of the hormone-sensitive pathways. How was it determined that the receptor contains all essential information for transmitting hormone action? For insulin, this conclusion was derived from studies of antibodies against the

receptor for insulin (produced "spontaneously" by some patients with autoimmune disorders[1]). These antibodies not only block binding of insulin to its receptor but also, *in the absence of insulin*, stimulate biochemical events that are typical of insulin action, including transport of glucose and amino acids, activation of glycogen synthase and pyruvate dehydrogenase, deactivation of phosphorylase, and increased synthesis of lipoprotein lipase. In addition, lectins, a group of plant proteins, are capable of binding to the insulin receptor and in the process generate the insulinlike programs. Thus it was the observations that ligands of diverse structure other than insulin can bind to receptor and also activate the target cell that suggested that it was the receptor rather than the ligand that contained all the information necessary for activation of the cell.

As noted, there are two fundamental events associated with interactions of hormones with their receptors (Exhibit 8–2). The receptor first recognizes and binds the hormone, and secondly, by binding of hormone, the information contained in the receptor is activated, which turns on events in the target cell. In addition, the hormone-receptor complex often serves other functions: as a reservoir for plasma hormone, regulator of receptor concentration and affinity, promoter of hormone and receptor internalization, regulator of postreceptor events, and other regulatory roles.

Historical Perspective

Hormones versus Receptors

Hormones and receptors were both conceptualized at the turn of the 20th century. Rapid progress occurred with the studies of hormones, but only the last quarter of the century has brought some depth to our understanding of receptor structure and function. Several factors have been responsible for this discrepancy in progress of our knowledge (Table 8–1).

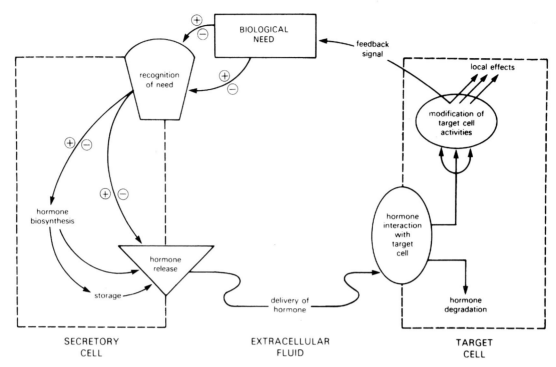

Figure 8–1. Overall scheme of an endocrine system. The keystone of an endocrine system is a biological need. Recognition of the need is carried out by a sensing or signaling system that often (although not always) is in the secretary cell itself. Often several needs are expressed through one type of endocrine secretory cell (e.g., plasma glucose, amino acids, fatty acids, and ketones regulate insulin secretion), and a single need may be expressed through multiple types of hormone-secreting cells (e.g., glucose regulates insulin, glucagon, GLP-1, and growth hormone). The sensing and signaling system, in recognizing the biological need, sends signals to stimulate or inhibit release of the hormone. Often there are several sensing systems and their multiple signals are integrated within the secretory cell. In addition, there may be independent signals to regulate hormone biosynthesis (and storage). Hormone, released into blood or extracellular fluid, is delivered to target cell and acts as the intercellular messenger from secretory cell to target cell. Hormone interaction with elements of the target cell leads to modification of cellular processes that are already present in the target cell. Most hormones produce a multiplicity of effects in any single target cell, only a minority of which are recognized outside the target cell (as feedback signals) to announce that the biological need has been met. Often hormone interaction with the target cell may lead to hormone degradation. Typically, defects on the left half of the illustration are lumped together as defects in hormone secretion, and defects on the right are grouped as target cell defects. From Roth J, Grunfeld C: Endocrine systems: Mechanisms of disease, target cells, and receptors. In Williams RH (ed): Textbook of Endocrinology, Ed. 6. Philadelphia: W.B. Saunders, 1981, pp. 15–74; with permission.

EXHIBIT 8–1 Information Transfer

I. Insulin and receptor ←/→ insulin-receptor complex → activation of target cell processes
II. Where is the information for activation? Insulin? Receptor? Both?
III. Classification
    A. Receptor has the information; hormone (or other ligand) only activates the program intrinsic to the receptor.
        1. Insulin receptor
        2. TSH receptor
        3. Acetylcholine receptor
        4. IgE receptor

    B. Ligand has the essential item; receptor serves to concentrate, process, or translate the ligand to intracellular site.
        1. Cholera toxin and *Escherichia coli* toxin (ADP-ribosylating enzymes)
        2. Low-density lipoproteins (cholesterol delivery)
        3. Transferrin (iron delivery)
        4. Viruses (nucleic acid delivery)
    C. Receptor and ligand both contribute information for cell activation.
        1. Egg and sperm
        2. Other cell-cell recognition systems

Abbreviations: ADP, adenosine diphosphate; IgE, immunoglobulin E; TSH, thyroid-stimulating hormone.

EXHIBIT 8–2   Function of the Hormone-Receptor Complex

Fundamental
    Recognition (binding)
    Activation (coupling)
Other
    Reservoir for plasma insulin
    Regulator of target cell sensitivity
    Regulator of receptor concentration and affinity
    Regulator of hormone degradation
    Regulator of receptor degradation
    Regulator of receptor internalization
    Mediator of hormone internalization
    Regulator of postreceptor events

TABLE 8–1   Comparison of Hormones and Cell Surface Receptors

	Hormones	Cell Surface Receptors
Highly concentrated in localized site for extirpation and purification	Yes	No
Soluble in simple solvents	Yes	No
Simple structure	Yes	No
Bioeffect when introduced in vivo or in vitro	Yes	No
Present in blood	Yes	No
Name of its own	Yes	No

From Roth J, Grunfeld C: Endocrine systems: Mechanisms of disease, target cells, and receptors. In Williams RH (ed): Textbook of Endocrinology, Ed. 6. Philadelphia: W.B. Saunders, 1981, pp 15–74; with permission.

Table 8–1 outlines the reasons why progress in our knowledge of the hormones has been much faster than progress in our knowledge of cell surface (and other) receptors. In fact, hormones or receptors that are exceptions to the rules act to emphasize the cogency of the rules. For example: (1) Hormones that have secretory cells that are diffusely distributed have been difficult to study in terms of function because surgical extirpation of all cells is impossible. Hormones that are not present in high concentrations in a gland have been difficult to purify. On the other hand, acetylcholine receptors, which are very highly concentrated in the electric organs of marine organisms, have been among the first receptors to be purified. (2) The cytoplasmic receptors for steroids, which are water-soluble, have been better characterized earlier than receptors for peptide hormones, which, when freed from the membrane, require the continuous presence of detergents in order to stay soluble. (3) The receptors for certain toxins are simple glycolipids; they were the first to have their structures determined. Most hormone receptors are large, complex proteins, typically with several subunits and are more complex than even the largest hormones. (4) The

hormones have an assay system intrinsic of their nature (the gland is extirpated and glandular extracts are injected into the hormone deficient animal), whereas assays for receptors require more sophisticated forms of reagents. (5) Those receptors that are normally present in blood cells have been more accessible to study, especially in humans. (6) That nearly all receptors are known only by the name of their partners may represent a subtle but potent barrier to their early study.

Because our understanding of the hormone has occurred at a much faster pace, our interpretation of endocrine diseases has emphasized the role of the hormone. Initially, whenever the biological effect of a hormone was excessive or deficient, it was ascribed to a corresponding increase or decrease of the hormone levels. Only much later came the realization that diseases could occur at other sites within the pathway of hormone action, and with it the concept of target cell insensitivity was born. For example, vasopressin deficiency (diabetes insipidus) was recognized long before vasopressin resistance (nephrogenic diabetes insipidus), parathyroid hormone deficiency before parathyroid hormone resistance (pseudohypoparathyroidism), growth hormone deficiency before growth hormone resistance (Laron dwarfism), and androgen deficiency before the corresponding hormone resistance state (testicular feminization). The story of insulin resistance will be considered in detail.

Evolution of Receptor Binding Techniques

To measure directly insulin binding to cells, Stadie and colleagues[2] used iodine- and sulfate-labeled insulin. The iodine-labeled insulin was bound to the tissue but the binding lacked the features of specificity, reversibility, and saturability, that is, competition by unlabeled hormone. Similar approaches were unsuccessful for nearly two decades—regardless of the hormone or target cell investigated. The poor biological activity of the labeled hormone, degradation of both hormone and receptor, and high nonspecific binding contributed to the failure.

The first successful methods developed to measure cell-surface receptors were for adrenocorticotropic hormone (ACTH) and angiotensin.[3–5] Essential to the success were, first, the preparation of radioactive hormone of high specific activity that possessed substantial biological activity and, second, handling of the target cell preparations to ensure low degradation of hormone and receptor as well as low nonspecific binding. To validate the methodology, it was demonstrated that analogs of the hormone competed for binding in proportion to their relative biological potency, while unrelated materials did not compete.

Methods for measuring the insulin receptors are similar to other competitive binding methods. A small amount of ^{125}I-labeled insulin is allowed to interact with receptors on whole cells or membrane-enriched cell fractions in the presence of a range of concentrations of unlabeled hormones competing for receptor binding. The binding reaction proceeds until steady-state or equilibrium is achieved. Reaction conditions (temperature, pH, ionic strength) are chosen to minimize degradation of both the receptor and hormone. Unlabeled hormones and hormone analogs are essential to define the most important characteristic of any receptor, that is, specificity. In the case of insulin it was demonstrated that there was a close correlation between the affinity of over 40 insulin analogs for the insulin receptor and their in vitro bioactivity.

Early Studies in Animal Models

Disease-related applications of these principles were first carried out in animal models of hyperinsulinemia with insulin resistance. It was observed that the concentration of insulin receptors per cell was decreased in many states of insulin resistance.

The animal model studied most extensively was that of the ob/ob mouse, an animal with a genetic deficiency in *leptin*, a hormone product of adipocytes that modulates appetite.[6] These mice have marked obesity, hyperinsulinemia, insulin resistance, and pancreatic β-cell hyperplasia. ^{125}I-insulin binding to receptors on

purified liver plasma membranes of obese mice was only 30% of that of thin littermates.[6] With intact hepatocyes from ob/ob mice, the insulin binding was reduced by 50%, the same degree of reduction as when whole liver homogenates were used. In addition, in the ob/ob mouse model, decreased insulin binding was also demonstrated for the receptors in plasma membranes from adipocytes, cardiac muscle, skeletal muscle, and thymic lymphocytes, suggesting that the regulation of insulin receptors might be similar in many or most tissues (except brain).

Analysis of the insulin binding data showed that the decreased binding was due to a decrease in the number of insulin receptors. Subsequently, it was realized that the decreased receptor concentration was dependent on chronic hyperinsulinemia (Fig. 8–2). Furthermore, multiple animal models, whether associated with genetic or acquired obesity, demonstrated this phenomenon. Hyperinsulinemia was associated with a loss of receptors. Moreover, reduction of the circulating levels of insulin by fasting or by destruction of the insulin-secreting cells (following administration of streptozotocin) led to an increase in the number of insulin receptors. Reduction in insulin level alone was sufficient to lead to the increased receptor concentration even in the presence of persistent obesity. Insulin thus turned out to be an important regulator of the concentration of its receptor.

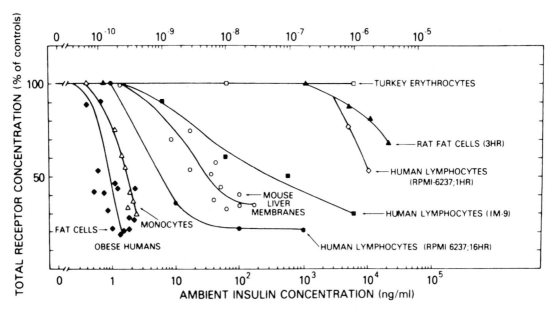

Figure 8–2.   Effect of ambient insulin concentration on the number of insulin receptors in various cell types. The inverse relationship between number of the receptors and ambient insulin concentrations is plotted for a diverse series of cell systems and cell types: fat cells and circulating monocytes from obese humans, liver membranes from obese mice, cultured human lymphocytes (IM-9, RPMI 6237), rat epididymal fat cells, and turkey erythrocytes. For humans, 100% receptor concentration represents the mean value obtained in thin normals; for the mice, 100% values represent the mean receptor concentration of thin mice; and for the remaining systems, 100% values represent the mean receptor number of cells not exposed to insulin. Adapted from Kosmakos FC, Roth J: Insulin-induced loss of the insulin receptor in IM-9 lymphocytes. A biological process mediated through the insulin receptor. J Biol Chem 255:9860–69, 1980; with permission.

Role of the Receptor in Human Disease

It has been known since the early part of this century that glucose stimulated the β-cells of the pancreas to make insulin, which then acted on target cells to promote glucose utilization. Since only glucose levels were measurable, hyperglycemic or hypoglycemic disorders were formulated simply in terms of insulin deficiency or excess. Only with the introduction of radioimmunoassay methodology for accurate measurement of circulating insulin levels by Yalow and Berson in 1960[7] did investigators become aware that the initial formulation was simplistic. A majority of hyperglycemic patients turned out to have normal or elevated circulating levels of biologically active insulin being delivered to their target cells. Since these cells fail to respond adequately to the hormone, a defect at the level of the target cell was implicated in these patients. Only that small proportion of diabetics who are truly insulin-dependent were found to be insulin-deficient. A similar, seemingly confusing pattern emerged when hypoglycemic states were studied. Insulin levels were elevated in patients with insulinomas. However, patients with nonislet cell tumors, anorexia nervosa, glucocorticoid deficiency, or growth hormone deficiency demonstrated hypoglycemia in combination with low plasma insulin levels.

Introduction of methods for measurement of the levels of insulin receptors in various disorders has allowed some insight into these apparently paradoxical situations. In many states of disordered glucose metabolism where hormone levels were discordant with the clinical conditions, it was the receptor that was altered and reflected the clinical state (Exhibit 8–3). Results of studies of the insulin receptor in various physiologic and disease states in humans are presented in Chapter 9.

Regulation of Receptor Status

Interaction of Hormone with Receptor. Hormone concentration [H], receptor concentration [R] or $[R_o]$, and the affinity (K) with which the hormone and receptor interact all have an essentially equal influence on formation of hormone-receptor complexes and therefore on activation of the target cell (Exhibit 8–4). This means that changes in plasma concentration of the hormone will be no more important than changes in receptor affinity or receptor concentration.

With the ability to measure directly hormone binding to its receptor came the realization that the receptor concentration and especially receptor affinity can change quickly, sometimes as rapidly as hormone concentrations. Many factors have been found capable of regulating the insulin receptors (Exhibit 8–5). De Meyts et al[8] demonstrated that the average affinity of the insulin receptors was decreased as the occupancy of the binding sites by insulin increased. This phenomenon, called *negative cooperativity*, showed that insulin could regulate the affinity of its own receptor. As suggested earlier, insulin is also able to influence the concentration of its receptor by the process of *down-regulation*. When cultured cells were exposed to various concentrations of insulin at 37 °C, extensively washed afterward, and then studied for ^{125}I-insulin binding, it was found that the concentration of receptors was decreased. The

---

EXHIBIT 8–3   Involvement of Insulin Receptors in Disorders of Glucose Tolerance and Insulin Sensitivity

I. Target cell dominates (i.e., plasma hormone
   concentration discordant with clinical state)
   A. Insulin resistance
      1. Moderate resistance
         (a) Clinical
            (1) Obesity
            (2) Type 2 diabetes, obese and thin
            (3) Acromegaly
         (b) Experimental animals
            (1) Glucocorticoid excess
            (2) Growth hormone excess
            (3) Uremia
      2. Extreme resistance
         (a) Immunologic (antireceptor antibodies)
            (1) Type B
         (b) Genetic (no autoimmunity)
            (1) Type A
            (2) Leprechaunism
            (3) Rabson-Mendenhall syndrome
   B. Insulin supersensitivity
      1. Anorexia nervosa

   2. Glucocorticoid deficiency
   3. Growth hormone deficiency
II. Hormone-dominated (i.e., plasma hormone
    concentration concordant with clinical state)
    A. Insulin deficiency
       1. Clinical
          (a) Type 1 diabetes
          (b) Pancreatic diabetes (e.g., chronic
              pancreatitis)
       2. Experimental animals
          (a) Streptozotocin-induced hypoinsulinemia
          (b) Hypoinsulinemic diabetic Chinese hamster
    B. Insulin excess
       1. Insulinoma
       2. Infants of diabetic mothers
       3. Other hypoglycemias in the newborn
       4. Chronic insulin excess in experimental animals
    C. Disorders of receptor design (specificity
       spillover)
       1. Infants of diabetic mothers
       2. Nonislet cell tumors with hypoglycemia

EXHIBIT 8–4   Hormone Interaction with Receptor-Quantitative Considerations

1. $H + R \rightleftarrows HR$

   $H = $ hormone
   $R = $ receptor
   $HR = $ hormone-receptor complex
   Free $ = $ Total $-$ Bound

2. Affinity $= K = \dfrac{[HR]}{[H][R]}$ $[HR] = [H_o] - [HR]$

   $[R] = [R_o] - [HR]$

   We have *expressed* K, the affinity or equilibrium constant, as the association reaction, $H + R \rightleftarrows HR$

3. $E = f([HR])$
   Magnitude of bioeffect, E, is some function f, of the size of the signal to the cell, [HR]

4. $[HR] = K[H][R] = \sim K[H][R_o]$

5. $E = f(K, [H], [R_o])$

6. Conclusion: Concentration of hormone, concentration of receptor, as well as affinity of receptor for hormone and affinity of hormone for receptor are effectively coequal determinants in signaling the cell.

EXHIBIT 8–5   Biologically Relevant Regulators of the Insulin Receptor

Insulin
Other hormones
pH; other ions
Ketone bodies
Exercise
Diet: calories, composition, fiber
Eating
Cell program: differentiation, maturation, growth, cell cycle, tumor transformation, viral infection
Drugs
Receptor affinity and concentration are both affected by insulin (homologous effect). The two best-studied hormones that affect insulin sensitivity are growth hormone, which largely affects receptor concentration, and glucocorticoids, which largely affect receptor affinity, at least in experimental animals. In humans, the situation is more complex.[9] The insulin receptor is very sensitive to pH, even within the range observed in vivo, and to a lesser extent to other common ions. Ketone bodies, especially β-hydroxybutyrate, have effects under some conditions. Some laboratories report that sulfonylureas and biguanides increase receptor concentration, but others disagree. In any case, these data should not be construed as a recommendation for the use of these drugs in patients. Exercise increases insulin binding to receptors. Insulin binding is very sensitive to diet; high calories, high carbohydrates, and high fat reduce receptor concentration. Dietary fiber, both soluble and insoluble, increases insulin binding to receptor. Eating causes a shift in the insulin binding curve. There may also be diurnal changes in insulin binding independent of eating and exercise. Any major change in cell program can also alter insulin binding, typically by altering receptor concentration. Not covered here is the ability of the insulin receptor to activate cellular events (intrinsic activity), which is also highly regulated (e.g., by hyperglycemia and by other hormones).

---

degree of receptor loss correlated with ambient insulin concentration (see Fig. 8–2). After removal of insulin from the medium, the receptor number increases rapidly and normal levels are seen within 18 to 24 hr. Insulin has to bind to its receptor for the hormone-mediated loss of the receptor to occur, but mere binding is apparently not sufficient. Thus, with lowering of temperature to 24 °C, insulin lost the regulatory ability on the receptor concentration. Inhibition of protein synthesis by agents such as cycloheximide also blocks the hormone-induced loss of receptors (and subsequent recovery of insulin receptors).

Insulin in some systems reduces the concentration of cell surface receptors by accelerating the rate of receptor degradation (thereby reducing the total cell content of receptors). In other systems insulin appears to favor the shift of receptors from the cell surface to the cell interior so that cell surface receptors are sparser but total receptors are largely unchanged. With some other hormones a reversible inactivation of receptors on the cell surface has also been described.

In summary, insulin receptors, exposed to both intracellular and extracellular fluids, are highly regulated in vivo by signals from both fluid compartments. In addition to insulin itself several other regulators are considered in more detail in Chapter 9.

Spare Receptors   Typically the maximal biological response to a hormone is achieved at hormone concentrations where not all of the receptors are occupied, a phenomenon referred to as showing "spare receptors." This means that with 90% spareness, 10% occupancy of

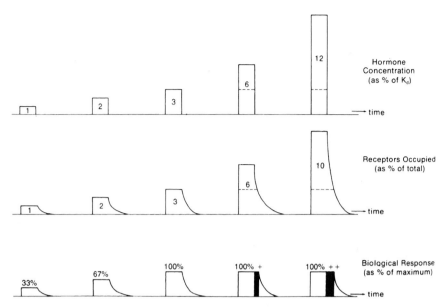

Figure 8–3. The effect of spare receptors on the duration of the biological response. In this diagram, we relate hormone concentration [H] to the concentration of occupied receptors [HR] to the biological response as a function of time. In each case the target cell was exposed briefly to hormone. In this system, the biological response, expressed per unit time, is maximal when [H] = 3U. Note that at [H] > 3U there is a further increase in receptor occupancy but no further increase in biological response per unit time, but the duration of the maximal response is prolonged (marked by the solid area), and the integrated biological response is increased. In this example we selected the dissociation of hormone from receptor as the only element in the decay process that was slow enough to be measured. Since the hormone in the medium and postreceptor events in the target cell also have finite decay rates, the effect in vivo would be even more marked than the effect we have schematically illustrated here. From Roth J, Grunfeld C: Endocrine systems: Mechanisms of disease, target cells, and receptors. In Williams RH (ed): Textbook of Endocrinology, Ed. 6. Philadelphia: W.B. Saunders, 1981, pp. 15–74; with permission.

the receptors by a hormone produces the maximal biological effect. It has to be understood, however, that the term is misleading. The 10% occupancy really means that all receptors are occupied but only 10% of the time. In addition, the degree of spareness depends on the ratio of receptor number to the capacity of the distal reaction to respond. Thus for a single cell the degree of spareness can vary from one response to another. This design of a very high concentration of receptors relative to other elements of the system (receptor affinity, hormone concentration) has several advantages. First, it permits wide shifts in the position of the biological response curve without changes in receptor affinity and rates of hormone dissociation; second, all of the distal capacity can be placed under hormonal regulation; third, each of the multiple responses of a cell can have its own dose response curve; and fourth, most of the secreted hormone will be receptor-bound even when the affinity of the receptor for the protein is low. This arrangement also adds a kinetic time dimension to the system as shown in Figure 8–3. Bursts of hormone secretion that increase hormone levels and thus levels of hormone-receptor complexes beyond the maximum capacity of the target cell to respond, while not increasing the magnitude of the effect above maximal, will prolong the duration of the effect.

The Insulin Receptor and Biologic Effects of Insulin

Mechanism of Insulin Action

The complete pathway of insulin action is being determined at last (Fig. 8–4).[10]

It is clear that phosphorylation/dephosphorylation processes plays an essential role in the action of insulin. In the case of glycogen metabolism, insulin acts to stimulate glycogen synthesis by activating phosphoprotein phosphatase; the latter enzyme dephosphorylates glycogen synthase and thereby activates the synthesis of glycogen. It also dephosphorylates phosphorylase, thereby inactivating the key enzyme in glycogen breakdown. In this example, insulin acts in a fashion opposite to glucagon by stimulating dephosphorylation. The actions of insulin are not, however, always reciprocal to glucagon and epinephrine. In some cases insulin stimulates protein kinases and thereby stimulates serine phosphorylation of various substrates. The general idea of regulation through a series of serine kinases and phosphatases is, however, similar for insulin as for other water-soluble hormones, including peptides and catecholamines.

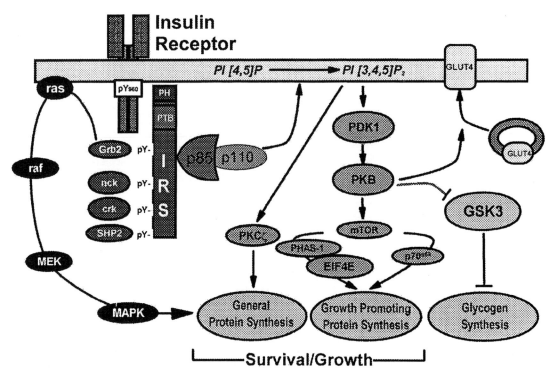

Figure 8–4. Simplified diagram of the insulin receptor signaling mechanism. The insulin receptor controls various enzyme pathways (including p70[s6k], MAP kinase, and glucose transporter translocation) largely through tyrosine phosphorylation of IRS proteins (in addition to IRS-1 pictured here, IRS-2, 3, and 4 have been identified) and Shc proteins. Abbreviations: pY, phosphorylated tyrosine; IRS-1, insulin receptor substrate-1; PH, pleckstrin homology domain; PTB, phosphotyrosine binding domain; p85 and p110, regulatory and catalytic subunits of phosphatidylinositol-3 kinase, respectively; Grb-2, Growth factor receptor-binding protein-2 (adapter molecule linking SOS, a guanine nucleotide exchange factor for p21[ras] to tyrosyl phosphoproteins such as growth factor receptors or IRS proteins); PKC, protein kinase C; PKB, protein kinase B; PHAS-I, insulin-stimulated heat- and acid-stable phosphoprotein; EIF-4E, initiation factor 4E; GSK-3, glycogen synthase-3; GLUT-4, glucose transporter-4; MEK, MAP kinase-kinase; MAP K, mitogen activated protein kinase. (From Ref. 10. White MF.)

Insulin-Induced Receptor Phosphorylation

Protein kinases that phosphorylate tyrosines (rather than serines or threonines) were described in the late 1970s. The earliest effects of insulin after the formation of the hormone-receptor complex are activation of a tyrosine-specific kinase and autophosphorylation of the receptor (actually, it is a transphosphorylation of one β subunit catalyzed by a specific domain in the other β subunit within the same heterotetramer).[11] Binding of insulin to receptor stimulates phosphorylation of the receptor itself both in intact cells and cell-free systems. Even though this "autophosphorylation" of the insulin receptor represents a very early post-binding event, it is not certain whether this step is the sole requirement for transmitting the hormone signal leading to the broad spectrum of insulin action.[10] The tyrosine phosphorylation of the receptor kinase makes it a much more powerful enzyme toward phosphorylation of other tyrosine residues within the receptor and other substrates.

The activation of tyrosine kinase is the initial event following binding of insulin to its receptor while phos-

phorylation of serine and threonine residues, a more classic event, is a later event requiring other cellular components. Protein kinase C activation resulting in phosphorylation of serines and threonines inhibits the tyrosine kinase activity of the insulin receptors and can be viewed as a feedback mechanism. Several other growth factors as well as some products of oncogenes have been demonstrated to stimulate phosphorylation of tyrosine residues. The precise role of this unusual group of kinases in regulation of cellular growth or differentiation is finally being elucidated. In the case of insulin the hormone-stimulated tyrosine kinase is actually an intrinsic part of the cytoplasmic domain of the smaller of the two subunits (β) of the insulin receptor. (The larger, or alpha, subunit binds the insulin.) The insulin receptor gene was cloned and sequenced in 1985. Its amino acid composition could then be deduced and enabled many workers to engage in elucidating an exact role of various receptor domains and individual amino acids in the transmembrane signaling of insulin action (Fig. 8–5). Some of the genetic mutations in the receptor structure believed to result in states of insulin resistance in patients are described

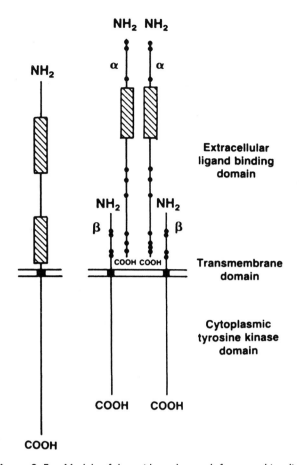

Figure 8–5. Models of the epidermal growth factor and insulin receptors. Insulin receptor (right) is a plasma membrane-spanning structure consisting of an α_2–β_2 complex. The β-subunits (95,000 daltons) serve a signaling role, possess tyrosine kinase activity, and are predominantly intracellular. The subunits are held together by disulfide bonds to form the symmetrical oligomer. The whole complex is anchored in the plasma membrane by a transmembrane domain of the β-subunit. Regions of high cysteine content (responsible for insulin binding) in the α-subunits are shown as hatched areas. The single cysteine residues (perhaps involved in formation of the receptor complex) are depicted as black circles. The structure of the epidermal growth factor is shown on the left for comparison. Adapted from Ullrich A, Bell JR, Chen EY, et al.: Human insulin receptor and its relationship to the tyrosine kinase family of oncogenes. Nature 313:756–761, 1985; with permission.

in Chapter 9. There are critical domains within the receptor's β subunit that ensure the proper propagation of the insulin signal. For example, there is an ATP binding domain, tyrosine kinase regulatory domain (three tyrosine residues, 1146, 1150, and 1151), tyrosine residue 960 in the immediate juxtamembrane position (its phosphorylation ensures appropriate tyrosine phosphorylation of IRS-1 and is also critical for endocytosis of the insulin receptor), and terminal (residues 1316, 1322) tyrosines that do not appear important for stimulation of glucose transport but might play a role in the mitogenic action of insulin.

It is generally accepted that the insulin receptor mediates the cellular actions of insulin. These include stimulation of membrane transport processes (ions, glucose, amino acids), stimulation of glycogen synthesis, lipogenesis, and protein synthesis, inhibition of lipolysis, proteolysis and glycogenolysis, and growth-promoting effects in certain cell types.[11]

In addition to itself, the tyrosine-specific kinase of the insulin receptor can utilize other intracellular substrates in vivo (such as the insulin receptor substrates 1,2, 3, and 4, Shc, Gab-1) and "artificial" substrates in vitro and has been shown to promote phosphorylation of these substrates on their tyrosyl residues.[12]

Even though insulin-stimulated phosphorylation of the insulin receptor has been established as a very early postbinding event, it is possible that endogenous substrates other than the receptor itself will be identified. Since the tyrosine kinase activity of the receptor remains tightly associated with the receptor itself, it is likely that this insulin-stimulated kinase is internalized along with the hormone-receptor complex. Hunter and Garvey[13] summarized the current hypotheses about insulin signal transmission beyond insulin binding and receptor autophosphorylation. The "substrate" hypothesis postulates that tyrosine phosphorylation of relevant cellular proteins propagates the insulin signal. The alternative, "association," hypothesis states that the tyrosine-phosphorylated β subunit mediates noncovalent interactions between the insulin receptor and cellular substrates. Judging from the knowledge gained from experiments with the first identified cellular protein serving as an endogenous substrate for the receptor, insulin receptor substrate 1 (IRS-1), both mechanisms are employed in target cells. IRS-1 possesses over 20 tyrosine residues that are phosphorylated by the activated β subunit. The substrate has no enzymatic activity by itself. However, it functions as a docking protein because it is capable of noncovalent interactions with other cellular proteins. One of the regions engaged with "charged" IRS-1 molecule is called Src homology-2 (SH-2) domain. Phosphotyrosine motifs of IRS-1 associate with SH-2 regions of several signaling molecules (for example, Grb-2, Syp, nck, crk, PI-3 kinase). All of the four IRS proteins identified to date share three domains: pleckstrin homology, phosphotyrosine, and carboxy-terminal. The pleckstrin and phosphotyrosine domains are critical for proper positioning of the insulin receptor relative to the IRS molecule. The carboxy-terminal region is involved in the docking with signaling molecules containing the SH-2 domains. With the additional identification of Shc molecule, which is likewise tyrosine phosphorylated by activated insulin receptor and can associate with the SH-2 containing signaling molecules, underlying molecular mechanisms for both the specificity and redundancy in insulin signal transduction can be investigated. For example, it has been postulated that the divergence in insulin action (i.e., insulin's role as a metabolic hormone vs. that of a mitogen) could occur at the level of IRS and Shc proteins. Propagation of the metabolic signal (for glucose transport, glycogen synthesis, antilipolysis, amino acid uptake, and so on) involves association of the specific tyrosine-phosphorylated residues of IRS with phosphatidylinositol-3 kinase (through its SH-2-containing p85 regulatory subunit). The activated PI-3 kinase, in turn, phosphorylates plasma membrane glycolipids in the 3-position. These phosphoinositides then are involved in activation of downstream signaling elements, such as phospholipid-dependent kinase 1 (PDK1), protein kinase B (PKB, also known as akt), glycogen synthase kinase3 (GSK3), and glycogen synthase. Protein kinase B (or at least one of its isoforms) appears to be essential in mediating the insulin-stimulated glucose transport.

Transduction of the mitogenic component of insulin action, in contrast, follows the Ras-mediated MAP kinase pathway. This route is analogous to that identified for many of the tyrosine-kinase containing growth factor receptors. The principal actors along the mitogenic arm of insulin signaling are a docking molecule called Grb-2, which associates, through its SH-2 domain, with specific phosphotyrosines of IRS protein(s), and through SH-3 domain with proline-rich portions of SOS, a guanine nucleotide exchange factor. SOS accelerates exchange of GTP for GDP in plasma membrane Ras, a small GTPase. The GTP-bound Ras, in turn, associates with Raf-1 kinase and initiates the MAP kinase signaling cascade, culminating in the phosphorylation of nuclear transcription factors and other events associated with the growth-promoting effects of insulin.

The technological progress in molecular biology has allowed detailed examination of the role the individual signaling elements play in mediating insulin action. The use of specific knockout and transgenic animal models has already led to some unexpected conclusions. For example, the targeted disruption of the IRS-1 gene in mice led to 50% reduction in intrauterine growth, impaired glucose tolerance, and a decrease in insulin and IGF-1-stimulated glucose uptake.[14] However, the fact that these mice lived and did not develop severe insulin resistance or diabetes provided evidence for duplication and/or redundancy of substrates capable of mediating insulin signaling. IRS-2 was identified as one of such substrates. With disruption of the IRS-2 gene, mice were born with impairment in both insulin signaling and pancreatic β-cell function.[15] These mice developed a progressively deteriorating glucose tolerance and eventually became diabetic. The phenotype in these animals with mild peripheral insulin resistance and β-cell deficiency at birth and subsequent β-cell failure and development of diabetes is akin to human type 2 diabetes mellitus. It is thus clear that IRS-1 and IRS-2 subsume specific, only partially interchangeable, roles,

in transmission of insulin signal. The exact determinants of the specific expression and/or subcellular location and interaction with other signaling molecules are still under study.

Receptor-Mediated Endocytosis

At a physiologic temperature insulin binds preferentially to specific microdomains of the membrane, such as microvilli and coated pits. In many cell types, the receptor-ligand complexes are then rapidly internalized by a process of adsorptive endocytosis (Fig. 8–6). The internalized material is enclosed in intracellular membrane-bounded structures including coated vesicles, noncoated vesicles, and lysosomal structures. Internalization of the insulin-receptor complexes is time and temperature dependent. It provides a simple mechanism coupling hormone binding to receptor-mediated hormone loss. Internalization thus serves as a degradative pathway removing insulin from the cell surface and delivering it to lysosomal proteases. There are, of course, other enzymes such as insulin proteases within endocytotic vesicles that can degrade the hormone. Internalization of the insulin signal occurs by removing the ligand from the cell surface.[16]

Hormone-induced receptor loss, so-called "downregulation," represents a new steady state of reduced

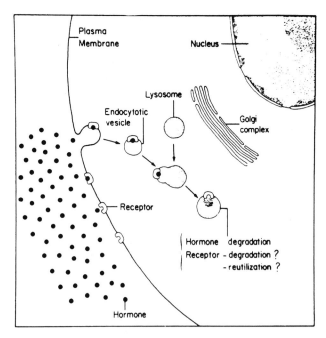

Figure 8–6. Internalization of polypeptide hormones. The hormone initially binds to a specific cell surface receptor. The hormone-receptor complex may then be redistributed in the plane of the membrane. The hormone is then internalized by the cell by adsorptive pinocytosis into a membrane-bounded vesicle that fuses with lysosomes. Inside the cell, the hormone is degraded and the membrane vesicle containing the receptor is recycled or degraded. Adapted from Ref. 16, with permission.

insulin binding. The hormone degradation and receptor regulation may be linked processes even though they do not necessarily occur at the same rate or same intracellular site. Specificity of the process of receptor-mediated endocytosis is provided by mobility of the hormone-receptor complex in the plane of the plasma membrane, allowing a specific ligand and its receptor to cluster in specific membrane domains and be selectively removed.

Characteristics of the Insulin Receptor

Plasma Membrane

Plasma membrane is an essential cellular structure involved in the hormone–target cell interactions. The components playing a role in the initial steps of action of peptide hormones—whether the receptors, transmembrane signals, or adenylate cyclase—are contained in the plasma membrane.

The two major components of the plasma membrane are lipids and proteins. The lipids, mainly cholesterol and phospholipids, insulate the intracellular space from the extracellular environment.

There are two groups of membrane proteins. Peripheral proteins, while associated with the membrane, can be removed by changing the aqueous medium (e.g., higher salt concentration) without disrupting the membrane itself. In contrast, integral proteins can be removed from their natural environment only by disrupting the membrane (e.g., by adding a detergent). Some examples of integral proteins include cell surface receptors, adenylate cyclase, and transport systems for various small molecules. The integral proteins that span the membranes have three distinct regions: (1) a portion of the molecule (to which carbohydrates are attached) that lies in the extracellular fluid, (2) a hydrophobic portion that keeps the proteins anchored in the membrane, and (3) a water-soluble segment facing the cytoplasm. The role of the carbohydrates, attached to the extracellular portion of the integral proteins, has not been precisely determined.

Structure of the Insulin Receptor

The insulin receptor is an "integral" membrane glycoprotein since detergents are necessary for its removal from membranes. From various techniques a model of the receptor structure has emerged: This complex glycoprotein has an apparent minimum molecular weight of 450,000 daltons composed of two larger, insulin-binding α subunits (with apparent molecular weight of 135,000 daltons each) and two smaller, tyrosine-kinase containing, β subunits (95,000 daltons each).

These subunits are held together by disulfide bonds, much as immunoglobulin subunits are (see Fig. 8–5). The receptor subunits are synthesized by both proteolysis and glycosylation of precursors. Both subunits are essential for insulin action, which is initiated by binding of insulin to specific domains of the α subunits and followed by postbinding events such as transphosphorylation of the receptor's β subunits (described above).

Biosynthesis of the Insulin Receptor

Biosynthesis of the insulin receptor involves a complex series of glycosylation and proteolytic steps. At least four glycosylated components of 210,000, 190,000, 135,000, and 95,000 daltons have been identified during the synthesis of the receptors.[17] Typical of other membrane glycoproteins, both major subunits contain complex and high mannose-type carbohydrate chains, suggesting a high mannose precursor. Biosynthetic processing has been estimated to take up to 6 hr after a short pulse of a labeled precursor (such as [³H] mannose). The 190,000-dalton component is the subunit of the receptor appearing earliest. It probably represents the high-mannose precursor of the receptor, which then undergoes carbohydrate maturation and proteolytic cleavage. This precursor is thought to be processed in two major steps. At first, some high-mannose chains are converted into the complex type; later, proteolytic cleavage of the protein-containing fully processed carbohydrate chain (210,000 dalton precursor) results in appearance of the two major receptor subunits (135,000 and 95,000 daltons). It is also possible that proteolytic cleavage of the 190,000 dalton component occurs first (into 115,000 and 80,000 dalton subunits) followed by terminal glycosylation of the products of proteolysis. This would make the 210,000 dalton component a precursor that escaped proteolytic cleavage, underwent glycosylation, and was inserted in the membrane. The formation and core glycosylation of the earliest receptor component (190,000 daltons) occurs in the endoplasmic reticulum and Golgi complex.[18] The mature α- and β-receptor subunits are subsequently inserted into the plasma membrane.

Turnover Rate of the Insulin Receptor Subunits

Turnover rates of the polypeptide subunits of the insulin receptor were directly measured utilizing biosynthetic (with [³⁵S]methionine) or cell surface labeling (with sodium ¹²⁵I and lactoperoxidase) and specific immunoprecipitation (with antireceptor antibody).[9] The two major receptor subunits—with apparent molecular weights of 135,000 and 95,000 daltons—turn over with half-lives of 9 to 12 hr. This turnover rate can be accelerated about threefold when the cells are grown in media containing concentrations of insulin that produce maximal down-regulation of the receptor.

It is clear from this discussion that processes involved in the biosynthesis and turnover of the insulin receptor are complex. Their study is essential in determining the precise nature and location of the defects identified in the various forms of insulin resistance. As expected, defects were found at each step of the biosynthetic and degradation pathways, leading to a subtly different type of insulin resistance at the clinical level (see Chapter 9).

References

1. Flier JS, Kahn CR, Roth J, et al.: Antibodies that impair insulin receptor binding in an unusual diabetic syndrome with severe insulin resistance. Science 190:63–65, 1975.

2. Stadie WC, Haugaard N, Vaughan M: The quantitative relation between insulin and its biological activity. J Biol Chem 200:745–751, 1953.

3. Pastan I, Roth J, Macchia V: Binding of hormone to tissue: The first step in polypeptide hormone action. Proc Natl Acad Sci USA 56:1802–1809, 1966.

4. Lefkowitz RJ, Roth J, Pricer W, et al.: ACTH receptors in the adrenal: Specific binding of ACTH- 125 I and its relation to adenyl cyclase. Proc Natl Acad Sci USA 65:745–752, 1970.

5. Goodfriend TI, Lin SY: Receptors for angiotensin I and II. Circ Res 26/27 (suppl 1):I-163–1–170, 1970.

6. Kahn CR, Neville DM, Jr, Roth J: Insulin-receptor interactions in the obese-hyperglycemic mouse. A model of insulin resistance. J Biol Chem 248:244–250, 1973.

7. Yalow RS, Berson SA: Immunoassay of endogenous plasma insulin in man. J Clin Invest 39:1157–1175, 1960.

8. De Meyts P, Bianco AR, Roth J: Site-site interactions among insulin receptors. Characterization of the negative cooperativity. J Biol Chem 251:1877–1888, 1976.

9. Fantus IG, Ryan J, Hizuka N, et al.: The effect of glucocorticoids on the insulin receptor: an in vivo and in vitro study. J Clin Endocrinol Metab 52:953–960, 1981.

10. White MF: The insulin signalling system and the IRS proteins. Diabetologia 40:S2–S17, 1997.

11. Schumacher R, Ullrich A: Insulin receptor. In Protein Kinase FactsBook CD-ROM, Academic Press, 1995, pp 1–5.

12. Zick Y, Whittaker J, Roth J: Insulin stimulated phosphorylation of its own receptor: Activation of a tyrosine specific protein kinase that is tightly associated with the receptor. J Biol Chem 258:3431–3434, 1983.

13. Hunter SJ, Garvey WT: Insulin action and insulin resistance: Diseases involving defects in insulin receptors, signal transduction, and the glucose transport effector system. Am J Med 105:331–345, 1998.

14. Araki A, et al.: Alternative pathway of insulin signalling in mice with targeted disruption of the IRS-1 gene. Nature 372:186–190, 1994.

15. Withers DJ, et al.: Disruption of IRS-2 causes type 2 diabetes in mice. Nature 391:900–904, 1998.

16. Gorden P, Carpentier JL, Freychet P, et al.: Internalization of polypeptide hormones: Mechanism, intracellular localization and significance. Diabetologia 18:263–274, 1980.

17. Hedo JA, Kahn CR, Hayashi M, et al.: Biosynthesis and glycosylation of the insulin receptor: Evidence for a single polypeptide precursor of the two major subunits. J Biol Chem 258:10020–10026, 1983.

18. Hedo JA, Simpson IA: Subcellular localization of the $M_r = 190K$ precursor of the insulin receptor in rat adipose cells. Diabetes 32 (suppl. 1):2A, 1983.

9

Insulin-Resistant Syndromes

The Role of the Insulin Receptor
and Its Signal Transduction Pathways

George Grunberger

Diabetes mellitus consists of a variety of syndromes with different etiologies. These syndromes can be broadly divided into two groups (Fig. 9–1): those associated with insulin deficiency and those associated with insulin resistance.[1,2] A combination of the two mechanisms, of course, exists in many patients (for example, those with type 2 diabetes).

In this chapter, we will consider hyperinsulinemic diseases characterized by insulin resistance. Several general characteristics, important diagnostically, apply to all diseases of insulin resistance:

1. Fasting plasma glucose may be normal or elevated. This is primarily determined by the magnitude of the basal insulin response.

2. Glucose tolerance may be normal or severely impaired. This is primarily determined by the magnitude of the insulin response to the carbohydrate or other secretagogue stimulus.

3. There is a decreased response to exogenously administered insulin. This is true whether one uses a standard insulin tolerance test or a more sophisticated measurement such as the glucose-insulin clamp, steady-state infusion technique, or forearm infusion; thus the resistance is usually manifested in the total body or in more isolated regions (forearm, thigh) depending on the technique used.

4. Usually one can achieve a qualitatively normal response using quantitatively larger concentrations of insulin.

Thus, endogenous hyperinsulinemia, with normal or elevated glucose concentrations, and resistance to exogenous insulin are characteristics common to all the syndromes we will consider.

Diseases That Mimic Insulin Resistance

Since hyperinsulinemia is characteristic of an insulin-resistant state, we must first consider syndromes of hyperinsulinemia that may mimic insulin resistance.

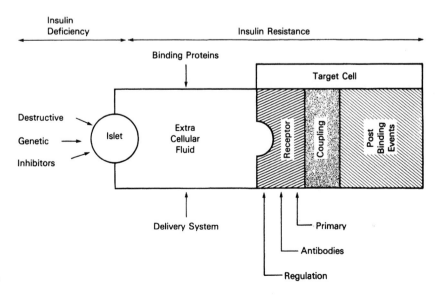

Figure 9–1. Schematic representation of mechanisms of insulin deficiency and resistance.

Genetic defects in the insulin molecule that render insulin less biologically active while retaining immunoreactivity are good examples. There are two syndromes that exhibit these characteristics: familial hyperproinsulinemia where a mutation in proinsulin[3] leads to defective conversion of proinsulin[3] and a second syndrome where an amino acid substitution in the β-chain of insulin renders the molecule biologically less potent.[4] These two syndromes are characterized by hyperinsulinemia, but the patients are not resistant to normal doses of exogenously administered insulin (see Chapter 18).

Diseases Associated with Defective Delivery of Insulin from Tissues or Plasma

Here we consider two special groups of "insulin-dependent" diabetes. A group of patients has been described who appear to respond normally to intravenously administered insulin but are resistant to subcutaneously injected insulin.[5] This probably represents a heterogenous group of disorders. In some instances, insulin may be inactivated in the subcutaneous tissues or prevented from being absorbed in some other way.

In a second, rare group of patients, insulin may normally enter the extracellular space but is then bound to anti-insulin antibodies. While virtually all insulin-requiring patients make antibodies, only a minority make very high-capacity immunoglobulins that lead to severe resistance. Thirty-six cases with high antibody titers to beef insulin responded to sulfated beef insulin therapy.[6] On transfer of over 1,000 individuals from animal-source insulin to rDNA human insulin and followed for three years, none developed immunologic insulin resistence.[7] Sulfated beef insulin therapy for 1 year was associated with a virtual disappearance of T-cell and antibody responses to beef, pork, and human insulin in parallel with the appearance of insulin-specific CD8$^+$ suppressor T-cells.[8] In a study of 26 individuals with a history of beef insulin immunologic resistance who had been successfully treated with sulfated beef insulin, it was shown that when rechallenged with beef insulin, the amnestic response was blunted in those who had been treated with sulfated insulin for more than 6 weeks,[9] presumably related to the appearance of insulin-specific CD8$^+$ suppressor T-cells.[8] Intermittent insulin therapy should be avoided.[10] This problem has greatly diminished as the use of human insulin has become widespread. (See chapter 18.)

Diseases Associated with the Target Cell

When adequate amounts of insulin are synthesized, secreted into the extracellular space, and gain access to the target tissues, abnormal function is then attributed to the target cell.

Since the first step in insulin action is binding to specific cell surface receptors, we must first consider the receptor as a potential site of dysfunction. Studies in the past have revealed a number of general principles regarding the insulin receptor:

1. Using direct binding techniques, estimates can be obtained of both the affinity and concentration of cell surface receptors.

2. Affinity is a complex function and is determined both by multiplicity of binding sites and by negatively cooperative interactions.

3. The receptor is highly regulated. Temperature, pH, and ligand concentration are among the various factors that regulate the receptor.

4. At physiologic temperatures, both the ligand and receptor are internalized by the cell. This receptor-mediated process provides a mechanism to remove the ligand from the cell surface and terminate its signal and a mechanism that may regulate the concentration of receptors on the cell surface.[11]

In animal models, the insulin receptor has been studied in multiple target and nontarget tissues. In humans, however, blood cells have been most frequently studied because of their accessibility. The insulin receptor of the human monocyte mimics the receptor status of the major target tissues of the rodent under similar physiologic and pathophysiologic circumstances. Until recently, however, no common mechanism was apparent to explain these findings. In both the rat hepatocyte and human monocyte, insulin initially binds to the cell surface. In both cells the ligand is internalized in an analogous fashion. Thus, in both a target and nontarget tissue, insulin is processed in a similar manner.[12] This suggests that biological activity and receptor regulation are separate functions; however, when target and nontarget cells are exposed to a similar environment, their cell surface receptors are regulated in a similar fashion. The same general principles may apply to the erythrocyte, but in this cell regulation occurs in the nucleated precursor. It would thus be expected to be much less responsive in a quantitative sense but to behave qualitatively similarly to the monocyte.[13]

Structure-Function Relationship of Insulin Receptor

The gene for the human insulin receptor has been identified, cloned, and sequenced. This single gene codes for a product that is a precursor for the mature receptor. Proteolytic cleavage results in formation of two receptor subunits. The larger, α, has a molecular weight

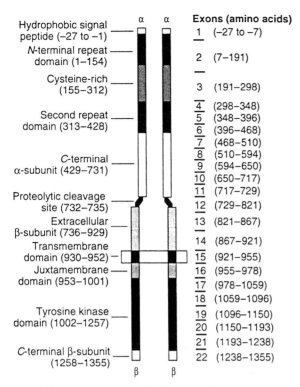

Figure 9–2. Structural domains in the insulin receptor. Key structural landmarks are marked on the left while the locations of the 22 exons are indicated on the right side of the insulin receptor scheme. Adapted from Taylor SI, et al.: Mechanisms of hormone resistance: Lessons from insulin-resistant patients. Acta Paediatr Suppl 399:95–104, 1994; with permission.

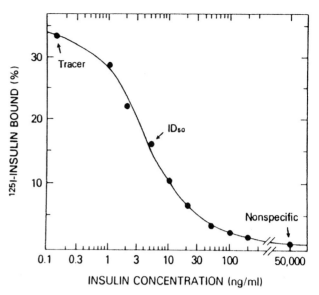

Figure 9–3. Competition-inhibition curve for [^{125}I]-insulin binding to cultured human lymphocytes. The cells were incubated with tracer amounts of ^{125}I-insulin and varying concentrations of unlabeled insulin. The percentage of the added ^{125}I-insulin bound to cells is plotted as a function of the concentration of unlabeled insulin. The arrows indicate points on the curve corresponding to ^{125}I-insulin binding in the presence of tracer concentration of the labeled hormone alone ("tracer"), in the presence of concentration of unlabeled insulin required for 50% inhibition of binding ("ID$_{50}$"), and in the presence of insulin concentration causing maximal inhibition of binding ("nonspecific"). Adapted from Ref. 14, with permission.

of –135,000 daltons and is located entirely extracellularly. Its main function is binding insulin. The smaller, β-subunit (–95,000 daltons) is embedded in the plasma membrane and serves chiefly for signal transduction. Its cytoplasmic portion contains a tyrosine kinase domain (Fig. 9–2). On binding of insulin to the α-subunit, the β-subunit undergoes autophosphorylation, which amplifies the activity of the receptor tyrosine kinase toward other substrates (as described in more detail in Chapter 8). The crystal structure of the insulin receptor has been presented, confirming previous, indirect, data.

Knowledge of characteristics of the receptor subunits is clinically relevant, since their activities are regulated in various physiologic and pathologic states. Modulation of the binding and phosphorylation activities of insulin receptors from cells of patients with type 2 diabetes mellitus serves as an excellent example (see later).

Analysis of Insulin-Binding Data

Whole cells or membranes are usually incubated with a small amount ("tracer") of ^{125}I-insulin and increasing concentrations of unlabeled insulin to construct a competition-inhibition curve (Fig. 9–3). Nonspecific or

nondisplaceable binding (i.e., the binding measured in the presence of the highest unlabeled insulin concentration used) is subtracted from each result to yield the percentage of ^{125}I-insulin bound specifically to the insulin receptors. These primary data may be transformed to derive other useful information regarding the receptor status. The most common method is the Scatchard analysis, where the ratio of bound to free insulin is plotted against the concentration of insulin bound to cells. Scatchard plots for insulin binding have a characteristic curvilinear shape (see Fig. 9–3). This has been interpreted as indicating either negative cooperativity (interactions among the receptor sites so that the affinity of the receptors for the hormone progressively decreases as more sites are occupied by insulin) or the presence of two separate classes of receptors—one with a high affinity for insulin but low capacity and others with a low affinity and high capacity. These concepts are not mutually exclusive. Other derived parameters include ID$_{50}$ (see Fig. 9–3), total number of receptors [R$_o$] (Fig. 9–4), and the average affinity profile (average affinity for insulin plotted as a function of receptor occupancy) (Fig. 9–5). All the derived data must be treated with caution because they only represent various mathematical transformations of the primary results [i.e., the competition curve (see Fig. 9–3)].

SCATCHARD PLOT

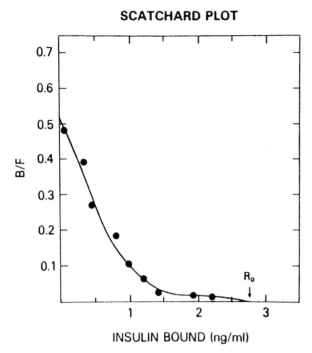

Figure 9–4. Scatchard plot of the binding data in Figure 9–3. The ratio of bound to free ^{125}I-insulin (B/F) is plotted as a function of the concentration of insulin (labeled plus unlabeled) bound to cells. R$_o$ refers to X-axis intercept used to calculate the receptor concentration. Adapted from Ref. 14, with permission.

AFFINITY PROFILE

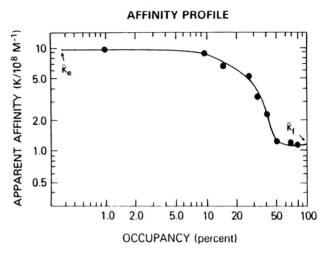

Figure 9–5. The negative cooperativity model of analyzing the curvilinear Scatchard plot. Apparent affinity of the receptor is plotted as a function of receptor occupancy. *Abbreviations:* K$_e$, affinity of the empty receptor; K$_f$, affinity of the filled receptor. Adapted from Ref. 14, with permission.

Analysis of Insulin Receptor Phosphorylation Data

Although the precise molecular details of transduction of the insulin signal are still being unraveled, a cascade of phosphorylation and dephosphorylation events is thought to play a key role in coupling of insulin binding to its action. As outlined in the previous chapter, the β-subunit of the insulin receptor possesses a tyrosine protein kinase domain. Our ability to measure the function of the receptor's β-subunit (i.e., its tyrosine kinase activity) has enabled investigators to assess alterations of the receptor function at a step distal to insulin binding in a variety of pathologic states. By measuring functions of both the α- and β-subunits of the insulin receptor from patients' cells, the site of clinical insulin resistance can be placed at either a prereceptor, receptor-binding, receptor-phosphorylation (postbinding), or a postreceptor level. This knowledge can potentially lead to development of logical treatment strategies. The activity of the receptor's β-subunit is typically assessed by two types of assays. In the first, the ability of insulin to increase phosphorylation of the β-subunit of its own receptor is measured. In these studies the insulin receptor serves both as a kinase and as a substrate. This is usually accomplished by incubation of an aliquot of sol-

ubilized purified insulin receptors from the tissue of interest with several concentrations of insulin. Phosphorylation reaction is then initiated, and phosphorylated proteins are analyzed by sodium dodecyl sulfate-polyacrylamide gel electrophoresis. The phosphorylated β-subunit is visualized by autoradiograph of the gel. Alternatively, immunoblotting of proteins with anti-phosphotyrosine antibodies can be used. In the second type of an assay, only the ability of the insulin receptor as a kinase is determined. This is accomplished by using an exogenous substrate with a high affinity for the tyrosine kinase of the receptor. Procedures are similar to those outlined for phosphorylation of the endogenous substrate, except that ^{32}P content incorporated into the exogenous substrate rather than into the receptor itself is calculated. Using the above approaches, the maximal stimulation of the receptor tyrosine kinase activity by insulin as well as insulin sensitivity (concentration dependence) can be assessed in a tissue obtained from patients with a given clinical condition. Since insulin binding to the same receptors is customarily measured at the same time, insulin-stimulated tyrosine kinase activity per receptor can be expressed.

Correlation of Insulin Binding to Bioactivity in Insulin-Resistant Syndromes

The binding of insulin to its receptor is determined by the number of receptor sites available and the affinity of these sites for the ligand. Although the relationship of insulin binding to action is complex (due to spare receptors as well as other considerations), the amount of insulin bound is a major determinant of biologic responsiveness to the hormone. Postbinding steps such as activation of the intrinsic receptor tyrosine kinase are also important, and their nature is finally being unraveled (see Chapter 8).

The most frequently studied freshly isolated insulin responsive cell is the adipocyte. This cell has been studied primarily in insulin-resistant states characterized by abnormalities of receptor regulation such as obesity, type 2 diabetes, and similar disorders. In general, two types of defects have been recognized: decreased sensitivity of the cell to insulin (a typical receptor-related defect) and decreased capacity of the cell to respond (a typical postreceptor defect).

In syndromes of extreme resistance the cultured skin fibroblast is the only insulin-responsive tissue that has been studied in detail. These cells maintain a normal diploid chromosome complement during in vitro cultivation and reflect the genetic makeup of the patient from whom they are derived. In addition, this cell manifests many of insulin's biological effects. Human fibroblasts are complex, however, in that they express not only classic insulin receptors but also receptors for several of the insulinlike growth factors. It is known that insulin has a weak affinity for the growth factor receptors, and the growth factors have a very low affinity for the insulin receptor. Thus, binding to multiple sites may be difficult to distinguish from an abnormal receptor.

The simplest view of the fibroblast system would be to suggest that classic insulin effects are mediated via the insulin receptor and that classic growth effects are mediated via the growth factor receptor. The data available, however, are difficult to interpret in this simplistic way and raise the question of overlapping systems interacting with different receptors.

Disorders Affecting the Insulin Receptor

Insulin binding to its receptor has been studied under various physiologic and pathologic conditions. Quantitative studies have involved human circulating cells such as monocytes and erythrocytes and target tissues such as the liver, fat and muscle, placental cells, and cultured cells such as fibroblasts and transformed lymphocytes.

Various physiologic conditions such as diurnal rhythm, diet, age, exercise, and the menstrual cycle affect insulin binding; in addition, many drugs perturb the receptor interaction.[14]

Diseases affecting the insulin receptor can be divided into five general categories:

1. Receptor regulation: This involves diseases characterized by hyperinsulinemia or hypoinsulinemia. Significant hyperinsulinemia in the basal state can lead to receptor downregulation as in obesity, type 2 diabetes, acromegaly, and islet cell tumors. Hypoinsulinemia such as seen in anorexia nervosa or type 1 diabetes may lead to elevated insulin binding.

2. Antireceptor antibodies: These immunoglobulins bind to the receptor and competitively inhibit insulin binding. They may act as agonists, antagonists, or partial agonists.

3. Genetic diseases that produce fixed alterations in the receptor structure in both freshly isolated and cultured cells.

4. Diseases of receptor specificity where insulin may bind with different affinity to its own receptor or related receptors, such as receptors for insulinlike growth factors.

5. Diseases of affinity modulation where physical factors such as pH, temperature, ions, and so forth may modify insulin binding.

6. Defective tyrosine kinase as a result of faulty intrareceptor coupling or intrinsic kinase defect.

Diseases of Receptor Regulation

In obesity alone, or associated with type 2 diabetes, insulin binding is frequently decreased; receptor concentration is inversely proportional to the degree of hyperinsulinemia. Reduced binding can be explained entirely by a decreased number of receptors (Figs. 9–6 and 9–7). The remaining receptors display normal binding characteristics. Treatment of the elevated insulin concentration by diet or diazoxide (to inhibit insulin secretion) corrects the binding abnormality in spite of the persistence of significant obesity[15] (Fig. 9–8).

Thus, the abnormality in insulin binding in obesity, type 2 diabetes, acromegaly (i.e., the reduced receptor concentration), insulinoma, and other disorders is due to a reversible defect in receptor regulation. The receptor per se is normal with respect to its affinity and other physiochemical characteristics. In these disorders, defects beyond the binding site may also exist. Additional defects may relate to intracellular control sites, putative insulin mediators, and abnormalities of intracellular enzymes.

Defects in the receptor tyrosine kinase activity have been documented in erythrocytes, monocytes, adipocytes, and hepatocytes from patients with type 2 diabetes (Fig. 9–9). Similar decrease in phosphorylating activity of the insulin receptor has been observed in skeletal muscle of obese subjects with or without type 2 diabetes.[16–19] Importantly, the kinase defect, at

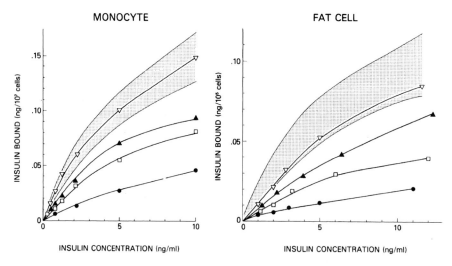

Figure 9–6. ^{125}I-Insulin binding capacity to monocytes and fat cells from obese patients. Cells were taken from the patients and incubated with 0.2 ng/ml ^{125}I-insulin. Bound insulin is graphed as a function of insulin in the incubation assay. The stippled areas represent the normal ranges ±SD. This type of plot takes data directly from the competition-inhibition curve and thus represents primary and not derived data. Adapted from Blecher M, Bar RS: Receptors and Human Disease. Baltimore: Williams & Wilkins, 1981; with permission.

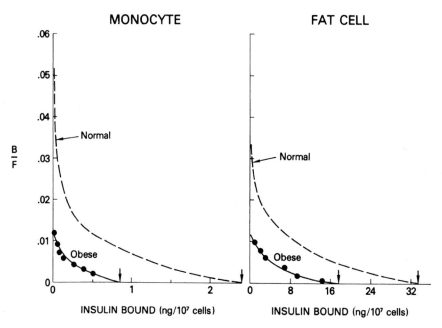

Figure 9–7.   Scatchard plots of binding data from Figure 9–6. B/F represents the ratio of bound to free hormone, lines represent mean data from studies in normal subjects. The arrows designate the maximal binding capacity that allows calculation of receptor concentrations. Adapted from Blecher M, Bar RS: Receptors and Human Disease. Baltimore: Williams & Wilkins, 1981; with permission.

least in some patients, is not fixed. Similar to the regulation of the α-subunit, the receptor phosphorylation defect appears to be reversible. However, although the regulation of the tyrosine kinase seems to be correlated with the state of the glycemic control, receptor down-regulation is related more to insulin resistance itself.

Acromegaly

In addition to the elevated levels of circulating growth hormone, some acromegalic patients exhibit moderate

insulin resistance associated with hyperinsulinemia with or without hyperglycemia. As in the obese and diabetic subjects, there is a correlation between the increased basal plasma insulin concentration and decreased number of insulin receptors in acromegaly. A direct relationship between plasma growth hormone and plasma insulin levels has also been demonstrated. Significantly, in acromegalic subjects there exists an adjustment of the receptor affinity that fully or partially offsets the effect of the decreased receptor number. In most acromegalic patients, therefore, the combination of decreased receptor concentration and increased

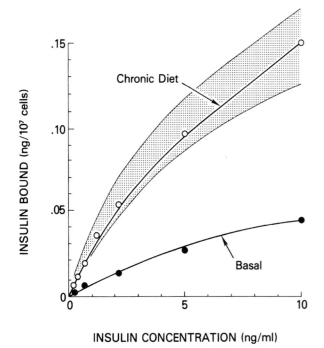

Figure 9–8. The effect of a chronic, low-calorie diet on insulin binding to circulating monocytes in an insulin-resistant obese patient. In the basal state, insulin binding was decreased over a wide range of insulin basal concentrations. After 10 weeks of a 600-calorie diet, insulin binding normalized over the entire range of insulin concentrations. Adapted from Blecher M, Bar RS: Receptors and Human Disease. Baltimore: Williams & Wilkins, 1981; with permission.

affinity of the receptor for insulin results in normal insulin binding. Acromegalic patients with hyperglycemia do not show the affinity shift; their insulin binding is generally low.

Glucocorticoid Excess

Hypercortisolism resulting from exogenous administration or endogenous overproduction of corticosteroids is associated with moderate insulin resistance. Decreased insulin binding, due to a marked decrease of receptor affinity, has been demonstrated in rat liver membranes as well as adipocytes exposed in vivo to higher ambient steroid concentration. Studies in peripheral blood cells of patients have been more difficult to interpret. This may be due to competing influences on the receptor. For instance, glucocorticoids induce the insulin receptor of cultured human lymphocytes. This leads to an increase in receptor number. On the other hand, glucocorticoids increase insulin secretion in patients with either exogenous or endogenous hypercortisolemia. This would be expected to down-regulate the receptor. Hence, it is not surprising to find no change in insulin receptor concentration on blood cells or changes that do not reflect the metabolic condition but instead reflect a change in the distribution of circulating white and red blood cells induced by the steroid.

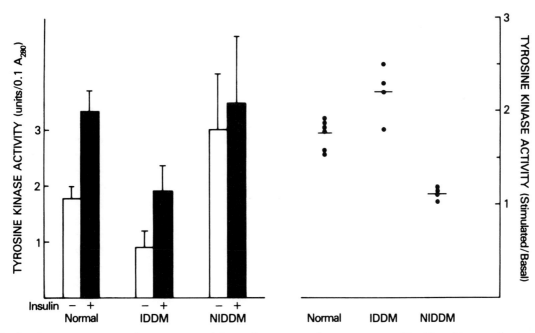

Figure 9–9. Insulin-sensitive tyrosine kinase activity of the insulin receptors from monocytes of healthy subjects and patients with diabetes mellitus (IDDM or NIDDM). (Left) Partially purified insulin receptors from freshly isolated monocytes were incubated with (+) or without (−) insulin (10 nM). Phosphorylation of an exogenous substrate, poly $(Glu^{80}Tyr^{20})$, was then carried out. (Right) Results of the same experiments are replotted to express the ratio of insulin-stimulated to basal tyrosine kinase activities. Insulin receptors from cells of patients with NIDDM showed impaired insulin effect. Receptors from monocytes of subjects with IDDM showed lower absolute kinase activity, but the stimulatory effect of insulin was retained. Adapted from Grunberger G: Insulin receptors in cultured and circulating human monocytes. In Insulin Receptors, Part B. Kahn, CR, and Harrison, LL (eds.). New York: Alan R. Liss, 1988; with permission.

Polycystic Ovarian Syndrome

Insulin resistance in the patients with polycystic ovarian syndrome (PCOS) has also been linked to defects in insulin receptor signal transduction.[20] PCOS is thought to result from defects in insulin signaling and ovarian steroid synthesis. In skeletal muscle and cultured fibroblasts from patients with PCOS the β subunits of the insulin receptor are excessively phosphorylated on their serine residues. This, in turn, results in decreased insulin-stimulated tyrosine autophosphorylation and tyrosine kinase activity of the receptor for artificial substrates. Since the structure of the insulin receptor in this disorder is normal, this serine phosphorylation of the receptor could be the primary defect. Serine phosphorylation (either by protein kinase C or in response to tumor necrosis factor-α) of either the insulin receptor, IRS-1, or IRS-2 can desensitize insulin signaling. In clinical trials, measures directed at improvements in insulin signaling (weight reduction, use of metformin or troglitazone) have successfully ameliorated patients' hyperandrogenism and insulin resistance.[21–23]

Disease States Associated with Carbohydrate Intolerance

A number of clinical syndromes are associated with glucose intolerance. In general, states such as cirrhosis, insulinoma, and a variety of neuromuscular syndromes are associated with mild to moderate insulin resistance. A summary of insulin receptor status in some of these syndromes is listed in Reference 14.

Molecular Biology of the Insulin Receptor

The tools of modern molecular biology have allowed investigators to pursue the mechanisms of insulin resistance in greater detail. Availability of the cloned human insulin receptor and specific cDNA probes has permitted qualitative and quantitative analysis of the insulin receptor gene and its transcription and translation into the final product. In analogy with the work of Brown and Goldstein[24] with the LDL receptor, a variety of theoretical defects were postulated for the processing of the insulin receptor gene (Fig. 9–10). Over the past decade these theories have been confirmed in dozens of patients. Work especially with cells from patients with extreme insulin resistance such as leprechaunism, Rabson-Mendenhall, and type A has revealed examples of specific molecular defects in the insulin receptor gene that cause these genetic syndromes (Figs. 9–11 through 9–15).[25] These receptor mutations have been divided into five categories. Thus, in some cases of extremely

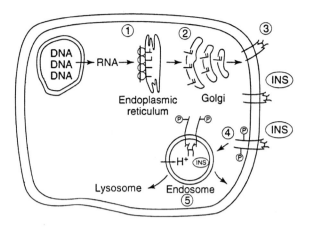

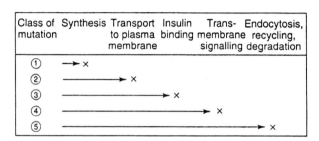

Figure 9–10. Classification of mutations in insulin receptor gene. Several theoretical possibilities have been proposed for mutations in the insulin receptor gene that could result in reduced receptor mRNA synthesis, impaired transport of the newly synthesized receptors to the plasma membrane, altered insulin binding to the plasma receptors, or decreased receptor tyrosine kinase activity. From Ref. 24, with permission. Photograph courtesy of Dr. Simeon I. Taylor.

low insulin binding very low levels of the receptor mRNA were found, indicating drastic reduction in receptor synthesis. Other specific gene mutations apparently prevent transport of newly synthesized receptors to the plasma membrane. Yet another type of mutation produces a defect in the receptor tyrosine kinase activity by preventing normal processing of the proreceptor into mature receptor subunits or by deletion or point mutation in the tyrosine kinase domain itself. The patients with two mutant alleles of the insulin receptor gene appear to have the most severe insulin resistance. Heterozygotes with a single mutation in the tyrosine kinase domain of the insulin receptor seem to be more insulin resistant than those who are heterozygotes for a null allele. It is possible that receptor mutations in the tyrosine kinase domain cause insulin resistance by a dominant mechanism. In contrast, patients heterozygous for a missense mutation in the receptor's extracellular domain are less insulin resistant, suggesting that these mutations may cause insulin resistance by a recessive mechanism.

Populations with type 2 diabetes have been screened for mutations in the gene for insulin receptor with only

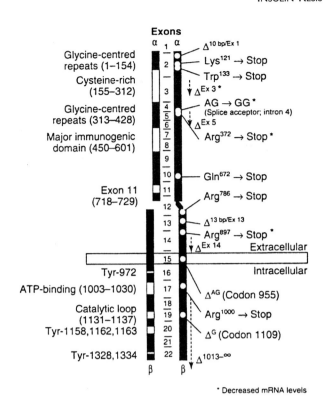

Figure 9–11. Examples of class 1 mutations in the insulin receptor gene reported in patients with insulin resistance. See Figure 9–10 for the overall scheme. From Ref. 25, with permission.

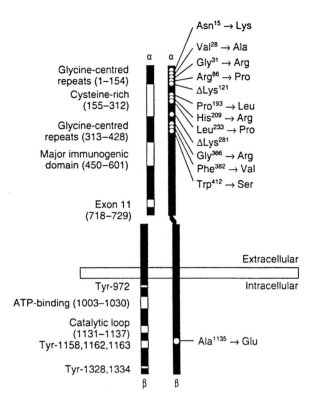

Figure 9–12. Examples of class 2 mutations in the insulin receptor gene reported in patients with insulin resistance. See Figure 9–10 for the overall scheme. From Ref. 25, with permission.

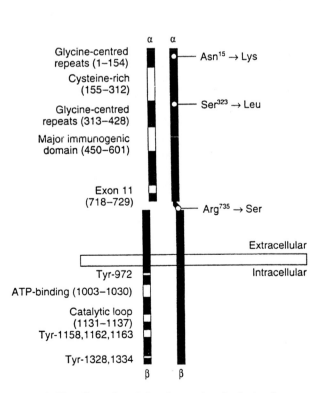

Figure 9–13. Examples of class 3 mutations in the insulin receptor gene reported in patients with insulin resistance. See Figure 9–10 for the overall scheme. From Ref. 25, with permission.

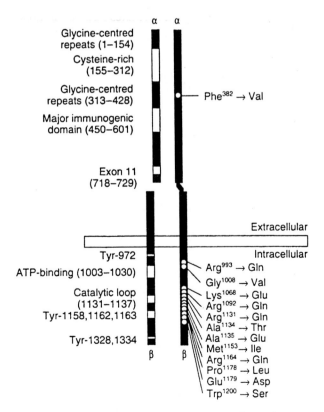

Figure 9–14. Examples of class 4 mutations in the insulin receptor gene reported in patients with insulin resistance. See Figure 9–10 for the overall scheme. From Ref. 25, with permission.

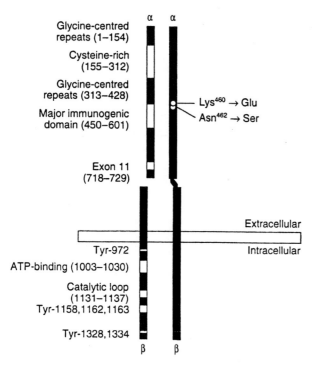

Figure 9–15. Examples of class 5 mutations in the insulin receptor gene reported in patients with insulin resistance. See Figure 9–10 for the overall scheme. From Ref. 25, with permission.

occasional positive findings (Table 9–1). The screening strategy has typically involved the molecular scanning technique of single-stranded conformational polymorphism and direct sequence analysis of the insulin receptor gene; pooled and multiplex single nucleotide primer extension method has also been used in large-scale population studies.[26,27]

In addition to the obvious choice of the insulin receptor gene, other candidate genes for insulin resis-

TABLE 9–1 Mutations in the Insulin Receptor Gene in Patients with Type 2 Diabetes Mellitus (Selected Cases)

- Type 2 DM screening (Italy): In 1/103 single nucleotide substitution in codon 1152 (exon 20) → Arg1152Gln - ins binding normal, IR autophosphorylation normal, but tyrosine kinase eliminated
- Type 2 DM screening (Japan): 3/51 heterozygous missense Thr831Ala (exon 13); 1 pt heterozygous missense Tyr1334Cys (exon 22)
- Two type 2 diabetes and insulin resistance patients: Normal IR gene but expression of nuclear-binding proteins for the 5' regulatory region of IR gene markedly reduced
- Screening of 18 familial type 2 diabetes pedigrees tyrosine kinase domain (exons 13–20): Val985Met mutation (exon 17) in one family; this substitution seen in three individuals in three generations

tance have been analyzed[28]; a complementary approach in search for responsible genes has been positional cloning using random DNA markers present throughout the genome. It has to be emphasized that in addition to type 2 diabetes, insulin resistance also confers increased susceptibility to atherosclerotic cardiovascular disease, hypertension, ovarian hyperandrogenism, and possibly other pathologic conditions.

Maturity-onset diabetes of the young (MODY), a monogenic subgroup of type 2 diabetes mellitus, is inherited as an autosomal dominant syndrome. "It is genetically heterogeneous, but several different MODY genes have been identified on chromosomes 20q12-q13.1 (*MODY1*), 7p15-p13 (*MODY2*), 12q24.2 (*MODY3*), 13q12.1 (*MODY4*) and 17cen-q21.3 (*MODY5*). The MODY genes encode hepatocyte nuclear factor-4α (MODY3), insulin promoter (MODY1), glucokinase (MODY2), hepatocyte nuclear factor-1α (MODY3), insulin promoter factor-1 (MODY4), and hepatocyte nuclear factor-1β (MODY5). Nonsense and missense mutations in these transcription factor have been reported as causes of MODY1, MODY3, and MODY4 subtypes to date. There are suggestions that additional loci can cause MODY because some families do not have mutations in the five known MODY genes."

Syndromes of Extreme Insulin Resistance Associated with the Target Cell

Acanthosis nigricans is found in a high proportion of patients with extreme insulin resistance but it is not an invariant finding (Exhibit 9–1). Acanthosis nigricans is an abnormality of skin characterized by a papillomatous hyperkeratosis with deposition of melanin. It typically occurs in the axilla but can be seen on other intertriginous areas, the back, the lips, and in extreme cases can involve the entire skin surface (Figs. 9–16 and 9–17). The condition is nonspecific, occurring commonly in obesity, endocrine diseases such as Cushing's disease and acromegaly, and may be a skin marker of abdominal malignancy (see Chapter 45).

EXHIBIT 9–1 Syndromes of Extreme Insulin Resistance (In Order of Increasing Likelihood of Insulin Receptor Gene Mutations)

Lipoatrophic diabetes
Insulin resistance with acanthosis nigricans (type B) due to antireceptor antibodies
Insulin resistance with acanthosis nigricans (type A)
Rabson-Mendenhall syndrome
Leprechaunism (Donohue syndrome)

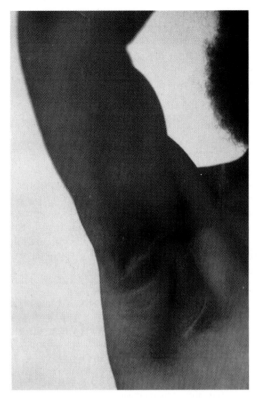

Figure 9–16. A typical lesion of acanthosis nigricans in a patient with type B insulin resistance and autoantibodies to the insulin receptor.

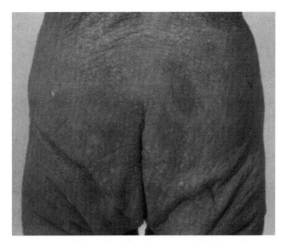

Figure 9–17. Unusual presentation of acanthosis nigricans involving essentially the entire body in another patient with the type B insulin resistance syndrome with autoantibodies to the insulin receptor.

Specific Syndromes

Lipoatrophic Diabetes

This syndrome is characterized by insulin resistance and lipoatrophy. The lipoatrophy may involve the entire body or may spare certain areas such as the face. Usually, these patients have severe hypertriglyceridemia (typically of the type V variety). The hyperlipemia in turn may lead to a fatty liver and cirrhosis. Hyperglycemia is variable in this syndrome, but most patients exhibit glucose intolerance. Hepatomegaly, acanthosis nigricans, and polycystic ovaries are also commonly seen in this syndrome. Insulin binding was initially reported to be low in circulating monocytes of patients with congenital lipodystrophy. Later, when a spectrum of these patients was considered, results of binding revealed heterogeneity. About half of the patients have low binding, but others have normal or even elevated insulin binding to peripheral blood cells. To the extent that binding has been studied in vitro in fibroblasts, binding is usually normal. Thus, binding abnormalities in lipoatrophic diabetes do not appear to be on a genetic basis. Although genetic polymorphism has been described in this disorder, in general, it appears that the receptor defect is that of regulation, as was seen in obesity and type 2 diabetes.

Autoantibodies to the Insulin Receptor (Type B Syndrome)

This syndrome was initially described in three female patients and shown to be associated with a plasma inhibitor of insulin binding.[29] Subsequently, about 20 patients have been studied. Most have been women of variable age; only two are male patients in the sixth decade of life. Patients exhibit acanthosis nigricans, and in one patient this disorder involved the entire body (see Fig. 9–17). Almost all patients have fasting hyperglycemia, and in these patients up to 100,000 U insulin/day may be required to normalize the blood glucose.

All of these patients have features typical of autoimmune diseases, such as pancytopenia and increased erythrocyte sedimentation rate (Exhibit 9–2). In some patients, a lupus or Sjögren-like syndrome is present with arthralgias, proteinuria, parotid enlargement, and positive antinuclear antibody. About half the patients have anti-DNA antibodies, but positive lupus preparations are uncommon.

In patients with suggestive clinical features the diagnosis is confirmed by demonstrating an inhibitor of insulin binding to an appropriate cell with insulin receptors or by an immunoprecipitation procedure. The circulating inhibitor has been shown to be a polyclonal immunoglobulin behaving as an antibody to the insulin receptor.

These antireceptor autoantibodies mimic insulin action in vitro. Furthermore, we have studied one patient who only manifested hypoglycemia.[30] Additional cases presenting solely with severe hypoglycemia have been reported since. Administration of corticosteroids resulted in a prompt increase in plasma glucose levels in all of these patients. Thus, autoantibodies to the insulin receptor must be considered in

EXHIBIT 9–2   Syndromes of Extreme Insulin Resistance with Acanthosis Nigricans

1. Extremely high basal and stimulated plasma insulin concentrations are present
2. Extreme resistance to exogenously administered insulin is present
3. Absence of any other known form of insulin resistance
4. Glucose tolerance can be normal or hyperglycemia with ketosis can be present

Type A	Type B
1. No immunologic features	1. Autoimmune features
2. Young women	2. Older, mostly women
3. Amenorrhea[a]	3. Elevated erythrocyte sedimentation rate
4. Hirsutism[a]	4. Leukopenia, antinuclear antibodies
5. Masculinization[a]	5. Alopecia, arthralgias, nephritis
6. Polycystic ovaries	6. Presence of other autoimmune disease
7. Insulin receptor binding decreased due to lowered receptor concentration	7. Antireceptor antibodies (bind to insulin receptor, block insulin binding, either impair or mimic insulin action)
8. In a variant form, insulin binding normal	8. Both insulin resistance and hypoglycemia possibly seen during clinical course
	9. Remissions or death possible

[a]When type B occurs in premenopausal women, these features can be seen also in that syndrome.

the differential diagnosis of hypoglycemia. Most patients, however, demonstrated hyperglycemia and insulin resistance. Studies using passive transfer of the antireceptor serum to the rat helped to clarify this paradox. When the antireceptor serum is injected into the starved rat, delayed and persistent hypoglycemia occurs. In contrast, when high doses of antireceptor serum are injected into the fed rat a diabetic syndrome is induced. Thus, both in cultured cells and in vivo in the rat a desensitization phenomenon occurs. Why this desensitization does not occur in all patients is unclear.

Insulin binding is qualitatively abnormal in circulating monocytes (Fig. 9–18) and erythrocytes from these patients, and in one patient decreased binding to freshly isolated adipocytes has been demonstrated.

Abnormal insulin binding results from antibody binding on or near the insulin receptor. This yields a competition curve that has decreased specific tracer binding but also a marked increase in the amount of insulin necessary for 50% competition of binding.

The net outcome is a major alteration in the affinity of the receptor for insulin. This abnormality can be reversed by removal of the circulating antibody by plasma exchange or by an acid wash procedure, indicating that the underlying receptor is normal. Furthermore, insulin receptors on cultured cells from these patients exhibit normal binding.

Analysis of the function of the β subunit of the receptor from cells of patients with the type B syndrome revealed a generally proportional decrease of the receptor kinase activity and insulin binding. There-

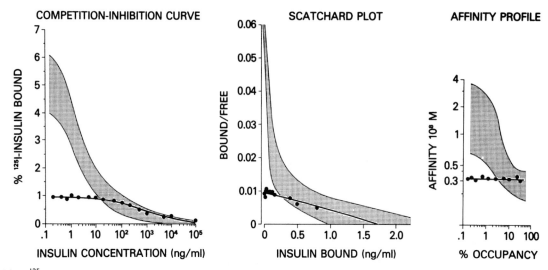

Figure 9–18.   ^{125}I-Insulin binding to monocytes of a patient with the type B syndrome of extreme insulin resistance and acanthosis nigricans. Competition-inhibition curve is at the left, Scatchard plot in the middle, and affinity profile at the right. The stippled areas represent the mean ± SD for the competition-inhibition curves and the range of normal for the Scatchard plots and average affinity profile.

fore the phosphorylating activity expressed per receptor appears to be normal.

Several therapeutic approaches have been suggested over the years directed at immunomodulation in these patients. A combination of a short-term suppression of autoantibodies with plasmapheresis and cyclophosphamide, followed by a chronic maintenance approach with cyclosporin A and azathioprin, offers a promise of prevention of relapses.[31]

Type A Insulin Resistance

This syndrome was originally described in young nonobese women with extreme hyperinsulinemia, variable resistance to exogenous insulin, hirsutism, polycystic ovaries, and android habitus.[32] All have had acanthosis nigricans. Only about one-third, however, have fasting hyperglycemia. Most have glucose intolerance, but some patients have normal glucose tolerance, and these patients demonstrate the greatest degree of basal and glucose-stimulated hyperinsulinemia.

All of these patients have had elevated plasma testosterone values usually associated with normal concentration of gonadotropins, and all have had polycystic ovaries. Elevated testosterone step-up in ovarian venous effluent was found in patients studied. Testosterone values have been easily suppressed by estrogen administration. This, however, does not alter the insulin resistance.

Several types of insulin receptor defects have been described. Typically, insulin binding to freshly obtained circulating monocytes and erythrocytes has been decreased (Fig. 9–19). Less commonly, in two patients insulin binding has been completely normal (these patients have been sometimes labeled as having type C extreme insulin resistance). Thus, insulin resistance is a fixed feature of the type A syndrome, but insulin binding is either low or normal. Typically, insulin binding does not increase when subjects are deprived of food for 48–72 hr, as is seen in states of down-regulation. More recently, insulin binding has been studied in cultured fibroblasts and cultured transformed B-lymphocytes from these patients and found to be low in those patients with low monocyte binding.

Studies of the function of the β-subunit of the monocyte receptors showed concomitant decrease of the receptor autophosphorylation and tyrosine kinase activity with the binding activity in patients with low insulin binding. Interestingly, in one of the patients with normal insulin binding, insulin receptor autophosphorylation and tyrosine kinase activity from circulating monocytes and erythrocytes as well as cultured fibroblasts were greatly decreased (Fig. 9–20).[33] Uncoupling of the receptor binding and phosphorylation thus exists in cells of some patients with type A syndrome.

A variant of this syndrome has been seen in a brother and sister who also exhibited muscle cramps, and a family with features of this syndrome has also been described. Another variation of this syndrome seen with precocious puberty, pineal tumors, and developmental defects is referred to as the Rabson-Mendenhall syndrome (see below).

The tools of modern molecular biology have allowed us to decipher defects in some of these patients at the level of the gene for their insulin receptor (Table 9–2). Although initially the type A and B syndromes were

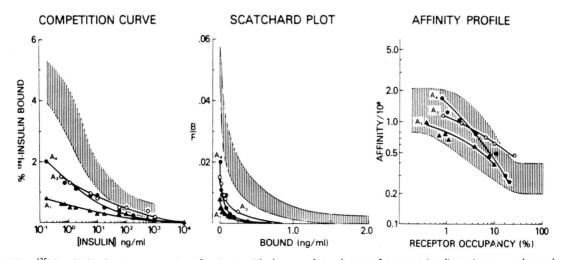

Figure 9–19.   ^{125}I-Insulin binding to monocytes of patients with the type A syndrome of extreme insulin resistance and acanthosis nigricans. Competition-inhibition curves from studies of monocytes from three patients are at the left, scatchard plots (bound to free hormone versus bound hormone) in the middle, and average affinity profile (average affinity versus percent receptor occupancy) at the right. The hatched areas represent the mean ± SD for the competition-inhibition curves and the range of normal for the Scatchard plots and average affinity profiles. Adapted from Bar RS, Muggeo M, Kahn CR, et al.: Characterization of the insulin receptors in patients with the syndromes of insulin resistance and acanthosis nigricans. Diabetologia 18:209–16, 1980; with permission.

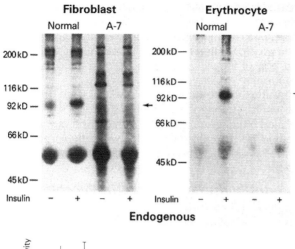

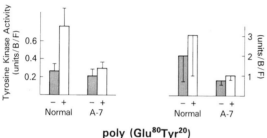

Figure 9–20. Insulin-stimulated phosphorylation of insulin receptor and an exogenous substrate poly $(Glu^{80}Tyr^{20})$ by partially purified insulin receptors from freshly obtained erythrocytes and cultured skin fibroblasts of healthy individuals (normal) and a patient with type A extreme insulin resistance (A-7). (Top) Autophosphorylation experiments were carried out in the presence $(+)$ or absence $(-)$ of insulin (100 nM). Arrows indicate the position of the phosphorylated β-subunit of the insulin receptor. Note the absence of stimulation of receptor autophosphorylation in the case of patient A-7. (Bottom) Insulin stimulated tyrosine kinase activity of 8 normal fibroblasts and 15 erythrocytes were compared with that of cells from patient A-7. Note the wide variation (large standard deviation) of absolute values of kinase activities among the healthy subjects. However, in each individual case, there was at least 80% stimulation of kinase activity by insulin. In the type A patient insulin stimulated the receptor kinase activity by less than 25% in every experiment. Adapted from Grunberger G, Comi RJ, Carpentier J-L, et al.: Insulin receptor tyrosine kinase activity is abnormal in circulating and cultured fibroblasts but normal in transformed lymphocytes from type A insulin-resistant patient. J Lab Clin Med 112:122–132, 1988; with permission.

described as distinctly different, we now know that patients with typical clinical and laboratory features of the type B syndrome may manifest the major features of the type A syndrome, including polycystic ovaries, elevated plasma testosterone, and hirsutism. Thus, it is apparent that the type A and B syndromes have overlapping phenotypic features (see Exhibit 9–2). Furthermore, it is clear that all of the syndromes of severe insulin resistance and acanthosis nigricans have many common clinical features (Fig. 9–21). The genetic or acquired factors, or both, that are responsible for the

TABLE 9–2 Mutations in the Insulin Receptor Gene in Patients with Type A Extreme Insulin Resistance (Selected Cases)

- Two missense mutations: Asp59Gly, Leu62Pro (reducing/binding by 90%)
- Five daughters inherited (four clinically affected with type A) paternal allele with deletion of exon 3
- Heterozygous point mutation: Arg174Gln (normal ins binding, decreased IR autophosphorylation)
- Homozygous point mutation: Arg252His (decreased receptor expression)
- Heterozygous for Gly1008Val (exon 17)
- Heterozygous for Trp1193Leu (exon 20)
- Compound heterozygote: Paternal—missense → premature termination at Arg981; maternal—nonsense → premature termination after amino acid 988
- Compound heterozygote: Paternal—A-T substitution in nucleotide 3205 → Ileu996Phe substitution; maternal—shorter receptor mRNA transcripts containing in-frame deletion of exon 2

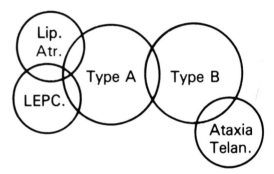

Figure 9–21. Overlapping phenotypic features of insulin resistance and acanthosis nigricans. *Abbreviations:* Ataxia telan., ataxia-telangiectasia; LEPC., leprechaunism; Lip. Atr., lipoatrophic diabetes.

various overlapping phenotypic features of these diseases are still being dissected.

Rabson-Mendenhall Syndrome

This autosomal recessive syndrome was described in 1956 in a family with hyperplasia of pineal gland and diabetes mellitus. Further characteristic features are low birthweight, thickened nails, hirsutism, acanthosis nigricans, dental precosity and dysplasia, polycystic ovaries, abdominal protuberance, and phallic enlargement. Most affected children die of ketoacidosis and intercurrent infections associated with extreme insulin resistance. Rabson-Mendenhall syndrome appears to lie between the type A syndrome and leprechaunism on the spectrum of severity of insulin receptor dysfunction (Table 9–3).

Leprechaunism (Donohue syndrome)

Leprechaunism is a complex congenital syndrome. These infants are small for gestational age and continue

TABLE 9–3 Mutations in the Insulin Receptor Gene in Patients with Rabson-Mendenhall (Selected Cases)

- Compound heterozygote: In-frame additional 12 bp in exon 3, coding for Leu-His-Leu-Val (located between amino acids 261 and 262); other allele-Arg86 in exon 2 changed into stop codon
- Two patients with homozygous Ser323Leu mutation
- Compound heterozygote: missense—Ser323Leu mutation; nonsense—truncation before transmembrane domain

TABLE 9–4 Mutations in the Insulin Receptor Gene in Leprechaunism (Selected Cases)

- Homozygous, missense mutation (in exon 2, Ile119Met)
- Homozygous, nonsense (Lys121Amber), null IR phenotype
- Compound heterozygous: de novo—2 bp deletion, exon 15; paternal—silent polymorphism, exon 17
- Homozygous missense mutation Asp707Ala
- Compound heterozygote; maternal allele: G to A transition in first nucleotide in intron 13; paternal: in-frame deletion of bp 1159-1161 in exon 3 (absence of Asn281)
- Deletion of 3 nucleotides, loss of Lys121 in binding domain
- Homozygous, exon 13; 13 bp deletion, replaced by 5 bp
- Homozygous, missense Arg1092Gln in TK domain
- Nonsense in one allele, exon 14
- Homozygous, missense, Arg86Pro
- Homozygous, missense, Trp412Ser (impairs prorereceptor processing)
- No mutations in receptor gene but 5′ flanking region has two polymorphic sites (−603, −500)
- Homozygous, nonsense, exon 12, C to T substitution at bp 8212, creating premature stop codon
- Compound heterozygote: Maternal allele—exon 18, Trp1092Arg; paternal—exon 20, Glu1179Lys
- Compound heterozygote: Maternal allele—exon 3, Cys274Tyr; paternal—exon 20, Arg1174Trp

to grow slowly in extrauterine life. They have a characteristically abnormal appearance with such features as low-set ears, saddle nose deformity, hypertrichosis, decreased subcutaneous fat, and, occasionally, acanthosis nigricans (Fig. 9–22). Curiously, in these infants a tendency to fasting hypoglycemia coexists with extreme resistance to insulin. Typically, the patients die within the first year of life, although an occasional child may live significantly longer.

Insulin binding studies have revealed significant heterogeneity. Leprechaunism appears to be caused by defects in the insulin receptor. Close to 20 kinds of mutations in the insulin receptor gene have been reported in patients with leprechaunism thus far (Table 9–4).

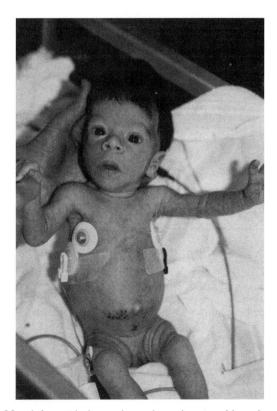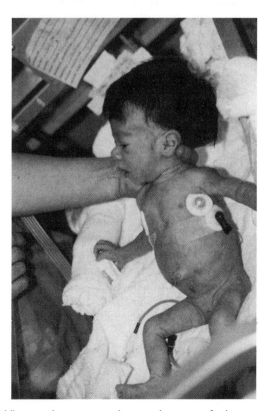

Figure 9–22. Infant with the syndrome leprechaunism. Note the saddle nose, low-set ears, decreased amount of subcutaneous fat, and the umbilical hernia. (A) Front view; (B) side view. Photographs courtesy of Dr. S.I. Taylor.

To demonstrate the recent explosion in our knowledge and understanding of the causes of extreme insulin resistance, the report of Takahashi et al. can serve as an illustration.[34] They described a boy with typical clinical features of leprechaunism. This patient was a product of a consanguineous marriage. His parents had features of type A syndrome of insulin resistance, while his brother with features of leprechaunism died at age 7; two other brothers were clinically normal. The structure and function of the insulin receptor from the proband and parents were studied in Epstein-Barr transformed cultured lymphocytes. The number and affinity of the patients' insulin receptors were normal, while the autophosphorylation and tyrosine kinase activity of his insulin receptors were severely impaired. Direct sequencing analysis revealed that the proband was homozygous for a missense mutation in the tyrosine kinase domain of the receptor (Arg1092Glu); the parents were heterozygous for the mutation. Next, the mutant insulin receptor (corresponding to the patient's) was expressed in Chinese hamster ovary cells to assess its effect on insulin action. Insulin-stimulated glucose uptake, DNA synthesis, and glycogen activation were all markedly impaired in the cells expressing the patient's mutant receptor. The results were consistent with the tyrosine kinase defect of the receptor and suggested that it was responsible for his growth retardation and diabetes mellitus. Insulin receptor number was normal in the proband's cultured skin fibroblasts, but insulin-stimulated phosphorylation of IRS-1 and glucose uptake were again severely impaired. In contrast, IGF-1-stimulated phosphorylation of IRS-1 and glucose uptake in the patient's cells were normal. This finding led to initiation of treatment by recombinant human IGF-1. This therapy was effective in markedly improving fasting plasma glucose, glycated hemoglobin, and serum insulin levels. The patient has remained on the IGF-1 therapy over the past 4 years without any complications. During the family's fifth pregnancy, the genotype of the fetus was determined as being heterozygous for the insulin receptor mutation and predicted not to have clinical leprechaunism at birth. The newborn was indeed a heterozygote and did not show the phenotype of the syndrome.

Beyond the Insulin Receptor

Even though this chapter has been focused on the role of the insulin receptor itself as a cause of some of the insulin-resistant conditions, our understanding of insulin signal transduction has advanced significantly over the past decade (reviewed in Ref. 35 and in Chapter 8). As a result of these advances, attempts have been made to discover the underlying molecular defects in those insulin resistant patients whose insulin

TABLE 9–5 Mutations in Genes Involved in Insulin Signaling (Selected Cases)

- Insulin receptor substrate-1(IRS-1): 11 variant sequences found in type 2 diabetes
- IRS-1: Gly972Arg substitution more prevalent in impaired glucose tolerance and late-onset type 2 diabetes (Japan); heterozygous form potentiates obesity-associated insulin resistance (Denmark)
- IRS-1: Molecular scanning of the gene by PCR-SSCP (England) in severe insulin resistance—six variant patterns (four silent polymorphisms at codons 90, 235, 805, 894), one nonconservative mutation (Gly972Arg), and a missense mutation (Met614Val)
- IRS-2: frequent Gly1057Asp polymorphisms; no association with type 2 diabetes (Denmark)
- IRS-4: SSCP scanning of the gene (Denmark)—five amino acid polymorphisms common; not associated with either type 2 diabetes or insulin resistance
- Rad ("Ras associated with diabetes"): From subtraction cloning of skeletal muscle mRNA in type 2 diabetes
- Hexokinase II: Two silent polymorphisms found among 34 most insulin resistant patients with type 2 diabetes (England)
- Glucokinase (hexokinase IV): Many mutations (heterozygotes with nonsense mutations, missense mutations, deletions) identified among patients with MODY2
- Glycogen synthase: Restriction fragment length polymorphisms in type 2 diabetes (Finland, France); simple tandem repeat polymorphism (Japan)
- Protein phosphatase type 1: Missense mutation in 1/30 type 2 diabetes (Denmark)
- Mitochondrial genes: Mutation in leucine tRNA in families with maternally transmitted late-onset DM and nerve deafness; mutation in lysine tRNA in family with maternally transmitted DM, deafness, and myoclonic epilepsy with ragged red fibers; 10.4-kb deletion on mitochondrial DNA in another subtype of maternally transmitted DM and nerve deafness

receptor structure or function could not explain their clinical conditions. Attention has been mainly directed at genes encoding proteins involved in glucose metabolism and insulin action, such as those regulating the gene transcription of the glycolytic and gluconeogenic enzymes, the insulin-sensitive glucose transporters, glucokinase, and the proteins implicated in the early postreceptor steps of the insulin signal transduction (Table 9–5).[36,37]

Conclusions and Future Directions

We have surveyed a spectrum of clinical disorders. Some of these syndromes have been recognized for over 5,000 years and some for less than a couple of decades. With the recent explosion in our understanding of the insulin-initiated cascade of insulin signal transduction, we are now finally in a position to understand the fine molecular details of the pathophysiology of this heterogeneous class of diseases associated with insulin resistance.

Furthermore, it will be necessary to understand factors other than insulin that interact with the receptor to trigger its program. For instance, autoantibodies, monoclonal antibodies, and plant lectins can subserve this function.

Finally, it will be important to understand the multiple other phenotypic features that affect patients with insulin-resistant syndromes. These include abnormalities of the skin, ovaries, plasma lipids, immune system, and other features that may further elucidate primary etiologic factors in these diseases.

References

1. Porte D, Sherwin RS (eds): Ellenberg and Rifkin's Diabetes Mellitus. Theory and Practice, Ed. 5. Stamford, CT: Appleton & Lange, 1997.

2. Report of the Expert Committee on the Diagnosis and Classification of Diabetes Mellitus. Diabetes Care 20: 1183–1197, 1997.

3. Gabbay KH, DeLuca K, Fisher JN, et al.: Familial hyperproinsulinemia: an autosomal dominant defect. New Engl J Med 294:911–915, 1976.

4. Kanazawa Y, Kayashi M, Ikeuchi M, et al.: Familial proinsulinemia: a possible cause of abnormal glucose tolerance. Eur J Clin Invest 8:327(A), 1978.

5. Paulsen EP, Courtney JW, Duckworth WC: Insulin resistance caused by massive degradation of subcutaneous insulin. Diabetes 28:640–645, 1979.

6. Davidson JK, Debra DW: Immunologic insulin resistance. Diabetes 27:307–318, 1978.

7. Davidson JK: Transferring patients with insulin dependent diabetes mellitus from animal-source insulins to recombinant DNA human insulin. Clin Therapeutics 11:319–330, 1989.

8. Naquet P, Ellis J, Kenshole A, Semple JW, et al.: Sulfated beef insulin treatment elicits CD8+ T-cells that may abrogate immunologic insulin resistance in type 1 diabetes. J Clin Invest 84:1479–1487, 1989.

9. Davidson JK, Fineberg SE, DeMeyts P, et al.: Immunological and metabolic responses of patients with history of antibody induced beef insulin resistance to treatment with beef, pork, human, and sulfated beef insulin. Diabetes Care 15:702–704, 1992.

10. Shipp JC, Cunningham RW, Russell RO, et al.: Insulin resistance: clinical features, natural course and effects of adrenal steroid treatment. Medicine 44:165–186, 1967.

11. Gorden P, Carpentier J-L, Freychet P, et al.: Internalization of polypeptide hormones: Mechanism, intracellular localization and significance. Diabetologia 18:263–274, 1980.

12. Grunberger G, Robert A, Carpentier JL, et al.: Human circulating monocytes internalize ^{125}I-insulin in a similar fashion to rat hepatocytes: Relevance to receptor regulation in target and nontarget tissues. J Lab Clin Med 106:211–217, 1985.

13. Dons RF, Ryan J, Gorden P, et al.: Erythrocyte and monocyte insulin binding in man: a comparative analysis in normal and disease states. Diabetes 30:896–902, 1981.

14. Grunberger G, Taylor SI, Dons RF, et al.: Insulin receptors in normal and disease states. Clin Endocrinol Metab 12:191–219,1983.

15. Olefsky JM: Insulin binding to adipocytes and circulating monocytes from obese patients. J Clin Invest 57: 1165–1172, 1976.

16. Comi RJ, Grunberger G, Gorden P: The relationship of insulin binding and insulin-stimulated tyrosine kinase activity is altered in type II diabetes. J Clin Invest 79:453–462, 1987.

17. Freidenberg GR, Henry RR, Klein HH, et al.: Decreased kinase activity of insulin receptors from adipocytes of non-insulin dependent diabetic subjects. J Clin Invest 79:240–250, 1987.

18. Caro JF, Ittoop O, Pories WJ, et al.: Studies on the mechanism of insulin resistance in the liver from humans with noninsulin-dependent diabetes: Insulin action and binding in isolated hepatocytes, insulin receptor structure, and kinase activity. J Clin Invest 78:249–258, 1986.

19. Caro JF, Sinha MK, Raju SM, et al.: Insulin receptor kinase in human skeletal muscle from obese subjects with and without noninsulin dependent diabetes. J Clin Invest 79:1330–1337, 1987.

20. Dunaif A, Xia J, Book CB, et al.: Excessive insulin receptor serine phosphorylation in cultured fibroblasts and in skeletal muscle. A potential mechanism for insulin resistance in the polycystic ovary syndrome. J Clin Invest 96:801–810, 1995.

21. Kiddy DS, Hamilton-Fairley D, Bush A, et al.: Improvement in endocrine and ovarian function during dietary treatment of obese women with polycystic ovary syndrome. Clin Endocrinol 36:105–111, 1992.

22. Nestler JE, Jakubowitz DJ: Decreases in ovarian cytochrome P450c17a activity and serum free testosterone after reduction of insulin secretion in polycystic ovary syndrome. New Engl J Med 335:617–623, 1996.

23. Dunaif A, Scott D, Finegood D, et al.: The insulin sensitizing agent troglitazone improves metabolic and reproductive abnormalities in the polycystic ovary syndrome. J Clin Endocrinol Metab 81:3299–3306, 1996.

24. Brown MS, Goldstein JL: A receptor-mediated pathway for cholesterol homeostasis. Science 232:34–47, 1986.

25. Taylor SI, Accili D, Haft CR, et al.: Mechanisms of hormone resistance: Lessons from insulin-resistant patients. Acta Paediatr Suppl 399:95–104, 1994.

26. Krook A, Stratton IM, O'Rahilly S: Rapid and simultaneous detection of multiple mutations by pooled and multiplex single nucleotide primer extension: Application to the study of insulin-responsive glucose transporter and insulin receptor mutations in non-insulin-dependent diabetes. Hum Mol Genet 1:391–395, 1992.

27. Krook A, Kumar S, Laing I, et al.: Molecular scanning of the insulin receptor gene in syndromes of insulin resistance. Diabetes 43:357–368, 1994.

28. Moller DE, Bjorbaek C, Vidal-Puig A: Candidate genes for insulin resistance. Diabetes Care 19:396–400, 1996.

29. Flier JS, Kahn CR, Roth J, et al.: Antibodies that impair insulin receptor binding in an unusual diabetic syndrome with severe insulin resistance. Science 190:63–65, 1975.

30. Taylor SI, Grunberger G, Marcus-Samuels B, et al.: Hypoglycemia associated with antibodies to the insulin receptor. New Engl J Med 307:1422–1426, 1982.

31. Eriksson JW, Bremel T, Eliason B, et al.: Successful treatment with plasmapheresis, cyclophosphamide, and cyclosporin A in type B syndrome of insulin resistance. Diabetes Care 21:1217–1220, 1998.

32. Kahn CR, Flier JS, Bar RS, et al.: The syndromes of insulin resistance and acanthosis nigricans. Insulin receptor disorders in man. New Engl J Med 294:739–745, 1976.

33. Grunberger G, Zick Y, Gorden P: Defect in phosphorylation of insulin receptors in cells from an insulin-resistant patient with normal insulin binding. Science 223:932–934, 1984.

34. Takahashi Y, Kadowaki H, Momomura K, et al.: A homozygous kinase-defective mutation in the insulin receptor gene in a patient with leprechaunism. Diabetologia 40:412–420, 1997.

35. Hunter SJ, Garvey WT: Insulin action and insulin resistance: Diseases involving defects in insulin receptors, signal transduction, and the glucose transport effector system. Am J Med 105:331–345, 1998.

36. Muller-Wieland D, Streicher R, Siemeister G, et al.: Molecular biology of insulin resistance. Exp Clin Endocrinol 101:17–29, 1993.

37. Genetics of endocrine disorders and diabetes mellitus. In Handbook of Endocrinology, Ed. 2. Gass, GG, and Kaplan, HM (eds.). Boca Raton, FL: CRC Press, 1996, pp. 331–345.

10

Diabetes Programs
of the Division of Diabetes, Endocrinology, and Metabolic Diseases, NIDDK, NIH

Richard C. Eastman, Joan T. Harmon, Catherine C. Cowie,
Sanford A. Garfield, Charles A. Wells, Judith Fradkin,
and Maureen I. Harris

Introduction

The Division of Diabetes, Endocrinology, and Metabolic Diseases (DDEM), NIDDK, has responsibility for extramural programs related to diabetes mellitus and its complications, endocrinology and a variety of endocrine disorders, and metabolism and metabolic diseases, including cystic fibrosis. The Institute provides approximately $230,000,000 in 1998 to scientists in medical schools, universities, and other research institutions throughout the country, and around the world, including private industry. Support for basic and clinical biomedical research, epidemiological and behavioral studies, and clinical trials is provided through investigator-initiated research grants, new investigator awards, program project and center grants, cooperative agreements, contracts, and Small Business Innovative Research awards (see Appendix). The division also supports a variety of career development and training awards as well as a limited number of resource and research and development contracts. In addition, the division provides leadership in coordinating activities throughout the National Institutes of Health (NIH) and various other Federal agencies.

In 1975 the National Commission on Diabetes was established under the NIH, in accordance with the National Diabetes Mellitus Research and Education Act.[1,2] The Commission, comprised of six nongovernment scientists, four persons from the general public, and the Directors of seven of the National Institutes of Health met throughout 1975, conducting intensive investigations on all aspects of diabetes mellitus and related topics with input from hundreds of people in the diabetes community. A long-range plan was developed consisting of specific recommendations to components of the health care community for the utilization and organization of national health resources. In 1976, the NIDDK's budget for diabetes and related research was approximately $19 million. Fueled by the provisions of the National Diabetes Mellitus Research and Education Act, the amount expended on diabetes research by the NIDDK has grown to $230,000,000 and NIH wide diabetes spending to $387,236,000. The following chapter summarizes several of the major new programs that have developed over the last two decades, in response to the 1975 initiative. Future directions for research are also indicated.

Diabetes Centers Program

The Diabetes Centers Program supported by the NIDDK includes two types of centers, Diabetes Research and Training Centers (DRTCs), and the Diabetes and Endocrinology Research Centers (DERCs), which have been in existence since 1973. The Diabetes Centers are located throughout the country and support the conduct of basic and clinical research in diabetes and related conditions (Table 10–1). They also engage in efforts to translate current diabetes knowledge to professional behavior and patient care.

The National Commission's original rationale for the creation of the DRTCs was the rapid development of new diabetes research information concerning the underlying pathophysiology of diabetes, its treatment, and prevention of complications. However, the Commission concluded that a significant and widening gap existed between the accumulation of increasing knowledge and the quality of diabetes care. The DRTCs were created to support ongoing basic and clinical research through shared core resources which define the DERCs. In addition the DRTCs support research into the mechanisms of information transfer and the development of diabetes outreach programs into the community. To accomplish this, the centers are expected to develop, test, and evaluate innovative programs directed at health-care professionals involved in the care and treatment of patients with diabetes.

An integral feature of all DRTCs is a model training–education–treatment demonstration facility commonly called a Model-Demonstration-Unit (MDU).

TABLE 10–1   Diabetes Centers Located Throughout the Country

Diabetes Research and Training Centers

  Albert Einstein College of Medicine
  Bronx, New York

  University of Chicago
  Chicago, Illinois

  Indiana University School of Medicine
  Indianapolis, Indiana

  University of Michigan
  Ann Arbor, Michigan

  Vanderbilt University School of Medicine
  Nashville, Tennessee

  Washington University School of Medicine
  St. Louis, Missouri

Diabetes and Endocrinology Research Centers

  University of Washington
  Seattle, Washington

  University of Iowa
  Iowa City, Iowa

  Joslin Diabetes Center
  Boston, Massachusetts

  University of Massachusetts
  Worcester, Massachusetts

  University of Pennsylvania School of Medicine
  Philadelphia, Pennsylvania

  Yale University School of Medicine
  New Haven, Connecticut

This important DRTC element contributes toward carrying out the center activities mentioned above. As an example, one Model Demonstration Unit provides patients having well-characterized diabetes for participation in a variety of research projects. These patients are supported while research protocols are being carried out. The unit also provides clinical and research training to physicians, allied health personnel and students.

The DRTCs are also distinguished by their Demonstration and Education (D&E) Divisions whose central purpose is to address barriers between ideal diabetes care and routine practice. This is accomplished through the support of individuals with expertise in the behavioral and social sciences to conduct translational research. Translation research is defined as investigation that tests strategies to overcome barriers to the adoption of new science into routine clinical practice. Translation in this context involves the communication of knowledge, creation of incentives for change, and surmounting obstacles to change.

DRTCs and DERCS are required to have a substantial base of ongoing, independently supported, high-quality research in diabetes and related metabolic and endocrine disorders. Support is used to operate core facilities (shared resources), pilot and feasibility studies, and an enrichment program. Centers are built on the core concept. The cores augment research efforts by providing a needed service to centers members. The cores furnish research techniques, measurements and assays, specialized instrumentation, technical expert consultation, or other services to investigators. This support enhances research progress by providing a service at lower cost and often higher quality than if investigators were to perform the same activities individually. Examples of typical biomedical research cores in Centers are a radioimmunoassay core, tissue culture core, molecular biology core, peptide sequencing core, and an instrumentation core (for large, complex, or expensive equipment that a single investigator would be unable to acquire).

The funding of these shared resources, the availability of funds for pilot and feasibility studies, and a modest enrichment program have allowed the Centers to develop new, unique, and highly desirable features. For example, not only do the biomedical cores provide a valuable resource for special measurements, determinations, and techniques for funded investigations, but they are also a source for consultation, collaboration and training in specialized methodologies.

All of the NIDDK-supported Diabetes Centers including the DRTCs provide the structure and resources needed to conduct high-quality research in diabetes and its management, to generate competent professional personnel in research and patient care, and to translate advances in diabetes research into improved patient care. The Centers are, in fact, a microcosm of the entire Diabetes Plan proposed by the National Commission on Diabetes. Their research and training programs are designed to provide, through the support of new research, new information and educational programs, and a more coordinated approach to the problem of diabetes.

Competition and Funding of the Diabetes Centers Programs

Applications for diabetes centers are accepted only in response to Request for Applications (RFAs) announced in the "NIH Guide for Grants and Contracts," available through the Internet by going to the NIH home page (http:\\www.nih.gov). Applicants must have an established research base with a strong central focus on diabetes and associated endocrinology and metabolism. Proposals may be submitted by applicants at domestic for-profit and nonprofit organizations, public and private, such as universities, colleges, hospitals, and eligible agencies of the Federal Government. Foreign institutions, however, are not eligible to apply. Direct cost award levels are currently capped at $1,250,000 per year for DRTCs and $750,000 per year for the DERCs with all diabetes center awards made for 5-year grant periods.

Applications are submitted to the NIH Division of Research Grants and are reviewed through the NIDDK Review Branch. Applications are evaluated for scientific and technical merit by an appropriate peer review group using the review criteria detailed in the RFA. Major review considerations in evaluating the strength of center investigators biomedical research at both center types are: (1) the strength of focus on diabetes, and (2) the likelihood for meaningful collaboration among center members. For the D&E component of DRTC proposals, major consideration is given to existing or planned activities to overcome barriers to translating research knowledge into improved diabetes health care.

National Diabetes Information Clearinghouse

To provide a mechanism to collect, evaluate, and disseminate information about the prevention, diagnosis, and treatment of diabetes, the Commission proposed an information clearinghouse. The National Diabetes Information Clearinghouse (NDIC) was established in 1978 in response to the mandate of the Commission. In the ensuing 20 years, the NDIC has evolved several channels of communication to health professionals, patients and the public, taking advantage of advancements in communications technology. Today, these channels include a home page on the Internet, mass media campaigns aimed at prevention and treatment of diabetes, three series of booklets, brochures and fact sheets targeted to different diabetes audiences, and a toll-free telephone number. The newsletter *Diabetes Dateline* continues to highlight research, clinical, and education advances for the diabetes community. Since its inception, the NDIC has answered more than 200,000 direct requests from the public and health professionals and distributed more than 2 million publications.

As diabetes moves into the new millenium, the NDIC is providing the foundation for a National Diabetes Education Program, a nationwide effort led by the NIDDK and the Centers for Disease Control and Prevention. The NDIC will perform all dissemination and fulfillment for the education program in continuation of its Congressional mandate "to enhance the knowledge and understanding of diabetes on the part of health professionals, patients and the public through the effective dissemination of information."

National Diabetes Data Group

To provide accurate statistics on diabetes that support public health policy, a data group was established to col-

lect and coordinate epidemiological information for analysis. The resulting data is published to assist investigators, other agencies of the Government, and the general public. NIDDK staff have authored or co-authored over 100 publications related to the mission of NIDDK and the National Diabetes Data Group (NDDG) since 1979.[97]

Another major activity of the NDDG has been the publication of *Diabetes in America*, published in two editions, the most recent in 1995. *Diabetes in America* is designed to carry out the mandate of the National Diabetes Commission to facilitate research on the epidemiological and clinical aspects of diabetes, and to develop reliable and accurate information on the scope and impact of diabetes in the U.S. population.[22] The most recent edition was also designed to serve as a reliable scientific resource for assessing the scope and impact of diabetes and its complications, to determine health policy and priorities in diabetes, and to identify new areas of need in research.

In addition to editing and publishing *Diabetes in America*, the NDDG has played an important role in devising the classification and criteria for the diagnosis of diabetes. The group first published a classification and diagnostic criteria in 1979, and participated in the recent revision of the criteria and classification by an expert committee of international scientists.[97,98]

The NDDG collaborates with other federal and nonfederal groups to foster and coordinate epidemiological data collection in diabetes, to modify data collection systems to ensure that timely and accurate information is obtained, and to promote standardization so that comparative studies can achieve their full potential for describing the scope and impact of diabetes in the United States. The NDDG works closely with the National Center for Health Statistics in design and conduct of their national surveys. The NDDG was also important in developing a portfolio of NIDDK grants through which research on diabetes in community populations is supported.

Diabetes Mellitus Interagency Coordinating Committee

The Commission also recommended that a Diabetes Mellitus Interagency Coordinating Committee (DMICC) be formed to establish Federal inter- and intra-agency linkages. Congress created the DMICC to (1) better coordinate the research activities of all the national research activities relating to diabetes mellitus, and (2) coordinate the aspects of all Federal health programs and activities relating to diabetes to assure their adequacy and technical soundness and provide for full communication. Recently, the DMICC established the National Diabetes Education Program.

National Diabetes Education Program

One of the most significant recommendations of the National Diabetes Commission was that NIDDK conduct a clinical study to assess the effect of treatment of type 1 diabetes on the development, and progression of the microvascular and macrovascular complications of diabetes. The Diabetes Control and Complications Trial (DCCT) was a randomized multicenter clinical trial sponsored by NIDDK at 29 institutions in North America. The DCCT was conducted in four phases. Phase I, devoted to planning, commenced in 1982. Phase II, a limited feasibility study, began in August 1983 with randomization of the first patient. In 1985, it was determined that the feasibility of recruitment, efficacy and acceptability of the treatment methods, and the accuracy and precision of important study measures, had all been sufficiently well established to warrant initiation of the full-scale trial. Recruitment was resumed, and eventually 1441 patients were randomized. The DCCT was highly successful. Not only were recruitment targets met in a timely fashion, but attrition was less than 5%, and more than 95% of all scheduled endpoint measures obtained.[99]

The DCCT was terminated 1 year ahead of schedule because the study demonstrated a highly clinically significant reduction in the risk of development and progression of microvascular and neuropathic complications. Intensive therapy reduced the risk of developing retinopathy by 76%, slowed progression of retinopathy by 53%, reduced risk of developing nephropathy by 44%, slowed progression of nephropathy by 56%, and reduced the risk of developing neuropathy by 60%.[99]

Prior to the conclusion of the DCCT, members of the D&E Divisions of the DRTCs began discussing the difficult problem of translating the results of the DCCT to clinical practice. It was recognized that direct application of the DCCT intervention to clinical practice would be difficult, and previous experience from other studies made it clear that simply announcing the results of the trial would produce little change in community practice patterns. At the behest of the diabetes division, the D&E Directors of the DRTCs/undertook a formal analysis of the translation strategies and research that would be needed to translate the DCCT into clinical practice.

This report, entitled "Metabolic Control Matters" and an updated set of recommendations entitled "Making Metabolic Control Matter" set forth the need for coordinating the many components of a DCCT translation program.[100] The report was based on expert opinion that the DCCT results should be applied to type 2 diabetes.[101] Subsequently, data from observational trials and a clinical trial have greatly strengthened this

recommendation.[102,103] A major conclusion reached in these reports is that a National Diabetes Education Program (NDEP) was needed. An NDEP would provide a framework for collaboration between Federal agencies and state health departments as well as multiple professional, voluntary health, minority, national, and other public and private sector organizations including industry (e.g., managed care, pharmaceutical companies, businesses, and others). It would be an umbrella program to coordinate national efforts to reduce the burden of diabetes.

During 1995 a plan was developed with the Division of Diabetes Translation at CDC to plan an NDEP. A Planning Committee was appointed and charged to explore the potential activities of an NDEP. Meetings were held to elicit input from four key constituency groups that included:

- primary care providers (e.g., physicians, certified diabetes educators, and dietitians);

- payers and purchasers of health care (e.g., insurance industry, managed care-organizations, employer purchasers, and government health programs);

- consumers and patient-advocates (e.g., persons with diabetes, organizations representing target populations such as African-Americans, Native-Americans, Asians, and the elderly); and

- public health providers (e.g., state and territorial diabetes control programs, public health educators, and public health nutritionists).

Using input from these planning meetings, a mission statement, goal, and objectives for the NDEP were drafted. The mission states that, "the NDEP is a collaborative effort to improve the treatment and outcome of people with diabetes, promote early diagnosis, and ultimately, prevent the onset of this disease." Based on existing scientific evidence, the NDEP will focus on the implementation of secondary and tertiary prevention strategies proven effective in preventing or delaying progression of the debilitating and costly medical complications related to diabetes.

Broad target audiences were identified for the NDEP, including the general public, patients and their families, health professionals, policymakers, and payers. The goal of the NDEP is "to reduce the morbidity and mortality of diabetes and its complications." Based on the work of the planning committee and a wide range of interested groups, the NDEP moved from its planning stage to the implementation stage with the formal announcement of the National Diabetes Education Program at the 1997 annual meeting of the American Diabetes Association.

Diabetes Research Programs

Type 1 Diabetes Research Program

This program emphasizes support of investigator-initiated basic and clinical research relating to type 1 diabetes, endocrine function of the pancreas including insulin secretion, and islet transplantation. Studies focus on: (1) the etiology, pathogenesis, prevention, diagnosis, treatment, and cure of type 1 diabetes; (2) the immunobiology of autoimmune diseases as it relates to type 1 diabetes; (3) the genetic basis of type 1 diabetes; (4) identification of specific markers that characterize individuals predisposed to type 1 diabetes; (5) the viral etiology of type 1 diabetes; (6) the environmental factors that relate to pathogenesis of type 1 diabetes; (7) the growth and differentiation of the pancreatic endocrine cells; (8) physiological regulation of pancreatic secretion of hormones, especially insulin; (9) molecular mechanisms of the pancreatic endocrine cell response to glucose and other secretogogues; (10) development of methods to prevent type 1 diabetes in high-risk individuals; (11) beta cell, islet, or pancreas transplantation; (12) the development of other approaches to achieve euglycemia; (13) the development and utilization of animal models for type 1 diabetes to further our understanding of this disease; and (14) type 1 diabetes in minority populations.

Type 2 Diabetes Research Program

The Type 2 Diabetes Research Program supports investigator-initiated basic and clinical research in type 2 diabetes, impaired glucose tolerance, and insulin resistance. The majority of individuals who suffer from diabetes have type 2 diabetes. Type 2 diabetes affects approximately 14–16 million Americans. The disease severely impacts on African-Americans, Hispanic-Americans, Native-Americans, Native-Hawaiians, and Asian-Americans. Identification of genetic and environmental factors underlying type 2 diabetes is a major goal of the type 2 Diabetes Research Program. Studies focus on: (1) the etiology, pathogenesis, prevention, diagnosis, American minority populations that are so severely impacted by type 2 diabetes; (3) the identification of genetic and environmental factors underlying type 2 diabetes; (4) the biochemistry and cell biology of insulin intolerance, insulin resistance, and type 2 diabetes; (5) the mechanisms of action of insulin and insulinmimetic agents; (6) the insulin receptor structure and function, postreceptor signaling and insulin-dependent regulation of cellular processes; (7) the glucose transporters; (8) the cellular uptake of other sugars, amino acids, and macromolecules relevant to diabetes; (9) the metabolism of carbohydrates and proteins in relation to diabetes including mathe-matical models of metabolism; (10) the relationship of exercise and obesity to diabetes; (11) the relationship of gestational diabetes to type 2 diabetes; (12) prevention of impaired glucose tolerance and type 2 diabetes, particularly in high-risk populations; and (13) the development and utilization of animal models to further our understanding of type 2 diabetes.

Diabetes Epidemiology Research Program

The Diabetes Epidemiology Research Program provides research grant and contract support for studies on the epidemiology of diabetes and its complications in type 1 diabetes and type 2 diabetes. This research focuses on study of the distribution and determinants of diabetes in various populations, including community-based groups and the general US population. It includes studies on the genetic and environmental factors that determine type 2 diabetes; the demographic patterns of diabetes, as well as the geographic and temporal variations in the disease, and variations in disease frequency by race, socioeconomic status, metabolic factors, and other determinants; studies on the etiology of diabetes including identification of risk factors determining susceptibility to diabetes and variations in the distribution of risk factors within populations and within individuals; research on the etiology and pathogenesis of diabetes complications in well-defined populations to define and quantitate the complications of diabetes; and the genetic, lifestyle, and environmental factors that predispose people with diabetes to complications. Special emphasis is placed on studies of US minority populations in which the prevalence and severity of type 2 diabetes and its complications is substantially elevated.

Diabetes Complications Research Program

This program focuses on research related to diabetic complications and to the effects of diabetes on organ systems, including but not limited to: the kidney, eye, nervous system, vascular system, and reproductive system. Areas of interest include the acute as well as the chronic complications of diabetes and includes fetal development in diabetes. The key areas related to pathogenesis encompass, but are not limited to: (1) the genetic factors influencing susceptibility to complications; (2) the interplay between diabetes and risk factors such as hypertension, dyslipidemia, and smoking in pathogenesis of complications; (3) the polyol pathway, and nonenzymatic glycation of proteins; and (4) use of aldose reductase inhibitors, aminoguanidines, and other agents to prevent complications. Research on mechanical methods of insulin administration, including glucose sensors, pumps, and integrators, also constitute a focus of this program. In addition, efforts are supported to investigate the link between behavior and physical health as related to diabetes, including bio-behavioral mechanisms; identification and distribution of psychosocial risk factors in behaviors and social interventions to prevent diabetes or its complications.

Not only does diabetes mellitus significantly affect minority populations, but its complications are disproportionately increased in minorities. A particular emphasis is placed on understanding the etiology, complications, and sequelae of diabetes in minority populations. The Diabetes Research Section encourages research on these issues in representative affected minority populations.

World Health Organization (WHO) Collaborating Center for Diabetes

This center, sponsored by DDEM, provides guidance in developing international research and training in diabetes through NIH research grants and contracts; conducts collaborative research on diabetes and its complications with international scientists; promotes interchange of scientific and health information among WHO member countries and among individual scientists in the international arena; and provides expert advice and consultation to WHO and other international committees and agencies. See Appendix I.

Diabetes Prevention and Treatment Initiative

The DCCT demonstrated the significant benefits of glycemic control in delaying and preventing the complications of diabetes, but with a two- threefold greater risk of significant hypoglycemia. This highlighted the need for more efficient and safer ways of achieving euglycemia. In response to this need, NIDDK - announced the Diabetes Prevention and Treatment Initiative (Table 10–2). The initiative is broad in scope, encompassing basic research, applied research on therapeutics, and clinical trials.

Molecular Pathogenesis of Diabetes

A complete understanding of the molecular pathogenesis of diabetes is central to the goal of preventing and curing diabetes. Thus, the bulk of diabetes research grants funded by DEMD relate to the etiology and pathophysiology of type 1 and type 2 diabetes mellitus. With regard to type 1 diabetes mellitus, significant efforts are directed at the role of T cells and B cells in the pathogenesis of disease. In particular, investigators are trying to ascertain the initial trigger of the autoimmune destruction of the beta cell. This trigger may be an environmental component or a genetic component

TABLE 10–2   Components of the Diabetes Prevention and Treatment Initiative

Approaches to achieving Euglycemia
    Molecular pathogenesis of diabetes
    Search for the diabetes genes
    Pancreas transplantation
    Islet cell transplantation
    Beta cell replacement therapy
    Mechanical approaches
    Interventions to heighten tissue responsiveness to insulin
International Pancreas and Islet Transplant Registry
Clinical trials and studies
    Diabetes Prevention Program
    Diabetes prevention trial—Type 1 diabetes
    Epidemiology of diabetes intervention and complications
    Diabetes in minority populations

or a combination of both such as a super-antigen. Once the immune system has been activated, researchers are attempting to understand the series of steps including the homing of the lymphocytes to the islets, the invasion of the islet, and the final destruction of the beta cells by the cytotoxic T cells. Others are delving into the role of B cells, that is, are antibodies from the B cells only harbingers of the autoimmune attack or are the B cells directly involved in an early amplification of the disease process? Clearly islet-specific antibodies are extremely useful in ascertaining risk of disease in humans. Studies are continuing to improve this risk assessment by use of improved antibody assays and improved knowledge of the natural history of the disease as exemplified by antibody determinations, genetic evaluations, and metabolic evaluations.

In response to the need for expertise from outside the field to study type 1 diabetes, NIDDK has since 1993 cofunded the Diabetes Interdisciplinary Research Program (DIRP) with the Juvenile Diabetes Foundation International. The DIRPS represent a broad coalition of international investigators who are addressing many facets of the pathogenesis and treatment of type 1 diabetes.

The etiology of type 2 diabetes mellitus is being studied on multiple fronts including peripheral insulin resistance and beta cell abnormalities. Basic research is being conducted with investigator initiated research grants and diabetes center core facilities in both areas. To address our basic knowledge of peripheral loss of insulin responsiveness, researchers are examining the mechanism of insulin action from interaction with its receptor on the outer surface of the cell membrane to regulation of gene expression. A major focus is on signal transduction through the insulin receptor, including coupling to the MAP kinase pathway through tyrosine-phosphorylated substrate coupling proteins, such as IRS-1. Also included are studies on nutrient transporters with a primary focus on glucose transporters. These studies involve aspects of hormonal regulation, gene expression of glucose transporters, and structure/function studies on the transporter proteins. Additionally, studies are being conducted on the normal and abnormal biosynthesis and metabolism of carbohydrates, fats and amino acids, as well as the regulation and structure/function of enzymes involved in these metabolic pathways and the control that insulin has in the regulation of these pathways.

The abnormal functioning of the β cell in type 2 diabetes mellitus is being examined by multiple investigators. There is particular emphasis on the biochemical components involved in the glucose-stimulated insulin response of the β cell and regulation of insulin release by calcium. The role of the beta cell ATP-sensitive potassium channel, I_{KATP}, which is composed of the sulfonylurea receptor and an inward rectifying potassium channel, has been deduced. Functional alterations in this complex are being evaluated to ascertain their involvement in abnormal beta cell function.

A component of diabetes risk is attributable to genetic determinants. To varying degrees, this is true for type 1 and type 2 diabetes. Thus, a major component of the research is to identify the genes responsible for the development of diabetes. Approaches to identification of genes causing these multifactorial disorders include studies in humans and in relevant animal models. Identification of susceptibility genes in minority populations disproportionately affected by type 2 diabetes mellitus is an important focus of research. Once a gene has been identified, research on the role of these genes in determining the pathophysiology of the disease, and the role of the genotype in determining the phenotype of the disease can be undertaken. This research may use genotype/phenotype correlation studies in the human population, the development of animal models, or overexpression of the mutant protein to define the role of particular mutations.

Because of the role of genetics in diabetes, two requests for applications were sponsored. These were entitled "Genes Responsible for Insulin Dependent Diabetes Mellitus" and "Human Genes for Non-Insulin Dependent Diabetes Mellitus." The meritorious grants resulting from these solicitations address the identification of genetic determinants in three ways: collaborative efforts between several laboratories to accomplish a human genome-wide linkage analysis; individual laboratories conducting candidate gene studies; and individual laboratories utilizing animal models to identify diabetes-risk genes for which the human homology could be determined.

The search for the diabetes genes has been interesting and informative. As a result of these studies, we have gained a greater appreciation of the role for glucokinase in the β cell and the importance of this enzyme in maturity onset diabetes of the young (MODY). Additional recent findings have given us a new appreciation for the role of transcription factors in the pathogenesis of type 2 diabetes mellitus. Thus, genetic analysis has been most informative in divulging the metabolic and regulatory components that have a significant role in the pathogenesis of diabetes. However, we have also learned more regarding the genetic complexity of this disease. New findings indicate that mutations in single alleles of two different genes can cause a type 2-like syndrome. Thus, a glucose tolerant animal heterozygous for a mutation in the insulin receptor when crossed with a glucose tolerant animal heterozygous for a mutation in an insulin response element (IRS-1) gives rise to a glucose-intolerant animal that develops diabetes with increasing age. These results exemplify the genetic complexity of this disease and the challenge we face in developing strategies to identify genes involved in the many different varieties of diabetes. Similar conclusions can be drawn from genetic studies of type 1 diabetes mellitus.

These results heighten the importance of examining the genetic makeup of specific populations, especially those populations having a unique or particular form of diabetes. They also demonstrate the critical need for the investment in statistical genetics that may offer experimental designs to dissect interactions between genes thus allowing identification of susceptibility gene loci. From the ascertainment of a genetic locus, it is essential to focus on and identify the specific gene(s) involved.

Approaches to Achieving Euglycemia

While our ultimate research goal is to prevent the onset of diabetes, investigators are also pursuing means to modulate blood glucose levels in diabetic patients and to restore insulin-producing capacity. These approaches are potentially applicable to all individuals with diabetes mellitus, through transplantation of the whole pancreas, or of isolated islets, or β cells. Today, the only method that offers fine blood glucose control is pancreas transplantation.

Several decades ago, islet transplantation was proposed—instead of whole pancreas transplantation—in the hope of reducing surgical complexity by allowing intravenous injection of islets. Initial animal studies on islet transplantation were encouraging, but subsequent research using larger animals and humans resulted in lower success rates. Unfortunately, the initial promise held out for islet cell transplantation has not been realized. Thus, of the 270 adult islet transplants in people with type 1 diabetes performed by the end of 1995, only 10% did not require insulin injections for more than 1 week, and only 5% remained off insulin injections for more than 1 year. In light of these results, and realizing that islet transplantation may reinitiate the autoimmune attack on the transplanted β cells, many researchers are pursuing studies to interdict the autoimmune destruction of islet cells. While the "gold standard" for transplant success has been insulin-independence, that is, β cell replacement therapy may have a role even if complete insulin-independence is not achieved. Clinicians are observing a beneficial effect of islet transplantation in transplant recipients who have not become insulin-independent, but who have demonstrable insulin production by the transplanted islets. These patients require less exogenous insulin and show an improvement in metabolic control, which equates to fewer incidents of serious episodes of hypoglycemia, and which may lower the risk of long-term complications.

Considerable knowledge has accrued from the early studies of islet transplantation, including: improved procedures for handling the donor pancreas to optimize islet survival; improved methods for preparing large quantities of islets; the development of standardized solutions of enzymes to dissociate the islets from the other pancreatic tissue; ascertainment of effective transplant sites; pretransplant treatment methods to reduce the recipient's islet rejection; ascertainment of the minimum number of islets necessary to acquire insulin-independence (6000 per kg body weight); cryopreservation procedures for islets; and demonstration of the detrimental effects of immunosuppressive therapy on islet function and survival.

Replacement of β cells may also be envisioned using bioengineered beta cells, β cells grown in continuous or permanent culture, and animal islets. The bioengineered β cells would be transfected cells whose origins were not beta cells. To be able to succeed in this endeavor, it is essential to establish which β cell components are required for glucose-stimulated insulin secretion as well as the regulation of these components. These components would, of course, include the internal β cell machinery, but it may also include interactions between beta cells and interactions between β cells and the extracelluar matrix. The cultured β cells require the identification and production of growth and differentiation factors that will enable the propagation of either fetal or adult β cells. Animal islets, while offering an ample supply of islets, offer additional complications and potential dangers, such as the transmission of animal diseases to humans.

Immune isolation procedures are presently being proposed in conjunction with β cell replacement procedures to obtain a successful cellular approach to achieving euglycemia. As in the case of β cell replacement there are several methods of isolating β cells from the immune system. These include implantation in an immune-privileged site, encapsulating in an immune protective membrane, and co-transplantation of beta cells with transfected myoblasts secreting agents (TNF or Fas-L) that will induce apoptosis of the cytotoxic lymphocytes. All of these methods must be tested and developed.

Inherent in many of the approaches to achieving euglycemia is the need to produce a self-renewing population of β cells. This would allow for potential treatments for diabetes by replacement of β cells by transplantation, implantation in an immune-privileged site, or by encapsulation in an immune protective membrane. These potential applications have been hampered by our lack of knowledge of the developmental biology of β cells. The natural growth and differentiation factors for islet cells have not been fully elucidated. In addition, the isolation of a self-renewing stem cell and identification of markers that can follow the movement and development of the β cell from the duct cell are critical for our understanding. These markers will also be important in charting the development of other islet cells and in establishing the architecture of the islet. Several transcription factors have been isolated that are β-cell specific. In particular, the IDX-1 homeodomain protein and hepatic nuclear factor, HNF-4, seem to be required for pancreas development or β-cell differentiation. These transcription factors may provide the key to dissect additional factors necessary for the beta cell growth and differentiation. Identification of the master control genes of the β cell would enormously improve our ability to produce a self-renewing population of β cells.

Finally, in addition to acquiring basic information on the cell biology of the β cell, it is critically important to establish methods to measure beta cell number or mass *in vivo*. In type 1 diabetes mellitus, it is assumed that the clinical onset of disease occurs when 90% of the β cells have been destroyed. Unfortunately, there is no method available today that can measure β-cell number noninvasively, that is, without pancreas biopsy or pancreatectomy. Therefore, we are not able to measure disease progression nor are we able to measure implant survival.

Present support in this area is almost entirely via investigator initiated research grants or program project grants with the remaining support via the core facilities at the various diabetes centers. The portfolio encompasses basic and clinical research. It includes β-cell-specific transcription factors involved in the control of insulin synthesis and in the regulation of islet cell development from progenitor cells. There are a number of grants which specifically address the biochemistry of β-cell function incorporating aspects of the glucose sensing apparatus and the machinery utilized to synthesize and secrete insulin. Embodied in the essential machinery grants are studies of the sulfonylurea receptor, another member of the ABC transporter family, and studies of cation channels related to cell signaling. Results from these basic studies have been applied to the bioengineering of cells capable of glucose-regulated insulin secretion.

The clinical studies consist of studies examining approaches to β-cell replacement including islet cell transplantation. In particular, one investigator is studying islet transplantation in animals and in humans, developing transplant tolerance induction methods using donor bone marrow cells. Other studies are examining transplant tolerance induction by implantation of donor tissue into the thymus or into immune privileged sites such as the testes. Results from the latter studies have allowed innovative proposals on the co-transplantation of beta cells with bioengineered cells which secrete the Fas-L to protect the β cells from immune destruction. The immunology of graft rejection is also being studied.

Mechanical and biomechanical approaches are an appealing alternative strategy to achieving euglycemia. Insulin pump technology has advanced significantly in recent years, and much experience has been gained with both external and implantable insulin pumps. What is clearly needed, however, is a continuous glucose sensor that can provide the necessary glucose input data to close the feedback loop and provide autoregulation of blood glucose. Sensor technology has also advanced in recent years, and intravascular devices are available that can continuously monitor glucose in animals for prolonged periods. Minimally invasive or noninvasive techniques are obviously appealing, but to date technologies using reflectance and transmission technologies and microdialysis have failed to produce a device suitable for routine patient use. This area of applied research remains a high priority of the treatment initiative.

International Pancreas and Islet Transplant Registry

In recent years there has been an expansion of research involving whole and segmental pancreas transplantation for the treatment of diabetes mellitus. To assist the research community in the evaluation of progress in this area of transplantation, the NIDDK established the International Pancreas and Islet Transplant Registry by a contract mechanism. This contract was awarded to Dr. David E.R. Sutherland at the University of Minnesota in 1989 and was renewed in 1994 (see Chapter 21). During the second year of the contract, the scope of the contract was expanded to allow the evaluation of the efficacy of pancreas transplantation on the secondary complications of diabetes (the Secondary Complications Study, SCS). While this expansion of the contract has been in force for several years, it has been the experience of the contractor that collection of secondary complications data from the transplant centers has been difficult and quite often incomplete. This may be due to the lack of insurance coverage for post-transplant testing comparable to that of pretransplant testing (cardiovascular studies, nerve conduction tests, renal function tests such as creatinine clearance, etc.). Also, patients often are followed after transplant in their home state, which frequently is different from that of the transplanting institution, making access to follow-up data more complex. To aid in the acquisition of reliable and complete data, the Health Care Financing Administration (HCFA) is joining the NIDDK and will support the clinical costs associated with simultaneous pancreas-kidney transplantation (SPK) as well as the follow-up tests to determine the benefits of the procedure. HCFA anticipates being able to acquire the necessary data to determine if there is sufficient justification to support SPK.

Interventions to Heighten Tissue Responsiveness to Insulin

Because the majority of people with diabetes (type 2 diabetes mellitus) are able to secrete appreciable amounts of insulin, novel approaches are necessary to increase the effectiveness of their own insulin or enhance the utilization of energy stores. Thus, innovative strategies are required to reduce peripheral insulin resistance, reduce insulin clearance, or design a more effective insulin molecule. Recently, several new pharmaceuticals, for example, troglitazone and metformin, have demonstrated the potential for development of other agents to rectify peripheral insulin resistance or regulate liver glucose production. Alternatively, agents may be found to stimulate energy utilization, thus negating the need to store glucose or other energy sources. These future therapies may be advantageous for individuals with either type 1 or type 2 diabetes because lower levels of insulin might be therapeutic under these circumstances. Additional emphasis in this direction should offer treatment options to both people with type 1 and type 2 diabetes.

Clinical Trials

Clinical trials are an important component of the initiative, because they have the most immediate potential to affect clinical practice. Trials supported by the NIDDK are supported by one of several mechanisms. Pilot and feasibility studies and single-center trials involving relatively small numbers of patients, and with total cost budgets less the $500,000, are usually supported by investigator initiated RO-1 research project grants. Large-scale trials with multiple centers and greater fiscal requirements are conducted under contracts or cooperative agreements (UO-1 mechanism).

The Diabetes Control and Complications Trial, for example, was done to definitively determine the role of glycemic control in the prevention of complications of diabetes. Efficacy trials like the DCCT are a critical first step in establishing the scientific basis for public health decisions. In 1991, with the end of the DCCT in sight, the division began to plan for the next generation of clinical trials and studies. It was the goal from the outset to broaden the clinical trial effort to include both types of diabetes, and to have more than one major trial underway simultaneously.

Diabetes Prevention Program

Between 1991 and 1993 NIDDK sought advice on future clinical trials from leaders in diabetes research, the National Diabetes Advisory Board, and an ad-hoc advisory committee. It was concluded that a primary prevention trial for type 2 diabetes was an important next step to reduce the excess morbidity and mortality from type 2 diabetes in the US population. Preliminary analyses indicated that such a trial could be conducted in a reasonable period of time (7 years including planning, implementation, analysis, and reporting) with the funds available to NIDDK.

During the planning stages of the trial, NIDDK adapted the DCCT chronic disease model of type 1 diabetes, to allow analysis of prevention of type 2 diabetes. Additional programming was added to model progression from impaired glucose tolerance to type 2 diabetes.[104] In addition, the model was programmed to allow comparisons of the benefits and cost-effectiveness of tertiary interventions for complications (i.e., photocoagulation, use of ACE inhibitors for gross proteinuria, preventive footcare), secondary prevention (glycemic control as in the DCCT), and primary prevention. Thus, the potential cost-effectiveness of primary prevention of type 2 diabetes could be considered in the context of other proven treatments for the disease.

The analysis indicated that delaying the onset of type 2 diabetes would have a clinically significant effect on the lifetime risk of microvascular complications and neuropathy when compared to optimal treatment of diabetes without primary prevention. Furthermore, a significant effect on survival was predicted.[104] These benefits were seen despite the fact that no direct effect of delaying diabetes on cardiovascular disease morbidity or mortality was assumed for these analyses.

A detailed cost-effectiveness analysis of primary prevention showed that primary prevention would be cost-effective over a wide range of assumptions. For example, an intervention that reduced the annual risk of diabetes by 40% would cost $13,740 per QALY (quality-adjusted life-year) gained, which is in the range of interventions that are considered highly cost-effective.[104] The analysis was robust, in that cost-effectiveness was reasonable over a wide range of assumptions regarding costs, progression rates to diabetes, efficacy of the interventions, screening costs, intervention costs, quality-of-life adjustments, compliance, and economic parameters.[104]

In the Fall of 1992 the division published an RFA for a primary prevention trial for type 2 diabetes. A special study section convened by NIDDK conducted primary preview, and approved 65 applications. From this pool, UO-1 awards were made to the first 21 centers. In addition, administrative actions were taken to support centers at the NIDDK facility in Sacaton, Arizona, with satellite centers at two other sites in American-Indian communities. In addition, a satellite center was established in Hawaii. Between July 1993 and November 1995 a consensus protocol was developed and unanimously approved by the steering committee. Patients are eligible for the trial who have a fasting plasma glucose greater than 95 mg/dL, and who have impaired glucose tolerance. Patients are randomized to a standard lifestyle arm, intensive lifestyle arm, and two drug arms (placebo-controlled administration of metformin and troglitzone). The primary endpoint is progression to diabetes. Secondary endpoints include assessments of cardiovascular disease risk factors, surrogate measures, and events. Studies of insulin secretion are also conducted during the course of the trial.

Recruitment for the DPP began in June of 1996, and to date is maintaining an excellent recruitment record in terms of numbers of patients and minority participation. The recruitment phase is planned for 3 years, and the total duration of the trial is planned for 6 years. The arm with troglitizone was terminated in 1998 because a patient developed liver failure and subsequently died after liver transplantation. Conclusion of the trial is expected by the year 2002.

The DPP is funded by a consortium of public and private funds, with the division serving as the principal supporter ($\sim 85\%$ of the funds). Additional support is made by other NIH institutes and offices, the American Diabetes Association, and industry.

Diabetes Prevention Trial-Type 1 Diabetes

In 1990, the NIDDK, NIAID, and NICHD cosponsored a workshop on "Clinical Trials of Immunosuppression for Prevention of Insulin Dependent Diabetes Mellitus." The workshop participants reached consensus that there were measurable parameters that could identify a group of individuals at high risk of type 1 diabetes and that further clinical studies were timely and warranted to explore the ability of immunomodulation to alter the natural history of type 1 diabetes. Subsequent to the workshop, several clinical trial proposals were submitted to the NIH, however, the immunosuppressive agents proposed were very nonspecific in nature. To generate more specific proposals, as recommended by the original workshop participants and the National Diabetes Advisory Board, a program announcement was released entitled "Prevention of Insulin Dependent Diabetes Mellitus by Immunomodulation."

The program announcement resulted in three investigator-initiated (RO1) research applications that were deemed to be of scientific value. The proposals were submitted by major centers involved in studies on the immunology of type 1 diabetes, immunomodulation, and family screening programs. The applications were reviewed initially by an NIDDK Ad Hoc Study Section and secondarily by the NIDDK Advisory Council in the spring of 1993. The NIDDK Advisory Council noted that the individual studies were timely because of the growing pressure in clinical practice to try unproven therapies in high-risk patients outside the framework of a clinical trial. Three UO1 cooperative agreements were awarded in September 1993 for a period of 5 years. Ten clinical centers and 339 affiliates and satellites are supported. A third UO1 cooperative agreement was awarded to support all data coordination, collection, and analysis, as well as to provide all laboratory support to the study. The trial is jointly supported by the NIDDK, NIAID, NICHDD and voluntary agencies (American Diabetes Association and Juvenile Diabetes Foundation International), and industry.

The major objective of Diabetes Prevention Trial-Type 1 Diabetes (DPT-1) is to determine whether early intervention by antigen-based therapies in nondiabetic relatives of persons with type 1 diabetes can delay the development of type 1 diabetes as a clinical disease. First-degree relatives of probands with type 1 diabetes have more than a tenfold risk of type 1 diabetes compared with the general population. Impending type 1 diabetes can often be identified through the detection of autoantibodies directed against self-antigens of the pancreatic β cells. Initial screening is being conducted by determining the presence of islet cell autoantibodies (ICA). Those individuals found to have ICA are then staged into different categories of risk of type 1 diabetes, depending on their point of progression to the clinical disease. This further assessment of risk of type 1 diabetes in nondiabetic relatives is based on a number of factors, including: genetic susceptibility, the presence of insulin autoantibodies (IAA), and the degree of loss of first phase plasma insulin response (FPIR) during an intravenous glucose tolerance test. "High Risk" relatives are those that have been predicted to have a greater than 50% probability of developing type 1 diabetes within the next 5 years based on being positive for ICA and having a low FPIR. "Intermediate Risk" relatives are those that have been predicted to have a 25–50% risk of type 1 diabetes during the next 5 years based on being positive for ICA and also for IAA, but having a normal FPIR. Relatives at lower risk lack IAA and have a normal FPIR. The purpose of dividing subjects into different predictive risk groups is that different intervention strategies are best applied to them because of their stage of natural history. In addition, the invasiveness of the therapeutic approaches to be tested needs to be appropriately reconciled with the estimated risk of type 1 diabetes in the different risk groups.

In the "High Risk" group, the protocol is designed to determine whether parenteral insulin therapy, consisting of annual courses of continuous intravenous insulin, with accompanying chronic subcutaneous insulin, will delay their expected development of clinical type 1 diabetes. Subjects are being randomized to either *the experimental treatment group* or *closely monitored (control) group* who will be closely monitored and offered treatment at the earliest sign of clinical diabetes. The intervention protocol for the "Intermediate Risk" group is designed to determine whether presentation of an islet cell autoantigen (i.e., orally ingested insulin) to the immune system via the intestinal mucosa can induce immunological tolerance, thereby delaying the development of type 1 diabetes. Subjects are being randomized to either the *experimental treatment group* or *placebo-controlled group*. Subjects who are ICA positive but who are at lower risk of type 1 diabetes are not being enrolled into the study but are being followed for progression to intermediate or high risk with the opportunity for enrollment at that stage. The goal of DPT-1 is to enroll 340 "High Risk" and 490 "Intermediate Risk" subjects. Subjects were first randomized to the "High Risk" protocol in December 1994 and to the "Intermediate Risk" protocol in September 1996. To date, recruitment is going well. The trial is expected to conclude early in the next decade.

Epidemiology of Diabetes Intervention and Complications. Epidemiology of Diabetes Intervention and Complications (EDIC) is a longitudinal epidemiological study of the later evolution of severe microvascular and macrovascular complications in the DCCT cohort of subjects with type 1 diabetes. At the conclusion of the DCCT in 1993, the Study Group and the NIDDK believed there was an excellent opportunity to address a number of deficiencies in our knowledge of the later evolution of the complications of type 1 diabetes, particularly related to nephropathy and macrovascular disease. There is a remarkable paucity of data on complications in type 1 diabetes, other than for retinopathy, regarding their occurrence, pathogenesis, associated risk factors, interactions (including co-occurrence), and effective treatments. No study has prospectively examined the course of diabetic nephropathy in a population of type 1 diabetic patients for a period long enough to characterize its progression and examine risk factors, including glycemia, diabetes treatment, blood pressure, and dietary and genetic factors. Current understanding of the development and progression of diabetic nephropathy is predicated on cross-sectional and retrospective analyses and brief interventional studies that have examined short-term surrogate outcomes rather than the hard outcomes of clinical nephropathy. Despite the major impact of macrovascular diseases on the type 1 diabetic population, almost no long-term, large-scale studies have been performed in type 1 diabetes. There are no current studies to determine whether risk factors for macrovascular disease identified in studies of nondiabetic and type 2 diabetic populations pertain in type 1 diabetes. The DCCT cohort afforded the opportunity to study the long-term complications of Type 1 diabetes due to the cohort's large size, detailed and comprehensive characterization of the development of early vascular disease, and the concurrent measures of metabolic control and other putative risk factors over an average 6.5-year period.

In early 1993, DCCT patients completed a closeout assessment. EDIC was launched in April 1994 and during 1994 all patients still alive were approached to complete the first-year assessment, with annual assessments thereafter. EDIC is now in its third year of follow-up with plans for follow-up into 2006. More than 90% of the former DCCT participants are participating. The EDIC study is strictly observational in that subjects are no longer randomized to their original glycemic treatment group; however, all EDIC subjects have been encouraged to practice intensive diabetes management. During EDIC, all subjects receive their diabetes care from community rather than study sources, although many continue to be followed by DCCT investigators.

With the transition from the DCCT to EDIC, funding for the study was changed from a UO1 cooperative agreement mechanism to a contract mechanism. A contract was believed by NIDDK to be the most efficient and expeditious mechanism for ensuring a smooth passage to EDIC for the DCCT study group. EDIC is supported predominently by the division, with a small contribution from industry.

Minority Health Issues and Research.   Minority health with respect to diabetes is a special concern of the NIDDK. Minority populations have a higher risk of developing diabetes, developing diabetes at an earlier age than the non-Hispanic White population, and in many communities suffer much higher rates of complications, such as blindness, amputations, and kidney failure. The division has stimulated research by minority investigators and on minority populations by publication of two RFAs for planning grants, and two subsequent RFAs for follow-up RO-1 grants. The division actively promotes research on diabetes in minority populations in the basic and clinical research portfolios, as well as in the large-scale clinical trials. For example, the minority recruitment goals for DPP and DPT-1 are based on assessment of the impact of diabetes on minority populations. For the DPP, the goal is 50% minority participation, and for DPT-1 is participation in proportion to the population burden of type 1 diabetes in minority populations.

References

1. National Diabetes Mellitus Research and Education Act. Public Law 93-354 (July 23, 1974).

2. Davidson JK: Diabetes milestone: Public Law 93-354. ADA Forecast 27:4–11, 1974.

3. Arthritis, Diabetes, and Digestive Disease Amendments of 1976, Public Law 94-562 (October 19, 1976); and Health Programs Extension Act of 1980, Public Law 96-538 (December 17, 1980).

4. Department of Health, Education and Welfare: Report of the National Commission on Diabetes to the Congress of the United States, Vol. 1. *In* The Long-Range Plan to Combat Diabetes, National Institutes of Health (NIH) Publication 76-1018. Washington, DC: Government Printing Office, 1976, pp. 31–36.

5. NDAB Long-Range Plan to Combat Diabetes—1987; National Institutes of Health Publication 88-1587. Washington, DC: Government Printing Office, 1988.

6. Roman SH, Harris MI: Management of diabetes mellitus from a public health perspective. *In* Hirsch I and Riddle M (eds): Current Therapies for Diabetes, Philadephia: W.B. Saunders Co. (in press).

7. Harris MI, Eastman RC, Cowie CC, et al.: Comparison of diabetes diagnostic categories in the U.S. population according to 1997 ADA and 1980–1985 WHO diagnostic criteria. Diabetes Care 20:1859–1862, 1997.

8. Harris MI, Zimmet PZ: Classification of diabetes mellitus and other categories of glucose intolerance. *In* Alberti KGGM, Zimmet P, DeFronzo RA and Keen H (eds): International Textbook of Diabetes Mellitus, 2nd ed. New York: John Wiley & Sons, 1997, pp. 9–24.

9. Eastman RC, Cowie CC, Harris MI: Undiagnosed diabetes or impaired glucose tolerance and cardiovascular risk (editorial). Diabetes Care 20:127–280, 1997.

10. Cowie CC, Harris MI: Ambulatory medical care for non-Hispanic whites, African Americans, and Mexican Americans with NIDDM in the U.S. Diabetes Care 20:142–47, 1997.

11. Harris MI, Eastman RC: Early detection of undiagnosed non-insulin-dependent diabetes mellitus. JAMA 276:1261–1262, 1996.

12. Harris MI: Epidemiology of NIDDM. *In* Proceedings of the Second Japan-US Diabetes Epidemiology Training Course. Japan Diabetes Foundation Publication Series No. 5, 1996, pp. 15–21.

13. Harris MI: Definition, classification, and diagnostic criteria for diabetes mellitus. *In* Proceedings of the Second Japan-US Diabetes Epidemiology Training Course. Japan Diabetes Foundation Publication Series No. 5, 1996, pp. 3–10.

14. Harris MI: The burden of undiagnosed diabetes. Reducing the Burden of Diabetes J, 6:5–7, 1996.

15. Harris MI: NIDDM: Epidemiology and Scope of the Problem. Diabetes Spectrum 9:26–29, 1996.

16. Harris MI: Impaired glucose tolerance—prevalence and conversion to NIDDM. Diabetic Med 13:S9–S11, 1996.

17. Harris MI: Medical care for patients with diabetes: Epidemiologic aspects. Annals Intern Med 124:117–122, 1996.

18. Klein R, Rowland ML, Harris MI: Racial/ethnic differences in age-related maculopathy. Ophthalmology 102:371–381, 1995.

19. Harris MI: Epidemiologic studies on the pathogenesis of non-insulin-dependent diabetes mellitus (NIDDM). Clin Invest Med 18:231–239, 1995.

20. Harris MI: Health insurance and diabetes. In Harris MI, Cowie CC, Reiber G, Boyko E, Stern M, Bennett P (eds): Diabetes in America, 2nd ed. Washington DC: U.S. Government Printing Office, 1995, pp. 591–600.

21. Cowie CC, Harris MI: Physical and metabolic characteristics of persons with diabetes. In Harris MI, Cowie CC, Reiber G, Boyko E, Stern M, Bennett P (eds): Diabetes in America, 2nd ed. Washington, DC: U.S. Government Printing Office, 1995, pp. 117–164.

22. Harris MI: Classification, diagnostic criteria, and screening for diabetes. In Harris MI, Cowie CC, Reiber G, Boyko E, Stern M, Bennett P (eds): Diabetes in America, 2nd ed. Washington, DC: U.S. Government Printing Office, 1995, pp. 15–36.

23. Harris MI, Cowie CC, Reiber G, et al. (eds): Diabetes in America, 2nd ed. NIH Publication No. 95-1468. Washington, DC: U.S. Government Printing Office, 1995.

24. Harris MI: Frequency of oral glucose tolerance testing in the U.S. Diabetes Care 18:134–135, 1995.

25. Harris MI, Robbins DC: Prevalence of adult-onset IDDM in the U.S. population. Diabetes Care 17:1337–1340, 1994.

26. Cowie CC, Howard BV, Harris MI: Serum lipoproteins in African Americans and Whites with non-insulin-dependent diabetes in the US population. Circulation 90:1185–1193, 1994.

27. Cowie CC, Harris MI, Eberhardt MS: Frequency and determinants of screening for diabetes in the U.S. Diabetes Care 17:1158–1163, 1994.

28. Eastman RC, Siebert CW, Garfield S, et al.: What you can do to lessen the burden of diabetes for your patients. Resident Staff Physician 40:15–19, 1994.

29. Coonrod BA, Betschart J, Harris MI: Frequency and determinants of diabetes patient education among adults in the U.S. population. Diabetes Care 17:852–858, 1994.

30. Harris MI, Eastman RC, Siebert C: The DCCT and medical care for diabetes in the U.S. Diabetes Care 17:761–764, 1994.

31. Cowie CC, Port FK, Rust KF, et al.: Differences in survival between black and white patients with diabetic end-stage renal disease. Diabetes Care 17:681–687, 1994.

32. Harris MI, Cowie CC, Eastman RC: Health insurance coverage for adults with diabetes in the U.S. population. Diabetes Care 17:585–591, 1994.

33. Harris MI, Modan M: Screening for NIDDM: Why is there no national program? Diabetes Care 17:440–444, 1994.

34. Modan M, Harris MI: Fasting plasma glucose in screening for NIDDM in the U.S. and Israel. Diabetes Care 17:436–439, 1994.

35. Eastman RC, Siebert CW, Harris M, et al.: Clinical Review 51. Implications of the Diabetes Control and Complications Trial. J Clin Endocrinol Metab 77:1105–1107, 1993.

36. Gorden P, Harris MI, Silverman R, et al.: A paradigm to link clinical research to clinical practice: The challenge in non-insulin dependent diabetes mellitus. In Ostenson CG, Efendic S, Vranic M (eds): New Concepts in the Pathogenesis of NIDDM. Proceedings of the 2nd Toronto-Stockholm Symposium on Perspectives on Diabetes Research. New York: Plenum Pub. Corp., 1993, pp. 303–310.

37. Harris, MI: Characteristics of the preclinical state in type 2 diabetes. In Nattras M (ed): Proceedings of the 3rd International Symposium on Type 2 Diabetes Mellitus. Bussum, Netherlands: Medicom Europe, 1993, pp. 62–65.

38. Brechner RJ, Cowie CC, Howie LJ, et al.: Ophthalmic examination among adults with diagnosed diabetes mellitus. JAMA 270:1714–1718, 1994.

39. Harris MI, Eastman R, Cowie CC: Symptoms of sensory neuropathy in adults with NIDDM in the U.S. population. Diabetes Care 16:1446–1452, 1993.

40. Eastman RC, Silverman R, Harris M, et al.: Lessening the burden of diabetes: intervention strategies. Diabetes Care 16:1095–1102, 1993.

41. Harris MI, Cowie CC, Howie LJ: Self monitoring of blood glucose by adults with diabetes in the U.S. population. Diabetes Care 16:1116–1123, 1993.

42. Tuttleman M, Harris MI: Attitudes and behaviors of primary care physicians regarding tight control of blood glucose in patients with IDDM. Diabetes Care 16:765–772, 1993.

43. Cowie CC, Harris MI, Silverman RE, et al.: Effect of multiple risk factors on difference between Blacks and Whites in the prevalence of non-insulin-dependent diabetes mellitus in the United States. Am J Epidemiol 137:719–732, 1993.

44. Harris MI: Undiagnosed NIDDM: Clinical and public health issues, the 1992 Kelly West lecture. Diabetes Care 16:642–652, 1993.

45. Harris MI: Diabetes in Blacks, Whites, and Hispanic populations from U.S. national surveys. In Proceedings of the Symposium on Diabetes in Minorities. Washington, DC: U.S. Government Printing Office, 1993, pp. 24–28.

46. King H, Rewers M, and the WHO Ad Hoc Diabetes Reporting Group: Global estimates for prevalence of diabetes mellitus and impaired glucose tolerance in adults. Diabetes Care 16:157–177, 1993.

47. Harris MI, Klein RE, Welborn TA, et al.: Onset of non-insulin-dependent diabetes occurs at least 4-7 years before clinical diagnosis. Diabetes Care 15:815–819, 1992.

48. Harris MI, Zimmet PZ: Classification of diabetes mellitus and other categories of glucose intolerance. In Alberti KGGM (ed): International Textbook of Diabetes Mellitus. New York: John Wiley & Sons Limited, 1992.

49. King H, Rewers M, and the WHO Ad Hoc Diabetes Reporting Group: Diabetes and impaired glucose tolerance in women aged 20-39 years. World Health Stat 45:321–327, 1991.

50. King H, Rewers M, and the WHO Ad Hoc Diabetes Reporting Group: Diabetes in adults is now a Third World problem. Bull World Health Organ 69:643–648, 1991.

51. Flegal KM, Ezzati TM, Harris MI, et al.: Prevalence of diabetes in Mexican Americans, Cubans, and Puerto Ricans from the Hispanic Health and Nutrition Examination Survey, 1982–84. Diabetes Care 14:628–638, 1991.

52. Harris MI: Epidemiological correlates of diabetes in Hispanics, Whites, and Blacks in the U.S. population. Diabetes Care 14 (Suppl 3):639–648, 1991.

53. Harris MI: Hypercholesterolemia and glucose intolerance in the U.S. population. Diabetes Care 14:366–374, 1991.

54. Harris MI: Screening for undiagnosed diabetes: Results from the U.S. and Mauritius. Bull Int Diabetes Fed 35:8–10, 1991.

55. Harris MI: The epidemiology of diabetes mellitus among the elderly in the United States. Clin Geriatr Med 6:703–719, 1990.

56. Harris MI: Non-insulin-dependent diabetes mellitus in black and white Americans. Diabetes/Metab Rev 6:71–90, 1990.

57. Harris MI: Screening for undiagnosed noninsulin-dependent diabetes. In Alberti KGGM (ed): Proceedings of the Symposium on Research and Clinical Frontiers in Diabetes. Amsterdam: Elsevier Science Publishers BV, 1990, pp. 16–19.

58. Harris MI: Testing for blood glucose by office-based physicians in the U.S. Diabetes Care 13:419–426, 1990.

59. Harris MI: Importance of classification and diagnostic criteria for diabetes. In Diabetes 1988, Proceedings of the 13th Congress of the International Diabetes Federation. Amsterdam: Excerpta Medica, 1989, pp. 6A–12A.

60. Modan M, Harris MI, Halkin H: Comparative evaluation of World Health Organization and National Diabetes Data Group criteria for impaired glucose tolerance: Results from two national samples. Diabetes 38:1630–1635, 1989.

61. Harris MI: Impaired glucose tolerance in the U.S. population. Diabetes Care 12:464–474, 1989.

62. Perez-Stable EJ, McMillan MM, Harris MI, et al.: Self-reported diabetes in Mexican-Americans: Hispanic Health and Nutrition Examination Survey, 1982–84. Am J Public Health 79:770–772, 1989.

63. Kleinman JS, Donahue RP, Harris MI, et al.: Mortality among diabetics in a national sample. Am J Epidemiol 128:389–401, 1988.

64. Harris MI: Classification and diagnostic criteria for diabetes mellitus and other categories of glucose intolerance. Primary Care Clin 15:205–225, 1988.

65. Harris MI: Gestational diabetes may represent the discovery of preexisting glucose intolerance. Diabetes Care 11:402–411, 1988.

66. Kovar MG, Harris MI, Hadden WC: The scope of diabetes in the United States population. Am J Public Health 77:1549–1550, 1988.

67. Harris MI, Hadden WC, Knowler WC, et al.: Prevalence of diabetes and impaired glucose tolerance and plasma glucose levels in the U.S. population. Diabetes 36:523–534, 1987.

68. Hadden WC, Harris MI: The prevalence of diagnosed diabetes, undiagnosed diabetes, and impaired glucose tolerance in U.S. adults aged 20–74 years. NCHS Vital and Health Statistics Series 11, No. 237. Washington, DC: U.S. Government Printing Office, 1987.

69. Harris MI: Diabetic women and childbearing (letter). Diabetes Care 9:213–214, 1986.

70. Harris MI: Selection bias (letter). Diabetes Care 9:94, 1986.

71. WHO Study Group: Diabetes Mellitus, Report of a WHO Study Group. WHO Technical Report Series #727, Geneva, Switzerland, 1985.

72. Harris MI, Hadden WC, Knowler WC, et al.: International criteria for the diagnosis of diabetes and impaired glucose tolerance. Diabetes Care 8:562–567, 1985.

73. Entmacher P, Sinnock P, Bostic E, et al.: Economic impact of diabetes. In Diabetes in America. NIH Pub. No. 85-1468, U.S. Washington, DC: Government Printing Office, 1985.

74. Harris MI, Entmacher P: Mortality from diabetes. In Diabetes in America. NIH Pub. No. 85-1468, U.S. Government Printing Office, 1985.

75. Harris M: Ambulatory medical care for diabetes. In Diabetes in America. NIH Pub. No. 85-1468, Washington, DC: U.S. Government Printing Office, 1985.

76. O'Sullivan JB, Harris MI, Mills JL: Maternal diabetes in pregnancy. In Diabetes in America. NIH Pub. No. 85-1468, Washington, DC: U.S. Government Printing Office, 1985.

77. Drury TF, Danchik KM, Harris MI: Sociodemographic characteristics of adult diabetics. In Diabetes in America. NIH Pub. No. 85-1468, Washington, DC: U.S. Government Printing Office, 1985.

78. Harris M: Prevalence of noninsulin-dependent diabetes and impaired glucose tolerance. In Diabetes in America. NIH Pub. No. 85-1468, Washington, DC: U.S. Government Printing Office, 1985.

79. Harris M: Classification and diagnostic criteria for diabetes and other categories of glucose intolerance. In Diabetes in America. NIH Pub. No. 85-1468, Washington, DC: U.S. Government Printing Office, 1985.

80. Harris M, Hamman R (eds): Diabetes in America. NIH Pub. No. 85-1468, Washington, DC: U.S. Government Printing Office, 1985.

81. LaPorte RE, Tajima N, Akerblom HK, et al.: Geographic differences in the risk of insulin-dependent diabetes mellitus, the importance of registries. Diabetes Care 8 (Suppl. 1):101–107, 1985.

82. Harris MI: The death rate decline for diabetes. Metropolitan Life Stat Bull 66:10–11, 1985.

83. Harris MI: Epidemiologic characteristics of impaired glucose tolerance in the U.S. population. In Baba S, Gould MK, Zimmet P (eds): Diabetes Mellitus, Recent Knowledge on Aetiology, Complications, and Treatment. New York: Academic Press, 1984, pp. 102–106.

84. Baynes JW, Bunn HF, Goldstein D, et al. for the National Diabetes Data Group: Report of the expert committee

on glucosylated hemoglobin. Diabetes Care 7:602–606, 1984.

85. Harris M: Classification of diabetes and its diagnostic criteria. *In* International Symposium on Diabetes Mellitus. Japan: Tohoku Univ. Press, 1984, pp. 92–99.

86. Bennett PH, Harris MI, Murphy RS: Geographic and ethnic differences in diabetes frequency in the Americas. *In* Diabetes 1982, Proceedings of the 11th Congress of the International Diabetes Federation. Amsterdam: Excerpta Medica, 1983, pp. 131–136.

87. Harris M: The prevalence of diagnosed diabetes, undiagnosed diabetes, and impaired glucose tolerance in the U.S. *In* Melish JS, Hanna J, Baba S (eds): Genetic-Environmental Interactions in Diabetes Mellitus. Amsterdam: Excerpta Medica, 1982, pp. 77–82.

88. Harris M: The public health impact of diabetes. *In* Eschwege E (ed): Advances in Diabetes Epidemiology. New York: Elsevier, 1982, pp. 17–20.

89. Harris M: Classification and diagnosis of diabetes mellitus. *In* Schnatz JD (ed): Diabetes Mellitus: Problems in Management. Menlo Park, CA: Addison-Wesley, 1982, pp. 6–10.

90. Drury T, Harris M, Lipsett L: Prevalence and management of diabetes. *In* Health, U.S. DHHS Pub. No. (PHS) 82–1232, Washington, DC.: U.S. Government Printing Office, 1982.

91. Harris M: Selected Statistics on Health and Medical Care Aspects of Diabetes. NIH Printing Office, 1981.

92. Harris M, Leslie RDG: Chlorpropamide-alcohol flushing and diabetes. Diabetologia 21:422–424, 1981.

93. Lilienfeld A, Hamman R, Bennett P, et al.: Research needs in the epidemiology of diabetes. Am J Epidemiol 113:105–112, 1981.

94. Harris MI: The changing prevalence of diabetes. Diabetes Dateline, Vol. 1, No. 5, November/December, 1980.

95. Harris MI: From the NIH: New standards for classification and diagnosis of diabetes. J Am Med Assoc 243:2296–2297, 1980.

96. Drury TF, Harris MI, Burnham C: Background, objectives, and significance of a proposed followback survey of diabetics ascertained through household health interviews. J Am Stat Assoc 1979, pp. 63–73.

97. National Diabetes Data Group: Classification and diagnosis of diabetes mellitus and other categories of glucose intolerance. Diabetes 28:1039–1057, 1979.

98. The Expert Committee on the Diagnosis and Classification of Diabetes Mellitus. Report of the Expert Committee on the Diagnosis and Classification of Diabetes Mellitus. Diabetes Care 20:1183–1197, 1997.

99. The Diabetes Control and Complications Research Group: The effect of intensive diabetes treatment on the development and progression of long-term complications in insulin-dependent diabetes mellitus. New Engl J Med 329:977–986, 1993.

100. Fisher EB, Heins JM, Hiss RG, et al.: Metabolic Control Matters. U.S. Dept. of Health and Human Services, Public Health Service, National Institutes of Health, National Institute of Diabetes and Digestive and Kidney Diseases. NIH Publication No. 94-3773, 1994.

101. American Diabetes Association: Metabolic control matters: Nationwide translation of the Diabetes Control and Complications Trial: Analysis and recommendations. Clin Diabetes 11:91, 95–96, 1994.

102. Klein R: Hyperglycemia and mircovascular and macrovascular disease in diabetes. Diabetes Care 18:258–268, 1995.

103. Ohkubo Y, Kishikawa H, Araki I, et al.: Intensive insulin therapy prevents the progression of diabetic microvascular complications in Japanese patients with non-insulin-dependent diabetes mellitus: A randomized prospective 6-year study. Diabetes Res Clin Pract 28:103–117, 1995.

104. Eastman RC, Javitt JJ, Herman WH, et al.: Prevention strategies for non-insulin-dependent diabetes mellitus: an economic perspective. *In* LeRoith D, Taylor SI, Olefsky JM (eds): Diabetes Mellitus: A Fundamental and Clinical Text. New York: Lippincott-Raven Publishers, 1996, pp 621–630.

Appendix

Mechanisms of Research Support

Research Project Grant. The Research Project Grant (RPG) is an investigator-initiated research grant awarded to public and private organizations and institutions, governments and their agencies including other Federal institutions), foreign institutions, and international organizations, to provide support for a discrete, specified research project to be performed by a named principal investigator. Detailed information and eligibility criteria may be found in the Grants Policy Statement, which is generally available in the grants and contracts office of the institution or can be obtained from the Division of Research Grants, National Institutes of Health, 6701 Rockledge Drive, Room 1040-MSC 7710, Bethesda, MD 20892-7710 [20817 for overnight service].

MERIT Award. Investigators who have demonstrated superior competence and outstanding productivity during their previous research endeavors may be selected to extend an initial 5-year research project grant award for an additional 3 years based on an expedited review. The Method To Extend Research In Time (MERIT) Awards are selected by NIH staff in consultation with the National Advisory Councils, from competing research applications. (Investigators may not apply for merit awards.)

FIRST Award. The objective of the First Independent Research Support and Transition (FIRST) Award is to provide a sufficient initial period of research support for newly independent biomedical investigators to develop their research capabilities and demonstrate the merit of their research ideas. These grants are intended to underwrite the first independent investigator efforts of an individual; to provide a reasonable opportunity for him/her to demonstrate creativity, productivity, and further promise; and to help effect a transition toward the traditional types of NIH research project grants. The principal features are: (1) new investigators may receive awards for a period of up to 5 years; (2) the maximum level for these awards is $350,000 for a 5-year period; and (3) the award will permit optional carry-over of unobligated balances from one budget period to the next.

Small Business Innovation Research Program. An amendment to the Small Business Act now requires certain Federal agencies, including the NIH, to set aside funds to promote technological innovation within the American small business community. The purpose of the legislation is to give small business an increased role in the Federal research and development (R&D) efforts as well as to attract private capital to commercialize the results of federally funded research.

The Small Business Innovation Research (SBIR) program consists of three phases: phase I—the establishment of the technical merit and feasibility of research and development ideas that may lead to commercial products or services (up to 6 months); phase II—the in-depth development of research and development ideas proposed in phase I (up to 5 years); and phase III—the promotion of commercialization of the results of the R&D funded by Federal agencies or use of non-SBIR contracting for products or processes as developed for use by the US Government.

The implementation of this program is principally through the research grant mechanism. Applications will be considered in any area within the mission of the division, although special programmatic interests have been developed as guidelines for those interested in applying for support.

Program Project Grant. This grant mechanism provides support for a broadly based, multidisciplinary, often long-term targeted research program consisting of coordinated research activities and projects led by established investigators. Program projects are directed toward well-defined research goals and generally involve the organized efforts of a number of individuals who are conducting research projects designed to elucidate various aspects or components of a central theme. The program project grant can provide support for certain basic resources used by groups in the program, including clinical components, the sharing of which facilitates the total research effort. Eligibility criteria are the same as for the traditional research project grant. Specific guidelines are available from the appropriate research program directors. Consultations with program staff prior to submission of an application are highly recommended.

Center Grant. Core Center grants supported by the Division are based on the concept of providing shared resources (cores) for a group of established investigators who are conducting independent programs of active, high-quality research. The center grant provides a mechanism for integrating, coordinating, and fostering interdisciplinary research among these investigators. Centers also provide funding for shared resources, limited support for pilot and feasibility studies, and funds for program enrichment. The pilot and feasibility studies are small research projects of limited duration. Their purpose is to enable investigators who are new to the program area to become independent or to support new research directions for established investigators. Core Centers are supported in the Diabetes Centers. Applications for center grants are accepted only in response to specific solicitations issued through Requests for Applications (RFA).

Cooperative Agreement. A cooperative agreement reflects an assistance relationship between the NIH and a recipient, but with substantial programmatic involvement by the NIH. The NIH assists, supports, or stimulates the recipients, and is involved substantially with recipients in conducting projects similar in program intent to those for grants, with the NIH playing a "partner" role in the effort. These are often designed to carry out specified clinical trials. Applications for Cooperative Agreements are accepted only in response to Requests for Applications.

Training and Career Development Opportunities

National Research Service Awards. Three types of National Research Service Awards (NRSA) are available under this program: institutional training grants, individual postdoctoral fellowships, and senior research fellowship awards.

Training grants are awarded to domestic nonprofit, private, and non-Federal public institutions to support costs of training students in biomedical research at the predoctoral and postdoctoral levels. A postdoctoral program must offer the opportunity for individuals to broaden their scientific backgrounds. These awards, however, are not made to support study leading to the M.D., D.O., D.D.S., or similar professional degrees nor are they to support non-research clinical training.

Postdoctoral fellowship awards are made directly to qualified individuals who have received a Ph.D., M.D., or equivalent degree for specified research training programs. The award provides the opportunity to carry out supervised research to enable biomedical scientists, clinicians, and others to broaden their scientific backgrounds and expand their potential for research in health-related areas. Prior to submission, an applicant must arrange for an appointment to an appropriate institution and acceptance by a sponsor who will supervise the training and research experience. The institutional setting may be a domestic or foreign nonprofit, private or public institution, including the NIH.

Senior fellowships provide the opportunity for experienced scientists to make major changes in the direction of their research careers, to broaden their research capabilities, or to enlarge their command of an allied research field. Candidates must have received a doctoral (Ph.D., Sc.D., D.Eng., M.D., D.D.S., D.O., D.V.M., O.D.), or equivalent degree, foreign or domestic, and must have had at least 7 subsequent years of relevant research or professional experience by the time the award is made. Senior fellowships will normally be awarded for a period of 12 months. Continued support beyond the first year is contingent upon the research training plan, satisfactory progress, and the availability of funds. The total period of the award will not exceed 24 months. These awards are not made for study leading to any of the professional degrees (M.D., O.D., D.D.S., etc.) or for residency or other clinical training.

Career Development Awards. NIDDK supports a program of career development awards available to newly trained or independent Ph.D. and M.D. scientists in the early and formative periods of their careers.

Mentored Clinical Investigator Award. This grant mechanism is designed to provide a first research experience that meets the needs of newly trained clinicians to develop independent research skills and experience in a fundamental area of biomedical science. Candidates having completed at least 1 postgraduate year and up to 7 years of clinical training by the time the award is made can apply by submitting an application consisting of an enhanced training component in basic or clinical science, to be followed by a comprehensive research plan under the supervision of a qualified mentor. The overall objective of this program is to provide the opportunity to develop into independent biomedical investigators. The award is intended to facilitate transition from postdoctoral or postclinical training to a career as an independent investigator. Five years of salary support and a limited budget for research expenses are provided. Candidates normally submit a comprehensive research plan of from 3-5 years allowing for release from clinical responsibilities to permit focus on development of their research. Consultation with Program/Institute staff is recommended before submitting an application.

Independent Investigator Award. The Independent Investigator Award is a salary grant (up to 5 years) to enable investigators (Ph.D. and/or M.D.) who have demonstrated outstanding research potential to further develop their research careers. This award is available for persons who have demonstrated independent research accomplishments but who need additional time in a productive scientific environment. Applications will be accepted only from applicants who are principal investigators on a regular research grant supported by NIDDK and are still categorized as junior faculty. Alternatively, an applicant may submit a regular research grant application and an Independent Investigator application concurrently. This award is not intended for the untried, or unfunded Investigator, and is not intended simply to substitute one source of salary support for another for an individual who is already conducting full-time research, or as a mechanism for substituting for institutional support.

For further information, contact: Applications and general information regarding NIH grants policy and procedure can be obtained from the Office of Grants Inquiries, Division of Research Grants, Rockledge 2 Building, 6701 Rockledge Drive, Room 1040-MSC 7710, Bethesda, MD 20892-7710 or 20817 for overnight delivery.

Section II.
Screening and Diagnosis

11

Screening
for Diabetes Mellitus

John K. Davidson

Historical Perspective

Between 1902 and 1907, Barringer (1909)[1] screened 71,729 insurance applicants for urine "sugar," and found a positive test in 2.8% with 0.9% having more than 1% "sugar" in the urine. In retrospect, it seems likely that many of these individuals were false-positive screenees who did not have diabetes, but who had either renal glucosuria, a nonglucose mellituria, or the presence in the urine of some other substance that could reduce copper sulfate in an alkaline solution (see Chapters 13 and 22).

During World Wars I and II, over 10 million inductees were screened for glucosuria and diabetes.[2,3] Wilkerson and Krall[4] screened 3,516 of the 4,983 inhabitants (70.9%) of Oxford, Massachusetts, using urine and blood sugar and dextrose tolerance tests, and found 40 known diabetics and 30 newly diagnosed diabetics for an overall prevalence of 2%.

During the next 30 years, automated techniques for blood sugar measurement became widely available and the unit cost per test decreased significantly. As a result, mass indiscriminate screening for diabetes became widespread and soon it was expanded to multiphasic (diabetes, hypertension, glaucoma, anemia, and so forth) screening.[5,6] Between 1950 and 1975, such screening activities were carried out in many communities, states, industries, employee groups, health fairs, and the like.[7–20]

Kurlander et al.[21] calculated the sensitivity (positive when diabetes is present) and specificity (negative when diabetes is absent) of urine (Clinitest) and blood tests (Somogyi-Nelson, Wilkerson-Heftmann with an arbitrary upper limit of normal cut-point of 130 mg/dL) that were available in the early 1950s. The Clinitest method failed to detect more than half of those subsequently diagnosed as diabetic (false-negatives), and many nondiabetics had a positive Clinitest (false-positives), thus both sensitivity and specificity for Clinitest were low. The blood tests were not sensitive (only 61% of individuals subsequently diagnosed as diabetic

had a blood sugar level greater than 130 mg/dL), but they were relatively specific (97.4% of the nondiabetics were correctly classified as true-negatives).

During the early 1970s, the pitfalls inherent in both mass indiscriminate screening and in the use of overly sensitive criteria to establish the diagnosis (resulting in many false-positive diagnoses) began to become apparent.[22–26] (See Exhibit 12–2). Since 1975, the importance of establishing the sensitivity, specificity, and predictive value of a positive test for the presence of diabetes and for a negative test for the absence of diabetes has become well known.[27] (See Table 11–1 and 11–2 for a comparison of the sensitivity, specificity, and predictive value of a positive test, and the predictive value of a negative test for Clinitest and random quantitative urine glucose measurements.) It is clear that as urine glucose methodology has improved, sensitivity and specificity have increased considerably. Also, raising the upper limit of normal cut-points during a glucose tolerance test (GTT) can increase the specificity of the test and can eventually eradicate false-positive diagnoses (see Exhibit 12–2).

When cost analysis of screening programs was initiated,[28] the lack of cost-effectiveness of many screening programs for diabetes became obvious.[22,25] Whether or not mass indiscriminate blood sugar screening after a glucose load was justified on the basis of cost-benefit and patient-benefit was evaluated in 5-yr controlled follow-up studies of individuals who participated in the Cleveland, Ohio, screening program.[12,16,29–31] A total of 600,000 individuals were screened in this program, which began in 1964. Half of the positive screenees in 1969 were negative on retest in 1974.

In the wake of the 1971 University Group Diabetes Program (UGDP) report, the Cleveland investigators concluded that the psychologic risks of a false-positive diagnosis and the physical risks of treating a nonexistent disease with medication (i.e., tolbutamide) far outweighed the potential benefits of early diagnosis and treatment. After 1978, the Cleveland diabetes detection

TABLE 11–1 Formulas for Calculation of Sensitivity, Specificity, and Predictive Value of a Positive Screening Test (RUG >25 mg/dL) for the Presence of Diabetes Mellitus (GTT Sum >800 mg/dL or FPG >140 mg/dL) and Negative Screening Test (RUG 3–25 mg/dL) for the Absence of Diabetes Mellitus (GTT Sum <800 mg/dL)

Sensitivity is positivity in disease (or RUG >25 mg/dL when GTT sum >800 mg/dL).

$$\text{Sensitivity} = \frac{\text{True-positives}}{\text{True-positives} + \text{false-negatives}} \times 100 = \frac{68}{68 + 0} \times 100 = 100\%$$

Specificity is negativity in health (or RUG ≤25 mg/dL when GTT sum <800 mg/dL)

$$\text{Specificity} = \frac{\text{True-negatives}}{\text{True-negatives} + \text{false-positives}} \times 100 = \frac{4{,}046^a}{4{,}046^a + 27} = \frac{4{,}046}{4{,}073} \times 100 = 99.3\%$$

Predictive value of a positive result (RUG >25 mg/dL) for diabetes mellitus (GTT sum >800 mg/dL)

$$\text{Predictive value (+)} = \frac{\text{True-positives}}{\text{True-positives} + \text{false-positives}} \times 100 = \frac{68}{68 + 27} \times 100 = 72\%$$

Predictive value of a negative result (RUG 3–25 mg/dL) for absence of diabetes mellitus (GTT sum <800 mg/dL)

$$\text{Predictive value (−)} = \frac{\text{True-negatives}}{\text{True-negatives} + \text{false-negatives}} \times 100 = \frac{450^a}{450^a + 0} = \frac{450}{450} = 100\%$$

[a] 450 persons were randomly selected from 4,046 individuals in the 3 to 25 mg/dL RUG group for a follow-up GTT. The findings for the 450 have been extrapolated to the entire group of 4,046.

Abbreviations: FPG, fasting plasma glucose; other abbreviatons as in text

[*Source:* Galen RD, Gambino SR: Beyond Normality: the Predictive Value and Efficiency of Medical Diagnosis. New York: John Wiley & Sons, 1975, pp. 115–119.]

TABLE 11–2 Sensitivity, Specificity, Predictive Value (in Percent) of a Positive Test and Predictive Value of Negative Test

Percent	Clinitest	Random Urine Glucose[a] <25 mg/dL
Sensitivity	77.3	100.0
Specificity	98.2	99.3
Sum of sensitivity plus specificity	175.5	199.3
Predictive value of a positive test for the presence of diabetes	33.3% (1 in 3)	71.6% (7+ in 10)
Predictive value of a negative test for the absence of diabetes	99.7	100.0

[a] Positive = RUG >25 mg/dL; negative = RUG 3–25 mg/dL

program was reduced in size to make it more cost-effective. *Discriminate screening* replaced *indiscriminate screening*, with screening activities being directed at those who requested it, those who were pregnant, those who were over 40 years of age, those who were obese, and those with a family history of diabetes.[32]

Ideas About Screening (1990)

Screening for diabetes (especially as conducted by community and/or voluntary health agencies without appropriate physician supervision) was controversial for the following reasons: (1) lack of consensus on definitions of the different types of diabetes and criteria for their diagnosis; (2) lack of accurate information about the prevalence of diagnosed and undiagnosed non-insulin-dependent diabetes mellitus (NIDDM) in different populations; (3) failure to appreciate the morbidity that persons with undiagnosed NIDDM incur before diagnosis; (4) lack of understanding regarding the identity, magnitude, and effect of risk factors for complications of NIDDM; and (5) lack of methods to reduce, eliminate, or modify the risk factors responsible for the development and progression of the chronic complications of NIDDM.[33]

During the decade of the 1980s, each of these controversies diminished in intensity, so that for the 1990s the American Diabetes Association (ADA) recommended routine screening (preferably under the direct supervision of a physician) of all who have one or more risk factors for NIDDM[40] (Exhibit 11–1). The ADA Committee believed that early diagnosis and appropriate treatment are essential because much evidence has accumulated indicating that weight loss from reduced caloric intake and increased exercise not only lowers elevated plasma glucose levels in those with NIDDM, but also has major ancillary cardiovascular health benefits[33] (Exhibit 11–2).

In 1998 The American Diabetes Association revised its diagnostic criteria for diabetes mellitus as noted in Exhibit 12–3. The criteria for screening for and diagnosis of gestational diabetes mellitus were not changed (see Chapters 40 and 41).

EXHIBIT 11-1   The 1989 and 1998 American Diabetes Association Position Statement on Screening for Diabetes[a]

I. Prevalence of undiagnosed diabetes
   It is estimated that six million Americans have undiagnosed diabetes, nearly all of whom have NIDDM.

II. Risk factors for NIDDM
   A. Family history of diabetes
   B. >20% above ideal body weight (obesity)
   C. Age >40 years
   D. Certain races (American Indians, blacks, Hispanics)
   E. Previously noted hyperglycemia (stress-related or drug-related)
   F. Hypertension
   G. Hyperlipidemia (cholesterol >240 mg/dL and/or triglycerides >250 mg/dL)
   H. In a nonpregnant woman, a history of gestational diabetes or of delivery of a baby weighing more than 9 lb (4.1 kg)

III. Objectives of diabetes screening programs
   A. Much support has been collected during the last 20 years for the hypothesis that the *high morbidity and mortality associated with the chronic complications of NIDDM* can be reduced or prevented by early detection and appropriate treatment.
   B. The relatively innocuous treatment program for most cases of NIDDM (decreased caloric intake and increased exercise to produce weight loss) has ancillary cardiovascular health benefits in addition to its now generally recognized ability to lower the plasma glucose level to normal in many individuals with NIDDM.

IV. Recommendations for diabetes screening programs
   A. It is preferable to screen for NIDDM with close supervision by a physician in his/her office, clinic, or hospital.
   B. Community screening programs, which are *not* under the close supervision of a physician, should

identify individuals (by a written or verbal questionnaire) who have one or more risk factors for NIDDM (see II above). All individuals with symptoms or signs suggestive of diabetes should be referred promptly to a physician for testing, as noted below in IV C and D.
   C. In men and nonpregnant women, a fasting plasma or serum glucose level ≥ 126 mg/dL × 2 is diagnostic of NIDDM. A fasting plasma glucose ≥ 110 mg/dL may require further testing.
   D. About 3% of pregnant women develop gestational diabetes. All pregnant women should be referred to a physician for a screening and/or glucose tolerance test and appropriate follow-up (see Exhibit 12-3).

V. A. Personnel conducting *community screening programs* must be adequately trained and must demonstrate competency in the testing procedure used.
   B. When individuals are referred from a *community screening program to a physician*, a list of diabetes risk factors, plasma and/or random urine glucose results, and methods of measurement should be transmitted in writing.

VI. Individuals who have diagnosed diabetes and those who are less than 20 years old should not be screened in community programs.

VII. A. Careful and strict infection control methods (particularly those designed to prevent HIV transmission[b]) should be utilized routinely.
   B. *Author's Note:* Random urine glucose screening (see Figs. 11-1 and 11-2) is noninvasive (thus avoiding HIV transmission), quantitative, sensitive, specific, rapid, and inexpensive. It can be used effectively as the initial test in a comprehensive screening program for NIDDM.

[a] Adapted from Position Statement of the American Diabetes Association: Screening for diabetes. Diabetes Care 12:588–590, 1989, and American Diabetes Association: Screening for Type 2 Diabetes. Diabetes Care 21(suppl. 1):520–522, 1998. With permission.

[b] Adapted from Centers for Disease Control: Recommendations for prevention of HIV transmission in health-care settings. MMWR 36 (Suppl 2):3–18, 1987. With permission.

Recommended Screening Methods (1998)

IDDM in those less than 20 years old has a low prevalence and incidence in the United States [*prevalence* 1 in 600 children, *incidence* 15 per 100,000 children (0.015%) per year]. In some countries (such as Finland) prevalence and incidence are higher, and in some countries (such as Japan) incidence is much lower [1 per 100,000 children (0.001%) per year]. Insulin-dependent diabetes mellitus (IDDM) in children usually develops over a short period of time (a few days to a few months) and is usually characterized by classic subjective and objective findings that should lead immediately to diagnosis and treatment.

Thus, it is *not* appropriate to screen asymptomatic individuals under age 20 years for hyperglycemia or glucosuria.[34,35]

Now screening is directed at those who have *undiagnosed NIDDM* (estimated at about 3% of the United States population above age 20 years) and at those who are pregnant and have *undiagnosed gestational diabetes mellitus* (estimated at about 3% of pregnant women). (see Chapters 40 and 41.)

Prior to 1969,[36-38] methods that were available for measurement of urine glucose were insensitive, semiquantitative, and nonspecific. In 1974, the ADA[39] recommended that screening for diabetes be done using plasma (or serum) glucose methods alone and that urine testing be abandoned because of the insensitivity and nonspecificity of Clinitest methods (Table 11-2).

EXHIBIT 11–2   Some Advances During the Last 15 Years That Can Decrease the Risks of Development of and Progression of the Chronic Complications of NIDDM to End-Stage Disease[a]

I. To be utilized before the chronic complications develop (secondary prevention)
  A. Development of the team approach (MD, RN, RD, DPM, others) for patient evaluation, education treatment, and follow-up utilizing methods listed in B, C, D, and E. See Chapter 14
  B. Better methods for control of hyperglycemia
   1. More effective diet and exercise therapy
   2. Better methods for self monitoring of blood glucose (SMBG)
   3. Better methods for measuring glycosylated hemoglobin
   4. rDNA human insulin, lispro insulin
   5. Better insulin delivery systems
  C. Better control of hypertension: drugs, diet
  D. Better control of hyperlipidemia: diet, drugs
  E. Increasing recognition of the risks of cigarette smoking and other tobacco use
II. Public Education
  A. American Diabetes Association and other national and international diabetes associations' public, patient, and professional education programs
  B. National high blood pressure education program
  C. National cholesterol education program
  D. Increasing public pressure against smoking in public places, transport vehicles, hospitals, doctors' offices, among others
  E. Surgeon General's reports on smoking and health and on the consequences of obesity
III. A. Continuing research to improve the treatment modalities noted in I B, C, D, and E, and to develop new treatment modalities with the goal of someday being able to "prevent" and "cure" diabetes
IV. To be utilized after chronic complications develop (tertiary prevention)
  A. Microangiopathy
   1. Retinopathy
    a. Better screening methods
    b. Laser photocoagulation
    c. Early vitrectomy
   2. Nephropathy
    a. Slowing progress to end-stage renal disease (ESRD) by controlling hypertension (especially angiotensin-converting enzyme inhibitors)
    b. Improved methods of measuring microalbuminuria (30–300 mg/24 hrs)
    c. Improved techniques of dialysis (especially peritoneal)
    d. Increasing frequency of renal transplant for ESRD
    e. Better immunosuppression (cyclosporine and others) and better survival of transplanted kidneys
  B. Macroangiopathy
   1. Coronary artery atherosclerosis
    a. Bypass surgery
    b. Angioplasty
    c. Better pacemakers
    d. Better diuretics to treat congestive heart failure
   2. Carotid artery atherosclerosis
    a. Bypass surgery
   3. Peripheral vascular disease
    a. Bypass surgery
    b. Angioplasty
  C. Neuropathy
   1. Peripheral
    a. Better podiatric care
    b. Special shoes to protect neuropathic feet from injury and infection (medicare pays)
    c. Better antibiotics
    d. More emphasis on education, foot evaluation on each visit, and *early* and *continuing conservative* care of foot ulcers to *prevent* amputation in all in whom adequate circulation is present or can be restored (IV B3 above)
    e. Excellent plasma glucose control (target range 80–150 mg/dL) will relieve neuropathic pain within 2 to 3 months in >80% of those with painful neuropathy
   2. Autonomic neuropathy
    a. Appears in many forms, which affect the cardiovascular, gastrointestinal, and genitourinary systems. Excellent plasma glucose control results in improvement in >80%, but this may require use of regular insulin four times daily or continuous subcutaneous insulin infusion (CSII)
    b. See Chapter 36 for other drug, procedure, or operative therapies that may be needed

[a] Adapted from Harris MI: screening for undiagnosed non-insulin dependent diabetes. *In* Alberti KGMM, Mazze RS (eds): Current Trends in Noninsulin Dependent Diabetes Mellitus. New York: Elsevier, 1989, pp. 119–131, and NIH, NIDDKD: Diabetes in America, 2nd ed. Washington, DC. U.S. Govt. Printing Office, 1995 (NIH publ. No. 95-1468).

In 1989 the ADA position statement on screening (Exhibit 11–1)[40] recommended that screening of asymptomatic individuals for NIDDM should be done on those over 20 years of age who had one or more risk factors for diabetes (Exhibit 11–1). Also, it recommended that screening be done under the direct supervision of a physician.

The desire to diagnose diabetes mellitus as early as possible resulted in another revision in 1998 of ADA criteria for the diagnosis of diabetes (NIDDM or type 2).

The new criteria (see Exhibit 12–3) discourage the use of the glucose tolerance test, and emphasize the importance of an elevated fasting plasma glucose [FPG $\geq$ 126 mg/dl (7.0 mmol/l) $\times$ 2 = Diabetes Mellitus]. A FPG $\geq$ 110 mg/dl and <126 mg/dl is classified as impaired fasting glucose. The physician may desire to initiate *non-pharmacologic therapy (diet and exercise)* as indicated in hopes that diabetes can be *prevented or* at least *delayed in appearance*. A sequential testing routine (Exhibit 11–5) beginning with RUG and proceeding to random (casual) and fasting plasma glucose levels is still a quick, efficient and inexpensive way to diagnose diabetes mellitus.

It is important to recognize that carefully planned and optimally executed screening and follow-up programs can provide significant benefits for newly diagnosed NIDDMs (Exhibit 11–2). The costs of a screening program in 1977 in a major teaching hospital are shown in Exhibit 11–3. Also, such screening programs can provide valuable epidemiologic data[41–45] on the prevalence, incidence, natural history, morbidity, and mortality of NIDDM in defined populations. Voluntary health agencies, such as the ADA, can increase public education by assisting in such screening programs.

The ADA (Exhibit 11–1) recommends that screening be done for NIDDM utilizing plasma glucose measurements by accurate methods (such as the polaragraphic glucose oxidase or a similar method) and *not* by frequently inaccurate, quickie meter methods that are used for self-monitoring of blood glucose (SMBG). Fasting and random plasma glucose levels are preferable, but occasionally a glucose tolerance test is needed (Exhibit 11–4).

Methods that involve collection of blood are invasive (risking human immunodeficiency virus (HIV)

and hepatitis B transmission to the collector[46]), expensive, and slow.

Since a quantitative random urine glucose (RUG) measurement has 99.3% specificity in detecting those with undiagnosed NIDDM, and the RUG is noninvasive (no risk of HIV or hepatitis B transmission), rapid, and inexpensive, it can be used to decrease significantly the costs and the number of plasma glucose determinations needed to satisfy the present ADA recommendations for screening (Exhibits 11–1 and 11–4).[47,48] If the RUG is >25 mg/dL, follow-up plasma glucose measurements (random, fasting, and possibly after a glucose load) are needed to classify the individual as diabetic or nondiabetic (Exhibit 11–4).

Problem Statement

How, when, and where should the population of those not known to have NIDDM be screened for the disease?

Plan

A sequential testing routine may be carried out in a physician's office, clinic, hospital, or any other medical facility that is adequately staffed by competent professionals, and who have equipment and supplies that are needed to measure *accurately* plasma and quantitative urine glucose levels (Figs. 11–1 and 11–2). Samples for random urine glucose measurements can be done on site or can be collected in the field and transported to a central laboratory. If samples are not infected, urine glucose levels are stable for up to 1 week.

The ADA campaign initiated in 1984 "to find the 5,000,000 with undiagnosed NIDDM" and the ADA campaign initiated in 1989 "to find the 6,000,000 with

---

EXHIBIT 11–3   Cost (in 1977 dollars) of Random Urine Glucose Screening of 4,141 Individuals for Diabetes Mellitus

Glucose analyzer (Beckman)	=	$ 5,000.00
Glucose oxidase for RUG = 4,141 $\times$ 25 cents	=	1,035.35
Technician—20% of time for 3 years	=	9,000.00
Facilities, utilities, and so forth for 3 years	=	1,200.00
Total cost for screening	=	$16,235.25
Follow-up testing for individuals		
With RUG >25 mg/dL (95 of 4,141) with random plasma glucose ($7 $\times$ 95)	=	665.00
Fasting plasma glucose ($21 $\times$ 64)	=	1,344.00
3-hr GTT ($25 $\times$ 2 $\times$ 31)	=	1,550.00
		$ 3,559.00
	Total cost =	$19,794.25

$$\text{Cost per person screened } (4{,}141) = \frac{\$16{,}235.25}{4{,}141} = \$3.92$$

$$\text{Cost per person screened } (4{,}141) \text{ plus follow-up testing for 95 individuals} = \frac{\$19{,}794.25}{4{,}141} = \$4.78$$

$$\text{Cost per each new person diagnosed as diabetic } (68) = \frac{\$19{,}974.25}{68} = \$291.09$$

EXHIBIT 11–4   Sequential Testing Routine to Detect and Diagnose Diabetes in the Nonpregnant Individual

I. Quantitative random urine glucose (RUG) screen:
  A. If 3-25 mg/dL (≥97% of asymptomatic screenees in the United States) → STOP. Diabetes has been ruled out
  B. If >25 mg/dL, go to II immediately

II. Random venous plasma (or serum) glucose:
  A. If ≥200 mg/dL and/or symptomatic and/or ketotic, initiate therapy immediately
  B. If ≥160 mg/dL, but not symptomatic or ketotic, go to III

III. Fasting venous plasma glucose:
  A. If ≥126 mg/dL × 2 = diabetes mellitus
  B. If ≥110 mg/dL but less than 126 mg/dL, and risk factors for diabetes present (Exhibit 11–1), *may* go to IV

IV. Glucose tolerance test (diet prepped, ambulatory, nonmedicated):
  A. Until 1998, if the FPG was <140 mg/dL, NIHDDG and WHO GTT criteria became the standards for making a diagnosis of diabetes or for ruling it out. Both required two abnormal GTTs to confirm the diagnosis

B. After a 75 g dose of glucose at time 0, a postglucose-load 2-hr glucose level ≥200 mg/dL is diagnostic of diabetes according to WHO criteria. NIH-DDG requires a 2-hr level ≥200 mg/dL plus at least one interval level (usually a $\frac{1}{2}$, 1, or $1\frac{1}{2}$ hour level ≥200 mg/dL

C. In the early 1990s, the author used the following criteria:
  1. If the sum of fasting and 1-, 2-, and 3-hour post-100 g glucose load plasma glucoses was >800 mg/dL × 2, the individual was diagnosed as *diabetic*.
  2. If the GTT sum was ≤800 mg/dL, the individual was classified as *nondiabetic*; if the GTT sum was 601 to 800 mg/dL, the individual was classified as *nondiabetic high-normal*.
  3. If the RUG was >25 mg/dL, and the GTT sum was ≤800 mg/dL, the screenee was classified as *random renal hyperglucosuric* (see Figs. 11–1 and 11–2).

Abbreviations: NIH-DDG, National Institutes of Health—Diabetes Data Group; WHO, World Health Organization.

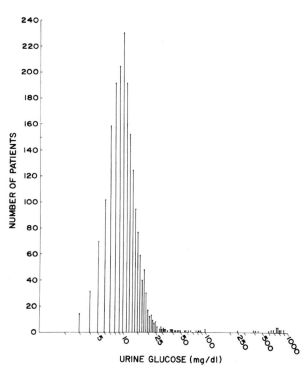

Figure 11–1.   Distribution of random (undiluted) urine glucose levels in 1,952 screenees (abscissa: log scale). (*Source:* Davidson JK, Reuben D, Sternberg JC, et al.: Diabetes screening using a quantitative urine glucose method. Diabetes 27:810–816, 1978. With permission.)

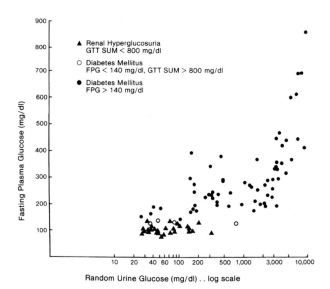

Figure 11–2.   Distribution of random urine glucose (RUG) levels in 95 (of 4,141) screenees whose RUG level was >25 mg/dL (abscissa: log scale) and comparison to the fasting plasma glucose level (ordinate). The highest RUG level in a renal hyperglucosuric was 317 mg/dL; all individuals with RUG levels higher than 317 mg/dL had diabetes mellitus. The lowest RUG level in those subsequently shown to have diabetes mellitus was 26 mg/dL. In the RUG range from 26 to 317 mg/dL, there were 27 screenees who had renal hyperglucosuria and 22 screenees who had diabetes mellitus [19 whose fasting plasma glucose (FPG) was >140 mg/dL, three whose FPG was <140 mg/dL and whose GTT sum was >800 mg/dL].

undiagnosed NIDDM" were unsuccessful because of some of the problems previously noted. Whether the campaign initiated in 1998 "to find the 6 to 8 million with undiagnosed NIDDM" will be successful may depend more on the education of the general public to seek periodic screening for diabetes than it does on physicians. See Chapters 10, 50, and 52 and Appendix I.

Cost-Effectiveness of a Hospital Diabetes Clinic Screening Program

The costs of a program that screened 4,141 individuals for diabetes over a 3-year period are shown in Exhibit 11–3. The screenees varied in age from 15 to 80 years, and none was known to have diabetes. Some were self-referred, some were hospital employees, and some were referred from the local diabetes association, public health agencies, and hospital clinics. The testing routine was sequential (Exhibit 11–4). The cost per person screened was $3.92 (1977 dollars), and the cost of each new case of diabetes diagnosed was $291.09. If similar screening programs were applied to all persons above age 20 years in the United States not known to have diabetes, the cost would be about 640 million dollars 1977 dollars. Three plasma glucose measurements per person would cost five times as much, and two GTTs per person would cost 15 times as much.

Follow-up of Screened Individuals

When rapid and efficient entry into the health care system for positive screenees is not planned in advance,

many problems can occur (Exhibit 11–1). At the present time, the most cost-effective screening program is a sequential one, starting with a quantitative urine glucose measurement (Exhibits 11–3 and 11–4) and progressing as far as necessary until diabetes is shown to be absent or present. Ideally, screening, diagnosis, and follow-up should take place in the same facility.

Audits

Audits of hospital, clinic, and physician office data will determine the costs and effectiveness of a specific screening program, and the prevalence and incidence of diabetes in a defined population. Audits are valuable in determining the sensitivity, specificity, and costs of various screening methods.

Research Considerations

More precise and cost-effective methods for detecting the undiagnosed diabetic are needed. An inexpensive self-testing method that gave a positive result when RUG was >25 mg/dL and a negative result at levels below that could be used to rule out a diagnosis of diabetes and would simplify the screening process.

It has been shown in research studies that glutamate decarboxylose-, insulin-, and islet-cell-antibodies with HLA typing can detect type 1 diabetes[49] in a general population (see Chapter 3), and that a combination of autoantibodies to insulin, GAD, and IC512bc/IA-2 can predict type 1 diabetes in first degree relatives.[50] Unfortunately, the high cost of currently available assays has limited their widespread use. No such tests are available for type 2 diabetes.

References

1. Barringer TB: The incidence of glycosuria and diabetes in New York City between 1902 and 1907. Arch Intern Med 3:295–298, 1909.

2. Spellberg MA, Leff WA: The incidence of diabetes mellitus and glucosuria in inductees. JAMA 129:246–250, 1945.

3. Blotner H: Studies in glycosuria and diabetes mellitus in selectees. JAMA 131:1109–1114, 1946.

4. Wilkerson HLC, Krall LP: Diabetes in a New England town: a study of 3,516 persons in Oxford Mass. JAMA 135:209, 1947.

5. Canelo CK, Bissell DM, Abrams H: A multiphasic screening survey in San Jose. Calif Med 71:409–413, 1949.

6. Breslow L: Multiphasic screening examinations: an extension of the mass screening technique. Am J Public Health 40:274–278, 1950.

7. Kenny AJ, Chute AL, Best CH: A study of the prevalence of diabetes in an Ontario community. Can Med Assoc J 65:233–241, 1951.

8. Kenny AJ, Chute AL: Diabetes in two Ontario communities: studies in case finding. Diabetes 2:187–193, 1953.

9. Olmstead WH, Drey NW, Agress H, et al.: Mass screening for diabetes: the use of a device for the collection of dried urine specimens and testing for sugar (St. Louis Dreypak). Diabetes 2:37, 1953.

10. Petrie LM, McLoughlin CJ, Hodgins TE: Mass screening for lowered glucose tolerance. Ann Intern Med 40:963–967, 1954.

11. McDonald GW, Hozier JB, Fisher GF, et al.: Large scale diabetes screening program for Federal employees. Public Health Rep 78:553, 1963.

12. Kent GT, Leonards JR: Mass screening for diabetes in a metropolitan area using finger blood glucose after a carbohydrate load. Diabetes 14:295–299, 1965.

13. Stein HJ, West KM, Robey JM, et al.: The high prevalence of abnormal glucose tolerance in Cherokee Indians of North Carolina. Arch Intern Med 116:842–845, 1965.

14. Millington JT, Tinsman CA: Diabetes screening in Pennsylvania. Pa Med 69:36, 1966.

15. West KM, Stein JH, Sanders TJ: Dextrostix estimates of blood glucose in mass screening for diabetes. Am J Public Health 56:2059–2064, 1966.

16. Kent GT, Leonards JR: Analysis of tests for diabetes in 250,000 persons screened for diabetes using finger blood after carbohydrate load. Diabetes 17:274, 1968.

17. Pell S, D'Alonzo CA: Diabetes in industry: prevalence, epidemiology, and prognosis in a large employed population. Arch Environ Health 17:425–435, 1968.

18. Welborn TA, Cullen KJ, Balazs N: Diabetes detection in mass health examinations: three-year experience from Busselton. Med J Aust 2:133–137, 1972.

19. Pyorala K, Lehtovirta E, Llomaki L: The relationship of obesity to prevalence and incidence of diabetes in Helsinki policemen. Acta Endocrinol Suppl (Copenh) 181:23–24, 1974.

20. Palumbo PH, Elvebaack LR, Chu CP, et al.: Diabetes mellitus: incidence, prevalence, survivorship and causes of death in Rochester Minnesota 1945–1970. Diabetes 25:566–573, 1976.

21. Kurlander AB, Iskrant AP, Kent ME: Screening tests for diabetes: a study of specificity and sensitivity. Diabetes 3:213, 1954.

22. Owen JA, Jr, Dennis BW, Hollifield G: Pitfalls in diabetes detection during the diagnostic study. South Med J 63:161–166, 1970.

23. Fleeson WP, Wenk RE: Pitfalls of mass chemical screening. Postgrad Med 48:59–64, 1970.

24. West KM, Wells RG, Burg BT: Case history of diabetes detection program: reappraisal of roles and methods of voluntary community programs. In Early Disease Detection. (Asymposium sponsored by the Ames Co., Division of Miles Laboratories, Inc.) Miami: Halos Associates, 1970, pp. 32–41.

25. Orzeck EA, Mooney JH, Owen JA, Jr: Diabetes detection with a comparison of screening methods. Diabetes 20:109–116, 1971.

26. West KM, Kalbfleisch JM: Sensitivity and specificity of five screening tests for diabetes in ten countries. Diabetes 20:239–296, 1971.

27. Galen RS, Gambino SR: Beyond Normality: the Predictive Value and Efficiency of Medical Diagnosis. New York: John Wiley & Sons, 1975, pp. 115–119.

28. Collen MF, Kidd PH, Feldman R, et al.: Cost analysis of a multiphasic screening program. N Engl J Med 280:1043–1045, 1969.

29. Genuth SM, Houser HB, Carter JR, et al.: Community screening for diabetes by blood glucose measurement: results of a five-year experience. Diabetes 25:1110–1117, 1976.

30. Houser HB, Mackay W, Venma N, et al.: A three year controlled followup study of persons identified in a mass screening program for diabetics. Diabetes 26:619–627, 1977.

31. Genuth SM, Houser HB, Carter JR, et al.: Observations on the value of mass indiscriminate screening for diabetic mellitus based on a five-year follow-up. Diabetes 27:377–383, 1978.

32. Herron CA: Screening in diabetes mellitus: report of the Atlanta Workshop. Diabetes Care 2:357–362, 1979.

33. Harris MI: Screening for undiagnosed non-insulin dependent diabetes. In Alberti KGMM, Mazze RS (eds): Current Trends in Noninsulin-Dependent Diabetes Mellitus. New York: Elsevier, 1989, pp. 119–131.

34. Rosenbloom AL, Allen CM: Mass urine glucose screening in children (Part II). Metabolism 22:323–326, 1973.

35. Gorwitz K, Thompson T, Howen GG: The prevalence of diabetes in school-age children. Diabetes 25:122–127, 1976.

36. Fine J: Glucose content of normal urine. Br Med J 1:1209–1214, 1965.

37. Kadish AH, Sternberg JC: Determination of urine glucose by measurement of oxygen consumption. Diabetes 18:467–470, 1969.

38. James RD, Chase GR: Evaluation of some commonly used semiquantitative methods for urinary glucose and ketone determinations. Diabetes 23:474–479, 1974.

39. American Diabetes Association: Detection and diagnosis of diabetes: plasma glucose procedures (brochure). New York: American Diabetes Association Detection and Education Program, 1974.

40. Position Statement of the American Diabetes Association: Screening for diabetes. Diabetes Care 12:588–590, 1989.

41. Remein QR, Wilkerson HLC: The efficiency of screening tests for diabetes. J Chronic Dis 13:6, 1961.

42. O'Sullivan JB, Wilkerson HLC, Krall LP: The prevalence of diabetes mellitus in Oxford and related epidemiologic problems. Am J Public Health 56:742, 1966.

43. O'Sullivan JB, Williams RF, McDonald GW: The prevalence of diabetes mellitus and related variables—a population study in Sudbury, Mass. J Chronic Dis 20:535–543, 1967.

44. West KM: Diabetes in American Indians and other native populations of the new world. Diabetes 23:841–855, 1974.

45. West KM: Epidemiology of Diabetes and Its Vascular Lesions. New York: Elsevier, 1978.

46. Centers for Disease Control: Recommendations for prevention of HIV transmission in health-care settings. MMWR 36 (Suppl 2):3–18, 1987.

47. Davidson JK, Reuben D, Sternberg JC, et al.: Diabetes screening using a quantitative urine glucose method. Diabetes 27:810–816, 1978.

48. Davidson JK: Random hyperglucosuria (RHG) and diabetes mellitus (DM). Fed Proc 40:741 (abstr 2917), 1981.

49. Hagopian WA, Sanjeevi CB, Kockum I, Landin-Olsson M, Karlsen AE, Sundkvist G, Dahlquist G, Palmer J, Lernmark A: Glutamate decarboxylase-, insulin-, and islet cell-antibodies and HLA typing to detect diabetes in a general population based study of Swedish children. J Clin Invest 95:1505–1511, 1995.

50. Verge CF, Gianani R, Kawasaki E, Chase H, Eisenbarth GS: Prediction of Type 1 diabetes in first degree relatives using a combination of insulin, GAD and IC512bc/IA-2 autoantibodies. Diabetes 45:926–933, 1996.

12

Diagnosis
of Diabetes Mellitus

John K. Davidson

Historical Perspective

Nineteen centuries ago Aretaeus wrote "Diabetes is a remarkable disorder, and not one very common to man. It consists of a moist and cold wasting of the flesh and limbs into urine, from a cause similar to that of dropsy, the secretion passes in the usual way, by the kidneys and bladder. The patients never cease making water, and the discharge is as incessant as a sluice let off. The disease is chronic in its character, and is slowly engendered, though the patient does not survive long when it is completely established, for the marasmus produced is rapid, and death speedy."

Three hundred years ago, Willis (1679)[1] discovered that the urine of patients with diabetes had a sweet taste. Dobson (1776) boiled to dryness 1 pint of urine from an individual with diabetes and obtained 1 ounce of crystalline material with the appearance and taste of brown sugar. Chevriel (1815) showed that urine and blood sugar were chemically similar to grape sugar (dextrose or glucose), and Bernard (1842–1848) demonstrated that glucose was stored in the liver as glycogen until it was broken down and released into the blood as glucose.

Bouchardat (1835–1875),[2] who had been trained in organic chemistry by Chevriel, was a pioneer in the study of the fermentive action of sugars and in the use of Biot's polariscopic method for the identification and measurement of sugars in the urine. Bouchardat was a superb clinician who taught patients how to test their urine for sugar, first with unslaked lime, then with a copper reagent (anticipating Fehling's test). He used these methods to measure the effects of carbohydrate ingestion on urine sugar excretion. Bouchardat noted that glucosuria was abolished or reduced in his patients because of inadequate food supplies, which produced weight loss during the siege of Paris (1870–1871). He then prescribed fasting, weight-reducing diets, and exercise to abolish or reduce glucosuria. In long-term studies he demonstrated conclusively that fat patients responded well to such therapy, whereas lean patients did not. Thus, he recognized more than 100 years ago that there were two relatively distinct types of diabetes. Allen (1913–1922)[3] carried out similar studies in the United States and confirmed Bouchardat's observations.

Fehling (1848) introduced the alkaline copper sulfate method as a urine glucose analytical procedure, and 48 years later it was applied to blood specimens after methods for removal of interfering substances were developed by Reid (1896). Since 1900, many advances in the methodology of glucose measurement in urine, blood, plasma, serum, and other body fluids have been made (see Chapter 13). The ability of monosaccharides to reduce cupric and ferric salts to cuprous and ferrous salts in alkaline solutions with resultant color changes that could be measured in a colorimeter were sufficiently developed by 1921 to play a critical role in the discovery of insulin.[4]

None of these methods was specific for glucose, and it was estimated that 10 to 30% of the reduction measured was due to other substances. In 1965,[5] the combination of an enzymatic method (glucose oxidase) and a polarographic electrode that measured the rate of oxygen consumption in the presence of glucose made it possible for the first time to measure specifically and quantitatively the glucose level in blood, plasma, and urine samples without interference by other substances. Not only has glucose measurement methodology become specific and quantitative, the sample volume needed has decreased over 200-fold (from 5 ml whole blood to 0.01 ml plasma) since the report of Bang (1913).[6]

Whole blood glucose was measured routinely until 1964, when the use of plasma or serum glucose[7,8] became preferable. The glucose content of whole blood is about 14% less than the glucose content of plasma, and plasma glucose content is about 15% greater than whole blood glucose. Since measured glucose levels in whole blood may be altered by anemia, polycythemia, and so forth, whole blood glucose measurements now are of historical interest only, excepting those who self-monitor capillary blood glucose levels (see Chapter 22).

Since the report of Hamman (1917),[9] measurement of blood sugar (plasma glucose) levels has become one of the most frequently performed laboratory procedures. In normal individuals, mean fasting and random plasma glucose levels are not significantly different, whereas 2-hr post-100-g carbohydrate meal levels are significantly higher and 2-hr glucose tolerance test (GTT) levels are higher still (Tables 12–1 and 12–2). A fasting plasma glucose level repeatedly greater than 140 ml/dL was universally accepted as being diagnostic of diabetes, whereas the utility of random and postcarbohydrate-load plasma glucose levels in making a diagnosis of diabetes continued to be a controversial matter.

TABLE 12–1   Outcome of Glucose Tolerance Tests (100-g Glucose Load) on 450 Asymptomatic Individuals in Age Range 15 to 80 Years Not Known to Have Diabetes Who Were Randomly Selected from 4,046 Screened Individuals with Random Urine Glucose Level from 3 to 25 mg/dL

	Glucose Tolerance Test (mg/dL)						
Time	Mean (m)	SD	SEM	M + 1 SD	M + 2 SD	M + 3 SD	Range
F	94	12.2	0.6	106.6	119	131	62–153
1 hr	137	42.6	2.0	179.6	222	265	49–271
1.5 hr	128	40.7	1.9	168.6	209	250	56–270
2 hr	120	36.3	1.7	156.0	192	229	50–265
3 hr	97	28.9	1.4	125.9	155	184	33–201

Sum of FPG and 1-, 2-, and 3-hr PGs
Mean   = 448
Range   = 254–785
SD   = 99.1
SEM   = 4.7
M + 1 SD = 546
M + 2 SD = 646
M + 3 SD = 745

Random Plasma Glucose (mg/dL)	2-hr Post 100-g Mixed Carbohydrate Meal (mg/dL)	Significance of Differences	
Mean = 96	Mean = 105	1. Fasting 94 versus random 96	p = 0.35 (NS)
Range = 60–161	Range = 54–225	2. 2-hr post-CHO meal 105 versus fasting 94	p < 0.0001
SD = 13.9	SD = 23.9	3. 2-hr post-CHO meal 105 versus random 96	p < 0.0001
SEM = 0.7	SEM = 1.1	4. 2-hr GTT 120 versus 2-hr post-CHO mean 105	p < 0.001
M + 1 SD = 110	M + 1 SD = 128.6		
M + 2 SD = 124	M + 2 SD = 152.4		
M + 3 SD = 138	M + 3 SD = 176		

Abbreviations: CHO, carbohydrate; NS, not significant; F, fasting; PG, plasma glucose; SD, standard deviation; SEM, standard error of the mean; other abbreviations as in text.

TABLE 12–2   Comparison (in mg/dL) of Fasting, Random, 1-hr-Post-100-g CHO Meal, and 2-hr GTT Levels (100-g Glucose Load) in 450 Individuals[a]

Classification	No.	%	Mean GTT Sum	Mean Fasting	Mean Random	Mean 2-hr Post-100 g CHO	Mean 2-hr GTT Post-100 g Glucose
All normals (sum <800 mg/dL)	450	100	448	94	96	105	120
All normals excluding high-normals (sum <600 mg/dL)	405	90	424	92	94	101	111
All high-normals (sum 601-800 mg/dL)	45	10	664	109	116	139	199

Abbreviations: as in text.
[a] See Exhibit 12–1 and Figure 12–8.

Glucose loading tests were introduced by Jarney (1918)[10]; Spence (1921) reported variations related to age; and Paullin (1922)[11] reported variations related to obesity. After the report of the results of 1,100 GTTs by John (1929),[12] the use of the test to detect those with undiagnosed diabetes expanded rapidly[13,14] as glucose loading tests became the most popular method of ascertaining whether or not diabetes should be diagnosed. Only in the last 30 years has the limited value of the GTT as a diagnostic procedure when applied to the general population become obvious, and only during the last 20 years have the disagreements related to its interpretation become readily apparent[15] (Fig. 12–1). Soskin,[16] Danowski,[17] Andres,[18] and others[19] had suggested that the diagnosis of diabetes was being made erroneously (false-positive diagnosis) in many individuals because the criteria used for interpretation were inappropriate.

In 1927 Lennox[20] had shown that there were large variations in blood sugar levels at 1 and 2 hr after a glucose load when the test was repeated in the same individual (*intraperson variation*). The lack of reproducibility of the test has been reported by numerous investigators since that time (Tables 12–3 and 12–4).[21–26] Mean absolute differences between test and retest varied from 17.2 to 35.1 mg/dL at 1 hr and from 12.2 to 31.3 mg/dL at 2 hr. *Interperson variation* during a GTT is even greater, as is demonstrated in Table 12–4. The Mayer group (1976)[24] was not prescreened to remove those who had glucosuria (many of whom would almost certainly have had undiagnosed diabetes). The Mayer group mean plasma glucose at 2 hr was 125

TABLE 12–3 Intraperson Variation of 1- and 2-hr GTT Determinations[21]

Mean Absolute Difference Between Test and Retest (mg/dL)		No. Tested	Glucose Load (g)	Reference
1 hr	**2 hr**			
35.1	31.3	28	1.5 g/kg body wt	Lennox (1927)[20]
29.9	20.4	35	100	Freeman (1942)
29.5	25.7	49	100	Unger (1957)
20.0	11.9	28	100	Hayner (1963)
—[a]	18	39	50	West (1964)
26	18	24, 26	70	
18	22	26, 50	1 g/kg body wt	
17.2	12.2[b]	334	100	McDonald (1965)
18.9	17.0	96	50	Sisk (1970)
25.2	17.7	96	100	
30.1	22.3	61	75	Rushforth (1975)[21]

[a] One hour not determined.

[b] Mean SD based on six determinations.

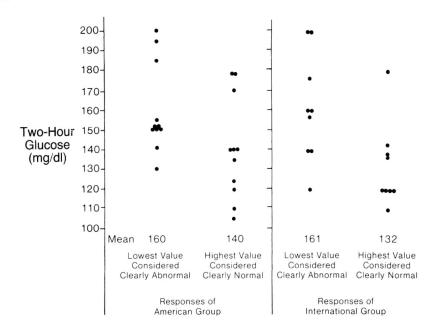

Figure 12–1. Differences in the lowest values considered clearly abnormal and the highest values considered clearly normal for the 2-hr GTT plasma glucose level by an American group and by an international group of diabetologists. (*Source*: Adapted from West KM: Substantial differences in diagnostic criteria used by diabetes experts. Diabetes 24:641–644, 1975. With permission.)

TABLE 12–4   Interperson Variation of 2-hr GTT Determinations

Author	No. and Procedure	Mean 2-Hr PG	SD	Mean+ 2 SD	Mean+ 3 SD
Mayer and coworkers (1976)[24]	1,674 individuals. Age 30–64 years. Not known to have diabetes. Not prescreened for diabetes. 100 g glucose load	125	63	252	315
Davidson (1981)[26]	450 individuals. Age 15–80 years. Not known to have diabetes. Prescreened by random urine glucose which was normal (3–25 mg/dL). 100 g glucose load	120	36	192	229

mg/dL with a standard deviation of 63 mg/dL. A pre-screened group (all of whom had a normal random urine glucose [RUG] of 3 to 25 mg/dL) had a group mean plasma glucose level at 2 hr of 120 mg/dL, with a considerably smaller standard deviation of 36 mg/dL.[25,26] Prescreening reduced the group standard deviation significantly by removing those with a RUG > 25 mg/dL, three fourths of whom were subsequently shown to have diabetes.[26]

Regardless of the other variables that may contribute to the outcome of a GTT the intraperson and interperson variables that determine the standard deviation of the population mean and the magnitude of that standard deviation are the dominant factors that determine the upper limits of normal for plasma glucose levels during a GTT. These variables may also differ in various defined populations and their subgroups. Also, it seems clear that the standard deviation of the mean will increase as the prevalence of diabetes increases.

Most populations have a prevalence of diabetes of less than 5%, and plasma glucose levels are distributed unimodally with a skew to the right.[27] (Fig. 12–2). In some population groups (Pima and other Indians,[21,22] Micronesians, and Polynesians[28–30]) in whom prevalence of diabetes exceeds 10%, plasma glucose levels during a GTT are distributed in an overlapping bimodal fashion (nondiabetic in first mode, diabetic in second mode) (Fig. 12–3). The percentage in the second mode increases from the second to the sixth decades,[21,22,30] signifying the increase in prevalence of diabetes with advancing age.

Although it was once thought that the increasing prevalence of glucose intolerance reflected physiologic events related to increasing age,[18,31] it now appears that it is primarily a pathologic event reflecting an increasing prevalence of non-insulin-dependent diabetes mellitus (NIDDM) in overfed populations.[30] Also, some overweight individuals with NIDDM can lose weight and their plasma glucose can return to and remain normal for at least 20 years thereafter, despite the fact that they are 20 years older.

Attempts to diagnose "diabetes" early while glucose tolerance was still "borderline," "equivocal," or only "slightly impaired" so that the disease could be treated aggressively in its earliest stages in hopes of preventing

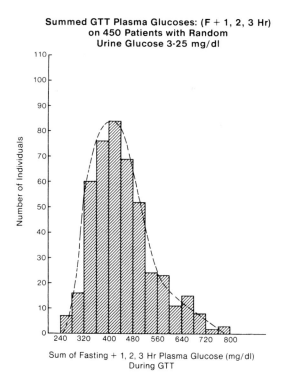

Figure 12–2. Histogram demonstrating distribution of summed GTTs in 450 individuals randomly selected from 4,046 individuals with a normal RUG level. The smoothed best-fit curve (dashed line) is a unimodal distribution skewed to the right. The prevalence of undiagnosed diabetes in this population was ascertained to be 1.6% (see Fig. 12–7).

or minimizing the morbidity and mortality thereunto related reached its zenith from 1950–1975.[13,14,32–37] This set the stage for the widespread use of criteria for the diagnosis of diabetes that were nonspecific and that resulted in a false-positive diagnosis of diabetes in many individuals who were subjected to a GTT even though their fasting, random, and postmeal blood glucose levels were perfectly normal. The beliefs and hopes of that time were expressed by Conn and Fajans[34] as follows:

We believe that most experienced students of clinical diabetes will agree with the following statements: (1) Diabetes mellitus can be defined as an abnormal metabolic state induced by deficient insulin activity. (2) At present, the most sensitive clinical index of the existence of this

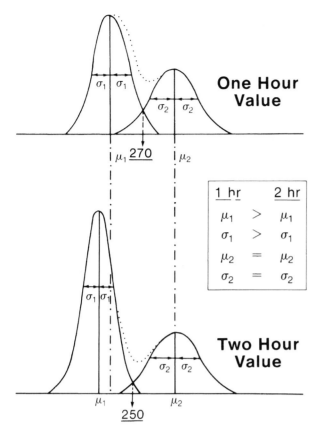

Figure 12–3. Bimodal distribution of 1- and 2-hr values during GTT.[21] The prevalence of diabetes in this population of Pima Indians exceeded 10%. μ_1 and μ_2 are the means of the 1- and 2-hr values for the nondiabetic and the diabetic populations, respectively, and σ_1 and σ_2 are their standard deviations. The optimal cut-point between the nondiabetic and the diabetic groups at 1 hr was 270 mg/dL, and at 2 hr was 250 mg/dL (see Fig. 12–4). (*Source:* Rushforth NB, Bennett PH, Steinberg AG, et al.: Comparison of the value of the two- and one-hour glucose levels of the oral GTT in the diagnosis of diabetes in Pima Indians. Diabetes 24:538–546, 1975. With permission.)

state is afforded by glucose loading tests. (3) Diabetes is genetically determined, and in whatever way the genetic determinant eventually brings about evidence of deficient insulin activity the basic abnormality has been present since conception. (4) The *prediabetic period* is defined as that period of time from conception to the demonstration of diminished insulin activity by whatever method is considered to be most sensitive in this respect at that time. This means that as more sensitive methods are discovered, the prediabetic period will become shorter. (5) The *prediabetic state* implies as yet undiscovered metabolic derangements which (a) lead eventually to insufficient insulin activity and (b) may give rise also to the generalized angiopathy which characterizes the syndrome. (6) A breakthrough in knowledge of mechanisms at work in the prediabetic state would offer great potential benefits to mankind. The area deserves concentrated research effort.

In the same article,[34] the following statements were made: "In young asymptomatic patients treated with

tolbutamide over long periods of time we have observed return of normal carbohydrate tolerance in some and marked improvement of tolerance in others. ... Perhaps an action of tolbutamide makes overworked beta cells better able to function under duress. If so, and if indeed the prediabetic state is characterized by a dynamic insular response (with eventual failure) to a diabetogenic influence, tolbutamide given in the prediabetic period might prevent or forestall the emergence of hypoinsulinism."

The enthusiasm for "early diagnosis" and treatment, and the use of the overly sensitive and nonspecific criteria to interpret GTTs, led to a false-positive diagnosis of diabetes in many individuals who did not have it and in whom the diagnosis would not have been made had less sensitive and more specific criteria been used (Exhibits 12–1 and 12–2).

Since 1975, several investigators have collected and analyzed data that suggested that the upper limits of normal for the 1- and 2-hr levels (and their sum) during a GTT should be increased significantly: Siperstein to 260 mg/dL at 1 hr and 220 mg/dL at 2 hr;[38] Rushforth to 270 mg/dL at 1 hr and 250 mg/dL at 2 hr;[21] and Köberling to 575 mg/dL for 1- plus 2-hr sum.[39]

Meanwhile, the effect of arbitrarily low cut-points in increasing the prevalence of diagnosed "diabetes" was becoming more apparent (Table 12–5).[40] In this study, diabetes was diagnosed during a GTT more than five times as often by a peak plasma glucose of 205 + mg/dL than by a 2-hr level of 160 + mg/dL. In retrospect, it appears that four of five diagnoses of diabetes using the most sensitive criterion (2-hr level, 205 + mg/dL peak) could have been false-positive diagnoses.

Concern related to the confusion generated by these and other studies led to the initiation of epidemiologic follow-up studies designed to determine the rate of progression from "borderline diabetes" or "impaired glucose tolerance" to "diabetes," and to its specific complications.[22,23] Although only 20 + years of experience with studies of this type are available, much has already been learned: that ≤3%/year progress from "borderline diabetes" to diabetes, that most revert to normal, and that many remain "borderline."[39,41,42] These studies suggest that an initial "borderline" test that is not clearly abnormal is of little value in individual subjects except to indicate that they may be at increased risk for the subsequent development of diabetes. The Bedford survey[42] did indicate a greater propensity for those with a "borderline" GTT to develop coronary heart disease, but it is not clear that other risk factors were not involved.

West[43] recommended that individuals previously classified as having "borderline diabetes" or "impaired glucose tolerance" because of nonspecific GTT criteria be classified as "high-normals," removing any suggestion that they had diabetes or were predestined to

EXHIBIT 12–1   Diagnostic Criteria for Diabetes Mellitus (National Diabetes Data Group)

Diabetes Mellitus in Nonpregnant Adults

Any one of the following are considered diagnostic of diabetes:

A. Presence of the classic symptoms of diabetes, such as polyuria, polydipsia, ketonuria, and rapid weight loss, together with gross and unequivocal elevation of plasma glucose.

B. Elevated fasting glucose concentration on more than one occasion:

Venous plasma ≥ 140 mg/dL (7.8 mmol/L)
Venous whole blood ≥ 120 mg/dL (6.7 mmol/L)
Capillary whole blood ≥ 120 mg/dL (6.7 mmol/L)

If the fasting glucose concentration meets these criteria, the oral glucose tolerance test (OGTT) is *not required*. Indeed, virtually all persons with fasting plasma glucose (FPG) > 140 mg/dL will exhibit an OGTT that meets or exceeds the criteria in (C) below.

C. Fasting glucose concentration less than that which is diagnostic of diabetes [(B), above], but sustained elevated glucose concentration during the OGTT on more than one occasion. *Both* the 2-hr sample *and* some other sample taken between administration of the 75 g glucose dose and 2 hr later must meet the following criteria:

Venous plasma ≥ 200 mg/dL (11.1 mmol/L)
Venous whole blood ≥ 180 mg/dL (10.0 mmol/L)
Capillary whole blood ≥ 200 mg/dL (11.1 mmol/L)

Impaired Glucose Tolerance (IGT) in Nonpregnant Adults

Three criteria must be met: the fasting glucose concentration must be below the value that is diagnostic for diabetes; the glucose concentration 2 hr after a 75 g oral glucose challenge must be between normal and diabetic values, and a value between $\frac{1}{2}$ hr, 1 hr, or $1\frac{1}{2}$ hr OGTT value must later be unequivocally elevated.

Fasting value:
Venous plasma < 140 mg/dL (7.8 mmol/L)
Venous whole blood < 120 mg/dL (6.7 mmol/L)
Capillary whole blood < 120 mg/dL (6.7 mmol/L)
$\frac{1}{2}$-hr, 1-hr, or $1\frac{1}{2}$-hr OGTT value:
Venous plasma ≥ 200 mg/dL (11.1 mmol/L)
Venous whole blood ≥ 180 mg/dL (10.0 mmol/L)
Capillary whole blood ≥ 200 mg/dL (11.1 mmol/L)
2-hr OGTT value:
Venous plasma of between 140 and 200 mg/dL (7.8 and 11.1 mmol/L)
Venous whole blood of between 120 and 180 mg/dL (6.7 and 10.0 mmol/L)
Capillary whole blood of between 140 and 200 mg/dL (7.8 and 11.1 mmol/L)

Normal Glucose Levels in Nonpregnant Adults

Fasting value:
Venous plasma < 115 mg/dL (6.4 mmol/L)
Venous whole blood < 100 mg/dL (5.6 mmol/L)
Capillary whole blood < 100 mg/dL (5.6 mmol/L)

2-hr OGTT value:
Venous plasma < 140 mg/dL (7.8 mmol/L))
Venous whole blood < 120 mg/dL (6.7 mmol/L)
Capillary whole blood < 140 mg/dL (7.8 mmol/L)
OGTT values between $\frac{1}{2}$-hr, 1-hr or $1\frac{1}{2}$-hr OGTT value later:
Venous plasma < 200 mg/dL (11.1 mmol/L)
Venous whole blood < 180 mg/dL (10.0 mmol/L)
Capillary whole blood < 200 mg/dL (11.1 mmol/L)
Glucose values above these concentrations but below the criteria for diabetes or IGT should be considered nondiagnostic.

Diabetes Mellitus in Children

Either of the following are considered diagnostic of diabetes:

A. Presence of the classic symptoms of diabetes, such as polyuria, polydipsia, ketonuria, and rapid weight loss, together with a random plasma glucose > 200 mg/dL.

B. In asymptomatic individuals, *both* an elevated fasting glucose concentration and a sustained elevated glucose concentration during the OGTT on more than one occasion. Both the 2-hr sample *and* some other sample taken between administration of the glucose dose (1.75 g/kg ideal body weight, up to a maximum of 75 g) and 2 hr later must meet the criteria below.

Fasting value:
Venous plasma ≥ 140 mg/dL (7.8 mmol/L)
Venous whole blood ≥ 120 mg/dL (6.7 mmol/L)
Capillary whole blood ≥ 120 mg/dL (6.7 mmol/L)
2-hr OGTT value and an intervening value:
Venous plasma ≥ 200 mg/dL (11.1 mmol/L)
Venous whole blood ≥ 180 mg/dL (10.0 mmol/L)
Whole capillary blood ≥ 200 mg/dL (11.1 mmol/L)

Impaired Glucose Tolerance in Children

Two criteria must be met: the fasting glucose concentration must be below the value that is diagnostic of diabetes, and the glucose concentration 2 hr after an oral glucose challenge must be elevated.

Fasting value:
Venous plasma < 140 mg/dL (7.8 mmol/L)
Venous whole blood < 120 mg/dL (6.7 mmol/L)
Capillary whole blood < 120 mg/dL (6.7 mmol/L)
2-hr OGTT value:
Venous plasma > 140 mg/dL (7.8 mmol/L)
Venous whole blood > 120 mg/dL (6.7 mmol/L)
Capillary whole blood > 120 mg/dL (6.7 mmol/L)

Normal Glucose Levels in Children

Fasting value:
Venous plasma < 130 mg/dL (7.2 mmol/L)
Venous whole blood < 115 mg/dL (6.4 mmol/L)
Capillary whole blood < 115 mg/dL (6.4 mmol/L)
2-hr OGTT value:
Venous plasma < 140 mg/dL (7.8 mmol/L)
Venous whole blood < 120 mg/dL (6.7 mmol/L)
Capillary whole blood < 140 mg/dL (7.8 mmol/L)

(*Source*: National Diabetes Data Group: Classification and diagnosis of diabetes mellitus and other categories of glucose intolerance. Diabetes 28:1029–1057, 1979. With permission.)

EXHIBIT 12–2 Criteria That Have Been Used for Interpretation of Oral Glucose Tolerance Tests in Nonpregnant Individuals[a]

Criterion	Prevalence of Diabetes (%)	Criterion	Prevalence of Diabetes (%)
Fasting venous plasma glucose repeatedly >140 mg/dL[44,45]	1.5	United States Public Health Service Wilkerson Point System[48]	
Davidson[26]		Fasting >130 mg/dL = one point	
FPG >140 mg/dL, or sum of fasting plus 1-, 2-, and 3-hr levels		1 hr >195 mg/dL = one half point	
		2 hr >140 mg/dL = one half point	
Diabetes mellitus if sum >800 mg/dL	1.6	3 hr >130 mg/dL = one point	
Nondiabetic if sum <800 mg/dL		Diabetes mellitus if point total is	
Nondiabetic *high-normal* if sum 601 to 800 mg/dL		two to three	6.0
		Equivocal if point total is $\frac{1}{2}$ to $1\frac{1}{2}$	
If the cut-point for the upper limit of normal is lowered, the prevalence of diabetes increases as follows:		Nondiabetic if point total is zero	
		World Health Organization[45]	
		Diabetes mellitus if one of the following:	
Sum >750 mg/dL	2.3	Fasting >140 mg/dL (three occasions)	
Sum >700 mg/dL	3.2	or 2 hr >200 mg/dL	6.0
Sum >650 mg/dL	6.6	National Institutes of Health Diabetes Data Group[44]	
Sum >600 mg/dL	10.2	Diabetes mellitus if one of the following:	
Danowski[17]		Fasting >140 mg/dL (three occasions)	
Sum of fasting, 0.5-, 1-, and 2-hr values		or 0.5 hr >200 mg/dL	
Diabetes mellitus if sum >805 mg/dL		or 1 hr >200 mg/dL or 1.5 hr	5.8
Equivocal if sum 501 to 805 mg/dL		>200 mg/dL and 2 hr >200 mg/dL	
Nondiabetic if sum ≤ 500 mg/dL		Impaired glucose tolerance if one of the following:	
Siperstein[38]			
Diabetes if 1 hr >260 mg/dL 2 hr >220 mg/dL	1.6	0.5 hr >200 mg/dL or 1 hr >200 mg/dL or 1.5 hr >200 mg/dL	
Köbberling[39]		and 2 hr >140 mg/dL	5.4
Diabetes if sum of 1-hr plus 2-hr values >575 mg/dL	1.6	Total for diabetes mellitus and impaired glucose tolerance	11.2
Rushforth and colleagues[21]	1.6	Positive by both United States Public Health Service (Wilkerson Point System) and National Institutes of Health Diabetes Data Group Criteria[44,48]	4.0
Mean upper limit of normal (male and female) 1 hr 270 mg/dL			
Mean upper limit of normal (male and female) 2 hr 250 mg/dL		Joslin Clinic[37]	
See Figures 12–3 and 12–4		Diabetes mellitus if all of the following:	
European Diabetes Epidemiology Study Group[19a,19b]		1 hr >190 mg/dL	
		2 hr >140 mg/dL	
Diabetes mellitus if one of the following:		3 hr >125 mg/dL	11.2
0.5 hr >285 mg/dL		Fajans-Conn[14]	
1 hr >255 mg/dL		Diabetes mellitus if all of the following:	
1.5 hr >255 mg/dL and 2 hr >200 mg/dL	2.5	1 hr >185 mg/dL	12.3
		(later age-adjusted to >195 mg/dL)	10.1
Nondiabetic if:		1.5 hr >165 mg/dL	
0.5-, 1-, and 1.5-hr values <185 mg/dL and 2-hr value <140 mg/dL		2 hr >140 mg/dL	
		British Diabetic Association[36]	
Borderline if between the above values		Diabetes mellitus if one of the following:	
Andes age-adjusted 2 hr GTT level[18]		0.5 hr >185 mg/dL or 1 hr >185 mg/dL	12.3
At age		and 1.5 hr >165 mg/dL and	
>20 years >180 mg/dL		2 hr >140 mg/dL	
>30 years >190 mg/dL		American Diabetes Association Criteria (1998)[48,49,50]	
>40 years >200 mg/dL		Diabetes mellitus if either:	
>50 years >210 mg/dL	3.4	FPG ≥ 126 mg/dL (7.0 mmol/L) × 2	
>60 years >220 mg/dL		or 2 hr post-75 g, glucose load >200 mg/dL	
>70 years >230 mg/dL		(11.1 mmol/L) × 2.	
>80 years >240 mg/dL			

[a] Venous plasma values in milligrams per deciliter.

Comparison of Upper Limits of Normal of Different Sets of Criteria for Interpretation of a Glucose Tolerance Test

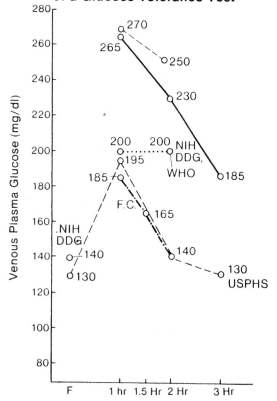

Figure 12–4. This figure illustrates the marked differences in recommended upper limits of normal during a GTT. One hour level varies from 185 mg/dL [Fajans-Conn (FC)[14]] to 265 mg/dL (Davidson[26]) and 270 mg/dL (Rushforth and colleagues[21]). Two-hour level varies from 140 mg/dL (F-C,[14] United States Public Health Service[48]) to 230 mg/dL (Davidson[26]) and 250 mg/dL (Rushforth and colleagues[21]). *Abbreviations*: DDG, Diabetes Data Group; FC, Fajans-Conn; NIH, National Institutes of Health; USPHS, United States Public Health Service; WHO, World Health Organization.

develop it. This approach could reduce to an absolute minimum the consequences of a false-positive diagnosis (anxiety, depression, restrictions on employment, insurance, and other activities, inappropriate treatment with drugs, and/or diet for a nonexistent disease, and so forth).

In the last 20 years, several expert committees have considered problems related to defining, diagnosing, and typing diabetes mellitus.[44–50] The National Institutes of Health Diabetes Data Group (NIH-DDG) and the World Health Organization (WHO) recommended that the upper limit of normal for the 75 g glucose load GTT at 120 min be increased to 199 mg/dL, with the NIH-DDG requiring at least one level ≥200 mg/dL between time zero and 120 min (30, 60, or 90 min) for a diagnosis of diabetes. Those with a 120 min level from 140 to 199 and with one other level between 30 and 90 min ≥200 mg/dL were to be classified as having *impaired glucose tolerance* (IGT). Although the classification of IGT is being widely used by epidemiologists, it is not being widely used by clinicians because of their concern about the consequences (as just discussed) of the classification being used erroneously and implying that the individual has "an abnormal GTT" and probably has early diabetes. It has been known since the early 1980s that "impaired glucose tolerance" in the general population has a variable natural history with the follow-up GTT results returning to normal, remaining the same, or progressing to clear-cut diabetes in ≤3%/year.

Despite reservations concerning the use of the IGT category, recommendations concerning the interpretation of the GTT by NIH-DDG and WHO criteria have been accepted almost universally by clinicians and researchers because for the first time a standardized set of measurements used in different laboratories and clinics worldwide could be directly compared.

In 1998, an American Diabetes Association Committee recommended *that the use of the glucose tolerance test be discouraged*, and that the diagnosis of NIDDM (type 2 diabetes) be based on *fasting plasma glucose levels. Diabetes mellitus* = fasting plasma glucose ≥126 mg/dL × 2 (7.0 mmol/L) × 2. The committee also recommended that a plasma glucose of ≥110 mg/dL (6.1 mmol/L) and ≤125 mg/dL (7.0 mmol/L) × 2 be classified *as impaired fasting plasma glucose (IFG).*[48,49]

TABLE 12–5 Effect of Varying Criteria on Prevalence of "Diabetes" in Random Sample of Bedford Population Undergoing Standard 50 g Oral Glucose Tolerance Test (converted from whole blood to plasma values, and rounded to closest 5 mg/dL)

	Percentage with "Diabetes" when Plasma Glucose (mg/dL) Is:			
Age	140+ at 2 hr	160+ at 2 hr	205+ Peak	Peak 205+ and 140+ at 2 hr
20–29	7.3	2.1	11.5	2.1
30–39	6.4	1.1	14.9	1.1
40–49	9.7	4.3	29.0	6.5
50–59	15.4	6.6	48.4	14.3
60–69	18.4	5.7	51.7	11.5
70+	40.2	22.0	61.0	34.1
Total	15.7	6.6	35.2	11.1

[*Source*: Adapted from Jarrett RJ, Keen H: Hyperglycemia and diabetes mellitus. Lancet 2:1009–1012, 1976. With permission.]

EXHIBIT 12–3   The 1998 American Diabetes Association Report on New Criteria for the Diagnosis of Diabetes Mellitus[48,49]

Normoglycemia	Impaired Glucose Metabolism (IGM)	Diabetes Mellitus*
FPG <110 mg/dL (6.0 mmol/L)	FPG ≥110 mg/dL and <126 mg/dL (IFG) (6.0–7.0 mmol/L)	FPG ≥126 mg/dL (7.0 mmol/L)
2-h PG** <140 mg/dL (<7.8 mmol/L)	2-h PG** ≥140 and <200 mg/dL (IGT) (7.8 mmol/L to 11.1 mmol/L)	2-h PG** ≥200 mg/dL (≥11.1 mmol/L)
		Symptoms and random plasma glucose ≥200 mg/dL (11.1 mmol/L)

* A diagnosis of diabetes mellitus must be confirmed, on a subsequent day, by measurement of FPG, 2-h PG or random plasma glucose (if symptoms are present). The FPG test is greatly preferred because of ease of administration, convenience, acceptability to patients, and lower cost. Fasting is defined as no caloric intake for at least 8 h. This test requires the use of a glucose load containing the equivalent of 75 g anhydrous glucose dissolved in water.

** 2-h postload glucose. *Abbreviations*: IGM–impaired glucose metabolism, IFG–impaired fasting glucose, IGT–impaired glucose tolerance.

Screening and Diagnosis Scheme for Gestational Diabetes Mellitus[50]

Plasma Glucose	50-g Screening Test	100-g Diagnostic Test
Fasting	—	105 mg/dL (5.8 mmol/L)
1-h	140 mg/dL (7.8 mmol/L)	190 mg/dL (10.6 mmol/L)
2-h	—	165 mg/dL (9.2 mmol/L)
3-h	—	145 mg/dL (8.1 mmol/L)

Screening for GDM may not be necessary in pregnant women who meet *all* of the following criteria: <25 years of age, normal body weight, no first degree relative with diabetes, *and* not Hispanic, Native American, Asian-, or African–American. The 100 g diagnostic test is performed on patients who have a positive screening test. The diagnosis of GDM requires any two of the four plasma glucose values obtained during the test to meet or exceed the values shown above.

Of course the committee's not-yet-proven hypothesis is that *lowering* the level of fasting plasma glucose necessary to diagnose diabetes mellitus or impaired fasting plasma glucose is desirable so that non-pharmacologic therapy (diet and exercise as indicated) can be started earlier to prevent or delay the appearance of the chronic complications (secondary prevention). Diet and exercise therapy can be started, if indicated, regardless of whether or not diabetes has been diagnosed. Because of the risks of side effects of pharmacotherapy in this situation, it should be undertaken only when significant hyperglycemia has not been controlled by diet and exercise alone, and *never* at the low levels of IFG noted.

The practitioner should always remember the *psychological and economic risks* to the patient of making a *false-positive diagnosis* of diabetes mellitus. Even the term *impaired fasting glucose* implies that diabetes may soon develop. That this is not true is clearly demonstrated by the fact that in Figure 12–5 *almost 2/3 of the individuals with high normal GTTs after 15 years of follow up had not developed diabetes.*

A study by the author that started in the mid-1970s[25,26] was designed to measure the upper limit of normal of plasma glucose levels during a 3-hr glucose tolerance test after a 100 g load of glucose at time zero (Figs. 12–5 through 12–11). The 450 individuals were selected at random from a mixed group of 4,046 blacks and whites, males and females, ages from 15 to 80 years. All had a normal RUG. All were instructed to eat 300 g carbohydrate per day for 3 days before the test and to fast for 15 hours before the test. Results are shown in Figure 12–2. Figure 12–7 illustrates how the outcomes were evaluated and how the 45 individuals in the "high normal" group (sum of GTT 601-800 mg/dL) were identified. These 45 individuals were followed for 15 years or until death (Fig. 12–5). In only 16 (35.6%) did the fasting plasma glucose exceed 140 mg/dL, or did the GTT sum exceed 800 mg/dL when the fasting plasma glucose was less than 140 mg/dL (a total of eight in each group). After 15 years follow-up, almost two-thirds (64.4%) had normal GTTs (37.7%) or had died without developing diabetes (26.7%). Over this period of time, the mean annual rate of progression of members of the group to diabetes was 2.4% per year. This slow rate of progression from "IGT" or "high normal GTTs" has been reported by a number of other investigators and provides a cautionary note concerning the risks of making an erroneous diagnosis of diabetes when it is based only on glucose tolerance test data that is not clearly abnormal in two tests and when the fasting plasma glucose is within normal limits.

A comparison of the different prevalence rates using different sets of criteria is shown in Exhibit 12–2. Of considerable interest is the fact that the most sensitive criteria (Joslin Clinic, Fajans-Conn, British Diabetic

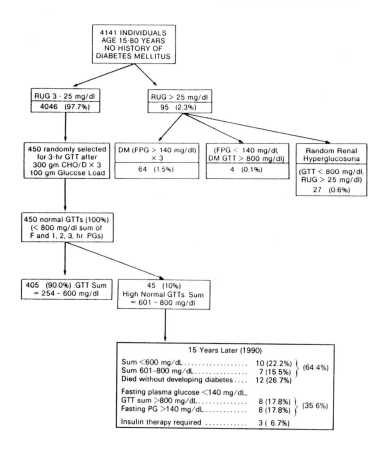

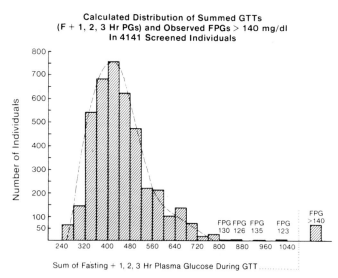

Figure 12–6. The assumption was made that the 450 randomly selected individuals from the population of 4,046 with a RUG of 3 to 25 mg/dL (Fig. 12–2) were representative of those in the nondiabetic segment (Exhibit 12–2). This figure is a composite of both the calculated nondiabetic and the observed diabetic individuals in the total population of 4,141 screened individuals. Of those with a RUG >25 mg/dL, 68 on follow-up testing were found to have diabetes. Sixty-four had a FPG level >140 mg/dL and 4 had a FPG <140 mg/dL and a GTT sum >800 mg/dL.

Figure 12–5. Distribution and follow-up of subgroups of 4,141 individuals who were screened for diabetes mellitus by measurement of RUG level. [*Source:* Davidson JK: Random hyperglucosuria (RHG) and diabetes mellitus (DM). Fed Proc 40:741 (abstr 2917), 1981.]

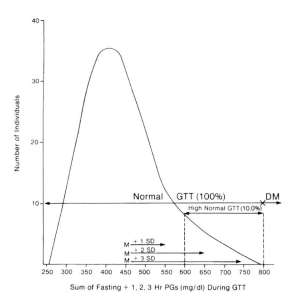

Figure 12–7. This smoothed normal curve was derived from Figure 12–2. The arrows show the cut-points for upper limits of normal for the mean plus 2 and plus 3 standard deviations of the mean. The prevalence of diagnosed diabetes in the population was 1.6%. The upper limit of normal cut-point was arbitrarily located at 800 mg/dL, and individuals with a GTT sum 601 to 800 mg/dL were classified as "high-normal."

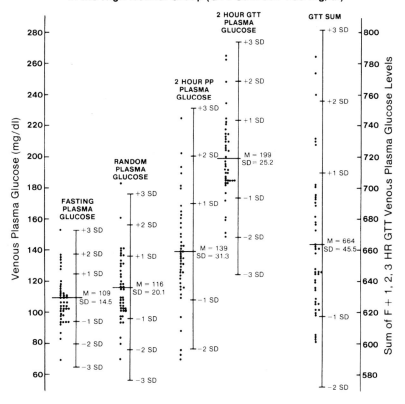

Comparison of Fasting, Random, 2 HR Post Prandial
(100 GM CHO), 2 HR GTT (100 GM Glucose), and
GTT Sum (F+ 1, 2, 3 HR) Plasma Glucose Levels for those
in the High Normal Group (GTT Sum 601-785 mg/dl)

Figure 12–8. The ranges, means, and standard deviations of the fasting, random, 2-hr post-100 g mixed-meal carbohydrate load, 2-hr GTT, and GTT sum plasma glucose levels of the 45 individuals in the "high-normal" group. See Exhibit 12–2.

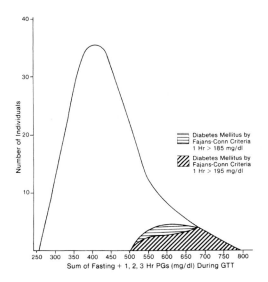

Figure 12–9. Forty-eight individuals (10.7%) were diagnosed erroneously by Fajans-Conn criteria using 185 mg/dL at 1 hr as upper limit of normal, and 38 individuals (8.5%) were diagnosed erroneously by Fajans-Conn criteria using 195 mg/dL at 1 hr as upper limit of normal. See Exhibit 12–2.

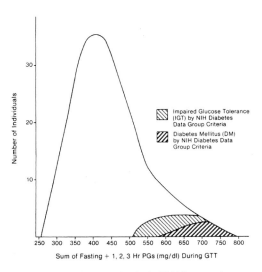

Figure 12–10. Nineteen individuals (4.2%) were diagnosed erroneously by NIH-DDG criteria and 24 (5.4%) were classified as "impaired glucose tolerance," making a total of 43 individuals (9.6%). See Exhibit 12–7.

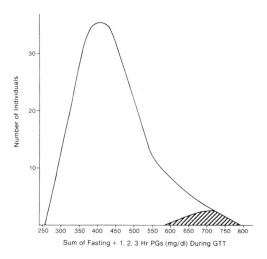

Figure 12–11. Twenty individuals (4.4%) were diagnosed erroneously by USPHS criteria. See Exhibit 12–1.

Association) resulted in a prevalence of diabetes that was seven times as great as was the prevalence using the least sensitive criteria (Rushforth, Köbberling, Siperstein, Danowski, Davidson, and the European Diabetes Epidemiology Study Group). Most of the "high normal" group were diagnosed as "diabetic" by Joslin Clinic, Fajans-Conn, and British Diabetic Association criteria. This despite the fact that after 15 years of follow-up, only slightly more than one-third diagnosed by the most sensitive criteria have developed diabetes that can be diagnosed by the least sensitive criteria.

When criteria of intermediate sensitivity (USPHS Wilkerson Point System, WHO, and NIH-DDG) were compared to the least sensitive criteria, the prevalence of diagnosed "diabetes" was almost four times as great. Prevalences by the Point System and WHO criteria were identical (6%), suggesting that prevalences of "diabetes" diagnosed by WHO and NIH-DDG criteria are still too high and may include some that will not progress to overt diabetes. The studies of Rushford et al.[21] and of Davidson[26] indicated that the GTT 2-hr level upper limit of normal should be 250 mg/dL or 230 mg/dL, respectively (Figs. 12–3 and 12–4).

Taken together, the studies of Rushforth et al.,[21,23] Davidson,[26] Zimmett and Whitehouse,[28–30] Köbberling and Berninger,[39] and others have confirmed that the recommended upper limit of normal fasting (139 mg/dL × 2–3) criterion will routinely avoid an erroneous diagnosis of diabetes. However, the prevalence of diagnosed diabetes by NIH-DDG and WHO GTT criteria is essentially the same as was the prevalence by USPHS Wilkerson Point System criteria 40 years ago, and it is four times as high as is the prevalence of diagnosed diabetes by the least sensitive criteria. This suggests that the upper limit of normal for the GTT at 2 hr should be increased from 199 mg/dL to the 230 to 250 mg/dL range. It also suggests that careful population follow-up studies

should be done to determine how many with "high normal" GTTs, IGT, and diabetes by NIH-DDG, WHO, and 1998 ADA criteria[45–50] progress over time to full-blown diabetes with chronic complications.

It is appropriate to follow individuals in the "high normal" (sum 601 to 800 mg/dL) at regular intervals, since they are at increased risk for developing clear-cut diabetes. About 17.8% progressed to a fasting plasma glucose (FPG) ≥ 140 mg/dL during 15 years of follow-up in the Davidson study previously noted.

Epidemiology of Chronic Complications

The prevalence and incidence are greater in those who are older, in those who are overweight, and in those who have a family history of diabetes. In the Pima Indian studies,[22,23] 30% of those in the diabetic mode had evidence of the specific vascular complications of diabetes (retinopathy and/or nephropathy), whereas these abnormalities were virtually absent in those in the non-diabetic mode (Fig. 12–3).

The Pima Indian and other studies have focused attention in the last 20 years on the natural history of NIDDM and the risk factors that contribute to the development and progression of the chronic complications of the disease. More effective treatment methods have been developed, and it is anticipated that both primary and secondary prevention strategies will be used more generally in the future.[52–55] See Chapters 2, 3, 10, 14, 50, 52, and Appendix I.

Pathophysiology

See Chapters 2, 3, 4, 5, 6, 7, 8, 9, 10, 14, 50, 52, and Appendix I.

Problem Statement.   Diagnosis of diabetes mellitus in a nonpregnant individual.

There are three subsets of the problem: (1) how to establish a diagnosis of diabetes mellitus in nonpregnant individuals (Table 12–6); (2) how to type it as NIDDM, or type 2, or as insulin-dependent diabetes mellitus (IDDM), or type 1 (Exhibit 12–4); and (3) how to identify associated problems that may be present (Exhibit 12–5). See Chapters 40 and 41 for criteria for diagnosis of gestational diabetes mellitus.

How to Establish a Diagnosis of Diabetes Mellitus in Nonpregnant Individuals

Classic IDDM usually presents with subjective and objective findings of short duration,[58,59] whereas clas-

TABLE 12–6   The Author's Recommended Criteria (1998),[48,49] for Establishing the Diagnosis of Diabetes Mellitus[a]

Nonpregnant Adults and Children	No. Measurements	
Fasting plasma glucose $\geq$ 126 mg/dL (7.0 mmol/L)	2 +	1 +
Random plasma glucose $\geq$ 200 mg/dL (11.1 mmol/L)	1	1 +
Postprandial plasma glucose $\geq$ 200 mg/dL (11.1 mmol/L)		1
Glucose tolerance test sum (fasting +1+2+3 hr) >800 mg/dL ($\geq$ 44.6 mmol/L)	2	
Glucose tolerance test 2-hr level >199 mg/dL (11.1 mmol/L) (WHO)	2	
Glucose tolerance test 2-hr level >199 mg/dL (11.1 mmo/L) + 1/2, 1, or 1 1/2 hr level >199 mg/dL (11.1 mmol/L) (NIH-DDG)	2	
Glucose tolerance test sum 601–800 mg/dL (33.5–44.6 mmol/L)	1 = High Normal	

[a] Pregnant women (gestational diabetes). See Chapters 40 and 41.

sic NIDDM is frequently asymptomatic and may have been present for 10 years or more when diagnosed.[60] Both may occur at any age, and present evidence suggests that adult-onset NIDDM progresses to IDDM at a rate of 1 to 2%/year, whereas childhood-onset NIDDM [formerly called "maturity-onset diabetes of the young" (MODY)] progresses at an even slower rate (about 10% in 17 years) to IDDM.[61]

MODY has been divided into 3 genetic defects of beta cell functions (1) chromosome 20:HNF-α (MODY 1) (2) chromosome 7, glucokinase (MODY 2) (3) chromosome 12, HNF-1 α (MODY 3). See Chapters 3 and 5.

For subjective and objective findings that may be present at the time of diagnosis or that may develop later, and for assessment of these findings, see Exhibit 12–6.

The most certain way to avoid an erroneous diagnosis of diabetes is to confine the diagnosis to those who have a FPG repeatedly $\geq$ 126 mg/dL and to those who have a GTT sum >800 mg/dL × 2 (Table 12–6). A random plasma glucose >140 mg/dL or a 2-hr plasma glucose >175 mg/dL after a mixed meal containing 100 g carbohydrate should have a follow-up FPG and/or a GTT. Those who have a "high-normal" GTT (sum 601 to 800 mg/dL) require periodic follow-up evaluation since about one in five will develop a FPG >140 mg/dL during a follow-up of 15 years.

The recommended glucose load has varied from 50 to 100 g for adults; WHO and NIH-DDG recommend 75 g. The recommended load for children is 1.75 g/kg, with a maximum of 75 g. The author has routinely used

EXHIBIT 12–4   Types of Diabetes Mellitus

Non-insulin-dependent diabetes mellitus (NIDDM, or type 2)[a–c]
  No history of diabetic ketoacidosis
  No history of hyperglycemic hyperosmolar state
  $\geq$ Ideal body weight
  Not pregnant[a]
  Fasting serum C-peptide 0.8 to 1.7 pmol/mL[56]
Insulin-dependent diabetes mellitus (IDDM, or type 1)
  Diabetic ketoacidosis
  Hyperglycemic hyperosmolar state
  History of diabetic ketoacidosis or hyperglycemic hyperosmolar state
  $\leq$ Ideal body weight and fasting plasma glucose consistently $\geq$ 126 mg/dL (7.0 mmol/L)
  Fasting serum C-peptide <0.5 pmol/mL[57]

[a] Individuals with NIDDM may become transiently insulin-dependent as a result of the stress of an acute or chronic illness (such as infection, trauma, surgery, or pregnancy (see Chapter 24), and may revert to non-insulin-dependence after the stress subsides.
[b] Over time, NIDDM (despite weight loss to level of ideal body weight) progresses to IDDM at a rate of about 1 to 2%/year.
[c] A therapeutic test that will differentiate IDDM from NIDDM can be carried out as follows: a total fast for 1 week with fluid intake of 3 L or more per day. In NIDDM, PG will fall to normal or near-normal, and carbon dioxide content will not fall below 15 mEq/L. In IDDM, plasma glucose will not fall to normal and carbon dioxide content may fall below 15 mEQ/L, necessitating insulin therapy. See Chapter 15 for details of fasting routine.

a 100 g pure glucose load for those more than 15 years old. The routine for a valid GTT is noted in Exhibit 12–7; and the variables that determine GTT outcomes are listed in Exhibit 12–8.

Assessment

How to Type Diabetes as NIDDM (Type 2) or IDDM (Type 1)

If an individual has a FPG >126 mg/dL, is above ideal body weight, is not pregnant, and is not in ketoacidosis or a hyperglycemic hyperosmolar state, it is very likely that the type of diabetes is NIDDM (type 2). If the individual is in ketoacidosis or is below ideal body weight, the type of diabetes is probably IDDM (type 1). A fasting and/or stimulated serum C-peptide measurement can help differentiate the two types (Exhibit 12–4). If the type of diabetes is still in doubt in those who are overweight, a 1-week total fast will determine whether the type is NIDDM or IDDM (Exhibit 12–4).

Identification of Other Problems Related to Diabetes:

See Exhibit 12–5.

EXHIBIT 12–5   Problems that May Be Associated with an Abnormal Glucose Tolerance Test or with Fasting Hyperglycemia

I. *Pancreatic B-cell disease* (transient diabetes in newborn, congenital absence of islets of Langerhans, viral infection, cytomegalovirus, congenital rubella, cystic fibrosis, hemochromatosis, hemosiderosis due to iron overload (repeated transfusions, excess dietary iron), pancreatic fibrosis (and calcification) due to protein-calorie malnutrition and/or cassava (?cyanide) ingestion ("diabetes of the tropics"), chronic pancreatitis (may be secondary to excess ethanol ingestion), or surgical removal, trauma, neoplasm, or bacterial or fungal infections of the pancreas,

II. *Malnutrition*
   A. Excess caloric intake leading to excess body weight and non-insulin-dependent diabetes mellitus (NIDDM). Available data indicate that >90% of those who develop diabetes are above ideal body weight at the time of diagnosis
   B. Inadequate protein and calorie intake leading to undernutrition and semistarvation
   C. Dependence on foods containing cassava (manioc, manihot, tapioca) leading to "diabetes of the tropics" (?) due to cyanide poisoning and pancreatic damage [see (I) above]

III. *Hepatic cirrhosis, chronic hepatitis, status-postportalcaval venous shunt*

IV. *Hormone excess*
   A. *Endogenous* (pheochromocytoma, glucagonoma, somatostatinoma, aldosteronoma, acromegaly, hyperthyroidism, tumors producing excess amounts of glucocorticoids, progestins, or estrogens, hypothalamic lesions)
   B. *Exogenous* [adrenocorticotropin, glucagon, cortisone, cortisol, prednisone, somatotropin, thyroid hormones, calcitonin, estrogens, medroxyprogesterone (in oral contraceptives), prolactin, epinephrine, norepinephrine]

V. *Hormone deficit* [isolated growth hormone deficiency (type 1, type 2), multitropic pituitary deficiency, Laron dwarfism, hypothalamic lesions, hypoparathyroidism with hypocalcemia]

VI. *Insulin receptor abnormalities* (congenital lipodystrophy with virilization and acanthosis nigricans, immune disorder with insulin-receptor antibody)

VII. *Drugs and other chemical agents*
   A. *Diuretics and antihypertensive agents* (thiazides, furosemide, metolazone, diazoxide, clonidine, chlorthalidone, bumetanide, clopamide, clorexolone, ethacrynic acid); hyperglycemic response may be independent of fluctuations in serum K^+
   B. *Psychoactive agents* (chlorprothixene, haloperidol, lithium carbonate, chlorpromazine, perphenezine, amitriptyline, desipramine, doxepin, imipramine, nortriptyline, marijuana)
   C. *Neurologically active agents* (phenytoin, isoproterenol, levodopa, fenoterol, propranolol)
   D. *Analgesics* (indomethacin, acetaminophen, aspirin, morphine)
   E. *Antineoplastic agents* (alloxan, L-asparaginase, streptozotocin, cyclophosphamide, megestrol acetate)
   F. *Miscellaneous* [isoniazid, nicotinic acid, carbon disulfide, cimetidine, edetic acid, ethanol, heparin, mannoheptulose, nalidixic acid, nickel chloride, niridazole, pentamidine, phenolphthalein, rodenticide (Vacor), thiabendazole]

VIII. *Genetic syndromes* (glycogen storage disease type I, acute intermittent porphyria, hyperlipidemia, hyperglycerolemia, ataxia-telangiectasia, myotonic dystrophy, Mendenhall's syndrome, lipoatrophic syndromes, optic atrophy and diabetes mellitus, diabetes insipidus with nerve deafness, muscular dystrophies, late-onset proximal myopathy, Huntington's chorea, Machado's disease, Herrmann syndrome, pseudo-Refsum's syndrome, Prader-Willi syndrome, achondroplasia, steroid-induced ocular hypertension, epiphyseal dysplasia and infantile-onset diabetes, Down's syndrome, Turner's syndrome, Klinefelter's syndrome), Wolfram's syndrome, Friedreich's Ataxia, Laurence-Moon-Biedl Syndrome, Type A Insulin Resistance, Leprechaunism

IX. *Stiff Man's Syndrome*

X. *Mody*

Follow-up

It is important to remember that, during stress (infection, and so forth), NIDDM may become transiently insulin-dependent (see Chapters 17, 18, and 24), and that even in those who attain and maintain ideal body weight, adult-onset NIDDM progresses to IDDM at a rate of about 2 to 5% per year.

Other Considerations

If an individual has subjective or objective findings of "reactive hypoglycemia," the GTT should be extended to 6 hr and the time and nature of all subjective and objective findings during the test should be recorded by the patient and other observers and compared with the plasma glucose levels. Although it was once thought that "reactive hypoglycemia" (as defined by a plasma glucose level <50 mg/dL during a GTT) may provide a hint that could lead to the early diagnosis of "diabetes,"[62] many subsequent studies have shown that this is not the case.[63,84] Many normal asymptomatic individuals attain plasma glucose levels below 50 mg/dL (some below 40 mg/dL) between 3 and 6 hr after a glucose load (Table 12–7). "Reactive hypo-

EXHIBIT 12–6   Clinical Manifestations and Assessment

I. Clinical manifestations
When initially detected, most individuals with NIDDM are asymptomatic, whereas many with IDDM are symptomatic. Findings that may be present include:

A. *Subjective*
- Polyuria
- Polydipsia
- Polyphagia
- Weakness
- Pruritus
- Dry mouth
- Leg cramps or pains
- Burning feet
- Family history of diabetes
- Large babies (more than 9 pounds)
- Complicated pregnancy (abortions, toxemia, hydramnios, or stillborns who have congenital defects or large pancreatic islets on autopsy)
- "Reactive hypoglycemia" was once thought to be a hint that could lead to a diagnosis of diabetes,[62] but this view is now assessed as being incorrect.[63] See Table 12–7.
- Vascular disease
- Impotence

B. *Objective*
Physical examination. Physical findings that may be present include:
- Above ideal body weight
- Visual abnormalities (changing visual acuity, cataracts)
- Microangiopathy (retinopathy, glomerulosclerosis)
- Arteriopathy (cerebral, coronary, peripheral)
- Hypertension
- Neuropathy (peripheral, spinal cord or roots, autonomic nervous system, cranial nerves)
- Amyotrophic lateral sclerosis
- Genitourinary abnormalities (Candida vulvovaginitis, Candida balanitis, bacterial bladder or kidney infection, renal failure, nephrotic syndrome)
- Dupuytren's contracture (usually begins as a nodular plaquelike thickening of the palmer fascia overlying the tendons on the ulnar side of the hand; flexion contracture of one or more fingers may occur)
- Xanthomatosis
- Skin abnormalities (necrobiosis lipoidica diabeticorum, granuloma annulare, alopecia, pyogenic or fungal infections)
- Foot abnormalities (dermatophytosis, onychomycosis, trophic ulcers, arterial insufficiency, gangrene)
- Periodontal disease
- Many infections, including tuberculosis and mucormycosis

C. *Laboratory findings that may lead to a diagnosis of diabetes mellitus include:*
- Random urine glucose >25 mg/dL
- Random venous plasma glucose ≥126 mg/dL (7.0mmmol/l)
- Two-hour post-100 g carbohydrate meal venous plasma glucose >175 mg/dL
- Hyperlipidemia, hyperlipoproteinemia, azotemia, hyperuricemia, and albuminuria

II. Assessment
The diagnosis of diabetes should be confirmed by the criteria listed in Table 12–6. It may be associated with one or more of the problems listed in Exhibit 12–5. These problems should be identified at the highest possible level of resolution. The diabetes should be typed, as noted in Exhibit 12–4.

---

glycemia" is now believed to be a "nondisease" physiologic response (catecholamine release, and so forth) related to metabolic homeostatic mechanisms as they shift from the "fed" to the "fasted" state. Many emotionally unstable individuals have similar symptoms not related to abnormally low levels of plasma glucose, and some overly sensitive individuals react emotionally to these physiologic changes. Their symptoms may be attributed erroneously to "reactive hypoglycemia,"[63] which is a socially acceptable diagnosis, rather than to a more likely but less socially acceptable psychiatric diagnosis, such as anxiety, hyperventilation, depression, and hysteria.

Alimentary hypoglycemia may occur in patients who have had a gastrectomy, gastroenterostomy, pyloroplasty, or vagotomy. It is characterized by subjective and objective findings of hypoglycemia 2 hr after eating.[63] Excessive secretion of insulinotropic gut factors (gastrointestinal polypeptide) has been postulated to be the underlying mechanism. Although the oral GTT is abnormal when this problem exists, the IV GTT is normal[68–71] (Fig. 12–12).

Alimentary hypoglycemia should be distinguished from the *dumping syndrome* which may also follow the surgical procedures just noted but in which subjective and objective findings occur within an hour of eating. The dumping syndrome is not associated with hypoglycemia, but is secondary to a contraction of the plasma volume due to an osmotically induced fluid shift into the gastrointestinal tract.[63,84]

The cortisone-primed GTT has resulted in many false-positive diagnoses of "diabetes" (positive equals a 2-hr plasma glucose level >160 mg/dL) and is no longer used.[32,77] The tolbutamide response test[78] is not specific, may be dangerous because of prolonged severe hypoglycemia, and should not be used as a

EXHIBIT 12–7   Routine for a Valid Glucose Tolerance Test

1. Do only on those whose fasting venous plasma glucose (FPG) level is <126 mg/dL.
   Before a glucose load is given, measure FPG. If it is >126 mg/dL, cancel the GTT.
2. Do on ambulatory outpatients only.
   Do not do on patients who are hospitalized, or on patients who have an acute or chronic illness that can affect the test.
3. Discontinue all drug therapy that can affect the test for at least 3 days prior to the test. (See Exhibit 12–5)
4. Have patient eat ≥ 300 g carbohydrate/day for 3 days prior to the test. A simple way to accomplish this objective is to add 12 slices of bread (180 g carbohydrate) to the patient's standard diet. Many diabetologists are of the opinion that a carbohydrate intake of ≥ 150 g/day for 3 days prior to the test is suffficient.
5. Fast 14 to 15 hr (from 6 P.M. of the day preceding the test to 8 to 9 A.M. of the day of the test).
6. Give 100 g orange or lemon-flavored pure glucose as 25% solution (400 mL) after establishing that the fasting venous plasma glucose level is ≤ 126 mg/dL. Have the patient drink it within 5 minutes. The first

swallow is time zero. Nausea and vomiting rarely occur. Should they occur, the test should be terminated.

7. Collect samples at 1, 2, and 3 hr. Extend the test by collecting samples at 4, 5, and 6 hr if the patient has complained of "reactive hypoglycemia." Have patient record all symptoms and an observer record all signs during the test to determine whether they coincide with the lowest observed plasma glucose level. See Table 12–7.
8. Have patient abstain from tobacco, coffee, tea, food, and alcohol during the test.
9. Have patient sit upright and quietly during the test. Slow walking is permitted, but vigorous exercise should be avoided.
10. Venous blood is preferable, collected in a gray-top tube containing fluoride and an anticoagulant so that plasma can be harvested.
11. Analyses should be done by a method specific for glucose (glucose oxidase is widely available).
12. The test should be interpreted by appropriate criteria (see Table 12–6) so that an erroneous diagnosis will not be made.

diagnostic procedure for diabetes. The mean width of the muscle capillary basement membrane is of no value in establishing the diagnosis of diabetes, but it is related both to duration of hyperglycemia and to age.[79]

A glycosylated hemoglobin (HbA_{1c}) measurement is of little value in establishing the diagnosis of diabetes, but it may be of some value in suggesting the length of time it was present before diagnosis.[80,81] Fasting and stimulated serum C-peptide[56,57] or serum insulin levels, or both, may be useful in differentiating NIDDM from IDDM (Exhibit 12–4).

It has been shown in research studies that decarboxyclase-, insulin-, and islet-cell antibodies with HLA typing can detect type 1 diabetes in a general population (see chapter 3), and that a combination of autoantibodies to insulin, GAD, and IC5 12GC/IA-2 can predict type 1 diabetes in first degree relatives. Unfortunately the high costs of currently available assays has limited their widespread use. No such tests are available for type 2 diabetes.[82,83] (See Chapter 3).

Audit

A continuing audit can familiarize physicians and other professionals with the utility of various tests

in establishing the diagnosis of diabetes and will acquaint them with prevalence, incidence, and natural history of diabetes in the population(s) with which they work.

Research Considerations

Until 1997, there was universal agreement that a fasting plasma glucose ≥ 140 mg/dL was diagnostic of diabetes mellitus. In 1998, an American Diabetes Association committee changed the fasting (8hr) plasma glucose level diagnostic for diabetes mellitus to ≥ 126 mg/dL (7mmol/L) × 2.

Whether ≥ 126 mg/dL fasting plasma glucose is the appropriate cut level is yet to be determined. Also, long-term (20-30 yr.) epidemiologic follow up studies in many different ethnic populations need to be done to determine the natural history of NIDDM and the evolution of its complications in well-designed and carefully executed prospective epidemiologic studies.

The European Epidemiology Study Group stated in November 1998 that "on the available evidence from Europe the ADA decision would appear to be very unwise."[19b]

EXHIBIT 12–8   Variables Responsible for GTT Outcomes

I. *Intraperson*
  A. Diet-prep versus no diet prep[64,65]   No diet prep may cause abnormal test
  B. Time of day for glucose load:
     1. Morning[65]
     2. Afternoon[66]   Afternoon levels frequently higher
     3. Exton-Rose 1 hr two-dose GTT[67]
  C. Effects of illness   May cause abnormal test
     1. Acute
     2. Chronic
  D. Effects of drug therapy-see Exhibit 12–4
  E. Route of glucose administration:
     1. Oral[65]
     2. IV[68-71]
  F. Effects of size of glucose load[72-74]   Levels higher with 100 g than with 50 g glucose
  G. Site of blood collection[75]   Capillary levels may be 20 to 30 mg/dL higher than venous
       levels during GTT

  H. Time of sample collection
  I. Plasma versus serum versus whole blood[7,8]   Plasma or serum ~15% higher than whole blood; whole
       blood ~14% lower than plasma or serum

  J. Sample preservation   Glucose falls from glycolysis by RBCs and WBCs if fluoride
       not added during plasma collection, or if serum not
       separated promptly and frozen
  K. Physical activity before and during test   May lower plasma glucose level
  L. Posture during test[76]   Reclining slows glucose absorption
  M. Smoking, coffee, tea, food, alcohol during test   All may elevate plasma glucose level
  N. Method of analysis:
     1. Specific for glucose (glucose oxidase or   Preferred
        hexokinase)
     2. Not specific for glucose   Avoid if possible
  O. Criteria for interpretation
     1. Cut-point for upper limit of normal should be
        high enough to avoid erroneous diagnoses (see
        Fig. 12–7)
     2. Epidemiologic research is underway to
        determine the prognostic value of GTT outcomes
        in predicting the rate of progression to fasting
        hyperglycemia and to the development of
        complications in NIDDM.[22,23]
        Presently available data suggest that the rate of
        progression from a "high-normal" GTT as shown
        in Figure 12–5 (sum of F + 1-hr + 2-hr + 3-hr
        post-100 g glucose load = 601-800 mg/dL) to a
        FPG >140 mg/dL is <2.5% per year.
  P. Age   Diabetes, especially NIDDM, much more prevalent after
       age 40 years

  Q. Sex[43]
  R. Race[43]
  S. Excess adiposity.[43] If individual's actual weight is
     141% of IBW, then 41% of weight is defined as
     excess adiposity. Excess adiposity is associated with
     up to a 20-fold increase in prevalence of diabetes.
     (In the study noted in Figure 12–5 the prevalence
     increased from 1.6% in those ≤100% IBW to 32.4%
     in those >200% IBW.)
  T. Pregnancy (see Chapter 40)
II. *Interperson*
  A. All of the above (I.A through I.T)
  B. Presence or absence of DM, especially NIDDM
  C. Family history of diabetes mellitus
  D. Antibody to B cells (IDDM)

Abbreviations: IBW, ideal body weight; RBC, red blood cell (count); WBC, white blood cell (count); other abbreviations as in text.

TABLE 12–7   Six-Hour Glucose Tolerance Tests in 43 Normal Individuals[84]

		Time in Minutes After 100 g Pure Glucose Load								
	Fasting	30	60	90	120	180	240	300	360
Mean	92	127	122	111	104	71	62	67	70
Range	78–115	81–172	78–171	52–162	74–138	40[a]–115	39[b]–101	43[c]–86	55–91
SD	±8	±22.1	±24.6	±26	±20.9	±19.6	±13.2	±9.7	±9.3

[a] At 180 min: one individual 40, one 42, one 48, and one 49 mg/dL (four <50 mg/dL).

[b] At 240 min: one individual 39, one 41, one 43, two 45, two 46, and two 48 mg/dL (nine <50 mg/dL).

[c] At 300 min: tone individual 43, one 46, and three 48 mg/dL (five <50 mg/dL).

Thus 18 of 51 normal individuals (35.3%) attained glucose level <50 mg/dL without symptoms during a 6-hr GTT.

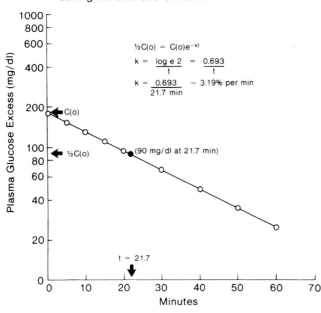

Calculation of Rate of Disappearance
of Excess Plasma Glucose
during Intravenous Glucose Tolerance Test

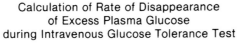

Figure 12–12. Calculation of rate of disappearance (percent per minute) of *excess plasma glucose.* C(o) = plasma glucose level 4 min after glucose injection, minus the initial fasting plasma glucose level. Four minutes was allowed for intermixing of the glucose in the plasma compartment, $\frac{1}{2}$ C(o) is one half the C(o) value, i.e., in this example, 90 mg/dL versus 180 mg/dL. The time required to reach $\frac{1}{2}$ C(o) determines K, or the rate of disappearance of glucose from the plasma in percent per minute. Rate of disappearance after 25 g glucose IV in nondiabetics was 3.00 to 4.81%/min, in mild diabetics it was 0.93 to 2.46%/min and in severe diabetics it was 0.23 to 1.64%/min.[68] Ganda and colleagues[71] noted no significant difference in the reproducibility of the oral GTT versus the IV GTT, with only about 50% of the tests in normal subjects and in the offspring of conjugal diabetic parents being considered "reproducible." (*Source*: Amatuzio DS, Stuzman FL, Vanderbilt MJ, et al.: Interpretation of the rapid intravenous glucose tolerance test in normal individuals and in mild diabetes mellitus. J Clin Invest 32:428–435, 1953. With permission.)

References

1. Willis T: Of the diabetes or pissing evil. Pharmaceutic Rationalis. London: T. Dring, C. Harper, J. Leight, 1679, Chap. 3, Part 1.

2. Bouchardat A: De la Glycosurie ou Diabèt Sucre, Vol. 2. Paris: Germer-Bailliere, 1875.

3. Allen FM: Glycosuria and Diabetes. Cambridge, MA: Harvard University Press, 1913.

4. Banting F: The history of insulin. Edin Med J 36:1–2, 1929.

5. Kadish AH, Hall D: A new method for the continuous monitoring of blood glucose by measurement of dissolved oxygen. Clin Chem 11:869–875, 1965.

6. Bank I: Der Blutzucker. Wiesbaden: 1913.

7. McDonald GW, Fisher GF, Burnham CE: Differences in glucose determinations obtained from plasma or whole blood. Pub Health Rep 79:515–521, 1964.

8. Zalme E, Knowles HC: A plea for plasma sugar. Diabetes 14:165–166, 1965.

9. Hamman L, Hirschman II: Studies on blood sugar. Arch Intern Med 20:761–808, 1917.

10. Jarney NW, Isaacson VI: A blood sugar tolerance test. JAMA 70:1131–1134, 1918.

11. Paullin JE, Sauls HC: A study of the glucose tolerance test in the obese. South Med J 15:249–253, 1922.

12. John HF: A summary of findings in 1100 glucose tolerance estimations. Endocrinology 13:388–392, 1929.

13. Mosenthal HO, Barry E: Criteria for an interpretation of normal glucose tolerance tests. Ann Intern Med 33:1175–1194, 1950.

14. Fajans.SS, Conn JW: The early recognition of diabetes mellitus. Ann NY Acad Sci 82:208–218, 1959.

15. West KM: Substantial differences in diagnostic criteria used by diabetes experts. Diabetes 24:641–644, 1975.

16. Soskin S: Use and abuse of the dextrose tolerance test. Postgrad Med 10:108–116, 1951.

17. Danowski TS, Aarons JH, Hydovita JD, et al. Utility of equivocal glucose tolerances. Diabetes 19:524–526, 1970.

18. Andres R: Aging and diabetes. Med Clin North Am 55:835–846, 1971.

19a. European Diabetes Epidemiology Study Group (EDESG): A brief account of the European Diabetes Epidemiology Study Group and its activities. Diabetologia 6:453–454, 1970.

19b. The European Diabetes Epidemiology Study Group: Epidemiological considerations related to the new diagnostic criteria. Diabetologia 41:p. 50–51, 1998.

20. Lennox WG: Repeated blood sugar curves in non-diabetic subjects. J Clin Invest 4:331–352, 1927.

21. Rushforth NB, Bennett PH, Steinberg AG, et al.: Comparison of the value of the two- and one-hour glucose levels of the oral GTT in the diagnosis of diabetes in Pima Indians. Diabetes 24:538–546, 1975.

22. Rushforth NB, Miller M, Bennett PH: Fasting and two-hour post-load glucose levels for the diagnosis of diabetes. The relationship between glucose levels and complications of diabetes in the Pima Indians. Diabetologia 16:373–379, 1979.

23. Bennett PH: Recommendations on the standardization of methods and reporting of tests for diabetes and its microvascular complications in epidemiologic studies. Diabetes Care 2:98–104, 1979.

24. Mayer KH, Stamler J, Dyer A, et al: Epidemiologic findings on the relationship of time of day and time since last meal to glucose tolerance. Diabetes 25:936–943, 1976.

25. Davidson JK, Reuben D, Sternberg JC, et al: Diabetes screening using a quantitative urine glucose method. Diabetes 27:810–816, 1978.

26. Davidson JK: Random hyperglucosuria (RHO) and diabetes mellitus (DM). Fed Proc 40:741 (abstr 2917), 1981.

27. Hayner NS, Kjelsberg MO, Epstein FH, et al: Carbohydrate tolerance and diabetes in a total community, Tecumseh, Mich. Diabetes 14:413–423, 1965.

28. Zimmet P, Whitehouse S: Bimodality in glucose tolerance—the phenomenon and its possible significance. Diabetologia 13:441, 1977.

29. Zimmet P: When is diabetes?—a new look at diagnostic criteria for diabetes mellitus. Aust NZ J Med 10:346–350, 1980.

30. Zimmet P, Whitehouse S: The effect of age on glucose tolerance: studies in a Micronesian population with a high prevalence of diabetes. Diabetes 28:617–623, 1979.

31. Davidson MB: The effect of aging on carbohydrate metabolism: a review of the English literature and a practical approach to a diagnosis of diabetes mellitus in the elderly. Metabolism 28:688–705, 1979.

32. Fajans SS, Conn JW: An approach to the prediction of diabetes mellitus by modification of the glucose tolerance test with cortisone. Diabetes 3:296–304, 1954.

33. Fajans SS, Conn JW: Tolbutamide-induced improvement in carbohydrate tolerance of young people with mild diabetes mellitus. Diabetes 9:83–88, 1960.

34. Conn JW, Fajans SS: The prediabetic state: a concept of dynamic resistance to a genetic diabetogenic influence. Am J Med 31:839–850, 1961.

35. Fajans SS: Early stages of diabetes: definitions and present concepts. In Fourth International Algarue Symposium on Diabetes (1978). New York: Plenum Press, 1979, pp. 7–11.

36. Fitzgerald MG, Keen H: Diagnosis and classification of diabetes. Br MedJ 1:1568, 1964.

37. Marble A, In Marble A, White P, Bradley RP, et al. (eds): Joslin's Diabetes Mellitus, 11th ed. Philadelphia: Lea & Febiger, 1971, pp. 202–208.

38. Siperstein MD: The glucose tolerance test: a pitfall in the diagnosis of diabetes mellitus. Adv Intern Med 20:297–323, 1975.

39. Köbberling J, Berninger D: Natural history of glucose tolerance in relatives of diabetic patients. Low prognostic value of the oral glucose tolerance test. Diabetes Care 3:21–26, 1980.

40. Jarrett RJ, Keen H: Hyperglycemia and diabetes mellitus. Lancet 2:1009–1012, 1976.

41. Sayegh HA, Jarrett RJ: Oral glucose tolerance tests and the diagnosis of diabetes. Results of a prospective study based on the Whitehall Survey. Lancet 2:431–433, 1979.

42. Jarrett RJ, McCartney P, Keen H: The Bedford Survey: ten year mortality rates in newly diagnosed diabetics, borderline diabetics and normoglycemic controls and risk indices for coronary heart disease in borderline diabetics. Diabetologia 22:79–84, 1982.

43. West K: Epidemiology of Diabetes and its Vascular Lesions. New York: Elsevier, 1978, pp. 224–274.

44. National Institutes of Health Diabetes Data Group: Classification and diagnosis of diabetes mellitus and other categories of glucose intolerance. Diabetes 28:1039–1057, 1979.

45. World Health Organization: Impaired glucose tolerance and diabetes—WHO criteria. Br Med J 281:1512–1513, 1980.

46. World Health Organization: Diabetes mellitus - Report of a WHO study group. WHO Technical Report Series, No. 727, Geneva, Switzerland, 1985.

47. Ad Hoc Committee on Diagnostic Criteria for Diabetes Mellitus, Clinical and Scientific Section, Canadian Diabetes Association: Acceptance of new criteria for diagnosis of diabetes mellitus and related conditions by the Canadian Diabetes Association. Can Med AssocJ 126:473–476, 1982.

48. Report of the Expert Committee on the Diagnosis and classification of Diabetes Mellitus: *Diabetes Care* 21: (Suppl. 1): S5-S19, 1998.

49. American Diabetes Association: Screening for Type 2 Diabetes: *Diabetes Care* 21: (Suppl. 1): S20-S22, 1998.

50. American Diabetes Association: Gestational Diabetes: *Diabetes Care* 21: (Suppl. 1): S60-S61, 1998.

51. Wilkerson HLC, Hyman H, Kaufman M, et al.: Diagnostic evaluation of glucose tolerance tests in nondiabetic subjeas after various levels of carbohydrate intake. N Engl J Med 262:1047–1053, 1960.

52. Keen H, Jarrett RJ, McCortney P: The ten-year follow-up of the Bedford survey (1962–1972): glucose tolerance and diabetes. Diabetologia 22:73–78, 1982.

53. Dwyer MS, Melton LJ, Ballard DJ, Palumbo PJ, Trautmann JC, Chu CP: Incidence of diabetic retinopathy and blindness: a population-based study in Rochester, Minnesota. Diabetes Care 8:316–322, 1985.

54. WHO Multinational Study of Vascular Disease in Diabetics: Prevalence of small vessel and large vessel disease in diabetic patients from 14 centres. Diabetologia 28:615–640, 1985.

55. Concensus Statement, American Diabetes Association: The role of cardiovascular risk factors in prevention and treatment of macrovascular disease in diabetes. Diabetes Care 12:573–579, 1989.

56. Ganey WT, Olefsky JM, Rubenstein AH, Kolterman OG: Day-long serum insulin and C-peptide profiles in patients with NIDDM: correlation with urinary C-peptide excretion. Diabetes 37:590–599,1988.

57. Maakso M, Ronnemaa T, Sarlund H, Pyorala K, Kallio V: Faaors associated with fasting and postglucagon plasma C-peptide levels in middle-aged insulin-treated diabetic patients. Diabetes Care 12:83–88, 1989.

58. Rosenbloom AL: Criteria for interpretation of oral glucose tolerance tests in children and insulin responses with normal and abnormal tolerance. Metabolism 22:301–305, 1973.

59. Rosenbloom AL, Drash A, Guthrie RV: Conference summary. Chemical diabetes in childhood. Metabolism 22:413–419, 1973.

60. Anderson TW: The duration of unrecognized diabetes mellitus. Diabetes 15:160–163, 1966.

61. Hager A: Asymptomatic diabetes in childhood and adolescence. Acta Paediatr Scand (suppl) 270:103–105, 1977.

62. Conn JW, Seltzer HS: Spontaneous hypoglycemia. Am J Med 19:460–478, 1955.

63. Hogan MJ, Service FJ: Reactive hypoglycemia. In Service FJ (ed): Hypoglycemic Disorders: Pathogenesis, Diagnosis and Treatment. Boston: G.K Hall, 1983, pp. 165–173.

64. Seltzer HS: Diagnosis of diabetes. In Ellenberg M, Rifkin H (eds): Diabetes Mellitus: Theory and Practice. New York: McGraw-Hill, 1970, pp. 436–507.

65. Committee on Statistics of the American Diabetes Association. Standardization of the oral glucose tolerance test. Diabetes 18:299–307, 1969.

66. Roberts HJ: Afternoon glucose tolerance testing: a key to the pathogenesis, early diagnosis and prognosis of diabetogenic hyperinsulinism. J Am Geriatr Soc 12:423–472, 1964.

67. Exton WG, Rose AR: The one-hour, two-dose dextrose tolerance test. Am J Clin Pathol 4:381–399, 1934.

68. Amatuzio DS, Stuzman FL, Vanderbilt MJ et al.: Interpretation of the rapid intravenous glucose tolerance test in normal individuals and in mild diabetes mellitus. J Clin Invest 32:428–435, 1953.

69. Amatuzio DS, Rames ED, Nesbitt S: Practical application of the rapid intravenous glucose tolerance test. J Lab Clin Med 48:714–720, 1956.

70. Nadon GW, Little JA, Hall WE, et al.: A comparison of the intravenous glucose tolerance test in nondiabetic and diabetic subjects. Can Med Assoc J 91:1350–1353, 1964.

71. Ganda OP, Day JL, Soeldner JS, et al.: Reproducibility and comparative analysis of repeated intravenous and oral glucose tolerance tests. Diabetes 27:715–725, 1978.

72. Sisk CW, Burnham CE, Stewart J, et al.: Comparison of the 50 and 100 gram oral glucose tolerance test. Diabetes 19:852–862, 1970.

73. Chandalia HB, Boshell BR: Diagnosis of diabetes. The size and nature of carbohydrate load. Diabetes 19:863–869, 1970.

74. van's Laar A: Comparison of the 50 and 100 gram oral glucose tolerance test in patients with borderline glucose tolerance. Diabetologia 8:71 (abstract), 1972.

75. Burgi W: Oral glucose tolerance test: significant differences between capillary and venous tolerance cunes. Schweiz Med Wochenschr 104:1698–1699, 1974.

76. Lewis RA, Said D: Influence of posture on oral glucose tolerance test. In Demole M (ed): Medicine et Hygiene. Proc 4th Congr Int Diab Fed. Geneva: Vol. 1, pp. 231, 1961.

77. Fajans SS, Conn JN: Comments on the cortisone-glucose tolerance test. Diabetes 10:63–67, 1961.

78. Unger RH, Madison LL: A new diagnostic procedure for mild diabetes mellitus. Evaluation of an intravenous tolbutamide response test. Diabetes 7:455–461, 1958.

79. Williamson JR, Kilo C: Current status of capillary basement membrane disease in diabetes mellitus. Diabetes 26:65–72, 1977.

80. Dunn PJ, Cole RA, Soeldner JS, et al.: Reproducibility of hemoglobin A_{1c} and sensitivity to various degrees of glucose intolerance. Ann Intern Med 91:390–396, 1979.

81. Engelgau MM, Thompson TJ, Herman WH, Boyle JP, Aubert RE, Kenny SJ, Badran A, Sous ES, Ali MA: Comparison of fasting and 2-hour glucose HbA_{1c} levels for diagnosing diabetes: diagnostic criteria and performance revisited. *Diabetes Care* 20:785–791, 1997.

82. Hagopian WA, Santeevi CB, Landin-Olsson M, Karlsenae, Sundkvist G, Palmer J, Lernmark A: Glutamate Decarboxylase-, Insulin-, and Islet Cell-Antibodies and HLA Typing to Detect Diabetes in a General Population Based Study of Swedish Children. *J Clin. Ivest* 95:1505–1511, 1995.

83. Verge CF, Gianani R, Kawasaki IE, Chase H, Eisenbarth GS: Prediction of Type 1 Diabetes in First Degree Relatives using a Combination of Insulin, GAD, and IC5 12bc/IA-2 Autoantibodies. *Diabetes*: 926–933, 1996.

84. Hypoglycemic Disorders. *In* Service, JF (ed): Endocrinology and metabolism clinics. W.B. Saunders, Philadelphia, 1999.

13

Methodology of Measuring Glucose, Glycated Serum Proteins and Hemoglobin, and Lipids And Lipoproteins

Gerald R. Cooper, Richard E. Mullins, Gary L. Myers, and Eric J. Sampson

Energy generated by an individual originates from ingested carbohydrates, lipids, and proteins. As a practical matter, most rapidly a.vailable energy is considered to come from carbohydrates, and most long-term energy from lipids. Glucose is formed mainly after the digestion of carbohydrates, and with the help of insulin, it is burned for fuel. Excess ingested glucose is automatically transferred to the liver or body fat and stored until it is needed. Triglyceride (TG) in serum lipoproteins and in stored fat is metabolized to generate energy over extended periods and to some extent is converted to glucose to give an endogenous source of fuel. In people with diabetes, whose insulin is deficient or ineffective, glucose is not used conventionally as fuel; it remains unused, builds up in concentration, and often affects the concentration and metabolism of lipids and lipoproteins. It is helpful therefore to determine and follow glucose levels in persons with suspected or known diabetes. It is also helpful to follow the TG levels of these people because the TG level of people with diabetes also tends to be elevated. A better understanding of metabolic and other disease risk factors is gained if these basic glucose and TG determinations are supplemented with measurements of related glycosylated hemoglobin, glycated serum proteins, and lipoproteins (see Chapters 23 and 39). This chapter presents basic analytic principles, desirable preanalytic conditions, and interpretation guidelines for the major clinically useful laboratory diagnostic procedures for diabetes. It also contains a discussion of how accurate these procedures are in identifying cases of diabetes.

Glucose Methodology

Historical Perspective

For over 100 years, various methods have been used to measure glucose in biological fluids, but the search for more specific, sensitive, and simple methods continues because of the ongoing need to investigate the cause(s) of diabetes and how to control it. When the second edition of this book was published, oxidation-reduction procedures were the described methods of measuring glucose,[1] but now enzymatic methods are preferred.

The enzymatic methods in which glucose oxidase and hexokinase are used are now considered the most accurate, precise, and easy-to-perform methods by which clinical and research laboratories can measure glucose. In the first enzymatic method, yeast was used to ferment glucose in biological fluids, and the differences between reducing sugars were measured before and after fermentation. On the basis of Miller's discovery in 1928[2] that glucose oxidase reacted in a specific manner with D-glucose, Keilin and Hartree[2] in 1948 applied the oxidation of glucose by glucose oxidase to the manometric determination of glucose in biological fluids. The current photometric measurement was made possible by coupling the glucose oxidase enzyme with another enzyme that catalyzes the reaction of hydrogen peroxide with a chromogenic oxygen receptor.[3] With this method, special equipment is used to measure the glucose oxidase reaction in a polarographic oxygen electrode, and paper strips impregnated by glucose oxidase reagents are used to measure glucose in blood, serum, and urine. An evaluated selected glucose oxidase method was published by Fales in 1963.[4]

In 1965, Stein coupled the hexokinase enzyme with glucose-6-phosphate dehydrogenase to measure glucose.[5] Reported successful applications of this method to the analysis of glucose in body fluids led to its publication by Neese[6] as a practical direct method and by Neese and coworkers as a proposed reference method.[7] In 1973, Cooper[8] compared the analytic problems and interferences arising from representative enzymatic and colorimetric glucose methods, and in 1977, Passey[9] compared the results obtained by the two analytic techniques.

Sampling

The analytic results are only as valid as the specimen used for analysis. Proper patient preparation is needed to control patients' physiological variables. Because food intake influences blood glucose levels, most patients are asked to follow their usual diets for several days before the blood specimen is collected. Information about medications must be obtained to determine if interferences are likely in the specimen. The sample must be processed in a suitable manner for the analytic method being used. The specimen's identification must be maintained without any transcription errors from the time the specimen is collected to the time the results are reported. The National Committee for Clinical Laboratory Standards has published standard procedures for collecting blood.[10]

Blood specimens are collected under defined conditions and at set times while the patient is either fasting or on a tolerance test schedule. Urine specimens may be collected at any time, but the time should be noted. Because bacterial contamination of samples rapidly affects glucose levels, all collection equipment must be sterile or chemically clean, and aseptic techniques must be used in collecting and processing samples for analysis. Hemolysis of the specimen is to be avoided.

Fasting whole blood specimens usually are drawn 12 to 14 hr after a patient's overnight fast. The patient should not smoke tobacco before the glucose sampling because this can affect the outcome of the test. Drinking small amounts of water does not adversely affect the test results. The fasting specimen is most conveniently collected in the morning before the patient eats or drinks anything. The proper collection of fasting serum or plasma specimens has become quite important because the increased specificity and sensitivity of glucose analytic measurements now permits the clinical interpretation of even small differences in glucose levels.

Preferably, the glucose tolerance test should be performed only on noninstitutionalized patients engaged in their normal day-to-day activities. For 3 days before the test, the patient should eat about 300 g carbohydrates and up to 2, 500 calories/day. The test is usually performed in the morning after the patient has fasted overnight. After blood and urine specimens are collected, the patient is given a known quantity, such as 100 g of glucose in 400 mL of cold, flavored water. Blood is collected at precisely set intervals, such as 0.5, 1, 2, 3, and occasionally 4 and 5 hr. The patient must not eat or drink anything or smoke tobacco during the test.

In a practical tolerance test that is widely used, a 2-hr postprandial glucose level is measured. The patient is asked to eat a breakfast consisting of approximately 100 g carbohydrates, 30 g protein, and 30 g fat. The blood specimen is collected 2-hr after the meal is finished. An alternate technique of giving the glucose challenge is to have the fasting patient drink 50 g of glucose in 200 mL of flavored water over a period not exceeding 10 min. The blood specimen is collected 2 hr after the patient finishes the drink.

For the evaluation of suspected reactive hypoglycemia, the mixed-meal challenge is preferred over the usual glucose solution challenge, and the patient should be tested 5 hr after eating.[11]

A whole blood specimen may be analyzed as a whole blood sample, but preferably it is processed to provide serum or plasma samples for analysis; urine specimens can be analyzed directly.

Whole Blood

Whole blood samples are seldom used for analysis, but when they are, they are collected either in the disodium salt of ethylenediaminetetraacetic acid (EDTA) and analyzed immediately or in a tube containing a glycolytic enzyme inhibitor, such as sodium fluoride, if analysis is expected to be delayed. Whole blood samples are susceptible to contamination, and they have a larger variation in sample measurement than other types of specimens. It is extremely important to mix the sample thoroughly, but gently, just before the assay. Anticoagulants and preservatives must not be used in concentrations high enough to affect the analytic procedures. Glucose values are usually about 15% lower in whole blood than they are in serum or plasma.[12]

Serum

Whenever practical, serum is the sample of choice for measuring glucose. An effort should be made to separate the clot as soon as possible and to obtain nonhemolyzed serum. Freshly drawn whole blood collected in a sterile dry tube is permitted to clot, a process that normally requires 15 to 25 min at room temperature. The serum should be separated from the clot of blood cells within 30 min.

Plasma

Plasma is obtained by centrifugation of anticoagulated whole blood. The main difference between serum and plasma is that plasma contains fibrinogen, which the anticoagulants do not allow to form a fibrin clot. Plasma has at least two advantages over serum: no delay is necessary to obtain plasma by centrifugation of whole blood, and more plasma than serum can be obtained from a given volume of whole blood. Many anticoagulants and combinations of anticoagulants are used by clinical laboratories, but problems arise from some. For instance, sodium fluoride in concentrations above 7.5 mg/mL increases the tendency of blood to undergo hemolysis and affects the results of some glucose oxidase procedures.

Urine

Urine glucose analysis, either qualitative or quantitative, is usually done on a random specimen, unless the analysis is done with a glucose tolerance test. Preferably, the urine specimen should be analyzed within 30 min after it is voided. If this is not possible, the specimen can be refrigerated (at about 2°C) for up to 12 hr or frozen for up to 1 week, without harm. Repeated freezing and thawing should be avoided.

Sampling Errors

Because errors can be caused by lack of information about sampling, results must be interpreted with care. Phlebotomy sites, interferences, and bacterial contamination can affect the analytic results. Venous and capillary blood samples should be distinguished and not used interchangeably because these two types of specimens have different values. Serum and plasma specimens should not be called blood samples in reports or publications, because "normal" glucose levels in whole blood are different from those in serum and plasma. Care must be taken to minimize hemolysis and the time that the serum or plasma is in contact with blood cells because glycolysis (the utilization of glucose by enzymes in the blood cells) increases while the serum or plasma remains in contact with cells of decreasing viability. Serum or plasma should not be stored at refrigerator temperatures longer than 3 days. When specimens are to be stored for longer periods, they should be placed in containers slightly larger than volume of the sample, the containers should be sealed tightly, and the specimens frozen. Bacterial contamination, particularly, can cause loss of glucose during storage.

Analytic Methods

The basic analytic methods for determining the amount of glucose in whole blood, serum, plasma, or urine involve enzymatic, colorimetric condensation, and colorimetric oxidation-reduction reactions.[8] The enzymatic methods, in which either glucose oxidase, glucose dehydrogenase, or hexokinase reagents are used, have replaced the other methods both as routine methods and as reference methods in clinical chemistry laboratories. The enzymatic methods have been used extensively for home glucose testing. Different enzymatic procedures have various advantages and disadvantages; some are more appropriate for use in clinical laboratories, some for use in physician offices, and some for self-monitoring in the home.

Glucose Oxidase

The enzyme glucose oxidase (EC 1.1.3.4) converts D-glucose into gluconic acid and hydrogen peroxide (H_2O_2).[4] The H_2O_2 is broken down in the presence of a chromogenic O_2 receptor by peroxidase (EC 1.11.1.7), yielding a chromogen whose color intensity is proportional to the amount of original glucose in the sample. False-positive results may be obtained if oxidizing agents other than H_2O_2 are in the sample and can react in the peroxidase system upon chromogens such as O-dianisidine. Body fluids without prior protein precipitation may give false high values. Chlorine in tap water can also cause a false positive. False results may occur if reducing agents other than O-dianisidine can compete in the peroxidase system, if substances exist in the sample that can reduce the colored oxidized chromogen, or if certain enzymes such as catalase or mutarotase contaminate the glucose oxidase reagent. Glucose oxidase levels can be decreased by elevated levels of reducing agents such as uric acid, ascorbic acid, glutathione, cysteine, bilirubin, thymol, and catechols in serum or urine. In urine, elevated levels of uric acid markedly inhibit the enzyme reaction, whereas only large therapeutic doses of ascorbic acid produce levels sufficient to inhibit the enzyme reaction. Some anticoagulants and preservatives, such as sodium fluoride and thymol, inhibit the reaction of enzymes; therefore, such additives must be removed or decreased to a compatible concentration in the preparation of a protein-free filtrate.

Hexokinse

The enzymes hexokinase (EC 2.7.1.1; adenosine triphosphate [ATP]: D-hexose-6-phosphotransferase) and glucose-6-phosphate dehydrogenase (EC 1.1.149; D-glucose-6-phosphate: NAA $[P]^+$ oxidoreductase) are coupled to accomplish phosphorylation, catalytic dehydrogenation, and hydrolysis to form 6-phosphogluconic acid from D-glucose. Hexokinase in the presence of ATP and Mg^{2+} reacts with glucose to form glucose-6-phosphate adenosine diphosphate (ADP).[6] The glucose-6-phosphate dehydrogenase in the presence of NADP reacts with glucose-6-phosphate to form 6-phosphoglucolactose, nicotinamide-adenine dinucleotide phosphate hydrogenase (NADPH), and H^+. For each mole of glucose reduced, one mole of NADPH is formed that can be measured spectrophotometrically. When this procedure is used as a direct method, in lieu of deproteinization, a specimen blank is used to correct for interfering substances. This method is especially suitable for small laboratories, even though the reagents are expensive, because it is simple, it requires small sample and reagent volumes, and it can be used with urine specimens as well as blood specimens.

Whole blood samples should be deproteinized as soon as possible to prevent the effects of hemolysis. The deproteinized filtrate should be stored at refrigerator temperatures to prevent hydrolysis of polysaccharides. Lipemic and icteric samples should be corrected by a serum blank. Fructose and mannose act as interfering materials in samples because they can be converted to glucose-6-phosphate. Invertase must be absent if sucrose is in the sample. At the usual concentrations, the common blood anticoagulants heparin, fluoride, oxalate, and EDTA exert no interfering actions; likewise, ascorbic acid and uric acid cause no interference. The hexokinase method is affected by increased background ultraviolet absorption of the sample and the inhibitory effect of another hexose, especially fructose.

Glucose Dehydrogenase (B–D Glucose: NAD-Oxidoreductase EC 1.1.1.47)

This enymatic method is mentioned because it has great potential as a routine glucose method. It is a one-step method based on the glucose dehydrogenase reaction with D-glucose and NAD to form D-gluconolactone and NADH and H[+]. It can be used either as an endpoint or a kinetic procedure, with or without deproteinization, and it can be adapted easily for use with automated instrumentation. Results obtained by this method with deproteinization are similar to those obtained by the hexokinase method.[13]

Accuracy Base for Glucose Measurements

The accuracy base for glucose measurements includes Standard Reference Material (SRM917), (D-glucose of 99.9% purity), from the National Institute of Standards and Technology (NIST),[14] an American Association for Clinical Chemistry-Center for Disease Control and Prevention (AACC)(CDC) hexokinase reference method,[7] a NIST definitive method based on isotope dilution-mass spectrometry,[15] and NIST SRM 909, (a freeze-dried human serum standard reference material).[14] To confirm that the method being compared with the reference or designated comparison method has acceptable traceability, users of the method should follow an evaluation protocol for method comparision and bias estimation that includes use of patient samples.[16]

Two other definitive methods have been proposed in an effort to simplify steps in the analytic procedure. One uses mass spectrometric measurements of the methyloxine trimethysilyl derivative of glucose.[17] The other uses isotope dilution-mass spectrometry with [13]C[6] glucose as the internal standard.[18] Both methods

have a precision in the range of 0.3 to 0.6%, which is similar to the glucose precision range of the NIST definitive method.

The hexokinase procedure has become the method most widely accepted as the international and national glucose reference method.[7] This coupled hexokinase and glucose-6-phosphate dehydrogenase procedure was subjected to studies on optimization of reaction conditions, the evaluation of candidate hexokinase modified approaches, interferences, and transferability testing at the CDC. The studies were sponsored by the Glucose Subcommittee of the Standard Committee, American Association for Clinical Chemistry. Linearity was observed to a glucose concentration of 6.00 g/L or 33.3 mmol/L. Standard deviations in results obtained by the hexokinase method were as low as less than 0.02 g/L (or 2 mg/dL). The average recovery for modified hexokinase methods ranged from 99.3 to 100.5%. Of 19 substances suspected of interference, only maltose, glucose-1-phosphate, fructose, fructose-6-phosphate, and glutathione showed a determinable effect on any of the hexokinase techniques. Glutathione is essentially confined to erythrocytes, which are removed to form serum or plasma as a sample for measurement. The addition of hemolysate to serum, to a hemoglobin level of 200 mg/dL, had no measurable influence on the results of the hexokinase method. Deproteinization was desirable, as was confirming that phosphoglucose insomerase did not contaminate the reagent enzymes.

Detection and Monitoring of Diabetis Mellitus

Community Screening Program

Screening programs for diabetes are conducted to identify individuals in the early stage of diabetes, particularly people without symptoms. Members of high-risk groups, such as people with a family history of diabetes, obese people, people with impaired glucose tolerance, people with hypertension or hyperlipidemia, and people more than 40 years old are encouraged to have their serum glucose levels monitored regularly.[19] The screening test is a fasting serum or plasma glucose test. Participants in screening found to have a plasma glucose level above 126 mg/dL should be referred for diagnostic evaluation. If participants have ingested food or drink other than water within 3 hr before the testing, a random plasma glucose level above 160 mg/dL is considered a positive result. Pregnant women with a positive community screening result for blood glucose, should be referred to a physician for an oral glucose tolerance test. Personnel conducting community screening programs must be properly trained and must demonstrate that they are able to perform the testing procedure.[19]

Testing at Hospital Bedsides and in Physician's Offices

Glucose monitoring at hospital bedsides or in physician offices, is useful primarily for managing of the diabetic patients and not for diagnosing diabetes. This monitoring procedure is usually performed by nurses who must be well-trained. Glucose monitoring at hospital bedsides or in physician offices requires a clearly written procedure manual, effective quality-control directions, a maintenance schedule for the instruments, and medical personnel who are competent to perform the testing. A study involving 187 hospitals with 4517 test comparisons showed that 75% of capillary samples tested with bedside glucose meters had values within 15% of simultaneously drawn venous samples tested in the hospital's laboratory.[20]

Evaluations have indicated that it is difficult for nurses, physicians, and other non-laboratory healthcare professionals to obtain and maintain the skills necessary to properly operate and maintain the portable glucose analyzers.[21] A small community hospital that used a glucometer on the nursing floor and the Hitachi 705 in the central laboratory, had yearly correlation coefficients of 0.85, 0.70, and 0.84 for values obtained by the two instruments over three consecutive years.[22] Because of the relatively high cost of training nurses in the procedure and maintaining nursing staff competency, the hospital decided to assign responsibility for bedside glucose testing to 11 phlebotomists, with 12 medical technologists serving as backups. After initiation of this plan, the correlation coefficients for two quarters rose substantially to 0.96 and 0.97.[22]

The National Committee for Laboratory Standards has prepared a guideline for method comparison and bias estimation for analyses of patient samples.[16]

Glucose Self-Monitoring at Home

The majority of out-of-laboratory glucose testing is done at home by patients with diabetes.[23] Of 171 diabetics using self-monitoring, 50% used incorrect techniques and produced results differing more than 10% from laboratory values.[23] Immediately following re-education, all performed adequately, but about 6 weeks later about 40% demonstrated unsatisfactory performance. The most common self-monitoring errors include inexact timing, incorrect sampling, improper hand cleaning, improper wiping, and use of outdated or incorrect strips. These findings have serious implications, because physicians and nurses depend on patient-generated data when changing medication and hypoglycemia prevention regimens.[23]

The American Diabetes Association has published recommendations related to quality assurance for home glucose self-monitoring.[24]

Glucose self-monitoring systems are based on a glucose oxidase colorimetric reaction that occurs when a drop of blood is added to a reagent strip. The developed color can be read visually or by a reflectance meter.

A conference sponsored by the American Diabetes Association reviewed the epidemiological, clinical, and laboratory aspects of self-monitoring of blood glucose.[24] Overall, 33% of patients with diabetes self-monitored their blood glucose. Intervention programs increased the proportion of people with diabetes who self-monitored. Intensive therapy programs for insulin-deficient patients depend on the blood glucose levels of patients being measured at least four times a day. A lesser frequency of testing may suffice for most patients with non-insulin dependent diabetes mellitus, and for most other patients once their therapy is optimized and glycemic control has stabilized. Therapy regimens are designed to prevent hypoglycemia and severe hyperglycemia. The performance goal of all current self-monitoring glucose systems should be to achieve total errors of less than 10%. The goal for the future should be to make self-monitoring glucose systems with an analytic error of ±5%.[24] To minimize lack of competency among people using these systems, manufacturers are encouraged to continue efforts to make fail-safe analytic systems (see Chapter 22).

Patients with diabetes are encouraged to monitor their glucose levels at home, especially to prevent and control hypoglycemia and gestational diabetes. Tighter metabolic control delays the development and progression of retinopathy, nephropathy, and neuropathy in patients with insulin-dependent diabetes mellitus, but it often is associated with increased frequency of treatment-induced hypoglycemia.[25] Glucagon and epinephrine counter-regulatory systems are usually activated at a glycemic threshold of about 68 mg/dL (3.8 mmol/L). This threshold is above the threshold both for symptoms of hypoglycemia of about (54 mg/dL [3.0 mmol/L]), for symptoms of cognitive dysfunction about (49 mg/dL [2.7 mmol/L]).[25]

Patients with glucose levels as high as 70 mg/dL (3.9 mmol/L) or even slightly higher, may need to eat more frequently, change their insulin dose, or control the amount (more or less depending on each patient's need) of exercise they do.[25] A study of the accuracy of plasma glucose measurements in the hypoglycemic range found that two portable glucose analyzers were capable of precise measurements; however, their results had a negative mean bias when compared with results from the reference hexokinase method of 7.5 and 3.3% for sera with a mean concentration near 50 mg/dL (2.8 mmol/L).[26] In a day-to-day precision study, a portable machine produced results with a CV of 5.2% when analyzing serum with glucose levels about 70 mg/dL (3.9 mmol/L), and a CV of 5.4 when analyzing serum with a glucose concentration of about 39 mg/dL (2.2 mmol/L). Results of analyses by the hexokinase method had a CV of 1.5% for serum with a mean glucose level of 85 mg/dL (4.7 mmol/L). Any interpretation of glucose measurements in the hypoglycemic range should account for methodological differences.[26]

Because any child of a woman with gestational diabetes is at significant risk for fetal macrosomia and other neonatal morbidities, all women should be monitored for onset of carbohydrate intolerance during pregnancy.[27] Pregnant women who have not been identified as having glucose intolerance before the 24th week of pregnancy should have a screening test with 50 g of oral glucose solution, usually while not fasting. Anyone with a value greater than 7.8 mmol/L (140 mg/dL) on the screening test, should be followed up with a diagnostic glucose tolerance test, for which a positive test result requires that two or more of the venous plasma glucose concentrations from a fasting subject exceed 5.8 mmol/L (105 mg/dL), that a 1-hr value exceeds 10.6 mmol/L (190 mg/dL), that a 2-hr value exceeds 9.2 mmol/L (165 mg/dL) or that a 3-hr test exceeds 8.1 mmol/L (145 mg/dL).[27]

Pregnant women whose self-monitored fasting glucose plasma levels exceeded 5.8 mmol/L (105 mg/dL) or whose postpostprandial levels exceeded 6.7 mmol/L (120 mg/dL) are at greater risk of having a child born dead or one who dies shortly after birth than are mothers with lower plasma glucose levels.[27] In one study a 75 g, 2-hr single-value glucose tolerance test was as effective as the standard 100-g, 3-hr multiple value oral tolerance test in detecting pregnant women who will have adverse pregnancy outcomes.[28] Fasting and nonfasting 50-g, 1-hr oral glucose levels in women with gestational diabetes averaged 10.5 mmol/L (189 mg/dL) and 11.0 mmol/L (198 mg/dL), respectively, whereas women without diabetes had levels of 7.8 mmol/L (140 mg/dL) and 6.7 mmol/L (120 mg/dL).[28]

Portable Glucose Instruments

Portable instruments for glucose measurement mostly measure reflectance absorbance or make amperometric measurements of capillary glucose levels. The portable instruments are usually designed to provide the same results as those obtained from venous plasma samples rather than the 15% lower glucose levels typically measured in whole blood. Enzymatic reagents contain either glucose oxidase, hexokinase, or glucose dehydrogenase for the chemical reaction with serum glucose.[26] Portable instruments for glucose testing are used mainly for bedside testing by nurses in a hospital setting, for home testing conducted by patients under living conditions, and for office testing conducted by the staff of a physician or a clinic.

In an accuracy evaluation of bedside glucose monitoring in 181 institutions, the College of American Pathologists gathered 4517 quality-control results, and found that approximately 58% of the bedside results were within 10% and that 78% were within 15% of the corresponding clinical laboratory result.[20] Precision expressed as CV was less than 10% in 90% of 15,950 quality-control results reported by 569 institutions,[20] three whole-blood meters used to test samples with a wide range of hematocrit and glucose values produced readings that exceeded the 15% maximum acceptable error for 35, 27, and 43% of the samples. Only about 25% of the measurements of these instruments fell within 5% of the measurement obtained by the designated comparison method, and each instrument exhibited a different bias with hematocrit.[29] Trained technologists found that three of five glucose meters demonstrated less than acceptable ±15% accuracy and ±10% CV precision and that only two of five produced acceptable results when operated by patients at home.[30] A glucose oxidase method that measures electron flow produced results of linearity with a mean bias of −0.044 mmol/dL (0.8 mg/dL) and bias of 0.327 mmol/L (6.5 mg/dL) and a CV of from 3 to 6%.[31]

An evaluation of five portable glucose meters found one was technically superior but had no data management capabilities, one had a high variance and low bias, one showed bias affected by hematocrit and glucose concentration, one had a negative hematocrit bias and limited linear range, and one showed greater imprecision in the low glucose range and a correlation that varied with capillary, venous or arterial blood.[32] This led to the recommendation that the clinicians should consider the limitations of the meter they use when interpreting results obtained with portable glucose monitors.[32] A glucose dehydrogenase reaction with hemolyzed blood that uses dual-wavelength photometric measurement decreased the effect of hematocrit and was found applicable in neonatal intensive care units.[33] Certain glucose monitors exhibit a biased positive mean error when the measurement is performed within 4 hr of when the patient last ate.[34] Novel multiple-analyte portable simultaneous assays including glucose assays based on the glucose oxidase method (in which measurements are made amperometrically) and assays that use biosensors that are thin-film electrodes micro fabricated on silicon chips are now proving to be less dependent on operator skill.[35]

The Concensus Development Conference on Self-Monitoring of Blood Glucose recommends that the goal of device manufacturers should be to make future portable glucose monitors capable of producing results with an analytic error of ≤5%.[24]

Comparison of Glucose Test Results Produced by Various Methods Used in Clinical Laboratories

To compare the glucose test results produced by various methods we examined results of studies on reference materials and specimens from observed populations (normal and abnormal values). One study evaluated the precison of 10 methods, with the hexokinase method serving as the reference method.[9] The 10 methods examined generally produced results with <3.0 mg/dL within-run standard deviation for samples in the normal range and 6.0 mg/dL for samples in the abnormal range. The automated glucose-oxidase oxygen-rate method generally produced results with smaller standard deviations than did the other methods (see Chapters 11 and 12). For measurements of reconstituted lyophilized control serum, results by the hexokinase reference method had the smallest standard deviation. Results of assays on 185 to 263 patient samples were used to compare standard deviation, y-intercept, slope, and bias of means. A bias >5 mg/dL from the manual hexokinase reference method was noted when the neocuproine, glucose oxidase, and alkaline ferricyanide methods were used. Y-intercepts >5 mg/L were observed when the *o*-toluidine, neocuproine, and alkaline ferricyanide methods were used.

The glucose concentration range of plasma specimens collected from 64 fasting "normal" donors (33 males, 31 females; 8 to 62 years old) by the proposed hexokinase reference method was 70 to 105 mg/dL.[6] A similar range of "normal" values has also been observed with most glucose oxidase methods. Slightly higher ranges are generally found for observed populations when other than enzymatic methods are used.

Methodology of Glycated Serum Protein and Glycated Hemoglobin Measurements

Historical Perspective

Fructosamine is the general name for the stable, rearranged product of glucose and a protein amino group. However, in the recent literature this name has been reserved for glycated serum proteins. Glycated hemoglobin is referred to either as HbA1c, indicating that hemoglobin has been glycated on the *N*-terminal valine of the b-chain, or as glycohemoglobin (Ghb), indicating that the hemoglobin molecule has been glycated at any of several possible lysine *e*-amino sites.

A minor component of hemoglobin with fast chromatographic mobility was first reported in 1958 by Schroeder and coworkers.[36] This component was called

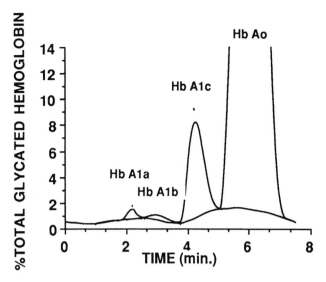

Figure 13–1. Chromatographic elution pattern of HPLC hemoglobins from HPLC ion-exchange column (Bio-Rex 70). Eluate was monitored at 414 nm.

HbA1c for its position in ion-exchange chromatographic elution patterns as seen in Figure 13–1. It was found to be a normal and constant component of red blood cells and accounted for 5 to 7% of the hemoglobin. It was not until 10 years later that Rahbar[37] and Trivelli et al.,[38] independently reported that erythrocytes from people with diabetes contained elevated quantities of HbA1c. Shortly thereafter Brookchin and Gallop[39] identified HbA1c as the addition product of a hexose to the *N*-terminal valine of the b-chain of hemoglobin. Koenig and Cerami[40] discovered that a protein similar to HbA1c appeared in increased amounts in the blood of mice after the onset of diabetes and noted that the modification appeared to be post-translational. It was subsequently discovered that many proteins, including albumin and other serum proteins, undergo analogous nonenzymic glycation reactions.

The reaction of reducing sugars with amino acids has been known as the "Maillard reaction" or the "Browning reaction" since the report in 1912 by L.C. Maillard.[41] The same multistep process is responsible for the formation of nonenzymically glycated proteins. Figure 13–2 illustrates the steps in this process, which involves the condensation of an unprotonated amino group (from a protein) with the aldehyde group of a reducing sugar. The products of this first step are a Schiffbase and one molecule of water. The Schiffbase is unstable and most of it decomposes to the original reactants (protein and sugar). However, a small portion of the Schiffbase undergoes an Amadori rearrangement to form a stable ketoamine.[42]

The Maillard reaction continues past the stages in Figure 13–2 to produce glucose-derived cross-links between proteins. These products are known to accumulate with age in long-term proteins (collagen,

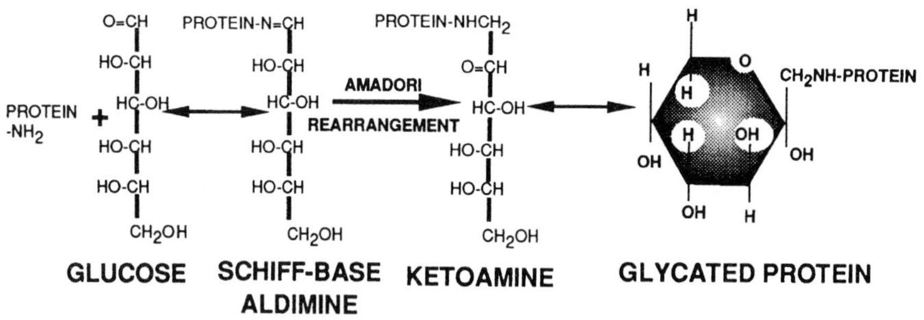

Figure 13–2. Multistep reaction of glucose aldehyde group with protein amino group to form intermediate Schiffbase, followed by Amadori rearrangement to form stable ketoamine.

glomerular basement membrane, and lens crystallins). The appearence of these advanced Amadori rearrangement products has been shown to be related to the aging process and the complications of chronic diabetes.[43–48]

At least three factors contribute to the degree of glycation of a specific protein. The first is the duration of the reaction. The longer the reaction is allowed to proceed, the more product will be formed. Thus proteins such as collagen and crystallins with half-lives of years will become more glycated than hemoglobin (half-life of 120 days),[49] albumin (half-life of 20 days), or transferrin (half-life of 8 days). The second factor is the number of potential glycation sites in a particular protein. Glycation sites are primarily the N-terminal amino group of the protein chain and the e-amino group of lysine. The third factor is the concentration of the product (glycated protein), which is related to the concentration of the reactants (glucose and the available amino group of the protein).

Methods of Analysis for Glycohemoglobin and Glycated Serum Proteins

Ion-Exchange Chromatography (HbA1c)

Different assay techniques make use of structural changes and properties introduced into the molecule on glycation. The reaction results in the slight alteration of the pI of the protein when an amino group is glycated.[50] Because of the different pKa of a-amino and e-amino groups, only glycation of the a-amino valine on HbA results in a charge difference at the pH of most assays. At physiological pH, HbA1c is less positively charged than HbA. Glycation at a lysine also produces a slight pI change; however, at the pH of analysis of the glycated proteins (near neutrality), both the reacted and unreacted amino groups possess a positive charge. Therefore, methods that depend on the charge difference between glycated and native proteins may, depending on the pH of analysis, quantitate only proteins glycated at the a-amino site. Proteins glycated at e-amino groups

are included in the not glycated fraction. Methods relying on this property of glycation are electrophoresis, ion-exchange chromatography, and isoelectric focusing.

Hemoglobin is unusual in that the primary glycation site is the N-terminal (a-amino group). The primary glycation site of other proteins is an e-amino group. For this reason, there are few assay procedures for measuring glycated serum proteins by ion-exchange or electrophoresis and many procedures for quantitating glycated hemoglobin by these methods.

The original method for quantitating HbA1c involved the use of ion-exchange chromatography. A modfied version of this method by Trivelli et al.[38] serves as the reference method. The method requires a 24-hr analysis time and is unsuited for use in the clinical laboratory. Ion-exchange methods in general are temperature dependent. In the analysis of HbA1c, each 1°C above 23°C increases the HbA1c by 1%.[51]

In attempting to make ion-exchange chromatography usable in the clinical laboratory, analysts use many procedures that measure "fast hemoglobins" as a group. These include HbAI in total, Schiffbase and labile HbA1c, as well as HbF. Because there is a rapid equilibration between blood glucose and hemoglobin in the first step of the glycation reaction (Fig. 13–2), Schiffbase concentrations fluctuate almost as rapidly as blood sugar concentrations. Therefore, care must be taken to eliminate the labile fraction of glycated hemoglobin before analysis, and several methods have been reported to do this.[52–55] However, simple incubation of the hemolysate at 37°C and a pH 5 to 6, for 30 min prior to analysis promotes decomposition of the labile Schiffbase.

Many commercial kits are available for the analysis of HbA1c by ion-exchange chromatography. Most have modified the procedure to eliminate the drawbacks just discussed, Bio-Rad (Hercules, CA), for example, uses minicolums packed with Bio-Rex 70 and provides a special hemolysis solution that eliminates the labile Schiffbase. Also included are three calibrators that compensate for day-to-day temperature fluctuations in the laboratory. This kit method is a three-buffer gradient procedure that separates HbA1c from other fast hemoglobins. This method has retained a time frame acceptable to clinical laboratories and requires approximately 3 hr to assay 20 samples plus calibrators. It typically produces results with CVs of 6 to 9%. Manual minicolumn methods require capturing the measured fraction in a test tube and quantitating the hemoglobin present by absorbance at 414 nm. This value is then compared with the absorbance at 414 nm of a dilution of the unfractioned hemolysate to determine the percentage of glycated hemoglobin.

Hands-on time is still a major drawback to all manual minicolumn methods. Automated high-performance liquid chromatography (HPLC) methods combine the technique of ion-exchange chromatography with precision and automation. Several companies provide turnkey instruments for the automated analysis of HbA1c. Among them are Bio-Rad Clinical Division (Hercules, CA); LKB Instruments (Gaithersburg, MD); and Pharmacia (Piscataway, NJ). Results of HPLC analysis of HbA1c have an interassay CV of 1 to 3%.

Electrophoresis (HbA1c)

Several agar gel electrophoretic methods have been reported as possible means of overcoming the temperature dependence of ion-exchange chromatography for measurement of HbAI.[56-57] In 1983, Ambler et al.[58] introduced "mobile affinity electrophoresis." This technique incorporates dextran sulfate into the mobile phase. The dextran sulfate binds preferentially to the unglycated hemoglobin and increases its mobility. Helena Laboratories (Beaumont, TX) markets an automated method for determination of HbAI by electrophoresis. CVs are <5% for both the manual and automated systems. However, all of these methods quantitate total HbAI and are not specific for HbA1c.

Isoelectric Focusing (HbA1c)

The isoelectric points of HbA and HbA1c are different by only 0.01 pH units.[50] In 1971, the laboratory of M.F. Bunn reported using this difference to separate glycated hemoglobin species by isoelectric focusing.[59] With isoelectric focusing, and the use of pH gradients of 0.1 units over the width of a polyacrylamide gel, several of the glycated hemoglobin species can be separated.[50,60] As seen in Figure 13–3, mono and diligated HbA1c and mono and diglycated Schiffbase can be resolved. Bands corresponding to hemoglobin glycated at lysine e-amino groups have not been identified. This method provides a unique opportunity to study the kinetics in the formation of glycated hemoglobin in that it allows quantitation of all the species in the multistep reaction in one assay. In addition, hemoglobins F, S, and A2 can be separated by this technique. These methods produced results with CVs of approximately 8% (Mullins RE: unpublished results). This technique does not lend itself

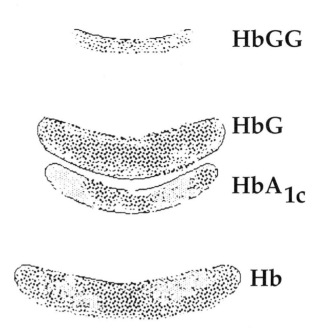

Figure 13–3. Isoeletric focusing banding pattern of glycated hemoglobins using Ampholine PAG precast HbA1c focusing gels (LBK-Productor, Bromma, Sweden). Erythrocytes were incubated in phosphate buffered saline containing 500 mmol/L glucose for 3 hr at 37°C to produce Schiffbase. The cells were collected and lysed with equal volume of water. Four microliters of hemolysate were placed on the gel and focused for 60 min at constant power of 20 W followed by 30 min at constant power of 30 W. Hb: native hemoglogin; HbG labile fraction; HbGG: double glycated labile fraction.

to routine use in the clinical laboratory because of its expense and the time required for analysis.

Immunochemical Techniques (HbA1c)

It has taken many years to produce reliable assays for HbA1c using anti-HbA1c antibodies. Boehringer-Mannheim, Bayer, and Roche all introduced assays in 1995. Each assay uses an antibody directed to the glycated n-terminal valine of the beta chain of hemoglobin to determine the HbA1c level and provides a spectrophotometric determination of total hemoglobin. These assays lend themselves to automation and a high degree of precision. They may become the methods of choice in the future.

Affinity Chromatography (GHb and Fructosamine)

In addition to altering the charge of a protein, glycation also introduces a bulky six-carbon chain with many hydrogen bond donors and acceptors into a space that formerly housed only a compact amino group. The glucose moiety contains 1, 2-cis-diols on carbons 4 and 5. At alkaline pH, boronate has a high affinity for this configuration of hydroxyls.[61] An affinity column for glycated proteins can be created by immobilizing

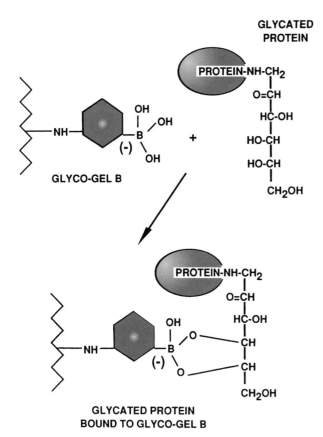

GLYCO-GEL B

GLYCATED PROTEIN

GLYCATED PROTEIN BOUND TO GLYCO-GEL B

Figure 13–4. Separation of glycated proteins from nonglycated proteins by phenylboronate affinity chromatography. The phenylboronate is immobilized onto an agarose matrix and binds 1,2-*cis*-diols found on glycated proteins. The bound glycated protein can be displaced by a competing 1,2-*cis*-diol.

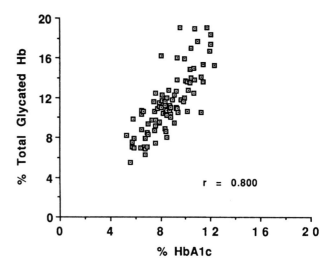

Figure 13–5. Relationship of glycated hemoglobin values from affinity chromatography to HbA1c values from ion-exchange chromatography.

m-aminophenylboronic acid onto agarose. Brownlee et al.[62] used this technique to measure glycated peptides in urine in 1980, and Mallia et al.[63] in 1981, Klenk et al.[64] in 1982, and Abraham et al.[65] in 1983 applied this procedure to the separation of glycated hemoglobins. In 1984, the laboratories of Gould and Yascoff independently reported using this technique to isolate and quantitate glycated proteins from serum and plasma.[66,67]

The mechanism of this separation is illustrated in Figure 13–4. Glycated proteins can be separated from nonglycated proteins by passing the mixture down a column containing the immobilized phenylboronic acid. Nonglycated proteins will pass through the matrix while glycated proteins will be retained. The glycated proteins can be recovered by washing the column with a solution containing a competing 1, 2-*cis*-diol (sorbitol) or by changing the pH of the eluting buffer. This method has the advantage of being able to quantitate many types of glycated protein. Protein in the fractions (bound fraction equals glycated protein; unbound fraction equals nonglycated protein) can be quantitated by a number of techniques. Mullins and colleagues reported measuring serum fructosamine (total glycated serum protein) by absorbance at 280 nm, glycated albu-

min by reaction with bromocresol green, and other glycated specific proteins by rate nephelometry and by densitometric scanning of electrophoretic and isoelectric focusing gels.[68] Because the separation conditions are mild and nondenaturing, functional tests may also be used to quantitate isolated glycated enzymes (Mullins, RE: unpublished results).

Hemoglobin fractions from the minicolumn are measured by absorbance at 414 nm. Abraham reported that the bound fraction containing glycated hemoglobin consisted of 10% HbAIa + b, 52% HbA1c, and 38% HbAO-like glycated hemoglobins.[65] It is apparent that HbA1c is the major glycated hemoglobin; however, as already stated, there are several other glycated species present that are not quantitated in assays specific for HbA1c.

Affinity chromatography agrees well with ion-exchange methods for measuring glycated hemoglobin as shown in Figure 13–5. The normal diabetic ranges are increased for GHb compared with HbA1c because more species of glycohemoglobin are being measured. Within-run CVs for the affinity chromatography procedures are 6 to 9%. [Time for analysis of 20 samples is approximately 2 hr]. Measured levels of glycated serum proteins, glycated albumin, and glycohemoglobin in the diabetic population are all significantly higher when these substances are measured by this technique.[62,65–67,69,70]

5-Hydroxymethyllfurfuraldehyde/ 2-Thiobarbituric Acid Procedure (GHb and Fructosamine)

Acid treatment of glycated proteins at high temperatures hydrolyzes the sugar moiety and produces 5-hydroxymethlyfurfuraldehyde (HMF).[71–73] HMF absorbs in ultraviolet light; however, sensitivity is increased when HMF is reacted with 2-thiobarbituric acid (TBA) to produce a new product with maximal absorbance at 443 nm. This technique can apply to a wide range of protein species. There are reports of it being used for the analysis of GHb,[74–79] albumin,[80–83] serum fructosamine,[84] and crystallins,[85] and for the filter paper collection of capillary blood.[86]

This method can be precise, with CVs reported to be <5%[78]; however, it has some major drawbacks. It requires long incubations of protein in acid to generate HMF (2 to 12 hr at 100°C). The HMF formed in the reaction is heat labile. Free glucose interferes with the test and must be removed by dialysis or protein precipitation.[87–89] Results are reported as moles HMF/mass of protein, which requires a protein determination of the sample. The reaction of TBA with HMF has been automated through the use of a Technicon AutoAnalyzer[90,91]; however, there has been no report of a procedure to automate the production of HMF.

Nitroblue Tetrazolium Reduction (Fructosamine)

This method, first described by Johnson et al.[92] in 1982, is based on the ability of fructosamines to reduce nitroblue tetrazolium (NBT) at alkaline pH. Serum fructosamine values have been shown by many investigators to be directly related to the time-average blood glucose value for the previous 2 to 3 weeks and are helpful in monitoring patients with diabetes.[92–96] The major advantages of this method are its low cost, ease of automation, and the short time required to conduct the assay and report the results. To date, this is the only test available that can practically provide a time-average glucose value while the patient remains in the physician's office.

The mechanism of NBT reduction by serum fructosamine is still unknown. The absorbance spectra of oxidized and reduced NBT are significantly different. Figure 13–6 illustrates the shift in absorbance. The procedure is simple and lends itself to automation, and it

has been adapted to many instruments.[97–104] It involves adding of 25 µL of serum or plasma to 200 µL of NBT reagent, incubating the solution at 37°C, and monitoring the absorbance at 550 nm at 10 and 15 min. The change in absorbtion at 550 nm between 10 and 15 min is proportional to the amount of fructosamine in the sample. The within-run precision of the assay is 2 to 3%. A 6-month interlaboratory study involving 33 laboratories using five different analyzers, plus a manual method, reported a CV of 54%.[102]

The time course of the reaction is shown in Figure 13–7. The change in reaction rate (slope) around 8 to 9 min should be noted. NBT can be reduced by other substances in blood. However, these interfering substances react rapidly and are consumed in the initial 10 min. Over the period from 10 to 15 min, fructosamines are the principal reactants. It should be emphasized that these interfering substances will falsely increase the fructosamine value if the incubation period is less than 10 min.[105–107] Baker et al.[98] investigated possible interference from 28 substances found in serum. However, they found that only heparin, cysteine, bilirubin, and urate produced significant interference when a 10-min preincubation step was used.[98] Glucose and the unstable Schiffbase do not affect the assay result. Hypoalbuminemia was reported to influence the test. However, several reports indicate that the results are unaffected when the albumin concentration is greater than 30 g/L.[94,95,108]

The NBT assay for fructosamine is calibrated by using 1-deoy-1-morpholinofructose (DMF, a synthetic ketoamine) in an albumin solution as primary standard.[75] An assayed serum pool is then used as the secondary standard for routine use. The method of calibrating of the NBT assay is presently a controversial point among users of the method. This controversy

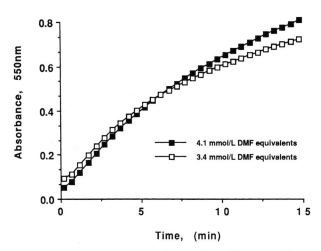

Figure 13–7. Increase in absorbance of nitroblue tetrazolium reagent on addtion of serum or plasma. The mixture contained 300 µL nitroblue tetrazolium reagent plus 20 µL serum. It was incubated at 37°C while being monitored at 550 mm. DMF, 1-deoxy-1-morpholinofructose.

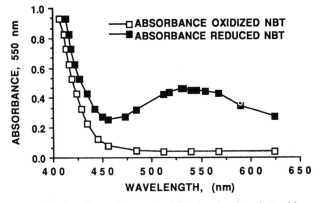

Figure 13–6. Spectral scan of oxidized and reduced nitroblue tetrazolium (NBT).

arises from two properties of the calibration procedure. The reduced NBT product has a different absorption spectrum in the presence of protein than it has the absence of protein. Thus, either protein- or serum-based calibrators are required. To complicate matters, bovine and human serum albumin behave differently in this procedure. Phillipou et al.[109] have proposed that this spectral difference is related to the low solubility of the resultant reduced NBT product, and they report that including Triton X-100 (20g/L) in the NBT reagent produces matching spectra. However, Kallner[110] indicates that the addition of detergent to the reagent increases the interference from urate. To date, no manufacturers include triton X-100 in the reagent. The other predicament is that DMF exhibits different reaction kinetics with NBT than those observed between glycated porteins and NBT.[109] As a result, there are an abundance of articles discussing the merits of standardizing the calibration of this assay.[98,99,109,111,112]

Serum is the matrix most often cited in the literature for determining fructosamine values by this method. In our experience, plasma produces results that are approximately 0.10 to 0.25 mmol/L lower than the corresponding serum sample because of the movement of cell water into the plasma phase in response to osmotic pressure from the anticoagulant. Obtaining an anticoagulated sample of blood by using sodium fluoride and rapidly separating the plasma from cells does have the advantage that a single sample can be used for HbA1c, GHb, fructosamine, and glucose determinations. Reference ranges need to be established for each sample type.

Hemoglobin Advanced Glycation End Product (Hb-AGE)

A new longer term measure of glucose control, advanced glycation end products (AGES) have a half-time of 45 days versus 35 days for HbA_{1c}, has been introduced to supplement the information obtainable with HbA_{1c}.[113] This test measures the further rearrangements and fragmentation reactions necessary to produce irreversible compounds from Amadori products such as HbA_{1c}. These AGES that are suspected of having toxic reactions, react with collagen, activate macrophages, and cause endothelial responses. The Hb-AGE is measured by a competitive enzyme-linked immunoadsorbent assay (ELISA) procedure on hemolysates delipidated with toluene by using a polyclonal anti-AGE antibody and alkaline-phosphatase-conjugated secondary antibody with added p-nitrophenol-phosphate for color development. The intra-assay and inter-assay CVs were 5 and 8%, respectively. This test is being evaluated to determine whether it can identify the 30–40% of people with type 1 diabetes who will have severe complications early in the course of the disease and whether it can predict the development of retinal, kidney, and heart diseases in patients with adult onset diabetes.

Standardization

Glycohemoglobin values, in the form of total glycated hemoglobin or HbA1c, and glycated serum protein values contain a plethora of information regarding the metabolic status of a patient. However, for this information to be useful to clinicians over a long period of time as a particular patient is followed, the values generated by laboratories must be similar month to month, year to year, and institution to institution. Each glycoprotein assay measures different species or groups of molecular species with different levels of accuracy and precision. Thus, although the assays discussed monitor similar molecules, they do not measure the same molecule.

Several prominent scientists have demonstrated the possibility and indeed the advantages of standardizing glycohemoglobin measurements.[114–116] Little et al.[114] first proposed standardization in 1986. As they stated, a major obstacle to standardization is the lack of an appropriate standard material. They described vast improvement in the agreement of different assays when the assays were standardized with a common calibrator. In 1992, after 3 years of conducting standardized glycohemoglobin assays, Boder et al.[115] reported long-term stability of the assays and a reduction in lot-to-lot variability.

Manufacturers and the scientific community should concur on one of several solutions to this need for a standard material. Possible solutions include developing a reference method or development of a pure standard or HbA1c and HBA0 with which to calibrate all methods. This need for standardization is now recognized by the American Association for Clinical Chemistry and the International Federation of Clinical Chemistry. A working group that includes manufacturers as well as scientists has been formed to find a solution to this problem (see Chapters 22 and 23).

Clinical Utility

If we assume that protein lifetimes and concentrations are relatively constant and that proteins reside in insulin-independent tissues, then the degree of glycation of a specific protein is directly related to the time-average concentration of blood glucose over the lifetime of that protein. Thus, the serum fructosamine (total glycated serum proteins) reflects integrated blood glucose concentration over the previous 2 to 3 weeks. Percent HbA1c is related to the time-average blood glucose concentrations over the prior 5 to 8 weeks. The integration of glucose concentrations over the lifetime of an individual is related to the accumulation of glycated collagen.

Each class of protein has been found to exhibit a higher degree of glycation in people with diabetes. Fur-

TABLE 13–1   Expected Values of Glycated Proteins in Diabetics and Non-Diabetics

Protein	Method	Nondiabetic	Diabetic
HbA$_1$	Ion-exchange	4.5–10.5%	
	Electrophoresis	4.5–9.2%	6–13%
HbA$_{1c}$	Ion-exchange	4.6–5.6%	
GHb	Affinity chromotography	4.0–9.8%	6.0–19.5%
	TBA		
Fructosamine	Affinity chromotography		
	TBA		
	NBT	1.4–2.9 mmol/L	2.1–5.7

Abbreviations: GHb, glycohemoglobin; HbA$_1$, hemoglobin A$_1$; HbA$_{1c}$, glycated hemoglobin; NBT, nitroblue tetrazolium; TBA, 2-thiobarbituric acid.

thermore, the degree of glycation is directly related to the degree of metabolic control or glycemic state of the individual. A person with chronic hyperglycemia, for example, produces more glycated proteins. Because of their easy access, GHb and serum fructosamine have proven to be of great benefit to physicians in monitoring patients with diabetes. The combination of GHb and fructosamine values provides a wide time window into the past glycemic state of an individual.

Reference ranges of each of the glycated proteins are listed in Table 13–1. The degrees of overlap between the diabetic and nondiabetic population should be noted. Many have proposed that these tools for monitoring glycemic control, particularly glycated hemoglobin values, have potential for use in screening or diagnostic tests for diabetes.[114–128] However, as pointed out by Forrest et al.,[129] only tests that exclude the labile fraction of glycated hemoglobin in the measurement are acceptable. Because of a wide overlap between diabetic and nondiabetic values, serum fructosamine does not appear to be valuable as a screening test.

Glycohemoglobin and fructosamine values can be used to help monitor patient adherence, and they provide a confirmation of, or call into question, self-monitored blood glucose results. A single or random glucose value provides little information to physicians about the glycemic state of the patient. For example, patients may present no sign of glycosuria and no hyperglycemia after only a few weeks on a low-calorie, low-carbohydrate diet. However, fasting glucose levels provide insight into the patient's immediate glycemic state, and fasting glucose levels in conjunction with serum fructosamine and glycohemoglobin levels, can indicate patients' average glucose levels over the past 2 to 3 weeks and 6 to 8 weeks, respectively.

The correlation between these three measures of metabolic control varies. If an individual is in "steady state," that is, has been at the present level of metabolic control for over 8 weeks, then the three parameters will agree very well with $r > 0.90$ between HbA1c and serum fructosamine levels (Mullins RE: unpublished results). If, however, the patient is in a state of flux, that is, moving from worse to better or from better to worse metabolic control, then the fructosamine value would be expected to reflect the mean level of control during the prior 2 to 3 weeks, whereas the HbA1c value would be expected to reflect the mean level of control during the prior 6 to 8 weeks.

Which Test to Use?

In light of the findings of the Diabetes Control and Complications Trial (DCCT),[130] HbA1c monitoring appears to be the method of choice. According to the DCCT Research Group, patients who maintained an HbA1c value below 6.05% had significantly fewer complications from diabetes.

Methodology of Lipid and Lipoprotein Measurements

Lipid measurements are important in understanding the course of diabetes and in monitoring the therapy of a person with the disease.[131] Each patient with diabetes has genetic lipid and lipoprotein metabolic changes that may occur when diabetes is out of control or is affected by environmental conditions. Lipid measurements help monitor the long-term energy metabolism of very low density lipoprotein (VLDL) or triglyceride (TG), just as glucose and related hormonal determinations monitor the short-term energy metabolism of carbohydrates (see Chapter 7).

Screening for Dyslipidemia

A person's lipid metabolic state usually is assessed after the first screening, after the lipid battery has been evaluated, and when indicated, after special follow-up procedures. The minimum screening necessary to detect most lipid abnormalities in serum is a quantitative determination of total and HDL cholesterol and an observation of the specimen's degree of opalescence. The lipid-lipoprotein battery that clinical chemistry laboratories are usually asked to perform to detect or confirm the presence of lipoprotein disorders is composed of quantitative total cholesterol (TC), TG, and high-density lipoprotein cholesterol (HDLC) measurements. Special follow-up studies may be requested in order to detect the presence of unique lipoproteins, such as intermediate-density lipoprotein (IDL) and apolipoprotein E isoforms in type III patients; a deficiency or unusual distribution of apolipoproteins, such as an apolipoprotein C-2 genetic defect in some patients with hypertriglyceridemia; and ineffective enzymes involved in lipoprotein metabolism (lipases and transferases). Chylomicrons, determined by visually examining the serum for a top layer of cream after the serum has been refrigerated overnight, are not associated with extensive atherosclerois, but they can increase atherosclerosis through persistent remnants. Assessing and monitoring lipoprotein disorders by laboratory methods requires an appropriate sample, a dependable method of known specificity, an effective quality-control system, and observed population values for use in interpreting the reported analytical results.

The following guidelines have been proposed for use by physicians screening for dyslipidemia.[132]

1. Use TC and HDLC as the primary screening tests for the general population.

2. Measure TC and HDLC in adults with a single sample at 5-year intervals beginning at age 20.

3. Measure TC in children with at least one parent having TC ≥ 6.24 mmol/L (≥ 240 mg/dL).

4. Measure lipoprotein panel (consisting of TC, HDLC, LDLC, and TG) for 12-hr fasting sample for the following patients:
   a. Adults with TC > 6.24 mmol/L (>240 mg/dL).
   b. Adults with TC of 5.20–6.23 mmol/L (200–229 mg/dL) and HDLC < 0.91 mmol/L(<35 mg/dL) or with two or more risk factors.
   c. Adults with TC < 5.20 mmol/L (<200 mg/dL) and HDLC < 0.91 mmol/L(<35 mg/dL).
   d. Children with TC > 5.200 mmol/L (>200 mg/dL) or a parent or grandparent with a history of coronary heart disease.

5. Conduct two or three serial lipoprotein analyses to get an average value for LDLC before starting the therapeutic regimen.

6. Remember that the predictive value of using TC to assess coronary heart disease risk is greatly improved when a person's TC level is considered along with other risk factors such as smoking, hypertension, obesity, sedentary life-style, genetic predisposition, male gender, age, and morbid conditions as diabetes, renal disease, and cerebrovascular or peripheral vascular disease (see Chapter 39).

Sampling

To best interpret analytic results, one also needs to know a subject's history including information on the patient's diet, medications, recent acute episodes of illness, and time of last food intake before the blood sample was collected for lipid and lipoprotein analysis. If possible, the subject should fast for 12 to 16 hr, have no medication or alcohol during the previous 24 hr, and be on a steady-state diet that does not cause weight gain or loss.

Special precautions should be used when collecting blood samples because lipoproteins are large molecules that cannot be transferred immediately between cells and body fluids,[133] as can smaller molecules. An excessive exchange of water between the tissue and blood can result from a tourniquet applied for more than 30 sec and from changes in posture.[134] A patient always should be in the same position when a blood sample is obtained and preferably, should be in a sitting or lying position for 10 min beforehand.[135]

Clinicians always should note whether arterial, capillary, or venous blood is sampled. Lipid and lipoprotein levels are lower in capillary blood than in venous blood,[136] and these levels also differ in paired serum and plasma samples.[137] For example, for a plasma specimen with a TC level near 200 mg/L, the plasma values would decrease approximately as follows, according to the anticoagulant used: heparin, 0.1%; EDTA, 3%; oxalate, 9%; and citrate, 14%.[138] To prepare plasma from blood, clinicians should fill each tube containing the anticoagulant to the same level to control the amount of water flowing from the blood cells into the plasma that contains the dissolved anticoagulant. During the preparation of serum, blood should be allowed to clot 30 min at room temperature before the serum is separated from the clot.

Lipid and lipoprotein analyses are best performed on "fresh" specimens because lipoproteins are relatively unstable. If lipoprotein analyses must be delayed, the lipoproteins should be isolated and then stored for cholesterol or apolipoprotein analysis. If an HDLC analysis must be delayed, the serum or plasma specimen should be stored at temperatures less than −60°C.

Analytic Methods

Total and isolated lipoprotein fractions are quantitatively estimated by measuring the cholesterol content. In the past, cholesterol was measured mainly by direct colorimetric methods, but now it is usually measured by enzymatic methods.[139] The enzymatic procedure is the method of choice because it is a direct method, it has potentially high specificity, and it requires only a small volume of reagents, thus compensating for the expensive enzyme preparation.

HDLC is measured in two steps; first, HDL is isolated, and then the cholesterol content of the isolated fraction is determined.[140] HDL is currently isolated with the use of different reagents: manganese-heparin, magnesium phosphotungstate, magnesium-dextran, calcium-dextran, calcium-heparin, and polyethylene glycol. The HDL isolated in the supernate is analyzed for cholesterol as a measure of HDL content.

TG measurements, which reflect the concentrations of VLDL, are now made mainly with enzymatic reagents.[141] Colorimetric and fluorometric TG procedures are also used in many clinical chemistry laboratories. The TG determination may be used as an independently reported lipid value and also may be used to calculate the concentration of VLDL cholesterol.[142]

The routine measurements of TC, HDLC, and TG can be followed up, when indicated, with measurements of apolipoproteins and enzymes and with special electrophoretic techniques to detect and evaluate lipoprotein metabolic disorders (see Chapter 39).

Compact Desktop Cholesterol Analytic Systems

Compact desktop analytic systems have become possible through remarkable developments in instrumentation and applicable enzymatic lipid methods. Capillary samples are usually used; however, results obtained with these can vary considerably from results obtained with venous samples taken at the same time.[143] The enzymatic methods employed in the compact analytic systems are the same methods that are used in conventional clinical chemistry laboratories.[144] Desktop analyzers provide more reliable results when operated by trained laboratory technicians than by personnel who do not have conventional laboratory training and experience.[145] The NCEP criteria for analytic performance by desktop analyzers are the same as those for conventional laboratory analyses.

The results of analyses by the desktop analyzers tend to be more variable than those of analyses done in conventional clinical laboratories. In analyses conducted on one widely used desktop analyzer, 15% of the TC values, 20% of the HDLC values, and 26% of the TG values differed by more than 10% from those determined in the lipid reference laboratory.[144] Five desktop analyzers were found not to meet the cholesterol analytic performance requirements of 3% CV and 3% bias, and three of the instrument analytic systems produced results with CVs and biases of 4 to 5%.[143] An evaluation of eight compact desktop analysis systems showed that the average bias was less than 3% for three of the desktop analytic systems; that the performance of three depended on reagent lot; and that three systems had CVs of less than 3%; and that two had CVs between 3 and 5% CV.[146] An assessment of the analytic performance of seven same-type compact desk-top analyzers for total cholesterol showed that they had different biases for different types of samples, and that the biases were lowest when the recommended type of sample was used.[147] An evaluation of five compact desktop analyzers with fresh plasma or serum specimens showed that two analyzers had biases of less than 2%, with the other three more than 5%, and that three analyzers had CVs of less than 3% for TC, with the other two exceeding 10%.[148] In classifications of specimens for total cholesterol, results from desktop analyzers agreed with results from the reference laboratory from 73 to 96% of the time.[148] Results of four screening organizations using three compact desktop analyzers agreed with reference laboratory results 100, 89, 72, and 67% of the time.[149] The majority of the fingerstick values tended to underestimate the reference cholesterol values, apparently because of insufficient operator training, inadequate quality-control procedures for field settings, and dilution of capillary blood by tissue fluid after the subject's finger was squeezed.[149] A workshop conducted by the National Heart, Lung, and Blood Institute recommended that the manufacturers and users of a compact desktop analytic system document its accuracy and precision, that the system be used only by properly trained operators, that a quality-control system be established, that the manufacturer's sample collection procedure be followed, and that results be compared at regular intervals with those of a reference method using serum.[150]

Analytic Reference Points and Goals

Reference methods are used to establish measurement reference points for TC[151] TG,[133] and HDLC.[133] These reference methods are used to label serum pools with accurate values so that the pools can be used as reference materials for routine analyses. When purified lipids such as cholesterol and TG are available for use as primary standards, standard curves are prepared from the analytic data. When purified standards are not available, the analytic system is calibrated with a serum pool labeled with a value determined by a reference procedure. The slope of the curve of the observed data with respect to the lipid concentration of different pools must be linear or of known and reproducible curvature for valid measurements.

Cholesterol measurements have excellent precision and a high potential for accuracy. Accuracy is based on a definitive isotope dilution-mass spectrometric method for total TC.[152] Accuracy and precision are aided by the use of a modified Abell–Levy–Brodie–Kendall method[151] as a reference method in research and reference laboratories (and by the use of precise enzymatic methods in clinical chemistry laboratories).[139] Certified purified preparations of cholesterol can be procured from the Office of Standards and Technology.[153]

The Laboratory Standardization Panel of the National Cholesterol Education Program (NCEP) recommends that the bias (the systematic deviation from the true value) of cholesterol measurement methods should be no greater than 3%. NCEP also recommends that the intralaboratory CV of cholesterol measurements should be less than 3%.[154]

The criteria for acceptable performance for the Centers for Disease Control-National Heart, Lung, and Blood Institutes (CDC-NHLBI) Lipid Standardization Program is 3% bias and CV for total cholesterol, 5% bias and 4.0% CV for HDL cholesterol, and 5.0% bias and CV for triglyceride.[155]

Reference Lipid and Lipoprotein Values

Both population-observed values[156] and physiological cut-points[157] can be used as reference values for interpreting reported lipid and lipoprotein serum concentration values. For clinical purposes, physiological cut-points are more widely used. In addition to reflecting the subjects' reported serum cholesterol level, the diabetes-risk classification for adults should reflect the presence or absence of other risk factors, including hypertension, cigarette smoking, severe obesity, and history of coronary heart disease (CHD) in the patient or premature CHD in a family member.

North American Lipid Research Clinics' Observed Population Values ("Normal" Values). In 1980, the Lipid Research Clinic (LRC) published observed lipid and lipoprotein prevalence values of 14 well-defined populations.[156] This information has provided reference population values obtained in standardized laboratories for use when lipid and lipoprotein analytic results are being interpreted. These reference population values for TC, TG, LDLC, and HDLC are expressed in percentiles, by age and sex, in Tables 13–2 and 13–3. The 50th percentile is closely equivalent to the mean, and the 5th and 95th percentiles are closely equivalent to the usually selected lower and upper limits of population values.

The results of the National Health Examination Survey, 1976–1980, were essentially the same as the LRC's results for TC[158] and HDLC.[159] Observed population distribution values provide the basis for selecting critical physiological cut-points for predicting risk for a certain disease and for comparing a reported result with the distributions' mean, mode, or 50th or other percentile value.

TC, TG, and HDLC Screening Cut-Points Recommended by NCEP. The NCEP Adult Treatment Panel recommends (for adults) that reported TC serum levels below 200 mg/dL (5.17 mmol/L) be classified as "desirable blood cholesterol," those 200 mg/dL (5.17 mmol/L) to 239 mg/dL (6.19 mmol/L) as "borderline high blood cholesterol," and those 240 mg/dL (6.21 mmol/L) and

above as "high blood cholesterol."[157] The desirable blood cholesterol cut-point is near the 50th percentile of LRC observed population values. The cholesterol cut-points primarily are used to make case findings of hypercholesterolemia and to refer adult men and women of all ages to preventive care or therapy.

Patients with desirable serum TC levels should undergo another serum cholesterol test within 5 years.[157] Patients with borderline high serum cholesterol levels should have a repeat test, and the average of the two test results should then be used to guide subsequent treatment decisions. Patients with high serum cholesterol levels who have definite CHD or two other CHD risk factors should be referred for serum lipoprotein analysis. They should undergo repeat testing at least once, but more if the second result is different from the first result by more than 30 mg/dL (0.78 mmol/L) because of the high individual variation in some people's test results.[160,161]

In tests for hypertriglyceridemia, triglyceride levels are classified as normal if <200 mg/dL (2.3 mmol/L), borderline if between 200–400 mg/dL (2.3 to 4.5 mmol/L), high if between 400–1000 mg/dL (4.5 to 11.3 mmol/L), and very high if >1000 mg/dL (11.3 mmol/L).

In tests for HDLC, a value below 35 mg/dL (0.9 mmol/L) is classified as a major risk factor for coronary heart disease and levels above 60 mg/dL (1.6 mmol/L) are called a negative risk factor,[157] which can cancel a positive risk factor.

LDLC Risk Treatment Cut-Points Recommended by NCEP. The NCEP recommends that decisions on whether to treat and what type of treatment to use should be based on LDLC classifications.[157] LDLC levels of <130 mg/dL (3.36 mmol/L) are classed as desirable, levels between 130–159 mg/dL (3.36 and 4.11 mmol/L) as borderline high risk, and levels ≥160 mg/dL (4.14 mmol/L) as high risk.[157] In considering the need to treat patients with high LDLC levels, physicians should also consider their HDLC level. Any level <35 mg/dL (0.91 mmol/L) is considered to be another risk factor and, thus, should influence clinical decisions about treatment.

The goal of treatment is to lower a patient's level of LDLC, which is considered an essential causative agent of CHD and which can be lowered by diet or drugs.[157] Before making treatment decisions, clinicians should conduct a complete history, physical examination, and basic laboratory tests, as well as LDLC evaluations to determine whether the high LDLC level is secondary to another disease or drug use and whether a familial lipid disorder is present.[131,157] Most lipoprotein disorders observed in medical clinics are secondary diseases, such as diabetes, pancreatitis, nephrosis, acute alcoholism, and hypothyroidism.[162] In treating patients with diabetes, clinicians should examine the patient data to

TABLE 13–2   Lipid and Lipoprotein Percentile Values (mg/dL) of Lipid Research Clinics-Observed Population (Males)

Age	No.	Total Cholesterol Percentiles							Triglyceride Percentiles							LDL Cholesterol Percentile							HDL Cholesterol Percentiles						
		5	10	25	50	75	90	95	5	10	25	50	75	90	95	5	10	25	50	75	90	95	5	10	25	50	75	90	95
0-4	238	114	125	137	151	171	186	203	29	33	40	51	67	84	99	—	—	—	—	—	—	—	—	—	—	—	—	—	—
5-9	1,253	121	130	143	159	175	191	203	30	33	40	51	65	85	101	63	69	80	90	103	117	129	38	42	49	54	63	70	74
10-14	2,278	119	127	140	155	173	190	202	32	37	45	59	78	102	125	64	72	81	94	109	122	132	37	40	46	55	61	71	74
15-19	1,980	113	120	132	146	165	183	197	37	43	54	69	91	120	148	62	68	80	93	109	123	130	30	34	39	46	52	59	63
20-24	882	124	130	146	165	186	204	218	44	50	63	86	119	165	201	66	73	85	101	118	138	147	30	32	38	45	51	57	63
25-29	2,042	133	143	159	178	202	227	244	46	54	70	95	136	199	249	70	75	96	116	138	157	165	31	32	37	44	50	58	63
30-34	2,444	138	148	167	190	213	239	254	50	58	75	104	149	213	266	78	88	107	124	144	166	185	28	32	38	45	52	59	63
35-39	2,320	146	157	176	197	223	249	270	54	62	81	113	170	251	321	81	92	110	131	154	176	189	29	31	36	43	49	58	61
40-44	2,428	151	163	182	203	228	250	268	55	64	86	122	174	248	320	87	98	115	135	157	173	186	27	31	36	43	51	60	67
45-49	2,296	158	169	188	210	234	258	276	58	68	89	124	174	253	327	98	106	120	141	163	186	202	30	33	38	45	52	60	64
50-54	2,138	158	169	187	210	235	261	277	58	68	87	124	180	250	320	89	102	118	143	162	185	197	28	31	36	44	51	58	63
55-59	1,621	156	167	189	212	235	262	276	58	67	87	119	170	235	286	88	103	123	145	168	191	203	28	31	38	46	55	64	71
60-64	905	159	171	188	210	235	259	276	58	68	87	119	169	235	291	83	106	121	143	165	188	210	30	34	41	49	61	69	74
65-69	750	158	170	190	210	233	258	274	57	64	83	112	149	208	267	98	104	125	142	170	199	210	30	33	39	49	62	74	78
70+	850	151	162	182	205	229	252	270	58	67	83	111	149	212	258	88	100	119	142	164	182	186	31	33	40	48	56	70	75

[*Source:* Lipid Research Clinics Population Studies Data Book, Prebalence Study, vol. 1, Bethesda, MD: Departmenti of Health and Human Services (PHS), National Institute of Health (NIH), National Heart, Lung, and Blood Institute, Publlication No. 80-1527, 1980. With permission.]

TABLE 13–3 Lipid and Lipoprotein Percentile Values (mg/dL) of Lipid Research Clinics-Observed Population (Females)

Age	No.	Total Cholesterol Percentiles							Triglyceride Percentiles							LDL Cholesterol Percentile							HDL Cholesterol Percentiles						
		5	10	25	50	75	90	95	5	10	25	50	75	90	95	5	10	25	50	75	90	95	5	10	25	50	75	90	95
0-4	186	112	120	139	156	172	189	200	34	38	45	54	77	96	112	—	—	—	—	—	—	—	—	—	—	—	—	—	—
5-9	1,118	126	134	146	163	179	195	205	32	36	44	55	71	90	105	68	73	88	98	115	125	140	36	38	47	52	61	67	73
10-14	2,080	124	131	144	158	174	190	201	37	44	54	70	90	114	131	68	73	81	94	110	126	136	37	40	45	52	58	64	70
15-19	1,911	120	126	139	154	171	190	200	39	44	52	66	84	107	124	60	67	78	93	110	127	135	35	38	43	51	61	68	73
20-24	778	122	130	143	160	182	203	216	36	41	51	64	84	112	131	—	62	80	98	113	136	—	—	37	43	50	60	68	—
25-29	1,329	128	136	151	168	187	209	222	37	42	51	65	86	116	145	70	73	87	103	122	141	151	37	40	47	55	64	73	81
30-34	1,569	130	139	154	172	193	213	231	39	44	54	69	91	123	151	67	76	89	108	126	142	150	38	40	46	55	64	71	75
35-39	1,606	140	147	163	182	202	225	242	40	46	57	73	101	137	176	76	81	96	116	139	161	172	34	38	44	52	63	74	82
40-44	1,583	147	154	170	191	214	235	252	45	51	62	82	111	155	191	77	89	105	120	145	164	174	33	39	48	55	64	78	87
45-49	1,515	152	161	177	199	224	247	265	46	53	65	87	119	171	214	80	90	105	127	150	173	187	33	39	46	56	66	78	86
50-54	1,257	162	172	192	215	241	268	285	52	59	74	97	135	186	233	90	102	118	141	169	192	215	37	40	49	59	70	77	89
55-59	1,112	173	183	204	228	253	282	300	55	63	79	106	149	204	262	95	103	126	148	176	204	213	36	39	47	58	68	82	86
60-64	723	172	186	203	228	254	280	297	56	64	80	105	150	202	239	100	105	130	151	172	201	234	36	43	49	60	73	85	91
65-69	593	171	183	208	229	256	280	303	60	66	84	112	153	204	243	97	104	128	156	189	208	223	34	38	46	60	71	79	89
70+	748	169	180	200	226	253	278	289	60	69	86	111	150	204	237	96	107	126	146	170	189	207	33	37	48	60	69	82	91

[*Source:* Lipid Research Clinics Population Studies Data Book, Prebalence Study, vol. 1, Bethesda, MD: Departmenti of Health and Human Services (PHS), National Institute of Health (NIH), National Heart, Lung, and Blood Institute, Pubblication No. 80-1527, 1980. With permission.]

detect any underlying lipid genetic disorder, such as type IIA or any tendency to type IV, which often is observed when the diabetes is out of control.[131]

Dietary treatment should always be the first therapy.[157] Dietary therapy is indicated for patients without CHD who possess two other risk factors and have an LDLC level above 160 mg/dL (4.14 mmol/L) and for patients with CHD who have two other risk factors and an LDLC level above 130 mg/dL (3.36 mmol/L). Drug treatment is recommended for patients without CHD who have two other risk factors and an LDLC level above 190 mg/dL (4.91 mmol/L) and for patients with CHD who have two other risk factors and an LDLC level above 160 mg/dL (4.14 mmol) (See Chapter 39).

To determine the effectiveness of dietary treatments on lipid levels (and whether patients are adhering to the diet) clinicians should measure lipid levels after 1, 3, and 6 months of therapy. They should prescribe a minimum of 6 months of intensive dietary therapy and counseling before initiating drug therapy. (See Chapters 15 and 16.) For patients with diabetes, treatment to control the disease must be instituted first, followed by treatment to control any familial lipid disorder. For instance, a person with diabetes also can have an underlying lipid disorder. The LDLC level should be measured at 1 and 3 months after drug therapy has begun. If the response to drug therapy is adequate, the patient should be seen every 4 months. For long-term monitoring, because the TC level is proportional to LDLC level, serum total cholesterol alone can be measured at most follow-up visits. The patient's LDLC level should be estimated once a year to confirm therapeutic success.

Interpretation Procedures

The NCEP screening and treatment cut-point guidelines outlined previously are now widely used to interpret a single lipid or lipoprotein result.[157] Interpretation can be extended to more depth through the use of percentile methods, projection models, or ratio considerations.

Interpretation by Percentiles.   Total cholesterol levels among children and young adults vary substantially with age and sex (Tables 13–2, 13–3).[156] Percentiles derived from observed population values may be used to interpret a reported TC or LDLC result in nonadult groups. The wide distribution of "normal" values in the "normal" range of observed population values, for

instance, between the 5th and 95th percentiles, is a relatively nonspecific and insensitive basis for interpreting a result. We express the position of a reported cholesterol value or other lipid or lipoprotein values relative to the observed range of population values, as shown in the example below (Table 13–4). Thus, a single cholesterol analytic result can be reported as equal to a certain percentile normal value and can be used to supplement interpretation by clinical cut-points. This approach also permits screening for hypolipidemia and hyperlipidemia on the basis of values outside the 5th and 95th percentiles, thus providing a more quantitative method of determining whether an individuals' lipid values are "normal" or "abnormal." The percentile ranking of a person's lipid level remains relatively constant with increasing age.[163,164] The lipid percentile of a person with controlled diabetes and a diabetic patient during fasting similarly can be determined for interpretation. The 75th percentile can be used as the cut-point for high lipid values for people of any age. For low HDLC levels, the 10th percentile could be used; this corresponds to the NCEP cut-point of 35 mg/dL (0.91 mmol/L) for adults. For TG, what the NCEH calls desirable values— those below 200 mg/dL (2.3 mmol/dL) for adults— corresponds to values below the 80th percentile; the borderline–high cut-point of 400 mg/dL (4.5 mol/L) corresponds to values below about the 97th percentile, and the very high cut-point of 1000 mg/dL (11.3 mmol/dL) corresponds to values near the 100th percentile. Thus, the 80th, 97th, and near 100th percentile for nonadults will correspond to desirable, high, and very high TG cut-points of adults and can be used to interpret nonadult results and further quantitate the risk range of patients' results.

For example, by comparing an analytic result with reference population percentiles in Tables 13–2 and 13–3, one can determine the concentration of lipid and lipoprotein and the corresponding percentile of an accepted reference normal distribution of population values. One can use percentiles from Table 13–2 to determine the population percentiles for the lipid analytic results of tests on a serum sample from a 46-year-old man with diabetes-related hypertriglyceridemia (Table 13–4).

As shown, this man has a TC level at the 70th percentile, a TG level at the 95th percentile, an LDLC level at the 35th percentile, and an HDLC level at the 50th percentile. Thus, the patient has a hyperlipoproteinemia

TABLE 13–4

	TC	TG	LDLC	HDLC
Value (g/L)	2.30	3.20	1.32	0.45
Percentile	70	95	35	50
NCEP Cut-point	Borderline	Borderline	Borderline	Desirable

associated with an elevated level of TG but not of LDLC. NCEP cut-points show that this patient's TC, TG, and LDLC levels are indicative to be borderline high risk, but that his HDLC level is not a high-risk value.

Interpretation by Projection Models. Future cholesterol levels can be estimated for persons at any age whose underlying true TC value has been measured.[163,164] This estimate can then be used to determine the age at which individuals can expect their serum lipid levels to reach borderline high, or high serum levels if they do not take action to prevent such elevation from happening. Nomograms demonstrate, for example, that a 30-year-old woman with a measured TC level of 155 mg/dL, (4.01 mmol/L) could expect her TC level to increase to 188 mg/dL (4.86 mmol/L) by age 50 and to reach a borderline high level by age 56.[164] Nomograms can be used to encourage young people to maintain desirable cholesterol levels and if necessary, to reduce those levels before they become elevated, through proper diet and exercise. The success of projection interpretation depends on determining a person's true underlying cholesterol or other lipid or lipoprotein level via the accurate laboratory analysis of multiple specimens taken at different times.[161]

Interpretation of Cardiovascular Risk Through the Use of Lipid Ratios. Although lipoprotein concentrations are interpreted as independent entities, they may be functionally related. If the lipoproteins are related and affect each other metabolically and functionally, the relative amounts expressed by ratios, as well as the concentration, could be important in determining the risk for cardiovascular disease of a person with diabetes.[165] Because LDL and HDL are the primary lipoproteins in serum associated with risk for cardiovascular disease, the ratio of the cholesterrol content of these two lipoproteins has been the most commonly used ratio. Some investigators prefer the HDLC-TC ratio.[166] The LDLC/HDLC ratio though is more popular because it is in whole numbers and can be compared with the once widely used beta/alpha-lipoprotein ratio determined by electrophoretic methods.[167]

The Framingham data indicate that the LDLC/HDLC ratio is a better indicator of coronary heart disease risk than either LDLC or HDLC alone.[165] Moreover, the 50th and 95th percentiles of these ratios among patients observed at the Lipid Research Clinic (LRC) could be used as desirable and high-risk cut-points, respectively. Desirable LDLC/HDLC ratios for adult men would be considered those less than 3.0, borderline risk ratios those between 3.0 and 5.5, and high-risk ratios those >5.5. The 50th and 95th percentiles of the distribution of this ratio in the LRC observed populations are presented by age and sex in Table 13–5.[165]

TABLE 13–5 LDLC/HDLC Ratio Percentiles[a] of Lipid Research Clinics Observed Populations

Age (yr)	Males			Females		
	No.	50th	95th	No.	50th	95th
5-14	412	2.0	3.0	353	2.0	3.0
12-24	415	2.5	4.0	363	2.0	3.0
25-34	656	2.5	5.0	386	2.0	3.0
35-70+	2,029	3.0	5.5	1,254	2.5	5.0

[a]The percentiles are rounded off to the nearest 0.5 value.

Interpretation of Lipid and Lipoprotein Values of Patients with Diabetes. The lipid and lipoprotein levels of patients with diabetes are often used to estimate their CHD risk because people with diabetes have a high incidence of CHD, and diabetes is recognized as a risk factor for CHD.[168,169] NCEP guidelines[157] are used widely now in such interpretation, and percentiles are used to supplement the interpretation when NCEP guidelines are not applicable.

Interpretation of Cholesterol Values of People with Diabetes. The classification of desirable, borderline, and high TC and LDLC risk levels are the same for persons with and without diabetes. The treatment decisions based on LDLC levels, however, are different for patients with diabetes. Because male sex and diabetes are two risk factors for CHD, men with diabetes are to reduce their LDLC level to less than 130 mg/dL (3.36 mmol/L).[157] Women with diabetes, should aim to reduce their LDLC level to less than 160 mg/dL (4.14 mmol/L) in the absence of CHD or another risk factor or to less than130 mg/dL (3.36 mmol/L) if definite CHD or another risk factor is present. Careful control of plasma glucose will reduce LDLC, HDLC, and VLDLC values, help maintain HDL values,[131] and minimize the development of complications.[130]

Interpretation of Hyperglycemia and Hypertriglyceridemia Test Results for Patients with Diabetes. The following data show lipid and lipoprotein results for two patients with diabetes, hyperglycemia, and hypertriglyceridemia, but no ketoacidosis. Cholesterol values are expressed in grams per liter. Fasting glucose values for both patients usually ranged above 300 mg/dL (16.5 mmol/L) (see Table 13–6).

TABLE 13–6

Sex	Age	TC	TG	LDLC	HDLC	LDLC/HDLC Ratio
F	51	7.65	37.8	2.08	0.17	12.3
F	22	5.45	33.4	1.13	0.14	8.1

In interpreting these results, one must consider that most of the TC comes from VLDLC, and this type of cholesterol apparently has much less risk associated with it than LDLC. The 51-year-old patient would be expected to have a high risk for CHD because her LDLC level of 2.08 g/L (5.38 mmol/L) is much higher than the 95th percentile of 1.74 g/L (4.50 mmol/L) in the LRC-observed populations and is also higher than the NCEP high-risk LDLC classification cut-point of 160 mg/dL (4.14 mmol/L). She also has a very low HDLC level, below the NCEP reduced level of 35 mg/dL (0.91 mmol/L), and a very high LDLC/HDLC ratio. HDLC is known to be highly involved in the metabolism of VLDLC, and its level falls when the VLDLC level is greatly elevated. The 22-year-old patient also has greatly elevated TC and TG levels. Her very low HDLC level is below the expected 5th percentile and also below the NCEP reduced level of 35 mg/dL (0.91 mmol/L) (Table 13–3), and her LDLC/HDLC ratio is above the expected 95th percentile of 3.0 (Table 13–4). Her LDLC level of 1.13 g/L (2.92 mmol/L) is less than the desirable adult cut-point of 130 mg/dL (3.36 mmol/L), but is the 75th percentile cut-point of the LRC observed population study. One possible reason for her very high TC level is that the lower-risk VLDLC associated with her high TG level could compensate partially for her high-risk reduced HDLC concentration and her high-risk LDLC/HDLC ratio.

Interpretation of Type V Hyperlipoproteinemia Results in Diabetes.

Type V hyperlipoproteinemia (hyperchylomicronemia) is characteristic of many patients with uncontrolled diabetes.[170] The following chart shows the mean results (g/L) reported for fasting hyperchylomiconemia subjects who received all appropriate medications and whose plasma, which stood overnight at 4°C, showed chylomicrons (see Table 13–7).

Of these 32 type V patients, 12 had pancreatitis or suspected pancreatitis, and 11 had xanthomatosis. The average age of male subjects was 43 years and of female subjects, 46 years. Both male and female subjects followed the same trends—their TC and TG levels were either greatly above the NCEP high serum cholesterol level or above the 95th percentiles (Tables 13–2 and 13–3); their LDLC levels were either below the NCEP desirable LDLC cut-point or below the 25th percentile (and often below the 5th percentile), and their HDLC levels were either below the NCEP reduced HDLC risk level or the 5th percentile of the LRC observed population. In this group of type V hyperlipoproteinemia subjects, the LDLC/HDLC ratio averaged below the desirable or 50th percentile for males and near the high cut-point or 75th percentile for females (Table 13–7). The ratio remained below the desirable cut-point for males and the borderline high-risk cut-point for females because both LDLC and HDLC levels were low, thus possibly decreasing the risk usually associated with a very low level of HDLC. The basic lipid pattern of the patients with diabetes cannot be determined until the hyperchylomicronemia is corrected.

Interpretation of High HDL Levels Among Subjects with Diabetes.

Nikkila and Hormila[171] reported that HDLC can be elevated in subjects with insulin-treated diabetes. They published the following mean data on lipid and lipoprotein levels (grams per liter) of 170 nonuremic, middle-aged subjects with diabetes who had been treated with insulin for at least 10 years. A control group consisted of nondiabetic subjects of the same age and sex who did not have diabetes. Standard deviations of the mean data were similar for both groups (see Table 13–8).

The TC, TG, and LDLC levels of patients with diabetes were similar to those observed in the control

TABLE 13–7

Sex	No.	TC	TG	VLDLC	LDLC	HDLC	LDLC/HDLC Ratio
M	19	3.48	19.9	2.83	0.57	0.22	2.59
F	13	3.65	13.6	2.38	1.00	0.27	3.70

TABLE 13–8

Subjects	Sex	No.	TC	TG	LDLC	HDLC	LDLC/HDLC Ratio
With Diabetes	M	84	2.59	1.22	1.78	0.59	3.02
Control	M	41	2.59	1.31	1.81	0.50	3.62
With Diabetes	F	86	2.78	1.02	1.97	0.68	2.90
Control	F	49	2.62	0.95	1.85	0.58	3.19

TABLE 13–9

Subjects	Sex	No.	TG	LDLC	HDLC	LDLC/HDL Ratio
With Diabetes	M	107	1.38	1.35	0.44	3.08
Control	M	847	1.35	1.42	0.46	3.10
With Diabetes	F	143	1.41	1.57	0.54	2.94
Control	F	1,215	1.13	1.55	0.58	2.67

group, but the HDLC levels tended to be slightly higher. These slightly increased HDLC levels are why the patients with diabetes had slightly lower LDLC/HDLC ratios. Males with diabetes had an average TC level above the NCEP high serum cholesterol cut-point of 2.40 g/L (6.21 mmol/L) and close to the 90th percentile of normal values for a 50-year-old man (Table 13–2); a TG level below the NCEP desirable triglyceride cut-point of 2.0 g/L (2.3 mmol/L) and near the 50th percentile; an HDLC level greatly above the NCEP-reduced HDLC risk cut-point (and near the 90th percentile), which is considered a negative risk factor for coronary heart disease; and a LDLC/HDLC ratio near the desirable cut-point or the 50th percentile of LRC population values. Females with diabetes had an average TC level of 2.78 g/L (7.19 mmol/L), which is above the NCEP high serum cholesterol cut-point of 240 mg/dL (6.21 mmol/L) and near the 95th percentile of normal values for a 50-year-old woman; a TG level below the NCEP desirable triglyceride cut-point of 200 mg/dL (2.3 mmol/L) and near the 50th percentile; an LDLC level above the NCEP high-risk LDLC cut-point of 130 mg/dL (3.36 mmol/L) and near the 90th percentile; an HDLC level greatly above the NCEP-reduced HDLC cut-point of 35 mg/L (0.91 mmol/L) and near the 75th percentile; and an LDLC/HDLC ratio in the NCEP borderline–high range and near the 60th percentile. From this study, Nikkila and Hormila[171] concluded that the average lipoprotein pattern of insulin-treated patients with chronic diabetes is no more atherogenic than that of a group of control subjects matched for age and sex and that these patients with

diabetes could be slightly less liable to coronary heart disease.

Interpretation of Results of Lipid Tests on Subjects with Diabetes in the Framingham Community Study. Results of a study in the Framingham community suggested that middle-aged people with diabetes have lower HDLC levels than do middle-aged people without diabetes.[172] One fifth of subjects in the diabetic group were receiving insulin, and the remainder were equally divided among three categories—those receiving an oral hypoglycemia agent, those on diet treatment, and those untreated. The mean data (grams per liter) reported for this community subgroup are as follows (standard errors of the mean are available in the original article).[172] (see Table 13–9)

The results were similar for both subjects with and without diabetes. Triglyceride levels for all groups were below the NCEP desirable triglyceride cut-point of 2.0 g/L (2.3 mmol/L) and near the 60th percentile range. The LDLC values were near the 65th percentile of observed population values (Fig. 13–2) and the high LDLC risk cut-point of 1.60 g/L (4.14 mmol/L) for females with diabetes but without another risk factor for CHD and above the high LDLC risk cut-point of 1.30 g/L (3.36 mmol/L) for women with diabetes and one or more risk factors for CHD. The LDLC values for men with diabetes were near the desirable LDLC risk cut-point and near the 50th percentile. Subjects with diabetes had a slightly lower HDLC level than those without.[172]

References

1. Cooper GR, Mullins RE, Stewart TC: Methodology of glucose, fructosamine, glycated hemoglobin and lipid measurements. *In* Davidson JK (ed): Clinical Diabetes Mellitus, 2nd ed. New York: Thieme Medical Publishers, 1991, p. 145.

2. Keilin D, Hartree EF: The use of glucose oxidase (notatin) for the determination of glucose in biological material and for the study of glucose producing system by manometric methods. Biochem J 42:230–238, 1948.

3. Huggett ASG, Nixon DA: Enzymatic determination of blood glucose. Biochem J 66:12, 1957.

4. Fales FW. Glucose (enzymatic). *In* Seligson D (ed): Standard Methods of Clinical Chemistry. New York: Academic Press, 1963, pp. 101–112.

5. Stein MW: D-Glucose. Determination with hexokinase and glucose-6-phosphate dehydrogenase. *In* Bergmeyer HU (ed): Methods of Enzymatic Analysis, 2nd ed. New York: Academic Press, 1965, p. 117.

6. Neese JW: Glucose, direct hexokinase method. *In* Faulkner WR, Meites S (eds): Selected Methods of Clinical Chemistry. Washington, DC: American Association for Clinical Chemistry, 1982, p. 241.

7. Neese JW, Duncan P, Bayse DD, et al.: Development and evaluation of a hexokinase/glucose-6-phosphate dehydrogenase procedure for use as a national glucose reference method. Department of Health, Education and Welfare (DHEW) Publication No. 77-8830, Atlanta: Centers for Disease Control, 1976.

8. Cooper GR: Methods for determining the amount of glucose in blood. Crit Rev Clin Lab Sci 4:101–105, 1973.

9. Passey RB, Gillum RL, Fuller JB, et al.: Evaluation and comparison of 10 glucose methods and the reference method recommended in the proposed product class standard (1974). In Cooper GR (ed): Selected Methods of Clinical Chemistry. Washington, DC: American Association for Clinical Chemistry, 1977, pp. 9–19.

10. National Committee for Clinical Chemistry Laboratory Standards. H3-A3 (Approved Standard): Standard procedures for the collection of diagnostic blood specimens by venipuncture, 3rd ed. Wayne, PA: National Institute for Clinical Laboratory Standards, 1991.

11. Hogan MJ, Service FJ, Sharbrough FW, et al.: Oral glucose tolerance test compared with a mixed meal in the diagnosis of reactive hypoglycemia: A caveat on stimulation. Mayo Clin Proc 58:491–496, 1983.

12. Burrin JM, Alberti KGMM: What is blood glucose? Can it be measured? Diabetic Med 7:199–206, 1990.

13. Vormbrock R: Comparison of Gluc-DH with the reference method for glucose determination. (Abstr. 438.) Clin Chem 29:1224, 1983.

14. National Institute for Standards and Technology: Standard Reference Materials Program: Glucose SRM 917a, Serum 909a. Gaithersburg, MD: National Institute for Standards and Technology.

15. White EV, Welch MJ, Sun T, et al.: The accurate determination of serum glucose by isotope dilution mass spectrometry—two methods. Biomed Mass Spectrum 9:395–404, 1982.

16. National Committee for Clinical Laboratory Standards: EP9—T Method comparison and bias estimation using patient samples. Wayne, PA: National Committee for Clinical Laboratory Standards, 1993.

17. Pelletier O, Arratoon C: Precision of glucose measurement in control sera by isotope dilution/mass spectrometry: Proposed definitive method compared with a reference method. Clin Chem 33:1397–1402, 1987.

18. Magni F, Paroni R, Bonini PA, et al.: Determination of serum glucose by isotope dilution mass spectrometry: Candidate definitive method. Clin Chem 38:381–385, 1992.

19. American Diabetes Association: Screening for diabetes. Diabetes Care 18 (suppl. 1):5–7, 1995.

20. Jones BA, Bachner P, Howanitz PJ: Bedside glucose monitoring. Arch Pathol Lab Med 117:1080–1087, 1993.

21. Nani AA, Poon R, Hinberg I: Quality of laboratory test results obtained by non-technical personnel in a decentralized setting. Am J Clin Pathol 89:797–801, 1988.

22. Missoula Community Medical Center: How a small community hospital laboratory improved its glucose-monitoring program. Lab Med 26:255, 1995.

23. Luxton GC. Diabetes monitoring with out-of-laboratory tests. Clin Biochem 26:19–20, 1993.

24. American Diabetes Association: Self-monitoring of blood glucose. Diabetes Care 18 (suppl. 1):47–52, 1995.

25. Cryer PE, Fisher JN, Shamoon H: Hypoglycemia. Diabetes Care 17:734–477, 1994.

26. Genter PM, Ipp E: Accuracy of plasma glucose measurements in the hypoglycemic range. Diabetes Care 17:595–598, 1994.

27. American Diabetes Association: Gestational diabetes mellitus. Diabetes Care 18 (suppl. 1):24, 1995.

28. Lewis GF, McNally C, Blackman JD, et al.: Prior feeding alters the response to the 50-g glucose challenge test in pregnancy. Diabetes Care 16:1551–1556, 1993.

29. Bain O, Deville PT, McPherson RA: Performance characteristics of three whole blood glucose monitors. Lab Med 22:470–474, 1991.

30. Bernbaum M, Albert SG, McGinnis J, et al.: Laboratory assessment of glucose meters does not predict reliability of clinical performance. Lab Med 25:32–324, 1994.

31. Mackinnon DT, Henderson AR: A laboratory assessment of the Miles Glucometer Elite blood glucose meter. Clin Biochem 27:501–505, 1994.

32. Nichols JH, Howard C, Loman K, et al.: Laboratory and bedside evaluation of portable glucose meters. Am J Clin Pathol 103:244–251, 1995.

33. Vadasdi E, Jacobs E: Hemocue B-glucose photometer evaluated for use in a neonatal intensive care unit. Clin Chem 39:2329–2332, 1993.

34. Vallera DA, Bissell MG, Barron W: Accuracy of portable blood glucose monitoring. Effect of glucose level and prandial state. Am J Clin Pathol 95:247–252, 1991.

35. Erickson KA, Wilding P: Evaluation of a novel point-of-care system, the c-STAT portable clinical analyzer. Clin Chem 39:283–287, 1993.

36. Allen DW, Schroeder WA, Balog J: Observations on the chromatographic heterogeneity of normal adult and fetal hemoglobin. J Am Chem Soc 80:1628, 1958.

37. Rahbar S: An abnormal hemoglobin in red cells of diabetics. Clin Chim Acta 22:296–368, 1968.

38. Trivelli LA, Ranney HM, Lai HT: Hemoglobin components in patients with diabetes mellitus. N Engl J Med 284:353–357, 1971.

39. Bookchin RM, Gallop PM: Structure of hemoglobin A_{1c} nature of the N-terminal b-chain blocking group. Biochem Biophys Res Commun 32:86–93, 1968.

40. Koenig RJ, Cerami A: Synthesis of hemoglobin A_{1c} in normal and diabetic mice: Potential model of basement membrane thickening. Proc Natl Acad Sci USA 72:3687–3691, 1975.

41. Maillard LC: Action des acides amines sur les sucres. Formation des melanoidines par voie methodique. C R Scad Sci 154:66–68, 1912.

42. Hodge JE: The Amadori rearrangement. Adv Carbohydr Chem 10:169–205, 1955.

43. Chiou SH, Chylack LT, Bunn HF, et al.: Role of nonenzymatic glycosylation in experimental cataract formation. Biochem Biophys Res Commun 95:894–901, 1980.

44. Chiou SH, Chylack LT, Tung WH, et al.: Nonenzymatic glycosylation of bovine lens crystallins. J Biol Chem 256:5176–5180, 1981.

45. Cohen M, Urdanivia E, Surma M, et al.: Increased glycosylation of glomerular basement membrane collagen in diabetes. Biochem Biophys Res Commun 95:765–769, 1980.

46. Hamlin CR, Kohn RR, Luschin JH: Apparent accelerated aging of human collagen in diabetes mellitus. Diabetes 24:902–904, 1975.

47. Kohn RR, Schnider SL: Glucosylation of human collagen. Diabetes 31 (suppl. 3):47–51, 1982.

48. McVerry BA, Fisher C, Hopp A, et al.: Production of pseudodiabetic renal glomerular changes in mice after repeated injections of glycosylated proteins. Lancet 1:738–40, 1980.

49. Kemp SF, Creech RH, Horn TR: Glycosylated albumin and transferrin: Short-term markers of blood glucose control. J Pediatr 105:394–398, 1984.

50. Righetti P: Isoelectric focusing in immobilized pH gradients. J Chromatogr 300:165–224, 1984.

51. Rosenthal MA: The effect of temperature on the fast hemoglobin test system. Hemoglobin 3:215–217, 1979.

52. Bisse E, Berger W, Fluckiger R: Quantitation of glycosylated hemoglobin. Elimination of labile glycohemoglobin during sample hemolysis at pH 5. Diabetes 31:630–633, 1982.

53. Dahl-Jorgensen K, Larsen AE: HbA$_1$ determination by agar gel electrophoresis after elimination of Labile HbA$_1$: A comparison with ion-exchange chromatography. Scand J Clin Lab Invest 42:27–33, 1982.

54. Nathan DM, Avezzano ES, Palmer JL: A rapid chemical means for removing labile glycohemoglobin. Diabetes 30:700–701, 1981.

55. Nathan DM, Dunn BS, Francis TB: Two commercial methods evaluated for eliminating the labile fraction from the assay for glycated hemoglobin (glycohemoglobin). Clin Chem 30:109–101, 1984.

56. Hayes EJ, Gleason RE, Soeldner JS, et al.: Measurement of HbA by liquid chromatography and by agar gel electrophoresis compared. Clin Chem 27:476–479, 1981.

57. Aleyassine H, Gardiner RJ, Blankenstein LA, et al.: Agar gel electrophoretic determination of glycosylated hemoglobin: effect of variant hemoglobins, hyperlipidemia and temperature. Clin Chem 27:472–475, 1981.

58. Ambler J, Janik B, Walker G: Measurement of glycosylated hemoglobin on cellulose acetate membranes by mobile affinity electrophoreses. Clin Chem 29:340–343, 1983.

59. Drysdale JW, Righetti P, Bunn HF: The separation of human and animal hemoglobins by isoelectric focusing in polyacrylamide gel. Biochim Biophys Acta 229:42–50, 1971.

60. Weykamp CW, Penders TJ: Mechanism and speed of reactions between haemoglobin and glucose; consequences for the measurement of glycosylated haemoglobins in patient material. Clin Chim Acta 125:341–350, 1982.

61. Weith HL, Wiebers JL, Gilham PT: Synthesis of cellulose derivatives containing the dihydroxyboryl group and a study of their capacity to form specific complexes with sugars and nucleic acid components. Biochemistry 9:4396–4401, 1970.

62. Brownlee M, Vlassara H, Cerami A: Measurement of glycosylated amino acids and peptides from urine of diabetic patients during affinity chromatography. Diabetes 29:1044–1047, 1980.

63. Mallia AK, Hermanson GT, Krohn RI, et al.: Preparation and use of a boronic acid affinity support for separation and quantitation of glycosylated hemoglobins. Anal Lett 14:649–661, 1981.

64. Klenk DC, Hermanson GT, Krohn RI, et al.: Determination of glycosylated hemoglobin by affinity chromatography. Clin Chem 28:2088–2094, 1982.

65. Abraham EC, Perry RE, Stallings M: Application of affinity chromatography for separation and quantitation of glycosylated hemoglobins. J Lab Clin Med 102:187–197, 1983.

66. Gould BJ, Hall PM, Cook JGH: A sensitive method for the measurement of glycosylated plasma proteins using affinity chromatography. Ann Clin Biochem 21:16–21, 1984.

67. Yascoff RW, Tavaarwerk GJM, MacDonald JC: Quantitation of nonenzymatically glycated albumin and total serum protein by affinity chromatography. Clin Chem 30:446–449, 1984.

68. Austin GE, Mullins RE, Morin LG: Non-enzymic glycation of individual plasma proteins in normoglycemic and hyperglycemic patients, Clin Chem 33:2220–2224, 1987.

69. Mahaffey EA, Buonanno AM, Cornelius LM: Glycosyated albumin and serum protein in diabetic dogs. Am J Vet Res 45:2126–2128, 1984.

70. Hall PM, Cook JGH, Gould BJ: An inexpensive, rapid and precise affinity chromatography method for the measurement of glycosylated haemoglobins. Ann Clin Biochem 20:129–135, 1983.

71. Gottschalk A: Some biochemically relevant properties of N-substituted fructosamines derived from amino-acids and N-arylglucosamines. Biochem J 52:455–460, 1952.

72. Keeney M, Bassette R: Rapid chemical changes in reconstituted dry milk. Science 126:511–512, 1957.

73. Keeny M, Bassette R: Detection of intermediate compounds in the early stages of browning reaction in milk products. J Dairy Sci 42:945–960, 1959.

74. Fluckinger R, Winterhalter KH: In virtro synthesis of hemoglobin A$_{1c}$. FEBS Lett 71:356–360, 1976.

75. Winterhalter KH: Determination of glycosylated hemoglobins. Methods Enzymol 76:732–739, 1981.

76. Fluckinger R, Gallop PM: Measurement of nonenzymatic protein glycosylation. Methods Enzymol 106:77–87, 1984.

77. Koch P, Sidloi M, Tonks DB: A new semi-automated method to determine glucose split off glycosylated hemoglobins in normal and diabetic bloods. (abstr.) Clin Chem 26:1048, 1980.

78. Nicol DJ, Curnow DH, Davis RE: Standardization of the colorimetric assay for glycosylated hemoglobin. Clin Chem 29:1694–1695, 1983.

79. Standefer JC, Eaton RP: Evaluation of a colorimetric method for determination of glycosylated hemoglobin. Clin Chem 29:135–140, 1983.

80. Dolhofer R, Wieland OH: Glycosylation of serum albumin: Elevated glycosylalbumin in diabetic patients. FEBS Lett 103:282–286, 1979.

81. Elbe AS, Thorpe SR, Baynes JW: Nonenzymatic glucosylation and glucose-dependent cross-linking of protein. J Biol Chem 258:9406–9412, 1983.

82. Ney KA, Colley KJ, Pizzo SV: The standardization of the thiobarbituric assay for nonenzymatic glucosylation of human serum albumin. Anal Biochem 118:294–300, 1981.

83. McFarland KF, Catalano EW, Day JF, et al.: Nonenzymatic glucosylation of serum proteins in diabetes mellitus. Diabetes 28:1011–1014, 1979.

84. Kennedy L, Mehl TD, Elder E, et al.: Non-enzymatic glycosylation of serum and plasma proteins. Diabetes 31 (suppl. 3):52–56, 1982.

85. Monnier VM, Cerami A. Nonenzymatic glycosylation and browning in diabetes and aging. Studies on lens proteins. Diabetes 31 (suppl. 3):57–63, 1982.

86. Little RR, Wiedmeyer HM, England JD, et al.: Measurement of glycosylated whole-blood protein for assessing glucose contol in diabetes: Collection and storage of capillary blood on filter paper. Clin Chem 31:213–216, 1985.

87. Yue DK, Morris K, McLennan S, et al.: Glycosylation of plasma protein and its relation to glycosylated hemoglobin in diabetes. Diabetes 29:296–300, 1980.

88. Ma A, Naughton MA, Cameron DP: Glycosylated plasma protein: A simple method for the elimination of interference by glucose in its estimation. Clin Chim Acta 115:111–117, 1981.

89. Murtiashaw MH, Young JE, Strickland AL, et al.: Measurement of nonenzymatically glucosylated serum protein by an improved thiobarbituric acid assay. Clin Chim Acta 130:177–187, 1983.

90. Menez JF, Meskar A, Lucas D, et al.: Glycosylated hemoglobin and serum proteins: semi-automated estimation (Letter) Clin Chem 27:1947–1948, 1981.

91. Moore JC, Outlaw MC, Barnes AJ, et al.: Glycosylated plasma protein measurement by a semi-automated method. Ann Clin Biochem 23:198–203, 1986.

92. Johnson RN, Metcalf PA, Baker JR: Fructosamine: A new approach to the estimation of serum glycoproteins. An index of diabetic control. Clin Chim Acta 127:87–95, 1982.

93. Baker JR, Metcalf PA, Holdaway IM, et al.: Serum fructosamine concentration as measure of blood glucose control in type I (insulin dependent) diabetes mellitus. B M J 290:352–355, 1985.

94. Baker JR, O'Conner JP, Metcalf PA, et al.: Clinical usefulness of estimation of serum fructosamine concentration as a screening test for diabetes mellitus. B M J 287:863–867, 1983.

95. Lim YS, Staley MJ: Plasma fructosamine in a measure of all glycated proteins [Tech. Brief]. Clin Chem 32:560, 1986.

96. Jury DR, Dunn PJ: Laboratory assessment of a commercial kit for measuring fructosamine in serum. Clin Chem 33:158–161, 1987.

97. Jones AF, Winkles JW, Thornalley PJ, et al.: Inhibitory effect of superoxide dismutase on fructosamine assay. Clin Chem 33:147–149, 1987.

98. Baker JR, Metcalf PA, Johnson RN, et al.: Use of protein-based standards in automated colorimetric determinations of fructosamine in serum. Clin Chem 31:1550–1554, 1985.

99. Howey JEA, Browning MC, Fraser CH: Assay of serum fructosamine that minimizes any matrix problems: use to assess components of biological variation. Clin Chem 33:269–272, 1987.

100. Redondo FL, Pascual T, Miravalles E, et al.: Automation of the "fructosamine assay" in the Hitachi 705 analyzer. Clin Chem 32:1149, 1986.

101. Lim YS, Staley MJ: Measurement of plasma fructosamine evaluated for monitoring diabetes. Clin Chem 31:731–733, 1985.

102. Baker J, Metcalf P, Tatnell M, et al.: Quality assessment of determination of serum fructosamine in 33 clinical chemistry laboratories. Clin Chem 32:2133–2136, 1986.

103. Mosca A, Carenini A, Zoppi F, et al.: Plasma protein glycation as measured by fructosamine assay. Clin Chem 33:1141–1146, 1987.

104. Bisse E, Rosenthal MA, Abraham EC: Plasma fructosamine levels determined by automated and manual methods. Clin Chem 32:1150, 1986.

105. Johnson RN, Baker JR: The alkaline reducing activity of glycated serum proteins and its relevance to diabetes mellitus. Clin Chem 32:368–370, 1986.

106. Hindle EJ, Roston GM, Gatt JA: The estimation of serum fructosamine: An alternative measurement to glycated haemoglobin. Ann Clin Biochem 22:84–89, 1985.

107. Lim YS, Staley MJ: A 10-min pre-incubation is required for measurement of fructosamine in plasma (Letter). Clin Chem 32:403–404, 1986.

108. Lloyd D, Marples J: Simple colorimetry of glycated serum protein in a centrifugal analyzer. Clin Chem 30:1686–1688, 1984.

109. Phillipou G, Seaborn CJ, Phillips PJ: Re-evaluation of the fructosamine reaction. Clin Chem 30:1686–1688, 1984.

110. Kallner A: Detergent enhances interferences of urate in determinations of fructosamine. Clin Chem 35:1803–1804, 1989.

111. Johnson R, Baker J: Assay of serum fructosamin: Internal vs. external standardization (Letter). Clin Chem 33:1955, 1987.

112. Farr G, Peacock MK, Ryall RG: Evaluation of purified globin as a primary standard for plasma fructosamine assays. Clin Biochem Rev 8:133, 1987.

113. Wolffenbuttel BHR, Giordano D, Founds HW, et al.: Long-term assessment of glucose control by haemoglobin-AGE measurement. Lancet 347:513–515, 1996.

114. Little RR, England JD, Wiedemeyer HM, et al.: Interlaboratory standardization of glycated hemoglobin determinations. Clin Chem 32:358–360, 1986.

115. Bodor GS, Little RR, Garrett N, et al.: Standardization of glycohemoglobin determinations in the clinical laboratory, three years of experience. Clin Chem 38:2414–2418, 1992.

116. Little RR, Wiedmeyer HM, England JD, et al.: Interlaboratory standardization of measurements of glycohemoglobins. Clin Chem 38:2472–2478, 1992.

117. Czech A, Taton J: Glycosylated hemoglobin assay and oral glucose tolerance test compared for detection of diabetes mellitus. Clin Chem 25:764–768, 1979.

118. Dods RF, Bolmey C: Glycosylated hemoglobin assay (HbA) as an indicator of therapy effects in different clinical types of diabetes. J Chronic Dis 36:803–810, 1983.

119. Fraser DM, Smith AF, Grays RS, et al.: Glycosylated haemoglobin concentrations in newly diagnosed diabetics before and during treatment. B M J 1:979–981, 1979.

120. Jovanovic L, Peterson CM: The clinical utility of glycosylated hemoglobin. Am J Med 70:331–338, 1981.

121. Forrest RD, Jackson CA, Yudkin JS: The glycohaemoglobin assay as a screening test for diabetes mellitus. The Islington Diabetes Survey. Diabetic Med 4:254–259, 1987.

122. Modan M, Halkin H, Karasik A, et al.: Effectiveness of glycosylated hemoglobin, fasting plasma glucose, and a single post load plasma glucose level in population screening for glucose intolerance: The Israel study of glucose intolerance, obesity, and hypertension. Am J Epidemol 119:431–444, 1984.

123. Verillo A, de Teresa A, Golia R, et al.: The relationship between glycosylated haemoglobin levels and various degrees of glucose intolerance. Diabetologia 24:391–393, 1983.

124. Cederholm J, Ronquist G, Wibell L: Comparison of glycosylated hemoglobin with the oral glucose tolerance test: A study in subjects with normglycemia, glucose intolerance and non-insulin-dependent diabetes mellitus. Diabetes Metab 10:224–229, 1984.

125. Simon D, Coignet MC, Thibult N, et al.: Comparison of glycosylated hemoglobin and fasting plasma glucose with post-load plasma glucose in the detection of the diabetes mellitus. Am J Epidemiol 122:589–593, 1985.

126. John WG, Richardson RW: Glucosylated haemoglobin levels in patients referred for oral glucose tolerance tests. Diabetic Med 3:46–48, 1986.

127. Albutt EC, Nattrass M, Northam BE: Glucose tolerance test and glycosylated haemoglobin measurement for diagnosis of diabetes mellitus-an assessment of the criteria of the WHO Expert Committee on Diabetes Mellitus 1980. Ann Clin Biochem 22:67–73, 1985.

128. Lester E, Fraser AD, Shepherd CA, et al.: Glycosylated haemoglobin as an alternative to the glucose tolerance test for the diagnosis of diabetes mellitus. Ann Clin Biochem 22:74–78, 1985.

129. Forrest RD, Jackson CA, Gould BJ, et al.: Four assay methods for glycated hemoglobin compared as screening tests for diabetes mellitus: The Islington diabetes survey. Clin Chem 34:145–148, 1988.

130. The Diabetes Control and Complications Trial Research Group: The effect of intensive treatment of diabetes on the development and progression of long-term complications in insulin-dependent mellitus. N Eng J Med 329:977–986, 1993.

131. Howard BV: Lipid metabolism in diabetes mellitus (review). J Lipid Res 28:613–628, 1987.

132. Hostetter AL: Screening for dyslipidemia. Practice Parameter. Am J Clin Pathol 103:380–385, 1995.

133. Hainline A Jr, Karon J, Lippel K (eds): Lipid Research Clinics Program: Manual of laboratory operation, lipid and lipoprotein analysis, 2nd ed. National Institute of Health (NIH) 75-628 (revised). Bethesda, MD: National Heart, Lung, and Blood Institute, 1982, pp. 157–64.

134. Cooper GR: Introduction to analysis of cholesterol, triglyceride and lipoprotein cholesterol: Reference values and conditions for analyses. In Faulkner WR, Meites S (eds): Selected Methods of Clinical Chemistry, Vol. 9. Washington, DC: American Association for Clinical Chemistry, 1982, pp 157–164.

135. Tan MH, Wilmshurst EG, Gleason RE, et al.: Effects of posture on serum lipids. N Engl J Med 289:416–419, 1973.

136. Kupke IR, Zuegner S, Gottshcalk A, et al.: Differences in lipid and lipoprotein concentrations of capillary and venous blood samples. Clin Chem Acta 97:279–283, 1979.

137. Lipid Research Clinics Program Laboratory Methods Committee of the National Heart, Lung, and Blood Institute. Cholesterol and triglyceride concentrations in serum-plasma pairs. Clin Chem 23:60–63, 1977.

138. Cooper GR, Roland DM, Eavenson E: Determination of total cholesterol with the Auto/Analyzer Automation in Analytical Chemistry, Technicon International Symposia Proceedings. New York: Mediad, 1964: 67.

139. Cooper GR, Duncan PH, Hazelhurst JS, et al.: Cholesterol, enzymic method. In Faulkner WR, Meites S (eds): Selected Methods of Clinical Chemistry, Vol. 9. Washington, DC: American Association for Clinical Chemistry, 1982, pp. 165–174.

140. Hainline A Jr, Cooper GR, Olansky AS, et al.: CDC Survey of High Density Lipoprotein Cholesterol Measurement: A report. Atlanta, GA: Centers for Disease Control, 1980.

141. McGowan MW, Artiss JD, Strandbergh DR, et al.: A peroxidase-coupled method for the colorimetric determination of serum triglycerides. Clin Chem 29:538–542, 1983.

142. Friedwald WT, Levy RI, Fridericson DS: Estimation of the concentration of low-density lipoprotein cholesterol in plasma, without the use of the preparative ultracentrifuge. Clin Chem 18:499–502, 1972.

143. Miller WG, McKenny JM, Conner MR, et al.: Total error assessment of five methods for cholesterol screening. Clin Chem 39:297–304, 1993.

144. Bachorik PS: Lipid and lipoprotein analysis with desktop analyzers. In Rifai N, Warnick GR (eds): Laboratory Measurement of Lipids, Lipoproteins, and Apolipoteins. Washington, DC: AACC Press, 1994, pp. 125–140.

145. Velsey R, Vandenbark M, Goitein RK, et al.: Evaluation of a laboratory system intended for use in physicians' offices. Reliability of results produced by health care workers without formal or professional laboratory training. JAMA 258:357–363, 1987.

146. Gregory LC, Duh SH, Christenson RH: Eight compact analysis systems evaluated for measuring total cholesterol. Clin Chem 40:579–585, 1994.

147. Rogers EJ, Misner L, Ockene IS, et al.: Evaluation of seven cholestech L.D.X. analyzers for total cholesterol determinations. Clin Chem 39:860–864, 1993.

148. Kaufman HW, McNamara JR, Anderson KM, et al.: How reliably can compact chemistry analyzers measure lipids? JAMA 263:1245–1249, 1990.

149. Naughton MJ, Luepker RV, Strickland D: The accuracy of portable cholesterol analyzers in public screening programs. JAMA 263:1213–1217, 1990.

150. National Heart, Lung, and Blood Institute: Summary of workshop recommendations regarding public screening for measuring blood cholesterol. October 1988. Arch Intern Med 149:2650–2654, 1989.

151. Duncan IW, Mather A, Cooper GR: The procedure for the proposed cholesterol reference method. Atlanta, GA: Centers for Disease Control, 1982.

152. Cohen A, Hertz HS, Mandel J, et al.: Total serum cholesterol by isotope dilution-mass spectrometry: A candidate definitive method. Clin Chem 26:854–860, 1980.

153. National Institute for Standards and Technology. Office of Standard Reference Materials: Cholesterol SRM No. 911a, Gaithersburg, MD: 20899.

154. National Heart, Lung, and Blood Institute. Current status of blood cholesterol measurement in clinical laboratories in the United States: A report from the Laboratory Standardization Panel of the National Cholesterol Education Program. Clin Chem 34:193–201, 1988.

155. Myers GL, Cooper GR, Winn CL, et al.: The Centers for Disease Control—National Heart, Lung, and Blood Institute Lipid Standardization Program. An approach to accurate and precise lipid measurements, Vol. 9. In Rifkind BM, Lippel K (eds): Cholesterol Screening. Clinics in Laboratory Medicine. Philadelphia: W.B. Saunders, 1989, pp. 105–154.

156. Lipid Research Clinics Population Studies Data Bood: Prevalence study, vol. 1. Bethesda, MD: National Institutes of Health (NIH), National Heart, Lung, and Blood Institute; 1980; Publication No. 80-1527.

157. National Cholesterol Education Program: Second report of the expert panel on detection, evaluation, and treatment of high blood cholesterol in adults. (Adult Treatment Panel II). JAMA 269:3015–3023, 1993.

158. Kalsbeek WD, Dral KM, Wallace RB, et al.: Comparing mean levels of total cholesterol from visit 2 of the Lipid Research Clinics Prevalence Study with the Second National Health and Nutrition Examination Survey. Am J Epidemiol 128:1038–1053, 1988.

159. Linn S, Fulwood R, Rifkind B, et al.: High density lipoprotein cholesterol levels among U.S. adults by selected demographic and socioeconomic variables. The Second National Health and Nutrition Examination Survey 1976–1980. Am J Epidemiol 129:281–284, 1989.

160. Demaker PN, Schrade RN, Jansen RT, et al.: Intraindividual variation of serum cholesterol, triglycerides, and high-density lipoprotein cholesterol on normal humans. Atherosclerosis 45:259–266, 1982.

161. Cooper GR, Myers GL, Smithe SJ, et al.: Standardization of lipid, lipoprotein, and apolipoprotein measurements. Clin Chem 34:B95–B105, 1988.

162. Fredrickson DS, Levy RI, Lees RS: Fat transport and lipoproteins—An integrated approach to mechanisms and disorders. N Engl J Med 276:32–44, 94–103, 148–156, 215–226, 273–281, 1967.

163. Caudill SP, Smith SJ, Cooper GR: Cholesterol-based personal risk assessment in coronary heart disease. Stat Med 8:295–309, 1989.

164. Caudill SP, Smith SJ, Cooper GR: Predicting future cholesterol levels for coronary heart disease risk assessment. MMWR 32:364–367, 1989.

165. Castelli WP, Abbott RD, McNamara PM: Summary estimates of cholesterol used to predict coronary heart disease. Circulation 67:730–734, 1983.

166. Green MS, Heiss G, Rifkind BM, et al.: The LRC prevalence study: The ratio of plasma HDL cholesterol to total and LDL lipoprotein cholesterol; age related changes, race and sex differences in selected North American populations. The Lipid Research Clinics Program Prevalence Study. Atherosclerosis 72:93–104, 1985.

167. Cooper GR, Bayse DD: Standardization of lipid and lipoprotein determinations for pediatric screening procedures. In Naito HK, Widhalm K (eds): Proceedings of Conference on Lipids and Lipoprotein Disorders of Childhood. New York: Alan R. Liss, 1985, pp. 1–17.

168. Wingard DL, Barrett-Conner E: Family history of diabetes and cardiovascular disease risk factors and mortality among euglycemic, borderline hyperglycemic, and diabetic adults. Am J Epidemiol 125:948–958, 1987.

169. Kannel WB, McGee DL: Diabetes and glucose tolerance as risk factors for cardiovascular disease: The Framingham Study. Diabetes Care 2:120–126, 1979.

170. Greenberg VH, Blackwelder WC, Levy RI: Primary type V hyperlipoproteinemia: A descriptive study in 32 families. Ann Intern Med 87:526–534, 1977.

171. Nikkila EA, Hormila P: Serum lipids and lipoproteins in insulin-treated diabetes: Demonstration and increased high density lipoprotein concentration. Diabetes 27:1078–1086, 1978.

172. Gordon T, Castelli WP, Hjortland MC, et al.: Diabetes, blood lipids, and the role of obesity in coronary heart disease risk for women. Ann Intern Med 87:393–397, 1977.

Section III.
Long-Term Mangagement

14

Integrated Team Approaches to Self-Management Education, Care, and Evaluation

Dawn W. Satterfield and John K. Davidson

Diabetes is a physiological and a cultural concern. Persons with diabetes conduct daily management and experience outcomes in a social environment. Their perceptions about these help to determine the actions they will take and the subsequent course of their health. Their communities, broadly defined as the surrounding social environment including the health-care system, influence their perceptions and those of members at risk for diabetes. These perceptions enable and reinforce behaviors that hold sway over health risks. Communities themselves are not unaffected, as resources prove inadequate to address the problems related to diabetes; frustration mounts as community members witness increasing rates, costs, and the loss of talents and wisdom of valued citizens to tragic outcomes of diabetes.

This social and physiological phenomenon, though ancient, was rare in the United States until 100 years ago.[1] Prior to this, the historical relationship of diabetes to times of prosperity and hardship was indisputable; type 2 diabetes tended to appear in people from prosperous circles.[2] Diabetes has dramatically escalated in the United States in recent years.[3] Type 2 diabetes is shortly expected to become epidemic in other countries including developing nations as, in the United States, people become less active and consume more refined sugars and saturated fats.[1] (See Chapters 2 and 6.) Although the relationship between socioeconomic status and diabetes is confounded by many variables and great diversity within populations, diabetes now disproportionately affects certain populations that, in general, tend to enjoy less socioeconomic advantages, including American Indians and Alaska Natives, African Americans, Hispanic/Latinos, and some Asian and Pacific Islanders.[4]

Documented originally in the Egyptian papyrus Ebers of 1500 B.C. as a disease of excess urinary output, diabetes, in later centuries, was named and a scientific understanding of the condition slowly emerged (see Chapter 1). The century of growing physiological and chemical understanding has been referred to as the "era of knowledge," the science of which contributed to the "era of insulin" revolving around the discovery of insulin, its use in treatment, and its refinement.[2,5] The medical communications published during the "era of insulin" contributed greatly to the evolving science and to diabetes care, including education; Krall and his colleagues[5] offer the monographs of Dr. Elliott P. Joslin and his collaborators (from 1912 to 1946) as some of the "best examples of medical communication in history." Recent history of diabetes is landmarked by the resolution of "the diabetic control controversy" proving the benefits of glycemic control in preventing complications of diabetes.[6,7]

Years after Dr. Joslin's early support of diabetes education by nurses and other professionals, the *team approach* became institutionalized and has significantly contributed to recent strides in quality care and education. In the face of evolving health-care changes, it should continue to be a pivotal force to promote health for people with and at risk for diabetes. Armed with epidemiological knowledge of diabetes' increase, growing appreciation of the cultural influence of social environments on health actions, and confirmation of the value of glycemic control in preventing complications, the next time period in the history of diabetes should reflect efforts to reach people and communities more directly and relevantly. Perhaps this period will someday be known as "the era of communication and community involvement." The team approach, integrated to embrace an even wider resource of liaisons and connect more holistically with communities, will be essential to its progress.

Historical Perspective of the Team Approach

Instructions for individual care of diabetes date back to antiquity. The consumption of cereal, milk, fruit, and wine was recommended by Aretaeus of Cappadocia centuries ago. (See Chapter 1). Rollo (1796)[8] and

Bouchardat (1883)[9] regarded intensive education as an integral part of diet therapy in their patients. Joslin provided guidance that influenced the acceptance of multidisiplinary team members as educators. By 1950, a number of other private clinics had formal diabetes teaching programs.

Runyan (1964)[10,11] early realized that university medical centers and their teaching hospitals, while excellent for people with severe and complex problems, functioned less effectively in caring for those with long-term chronic disorders. He placed nurses in decentralized clinics to manage chronic diseases (including diabetes) with established protocols and physician backup.[11-15] Patients found the continuous care accessible and individualized, unlike the overloaded emergency clinics that had provided them with care that was primarily episodic and crisis-oriented. Prospective studies showed that acute and chronic complications as well as hospitalizations were significantly reduced under the new arrangement.[15]

Miller (1969)[16] showed that a health-care system providing education, easy access to information (a 24-hr telephone answering service), and care delivered by a multidisciplinary team decreased morbidity more than threefold within 2 years after initiation of the changes. The hospitalization rate for this population dropped to a level comparable a sample group of patients at the hospital without diabetes.

Diabetes management at Atlanta's Grady Memorial Hospital (GMH) improved dramatically within 2 years after incorporation of the multidisciplinary team concept.[17-20] A decrease to one fourth of the 1974 incidence of severe diabetic ketoacidosis occurred (see Chapter 24). Since a podiatrist joined the team full time in 1974, amputations decreased to one half the 1973 rate (see Chapter 33). The hospital avoided millions in costs from preventable admissions since 1974.[20] The Diabetes Unit of GMH, since renamed Grady Health System (GHS), received the American Hospital Association's First National Patient Education Leader's Award for Outstanding Program Achievement in Patient Education Services to a Specific Target Population in 1972. In 1997, the unit, which continues to utilize nurse-managed clinics,[21] was awarded the Quality Improvement Award by the National Association of Public Health Hospitals and Health Systems.[22] The structure of the Grady diabetes unit is shown in Figure 14–1.

Mulhauser and associates,[23] Laron and coworkers,[24] Warren-Boulton and associates,[25] Chandalia,[26] and others reported similar outcomes after adopting a team approach to diabetes care and education. Interest in the success of the team approach for diabetes care and education, as well as the advocacy of organizations such as the American Diabetes Association (ADA) and the American Association of Diabetes Educators (AADE), which was established in 1973, helped influence Congress, to pass in 1974, the National Diabetes Mellitus Research and Education Act (Public Law 93-354),[27] which established the National Commission on Diabetes. The Commission published *A Long-Range Plan to Combat Diabetes* in 1975, which was funded by Congress to promote diabetes research and to translate research advances into clinical practice.[28] The National Diabetes Advisory Board (NDAB), the National Diabetes Data Group, the National Diabetes Information Clearinghouse, The Diabetes Research and Training

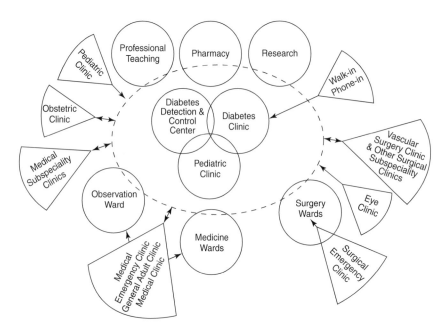

Figure 14–1. Venn diagram showing the interrelationships of the components of the Grady Memorial Hospital Diabetes Unit and flow patterns to and from other outpatient and inpatient hospital areas. [*Source:* Davidson JK, Alogna M, et al.: Assessment of program effectiveness at Grady Memorial Hospital. *In* Report of the National Commission on Diabetes, Vol. 3, Part 5. Diabetes Education for Health Professionals, Patients and the Public, Appendix 7. Department of Health,. Education and Welfare (DHEW) Publication No. National Institutes of Health (NIH) 76-1031, 1975, pp. 227–249].

Centers, and the Centers for Disease Control and Prevention's (CDC) Division of Diabetes Control (later renamed Division of Diabetes Translation) were all established. Outcomes of this initial support included a foundation of epidemiological information, guidelines for screening for diabetes, standard definitions and classifications of diabetes, and recommendations for prevention of major complications of diabetes.[29]

The use of the team approach and quality diabetes education are intertwined, and have been formally so since publication of the NDAB's "National Standards for Diabetes Patient Education Programs" in 1983,[30] which specifically tied the use of the team approach to the provision of quality diabetes education. AADE, ADA,[31,32] and other voluntary diabetes organizations have continued to promote the team approach and state-of-the-art care and education. It is now difficult to differentiate the effect of diabetes education from that of treatment.[33] The contribution of the team approach to the success of the DCCT is also unknown although its importance has been mentioned by a number of experts.[34–47] Indeed, the DCCT experience suggests that people seeking optimal metabolic control need team care although it has been acknowledged that the expertise and intensity of the DCCT team would be very difficult to duplicate in most settings.[34]

Shifts in the Team Approach to Diabetes Education and Care

Structure

Perhaps the majority of the team approaches used in diabetes care recently have been multidisciplinary. In such cases professionals retain their individual identities and perform in defined, consultative roles; commonly, a nurse serves as a "linchpin" in provisioning care and a physician directs the team.[48] Another option is the interdisciplinary approach, in which members share identity, leadership, and goals.[34,49,50] The most functional approach may vary by settings and goals; an interdisciplinary structure was most feasible for many of the DCCT sites.[34] The research in this area to date is quite scant; more information might help in developing programs.

The role of the patient in the team approach also needs further examination, particularly regarding empowerment to make informed choices about the intensity of the regimen.[47,51]

Liability

The legal ramifications of providing care as a team must also be considered especially in today's litigious environment. At issue are legal concerns centering around standards of care, quality of care and scopes of practice. Ratner and El-Gamassy suggest that thoughtful attention to the requirements of practice standards is particulary advisable in light of the "innovative" nature of diabetes team treatment, since adherence to those standards would ensure that health professionals were acting "reasonably" when in accordance with the national standards.[52] Certification of team members as certified diabetes educators (C.D.E.) by the National Certification Board for Diabetes Educators and recognition of programs based on the National Standards for Diabetes Self-Management Education Programs (such as through the ADA Recognition Program) are also advisable.

Education and Its Effectiveness

The past decade has witnessed a dramatic shift from an emphasis on models built on a knowledge-attitudes-belief triad to a focus on patient-centered perspectives, self-efficacy, self-management, and empowerment issues.[53] Recent meta-analyses of the diabetes education literature suggest that diabetes education programs generally produce positive patient outcomes with the greatest effects obtained in client knowledge.[54–57] In a 1992 meta-analysis of diabetes patient education research, that diabetes education was more effective with younger clients and improved metabolic control lasted at least 6 months.[56] Subsequently, Brown and Hedges tested a model that included metabolic control as an outcome and three predictors—knowledge, health beliefs, and compliance; health beliefs had direct and indirect effects on metabolic control.[57]

Most educators would agree that knowledge about diabetes is necessary but insufficient to stimulate the behavioral changes needed. Attitudes, beliefs, and similar characteristics all help explain behavior and some research in these areas has suggested change strategies to researchers, practitioners or persons with diabetes.[58–66] Patients awareness of and beliefs about the DCCT findings relative to their own self-management is another area where research may help by illuminating effective messages and strategies for communicating new knowledge.[67,68]

Basic learning principles (See Exhibit 14–1) have long been acknowledged as important in diabetes education; behavioral theory has in recent years been mentioned frequently in assessment and program planning literature.[69–72] In addition theory-based approaches that describe the involvement of local communities in planning strategies to promote diabetes-related health behaviors and that illustrate the integration of support needed have been reported.

EXHIBIT 14–1 Principles of Learning Important in Diabetes Education

1. Assessment of learning readiness before initiating teaching saves time in the long run.

2. Learning is more likely to occur if the learner perceives a need for the knowledge.

3. Learning is facilitated when a trusting partnership exists between the educator and the learner.

4. Active participation by the learner is essential for future recall of learned material.

5. Learning is retained longer when it is reinforced by immediate use.

6. Learning is facilitated when learners are aware of their progress.

7. Learning proceeds best when it is incremental.

8. Learning is facilitated when the material to be learned is related to what the individual already knows.

9. Mild anxiety can facilitate learning, but excessive fear can be incapacitating.

10. Health beliefs regarding susceptibility to disease, severity of disease, and perceived benefits of following prescribed therapy may influence interest in learning and changing behavior.

11. The expectation of personal success and mastery influences the likelihood an individual will engage in a particular behavior.

12. Persons who feel that they are in control of their own lives are more likely to take health action than those who express feelings of powerlessness.

13. Behaviors that are reinforced, or rewarded, tend to be learned and repeated, while those that are not reinforced may be extinguished.

14. Learning and life-style changes can be reinforced not only by professionals, but also by the individual and significant others (parent, spouse, other family members, friends).

15. Individuals may be able to change destructive behaviors (e.g., overeating) by altering the behaviors associated with the negative behaviors (e.g., snacking while watching television).

16. Individuals need opportunities to make a commitment (verbal confirmation, contract) to a behavioral change.

17. When individuals have not responded to efforts to help them learn, try using the skills of another professional.

(*Source*: Adapted from DuGas BW: Introduction to Patient Care. Philadephia W.B. Saunders, 1977, p. 258.)

National Diabetes Initiatives Influence Levels of Prevention

Scientific knowledge and national diabetes initiatives continue to influence the level of prevention at which most health-care occurs (see Exhibit 14–2). Studies in the 1970s and 1980s pointed to the value of early detection and treatment of retinopathy[75,76] and foot care education and early detection of lower extremity problems,[14,20,77–79] both resulting in at least a 50% reduction in blindness, and amputations, respectively.

These, along with reported success of the team approach, helped to shift diabetes care from an episodic approach to tertiary and secondary prevention. These levels of prevention are further supported by the DCCT and the Kumamato study, reporting the benefits of glycemic control in preventing complications.[6,7] Primary prevention of both type 1 and type 2 diabetes is being investigated in trials by the National Institute of Health (see Chapter 10).

State-of-the-art diabetes care emphasizes secondary and tertiary prevention; it is easy for primary prevention of diabetes to "get lost" in the faster-paced, symptom-

EXHIBIT 14–2 Objectives of a Prevention-Onented Approach to Diabetes Mellitus

Prevention Orientation	Obiectives
Primary prevention (applied to the general population.	To prevent hyperglycemia throughout a lifetime.
Secondary prevention (applied when diabetes mellitus is diagnosed; an estimated 10.3 million Americans have been diagnosed with diabetes; another 5.4 million have undiagnosed diabetes.	To prevent acute complications and to prevent or delay the appearance of chronic complications of diabetes mellitus.
Tertiary prevention (applied when acute or chronic complications of diabetes are detected. Diabetes is the leading cause of new cases of blindness, end-stage renal disease, and lower extremity amputations. Each year, about 28,000 people with diabetes develop kidney failure. About 67,000 people undergo diabetes-related lower extremity amputations each year).	To decrease mortality and morbidity resulting from acute and chronic complications of diabetes mellitus by preventing them, or by detecting and treating them early.

Source: Davidson JK: The Grady Memorial Hospital Diabetes Unit Ambulatory Care Program. *In* Assal JP, Berger M, Gay N, Canivet J (eds): Diabetes Education: How to Improve Patient Education. Amsterdam: Elsevier, 1983. pp. 286–297. National Diabetes Fact Sheet, 1997.

driven arena of the traditional acute care model.[81] What should most concern diabetes teams currently is that secondary prevention appears not to get nearly the attention in deserves among health care professionals. Standards of care for diabetes, for example, published annually by the American Diabetes Association,[82] are not being consistently followed in many health-care settings.[83,84] Behavioral Risk Factor Surveillance System (BRFSS) self reported data offer further evidence: An analysis of 469 enrollees with diabetes in a managed-care organization found that the majority reported receiving most preventive-care practices but two thirds had never heard of the term "hemoglobin A1c," an indication that diabetes education and provider attention to glucose control were insufficient. Furthermore, one fourth of these enrollees had not had their feet examined in the preceding year and nearly one fifth did not receive an annual dilated eye examination.[85] A BRFSS analysis for North Carolina that focused on the general population with diabetes also found low levels of knowledge of the term hemoglobin A1c (26% had heard of it) and performance (among adults) of a dilated eye examination in the preceding year (65%).[86]

Diabetes relevant objectives were included in *Healthy People 2000: National Health Promotion and Disease Prevention Strategies*, a set of 226 objectives established by the U.S. Office of Disease Prevention and Health Promotion based on a wide consensus-development process.[87] This national agenda to improve the nation's health is presently being updated for the objectives of the year 2010. Objective 17.14a, for example, is to increase to 75% the proportion of people with diabetes who receive formal patient education. Yet, in a representative sample of persons with diabetes in 1989, only 35.1% had attended a class or program about diabetes at some time during the course of their disease, 58.6% of those with type 1 diabetes, 48.9% of persons with insulin-treated type 2 diabetes, and just 23.7% of those with type 2 diabetes not treated with insulin.[88] A similar disparity between those treated with insulin and those not so treated has been noted in several other studies.[83–86]

Prior to its dissolution in 1994, the National Diabetes Advisory Board recommended the formation of a National Diabetes Education Program (NDEP) to educate, inform, and train targeted groups about self-care, clinical care, and community strategies to reduce the devastating unnecessary complications of diabetes. The NDEP, which is a joint initiative led by the CDC and NIH and guided by a steering committee, (i.e., representatives of national diabetes organizations, leading clinical researchers, and ex-officio members from the CDC, NIH, Health Care Financing Administration and Veterans Administration) was established in 1995. The NDEP plans to apply multidimensional approaches to improve the quality, continuity, and effectiveness of

diabetes care and education.[89,90] Communication will be focused at multiple levels, including persons with diabetes, health-care professionals, and third-party payers. The NDEP is building its plans on a foundation of "listening" to these audiences, both by studying the literature and conducting formative evaluation, a principle important to designing, refining and implementing relevant health communications.[90,91]

Another recent development is passage of the Balanced Budget Act of 1997, which includes three diabetes initiatives: (1) an increase in Medicare coverage to help beneficiaries achieve better control and prevent complications; (2) expanded research for type 1 diabetes; and (3) the funding of expanded services and community-based intervention programs in the Indian Health Service, including diabetes screening and primary prevention of type 2 diabetes.[92] This legislation has the potential to work synergistically with other efforts (e.g., voluntary agency initiatives, grassroots efforts and health care delivery programming) to reduce the burden of diabetes for individuals, families, and communities.

Developing Programs with Theory and Models in Mind

Theories and models can help explain behavior and suggest ways to promote behavioral change. Program planners use theories to shape the pursuit of answers to **WHY?** (e.g., why or why not are people following guidelines?); **WHAT?** (e.g., what information is needed before developing or organizing a program, or terms of evaluation, what should be monitored, measured, or compared?); and **HOW?** (e.g., how to shape program strategies to reach and impact people or groups). In short, theories guide the search for modifiable factors like knowledge, attitudes, self-efficacy, social support, and available resources, and pave the way for developing relevent health promotion interventions.[93,94]

Diabetes, perhaps because of its complexity and multiple levels of influence, presents special challenges in identifying and applying appropriate health promotion theories. Indeed, the literature reveals few unqualified successes. Perhaps, failure to consider the environmental setting in which people live and to build interventions grounded in theory account for some of the disappointing results. Furthermore, omitting theory can cause even successful programs to stand in isolation–without common ground for explanation. Such omissions can also result in a lack of specificity in the definition of constructs and variables important to particular cultures.[95] Those programs *most* likely to succeed, according to Glanz and Rimer,[93] are strategically planned and based on a clear understanding of the targeted health behavior and its environmental context.

A Practical Model of Diabetes Management and Education

It may be helpful for program planners to first take a "big picture" view of diabetes care and education. The need for a new direction for diabetes care and education, distinct from the biomedical model, that encompasses the multidimensionality of diabetes has been implicit in the diabetes literature of the past decade. Strowig[96] in 1982 called for an integrated concept of health and wellness and Dunn[97] in 1990 beseeched for new models and modes for diabetes care.

An evolving conceptual model of diabetes has been developed by Russell Glasgow[98] (see Fig. 14–2) that may be helpful in planning, evaluating, and disseminating programs that facilitate the attention of both patients and health-care teams to recommended guidelines for diabetes care. The model contains three primary levels: (1) social environment and contextual factors; (2) patient–health-care provider interactions, self-management behaviors, and short-term physiological outcomes, which constitute an ongoing feedback system; and (3) longer term health and quality-of-life outcomes. This model could remind those planning interventions of the importance of paying attention to a variety of factors, such as societal support or barriers for both persons with diabetes and members of their health-care team. It may help to reduce victim blaming (e.g., of the "noncompliant" individual with diabetes; of the "insensitive" provider) as program planners consider and plan for influence at multiple levels. Low-cost, system-wide actions appropriate at each level should suggest themselves to observant program planners as they consider the factors at work in their own settings.

The first level of the model which influences a patient's level of readiness to respond to diabetes education and care activities is composed of three cells: community and social context, patient characteristics, and clinic and program characteristics. Community and social context factors include work, family, neighborhood, general community support, and encouragement of recommended behaviors. These factors may increase or decrease a person's likelihood to engage in beneficial self-management. Patient characteristics include demographic and clinical history as well as psychological factors such as beliefs, expectations, and preferences. Clinic and program characteristics include continuity of care, as well as experiences in entering the system, such as when making a first appointment.

The second level refers to a "cycle of care" that influences whether and to what extent the individual with diabetes takes responsibility for her or his diabetes self-management.[99] It includes patient–health-care team communication, self-management behaviors, and short-term physiological outcomes with variables such as hemoglobin A1c levels, and cardiovascular risk factors (e.g., smoking status, blood pressure, and lipid profiles). The third level refers to long-term outcomes of care. Glasgow[96] points out that the major societal as

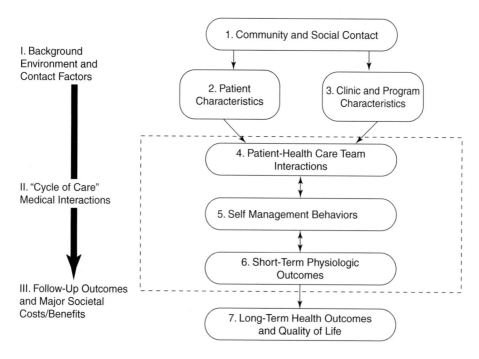

I. Background Environment and Contact Factors

1. Community and Social Contact

2. Patient Characteristics

3. Clinic and Program Characteristics

II. "Cycle of Care" Medical Interactions

4. Patient-Health Care Team Interactions

5. Self Management Behaviors

6. Short-Term Physiologic Outcomes

III. Follow-Up Outcomes and Major Societal Costs/Benefits

7. Long-Term Health Outcomes and Quality of Life

Figure 14–2. Practical model of diabetes management and education. (Russell Glasgow, of The Diabetes Educator)[98]

well as personal costs of poor diabetes care reside at this level. Agreeing with Kaplan[100] and others[101] he asserts that these outcomes must include behavioral functioning and quality-of-life.[53]

Metaphors for Diabetes Management

Metaphors often describe large truths in pithy fashion and even help unify people by the creation of *new* similarities.[102] Glasgow himself had used the metaphors of flying a modern, supersonic aircraft: while the pilot must be the person with diabetes, fortified with self-management skills and problem-solving ability, health-care providers serve as air traffic controllers who make critical recommendations based on their knowledge and experience.[53] We suggest the metaphor can be spun further—to visualize the roles of others invested in promoting health for people with diabetes, including family and community members, policy makers, and third-party payers. A large and supportive ground crew is needed to assure access to clear runways that are free of insurmountable barriers.

A concept of balance, in the day-to-day and hour-to-hour self-management decisions that affect physiological control and the larger integration of spiritual, emotional, physical, and mental aspects of life, is an important concept that could be expanded as a metaphor. Perhaps an eagle or other high-flying bird, would serve, a creature who meets challenges, maintains balance, and stays focused on its goals, with a "big picture" view of the outcomes desired. Beyond simple metaphors story telling in general may help educators and other interventionists to reach people effectively. Stories, which often reflect collective cultural wisdom, can offer a vision of hope and even help to reshape thinking.[103] Indeed, stories have been said to "clothe theory in humanity."[104]

Personal Models

Anderson[103] and others have long referred to the personal interpretation of having diabetes. Consistent with these observations is the theory of personal models, which refers to an individual's representations of their illness, including their diabetes-related knowledge and beliefs, as well as their emotional response to their experiences with diabetes.[104–106] Personal models may contribute unique information for predicting self-management, and assessing patients on key personal model constructs may help the diabetes care team identify fears and determine the appropriateness of various approaches for care and education.

Wellness

A concept of wellness that incorporates spiritual well being provides a framework for intervention planning. Views of the personal status regarding one's physical, emotional, social, spiritual, and mental health, impacted by diabetes in these areas, comes together to form one's wellness state. Empowerment and self-efficacy may help strengthen the wellness state by influencing the spiritual component of health, the core of the wellness model, notes Klepac.[107] Visual images such as the circle, used since ancient times to express the holistic integration of physical, mental, spiritual and emotional well being,[108] is sometimes applied to this concept.

Health Belief Model

The health belief model (HBM), as in the case with the theory of personal models and the wellness concept is usually viewed as intrapersonal ("within the individual"). This model has four constructs that together represent the perceived threat of a condition and the net benefits of recommended actions: perceived *susceptibility*, perceived *severity*, perceived *benefits* and perceived *barriers*.[109] Recently, *cues to action* and *self-efficacy* were added.[94] Assessments and programs based on the HBM have provided interesting findings.[112–116]

Stages of Change Model

The stages of change model contends that behavior change is a process rather than an event and that people are at varying levels of motivation, or readiness, to change. Five distinct stages are identified: *precontemplation, contemplation, decision/determination, action,* and *maintenance.* This model, which was based on Prochaska and Di Clemente's work on addictive behaviors[116] represents a stimulating area of research and program planning that might help a team to determine and plan approaches for their paients' readiness for action.

Theory of Reasoned Action and Planned Behavior

According to the theory of Reasoned Action and Planned Behavior, the best determinant of whether a person takes a health-related action is whether the person *intends* to take the action.[117] Intention is determined by the person's attitude toward the behavior (behavioral beliefs) and what the person thinks other people (e.g., by referents) would want him to do regarding the behavior (normative beliefs). Depending on the direction of the normative beliefs, program planners may want to try to alter the attitudes of important referents, add new "others" to a person's life, challenge a person's beliefs about what others think they should do.[118]

Social Cognitive Theory

Albert Bandura's social cognitive theory (originally called social learning theory) is an interpersonal health behavior theory that incorporates interaction with the social environment. It provides another framework for the educator to consider in program planning since it addresses both the psychosocial factors that determine health behavior and strategies to promote behavior change. Social cognitive theory assumes that people and their environments interact continuously; other key concepts include incentives, outcome expectations, and efficacy expectations.[119,120] Social cognitive theory which is frequently considered integral to diabetes program planning, helped to guide development of the *AADE's Core Curriculum for Diabetes Education*, third edition.[121]

Self-Efficacy Construct

Self-efficacy, a critical concept in social cognitive theory and now a construct of the health belief model, as well, is a judgment of one's capability to accomplish a certain level of performance and includes the confidence to overcome barriers.[119,120] Beliefs about whether making the behavior change will lead to a particular outcome are called *outcome expectations*. Self-efficacy determines the behaviors in which a person will engage, how long they will persist, and how much effort people will expend to reach their goals. Experience in mastering skills or knowledge, vicarious experience, verbal persuasion, and physiological state all contribute to self-efficacy beliefs.[119,120]

Studies have found relationships between self-efficacy and smoking cessation, weight loss, contraceptive use, maintenance of alcohol abstinence, and exercise adoption and maintenance.[122] In addition, using the Insulin Management Diabetes Self-Efficacy Scale and the Diabetes Self-Care Scale, Hurley and Shea found self-efficacy to be highly predictive of diabetes self-care behavior among adults[70] and Johnson found it useful in the delivery of community pharmacy-based diabetes education programs.[71] For conditions for which there are large gaps between knowing what to do (knowledge) and actually doing it (behavior) as is the case with diabetes, self-efficacy would seem very important to incorporate into program planning.

Three strategies for increasing self-efficacy are setting small, incremental goals; behavioral contracting, and monitoring and reinforcement.[93] Appropriate interventions including teaching and modeling specific behavioral and commincation skills for desired behavior (e.g., consistently performing self-monitoring blood glucose, engaging in physical activity or being careful about nutritional intake), focusing on the positive aspects of an incomplete performance (e.g., in record-keeping, losing weight), and teaching relaxation skills.[118] To help change negative outcome expectations, a program should clearly demonstrate the relationship between the desired behavior and the outcome, perhaps using creative teaching strategies (e.g., stories, role plays, drama).[123]

Social Support

Social support has been defined as the comfort, assistance, or information people receive from their social network.[124] Social support falls into four broad types of supportive behaviors or acts: (1) emotional support (e.g., empathy), (2) instrumental support (e.g., tangible aid) informational (e.g., advice), or appraisal (feedback).[125] Social support from family and friends has been found to significantly influence the participation of persons with Type 2 diabetes in certain self-care behaviors that affect glycemic control. These findings indicate the need to assess patient's sources of support when planning their care and education; mobilizing support early in the process is most desirable.[72]

Ecological Models

Ecological models seem to offer some of the best approaches for diabetes program planning, because they acknowledge the reciprocal relationship between individuals and their environments. These models can include intrapersonal factors (e.g., individual characteristics), interpersonal processes (e.g., formal and informal social network and support systems), institutional factors (e.g., social institutions), community factors (e.g., relationships between organizations or informal networks), and public policies (e.g. local, state, or national laws). The physical environment (e.g., geography, weather, land resources) also comes into play.[126] Several ecological models include a philosophy of empowerment, defined by Wallerstein as "a process of enabling individuals and communities to increase control over the determinants of health."[127] For example, such a philosophy is embodied in the Precede-Proceed model[127,74] and CDC's "Diabetes Today" program[129] both of which seem appropriate for populations that may have shown patience with outside experts but that possess within their own cultural heritage rich models of health that could improve the health status of their people. Both Precede-Proceed and Diabetes Today are based on the premise that enduring health behavior change should be voluntary and that the community's voice should be heard when programs and culturally relevant strategies are developed. In such models, evaluations begin as soon as implementation starts because the evaluation process in built on carefully chosen objectives. Accordingly evaluation helps to detect and correct problems early in the process.

Problem Statement

How Can an Effective Health-Care Delivery System or Health Promotion Program for Persons with Diabetes be Developed, Monitored, and Evaluated?

Program planners are encouraged to review the literature for lessons learned, use the "National Standards for Diabetes Self-Management Education Programs" and other published standards of care, and consider developing their program with the guidance of the ADA's Recognition Program or in some states, their state or territory's diabetes control program (see Chapter 52). Planners should build their research questions and their interventions on scientifically grounded theories and models, which will help to explain behavior, suggest strategies for change, and assist in setting program objectives, thereby providing the groundwork for evaluation. Adopting creative, action-oriented teaching strategies should also be considered.[123] Including lay health workers (e.g., community health workers, natural helpers), in the program may serve as a bridge between patients and systems that can help to promote health.[124,125,130,131]

Evaluation

Evaluation is part of the language of an accountable program planner. This ancient endeavor identifies what works and *what does not*.[132] Formative evaluation allows planners to modify a program to improve it. Carrying out an evaluation gives stakeholders the opportunity to know how their investment turned out (e.g., Did the program accomplish its goals? Did people benefit?) and to make decisions about additional support or replication in other communities. Evaluation results, when communicated in the literature, add to our understanding of effective strategies for diabetes care and prevention.

Evaluation has been defined as the comparison of an *object of interest* against a *standard of acceptability*[128]. The *objects of interest* address the "who" and "what" of program objectives. *Standards of acceptability* can be understood as the expected level of improvement in conditions stated in the objectives, ("how much" and "when").[128] Standards of acceptability for evaluation are chosen by the program planners, are often based on the scientific literature (e.g., parameters of glycemic control for DCCT participants), standards of care (e.g., ADA Clinical Practice Recommendations), or even arbitrary standards based on one's previous experience or reports of others' experience. The *Healtly People 2000* objectives include examples of standards of acceptability that can be applied as is or modified to use in com-

parisons (e.g., in before-and-after or between-groups). Measures for assessing behaviorally based standards of acceptability could be derived from validated questions in existing survey tools such as the CDC's Behavioral Risk Factor Surveillance System which is used by all state and terriorial health deparments,[133] or in other tested instruments.[59]

Outcome evaluation considers a program's distant or ultimate effect. Typically, outcome is described in terms of mortality, disease, or disability rates, but social indicators such as rates of elderly people able to live independently may be appropriate. A hypothetical example of outcome evaluation inspired by the *Year 2000* objective 17.10b might read as follows: "Reduce the rate of end-stage renal disease among people with diabetes in our tribal program from 2.0 per 1000 to 1.8 per 1000 by the year 2005." The 1983–86 national baseline for American Indians and Alaska Natives was 2.1 per 1000 and the federal target for the year was 1.9 per 1000.[87] Program directors should be able to calculate specific rates for an American Indian population from local data or with the assistance of the Indian Health Service. Because stakeholders may not be able to wait for the long-term outcomes of a program, however, it may be wise for programs to evaluate their behavioral or environmental objectives to determine the *impact* of the program in the short term (i.e., impact objectives). Stakeholders who are given help to understand the relationship between impact, and, outcomes should appreciate report of these findings and additional support may be forthcoming as a result.

Research Considerations

As the field of diabetes proceeds toward greater communication and enhanced community involvement members of the diabetes team need to consider a role that may seem foreign—that of researcher. Although the role may be unfamiliar, team members can be encouraged by the words of Michael and Sabo that practitioners are in a good position to make research a part of their practice because they are knowledgeable about the problems that need to be addressed.[134]

In what research initiatives might team members become involved? Authors have observed many innovative community-based programs that warrant further demonstration and publication of findings. In particular, programs developed in communities that use ecological approaches with local involvement and authority in decision-making and intervention planning merit attention.

Team members might also examine in an organized fashion the use of storytelling and culturally appropriate wellness concepts to promote positive personal or community models of diabetes and alter negative models; these models might be revealed. Community members should be asked for guidance.

The use of social support is another important research area; diabetes is becoming more common; there is a disparity between health professionals certified in diabetes education, and people in need of diabetes education, and a connection with community members may be critical. Innovative measures such as using community health workers (e.g., community health representatives, who serve tribal communities[135] promotors who serve Latino communities,[136] health workers in urban settings[131]) offer promise for culturally relevant, relational strategies that promote health. Evaluation and reports on such programs are very much needed.

Evaluation and reporting of the results of diabetes programs at all levels is critical to effective programming. Process evaluation, including identifying the characteristics of effective programs (e.g., team approach and structure) is still needed, along with reports of the impact and outcomes of such programs. The use of short-term interventions (e.g., nutrition intervention on fat consumption), client-provider relationships, and other aspects of interpersonal relationships are also intriguing research areas for the team to consider.

In conclusion, diabetes and the patients, families, and communities it affects constitute a multidimensional phenomenon. Feasible approaches to reducing the unnecessary losses imposed by this disease may include those that integrate emotional, spiritual, mental, and physical dimensions in an environmental context. Applying and evaluating holistic and scientifically grounded theoretical models can provide programs with more powerful, generalizable approaches to share with other providers and communities seeking answers to reduce the tragic toll of diabetes. In this era of growing knowledge, collaboration, and communication, the opportunities to develop and evaluate programs that promote health among people and populations affected by diabetes around the world are rich and far-reaching.

References

1. American Diabetes Association. News From Finland. Diabetes Forecast 62–66, 1997.

2. von Engelhardt E: Outlines of historical development. *In* Diabetes Its Medical and Cultural History. New York: Springer-Verlag, 1989, pp. 3–10.

3. U.S. Dept. Health and Human Services. Centers for Disease Control and Prevention: Trends in the Prevalence and Incidence of Self-Reported Diabetes Mellitus— United States, 1980–1994. Morbidity and Mortality Weekly Report 46:1014–1018, 1997.

4. U.S. Dept. Health and Human Services. Centers for Disease Control and Prevention: Chronic disease in minority populations: African-Americans, American Indians and Alaska Natives, Asians and Pacific Islanders, Hispanic Americans, 1994.

5. Krall LP, Levine R, Barnett D: The history of diabetes. *In* Kahn CR, Weir GC (eds): Joslin's Diabetes Mellitus, 12th ed. 1992.

6. The Diabetes Control and Complications Trial Research Group: The effect of intensive treatment of diabetes on the development and progression of longterm complications in insulin-treated diabetes mellitus. N Engl J Med 329:977–986, 1993.

7. Ohkubo Y, Kishikawa H, Araki E, et al.: Intensive insulin therapy prevents the progression of diabetic microvascular complications in Japanese patients wich non-insulin dependent diabetes mellitus: A randomized prospective 6-year study. Diabetes Res Clinical Pract 28:103-117, 1995.

8. Rollo J: A General View of the History, Nature, and Appropriate Treatment of Diabetes Mellitus, London: 1798.

9. Bouchardat A: De la glycosurie ou diabet sucre, Vol. 2. Paris: Germer-Bailliere, 1875.

10. Keenan T: *In* Runyan JW (ed): Problem-Oriented Primary Care, Ed 2. Philadelphia: Harper & Row, 1982, p. xi.

11. Runyan JW: The clinical nursing conferences. N Engl J Med 270:1411–1413, 1964.

12. Runyan JW: A program for the care of patients with chronic diseases. JAMA 1970;211:476–79.

13. Runyan JW, Vander Zwaag R, Joyner MB, et al.: The Memphis diabetes continuing care program. Diabetes Care 3:382–386, 1980.

14. Runyan JW: The Memphis chronic disease program. JAMA 231:264–267,1975.

15. Vander Zwaag R, Connor M, Dickson HD, Runyan JW: Cost of diabetes care. *In* Davidson JK (ed): Clinical diabetes: a problem oriented approach, 2nd ed., 1991 New York: Thieme Medical Publishers, Inc., pp. 717–722.

16. Miller LV, Goldstein J: More efficient care of diabetic patients in a county-hospital setting. N Engl J Med 286:1388–1391, 1972.

17. Davidson JK, Alogna M, Goldsmith M, et al.: Assessment of program effectiveness at Grady Memorial Hospital. In Report of the National Commission on Diabetes, Vol. 3, Part 5, Diabetes Education for Health Professionals, Patients, and the Public, Appendix 7. Department of Health, Education and Welfare (DHEW) Publication No. National stitutes of Health (NIH) 76-1031, pp. 227–249, 1975.

18. Davidson JK, Delcher HK, Englund A: Spin-off cost benefits of expanded nutritional care. J Am Diet Assoc 75:250–257,1979.

19. Davidson JK: The Grady Memorial Hospital Diabetes Unit Ambulatory Care Program. *In* Assal J, Berger M, Gay N, Canivet J, et al. (eds): Diabetes Education: How to Improve Patient Education. Excerpta Medical Amsterdam: Elsevier Science Publishers, 1983, pp. 286–297.

20. Davidson JK, Alogna M, Goldsmith M, et al.: Assessment of program effectiveness at Grady Memorial Hospital, Atlanta. *In* Steiner G, Lawrence PA, (eds): Educating Diabetic Patients. New York: Springer-Verlag, 1981.

21. Ziemer DC, Goldscmid MG, Musey VC, et al.: Diabetes in urban African Americans. III. Management of Type II Diabetes in a Municipal Hospital Setting. Am J Med 101:25–33, 1996.

22. Hosaka T: Grady Health Systems Diabetes Unit: Award-Winning Team Plan Improves Treatment, Lives. Atlanta Journal and Constitution 1997.

23. Mulhauser L, Jorgens V, Berger M, et al.: Bicentric evaluation of a teaching and treatment programme for type I diabetic patients; improvement of metabolic control and other measures of diabetes care for up to 22 months. Diabetologia 25:470–476, 1983.

24. Laron Z, Galatzer A, Shoshana A, et al.: A multidisciplinary comprehensive ambulatory treatment scheme for diabetes mellitus in children. Diabetes Care 2:342–348, 1979.

25. Warren-Boulton E, Anderson BJ, Schwartz NL, et al.: A group approach to the management of diabetes in adolescents and young adults. Diabetes Care 4:620–623, 1981.

26. Chandalia HB, Bagrodia J: Effect of nutritional counseling on the blood glucose and nutritional knowledge of diabetic subjects. Diabetes Care 2:353–356, 1979.

27. Davidson JK: Diabetes milestone: Public Law 93–354. ADA Forecast 27:4–11, 1974.

28. National Commission on Diabetes: The Long-Range Plan to Combat Diabetes 1974. Washington, D.C., U.S. Department of Health, Education, and Welfare, Public Health Service, National Institutes of Health. DHEW Publication No. (NIH) 76-1018.

29. Carter Center of Emory University: Closing the gap: The problem of diabetes mellitus in the United States. Diabetes Care 1985:8:391–406.

30. National Diabetes Advisory Board: National Standards for Diabetes Patient Education Programs. Diabetes Educ 9:11–14, 1984.

31. American Diabetes Association: National Standards for Diabetes Self-Management Education Programs and American Diabetes Association Review Criteria. Diabetes Care 19(Suppl 1): 1995.

32. Funnell MM, Haas LB: Technical review: National Standards for Diabetes Self-Management Education Programs. Diabetes Care 18:100–116, 1995.

33. Clement S: Diabetes self-management education. Diabetes Care 18:1204–1214, 1995.

34. Funnell MM: Integrated Approaches to the Management of NIDDM Patients. Diabetes Spectrum 9:55–59, 1996.

35. Lorenz RA, Bubb J, Davis D: Changing behavior: Practical lessons from the Diabetes Control and Complications Trial. Diabetes Care 19:648–652, 1996.

36. Fain JA: DCCT: Model of partnerships. (Editorial). Diabetes Educ 20:9, 1994.

37. American Diabetes Association Position Statement. Implications of the Diabetes Control and Complications Trial. Diabetes Care 21(Suppl 1):S88–S90, 1998.

38. The DCCT Research Group: Implementation of Conventional and Intensive Treatment in the Diabetes Control and Complications Trial. Diabetes Care 18:361–376, 1995.

39. American Association of Diabetes Educators Position Statement: Diabetes Control and Complications Trial (DCCT). Diabetes Educ 29:106, 108, 1994.

40. Dawson LY: DCCT and primary care: Prescription for change. Clin Diabetes (July/Aug):88, 90, 1993.

41. Dawson LY: DCCT: Team approach takes center stage. Diabetes Spectrum 6:222–24, 1993.

42. The DCCT Research Group: Expanded role of the dietitian in the Diabetes Control and Complications Trial: Implications for clinical practice. J Am Diet Assoc 93:758–64, 1993.

43. The DCCT Research Group: Resource utilization and costs of care in the Diabetes Control and Complications Trial. Diabetes Care 18:1468–1478, 1995.

44. McColloch DK, Glasgow RE, Hampson SE, et al.: A Systematic Approach to Diabetes Management in the Post-DCCT Era. Diabetes Care 17:765–769, 1994.

45. Santiago JB: Perspectives in diabetes: Lessons learned from the Diabetes Control and Complications Trial. Diabetes 42:1549–1554, 1993.

46. Etzwiler DD: Diabetes translation: A blueprint for the future. Diabetes Care 17:1–4, 1994.

47. Fisher EB Jr, Heins JM, Hiss RG, et al.: Metabolic control matters: National Wide Translation of the Diabetes Control and Complications Trial: Analysis and recommendations. Bethesda, MD: National Institutes of Health, 1993.

48. MacKinnon M: Diabetes: An overview. *In* MacKinnon M (eds): Providing Diabetes Care in General Practice, 2nd ed. London: Class Publishing, 1995.

49. Mazze R, Alkin J, Friedman J, et al.: Diabetes education teams. *In* Mazze R (ed): Professional Education in Diabetes. Rockville, MD: U.S. Department Health and Human Services, 1980, pp. 45–74.

50. Heins JM, Nord WR, Cameron M: Establishing and maintaining state-of-the-art diabetes patient education programs: Research and recommendations. Diabetes Educ 18:501–508, 1992.

51. Funnell MM, Anderson RM, Arnold MS, et al.: Empowerment: An idea whose time has come in diabetes education. Diabetes Educ 17:37–41, 1991.

52. Ratner RE: Legal aspects of the team approach to diabetes treatment. Diabetes Educ 16:113–116, 1990.

53. Glasgow RE, Osteen VL: Evaluating diabetes education: Are we measuring the most important outcomes? Diabets Care 15:1423–1432, 1992.

54. Padgett D, Mumford E, Hynes M, Carter R: Meta-analysis of the effects of educational and psychological interventions on management of diabetes mellitus. J Clin Epidemiol 41:1007–1030, 1988.

55. Brown SA. Studies of Educational Interventions and Outcomes in Diabetic Adults: A Meta-Analysis Revisited. Patient Education and Counseling 1990:16:189–215.

56. Brown SA: Meta-analysis of diabetes patient education research: Variations in intervention effects across studies. Res Nurs Health 15:409–419, 1992.

57. Brown SA, Hedges LV: Predicting metabolic control in diabetes: A pilot study using meta-analysis to estimate a linear model. Nurs Res 43:362–368.

58. Quakenbush PA, Brown SA, Duchin SP: The Influence of demographic and treatment variables on the health beliefs of adults with diabetes. Diabetes Educ 22:231–236, 1996.

59. Bradley C: Handbook of Psychology and Diabetes: A Guide to Psychological Measurement in Diabetes Research and Practice. Berkshire, England: Harwood Academic Publishers, 1994.

60. Peyrot M, Rubin RR: Structure and correlates of diabetes-specific locus of control. Diabetes Care 17:994–1001, 1994.

61. Anderson RM, Fitzergald JT, Oh MS: The relationship between diabetes-related attitudes and patients' self-family and friends. Diabetes Educ 22:465–470, 1996.

62. Kern RM, Penick JM, Hamby RD: Prediction of diabetic adherence using the BASIS-A inventory. Diabetes Educ 22:367–373, 1996.

63. Tamez EG, Vacalis TD: Health beliefs, the significant other and compliance with therapeutic regimens among adult Mexican American diabetics. Health Educ 20:24–31, 1989.

64. Tillotson LM, Smith MS: Locus of control, social support, and adherence to the diabetes regimen. Diabetes Educ 22:133–139, 1996.

65. Pham DT, Fortin F, Haibaudeau MF: The role of the health belief model in amputees' self-evaluation of adherence to diabetes self-care behaviors. Diabetes Educ 22:126–32, 1996.

66. Irvine AA, Saunders JT, Blank MB, Carter WR: Validation of scale measuring environmental barriers to diabetes-regimen adherence. Diabete Care 13:705–711, 1990.

67. Ruggerio L, Glasgow RE, Dryfoos JM, et al.: Diabetes self-management: Self-reported recommendations and patterns in a large population. Diabetes Care 20:368–376, 1997.

68. Thompson CJ, Cummings JFR, Chalmers J, et al.: How have patients reacted to the implications of the DCCT? Diabetes Care 19:876–879, 1996.

69. Massouth SR, Steele TMO, Alseth ER, et al.: The Effect of social learning intervention on metabolic control of insulin-dependent diabetes mellitus in adolescents. Diabetes Educ 15:518–521, 1989.

70. Hurley CC, Shea CA: Self-Efficacy: Strategy for enhancing diabetes self-care. Diabetes Educ 18:146–150, 1992.

71. Johnson JA: Self-efficacy theory as a framework for community pharmacy-based diabetes education programs. Diabetes Educ 22:237–241, 1996.

72. Wang CY, Fenske MM: Self-care of adults with non-insulin-dependent diabets mellitus: Influence of family and friends. Diabetes Educ 22:466–470, 1996.

73. Byrd T: Project Verdad: A community development approach to health. Hygie: Int J Health Educ 11:15–19, 1992.

74. Daniel M, Green LW: Application of the precede-proceed planning model in diabetes prevention and control: A case illustration from a Canadian aboriginal community. Diabetes Spectrum 8:74–84, 1995.

75. Diabetic Retinopathy Study Group: Photocoagulation treatment of proliferative diabetic retinopathy: Clinical application of Diabetic Retinopathy Study Findings. D.S. Report No. 8. Ophthalmology 88:583–600, 1981.

76. Ferris FL III: How effective are treatments for diabetic retinopathy? JAMA 269:1290–1291, 1993.

77. Edmonds ME, Blundell MP, Morris ME, et al.: Improved survival of the diabetic foot: The role of a specialized foot clinic. Quart J Med 60:763–771, 1986.

78. National Institutes of Health: Reiber GE, Boyko EJ, Smith DG: Lower extremity foot ulcers and amputations. In Harris M (ed): Diabetes in America, 2nd ed. NIH Publication No. 95-1468, Bethesda, MD: NIH, 1995.

79. Litzelman DK, Slemenda CW, Langefield CD, et al.: Reduction of lower extremity clinical abnormalities in patients with non-insulin dependent diabetes mellitus. Ann Intern Med 119:36–41, 1993.

81. Hiss RG, Greenfield S: Changes in the U.S. Health System that would facilitated improved care for NIDDM. Ann Intern Med 124:180–183, 1996.

82. American Diabetes Association. Clinical practice recommendations 1997. Diabetes Care 20(Suppl 1): 1997.

83. Kenny SJ, Smith PJ, Goldsmid MG, et al.: Survey of physician practice behaviors related to diabetes mellitus in the U.S. Diabetes Care 16:1507–1510, 1993.

84. Marrero DB: Evaluating the quality of care provided by primary care physicians to people with non-insulin dependent diabetes mellitus. Diabetes Spectrum 9:30–34, 1996.

85. Centers for Disease Control and Prevention: Diabetes specific preventive-care: Practices among adults in a managed-care population—Colorado, Behavioral Risk Factor Surveillance System. MMWR 46:1023–1028, 1995.

86. Centers for Disease Control and Prevention: Preventive-care knowledge and practices among persons with diabetes mellitus—North Carolina, behavioral risk factor surveillance system, 1994–1995. MMWR 46:1023–1028, 1997.

87. U.S. Dept. Health and Human Services, Public Health Service: Healthy People 2000: National Health Promotion and Disease Prevention Objectives. DHHS Publication No. (PHS) 91-50213.

88. Coonrod BA , Betschart J, Harris MI: Frequency and determinants of diabetes patient education among adults in the US population. Diabetes Care 17:852–858, 1994.

89. Ernst K: National Diabetes Education Program. AADE News 23:1, 3, 1997.

90. Leontos C, Wong F, Gallivan J, Lising M: National Diabetes Education program: opportunities and challenges. Am J Diet Assoc 98:73–75, 1998.

91. National Institutes of Health. Centers for Disease Control and Prevention. National Diabetes Education Program: Planning Strategy 1997.

92. Health Human Services (HHS) Targets Efforts on Diabetes (Fact Sheet). August, 1997.

93. Glanz K, Rimer BK: Theory at a glance: A guide for health promotion practice 1995, National Institutes of Health, National Cancer Institute.

94. Glanz K, Lewis FM, Rimer BK (Eds). Health Behavior and Health Education: Theory Research and Practice, 2nd ed. San Francisco, CA: Jossey-Bass, 1997.

95. Flores ET, Castro FG, Fernandez: Social theory, social action and influence research for cancer prevention among Latinos. J Nat Inst Monographs 18:101–108, 1995.

96. Strowig S: Patient education: A model for autonomous decision-making and deliberate action in diabetes self-management. Med Clin North Am 1982;66:1293–1307.

97. Dunn SM: Rethinking the models and modes of patient eduation. Patient Educ Couns 16:281–286, 1990.

98. Glasgow RE: A practical model of diabetes management and education. Diabetes Care 18:117–126, 1995.

99. Anderson LA: Health-Care Communication and Selected Pschosocial Correlates of Adherence in Diabetes Management. Diabetes Care 13:66–70, 1990.

100. Kaplan RM: Behavior as the central outcome in health care. Am Psychol 9:632–646, 1990.

101. Karolys P: Goals systems: An organizing framework for clinical assessment and treatment planning. Psychol Assess 5:273–290, 1993.

102. Lakeoff G, Johnson M: Metaphors to Live By. Chicago, IL: Univ Chicago Press, 1980.

103. Carter JS, Perez GE, Gilliland SS: Communicating through stories: experience of the Native American Diabetes Project. *Diabetes Educ* 25:179–188, 1999.

104. Feste C: Storytelling in diabetes education. Diabetes Educ 8:119–123, 1995.

105. Anderson RM: The personal meaning of having diabetes: Implications for patient behavior and education or kicking the Buchet theory. Diabetic Med 3:8–89, 1986.

106. Hampson SE, Glasgow RE, Foster LS: Personal Models of Diabetes Among Older Adults: Relationship to Self-Management and Other Variables. Diabetes Educ 21:300–307, 1995.

107. Standiford DA, Turner AM, Allen SR, et al.: Personal models of diabetes: Preadolescents and adolescents. Diabetes Educ 23:147–151, 1997.

108. Drozda DJ, Allen SR, Standiford DA, et al.: Personal illness models of diabetes: Parents of preadolescents and adolescents. Diabetes Educ 1997;23:550–557.

109. Klepac MJ: Theory and practical applications of a wellness perspective in diabetes education. Diabetes Educ 22:225–230, 1996.

110. Black Elk, B, as told to John G. Neihardt. Black Elk Speaks. Reprinted, University of Nebraska Press, Lincoln, NE, 1961.

111. Becker MH, Maiman LA, KirschtJP, et al.: The health belief model and prediction of dietary compliance: a field experiment. J Health Soc Behav 18:346–366, 1977.

112. Alogna M: Perception of severity of disease and health locus of control in compliant and noncomplaint diabetic patients. Diabetes Care 3:533–534, 1980.

113. Rabkin SW, Boyko E, Wilson A, et al.: A randomized clinical trial comparing behavior modification and individual counseling in the nutritional therapy of NIDDM; comparison of the effect on blood sugar, body weight and serum lipids. Diabetes Care 6:50–56, 1983.

114. Cerkoney KAB, Hart LK: The relationship between the health belief model and compliance of persons with diabetes mellitus. Diabetes Care 3:594–598, 1980.

115. Woolridge KL, Wallston KA, Graber AL, et al.: The relationship between health beliefs, adherence, and metabolic control of diabetes. Diabetes Educ 18:495–500, 1992.

116. Prochaska JO, Diclemente CC, Norcross JC: In search of how people change: Applications to addictive behaviors. Am Psychol 47:1102–1114, 1992.

117. Fishbein M, Ajzen I: Belief, Attitude, Intention and Behavior: An Introduction to Theory and Research. Reading, MA: Addison-Wesley, 1975.

118. Kreuter MW, Lezin NA, Kreuter MW, Green LW. Community Health Promotion Ideas That Work: A Field Book for Practitioners. Jones and Bartlett Publishers: Massachussetts, 1998.

120. Bandura A, *Social foundations of thought and action: a social cognitive theory*. Englewood Cliffs, N.J.: Prentice Hall, 1986.

121. American Association Diabetes Educators, Core Curriculum for Diabetes Education, Chicago, IL, 1999.

122. Strecher VJ, De Villis BE, Becker MH, Rosenstock IM: The role of self-efficacy in archiving health behavior changes. Health Educ 3:73–91, 1986.

123. AMC Cancer Research Center: Beyong the Brochure: Alternative Approaches to Effective Health Communication, 1994. (http://www.cdc.gov/cancer).

124. Wallston BS, Alagna SW, De Vellis BM, De Vellis RF: Social Support and Physical Health. Health Psychol 2:367–391, 1983.

125. Eng E, Young R. Lay health advisors as community change agents. Farm Community Health 15:24–40, 1992.

126. McLeroy KR, Bibeau D, Stecklen A, Glanz K: An ecological perspective on health promotion programs; *Health Educ Quar* 15:351–377, 1988.

127. Wallerstein N. Powerlessness, empowerment, and health: implications for health promotion programs. Am J Health Promotion.

128. Green LW, Kreuter MW. Health Promotion Planning: An Educational and Environmental Approach. Mountain View, CA: Mayfield Publishing Co., 1991.

129. Centers for Disease Control and Prevention. Division of Diabetes Translation. Diabetes Today: A Course on How to Build Skills to Plan and Implement Community-Based Programs for Persons with Diabetes. Atlanta, GA, 1997.

130. Israel B. Social networks and social support: implications for natural helper and community level interventions. Health Educ Q 12:65–80, 1985.

131. Berkley-Patton J, Fawcett SB, Paine-Andrews A, Johns L. Developing capacities of youth as lay health advisors: a case study with high school students. Health Educ Behav 24:481–494, 1997.

132. Peyrot M: Evaluation of patient education programs: How to do it and how to use it. Diabetes Spectrum 9:86–93, 1996.

133. Centers for Disease Control and Prevention: Assessing health risks in America: The behavioral risk factor surveillance system. (BRFSS), 4770 Buford Hwy, K-13, Atlanta, GA 30341.

134. Michael SR, Sabo CE: The challenge of conducting clinical research in diabetes care and education. Diabetes Educ 1995;22:23–27.

135. Landen, JB: Community health representatives: the vital link in Native American health care. IHS Primary Care Provider 17:101–102, 1992.

136. Brecho A, Londono M: Diabetes management: An intervention at the community level 1997 (Nov. 9–13). Abstract in session #3219. American Public Health Association 125th Annual Meeting and Exposition, Indiannopolis, Indianna.

15

Diet Therapy for Insulin-Dependent (Type I) Diabetes Mellitus

John K. Davidson

Historical Perspective

Before the clinical use of insulin (1922),[1] the only methods available to reduce the incidence and severity of diabetic ketoacidosis (DKA) in those with insulindependent diabetes mellitus (IDDM) were periodic short-term fasts, low-calorie diets, and exercise. Such therapy could prolong life for a few months or a few years in many individuals, but death due to diabetic coma or starvation was the inevitable outcome in essentially all. Diabetic ketoacidosis became "curable" and preventable when insulin therapy was introduced, and some individuals who developed IDDM during childhood were alive in 1989 because insulin therapy was available.

Yet, despite a marked decrease in mortality due to DKA by 1950, it was evident that normal growth and maturation did not occur in children with IDDM when metabolic control was unsatisfactory. Diabetic dwarfism was common in persistently hyperglycemic children whose linear growth velocity was subnormal.[2-5]

Growth charts have been used for 60 years to measure linear growth velocity (height) in boys and girls through age 18. National Center for Health Statistics (NCHS) growth charts[6] were introduced in 1976. By means of data collected every 3 to 6 months on these charts, physicians can assess whether linear growth velocity and weight gain are normal or abnormal (Figs. 15–1 and 15–2).

Excellent control of IDDM will sustain normal growth velocity. Subnormal growth can accelerate to normal and "catch-up" growth can occur when good or excellent metabolic control replaces poor metabolic control in those whose epiphyses are still open.[7] Identical twins with IDDM grow at a slower rate than paired nondiabetic twins.[8] Linear growth may accelerate when continuous subcutaneous insulin infusion (CSII) is substituted for conventional (subcutaneous) insulin therapy (CIT) and when metabolic control improves.[9]

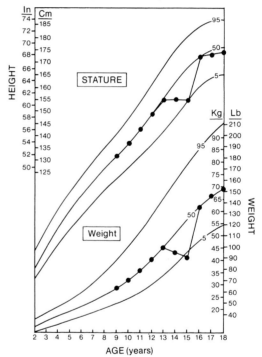

BOYS:
2 to 18 years, Physical Growth, NCHS Percentiles

Figure 15-1. Inadequate caloric intake (1,800 cal/day) with failure of linear (height) and weight growth in a male from age 13 to 15 years. During this 2-year period, height fell from the 50th to the 5th percentile and weight fell from the 50th to less than the 5th percentile. The caloric intake was increased to 3,500 cal/day and plasma glucose control was optimized. Weight increased by 45 pounds and height by 7 in. during the following year, with both height and weight returning to 50th percentile by age 16 years ("catch-up" growth).

Yet insulin therapy alone, including CSII, is unlikely to maintain normal growth and good metabolic control in the absence of a meal plan (i.e., diet) that contains adequate calories, protein, vitamins, minerals, and trace elements.[7,10-12]

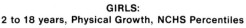

GIRLS:
2 to 18 years, Physical Growth, NCHS Percentiles

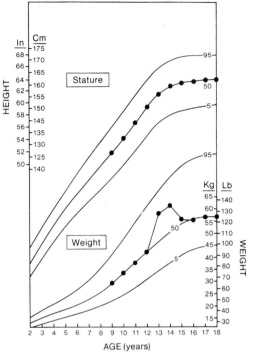

Figure 15-2. Caloric intake that exceeded basal, activity, and growth needs from age 12 to 14 years in a female. It was estimated that she had been eating about 2,700 cal/day, though only 2,200 calories had been prescribed. Height remained on the 50th percentile, but weight increased from the 50th to the 85th percentile. She was instructed on an 1,800-calorie diet and lost 13 pounds between age 14 and 15 years, and weight decreased to the 50th percentile. The diet prescription was increased to 2,100 calories, and weight remained on the 50th percentile.

Despite substantial contrary opinion, there is evidence that the emotional state is more stable, and there is less depression and anxiety in juveniles (ages 12 to 18 yr) in good to excellent metabolic control than in those in poor metabolic control.[13]

Failure to grow is not a problem in those who develop IDDM after age 20 years (see Chapter 16), since they are fully grown when the disease becomes evident.

All diets for those with IDDM, regardless of age, should contain adequate calories, protein, vitamins, minerals, and trace elements to attain and maintain ideal body weight.

Epidemiology

The incidence of failure to attain maximal or nearmaximal height in children with IDDM has decreased in developed countries in recent decades, but it is still common [it is estimated that 30 to 50% of children fall 2 to 3 inches (5 to 7.5 cm) or more short of maximum growth potential]. Growth failure is more prevalent in underdeveloped countries because of protein-calorie malnutrition, inadequate medical care, and poor metabolic control. More data are needed to assess the prevalence, incidence, and degree of subnormal growth in both developed and underdeveloped countries.

Pathophysiology

Growth failure can occur as a result of inadequate calorie, protein, vitamin, mineral, or trace element intake. Normal growth occurs when an adequate diet is combined with normal levels of growth hormone, endogenous insulin, somatomedin activity [(insulin-like growth factors 1 and 2) (IGF 1 and 2)], and possibly other growth factors.[14] Thus adequate amounts of foods of high biologic value and optimal replacement of the endogenous insulin deficit by exogenous insulin are essential if the maximal growth potential of a child with IDDM is to be attained.

Problem Statement: Diet Therapy for Insulin-Dependent Diabetes Mellitus [Subsets: (1) Age 0 to 18 Years at Diagnosis, (2) Age > 18 Years at Diagnosis]

The objectives of diet therapy for IDDM are noted in Exhibit 15–1. Diet therapy is combined and coordinated with insulin therapy (see Chapter 18) and exercise therapy (see Chapter 17). Before prescribing the diet, the data base shown in Exhibit 15–2 (subjective, objective)

EXHIBIT 15–1   Objectives of Diet, Insulin, and Exercise Therapy for Insulin-Dependent Diabetes Mellitus

1. Minimize hyperglycemia and ketonemia, and avoid DKA and significant hypoglycemia
2. In those 0 to 18 years of age, attain and maintain normal rate of growth and maturation (see Figs. 15–1 and 15–2).
3. In those >18 years of age, attain and maintain IBW (see Fig. 15–3 and Table 16–1).

4. Prevent or delay the development or progression of renal, retinal, neurologic, cardiovascular, and other complications of IDDM.
5. Modify the diet prescription as indicated to include the constraints imposed by the complications of diabetes and by associated problems (see Exhibit 16–10).

Abbreviations: DKA, diabetic ketoacidosis; IBW, ideal body weight.

Figure 15-3. Example of a 25-year-old man who had polyuria, polydipsia, polyphagia, and weight loss of 36 pounds in a 6-month period.

Objective:
Fasting plasma glucose 450 mg/dL

Height	71 in., medium frame
Weight	136 pounds
Ideal body weight (Hamwi)[18]	172 pounds

Assessment

Estimated *basal* calories	1,720
Estimated *activity* calories	860
Estimated calories to gain about 2 pounds/week	1,000
Total calories	3,580

Plan: 3,580 cal/day to gain 36 pounds in 18 weeks

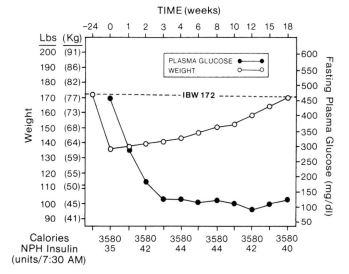

Calories	3580	3580	3580	3580	3580	3580
NPH Insulin (units/7:30 AM)	35	42	44	44	42	40

EXHIBIT 15–2   Data Base (Subjective, Objective) and Assessment of Nutritional Needs

I. *Subjective:* Birthweight and length; age at diagnosis and at present; growth rate (height, weight) before and after diagnosis, therapy [insulin: type(s), amount(s), time(s); diet: calories, protein, carbohydrate, fat, vitamins, minerals, trace elements, distribution into meals and snacks; exercise: type(s), amount(s), time(s)], height and weight of relatives (father, mother, siblings); school, work, and social activities, economic status, habits, history of complications (DKA, retinopathy, nephropathy, neuropathy, arteriopathy) and associated disease; emotional status (anxious, depressed, denial, locus of control, assertiveness)

II. Objective

A. *Physical examination:* weight (pounds or kilograms), height (inches or centimeters), frame (estimate from wrist circumference, finger size, elbow breadth, see Table 16–11), growth curves (height, weight), adiposity (estimate from skinfold thickness, palpation of abdomen and other parts of the body to estimate muscle mass and adiposity)

B. *Laboratory:* If ≤ 18 years old: wrist x-ray films (are epiphyses open or closed?), urine glucose, acetone, protein, hemoglobin A_{1c}, triglycerides, cholesterol, low-density lipoprotein, capillary basement membrane thickness

III. *Assessment*

A. *0 to 18 years old*

1. What is the estimated maximal growth potential? Estimate from length and weight at birth and height and weight of father and mother, and nondiabetic siblings of same sex.

2. Has linear growth velocity (NCHS growth curve) been subnormal (see Fig. 15–1), or normal? Has rate of weight gain been subnormal (see Fig. 15–1), normal, or greater than normal (see Fig. 15–2)? Is there a need for supplementary growth ("catch-up") calories, or for decreased calories to lose excess adiposity?

3. What is the estimated need for calories and protein (see Table 15–1), vitamins, minerals, and trace elements (see Table 15–2)?

4. Is metabolic control excellent, good, fair, or poor?

5. Should the insulin treatment routines and exercise pattern be changed? (See Chapters 17 and 18)

B. *≥ 18 years old:* What is the estimated ideal body weight (see Table 16–1)? Is patient underweight due to delayed diagnosis or poor control? Is there a need to change insulin treatment routine and/or exercise pattern? (see Chapters 17 and 18.)

Abbreviations: DKA, diabetic ketoacidosis; NCHS, National Center for Health Statistics.

---

should be collected and an assessment of the nutritional needs should be made. The initial plans for prescribing and for implementing diet therapy, and for educating the patient and family are noted in Exhibits 15–3 and 15–4, and Tables 15–1 through 15–4. Follow-up plans are noted in Exhibit 15–5.[15]

The American Dietetic Association introduced the term "medical nutrition therapy" (MNT)[21] primarily to encourage reimbursement for services that they render as members of the diabetes treatment team (MD, RN, RD, podiatrist, etc.) and to define those services for the third party payers. Many individuals with IDDM and NIDDM are unable to obtain needed services because third party payers are usually unwilling to provide them except occasionally on a very limited basis, or because they cannot afford them.

EXHIBIT 15–3   Initial Diet Therapy Plans for Insulin-Dependent Diabetes Mellitus

I. For those 0 to 18 years old
  A. Physician writes prescription for the diet
    1. Calories (see Table 15–1)
    2. Protein (g), carbohydrate (g), fat (g) (see Table 15–1, Exhibit 15–4); division into meals and snacks (see Table 15–4)
  B. Dietitian evaluates adequacy of nutrients in the prescription (see Tables 15–1 and 15–2), translates it into food exchanges (see Table 15–3), and divides exchanges into meals and snacks (see Table 15–4).
  C. If growth velocity is subnormal (poor metabolic control?, insufficient calories?) (see Fig. 15–1), increase calories ("catch-up calories") and adjust insulin administration routine and exercise pattern to attain and maintain normal growth velocity.
  D. If weight is abnormally high because of excess caloric intake (insulin-induced hypoglycemia?, nonadherence to diet?), reduce caloric intake so that weight returns to normal (see Fig. 15–2).
II. For those ≥ 18 years old
  A. If weight is ideal (see Exhibit 16–9) prescribe diet to maintain it (see Exhibit 16–9).
  B. If weight is below ideal, prescribe diet to attain and maintain IBW (see Fig. 15–3, Exhibit 16–9).
III. Initial education
  A. If the patient is <12 years old, the parent or guardian must assume primary responsibility for implementing the diet therapy plan. Most children ≥12 years old with parental support can assume more responsibility, and should be encouraged to do so (see section on adherence in this chapter). After independence is established and maturity is attained (>18 years old), primary responsibility rests with the patient.
  B. The patient and a responsible family member should be educated during the initial interview or shortly thereafter by the dietitian using *Diabetes Guidebook Diet Section*[17] or a similar publication. They should acquire a personal copy for continuing use at home and on return clinic visits. They should be taught how to measure food (see Exhibit 16–16), and should own a measuring cup, spoon, and ruler so that they can measure accurately the size of prescribed food servings. They should be taught how to read nutrition labels (see Table 16–7) and should memorize the referent exchanges (see Table 16–2), foods that should be avoided (see Exhibit 16–2), and foods that are allowed in reasonable amounts (see exhibit 16–3).
  C. Schoolteachers and coaches in athletic and physical exercise programs should be acquainted with the fact that the child has IDDM, and should share the responsibility for appropriate and regularly scheduled food intake during school hours and during school-related events involving exercise. Also, they should be prepared to recognize and treat hypoglycemia should it occur. If proper foods are not available in the school lunchroom, lunch (and snacks if needed) should be prepared at home and may be carried to school. As children mature and become independent, they can assume more responsibility for the regularity and consistency of food intake. This would include social snacks, meals with their peers, and food consumed during occasions such as evenings spent away from home and trips.

Abbreviations: IBW, ideal body weight; IDDM, insulin-dependent diabetes mellitus.

EXHIBIT 15–4   Calculation of Carbohydrate and Fat Intake for Those 0 to 18 Years of Age

After the estimated need of total calories and protein have been calculated (see Table 15–1), the estimated carbohydrate and fat intake may be calculated as follows:
  1. Protein (g) × 4 = protein calories
  2. Total calories minus protein calories = nonprotein calories; nonprotein calories to be divided between carbohydrate (4 cal/g) and fat (9 cal/g)
Example: A 14-year-old boy growing normally on the NCHS 50th percentile is 64.5 in. (164 cm) tall and weighs 112 pounds (51 kg). You estimate his caloric need as 2,700 calories, his minimal protein requirement as 0.45 g/pound (1 g/kg), or 51 g protein, which equals 204 calories (or about 8% of the total calories). 2,700 calories minus 204 calories = 2,496 nonprotein calories (or about 92% of the total calories). You may decide to prescribe more protein than the NRC Food and Nutrition Board recommends (see Table 15–1),in which case the additional protein calories should be subtracted from the calories allotted to carbohydrate and fat. If not, you may decide to divide the 2,496 nonprotein calories as follows: two thirds to carbohydrate (then 62% of the total calories would be carbohydrate), and one third to fat (then 30% of the total calories would be fat). Then the diet would contain 1,660 carbohydrate calories (415 g), 828 fat calories (92 g), and 204 protein calories (51 g), for a total of 2,692 calories. Of course, the diet prescription should not only meet the patient's minimal nutritional needs, it should be adjusted to his food likes and dislikes and life-style to the greatest extent possible. For example, you learn in the initial interview that the 14-year-old cited above likes meat, so you decide in consultation with the dietitian to increase the protein in his diet prescription from 51 g (8% of total calories) to 136 g (21% of total calories), and reduce his carbohydrate allowance to 338 g (49% of total calories), and leave his fat allowance at 90 g (30% of total calories). See Table 15–4. You complete the prescription by dividing the food exchanges into three meals and two snacks (20% breakfast, 30% lunch, 10% 3:30 P.M. snack, 30% supper, and 10% bedtime snack), and the dietitian translates the prescription into food servings. See Table 15–4.

Abbreviations: NCHS, National Center for Health Statistics; NRC, National Research Council.

TABLE 15–1   Caloric and Protein Requirements for Infants and Children

Age (years)	Caloric Needs[a]		Protein (g)
	Mean	Range	
0.0–0.5	Pounds × 52 (kg × 115)	95–145	Pounds × 1.0 (kg × 2.2)
0.5–1.0	Pounds × 47.7 (kg × 105)	80–135	Pounds × 0.9 (kg × 2.0)
1–3	1,300	900–1,800	Pounds × 0.8 (kg × 1.7)
4–6	1,700	1,300–2,300	Pounds × 0.7 (kg × 1.5)
7–10	2,400	1,650–3,300	Pounds × 0.5 (kg × 1.2)
11–14 M	2,700	2,000–3,700	Pounds × 0.45 (kg × 1.0)
F	2,200	1,500–3,000	Pounds × 0.45 (kg × 1.0)
15–18 M	2,800	2,100–3,900	Pounds × 0.36 (kg × 0.8)
F	2,100	1,200–3,000	Pounds × 0.38 (kg × 0.8)

[a] Caloric needs for children are based on medium intakes of children through age 18, followed in longitudinal growth studies. The caloric range represents the 10th through 90th percentiles of caloric consumption among children of these ages. [*Source:* Recommended Dietary Allowances 1989, Ed. 10. Washington DC: Food and Nutrition Board, National Research Council, National Academy of Sciences.[10] With permission.]

Adherence (or Lack of Adherence) to Diet Therapy

Thorough education and intensive follow-up of the patient (and involved family members) increases motivation, improves therapeutic adherence, and reduces long-term morbidity and mortality.[7,16,17] Socioeconomic stress (poverty and lack of access to good medical care), lack of family understanding and support, and lack of peer understanding and support can decrease therapeutic adherence. Continuing access to a knowledgeable health care team [MD, registered dietitian (RD), RN], a stable family setting that develops self-esteem, self-reliance, and independence, and supportive and knowledgeable peers (with and without IDDM) who encourage self-assertiveness during social events and during "rap" and camping sessions, will increase therapeutic adherence.

The physician, nurse, and dietitian can provide continuing support and education by appropriate monitoring of the level of metabolic control and updating therapeutic recommendations at regular intervals. They should maintain an atmosphere of friendly good humor and communicate candidly and confidentially with adolescents who have IDDM and who are reaching for maturity and emerging adulthood. Family dynamics are very important and should be followed carefully. Is there marital conflict? Sibling conflict? Are the parents consumed by their concern for the child's health? Are parents overindulgent? Overprotective? Sometimes a history obtained from someone outside

the family (teacher, minister, and so forth) may be helpful. Is there a history of accidents, sexual activity, or use of alcohol, drugs, or tobacco? Is the individual's school performance satisfactory? Are peer relationships good? The adolescent usually rejects some and possibly all of his parent's values as he moves toward independence. Do the parents and the patient understand this aspect of development, and the stresses it may create in family relationships? Does the adolescent like being around home, or does he prefer to be in school or in friends' homes? Why? Are there any somatic or emotional complaints that suggest a depressive reaction? If so, the physician should suspect that suicide is a possibility, and should take immediate and appropriate action to prevent it.

All of the influences noted above may contribute to an adolescent's level of adherence (or lack of adherence) to prescribed diet therapy.

The DCCT study[19,20] which was conducted by a team of professionals (MD, RN, RD, and others) utilized intensive insulin therapy (3-4 injections per day) or continuous subcutaneous insulin infusion to keep blood glucose levels (self blood glucose monitoring 4-8 times per day) as near normal as possible to show that "tight blood glucose control" was more effective than "conventional blood glucose control" in preventing or slowing the progression of the chronic complications of IDDM (retinopathy, nephropathy, neuropathy, etc.) It seems reasonable to conclude that dietitians made a significant contribution to this favorable outcome.

For 65 years there has been a small number of physicians that have advocated no dietary restrictions in the

TABLE 15–2 Food and Nutrition Board, National Academy of Sciences—National Research Council Recommended Dietary Allowances,[a] Revised 1989

Category	Age (years) or Condition	Weight[b] kg	Weight[b] lb	Height[b] cm	Height[b] in	Protein (g)	Fat-Soluble Vitamins Vita-min A (µg RE)[c]	Vita-min D (µg)[d]	Vita-min E (mg α·TE)[e]	Vita-min K (µg)	Water-Soluble Vitamins Vita-min C (mg)	Thia-min (mg)	Ribo-flavin (mg)	Niacin (mg NE)[f]	Vita-min B6 (mg)	Folate (µg)	Vita-min B12 (µg)	Minerals Cal-cium (mg)	Phos-phorus (mg)	Mag-nesium (mg)	Iron (mg)	Zinc (mg)	Iodine (µg)	Sele-nium (µg)
Infants	0.0–0.5	6	13	60	24	13	375	7.5	3	5	30	0.3	0.4	5	0.3	25	0.3	400	300	40	6	5	40	10
	0.5–1.0	9	20	71	28	14	375	10	4	10	35	0.4	0.5	6	0.6	35	0.5	600	500	60	10	5	50	15
Children	1–3	13	29	90	35	16	400	10	6	15	40	0.7	0.8	9	1.0	50	0.7	800	800	80	10	10	70	20
	4–6	20	44	112	44	24	500	10	7	20	45	0.9	1.1	12	1.1	75	1.0	800	800	120	10	10	90	20
	7–10	28	62	132	52	28	700	10	7	30	45	1.0	1.2	13	1.4	100	1.4	800	800	170	10	10	120	30
Males	11–14	45	99	157	62	45	1,000	10	10	45	50	1.3	1.5	17	1.7	150	2.0	1,200	1,200	270	12	15	150	40
	15–18	66	145	176	69	59	1,000	10	10	65	60	1.5	1.8	20	2.0	200	2.0	1,200	1,200	400	12	15	150	50
Females	11–14	46	101	157	62	46	800	10	8	45	50	1.1	1.3	15	1.4	150	2.0	1,200	1,200	280	15	12	150	45
	15–18	55	120	163	64	44	800	10	8	55	60	1.1	1.3	15	1.5	180	2.0	1,200	1,200	300	15	12	150	50

[a] The allowances, expressed as average daily intakes over time, are intended to provide for individual variations among most normal persons as they live in the United States under usual environmental stresses. Diets should be based on a variety of common foods in order to provide other nutrients for which human requirements have been less well defined. Designed for the maintenance of good nutrition of practically all healthy people in the United States.

[b] The median weights and heights of those under 19 years of age were taken from Hamill et al. (1979). The use of these figures does not imply that the height-to-weight ratios are ideal.

[c] Retinol equivalents. 1 retinol equivalent = 1 µg retinol or 6 µg β-carotene.

[d] As cholecalciferol. 10 µg cholecalciferol = 400 IU of vitamin D.

[e] α-Tocopherol equivalents. 1 mg d-α tocopherol = 1 α-TE.

[f] NE (niacin equivalent) is equal to 1 mg of niacin or 60 mg of dietary tryptophan.

Summary Table: Estimated Safe and Adequate Daily Dietary Intakes of Selected Vitamins and Minerals[a]

Category	Age (years)	Vitamins Biotin (µg)	Pantothenic Acid (mg)	Trace Elements Copper (mg)	Manganese (mg)	Fluoride (mg)	Chromium (µg)	Molybdenum (µg)
Infants	0–0.5	10	2	0.4–0.6	0.3–0.6	0.1–0.5	10–40	15–30
	0.5–1	15	3	0.6–0.7	0.6–1.0	0.2–1.0	20–60	20–40
Children and adolescents	1–3	20	3	0.7–1.0	1.0–1.5	0.5–1.5	20–80	25–50
	4–6	25	3–4	1.0–1.5	1.5–2.0	1.0–2.5	30–120	30–75
	7–10	30	4–5	1.0–2.0	2.0–3.0	1.5–2.5	50–200	50–150
	11+	30–100	4–7	1.5–2.5	2.0–5.0	1.5–2.5	50–200	75–250

[a] Because there is less information on which to base allowances, these figures are not given in the main table of RDA and are provided here in the form of ranges of recommended intakes.

[b] Since the toxic levels for many trace elements may be only several times usual intakes, the upper levels for the trace elements given in this table should not be habitually exceeded. [Source: Recommended Dietary Allowances, Ed 10. Washington, DC: Food and Nutrition Board, National Research Council, National Academy of Sciences, 1989. With permission.]

TABLE 15–3   Diet Prescription: 2,700 Calories—136g Protein, 338g Carbohydrate, 90g Fat, Divided 0.2, 0.3, 0.1, 0.3, 0.1[a]

Exchange Group	No. Exchanges	Carbohydrate (g)	Protein (g)	Fat (g)
Starch/bread	11	165	33	11
Meat (medium fat)	9	—	63	45
Vegetables	4	20	8	—
Fruit	7	105	—	—
Milk (skim)	4	48	32	4
Fat	6	—	—	30
Total		338	136	90

[a] Twenty percent breakfast (0.2), 30% lunch (0.3), 10% 3:30 p.m. snack (0.1), 30% supper (0.3), and 10% bedtime snack (0.1). See table 15–4.

treatment of IDDM.[22,23] *Clearly the inordinate difficulties in weighing food, or even of selecting items for rigidly restricted diets, should not be tolerated by patients or professionals in 1998.* Yet families with growing diabetic youngsters need to understand and utilize appropriate diet so that normal growth will occur and complications will be prevented or delayed. *It has become possible to relax dietary restrictions*[24,25] because of the availability of blood glucose monitors, multiple-injection insulin routines, rapid-acting insulins (lispro, etc.), and continuous subcutaneous insulin infusion (CSII). Learning and practicing good principles of nutrition should not be abandoned, however, because the success of the DCCT "tight control" group in minimizing both hyperglycemia and hypoglycemia was due at least in part to the practice of appropriate meal planning and consumption.[20]

Process and Outcome Audits

IDDM is a relatively distinct subset of diabetes mellitus. In order to define more precisely its natural history, morbidity, and mortality, and to monitor and evaluate the outcomes of different approaches to diet therapy and their cost-effectiveness, it will be necessary to collect and analyze morbidity and mortality data at regular intervals in the population of patients who have the disease. For example, the consequences of "loose" versus "tight" control of plasma glucose levels for the subsequent development of microangiopathy (retinopathy, nephropathy) and macroangiopathy in those with IDDM are unknown. Although there is continuing controversy in this area, most diabetologists attempt to attain and maintain the best attainable individual metabolic control (growth curves, hemoglobin A_{1c} levels, and a satisfactory range of plasma glucose levels over time) with diet, exercise, and insulin therapy.[16,17] Systematic audits permit the physician, dietitian, and nurse to identify deficiencies in patient and family education and behavior, and to act promptly to modify the strategy and processes of care and follow-up as needed.[19,20]

Research Considerations

Although much epidemiologic, biochemical, and pathophysiologic research has been completed, more is needed. This includes demographic, genetic, and environmental factors (especially viruses and autoimmune processes) that are related to the development of IDDM. More information is needed on the substrate,

TABLE 15–4   Distribution of Exchanges from Table 15–3 into Meals and Snacks

Exchanges	Breakfast	Lunch	Afternoon Snack	Supper	Bedtime Snack	Total No. Exchanges	Total Calories
Starch/bread	3	3	1	3	1	11	891
Meat (medium fat)	2	2	1	3	1	9	657
Vegetables		2		2		4	112
Fruit	1	2	1	2	1	7	420
Milk (skim)	1	1	$\frac{1}{2}$	1	$\frac{1}{2}$	4	356
Fat	2	2		2		6	270

EXHIBIT 15–5   Follow-up Diet Therapy for Insulin-Dependent Diabetes Mellitus for Those 0 to 18 Years Old

1. Record height and weight every 3 to 6 months (see Figs. 15–1 and 15–2).
2. Revise calories and protein intake to sustain normal growth velocity (see Table 15–1, Fig. 15–1) and to avoid excess adiposity, especially in teenage girls (see Fig. 15–2).
3. If a honeymoon period develops, adjust insulin dose to avoid hypoglycemia.[4]

4. Adjust meals and snacks to accommodate variable exercise patterns and to avoid hypoglycemia (20 to 40 g carbohydrate before nonroutine vigorous exercise and 10 to 15 g at hourly intervals during prolonged exercise—determine for each individual and each type of exercise).

hormone, somatomedin activity (IGF 1 and IGF 2) and receptor perturbations of IDDM, and how dietary components (different types and amounts of carbohydrates, proteins, and fats) relate to these perturbations and their consequences (chronic complications) during long-term follow-up.

What is "normal growth" for various sexes, races, national, and ethnic groups? How do food availability and socioeconomic status affect growth? How do insulin, growth hormone, and IGF 1 and 2 interrelate in determining growth velocity? Is it appropriate to relax dietary restraints for those on CSII therapy? What are the psychologic effects of various types of diets? How do patient and family psychodynamics influence adherence and how can they be altered to minimize nonadherent behavior? Is carbohydrate, protein, or a mixture of the two more effective in preventing insulin-induced hypoglycemia, or is timed consistency of food (especially complex carbohydrate) intake more important?

References

1. Banting FG, Best CH, Collip JB, et al.: The effect produced on diabetes by extracts of pancreas. Trans Assoc Am Phys 31:1–11, 1922.

2. Wagner R, White P, Bogan I: Diabetic dwarfism. Am J Dis Child 63:667, 1942.

3. Jackson RL, Kelly HG: Growth charts for use in pediatric practice. J Pediatr 27:215–229, 1945.

4. Jackson RL, Kelly HG: Growth of children with diabetes mellitus in relationship to level of control of the disease. J Pediatr 29:316, 1946.

5. Guest CM: The Mauriac syndrome: dwarfism, hepatomegaly, and obesity with juvenile diabetes mellitus. Diabetes 2:415, 1953.

6. National Center for Health Statistics Growth Charts, 1976: National Center for Health Statistics: Monthly Vital Statistics Report 25(3) [suppl (HRA) 76-1120]. Rockville, MD: Health Resources Administration, 1976.

7. Jackson RL, Holland E, Chatman ID, et al.: Growth and maturation of children with insulin-dependent diabetes mellitus. Diabetes Care 1:96–107, 1978.

8. Tattersall RB, Pyke DA: Growth in diabetic children: studies in identical twins. Lancet 2:1105, 1973.

9. Rudolph MCJ, Sherwin RS, Markowitz R, et al.: Effect of intensive insulin treatment on linear growth in the young diabetic patient. J Pediatr 101:333–339, 1982.

10. Recommended Dietary Allowances 1989, Ed. 10. Washington, DC: Food and Nutrition Board, National Research Council, National Academy of Sciences.

11. Meredith HV: Change in the stature and body weight of North American boys during the last 80 years. In Lipsett LP, Spiker CC (eds): Advances in Child Development and Behavior, vol. 1, New York: Academic Press, 1963, pp. 69–114.

12. Orinvolsky M, Nathan DM: Diets for insulin pump and multiple injection therapy. Diabetes Care 6:241–244, 1983.

13. Simonds JF: Psychiatric status of diabetic youth matched with a control group. Diabetes 26:921–925, 1977.

14. Phillips LS, Unterman TG: Somatomedin activity in disorders of nutrition and metabolism. Clin Endocrinol Metab 13:145–189, 1984.

15. Deckert T: The influence of supervision and endogenous insulin secretion on the course of insulin dependent diabetes mellitus. Acta Endocrinol 94 (suppl 238):31–38, 1980.

16. Molnar GD: Clinical evaluation of metabolic control in diabetes. Diabetes 27 (suppl 1):216–225, 1978.

17. Davidson JK, Goldsmith MP: Diabetes Guidebook: Diet Section, Ed. 4. Davicone, Inc., 1075 Lullwater Rd NE, Atlanta, GA 30307–1243, 1984.

18. Hamwi GJ. Therapy: changing dietary concepts. In Danowski TS (ed): Diabetes Mellitus: Diagnosis and Treatment, Vol. 1. New York: American Diabetes Association, 1964, pp. 73–78.

19. The Diabetes Control and Complications Trial Research Group: "The Effect of Intensive Treatment of Diabetes on the Development and Progression of Long-Term Complications in Insulin-Dependent Diabetes Mellitus." New Engl. J. Med 329:977–986, 1993.

20. The DCCT Research Group: Expanded role of the Dietitian in the Diabetes Control and Complications Trial: Implications for Clinical Practice. J Am Diet Assoc. 93:758–764, 1993.

21. American Diabetic Association's definition for nutrition screening and nutrition assessment. J Am Dietetic Association 94:838–839, 1994.

22. Stolte K. "Freie Diät biem Diabetes." Med Klinik 29:288–289, 1933.

23. Knowles H, Guest GM, Lampe J, et al. "The Course Of Juvenile Diabetes Treated with Unmeasured Diets." Diabetes 14:239–273, 1965.

24. Slama G, Haardt MJ, Jean-Joseph P, et al. Sucrose taken during mixed meal has no additional hyperglycemic effect over isocaloric amounts of starch in well-controlled diabetics. Lancet II:122–125, 1984.

25. Mulhauser I, Bott U, Overmann H, et al. Liberalized Diet in Patients with Type One Diabetes. J Int. Med 237:591–597, 1995.

16

Diet Therapy for Non-Insulin-Dependent (Type 2) Diabetes Mellitus

John K. Davidson

Historical Perspective

Aretaeus of Cappadocia (81–138 AD) recommended that diabetes be treated with milk, cereal, starch, fruit, and wine.

Seventeen centuries later, the English physician Rollo (1796)[1] was consulted by a "corpulent" Captain Meredith, who was 34 years old, had had symptoms of diabetes for 7 months, and was known among his fellow officers as a man with a ravenous appetite. Rollo found that he had glucosuria and started treatment with bleeding and an unpalatable diet containing milk, lime water, blood pudding and suet, rancid old game, pork, fats including butter, and small amounts of bread. When the urine became sugar-free, the diet was changed to include cabbage, lettuce, boiled onions, and radishes. Meredith became asymptomatic and aglucosuric and resumed his military career. Rollo was not only aware of the importance of stringently restricting food intake, he was also aware of the importance of modifying patient behavior concerning food intake patterns in order to "remove the disease, and the disposition to it."

Bernard (1848)[2] developed the hypothesis that *glucose overproduction* by the liver caused diabetes. Bouchardat (1871–1883), after observing the effects of starvation during the siege of Paris during the Franco-Prussian war, modified the Rollo diet by objecting to its rancidity; by substituting fats and alcohol for carbohydrates, and by individualizing diet therapy for each patient. The bread that he allowed had to be charred almost to a cinder before it was eaten. He started the use of fast days and showed the value of the intelligent use of exercise. He told a patient who asked for bread, "You shall earn your bread by the sweat of your brow."

Somewhat later, Cantani limited daily food intake to about 1 pound of cooked meat. If glucosuria persisted, he fasted patients. The treatment continued for 3 months, and if the patient was not then aglucosuric, it was extended to 6 or 9 months. He frequently put patients in locked rooms to be certain they adhered to the prescribed diet.

Von Noorden (1895) noted that a high-carbohydrate diet suppressed ketosis and prescribed a diet consisting principally of oatmeal. Naunyn (1899) developed the hypothesis that *glucose underutilization* caused diabetes. He prescribed a carbohydrate-free (high-fat) diet, and noted that it decreased glucosuria.

Various dietary schools quickly developed, and by the beginning of the 20th century their respective adherents were embroiled in heated controversies reflecting their dogmatism, contradiction, and confusion. Cantani and his German follower, Naunyn, championed carbohydrate-free diets, while those on the other extreme championed high-carbohydrate diets variously consisting of milk, oatmeal and other cereals, potatoes, and a number of other foods containing largely carbohydrates. By the early part of the 20th century, diet partisanship was so intense that some physicians were arguing the relative merits of different brands of oatmeal and the various ways of cooking them. As these controversies boiled, Naunyn gradually swung away from the Cantani school and developed diets that were more closely keyed to the needs and tolerances of individual patients, but he recognized the value of fast days and continued to use them. Von Noorden labeled these fast days "metabolic Sundays," thus endowing them with an aura of religious self-denial. Efforts to change deeply ingrained eating habits have continued to the present day in lay groups that operate under names such as Weight Watchers, Take Off Pounds Sensibly, Overeaters Anonymous, and Counting Calories for Christ. All of these groups try to curb excessive food intake by modifying patient behavior through response to education, self-restraint, and peer pressure.

Guelpa (1910) reported the effectiveness of 3- to 5-day fast periods alternating with 7- to 10-day periods of restricting food intake to no more than $2\frac{1}{2}$ pints of milk per day. This therapy resulted in marked weight loss, with many patients becoming emaciated and most becoming aglucosuric. An extension of the Guelpa semistarvation treatment was the Allen diet, developed during the second decade of this century by F. M. Allen (1919)[3] at the Rockefeller Institute for Medical Research. The Allen diet typically consisted of an initial 7-day fast, followed by caloric restriction for 9 days, with caloric intake rising from 64 on the first day to 504 on the 9th, a fast on the 10th day, 151 calories on the 11th, and an incremental increase in caloric intake to 1,031 on the 34th day, with the 17th, 24th, and 31st being fast days. After considerable weight loss, the urine usually became sugar-free, and the patient was discharged on a maintenance diet with a fast day (usually Sunday) every 2 weeks to "atone for any chance indiscretions." Allen encouraged patients to use foods that contained bulk but no calories, including calorie-free fluids, bran muffins, and coarse bran flakes commonly used in cattle feed.

Although Allen recognized that death from starvation was possible, Joslin (1923)[4] showed that such deaths were less common than were those from diabetic coma. Joslin prescribed and taught a restricted *weighed* diet (including short periods of fasting) for both the diabetic ketoacidosis (DKA)-prone and the non-DKA-prone. The experience of the Joslin Clinic was analyzed by Marks, a medical statistician of the Metropolitan Life Insurance Company, who found that life expectancy increased from the Naunyn diet era (1897–1914) to the Allen diet era (1914–1922) as follows: (1) from 1.3 to 2.6 years for the 10-year-old diabetic, (2) from 2.1 to 4.0 years for the 25-year-old diabetic, and (3) from 8.5 to 10.5 years for the 45-year-old diabetic.

Paullin (1922) was the first to demonstrate that abnormal glucose tolerance tests were common in those who were obese.

The science of metabolism was born in the late 18th century (1792) when Lavoisier, the father of modern chemistry, and LaPlace, a physicist, showed that "animal heat" resulted from the oxidation of carbon and hydrogen in the body, and that the amount of heat generated paralleled the quantity of carbon dioxide eliminated. Since that time, research in the basic sciences has converged with and has influenced profoundly the development and progress of clinical medicine. Prout (1834) developed the modern view that the three components of natural foods (albuminous or protein, saccharine or carbohydrate, and oleagins or fat) are essential in the animal diet, and Liebig (1842) established that it was not carbon and hydrogen that the body burned, but carbohydrate and fat.

Mayer (1844) published his revolutionary theory of heat together with his views on the *conservation of energy* [the sum total of energy in the universe remains constant but any one form (potential, mechanical, thermal, chemical, electrical) may be converted into another] and von Helmholtz (1845) formulated mathematically the Law of Conservation of Energy (the First Law of Thermodynamics).

Between 1850 and 1920, the heat of combustion of various foodstuffs was measured in the bomb calorimeter, and Pettenhoffer, Voit, Rubner, Atwater, Rosa, Benedict, and others, demonstrated that energy balance was maintained during the chemical interconversions of edible foods during animal metabolism.[5,6] Heat production (measured by direct calorimetry) was equivalent to consumption of oxygen and to production of carbon dioxide during respiratory exchange (indirect calorimetry). Dubois (1936)[7] and colleagues extended these concepts by measuring catabolic expenditure during the *basal metabolic state*, during *exercise*, at different environmental temperatures, and in various disease states.

The energy value of foods and the energy expenditure of the body are measured by *calories*. Initially, the metabolic *calorie* (as it related to biologic systems) was written with a capital "C" to designate a kilogram Calorie or a kilocalorie (still called a large Calorie, 1,000 small calories, a kilogram calorie, or a kilocalorie by some writers). A Calorie is the amount of heat expended to raise the temperature of 1 kg of water 1°C (from 15° to 16°C) at normal atmospheric pressure. By common usage, the large "C" has been dropped, and in this discussion, a *calorie* with a lower-case "c" is defined as a kilogram calorie, a large calorie, or a kilocalorie. The calorie (energy) content of foods has been shown to be: (1) for carbohydrates, about 4 cal/g, (2) for proteins, about 4 cal/g, (3) for fat, about 9 cal/g, and (4) for alcohol, about 7 cal/g. The calorie content for body tissues is: (1) for muscle, which contains about 75% water, about 400 cal/pound (about 880 cal/kg); (2) for fat, which contains about 15% water and fibrous tissue, about 3,500 cal/pound (about 7,700 cal/kg).

The modern science of nutrition deals with (1) the composition and energy content (calories), protein content (amino acids), and mineral and trace element contents of foods; (2) the requirements of these materials (kinds and amounts) by the growing and mature animal to prevent nutritional disease and to maintain health; and (3) the choice of foods that will meet these needs. Dietary intake of a number of substances that the body cannot manufacture from materials ordinarily available to sustain normal growth and adult health have been identified: (1) eight amino acids (isoleucine, leucine, lysine, methionine, phenylalanine, threonine, tryptophane, and valine) are essential in adults and children, and two others (arginine and histidine) are essential in growing children;[8] (2) vitamins; (3) minerals; and (4) trace elements. It was hypothesized by Hopkins (1912) that "accessory food factors, which cannot be made by the body, are needed to catalyze enzymatic reactions." Hawkins (1593) showed that oranges and lemons prevented scurvy in sailors, and Funk (1912) identified an antiberiberi substance (thiamine) in rice bran. Goldberger (1927) identified an antipellagra substance (niacin). By the mid-1950s, water-soluble and fat-soluble vitamins had been identified, characterized, and synthesized.[9] See Table 16–6 for 1989 Recommended Dietary Allowances (RDA) of vitamins, minerals, and trace elements.[10] Essential fatty acids may be mobilized from fat stores in overweight individuals and need not be ingested during weight reduction therapy.

The American Diabetes Association recommended in 1971 that the complex carbohydrate content of the diet be liberalized[11] and experts suggest carbohydrate comprise 55 to 60% of total calories (Exhibit 16–1).[12] The 1977–1978 Department of Agriculture reports that per capita consumption of sugars in the United States accounts for 48% of carbohydrate and 21% of total calorie intake.[13] Today, the major controversy over consumption of carbohydrate for people with diabetes is the type of carbohydrate—complex versus simple. Traditionally, simple sugars were avoided in the diet. Crapo was one of the first to test the physiologic effect of certain carbohydrate foods and found that their chemical composition did not match the expected metabolic response.[14] In fact, simple carbohydrate can no longer be distinguished as a separate group. *This has resulted in a relaxing of the rules prohibiting sucrose in the diet to allow modest amounts contingent on metabolic control.*[12] Fructose has been evaluated as a possible sweet-

ener for people with diabetes and although fructose does not worsen glycemic control, it may cause adverse effects on serum lipids, postprandial serum lactate, and rate of nonenzymatic glycosylation of proteins.[15] Also, most foods high in refined carbohydrate are also high in fat and calories and for overweight patients these foods should be avoided. The noncaloric sweetners (saccharin, aspartame and acelsulfame-K) can be used with no adverse effect on metabolic control.

Controversy continues on the daily protein requirement of otherwise healthy adults. Chittenden[16] showed that 25 g or less of high-quality protein (egg albumin, milk) maintained nitrogen equilibrium (intake = output) for several months. The Food and Agriculture Organization (FAO) and the World Health Organization (WHO) report (1975) recommended that protein allowance be based on a requirement of 0.35 g/kg of body weight per day to meet the needs of most adults. Some recommend an allowance of 0.6 g/kg/day of high quality protein. After correcting for 75% efficiency of utilization of protein in a mixed diet, the allowance for protein in the United States (1980) became 0.8 g/kg of body weight per day. This translates into 56 g for a 70 kg male and 44 g for a 55 kg female. A more generous allowance is recommended for pregnant women (add 30 g/day) and for lactating women (add 20 g/day). In growing children the allowances decrease gradually from 2.0 g/kg at ages 0.5 to 1 year to 0.8 g/kg at age 18 years.[10] Adults with protein depletion associated with acute or chronic illnesses add enough protein

---

EXHIBIT 16–1 Target Nutrition Goals for People With Diabetes[a,b]

Calories
Sufficient to achieve and maintain reasonable weight

Carbohydrate
May be up to 55–60% of total calories. Liberalized; individualized; emphasis on unrefined carbohydrate with fiber; modest amounts of sucrose and other refined sugars may be acceptable contingent on metabolic control

Protein
Usual intake of protein in most Americans is double the amount needed; exact ideal percentage of total calories is unknown. Usual recommendation for people with diabetes is 12–20% of total calories. Recommended daily allowance is 0.8 g/kg body weight for adults; intake is modified for children, pregnant and lactating women, the aged, and individuals with special medical conditions, e.g., renal complications

Fiber
Up to 40 g/day; 25 g/1000 kcal for low calorie intakes

Fat
Ideally <30% of total calories. However, this needs to be individualized because 30% may be unachievable for some individuals
Polyunsaturated fats, up to 10%
Saturated fats, <10%
Monounsaturated fats, remaining percentage (10–15%)

Cholesterol
<300 mg/day

Alternative sweeteners
Use is acceptable

Sodium
Not to exceed 3,000 mg/day; modified for special medical conditions

Alcohol
Occasional use; limit to 1–2 alcohol equivalents 1–2 times/wk

Vitamins/minerals
No evidence that diabetes causes increased need

[a] Each goal needs to be individualized. The above goals should serve as a guide for establishing short- and long-term goals. See individual sections for further discussion.

[b] Adapted from American Diabetes Association: Nutritional Recommendations and Principles for Individuals with Diabetes Mellitus: 1986 (Position Statement). Diabetes Care 10:126–132, 1987.

to sustain positive nitrogen balance. Some investigators recommend a minimum intake of high-quality protein of 0.5 g/pound (1.1 g/kg) per day. See Exhibit 16–10. This level appears to be generous. However, there is no convincing evi-dence that a generous intake of protein (up to 1 g/pound/day, 2.2 g/kg/day) is harmful in healthy adults.[10] The target nutrition goal for protein for people with diabetes is 0.8 g/kg/day for adults subject to modification for children, pregnant and lactating women, the aged, and individuals with special medical conditions, such as renal complications.[12] (See Exhibit 16–1). Some investigators have shown results that suggest that a low protein diet in early renal changes may delay progression of renal disease.

In The Diabetes Control and Complications Trial (DCCT), intensive therapy with "tight control" of the plasma glucose level reduced the occurrence of microalbuminuria (30-300 mg/24 hr) 39% and of gross albuminuria (>300 mg/24 hr) by 54% in comparison to the "conventional control" group.[17]

The understanding of undernutrition and its consequences (calorie deficiency with starvation and death,[18] protein or vitamin or mineral deficiencies with development of various nutritional deficiency states) and overnutrition and its consequences (obesity, diabetes, hypertension, hyperlipidemia, premature atherosclerosis with vascular occlusion and death)[19,20] has expanded and matured during the last four decades.

The concept of *lean body mass* was introduced by Behnke (1953)[21] as a hypothetical fat-free body with a relatively fixed composition. He proposed that this artificial entity contained 15% bone, 75% tissue (primarily muscle, skin, and other organs), and 10% essential fat (but he later revised the essential fat content downward to 2%). Fat has a specific gravity of 0.90, bone 1.56, and other tissue 1.06. If the body specific gravity is measured (by underwater weighing), the fat mass and lean body mass can be estimated. For instance, if the body specific gravity is 1.10, the lean body mass is about 100% and the fat mass about 0%, whereas if the body specific gravity is 1.00, the lean body mass is about 50%, and the fat mass about 50%. A hypothetical female weighing 180 pounds, with about 50% body fat would have about 315,000 calories stored in her adipose tissue, of which at least 280,000 calories (80 pounds) would be excess storage calories. This excess fat increases her risk of developing non-insulin-dependent diabetes mellitus (NIDDM).

Nutritional science has reached a level of sophistication that permits effective therapeutic modalities to be applied to prevent and to cure disorders related not only to undernutrition, but to disorders related to caloric overnutrition as well.

After the initial clinical use of insulin (1922), it became apparent that the hormone could prevent death from diabetic coma. For some years after its discovery, insulin therapy was looked on as a "cure" for diabetes; many prominent physicians felt that by attaining and maintaining normoglycemia one could prevent the acute complications, and, very likely, the chronic complications as well. Thus, the therapeutic desideratum of normoglycemia became firmly entrenched.

Himsworth (1936)[22] reported that those with diabetes at time of diagnosis had consumed more calories and fat than a similar group of individuals without diabetes. Newburgh (1942)[23] demonstrated that therapeutically induced weight loss, in those who were obese and had diabetes, frequently caused the glucose tolerance test to revert to normal. In 1944,[24] he reported that when compared to the mortality rate of those at normal weight, the death rate for those 50 pounds overweight was 56% greater and for those 90 pounds overweight was 116% greater.

Meanwhile, with the widespread use of insulin, the dogmas of carbohydrate and caloric restriction and starvation were progressively relaxed so that by 1950 many physicians, led by Tolstoi (1950),[25] had essentially discarded diet therapy and encouraged patients to eat a "normal" or "free" diet. Interestingly enough, Tolstoi still recommended that obese patients lose weight, but he condemned the weighed (Joslin) diet as "unendurable self-deprivation and punishment of patients by die-hard physicians."

In 1950, the American Diabetes Association and the American Dietetic Association introduced a list of *food exchanges* as a compromise between weighed (Joslin) diets and "free" (Tolstoi) diets.

Two classes of drugs that could be swallowed rather than injected (as was the case with insulin) were marketed in the 1950s: sulfonylureas in 1955 (Franks and coworkers), and biguanides (phenformin) in 1957 (Shapiro and associates). These therapeutic modalities of convenience were widely used until the University Group Diabetes Program Reports (1970–1971) questioned their safety and effectiveness. In 1977 phenformin was removed from the market in the United States as an imminent hazard to the public's health because of hundreds of reported lactic acidosis-related deaths. From 1974 to 1983, the sale of sulfonylureas in the United States dropped by more than 50% (see Chapter 20).

However, in 1984, the second-generation sulfonylureas glyburide and glipizide were approved by the Food and Drug Administration (FDA), creating a resurgent use of the oral hypoglycemic agents. In 1986, the oral hypoglycemics accounted for 21.5 million prescriptions, approximately 1% of all prescription drugs dispensed that year.[26] These new drugs are more potent than the original products and most have a longer duration of action. However, the greater effectiveness of the second-generation over the first-generation drugs has not been established. According to available data, 10 to 15% of patients respond to sulfonylureas.[27] Oral agents must not be used as a substitute for reduced caloric intake and weight loss (See Chapter 20).

Bloom (1958) reintroduced total fasting (1 to 6 days) as a therapeutic modality for obesity, and Duncan (1960) used it to treat those with diabetes who were obese. Stone and colleagues (1961–1963)[28] showed that dietary nonadherence rather than failure to take insulin usually was responsible for poor control of the blood glucose, and that a high carbohydrate diet lowered serum lipids. Karam et al. (1963)[29] demonstrated that many who had diabetes and obesity had higher serum insulin levels than those who were lean and did not have diabetes. Sims[30] et al. (1968)[30] produced experimental obesity in humans, and proved that increased adiposity increased serum insulin, plasma glucose, and serum lipids. Wing and co-workers[31] (1988) were able to obtain normal and near-normal blood sugar with a very low calorie diet in 18 obese patients with diabetes and stop diabetes medication and insulin in 93% of these patients. In a published debate with Lebovitz, Davidson reports 80% adherence rate and stresses that *conventional diet therapy* is almost universally ineffective but that *intensive diet therapy* has been shown to be successful in a majority of NIDDMs.[32]

Hamwi (1964)[33] introduced the formula now in widespread use for estimation of ideal body weight (IBW) in adults (Table 16–1). West[20] (1971) showed that increased prevalence of diabetes in different national, ethnic, and socioeconomic groups is correlated with excess body weight. Davidson (1971–1977) treated over 3,000 overweight hyperglycemic nonketotic individuals with a 1-week total fast and a follow-up low-calorie diet. No deaths occurred during the *short-term fast*, and

this therapy was more successful in lowering group mean plasma glucose levels than was either sulfonylurea or insulin therapy.[34] Bar and Roth (1972)[35] showed that an increased serum insulin level decreased the number of insulin receptors on insulin-sensitive cells and that fasting and weight loss decreased the serum insulin level and increased the number of insulin receptors. The 1986 NIH Consensus Development Conference on Diet and Exercise in NIDDM recognizes fasts of several days' duration in the therapy for NIDDM as safe and effective.[36]

The American Diabetes Association and the American Dietetic Association published a revised *Exchange List for Meal Planning* 1986[37] and a *Nutritional Guide for Professionals* (1988),[38] and recommended that those who are overweight limit caloric intake, increase exercise, and attain a reasonable weight.[12]

In order to prevent the negative nitrogen balance that occurs during a total fast, Bistrian[39] and colleagues started using long-term protein-sparing modified fasts to produce weight loss. It became popular and was prescribed in a variety of forms by many physicians. Similar diet formulas were sold over-the-counter and were used for prolonged periods by many thousands of individuals who were not under medical supervision. By 1979, 58 deaths of otherwise apparently healthy overweight patients on protein-sparing modified fasts of several months duration had been reported to the Centers for Disease Control. In some of these individuals, there was histologic evidence during autopsy of heart damage similar to that seen during fatal starvation. Thus, it appears that *long-term fasting*, even "protein-sparing" long-term fasting, if not safe and may terminate fatally.[40,41]

Of course, it is important to preserve lean body mass during weight reduction. This is accomplished

TABLE 16–1 Calculation of Ideal Body Weight[a]

Build	For Adults (Age >20 Years)		
	Women	Men	Children
Medium frame[a]	Allow 100 pounds (45.5 kg) for 5 ft (152 cm) of height, plus 5 pounds (2.27 kg) for each additional inch (2.54 cm)	Allow 106 pounds (48.2 kg) for 5 ft (152 cm) of height, plus 6 pounds (2.73 kg) for each additional inch (2.54 cm)	Chart grown pattern on National Center for Health Statistics Growth Charts (NCHS Growth Charts, 1976); graph every 3–6 months (see Chapter 15)
Small frame[a]	Subtract 10%	Subtract 10%	(See Chapter 15)
Large frame[a]	Add 10%	Add 10%	(See Chapter 15)

[a] At this time, frame size is *estimated* from bone structure as ascertained by examining the fingers and wrist. Those with thin fingers and small wrists have a small frame (about 10% of the population), those with average fingers and average wrists have a medium frame (about 75% of the population), and those with thick fingers and large wrists have a large frame (about 15% of the population). Elbow breadth (caliper measured) has been recommended by Metropolitan Life[40] (see tables 16–10 and 16–11) and may be the best anthropometric determinant of frame size.

[*Source:* Hamwi GJ: Therapy: changing dietary concepts. *In* Danowski TS (ed): Diabetes Mellitus: Diagnosis and Treatment, Vol. 1. New York: American Diabetes Association, 1964, pp. 73–78. With permission.]

easily during short-term fasting, since less than 2% of the lean body mass is lost during a 1-week fast. A positive nitrogen balance then can be reestablished on a 32 g protein intake (>75% of high biologic quality) during a followup 622-calorie diet (see Table 16–5).

West (1978)[20] stated "recent epidemiologic and laboratory studies show that a preventive and cure are clearly at hand for most diabetics; the cause is usually obesity and the prevention and often the cure is leanness." He suggested that excess calorie intake with resultant adiposity, rather than any specific dietary component (i.e., sugar, carbohydrate, fat) accounted for the increased prevalence of diabetes. Anderson[42-44] (see Table 16–9) suggested that high-fiber, high-carbohydrate diets could lower the plasma glucose, particularly water-soluble fiber, which represents an average of 32% for cereal products, 32% for vegetables, 25% for dried beans, and 38% for fruit of the total dietary fiber. Whether this effect correlated with fiber per se (and if so, what types in what amounts), or with a decrease in caloric intake (because of the satiating effects of the ingested low-caloric-density foods) with resultant weight loss has not been determined.

The National Diabetes Data Group[45] recommended that diabetes be reclassified as NIDDM, insulin-dependent diabetes mellitus (IDDM), and gestational diabetes mellitus (GDM). Davidson[46] reported that intensive continuing nutritional care (initial 1-week fast followed by low-calorie diet) over a 10-year follow-up period for those who have NIDDM is therapeutically safe and effective and is cost-effective.

The 1986 NIH Consensus Development Conference on Diet and Exercise in NIDDM suggests a fast of several days duration and very low calorie diets for several weeks as a successful method for immediate reduction in both weight and blood glucose levels.[36] The 1987 European Non-insulin-dependent Diabetes Policy Group placed dietary adjustments and reduction of overweight in the obese as the two principal means for achieving metabolic control in NIDDM.[48] Kronsbein et al.[49] demonstrated successful patient outcome with a structured treatment and teaching program using paramedical personnel. At 1 year follow-up, body weights decreased significantly, sulfonylurea use fell from 68 to 38%, and triglyceride concentrations improved.

Garfield[50] suggested the need for a collaborative controlled prospective study to determine the value of short-term fasts for initiation of and for follow-up treatment of diabetes, hypertension, and obesity. The University Group Diabetes Program reported almost identical mortality and morbidity rates for placebo, insulin standard, and insulin variable treatments of NIDDM, again demonstrating the lack of effectiveness of insulin therapy (and of the resultant lower plasma glucose level) in the treatment of NIDDM.

Epidemiology

Excess caloric intake and decreased exercise produce excess adiposity, and this in turn increases the prevalence of NIDDM (See Chapter 2).

Pathophysiology

Excess adiposity produces hyperinsulinemia which down-regulates insulin receptors on insulin-sensitive cells. The tissues become "resistant" to endogenous and exogenous insulin, and plasma glucose and serum lipids rise. Fasting and weight loss decrease the insulin level, and increase the number and affinity of insulin receptors. The tissues become more sensitive to endogenously produced insulin, and glucose and lipid levels decrease (See Chapters 2, 8, and 9).

Problem Statement and Plan for Diet Therapy for Non-insulin-Dependent Diabetes Mellitus

Nutritional therapy for NIDDM is safer and more effective than drug therapy in those who are above ideal body weight (see Table 16–1).[51] After collecting the data base noted in Chapter 2, Exhibit 2–1, professionals [MDs, registered dietitians (RDs), RNs] should devise a strategy and implement processes of care for each individual that will produce a predictable rate of weight loss and an estimated date when IBW will be attained (Exhibits 16–2 through 16–5; Fig. 16–1). Processes of care that are involved include: (1) a 1-week total fast (Exhibits 16–6 through 16–8); (2) *the writing of the diet prescription by the physician* (Exhibits 16–9 through 16–12); and (3) *the translation of the prescription by the dietitian into food exchanges*, which are divided into meals (Tables 16–2 through 16–5). The dietitian should also evaluate the diet prescription to be certain that the content of vitamins, minerals, and trace elements (Tables 16–6 and 16–7), and protein (Exhibit 16–10) meet minimal requirements. Note that the terms RDA and USRDA have different meanings (Table 16–6).

Prescribed diet therapy is more successful during long-term follow-up if the patient, during the initial evaluation, agrees informally to set a date when IBW will be attained (Fig. 16–1, Exhibit 16–5), and participates in the strategies of education and changes in eating habits noted in Exhibits 16–13 and 16–14.

The patient should be educated during the initial visit or shortly thereafter by the dietitian using *Diabetes Guidebook: Diet Section*[52] or a similar publication: *Exchange Lists for Meal Planning*, 1989; *Exchange Lists for Low-sodium Meal Planning*, 1989; *Exchange Lists for Low-*

EXHIBIT 16–2   Foods Whose Intake Should Be Strictly Limited

Sugar (sucrose)	Cough drops, regular
Fructose	Cough syrup, regular
Honey	Fruit drinks containing sugar or other natural sweeteners
Molasses	(i.e., Hi-C, Gatorade, Hawaiian Punch)
Jams and jellies	Chewing gum, regular
Gelatin, sweetened (Jello)	"Dietetic" foods that contain sucrose, mannitol, sorbitol,
Pies	dextrose, fructose, corn sweeteners, carob powder, or
Cakes	dextrins–for example: dietetic ice cream, dietetic candy,
Cookies	or dietetic cookies
Candy	Alcoholic beverages–unless your physician specifically
Ice cream, ice milk, sherbet	permits you to use them (see Exhibit 14–16)
Pastries, sweet rolls, doughnuts	Coffee lighteners and other nondairy products that contain
Soft drinks, regular	nutritive sweeteners, e.g., Coffee-mate, Cremora

EXHIBIT 16–3   Foods Allowed in Resonable Amounts

Coffee	Mint leaf
Tea	Parsley
Bouillon, fat-free—limit to two cubes per day	Soft drinks, dietetic, that do not contain sugar (e.g., Diet
Broth, fat-free	Coke, Diet Pepsi, Diet Shasta, Tab, and so forth)
Condiments: salt, pepper, mustard, onion flakes, garlic	Postum—limit to 2 tsp/day
powder, spices, herbs	Cocoa—limit to 1 tsp/day
Vinegar	Soy sauce
Lemon juice	Worchestershire sauce
Gelatin, plain (i.e., Knox)	Saccharin, aspartame (Nutrasweet), acesulfame-K (Sunette)
Gelatin, sweetened with artificial sweetener (e.g., D-Zerta	and low-calorie sweeteners containing $\leqq 4$
gelatin, Jell-O brand gelatin)	calories/serving (e.g., Sweet 'N Low, Equal, Sweet 10,
Vanilla and other flavoring extracts	Sweet One)
Garlic	

EXHIBIT 16–4   Objectives of Diet Therapy for Non-Insulin-Dependent Diabetes Mellitus

1. Abolish glucosuria and minimize hyperglycemia
2. Attain and maintain ideal body weight
3. Prevent or delay the development or progression of cardiovascular, renal, retinal, neurologic, and other complications
4. Adjust the diet prescription to include the constraints imposed by the complications of diabetes and by associated problems (see Exhibit 16–11).

sodium, Low-fat Meal Planning, 1989 and *Exchange Lists for Low-fat Meal Planning*, 1989.[37,53–55] He should acquire a personal copy for continuing use at home and on return clinic visits. He should be taught how to measure food (Exhibit 16–15) and should own a cup, spoons, and ruler so that he can measure accurately the size of prescribed food servings. He should be taught how to read nutritional labels (see Table 16–7), and he should memorize the referent exchanges (see Table 16–2), foods that should be avoided (see Exhibit 16–2), and foods that are allowed in reasonable amounts (see Exhibit 16–3). Those who use alcoholic beverages should learn that they contain many calories and promote overeating and weight gain (Exhibit 16–16).

Dietitians are indispensable members of the type 2 diabetes mellitus (NIDDM) treatment team. In 1994, the American Dietetic Association introduced the term "medical nutrition therapy" (MNT)[56] as a political ploy to highlight their contributions in educating patients (especially those with diabetes) to learn, practice, and attain optimal nutrition goals (Exhibit 16–1). Third party payers do not pay dietitians for their services. These financial restrictions make it impossible for many IDDMs and NIDDMs to access dietitians' services because of their inability or unwillingness to pay for them. This lack of access to care today will almost certainly lead to increased expenditures for chronic complications in the future.

EXHIBIT 16–5   Calculation of Estimated Rate of Weight Loss During Therapy with 1-Week Fast and Follow-up Low-Calorie Diet (512 Calories, then 1,024 Calories) in Individual Whose Actual Weight Is 176 Pounds (80 kg) and Whose Ideal Body Weight Is 120 Pounds (54.5 kg)

Plan: Prescriptions	Estimated Caloric Deficit of Prescribed Diets	Estimated Weight Loss on Prescribed Diets
7-day fast, follow-up visit(s) at intervals of 2 and 7 days	*Weight 5/11/81* 176 pounds (80 kg)	*Excess weight in pounds (kg)* +56 pounds (+25.5 kg) −10 pounds (−4.5 kg)
After fast 512 calories for 12 weeks (*see* Exhibit 16–6)	−1,500 cal/day × 12 weeks = −3 pounds/wk = −36 lb (−16.4 kg)	+46 pounds (+21.0 kg) −36 pounds (−16.4 kg)
1,024 calories for continued weight reduction for 5 weeks	−1,000 cal/day × 5 wk = −2 pounds/wk × 5 wk = −10 pounds (−4.6 kg)	+10 pounds (+4.6 kg) −10 pounds (−4.6 kg) 0 pounds (0.0 kg) = IBW
2,000 calories for maintenance for IBW	(See Figure 16–1)	

Patient goal: to attain IBW of 120 pounds (54.5 kg) 9/4/81

Exercise: _____

Medications: _____

_____

Other therapy: _____

Physician signature: _____

Patient signature (optional): _____

Other signature(s): _____

Abbreviations: IBW, ideal body weight.

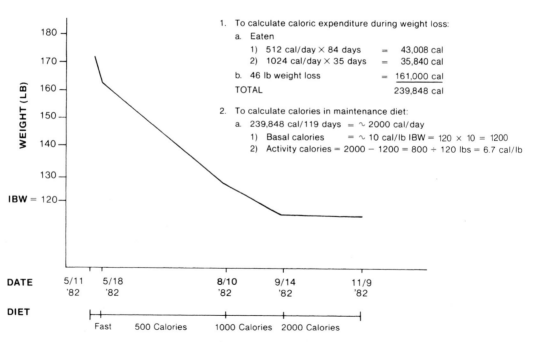

Figure 16–1.   (See Exhibit 16–5): This graph indicates the estimated rate of weight loss during a 1-week fast which is followed by a 512-calorie diet for 84 days and a 1,024 calorie diet for 35 days. When rate of weight loss is known over a period of time in those who are adherent to the prescribed diet, the calories needed to maintain ideal body weight can be estimated accurately.

EXHIBIT 16–6   Indications and Contraindications for a 1-Week Total Fast

I. Indications
   A. >50 pounds (22.7 kg) above ideal body weight
   B. Above ideal body weight and symptomatically hyperglycemic
   C. Above ideal body weight and persistently hyperglycemic on insulin or sulfonylurea therapy, no history of ketoacidosis
II. Contraindications
   A. Absolute
      1. Diabetic ketoacidosis (carbon dioxide content <20 mEq/L)
      2. Pregnancy
      3. Preinfarction angina, myocardial infarction within last 6 weeks, incipient gangrene, transient ischemic attacks with neurologic symptoms and/or signs
   B. Relative
      1. Renal failure (serum creatinine >1.5 mg/dL)
      2. History of psychosis
      3. History of gout (normalize serum uric acid level with probenecid therapy before fast is started)

EXHIBIT 16–7   Routine for 1-Week Total Fast

I. *For patients not on insulin therapy*
   A. Individual may fast as outpatient.
   B. Drink minimum of 100 oz. (3 L) of water per day, more if possible.
   C. Omit all other food and drink, including tea, coffee, diet soft drinks, and so forth.
   D. Continue normal exercise and work pattern.
   E. Discontinue diuretics, potassium supplements, other drugs being used for hypertension therapy (if appropriate).
   F. Discontinue sulfonylurea therapy.
   G. A mild tranquilizer and/or bedtime sedative may be useful in improving patient adherence in anxious patients (less than 20% of those being fasted).
   H. Have patient keep diary of urine glucose and acetone (8 A.M., 1 P.M., 6 P.M., and bedtime), weight (daily), and symptoms.
   I. Have patient report by phone to RN, registered dietitian (RD), or MD every 1 to 2 days.
   J. Have patient return on second day and seventh day for follow-up weight, plasma glucose, and evaluation.
   K. If outpatient fast is unsuccessful [weight loss <4 pounds (1.8 kg)], may hospitalize patient for inpatient fast.
II. *For patients on insulin therapy*
   A. Same as in I. B. through I. G. except that it is optimal to hospitalize the patient since 5 to 10% who have insulin therapy discontinued abruptly will develop diabetic ketoacidosis and insulin therapy must be restarted promptly. These individuals have IDDM.
   B. Discontinue insulin therapy abruptly, start fast same day.
   C. Measure weight (daily), blood pressure lying and standing (four times daily), plasma glucose (8 A.M. and 4 P.M. daily), urine glucose and acetone four times daily, carbon dioxide content and uric acid every 2 days.

EXHIBIT 16–8   Effects of a 1-Week Fast and of Refeeding a Hypocaloric Diet

I. *Effects of 1-week fast*
   A. Plasma glucose usually falls to normal or nearnormal; if it does not fall, or rises, diabetic ketoacidosis usually develops.
   B. Carbon dioxide content may fall as low as 16 mEq/L with fasting; if it falls as low as 15 mEq/L, restart insulin therapy and a hypocaloric diet (usually 622 calories—see Table 16–5).
   C. Hunger diminishes or disappears after 2 to 3 days and euphoria frequently develops. Weakness and/or vomiting occasionally occur.
   D. Blood pressure may drop and postural hypotension may develop; if it does, have patient assume erect stance carefully and slowly, and recline if dizziness or faintness occur. These changes are due to hypovolemia which is more marked if fluid intake is inadequate (i.e., <100 oz/day), the consequences of which are more marked in those with autonomic neuropathy.
   E. Uric acid may rise as high as 18 mg/dL, but acute gouty arthritis does not develop unless there was a history of gouty arthritis prior to the fast.
   F. Hematuria has not been observed; should it occur, uric acid renal stone formation should be considered.
   G. Mean weight loss in the hospital of those not on insulin therapy has been 12 pounds/week, range 5 to 22 pounds/week (5.5 kg/week, range 2.3 to 10 kg). Of those who have been on insulin (about 1,000 individuals) mean weight loss during the 1 week fast has been 14 pounds/week, range 8 to 25 pounds/week (6.4 kg/week, range 3.6 to 11.4 kg/week).

II. *Effects of refeeding a hypocaloric diet*
   A. Mean weight gain on refeeding in hospital has been 2 pounds/week, range −1 to +5 pounds/week (1 kg, range −0.5 to 2.3 kg).
   B. Plasma glucose rises modestly (usually 20 to 80 mg/dL), then levels and declines to normal or near-normal with continuing weight loss.
   C. Nausea and vomiting occasionally occur.
   D. Pancreatitis has not been observed.

EXHIBIT 16–9   Calculation of Caloric Requirements for Adults

Ideal body weight is calculated according to the method shown in Table 16–1. Caloric requirements are estimated as follows:

   _____ *Basal calories* [10 cal/pound (22 cal/kg) ideal body weight]

+ _____ *Activity calories* (about 3 cal/pound or 6.6 cal/kg ideal body weight for sedentary activity; about 5 cal/pound or 11 cal/kg ideal body weight for moderate activity; about 10 cal/pound or 22 cal/kg ideal body weight for strenuous activity)

– _____ *Calories to lose weight* (subtract 500 cal/day, or 3,500 calories/week, to lose 1 pound/week or 0.45 kg/week). Subtract more calories to lose more weight (see Fig. 16–1 and Exhibit 16–5)

+ _____ *Calories to gain weight* (add 500 cal/day, or 3,500 cal/week, to gain 1 pound/week or 0.45 kg/week). Add more calories to gain more weight.

= _____ Total calories

EXHIBIT 16–10   Distribution of Calories into Grams of Protein, Carbohydrate, and Fat for Nonpregnant, Nonlactating Individuals ≧ 18 Years of Age with Non-Insulin-Dependent Diabetes Mellitus

I. A. Recommended *minimum* protein (high-biologic-quality) intake (FAO, 1957):
   1. 0.16 g/pound (0.35 g/kg) estimated IBW equals:
      (a) About 20 g protein for 120 pounds (54.5 kg)
      (b) About 30 g protein for 180 pounds (81.8 kg)
   2. Protein malnutrition states: add enough protein to replete depleted body stores and to establish a positive nitrogen balance.
   B. *Generous* protein intake (NRC Food and Nutrition Board, 1989)
      0.50 g/pound (1.1 g/kg) estimated IBW equals:
      (a) About 60 g protein for 120 pounds (54.5 kg)
      (b) About 90 g protein for 180 pounds (81.8 kg)

II. Recommended carbohydrate intake: 65 to 100% of nonprotein calories
III. Recommended fat intake: 0 to 35% of nonprotein calories. Fat can be omitted completely during an aggressively implemented weight loss program, in which case essential fatty acids are provided from mobilization of adipose tissue. When fat is used, one third should be polyunsaturated, one third monounsaturated, and one third saturated.

Abbreviations: FAO, Food and Agricultural Organization (of United Nations Committee on Protein Requirement); IBW, ideal body weight; NRC, National Research Council.[10]

TABLE 16–2   Food Exchanges

Food Exchange	Values (in grams) for Exchanges			
	Carbohydrate	Protein	Fat	Calories
Starch/bread	15	3	1[a]	80
Meat				
Lean		7	3	55
Medium fat		7	5	75
High fat		7	8	100
Vegetable	5	2		25
Fruits	15			60
Milk				
Skim	12	8	1[a]	90
Low fat	12	8	5	120
Whole	12	8	8	150
Fats			5	45

[a] In the exchange list, trace is listed, calculated as 1 g. Dietitians should calculate using medium fat meat exchange.

[*Source:* Exchange lists for meal planning. New York: American Diabetes Association. Chicago: American Dietetic Association, 1986. With permission.]

EXHIBIT 16–11   Problems Requiring Modification of the Diet Prescription for Diabetes

Problem	Indicated Diet Modifications
I. A. Congestive heart failure	Limit sodium[52]; supplementary potassium if on diuretic
B. Hypertension	Limit sodium[52]; supplementary potassium if on diuretic
II. Diabetic nephropathy	
A. Nephrotic syndrome	Limit sodium[52]; increase protein intake of 0.8 g/kg IBW plus 1 g for each gram of protein lost in urine
B. Far-advanced azotemia (BUN >100 mg/dL, creatinine >5 mg/dL)	Restrict protein intake to 0.55 to 0.60 g/kg/day (0.35 g of high-biologic value protein kg/day). Marked restriction of protein intake (0.216 g/kg/day) plus 10 to 20 g essential amino acids or 0.28 g/kg/day with keto acids or hydroxy acid anologues may slow the progress of renal failure. Limit phosphorus intake. Give supplementary water-soluble vitamins and calcium.[60]
C. Hyperkalemia: K$^+$ >6 mEq/L	Limit potassium intake[52]
D. Inability to excrete water	Limit water intake
E. Hemodialysis	May require 1.2 to 1.4 g/kg/day (50% high biologic value)[60]
F. Peritoneal dialysis	Recommend 1.2 to 1.5 g/kg/day[60]
III. Liver failure	Limit protein to 20 to 40 g/day; may limit sodium[52]
IV. Hyperlipidemia	Limit fat and cholesterol intake[52]
V. Milk and/or lactose intolerance	Omit milk and other foods containing milk or lactose
VI. Food allergies (urticaria, and so forth)	Omit foods that produce allergy
VII. Diverticulitis, constipation	Increase intake of fiber (up to 35 g/day)
VIII. Autonomic neuropathy with diarrhea	Decrease intake of fiber: low-fiber diet, 2 to 3 g/day, or very low-fiber diet (<2 g/day)
IX. Caloric intake < 1,000 cal/day for more than 4 weeks	Give supplementary iron and folacin (or an appropriate multiple vitamin and mineral supplement)
X. Pregnancy, lactation	(See Chapters 40 and 41.) Give supplementary calcium, iron, and folacin (or an appropriate multiple vitamin and mineral supplement)

EXHIBIT 16–12   Contents of a Complete Diet Prescription

_____ Calories

_____ g protein, _____ g carbohydrate, _____ g fat

Divided (tenths)   _____

Limitations _____

Supplements _____

EXHIBIT 16–13   Professionals' Strategy for Successful Diet Therapy for Non-Insulin-Dependent Diabetes Mellitus

1. Use of the team approach (physician, dietitian, nurse, patient, and significant members of patient's family).
2. Routine use of a 1-week fast (if not contraindicated) to start diet therapy in the overweight patient. If fast is contraindicated, start with 622 calorie lactovegetarian diet (see Table 16–5).
3. Routine prescription of individualized diet, intensive education, and continuous follow-up (initially weekly, later at no longer than monthly intervals) until the patient attains IBW.
4. Routine instruction using a publication such as "Diabetes Guidebook: Diet Section"[52] with the patient bringing the manual to the physician's office on each follow-up visit.
5. Instruction of the family member who prepares meals so the meals will be prepared, measured, and served correctly.
6. Sharing with patients their weight and glucose levels at each follow-up visit.
7. Prescription of a maintenance diet and continued follow-up.
8. Repeat (2 to 7 days) fast for those who are partially adherent, the length of the fast being patterned to the degree of adherence—project rate of weight loss and plan time to attain IBW during initial evaluation.

Abbreviation: IBW, ideal body weight.

TABLE 16–3   Translation into Food Exchanges of a Diet Prescription for 1,200 Calories[a] Containing 160 g Carbohydrate, 70 g Protein, and 30 g Fat, Divided 0.3 (Breakfast), 0.3 (Lunch), 0.4 (Supper)[b]

List	Exchange Group (See Table 16–2)[a]	No. Exchanges	Carbohydrate (g)	Protein (g)	Fat (g)
1	Milk	2	24	16	2
2	Vegetable	4	20	8	
3	Fruit	3	45		
	Total carbohydrate from sources other than bread exchanges		89		
4	Bread				
	160 g carbohydrate in prescription				
	89 g from sources other than bread				
	71 g ÷ 15 = no. of bread exchanges	5	75	15	5
	Total protein from sources other than meat exchanges			39	
5	Meat				
	70 g protein in prescription				
	−39 g from sources other than meat				
	31 g ÷ 7 = no. meat exchanges	4	—	28	20
	Total fat from sources other than fat exchanges				27
6	Fat				
	30 g fat in prescription				
	−27 g from sources other than fat				
	18 g ÷ 5 = no. fat exchanges	1	—	—	5
Total grams			164	67	32
Percentage of calories[a]			54	23	24

[a] Of the 944 nonprotein calories, 70% are carbohydrate and 30% are fat.

[b] See Table 16–4 for distribution of exchanges.

TABLE 16–4   Distribution of Exchanges by Meals[a]

	Distribution		
Food Exchanges	0.3 Breakfast	0.3 Lunch	0.4 Supper
Starch/bread	1	2	2
Meat	1	1	2
Vegetable	—	2	3
Fruit	1	1	1
Milk	1	—	1
Fat	—	—	1
Total Calories	305	345	555

[a] See table 16–3.

TABLE 16–5   Two Low-Calorie Diets (622 Calories[a] and 1,244 Calories[b]) that Contain Only Skim Milk, Vegetables, and Fruits, and a High Content of Dietary Fiber

Food Exchanges	Total/Day	Carbohydrate (g)	Protein (g)	Fat (g)	Total Calories
1[a]					
Vegetable	4	20	8	0	112
Fruit	4	60	0	0	240
Milk, skim	3	36	24	3	270
Totals		116	32	3	622
2[b]					
Vegetable	8	40	16	0	224
Fruit	8	120	0	0	480
Milk, skim	6	72	48	6	540
Totals		232	64	6	1,244

[a] Average dietary fiber/day = 25 g (depending on choice of vegetable and fruit exchanges).

[b] Average dietary fiber/day = 50 g (depending on choice of vegetable and fruit exchanges).

TABLE 16–6   Recommended Dietary Allowance (RDA) for Vitamins and Minerals for Normal Adults (Nonpregnant and Nonlactating)[a]

Fat-Soluble Vitamins	Water-Soluble Vitamins	Minerals	Trace Elements
A(IU): 4,000–5,000 (800–1,000 retinal equivalents) D(IU): 5–10 μg E(IU): 8–10 mg–Tocopherol equivalent Vitamin K: 60 80 μg	Ascorbic acid: 60 mg Folate: 180–200 μg Niacin: 15–19 mg Riboflavin: 1.2–1.7 mg Thiamine: 1.0–1.5 mg B_6: 1.5–2.0 mg B_{12}: 3 μg Biotin: 0.1–0.2 mg Pantothenic acid: 4–7 mg	Calcium: 8–12 g Phosphorus: 8–12 g Iodine: 150 μg Iron: 10–15 mg Magnesium: 280–350 mg Zinc: 12–15 mg	Copper: 2.0–3.0 mg Manganese: 2.5–5.0 mg Fluoride: 1.5–4 mg Chromium: 0.05–0.2 mg Selenium: 55–70 μg Molybdenum: 0.15–0.5 mg

[a] The terms RDA (Recommended Dietary Allowance) and USRDA (United States Recommended Daily Allowance) have different meanings. RDAs were developed by the Food and Nutrition Board of the National Research Council (see reference 10) and are the average amounts of nutrients that individuals should consume over time (expressed as amount per day) to remain healthy. USRDAs were set by the Food and Drug Administration (FDA) and represent the FDA recommendations of the amount of protein, vitamin, mineral, etc., that people need each day to stay healthy.

[*Source:* Recommended Dietary Allowances, Ed. 10. Washington, DC: Food and Nutrition Board, National Research Council, National Academy of Sciences.]

EXHIBIT 16–14   Patients' Strategy for Modifying Eating Habits

1. Use a diary for recording diet, weight, urine glucose values (and acetone if fasting). Home blood glucose monitoring and weighing also may be helpful.
2. Practice frequent use of a measuring cup, spoons, and ruler at home.
3. Substitute water or noncaloric foods or drinks when hunger creates the urge to eat between meals or to eat excessively at meals.
4. Avoid compulsive or social eating and drinking, *especially* avoid alcoholic beverages (see Exhibit 16–16).
5. Avoid "dietetic" and "health" foods, many of which contain large numbers of calories.
6. Buy and store only the types and amounts of food called for by the diet plan, shop for food and plan menu 1 week in advance (weekly intervals).
7. Serve plates from which food is to be eaten with correctly measured amounts of food *before* they are placed on the table. Do not place serving dishes on the table; this increases the temptation to take additional (excessive) food.
8. Eat food only at the table on a regular schedule. Do not snack between meals, while watching television and so forth.
9. Choose foods that provide more satiety and bulk such as fresh fruits instead of fruit juices.
10. Avoid the preparation of food for others until adequate weight loss has taken place.
11. Exercise daily (see Chapter 17) if there are no contraindications (walking a few miles per day is ideal).

EXHIBIT 16–15   Measuring Food

Food servings are measured in *exchanges* (see Table 16–2). Each exchange in a food group contains about the same number of calories, and about the same number of grams[a] of protein, carbohydrate, and fat.

Food exchanges can be measured accurately with a measuring cup, a tablespoon, a teaspoon, and a plastic ruler. Though it is *not necessary*, patients who wish to weigh foods may do so.

 The measuring cup is used to measure milk, vegetables, fruits, juices, some bread exchanges, some meat exchanges, some fat exchanges, and some combined foods.

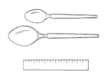 The tablespoon and teaspoon are used to measure fat exchanges, some bread exchanges, raisins, peanut butter, and some foods allowed in reasonable amounts.

The ruler is used to measure meat, fruit, and some bread and fat exchanges.

Once the patient has learned to measure food servings accurately at home, he can eat away from home and *estimate* the size servings of the various food exchanges that the diet prescription permits.

[a] The diet prescription is written in terms of *calories* and *grams*. A calorie is the amount of food energy which, when burned, will raise the temperature of 1 L (slightly more than 1 quart) of water from 15° to 16°C. One gram is equal to 1/1,000 kg, 1/28 oz., and 1/453 pound.

EXHIBIT 16–16   Caloric Content of Alcoholic Beverages

Alcohol provides 7 cal/g and its caloric content may cause a gain in weight. If diabetes is under control and the patient is at ideal body weight, most physicians permit moderate use of alcoholic beverages with a meal or snack. Sweet wines, liqueurs, beer, ale, and sweetened mixed drinks should be avoided because of their high sugar content. One can calculate the content of calories provided in a given volume of an alcoholic beverage by using the following formula:

$$0.8 \times proof \times ounces = calories \ (2 \times \% \ alcohol = proof)$$

Thus 4 oz. of dry wine containing 12% alcohol would provide approximately 77 calories. Eighty-proof whiskey, scotch, rum, gin, and vodka would provide 96 calories in 1.5 oz., whereas 100-proof alcoholic beverages contain 120 calories in 1.5 oz. Twelve ounces of low-calorie beer contains approximately 90 calories.

Follow-Up

Thorough education and intensive follow-up of the patient (and involved family members) improve therapeutic adherence and increase motivation. Follow-up visits should be at 2-week intervals until 50% or more of the excess weight has been lost and the plasma glucose level is normal or near-normal. Visits then may be at 4-week intervals until IBW is attained. Thereafter the diet should be revised so that IBW is maintained (see Exhibits 16–13 and 16–14, and Fig. 16–1). Visits then may be reduced to once every 2 to 3 months, and eventually to once every 3 to 6 months. If weight should plateau or increase before IBW is attained, the patient should repeat the fast and/or resume a low-calorie diet (see Table 16–9). After IBW has been attained, it may be maintained by an appropriately prescribed diet. Thereafter, should weight gain occur, a short-term fast (2 to 7 days) may be used again to attain and maintain IBW.

Adherence (or Lack of Adherence) to Diet Therapy

It is well known that conventional diet therapy as it has been used in the past to treat overweight individuals has had a very high failure rate. Many authors report failure rates >90%. For instance, after a mean follow-up of 12.5 years in the University Group Diabetes Program (UGDP) study, the group relative body weights (observed/desirable, Metropolitan Life Insurance Company tables)[57] were unchanged in the insulin variable treatment group (1.36 initial versus 1.36 final) and the insulin standard treatment group (1.33 initial versus 1.33 final), and was modestly lower in the placebo (no treatment other than conventional diet) group (1.34 initial versus 1.27 final).

As more knowledge of the nature and treatment of NIDDM has become available, it appears that conventional weight reduction therapy failed for a number of reasons, of which patient nonadherence was only one. In fact, it is probably not the most important reason for failure. Medication (insulin, sulfonylureas) used to lower the plasma glucose level can promote weight gain by increasing appetite and food intake (sometimes related to hypoglycemia), and by diminishing glucosuria. Many patients and some professionals believe that it is easier to attain and maintain normoglycemia (the essentially universal therapeutic desideratum) with medication than with aggressive continuing limitation of caloric intake. At the present time, inappropriate processes of care and/or inadequate patient education and follow-up appear to be the most common causes of patient nonadherence and diet therapy failure in NIDDM. Diabetes prevails in many ethnic groups. Nutrition counseling for these groups requires understanding and appreciation of cultural differences

TABLE 16–7 Nutrition Labeling[a]

Nutrients are listed for one serving	Nutrition Information (per serving) Serving size = 1 cup[b] Servings per container = two		
	Calories	110	Nutrients in
	Protein	1 g	metric weight
	Carbohydrate	25 g	as grams
	Fat	1 g	(1 ounce = 28 g)
	Sodium	30 mg	
	Percentage of USRDA[c]		
	Protein	2	Percentages of
	Vitamin A	25	USRDA
	Vitamin C	25	
	Thiamine	25	
	Riboflavin	25	
	Niacin	25	
	Calcium	4	
	Iron	4	

[a] The upper portion of the label shows the number of calories in a serving of the food and lists, in grams, the amount of protein, carbohydrate, and fat and sodium in one serving. Also, labels may show the amount of sodium, cholesterol, and sugar in a product. Those containing a significant amount of sugar should not be used.

[b] The serving size on nutrition labels frequently may differ from the serving size recommended on the exchange lists. For instance, in the above example, 110 calories containing 1 g protein, 25 g carbohydrate, and 1 g fat, should be equated to one bread and one-half fruit exchange.

[c] The lower portion of the label shows the percentage of the United States Recommended Daily Allowance (USRDA) for protein and seven vitamins and minerals provided in one serving. Add percentages for each nutrient consumed through the day. When the daily total approaches 100%, you are getting an ample supply of that nutrient. Be sure to discuss with the dietitian the proper way to use this information so that you do not deviate from your prescribed diet. Nutrition labeling can help you count calories and can help you save money by comparing the nutrient content, and the cost per serving of similar foods. The USRDAs are the amounts of protein, vitamins, and minerals people need each day to stay healthy. These allowances are set by the Food and Drug Administration. They are based on body needs for healthy adults. Set at generous levels, they provide a considerable margin of safety for most people above minimum needs for most nutrients. Nutrition labels list USRDAs by percentage per serving of food. For example, if the nutrition label says "Vitamin A . . . 25" that means a serving of the food contains 25% of the USRDA for vitamin A [*Source:* Davidson JK, Goldsmith MP: Diabetes Guidebook: Diet Section, Ed. 4. Atlanta: Davicone, 1984. With permission.]

for successful intervention.[58] The development of *aggressive diet therapy* in the 1970s, which was designed to produce maximal attainable weight loss in overweight individuals, has increased significantly the amount and duration of weight loss in those with NIDDM[59] (Table 16–8).

Aggressive diet therapy (including 1-week fasts, intensive education, and frequent follow-up visits) produced sustained significant weight loss (>10 pounds) in 87% of overweight individuals during an 8-year follow-up period at Grady Memorial Hospital (see Table 16–8). Since 1982, *adherence* to diet therapy in this program has been *defined by outcome*, which is related to the *ratio of observed to predicted weight loss* (when weight change is not secondary to poor plasma glucose control and glucosuria). Those whose observed weight loss in the prescribed time frame is >90% of that predicted are classified as *totally adherent* (about 20% of those treated in 1982); those who lost weight at a rate from 10 to 90% of the predicted rate are classified as *partially adherent* (about 60% of those treated in 1982), and those who gain weight, who do not lose weight, or who lose weight transiently then regain it, or who lose weight at a rate <10% of the predicted rate over time are classified as *nonadherent* (about 20% of those treated in 1982). Examples of each type of outcome are noted in Exhibits 16–17 through 16–19.

Lack of easy access to foods (especially foods of medium and high caloric density, i.e., bread, meat, fat, and alcohol), and the temptation thereunto related, will reduce caloric intake and increase the rate of weight loss in the *partially adherent*. The order of therapeutic effectiveness as measured by amount of weight loss in the partially adherent group is: inpatient fast > outpatient fast >622 calorie lactovegetarian diet >1,244 calorie lactovegetarian diet (both diets containing only skim milk, vegetable, and fruit exchanges) (see Table 16–5).

Persistently nonadherent individuals appear to be compulsive eaters who cannot (or will not) change their food (and calorie) intake patterns over the long term. Most individuals who have been obese since childhood are persistently nonadherent. Some who became obese during adult life are persistently nonadherent. The cause(s) of nonadherence in these groups is not known at present. The consequences of such behavior should be explained to these individuals and their families. Although available alternative therapies (insulin, sulfonylurea) may lower the plasma glucose level transiently, over the long term both insulin and sulfonylurea therapy promote weight gain, hyperinsulinemia, and sustained tissue resistance to insulin.

Demographic, social, and economic characteristics of patients have not been helpful in predicting who will adhere and who will not adhere to diet therapy. Patient adherence during long-term chronic disease therapy which may last for 50 years or longer (i.e., diabetes mellitus) differs from patient adherence during short-term acute disease therapy (during which medications, surgery, and so forth, are largely under the control of the physician). Some patients believe that *external controls* (physicians, religious beliefs, and so on) determine their health status and that *internal controls* (physician-initiated and patient-implemented lifestyle changes) have little or no influence on disease outcomes (morbidity, mortality). Participation in

TABLE 16–8　Mean Weight (MWt) and Mean Random Plasma Glucose (MPG) Changes in Cohort of 433 Patients in Whom Oral Agent Therapy Was Discontinued in 1970 and Who Were Alive and Active in the Grady Diabetes Clinic in 1979

	433 Individuals							
	MWt (Pounds)				**MPG (mg/dL)**			
	1970: 171.8 1979: 154.1 (↓ 17.7)				1970: 218 1979: 221 (↑ 3)			
	Diet Only (311 Individuals)[a]				**Diet and Insulin (122 Individuals)[b]**			
	MWt (Pounds)		**MPG (mg/dL)**		**MWt (Pounds)**		**MPG (mg/dL)**	
	1970: 178.4 1979: 158.1 (↓ 20.3)		1970: 211 1979: 213 (↑ 2)		1970: 155.6 1979: 144.3 (↓ 11.3)		1970: 236 1979: 242 (↑ 6)	
Stratification of 1979 PGs at Five Levels, and Comparison with 1970 PGs (While Still on Oral Agents) and with Wt Changes from 1970 to 1979	**N**	**1970 PG (mg/dL)**	**1979 PG (mg/dL)**	**PG Change (%)**	**MWt Change (Pounds) 1970-1979**	**N**	**1970 PG (mg/dL)**	**1979 PG (mg/dL)**	**PG Change (%)**	**MWt Change (Pounds) 1970-1979**
1979 PG < 150	83	182	116	−36.1	−25.0	26	222	123	−44.5	−19.9
1979 PG 151–200	68	224	172	−23.0	−18.3	17	188	169	−10.0	−8.4
1979 PG 201–250	58	223	223	0.0	−18.6	24	239	227	−5.0	−12.5
1979 PG 251–300	42	208	275	+31.9	−22.9	21	215	277	+28.8	−9.7
1979 PG > 300	60	221	356	+61.1	−18.6	34	278	358	+28.8	−7.3

[a]*In the diet only group*, 87% lost weight and 13% gained weight from 1970 to 1979. 1979 PG was lower in 151 individuals (48.6%), unchanged in 58 individuals (18.6%), and higher in 102 individuals (32.8%).

[b]*In the diet and insulin group*, 72% lost weight and 28% gained weight from 1970 to 1979. 1979 PG was lower in 67 individuals (54.9%) and higher in 55 individuals (45.1%).

weight loss-oriented lay groups and isolated psychologic and psychiatric evaluation and treatment have not increased weight loss in the nonadherent group at Grady Hospital. An understanding of the genetic, physical, hormonal, emotional, and environmental causes of nonadherence to diet therapy in those with NIDDM are at best rudimentary.[19,61–63]

Nutritive values of foods being used by various ethnic groups in different areas of the world need to be determined and made generally available to physicians, dietitians, nurses, and patients.[64] See section following on Research Considerations.

Process and Outcome Audits

Type 2 or NIDDM is a relatively distinct subset of diabetes mellitus. In order to define more precisely its subtypes, epidemiology, natural history, morbidity, and mortality, and to monitor and evaluate the therapeutic consequences (outcomes) of different processes of care (alternative therapies) and the cost-effectiveness of each, it will be necessary to collect and analyze data at regular intervals in the population of patients

who have NIDDM. Morbidity and mortality of NIDDM in various subgroups (overweight, normal weight, and so forth), and outcomes of alternative therapies in each subgroup, need to be determined during long-term follow-up.

Present evidence suggests that NIDDM in many overweight individuals (after sufficient weight loss) goes into a remission phase (normal glucose tolerance test) which lasts in some individuals for more than 15 years. Available data also suggest that each year about 1 to 2% of those with NIDDM progress to IDDM (i.e., at or below IBW on optimal diet and exercise therapy, and fasting plasma glucose consistently above 125 mg/dL).

As an example of audits of outcome of one type of therapy for NIDDM, it has been shown that 100% of those who fast as *inpatients* lose weight, an average of 12 pounds/week (range, 5 to 25 pounds), whereas those who fast as *outpatients* lose an average of 6 pounds/week (range, 0 to 20 pounds). A 1-week outpatient fast is a useful way to separate patients into adherent, partially adherent, and nonadherent groups, and alerts the physician, dietitian, and nurse to act promptly to identify deficiencies in patient and family

TABLE 16–9 Dietary Fiber in Food

	Amount	Weight (g)	Dietary Fiber (g)		Amount	Weight (g)	Dietary Fiber (g)
Bread and Crackers				*Meat, Milk, Eggs*			
Graham cracker	2 squares	14.2	1.4	Beef	1 oz.	28	0
Pumpernickel bread	$\frac{3}{4}$ slice	24	1.4	Cheese	$\frac{3}{4}$ oz.	21	0
Rye bread	1 slice	25	.8	Chicken/turkey	1 oz.	28	0
Wholewheat bread	1 slice	25	1.3	Cold cuts, frankfurters	1 oz.	28	0
Wholewheat cracker	6 crackers	19.8	2.2	Eggs	3 large	99	0
Wholewheat roll	$\frac{3}{4}$	21	1.2	Fish	2 oz.	56	0
				Ice cream	1 oz.	28	0
Cereals				Milk	1 cup	240	0
				Pork	1 oz.	28	0
All-Bran, 100%	$\frac{1}{3}$ cup	28	8.4	Yogurt	5 oz.	140	0
Bran Chex	$\frac{1}{3}$ cup	21	4.1				
Corn Bran	$\frac{1}{3}$ cup	21	4.4	*Rice*			
Corn Flakes	$\frac{3}{4}$ cup	21	2.6				
Grapenuts Flakes	$\frac{2}{3}$ cup	21	2.5	Rice, brown (cooked)	$\frac{1}{3}$ cup	65	1.6
Grapenuts	1 Tb	21	2.7	Rice, white (cooked)	$\frac{1}{3}$ cup	68	0.5
Oatmeal	$\frac{3}{4}$ pkg	21	2.5				
Shredded Wheat	1 biscuit	21	2.8	*Leaf Vegetables*			
Wheaties	$\frac{3}{4}$ cup	21	2.6				
				Broccoli	$\frac{1}{2}$ cup	93	3.5
Fruit				Brussels sprouts	$\frac{1}{2}$ cup	78	2.3
				Cabbage	$\frac{1}{2}$ cup	85	2.1
Apple	$\frac{1}{2}$ large	83	2.0	Cauliflower	$\frac{1}{2}$ cup	90	1.6
Apricot	2	72	1.4	Celery	$\frac{1}{2}$ cup	60	1.1
Banana	$\frac{1}{2}$ medium	54	1.5	Lettuce	1 cup	55	0.8
Blackberries	$\frac{3}{4}$ cup	108	6.7	Spinach, raw	1 cup	55	0.2
Cantaloupe	1 cup	160	1.6	Turnip greens	$\frac{1}{2}$ cup	93	3.5
Cherries	10 large	68	1.1				
Dates, dried	2	18	1.6	*Root Vegetables*			
Figs, dried	1 medium	20	3.7				
Grapes, white	10	50	0.5	Beets	$\frac{1}{2}$ cup	85	2.1
Grapefruit	$\frac{1}{2}$	87	0.8	Carrots	$\frac{1}{2}$ cup	78	2.4
Honeydew melon	1 cup	170	1.5	Potatoes, baked	$\frac{1}{2}$ medium	75	1.9
Orange	1 small	78	1.6	Radishes	$\frac{1}{2}$ cup	58	1.3
Peach	1 medium	100	2.3	Sweet potatoes, baked	$\frac{1}{2}$ medium	75	2.1
Pear	$\frac{1}{2}$ medium	82	2.0				
Pineapple	$\frac{1}{2}$	78	0.8	*Other Vegetables*			
Plum	3 small	85	1.8				
Prunes, dried	2	15	2.4	Beans, green	$\frac{1}{2}$ cup	64	2.1
Raisins	$1\frac{1}{2}$ Tb	14	1.0	Beans, string	$\frac{1}{2}$ cup	55	1.9
Strawberries	1 cup	143	3.1	Cucumber	$\frac{1}{2}$ cup	70	1.1
Tangerine	1 large	101	2.0	Eggplant	$\frac{1}{2}$ cup	100	2.5
Watermelon	1 cup	160	1.4	Lentils, cooked	$\frac{1}{2}$ cup	100	3.7
				Mushrooms	$\frac{1}{2}$ cup	35	0.9
High-Fiber Supplement				Onions	$\frac{1}{2}$ cup	58	1.2
				Tomatoes	1 small	100	1.5
Fibermed	2	35.4	10.0	Winter squash	$\frac{1}{2}$ cup	120	3.5
				Zucchini squash	$\frac{1}{2}$ cup	65	2.0

[*Source:* Anderson JW, Chen WL, Sieling B: Plant Fiber in Foods. Lexington, KY: HCF Diabetes Research Foundation, 1980. With permission.]

EXHIBIT 16–17   Example of a Totally Adherent Patient[a]

A 44-year-old white male heavy equipment operator who had been unable to work for 2 months because of severe leg pain, inability to sleep, and exertional chest pain, was referred by his primary care physician for evaluation and therapy.

Problems (7/15/82):
  I. Diabetes mellitus
    A. Painful peripheral neuropathy
    B. Stable angina pectoris
  II. Hypertension
  III. Obesity

Subjective: Diabetes diagnosed 1977 (weight 300 pounds) treated for 2 years with tolbutamide, then for 3 years with NPH insulin. Severe pain and numbness in legs and feet with inability to sleep, exertional chest pain after walking one block. Treatment on 7/15/82 consisted of 85 U NPH insulin nitroglycerin, reserpine, hydralazine, hydrochlorthiazide, codeine, oxycodone, zomepirac, and diazepam.

Objective: Fasting plasma glucose 320 mg/dL weight 304 pounds, height 71 in., large frame, decreased light touch and vibratory sense over feet, lower legs, and fingers, absent ankle and knee jerks, substernal pain and abnormal ECG after walking one block, blood pressure 140/88 mmHg.

Assessment: NIDDM being treated with insulin, painful peripheral neuropathy, stable exertional angina, hypertension, 112 pounds above IBW of 192 pounds.

Initial plan and therapy: Hospitalized in ambulatory care unit 7/20–8/1/82. Seven-day total fast, insulin discontinued abruptly, weight decreased from 298 to 276 pounds (22 pounds), fasting plasma glucose from 264 to 97 mg/dL, blood pressure (without medication) from 140/88 to 122/80 mmHg. On 7/28/82, 1,024-calorie diet consisting of skim milk, vegetables, and fruits was started. On 8/1/82,

weight 278 pounds, fasting plasma glucose 137 mg/dL, blood pressure 130/80 mmHg.

Follow-up: Clinic visits at monthly intervals. Progressive weight loss to IBW of 192 lb on 1/7/83. From 7/20/82 to 1/7/83 observed/predicted weight loss was:

$$\frac{\begin{array}{c}20 \text{ pounds (1-week fast + 2 days 1,024-calorie diet)}\\+ 86 \text{ pounds}\end{array}}{\begin{array}{c}20 \text{ pounds (1-week fast + 2 days 1,024-calorie diet)}\\+ 80.5 \text{ pounds}\end{array}}$$

$$\frac{\text{in 23 weeks (3.74 pounds/week) on 1,024 calories}}{\text{in 23 weeks (3.5 pounds/week) on 1,024 calories}} =$$

$$\frac{106 \text{ pounds}}{100.5 \text{ pounds}} = 104\% \text{ (see Fig. 16–2)}$$

He had resumed work as a heavy equipment operator in 11/82. For 3 months he had not had angina or neuropathic pain, nor had he taken medication for hypertension.

On 1/7/83 his fasting plasma glucose was 91 mg/dL and his blood pressure was 110/70. On 1/12/83, his glucose tolerance test sum was 515 mg/dL (fasting plus post-100-g glucose load 1-, 2-, and 3-hr plasma glucose levels), which is within limits classified as nondiabetic (sum <600 mg/dL).

On 1/7/83, he was placed on a 2,500-calorie diet to maintain IBW. On 5/10/83, his random plasma glucose was 92 mg/dL, weight 192 pounds, blood pressure 114/72. He had no angina, no neuropathic pain, and had taken no medication for eight months. He had been working regularly for 6 months. On 7/20/84, his weight was 192 pounds, and his random plasma glucose was 88 mg/dL. He was working full-time (see Fig. 16–2). On 1/20/89, his weight was 196 pounds and his random plasma glucose was 98 mg/dL

[a] Totally adherent is defined as the ratio of observed to predicted weight loss being ≥ 90%.

Abbreviations: ECG, electrocardiogram; IBM, ideal body weight; NPH, neutral protein Hagedorn; other abbreviations as in text.

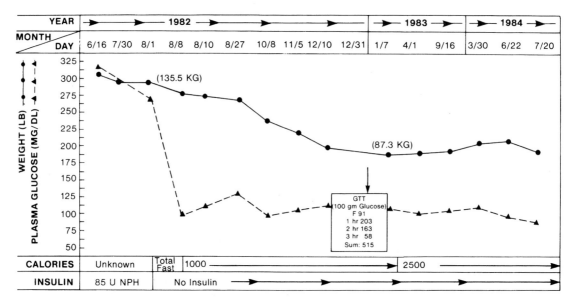

Figure 16–2. (See Exhibit 16–17): This graph shows the rate of weight loss in an individual who was totally adherent during a 1 week fast followed by a 1,024 calorie diet for 150 days (mean weight loss = 0.6 lbs/day). At ideal body weight, weight was maintained on 2,500 cal/day.

EXHIBIT 16–18   Example of a Partially Adherent Patient[a]

A 59-year-old white female restaurant manager had had diabetes for 19 years (since 1963), which had been increasingly hard to control despite larger doses of insulin during the last 2 years; the severity of her painful peripheral neuropathy had increased markedly during the last year and had produced insomnia and caused her to miss many work days. Her primary care physician referred her for evaluation and treatment.

Problems:

  I. Diabetes mellitus:
    A. Painful peripheral neuropathy
    B. Peripheral vascular disease
    C. Right carotid bruit
    D. Preproliferative diabetic retinopathy
  II. Hypertension
  III. Obesity

Subjective: Diabetes diagnosed 1963 (when at maximum weight of 230 pounds); treated with tolbutamide, then chlorpropamide until 1971, when NPH insulin therapy was started. Dose was increased progressively until it reached 110 UNPH each day in 5/82. During the last year her physician had difficulty in controlling her plasma glucose level with insulin therapy, and disabling painful peripheral neuropathy developed. Her hypertension had been treated with hydrochlorthiazide 100 mg/day since 1964.

Objective: Fasting plasma glucose 199 mg/dL, hemoglobin A_{1c} 12.2%, weight 207 pounds, height 64 in., medium frame decreased light touch and vibratory sense over feet, absent ankle jerks, blood pressure standing 180/80 mmHg, preproliferative diabetic retinopathy (microaneurysms, punctate hemorrhages, lipid exudates), absent dorsalis pedis pulses bilaterally, right carotid bruit.

Assessment: NIDDM being treated with insulin, painful peripheral neuropathy, right carotid bruit and bilaterally absent dorsalis pedis pulses, preproliferative diabetic retinopathy, hypertension, 87 pounds above ideal body weight of 120.

Initial plan and therapy: Hospitalized in ambulatory care unit 7/23–8/1/82. Seven-day total fast, insulin discontinued abruptly. Weight decreased from 207 to 193 pounds (14 pounds), fasting plasma glucose from 199 to 110 mg/dL, blood pressure (without medication) from 180/80 to 130/70. On 7/30/82, 512-calorie diet consisting of skim milk, vegetables, and fruits was started. On 8/1/82, weight 195 pounds, fasting plasma glucose 156 mg/dL, blood pressure (without medication) 140/76 mmHg.

Follow-up: Clinic visits at monthly intervals. Over a 30-week period (until 2/18/83) her weight decreased to 151 pounds, for a total weight loss of 56 pounds. Sporadically she would eat excessive amounts of food, including sweets. As a result, her follow-up plasma glucose levels were erratic, and varied with food intake during the previous 24 hr [105, 143, 180, 360 (after cake the previous evening), 260, and 144 mg/dL]. An outpatient 1-week total fast was prescribed on three occasions (she adhered during the first, but not during the second or third). Her observed/predicted weight loss during 30 weeks follow-up was:

$$\frac{12 \text{ pounds (1-week fast + 2 days 512 calories)} + 44 \text{ pounds in 30}}{12 \text{ pounds (1-week fast + 2 days 512 calories)} + 75 \text{ pounds in 30}}$$

$$\frac{\text{weeks (1.5 pounds/week) on 512 calories} + \text{three prescribed}}{\text{weeks (2.5 pounds/week) on 512 calories}}$$

$$\frac{\text{1-week fasts}}{} = \frac{56 \text{ pounds}}{87 \text{ pounds}} = 64\%.$$

Her weight remained on a plateau of 150 to 154 lb from 2/18/83 to 7/14/83. Yet her plasma glucose remained 159 to 208 mg/dL without insulin therapy, her blood pressure 130/70 to 140/80 without medication, neuropathic pain had subsided, and she was exercising and working regularly. Her body image concept dictated that she not lose more weight, and she refused to fast in the hospital or as an outpatient and she refused psychiatric consultation, even though she was still 30 pounds above her ideal body weight and she was still moderately hyperglycemic.

[a] Partially adherent is defined as the ratio of observed, to predicted weight loss being 10% to 90%.

Abbreviation: NPH, neutral protein Hagedom.

---

education and behavior, and to modify the strategy and processes of care and follow-up as needed.

Research Considerations

Significant epidemiologic research has been completed, but more is needed.[19–21] Many investigators have tried to develop methods that could determine accurately the amount of fat tissue and the amount of nonfat tissue ("lean body mass"). The only direct method for obtaining such data is autopsy tissue analysis, and this has been done on only a few cadavers. All methods applied to the living body are indirect, and none has been validated. Researchers estimate body fat by a densitometric method (underwater weighing), an inert gas (cyclo-propane) uptake method by adipose tissue, and measurement of body potassium in a total body counter. These methods are much too expensive and cumbersome for clinical use. Various anthropometric measurements designed to provide estimates of body fat content have been used and are under investigation [chest, waist, and wrist circumference, arm length, elbow breadth, caliper-measured skinfold thickness (triceps, biceps, subscapular, and suprailiac)], and thickness of subcutaneous fat tissue measured by ultrasound. Relative body weight, or the ratio of actual patient weight to population standard (mean) weight as related to height and frame, is now routinely used to estimate the amount of excess adiposity (Hamwi formula, Metropolitan Life Insurance Co. 1980,[65] Fogerty, Framingham,

EXHIBIT 16–19　Example of a Nonadherent Patient[a]

A 33-year-old white female hospital food service worker had had diabetes for 7 years (since 1975) and had been hospitalized on four occasions for acutely decompensated diabetes (plasma glucose >500 mg/dL, but without ketoacidosis). She had been treated with as much as 225 U NPH insulin daily. Her primary care physician referred her for evaluation and treatment.

Problems(7/22/82):

I. Diabetes mellitus
   A. Necrobiosis lipoidica right and left tibial regions, healed
   B. History of acutely decompensated diabetes × 4 (plasma glucose >500 mg/dL without ketoacidosis) despite therapy with 225 U NPH insulin daily
II. Status postcholecystectomy for stones, 1972
III. Hypertension
IV. Obesity

Subjective: Diabetes diagnosed 1975 (when at maximum weight of 250 pounds). NPH insulin therapy started at the time of diagnosis, with progressive increase in dose to 225 U insulin per day in 1981 and early 1982. She was on 125 U NPH insulin on 7/22/82. She had a cholecystectomy (gallstones) 1972, and had necrobiosis lipoidica in 1975 which had healed by 1980. She had hypertension, which had been treated with clonidine since 1980, and had been obese since childhood.

Objective: Weight 195 pounds, height 64 in., medium frame, blood pressure 160/90 mmHg, fasting plasma glucose 281 mg/dL, hemoglobin A_{1c} 15.4%, no detectable serum insulin-neutralizing antibody.

Assessment: Probable NIDDM being treated with insulin, hypertension, 75 pounds above ideal body weight of 120 pounds.

Initial plan and therapy: Hospitalized in ambulatory care unit 7/23–8/5/82. Seven-day total fast, insulin discontinued abruptly. Weight decreased from 195 to 183 pounds (12 pounds) and fasting plasma glucose from 281 to 182 mg/dL, and blood pressure from 160/90 to 120/80 (without medication). Because the carbon dioxide content dropped to 15 mEq/L and the fasting plasma glucose was still elevated on the seventh fast day, 20 U NPH insulin and a 512-calorie diet consisting of skim milk, vegetables, and fruits was started. Carbon dioxide content increased to 26 mEq/L, fasting plasma glucose to 201 mg/dL, and blood pressure to 140/85. She was discharged on 512-calorie diet and 20 U NPH insulin.

Follow-up: On 8/13/82, weight was 183 pounds, fasting plasma glucose 93 mg/dL. By 11/5/82, her weight was 198 pounds, fasting plasma glucose 177 mg/dL, and blood pressure 160/90 (on clonidine). To account for their weight gain, it was estimated that she had been eating about 3,300 calories/day during the 8/13–11/5/82 interval. She did not adhere to prescribed fasts or to the prescribed 512-calorie diet. She did not keep her appointment on 12/10/82. In 2/83, her primary cary physician hospitalized her for phlebothrombosis of the legs and initiated warfarin therapy. By 5/15/83, her NPH insulin dose was 75 U/day, fasting plasma glucose 265 mg/dL. On 7/8/83, her weight was 195 pounds, fasting plasma glucose 250 mg/dL, NPH insulin dose 125 U/day, blood pressure 160/90 (on clonidine). She refused psychiatric consultation. Compulsive eating appeared to be an integral part of her life-style, which was uncontrollable with contemporary knowledge. Yet it was clear that insulin therapy was incapable of reversing the hyperglycemic consequences of excessive caloric intake and obesity.

[a] Nonadherent is defined as the ratio of observed to predicted weight loss being <10%.

Abbreviations: NPH, neutral protamine Hagedorn; other abbreviations as in text.

---

and the English Consumer's Association). Unfortunately, recommended population standard weights differ for all five methods. For instance, for a male 70 in. tall of medium frame, the recommended standard weights are: (1) Hamwi, 166 pounds; (2) Metropolitan Life Insurance Company, 173 pounds[65] (see Tables 16–10 and 16–11), (3) Fogerty, 153 pounds; (4) Framingham, 176 pounds; and (5) English Consumer's Association, 143 pounds, or *a range among five recommended standards of 33 pounds!* No wonder there is so much controversy among professionals and so much confusion among patients with NIDDM about the individual's optimal body weight.[67,68]

In order to standardize weight (and adiposity) comparisons in the scientific literature, most investigators now express body weight as the body mass index.[67] BMI equals weight in kilograms divided by the square of the height in meters (W/H^2). Optimal BMI is 19–20

(smallest mortality). Some accept up to 25 as "normal," but 25–29.9 is overweight, and ≥30 is obese. Relative mortality rate increases progressively above 25, and so does the prevalence of type 2 diabetes.

% body fat can be calculated from BMI using the following formulas:

1. For men, the % fat $= 1.218 (W/H^2) - 10.13$

2. For women, the % fat $= 1.48 (W/H^2) - 7.17$

Some investigators use the pondral index (3/weight/height). There is little reason for clinicians to believe that either in their daily practice is superior to relative body weight (weight, height, frame) as a predictor of fatness. Much carefully planned prospective, longitudinal research from birth to morbidity (NIDDM) to death is needed. Also, the consequences of various levels of relative body weight for morbidity

TABLE 16–10 1980 Metropolitan Life Insurance Co. Height-Weight Tables

Men[a]					Women[b]				
Height		Small Frame Pounds	Medium Frame Pounds	Large Frame Pounds	Height		Small Frame Pounds	Medium Frame Pounds	Large Frame Pounds
Ft.	In.				Ft.	In.			
5	2	128–134	131–141	138–150	4	10	102–111	109–121	118–131
5	3	130–136	133–143	140–153	4	11	103–113	111–123	120–134
5	4	132–138	135–145	142–156	5	0	104–115	113–126	122–137
5	5	134–140	137–148	144–160	5	1	106–118	115–129	125–140
5	6	136–142	139–151	146–164	5	2	108–121	118–132	128–143
5	7	138–145	142–154	149–168	5	3	111–124	121–135	131–147
5	8	140–148	145–157	152–172	5	4	114–127	124–138	134–151
5	9	142–151	148–160	155–176	5	5	117–130	127–141	137–155
5	10	144–154	151–163	158–180	5	6	120–133	130–144	140–159
5	11	146–147	154–166	161–184	5	7	123–136	133–147	143–163
6	0	149–160	157–170	164–188	5	8	126–139	136–150	146–167
6	1	152–164	160–174	168–192	5	9	129–142	139–153	149–170
6	2	155–168	164–178	172–197	5	10	132–145	142–156	152–173
6	3	158–172	167–182	176–202	5	11	135–148	145–159	155–176
6	4	162–176	171–187	181–207	6	0	138–151	148–162	158–179

[a] Weights at ages 25–59 based on lowest mortality. Weight in pounds according to frame (in indoor clothing weighing 5 pounds, shoes with 1-in. heels).

[b] Weights at ages 25–59 based on lowest mortality. Weight in pounds according to frame (in indoor clothing weighing 3 pounds, shoes with 1-in. heels).

[*Source:* Height and Weight table. Metropolitan Life Insurance Co. Society of Actuaries: Build Study, 1979. Association of Life Insurance Medical Directors of America, 1980. With permission.]

TABLE 16–11 Elbow Breadth Measurements for Determination of Frame Size[a]

Men				Women			
Height in 1-in. Heels		Elbow Breadth		Height in 1-in. Heels		Elbow Breadth	
In.	Cm	In.	Cm	In.	Cm	In.	Cm
62–63	157–160	2.5–2.9	6.35–7.3	58–59	147–150	2.25–2.5	5.7–6.35
64–67	163–170	2.6–2.9	6.67–7.3	60–63	152–160	2.25–2.5	5.7–6.35
68–71	173–180	2.75–3	6.98–7.62	64–67	163–170	2.4–2.6	6.03–6.67
72–75	183–181	2.75–3.1	6.98–7.94	68–71	173–180	2.4–2.6	6.03–6.67
76	193	2.9–3.25	6.35–8.3	72	183	2.5–2.75	6.35–6.98

[a] Extend your arm and bend the forearm upward at a 90° angle. Keep fingers straight and turn the inside of your wrist toward your body. If you have a caliper use it to measure the space between the two prominent bones on either side of your elbow. Without a caliper, place thumb and index finger of your other hand on these two bones. Measure the space between your fingers against a ruler or tape measure. Compare it with these tables that list elbow measurements for medium-framed men and women. Measurements lower than those listed indicate you have a small frame. Higher measurements than those listed indicate that you have a large frame.

[*Source:* Height and Weight table. Metropolitan Life Insurance Co. Society of Actuaries: Build Study, 1979. Association of Life Insurance Medical Directors of America, 1980. With permission.]

and mortality outcomes for those with type 2 diabetes (NIDDM and its subtypes) need to be measured prospectively and longitudinally.[67,68]

Studies of demographic, genetic, physical, hormonal, emotional, and environmental factors that determine food intake patterns (calories, carbohydrate, sugars, fats) and exercise patterns (which in turn influence the prevalence of NIDDM and its complications in different sexes and races, and in different national, socioeconomic, ethnic, and religious groups) need to be undertaken. The rate of progression of NIDDM to IDDM and the cause(s) thereunto related (possibly inability of the B cells to divide during persistent hyperglycemia or increased susceptibility to B-cell destruction by viral infection or autoimmune processes?) need to be studied in detail.

A great deal of biochemical and pathophysiologic research has been done, but the eventual significance of much of it is controversial. For instance, there is disagreement as to whether those with diabetes should use sucrose and/or fructose in their diet.[65] Research indicates that various components of food and combinations of these components as well as the form in which food is ingested may be responsible for differences in glycemic responses to different foods.

There is still not universal agreement about how to determine the amount of sucrose and other sugars that can be used in the diet without producing undesirable hyperglycemic effects.[66,71] Now most physicians permit up to 10% of the daily carbohydrate intake in the form of glucose, fructose, and sucrose (i.e. 250 grams of carbohydrate prescribed permits up to 25 gm sugar). The frequent use of sugar containing prepared foods in today's diet makes it impossible to arrange a diet that is free of sugars. However, the blood glucose effects of dietary sugars should be evaluated (especially in IDDMs) by post-prandial SMBG occasionally (see Chapter 15).

New insulins (lispro, etc.) and continuous subcutaneous insulin infusion (CS11) techniques have permitted considerable relaxation of formerly rigid rules of prescribing content and timing of feedings. This freedom of patient food ingestion in the practice of Mühlhauser, Berger and colleagues[71] resulted in acceptable levels of metabolic control without requiring the patient to adhere to any of the classical dietary prescriptions. Needless to say, in NIDDMs who are overweight, caloric intake needs to be reduced to produce weight loss.

Jenkins (1982)[69] developed a glycemic index table in which he classified 60 different foods according to the extent to which they raise the 2-hr postprandial blood glucose compared with equivalent amounts of glucose *in nondiabetic subjects* (see Exhibit 16–20).

Factors that affect the rate of digestion and absorption such as food processing, fiber content,[69] enzyme inhibitors, protein-fat content, and other nutrient interactions appear to have an effect on the postprandial blood glucose response.

Further research is needed to investigate the effects of different carbohydrates ingested separately and in "mixed-meals" combination (with protein, fat, and/or various types and amounts of fiber) in patients with NIDDM or IDDM before altering the recommendations of the American Diabetes Association and the American Dietetic Association as reflected in the food exchange lists.[44]

Much research needs to be done on the substrate, hormone, receptor, and postreceptor intracellular events that precede the development of NIDDM in those who are overweight and in those who are not overweight. The effects of gaining and losing weight on the same parameters need detailed study. For instance, it has been shown that B-cell sensitivity to gastric inhibitory polypeptide decreases with age, and it may contribute to the glucose intolerance of patients with NIDDM.[70]

EXHIBIT 16–20   Glycemic Index: the Area Under the Blood Glucose Curve for Each Food Expressed as a Percentage of the Area After Taking the Same Amount of Carbohydrate as Glucose[a]

100%	*60 to 69%*	Oatmeal biscuits	Blackeyed peas
Glucose	Bread (white)	Peas (frozen)	Chick peas
	Rice (brown)	Yam	Apples (golden delicious)
80 to 90%	Muesli	Sucrose	Ice cream
Corn flakes	Shredded wheat	Potato chips	Milk (skim)
Carrots	Ryvita		Milk (whole)
Parsnips	Water biscuits	*40 to 49%*	Yogurt
Potatoes (instant, mashed)	Beets	Spaghetti (whole wheat)	Tomato Soup
Maltose	Bananas	Oatmeal	
Honey	Raisins	Potato (sweet)	*20 to 29%*
	Mars bar	Beans (canned navy)	Kidney beans
		Peas (dried)	Lentils
70 to 79%	*50% to 59%*	Oranges	Fructose
Bread (whole wheat)	Buckwheat	Orange juice	
Millet	Spaghetti (white)		*10 to 19%*
Rice (white)	Sweet-corn	*30 to 39%*	Soy beans
Potato (new)	All-Bran	Butter beans	Soy beans (canned)
Turnips	Digestive biscuits	Haricot beans	Peanuts

[a] Data from normal individuals. It should be noted that those with diabetes, especially if it is uncontrolled, would have plasma glucose responses that were both quantitatively and qualitatively different.

[*Source:* Jenkins DJA: Lente carbohydrate: a newer approach to the dietary management of diabetes. Diabetes Care 5:634–641, 1982. With permission.]

The ability of exercise to increase muscle mass and decrease adipose mass and its effects on substrate, hormone, and receptor levels need more study. The *safety*, *therapeutic effectiveness*, and *cost-effectiveness* of various *processes of care* (alternative therapeutic modalities) should be researched in detail (Exhibit 16–21).

A recent randomized controlled trial[72] demonstrated that a popular herbal compound containing hydroxyc-itric acid plus a low-energy diet was no more effective than placebo plus a low energy diet in producing weight loss in obese individuals. Considering the aggressive advertising and marketing campaigns of the companies that sell these products to millions of easily duped consumers, more studies of this type are needed. Ideally, products that are ineffective (and sometimes unsafe) should be removed from the market.

EXHIBIT 16–21 Processes of Care Used in the Treatment of Non-Insulin-Dependent Diabetes Mellitus Whose Outcomes (Safety, Therapeutic Effectiveness, and Cost-Effectiveness) Need Comprehensive Evaluation

I. A. Fasting: short-term (7 days), long-term (more than 7 days), and protein-sparing (7 days and more than 7 days)
   B. Various types of diets: low-caloric-density versus high-caloric-density diets, and so forth
   C. Various types and amounts of fiber
   D. Non-nutritive sweeteners (saccharine, cyclamates, aspartame, acesulfame-K, and so on)
   E. Non-nutritive and low-calorie beverage and food substitutes
   F. Inhibitors of carbohydrate breakdown and absorption (glucosidase inhibitors, and so on)
   G. Inhibitors of fat breakdown and absorption
   H. "Dietetic foods" with lower calorie content versus conventional foods with standard calorie content
   I. Nutritive sweeteners (fructose, sorbitol, mannitol, xylitol, and the like)
II. A. Psychiatric, psychologic, and environmental determinants of behavior. Can interventional psychiatric or psychologic therapy change behavior related to food intake? How? Side effects?
   B. Can behavior modification therapy and/or self-help groups change life-styles and eating habits over the long term? How? Side effects?
   C. Hypnotherapy: Is it safe: Is it effective?
III. A. The following drugs have been used to suppress appetite: amphetamines, benzphatamine, dextro-amphetamine, diethylpropion, fluoxetine hydrochloride, levamfetamine, methamphetamine, methylphenidate, phendimetrazine, phenmetrazine, and phentermine. What is the addictive and abuse potential and what are the side effects of each? Are any of them safe and effective over the long term in the treatment of overweight individuals?
   B. The following surgical procedures have been used: clamping jaws, stapling stomach, short-circuiting intestine (several versions). What are the complications of each? Are any of them safe and effective over the long term? If so, what are valid criteria for patient selection?

References

1. Rollo J: A general view of the history nature and appropriate treatment of diabetes mellitus. London: 1798.

2. Bernard C: Lecons sur diabete et la glycogenese animale. Paris: J.B. Baillère, 1877.

3. Allen FM, Stillman E, Fitz R: Total dietary regulation in the treatment of diabetes. New York: Rockefeller Institute for Medical Research, No. 11, 1919.

4. Joslin EP: Diabetic metabolism with high and low diets. Washington, DC: Carnegie Institute, Publication No. 323, 1923.

5. Rubner M: Die (Quelle) der Thierischen Warme. Ztshr Biol 73, 1894.

6. Atwater WO, Rose EB: A new respiration calorimeter. Bull. No. 63, Washington, DC: Department of Agriculture, 1899.

7. Dubois EF: Basal Metabolism in Health and Disease, Ed. 3, Philadelphia: Lea & Febiger, 1936.

8. Rose WC: The nutritive significance of the amino acids. Physiol Rev 18:109–136, 1938.

9. McCollum EV: The beginnings of essential nutrition. Nutr Rev 14:257, 1956.

10. Recommended Dietary Allowances 1989, Ed. 10. Washington, DC: Food and Nutrition Board, National Research Council, National Academy of Sciences.

11. Bierman EL, Albrink MJ, Arky RA et al.: Principles of nutrition and dietary recommendations for patients with diabetes mellitus. Diabetes 20:633–634, 1971.

12. Franz MJ, Barr P, Holler H, et al.: Exchange List: Revised 1986. J Am Dietetic Assoc 87:28–34, 1987.

13. Glinsmann WH, Irausquin H, Park Y: Evaluation of health aspects of sugars contained in carbohydrate sweeteners. Report of Sugars Task Force, Washington, DC: Food and Drug Administration, 1986.

14. Crapo PA, Kolterman OG, Waldeck RN: Postprandial hormonal responses to different types of complex carbohydrate in individuals with impaired glucose tolerance. Am J Clin Nutr 33:1723–1728, 1980.

15. Bantle J: Clinical aspects of sucrose and fructose metabolism. Diabetes Care 12:56–61, 1989.

16. Chittenden RH: Physiological Economy in Nutrition. New York: Frederick A. Stokes, 1907.

17. The Diabetes Control and Complications Trial Group: "The Effect of Intensive Treatment of Diabetes on the Development and Progression of Long-Term Complications in Insulin-Dependent Diabetes Mellitus. New Engl. J Med. 329:977–986, 1993.

18. Keys A, Brozek J, Henschel A, et al.: The Biology of Human Starvation, Vols. 1 and 2. Minneapolis: University of Minneapolis Press, 1950.

19. Bray G (ed): Obesity in Perspective, vol. 2, parts 1 and 2. Washington DC: Government Printing Office, 1975.

20. West KM: Epidemiology of Diabetes and Its Vascular Lesions. New York: Elsevier, 1978.

21. Behnke AR, Osserman EF, Walham WC: Lean body mass. Arch Intern Med 91:585, 1953.

22. Himsworth HP: Diabetes mellitus: its differentiation into insulin-sensitive and insulin-insensitive types. Lancet 1:127–130, 1936.

23. Newburgh LH: Control of the hyperglycemia of obese "diabetics" by weight reduction. Ann Intern Med 17: 935–942, 1942.

24. Newburgh LH: Obesity: I. Energy metabolism. Physiol Rev 24:18, 1944.

25. Tolstoi E: In Soskin's Progress in Clinical Endocrinology. New York: Grune & Stratton, 1950, p. 292.

26. Kennedy DL, Piper JM, Baum C: Trends in use of oral hypoglycemic agents 1964–1986. Diabetes Care 11:558–562, 1988.

27. Lebovitz HE: Second-generation sulfonylureas: What are they and what is their value? Clin Diabetes 6:84–85, 1984.

28. Stone DB, Connor WE: The prolonged effects of a low cholesterol, high carbohydrate diet upon the serum lipids in diabetic patients. Diabetes 12:127, 1963.

29. Karam JH, Grodsky GM, Forsham PH: Excessive insulin response to glucose in obese subjects as measured by immunochemical assay. Diabetes 12:197, 1963.

30. Sims EAH: Endocrine and metabolic effects of experimental obesity in man. Rec Prog Horm Res 29:457–496, 1973.

31. Wing RR, Salata R, Marcus T, et al.: A very low calorie diet (VLCD) plus behavior modification in the treatment of type II diabetes. Diabetes 37(Suppl 1):110A, 1988.

32. Davidson JK, Lebovitz HE: Debates in Medicine: Diet is the therapy of choice in adult non-insulin-dependent diabetes mellitus. Mosby: Yearbook Medical Publishers, Chicago 1991.

33. Hamwi GJ: Therapy: changing dietary concepts. In Danowski TS (ed): Diabetes Mellitus: Diagnosis and Treatment, vol. 1. New York: American Diabetes Association, 1964, pp. 73–78.

34. Davidson JK: Educating diabetic patients about diet therapy. Int Diabetes Fed Bull 20:1–5, 1975.

35. Bar RS, Roth J: Insulin receptor status in disease states of man. Arch Intern Med 127:474–481, 1977.

36. National Institutes of Health: Concensus development conference on diet and exercise in non-insulin-dependent diabetes mellitus. Diabetes Care 10:639–644, 1987.

37. Exchange Lists for Meal Planning. New York: American Diabetes Association; Chicago: American Dietetic Association, 1989.

38. Nutrition Guide for Professionals Diabetes Education and Meal Planning. New York: American Diabetes Association; Chicago: American Dietetic Association, 1988.

39. Bistrian BR: Recent developments in the treatment of obesity with particular reference to semistarvation ketogenic regimens. Diabetes Care 1:379–384, 1978.

40. Sours HE, Frattali VP, Brand CD, et al.: Sudden death associated with very low calorie weight reduction regimens. Am J Clin Nutr 34:453–461, 1981.

41. Apfelbaum M, Fricker J, Igoin-Apfelbaum: Low and verylow calorie diets. Am J Clin Nutr 45:1126–1134, 1987.

42. Anderson JW, Story L, Seeling B: Hypocholesterol effects of oat-bran or bean intake for hyperchoesterolemic men. Am J Clin Nutr 40:1146–1155, 1984.

43. Anderson JW, Bridges SR: Dietary fiber content of selected foods. Am J Clin Nutr 47:440–447, 1988.

44. Anderson JW: Fiber and diabetes. Diabetes Care 2(4):369–378, 1979.

45. National Diabetes Data Group: Classification and diagnosis of diabetes mellitus and other categories of glucose intolerance. Diabetes 28:1029–1057, 1979.

46. Davidson JK, Delcher HK, Englund A: Spin-off cost/benefits of expanded nutritional care. J Am Diet Assoc 75: 250–257, 1979.

47. Davidson JK, Zwaag RV, Cox CL, et al.: The Memphis and Atlanta continuing care programs for diabetes. II Comparative analyses of demographic characteristics, treatment methods, and outcomes over a 9–10 year follow-up period. Diabetes Care 7:25–31, 1984.

48. Alberti KGMM, Gries FA: Management of non-insulin dependent diabetes mellitus in Europe: A concensus view. Diabetes Med 5:275–281, 1988.

49. Kronsbein P, Muhlhauser I, Venhaus A: Evaluation of a structured treatment and teaching programme on noninsulin-dependent diabetes. Lancet 2:1407–1411, 1988.

50. Garfield E: Current comments: To fast or not to fast. A controversial question gets some scientific answers. Curr Contents 47:5–11, 1981.

51. Flood TM: Diet and diabetes mellitus. Hosp Prac, February 1979; 17:61–69.

52. Davidson JK, Goldsmith MP: Diabetes Guidebook: Diet Section, Ed. 4. Davicone, 1075 Lullwater Rd NE, Atlanta, GA 30307, 1984.

53. Guidelines for use of the Exchange Lists for low-sodium meal planning. Chicago: American Dietetic Association; New York: American Diabetes Association, 1989.

54. Guidelines for use of the Exchange Lists for low-sodium, low fat meal planning. Chicago: American Dietetic Association; New York: American Diabetes Association, 1989.

55. Guidelines for use of the Exchange Lists for low-fat meal planning. Chicago: American Dietetic Association; New York: American Diabetes Association, 1989.

56. ADA's definition for nutrition screening and nutrition assessment. J Am Diet Assoc 94:838–839, 1994.

57. Subcommittee on Nutrition, Committee on Public Health. Medical Society of the County of New York: New height-weight tables; importance of new (Metropolitan Life Insurance) criteria. JAMA 173:1576, 1960.

58. Maras ML, Adolphi CL: Ethnic tailoring improves dietary compliance. Diabetes Educator, 11:47–50, 1985.

59. Davidson JK: A new look at diet therapy. Diabetes Forecast, May-June:14–19, 1976.

60. Mitch WE: Nutrition and the kidney. Boston: Little Brown & Co., 1988.

61. Stuart RB, David B: Slim Chance in a Fat World: Behavioral Control of Obesity. Champaign, IL: Research Press, 1972.

62. Stunkard AJ, Craighead LW, O'Brien RO: Controlled trial of behavior therapy and their combination in the treatment of obesity. Lancet 2:1045–1047, 1980.

63. Rabkin SW, Boyko E, Wilson A, et al.: A randomized clinical trial comparing behavior modification and individual counseling in the nutritional therapy of non-insulin-dependent diabetes mellitus: comparison of the effect on blood sugar, body weight, and serum lipids. Diabetes Care 6:50–56, 1983.

64. Adams CF: Nutritive values of American foods in common units. Agriculture No. 456. Washington, DC: United States Department of Agriculture, Superintendent of Documents, Government Printing Office, 1975.

65. Height and weight table. Metropolitan Life Insurance Co. Society of Actuaries: Build Study, 1979. Chicago: Association of Life Insurance Medical Directors of America, 1980.

66. Bantle J: Clinical aspects of sucrose and fructose metabolism. Diabetes Care 12:56–61, 1989.

67. Flyer JS, Foster DW: Eating disorders: obesity, anorexia nervosa, and bulimia nervosa. *In* Williams Textbook of Endocrinology, Edition 9, p. 1061–1097, 1998. WB Saunders, Philadelphia.

68. Simopoulos AP, Van Itallie TB: Body weight, health, and longevity. Ann Intern Med 100:285–295, 1984.

69. Jenkins JA: Lente carbohydrate for diabetic individuals. Diabetes Care 5:634–641, 1982.

70. Elahi D, Andersen DK, Muller DC, et al.: The enteric enhancement of glucose-stimulated insulin release: the role of GIP in aging, obesity, and non-insulin-dependent diabetes mellitus. Diabetes 33:950–957, 1984.

71. Mühlhauser I, Bott U, Overman H, et al.: Liberalized diet in patients with type 1 diebetes. J Inter Med 237:591–597, 1995.

72. Heymsfield S, Allison D, Vasselli J, et al.: Garcinia Cambogia (Hydroxycitric Acid) as a potential antiobesity agent: a randomized control trial. JAMA 280:1596–1600, 1998.

17

Exercise and Stress
in Diabetes Mellitus

Mladen Vranic, Carol Rodgers,
John K. Davidson, and Errol Marliss

In the nondiabetic individual, exercise activates a series of physiologic responses that are directed toward ensuring adequate fuel supply for muscular activity, while at the same time maintaining the individual within tight physiologic metabolic control. This is achieved primarily by directing the flux of nutrients toward the active muscle group(s) and by increasing fuel mobilization from the liver and adipose tissue to compensate for the enhanced uptake of fuel by the working tissues. Although the principles that govern the response to exercise are similar in the diabetic individual, the actual responses may differ depending on the current degree of metabolic stress that the diabetic individual is experiencing. Factors that influence the degree of metabolic stress, including, but not limited to, the type of diabetes, the state of metabolic control, nutritional status, appropriateness of insulin treatment, level of physical fitness, and time of exercise in relation to last meal and/or pharmacologic drug intake, will all contribute to the nature of the response to exercise observed in the diabetic individual.

By definition, stress is any factor or variable that causes a deviation from homeostasis.[1] Stress may occur for only a short period, as in a single bout of exercise, or may be chronically imposed on the body, like the metabolic stress of diabetes. In instances of a chronic state of stress the body's defense mechanisms ultimately fail to preserve homeostasis, and further physiologic deterioration occurs. Stress activates a physiologic to pathophysiologic spectrum of responses, a portion of which resemble those evident during exercise-induced stress. However, unlike what occurs during exercise, fuel mobilization is no longer directed solely to the working muscles. In contrast, during stress fuel mobilization is multidirectional, often being directed toward repair processes, or ultimately to provide energy requirement for the brain. The increase in fuel mobilization of nutrients is usually greater than the increase in uptake, and hyperglycemia accompanies most stress situations. As with exercise-induced stress, the response to other forms of stress can vary according to the type and severity of the stress and are also affected by the underlying condition(s) of the subject. In diabetes, the response to stress may be deleterious, leading to decompensation of metabolic control (see Chapter 24).

Exercise

Historical Perspective

Physical exercise has been recognized as a valuable adjunct therapy in the treatment of diabetes mellitus since the late 18th century.[2-4] Over the last century, and in particular since the discovery of insulin, exercise has become one of the three basic principles for the management of diabetes.[5,6] Recently, the interrelationship between exercise and various aspects of metabolism have been more clearly delineated, particularly in relation to improvements in factors associated with metabolic control in type 2 diabetes. Interestingly, however, while some improvements have been noted in individuals with type 1 diabetes, the benefits of exercise on overall metabolic control have not been as clearly demonstrated and thus, unlike in the past, exercise is not currently regarded as a *necessary* component of the *management of metabolic control* for all individuals with type 1 diabetes. Exercise is, however, still *recommended* for individuals with diabetes, although the rationales for exercise as part of the treatment program differ between type 1 and type 2 diabetes. In type 2 its role in energy balance and overall lifestyle change is prominent, while for individuals with type 1 diabetes the challenge is to help the person perform optimally without extremes of variation in glycemia. Regardless of the type of diabetes, exercise also provides the benefits of improved cardiovascular fitness, weight control, stress reduction, and an increased overall state of well-being. For these reasons alone, recommending an active lifestyle in individuals with diabetes must be encouraged.

Introduction

Before discussing the metabolic responses that occur during exercise it is important to differentiate between acute and chronic exercise. Acute exercise refers to a single bout of exercise that in itself requires a variety of metabolic, circulatory, and temperature-controlling adaptations for the body to meet the acute oxygen and fuel requirements of the exercise bout and to minimize the deviations from normal homeostasis. These short-lived regulations vary with the type, intensity, and duration of exercise; muscles used; and a variety of environmental factors such as the physical condition and nutritional state of the individual. In contrast, chronic exercise, or physical training, results in system adaptations that reflect the body's means of optimizing its ability to respond to regularly imposed cumulative exercise stress. In addition to improvements related to cardiovascular and respiratory function the body also demonstrates an improved metabolic ability to produce energy through its primary metabolic pathways. These improvements can be noted across all physiologic systems of the body at rest, during submaximal exercise and during maximal exercise. Ultimately, chronic exercise training results in a bodily system that is both structurally and metabolically better able to deal with homeostatic stress.

Fuel Sources During Exercise

Muscular contraction requires energy. This energy is provided by the hydrolysis of the high-energy phosphate compound adenosine triphosphate (ATP). The body has three primary sources of ATP: (1) immediate/stored ATP and the ATP that is generated through either (2) nonoxidative or (3) oxidative sources of food fuel metabolism. The dominant energy source during a particular exercise bout or during a specific phase (e.g., onset, mid, or late) of an exercise period is determined by the rate and amount of ATP required. As exercise intensity increases the rate that ATP must be supplied increases. Similarly, as exercise duration increases the amount of ATP required increases.

The ATP stored in the muscle is one component of the body's immediate source of energy. Approximately 85 g of ATP are stored in muscle at rest. When hydrolyzed, ATP yields energy (-7.3 to -11 kcal$\cdot$mol^{-1} free energy) and the products adenosine diphosphate (ADP) and inorganic phosphate (PI).[7] To prevent an immediate depletion of muscle ATP a second, "immediate" source of energy exists. This source, creatine phosphate (CP), exists in quantities five to six times greater than ATP and provides a reserve of energy to enable the regeneration of ATP until other energy sources (nonoxidative and oxidative) can be more fully utilized. The final immediate energy source that enables the regeneration of ATP requires the enzyme adenylate kinase (myokinase in muscle) to catalyze the formation of ATP by combining two ADPs. Both the second and third sources help prevent complete ATP depletion by facilitating a high rate of ATP regeneration. Despite these rapid regeneration systems, however, there is only enough immediate energy in the muscle to provide for approximately 5–15 sec of maximal intensity contraction.[7]

Thus, although the rate (power) by which ATP is supplied by the immediate system is very high (36 kcal$\cdot$min^{-1}), its capacity, or the amount of ATP made available for conversion to energy, is extremely limited (11.1 kcal).[7] Since most of our daily activities readily exceed the amount of energy that is available through this immediate energy system, other systems of producing ATP with a greater capacitance must exist in the body. The nonoxidative and oxidative sources of energy, through the metabolism of nutrient sources of carbohydrate, fat, and protein, thus become the primary means by which the body generates ATP to provide the necessary energy to maintain body function at rest, as well as to meet the additional energy demands of exercise.

The nonoxidative and oxidative energy sources are named as such to reflect the oxygen requirements of each system. Production of energy through nonoxidative fuel metabolic pathways does not require the presence of oxygen. In contrast, oxidative pathways require the presence of oxygen to generate ATP. The body's nonoxidative nutrient source of energy is carbohydrate. Fat, carbohydrate, and protein can be metabolized through oxidative pathways. Since differences in the rate and capacity of ATP production also exist between the nonoxidative and oxidative energy pathways, the body's choice of food fuel is therefore also dependent on the rate of ATP production required and how much ATP is needed. While the breakdown of carbohydrate and the subsequent formation of ATP occur more rapidly than the breakdown of fat, fat provides much more ATP on a per gram basis (9.5 kcal$\cdot$g^{-1}).[7] Thus, when the amount of energy required is high but does not need to be provided rapidly, such as during rest, the oxidative metabolism of fat will be the predominant fuel source. In contrast, when energy must be provided quickly, but large quantities are not immediately required, nonoxidative metabolism of carbohydrate will be the main energy source.

Optimal energy provision during any given activity is a function of the overlap among the three primary energy source systems (immediate, nonoxidative, and oxidative) in accordance with the rate and the amount of ATP required (Fig. 17–1). Thus at rest, skeletal muscle relies predominantly (80%) on the oxidation of fatty acids and 20% on carbohydrate. With the onset of exercise, energy must be provided immediately and rapidly, and hence the immediate energy sources are nonoxidative metabolism of carbohydrate (glycogen) supplementing the ATP pool. During short-term high-

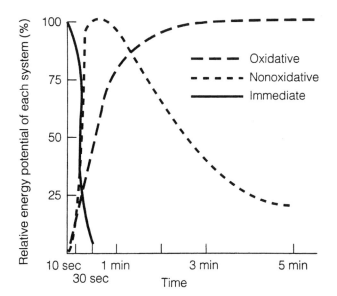

Figure 17–1. Energy sources for muscle as a function of activity duration. Schematic presentation showing how long each of the major energy systems can endure in supporting all-out work. Ref. 7.

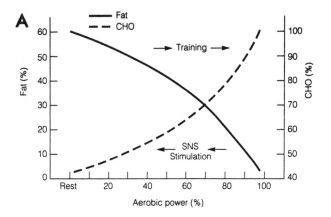

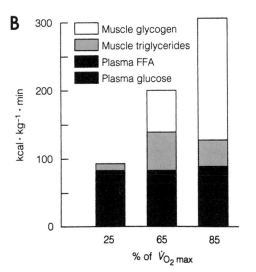

Figure 17–2. (A) The balance of carbohydrate and lipid use during exercise in explained by the "crossover concept." At low- to moderate-intensity exercise, carbohydrates and lipids both play major roles as energy substrates. However, when relative aerobic power output reaches 60–65%, then carbohydrates (CHO) become increasingly important and lipids become less important. Because of the crossover phenomenon, in most athletic activities glycogen stores provide the greatest fuel for exercise. Lipids become important energy sources during recovery. SNS refers to the sympathetic nervous system and the metabolic effects of epinephrine and norepinephrine. (B) Illustration of the crossover from lipid to carbohydrate dependency as exercise intensity increases from mild (25% VO$_2$ max). (Reproduced from Ref. 7)

intensity exercise when rapid ATP regeneration is required or when oxygen availability is limited, carbohydrates are the most efficient fuel and primary metabolic source of energy. In this situation muscle glycogen is the primary energy source (nonoxidative carbohydrate) supplemented with energy provided by the breakdown of circulating glucose from hepatic glycogenolysis. A very small portion of energy is also derived from oxidative sources. In contrast to heavy exercise, during mild and moderate exercise oxidative fuel sources predominate. The breakdown of glycogen, circulating glucose, and free fatty acid through oxidative pathways provides a high yield of ATP and enables the maintenance of exercise at this intensity for long periods of time. Differences in the degree of saturation between fatty acids and glucose predict that twice as much energy can be gained from the oxidation of 1 g of triglyceride as from 1 g of glycogen. In addition, while glycogen is stored with water, fat and water are immiscible; thus fats are stored in pure form. Hence, the economy of fat storage makes this the most efficient fuel for muscle activity of long duration. In contrast, the regeneration of ATP from immediate sources and the generation of ATP from glycolysis in the cytoplasm occur much more rapidly than the generation of ATP from fat oxidation in the mitochondria. Moreover, the oxidative metabolism of carbohydrates in the mitochondria requires less oxygen for metabolism than fats, since glucose carbon atoms are already partially oxidized compared with the highly saturated carbon skeleton of fat. Thus immediate sources are carbohydrate dominant in oxygen-limited situations (anaerobic) and in situations when ATP needs to be provided at a high rate so that activity can be initiated and maintained. However, if

the individual is to prolong the duration of the exercise bout the generation of ATP through the oxidation of fatty acids must be increased. For this to occur, the intensity of exercise must simultaneously decrease since the generation of ATP from fatty acid oxidation, although more efficient, is less rapid. Thus, energy provision during exercise is optimal at any given intensity and duration due to the coordinated integration of the three primary sources of energy provision in the body. While at any given intensity one energy source will be dominant, and at least one of the two other energy sources will also contribute (Fig. 17–2). This overlap of energy source contribution also helps prolong the onset of fatigue. The increased oxidation of lipids during the mid-later stages of moderate intensity exercise decreases the amount of energy that must be derived from the breakdown of muscle glycogen, the depletion of which has been shown to be a primary cause of muscular fatigue during exercise that is not limited by the cardiopulmonary system. By decreasing the "dominance" of energy provision by glycogen through increased fat oxidation and an increase in the channeling of glycerol, lactate, alanine, and other amino acids into the gluconeogenic pathway, muscle glycogen as an energy source can be "spared" until later in the exercise bout, delaying the onset of muscular fatigue and concomitantly prolonging the duration of the exercise bout. This "crossover" point, or the time when fat and carbohydrate "switch" as predominating energy sources, is determined by exercise intensity and is controlled by hormonal and neural signals in response to changes in the energy state (e.g., ATP/ADP ratio) of the body.[8,9] This "crossover" point occurs later in chronically exercising individuals and reflects training adaptations that enhance the body's ability to use lipid as a primary energy source at higher intensities of exercise (Fig. 17–2).

The contribution of protein to ATP generation becomes most apparent when exercise continues for a very prolonged period of time, as one approaches total exhaustion, and/or when prolonged exercise is carried out in a "starved" state. During these periods the oxidation of branched chain amino acids (leucine, isoleucine, valine) and ketone bodies is increased in order to maintain plasma glucose levels and the overall functioning of the individual.

Carbohydrate as a Source of Fuel (Fig. 17–3). When one considers the role of carbohydrate metabolism in providing energy during exercise, two primary areas need to be addressed: (1) fuel for energy supply and (2) maintenance of plasma glucose levels. The energy needs of the muscle are met by the metabolic breakdown of glucose and glycogen, while plasma glucose homeostasis is maintained through alterations in hepatic glucose production. Simply described, the uptake of glucose must be increased from resting levels during exercise so that enough fuel (glucose and glycogen) is available to be broken down to provide energy. To maintain plasma glucose levels this increase in glucose uptake must be "matched" by the input of glucose via an increase in hepatic glucose production. During low- and moderate-intensity exercise the increase in glucose uptake and the increase in hepatic glucose production are matched.[10] However, during high-intensity exercise (see description later in text), the increase in hepatic glucose production has been shown to exceed the rise in glucose use, as reflected by an increase in plasma glucose levels.

Regulation of Hepatic Glucose Production (Fig. 17–4). Changes in the rate of hepatic glucose production (HGP) are mediated through both hormonal (insulin, glucagon, catecholamines, cortisol, growth hormone) and neural processes. The influence of each of these mechanisms is determined by the duration and intensity of exercise. Although there continues to be considerable debate concerning the actual signals that mediate these hormonal and neural changes, it is their precise interplay that enables changes in intermediary

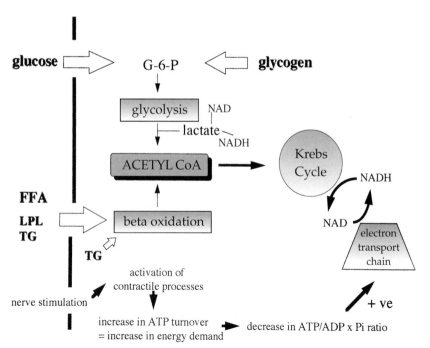

Figure 17–3. Pathways regulating glucose transport in skeletal muscle during exercise.

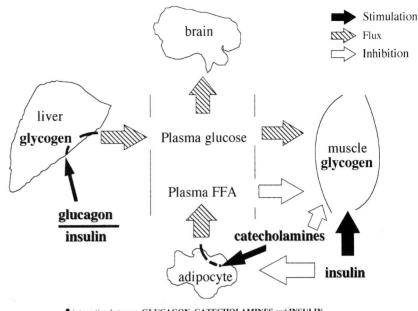

Figure 17–4. Hormonal control and the interaction between the brain, liver, muscle, and fat cell in control of glucose homeostasis. It is indicated that glucagon/insulin interaction controls hepatic glucose production. Epinephrine and insulin have opposite effects in control of peripheral glucose uptake, and an important effect is indirect through control of lipolysis in adipocytes (FFA-glucose cycle).

• interaction between **GLUCAGON, CATECHOLAMINES** and **INSULIN** determines the fuel contribution of liver and muscle glycogen to exercising muscle

metabolism of the liver so that HGP can be adjusted in accordance with changes in the energy demand of the active tissue. Thus, when one examines the hormonal response to exercise it is more important to examine the changes in hormone ratios or relationships (e.g., insulin/glucagon; insulin/epinephrine) than changes in individual hormones.

During resting conditions HGP is regulated by circulating insulin and glucagon levels such that a decrease in plasma glucose concentration stimulates an increase in the secretion of glucagon by the pancreas that elicits an increase in hepatic glucose production so that plasma glucose concentration can be restored to normal. In contrast, an increase in plasma glucose concentration stimulates an increase in insulin secretion by the pancreas that simultaneously decreases HGP and enhances muscle glucose uptake until plasma glucose levels are returned to normal. During moderate-intensity exercise a similar pattern of glucoregulation predominates.[11] It is interesting to note, however, that exercise is accompanied by a fall in plasma insulin levels, which is compensated by an increase in blood flow and an increase in glucagon (Fig. 17–5). Although this alteration might seem counterproductive in light of the need for an increase in glucose uptake by the working muscle, in fact this hormonal response only further highlights the dominance of the liver in glucoregulation and the importance of factors other than insulin in stimulating muscle glucose uptake during exercise.

The most important facet of the hormonal response is that the interrelationship between the levels of insulin and glucagon during exercise stimulate glucose production and maintain plasma glucose levels, thus

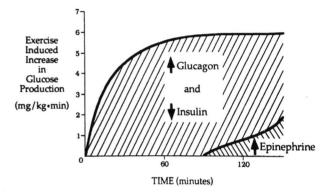

Figure 17–5. Schematic representation of the rise in glucose production during moderate-intensity exercise and the impact of the fall in insulin and the rise in glucagon and epinephrine to this response. (Reprinted from Ref. 10)

preventing hypoglycemia despite the increased glucose uptake by the working tissue(s).[12] The increase in pancreatic glucagon secretion causes an increase in hepatic glycogenolysis that is augmented by the potentiation effect on the liver of glucagon by the fall in insulin concentration.[13,14] As exercise duration becomes more prolonged the increase in glucagon secretion becomes particularly important in stimulating hepatic gluconeogenesis through the channeling of a greater portion of the 3-carbon molecules taken up by the liver into glucose.[14–16] Thus, the rise in glucagon acts by stimulating both hepatic glycogenolysis and gluconeogenesis, while the decrease in insulin has its impact mainly through the stimulation of hepatic glycogenolysis.

The role of each of the pancreatic hormones in hepatic glucose production has been determined primarily by examining the impact of each hormone under isolated, suppressed conditions.[17,18] Studies in dogs showed that somatostatin-induced glucagon suppression reduces hepatic glucose production and leads to a fall in blood glucose that is normalized by glucagon replacement.[18] These studies were subsequently extended to enable quantification of the role of glucagon by clamping glucose levels in conjunction with the somatostatin-induced glucagon suppression so the effect of the counterregulatory response to hypoglycemia could be eliminated.[17] Glucagon was responsible for over 60% of the total glucose production during moderate exercise. This percentage is similar to that observed under resting conditions in dogs[19] and humans[20]; however, since hepatic glucose production is many times greater during exercise, the absolute role of glucagon is also greater. During exercise in humans, the glucagon/insulin ratio controls HGP, particularly during the early stages of exercise. While peripheral glucagon levels do not increase, the decrease in insulin creates a hormonal ratio that the body perceives as an "increase" in glucagon. An actual plasma increase in glucagon only occurs during the later stages of prolonged exercise, and it is important to remember that peripheral glucagon levels do not accurately reflect portal levels. When the glucose level falls cortisol and the catecholamines initiate a series of counterregulatory mechanisms that can compensate for approximately 40% of the deficit in hepatic glucose production created by glucagon deficiency.

The studies described here outline the role of glucagon during exercise; however, they fail to differentiate between the role of basal glucagon and the role of the increased load of glucagon released into the circulation during exercise. By modifying the experimental protocol(s) and using the pancreatic clamp technique (somatostatin plus glucagon and insulin replacement) to simultaneously prevent the changes in glucagon and insulin, plasma glucose fell from 25 to 50 mg/dL over a 1 hr period.[21–23] This fall in blood glucose occurs despite a large compensatory release in catecholamines and emphasizes the importance of the actual increase in glucagon and decrease in insulin in the maintenance of glucose homeostasis during exercise. Furthermore, additional clamp studies designed to selectively isolate the specific role of the change in insulin and the change in glucagon, which were performed in moderately exercising dogs,[24,25] have shown that the exercise-induced increment in glucagon controls approximately 60% of the exercise-induced increment in glucose production.[25] This is consistent with findings in humans showing that the rise in glucagon is necessary for glucose homeostasis during moderate exercise.[21] Studies in the dog have also shown that the rise in the glucagon/insulin ratio is necessary for the full increment in both hepatic glycogenolysis and gluconeogenesis.[25] This stimulatory

effect of glucagon on gluconeogenesis is due to an accelerated rate of gluconeogenic precursor extraction by the liver and enhanced channeling of precursor to glucose within the liver.

The role of the decrease in insulin levels during moderate exercise[26] was studied in dogs by infusing insulin in the portal vein to prevent its fall during a glucose clamp.[24] This resulted in an impaired increase in glucose production due to an attenuation of glycogenolysis. The fall in insulin controlled 55% of the increase in glucose production. Studies in human subjects have shown that prevention of the exercise-induced fall in insulin using the pancreatic clamp technique caused a more expeditious fall in blood glucose.[21] Furthermore, in the dog, when the fall in insulin was prevented and glucose levels were not clamped, counterregulation (as evidenced by excessive glucagon, cortisol, and catecholamine increases) prevented severe hypoglycemia by stimulating hepatic glycogenolysis and gluconeogenesis.[27] This suggests that effective counterregulation is able to partially compensate for the absence of the exercise-induced decrease in insulin and minimize the fall in glucose. Recently, it has been shown that hepatic glucose production remains the same when insulin levels fall and glucagon levels are maintained at basal.[13] This finding isolates the role of insulin even further and suggests that the fall in insulin acts solely by sensitizing the liver to the effects of glucagon. Therefore, interaction between insulin and glucagon is most critical,[17,18,28] and a stronger correlation is observed between HGP and the ratio between glucagon and insulin, than between the individual changes in these hormones and HGP.[12,17,18,26,29]

Hepatic glucose production during exercises presumably controlled by hepatic nervous stimulation and/or hormonal stimulation. Much of the early work focused on defining which of these stimuli was the primary regulator; however, it is now believed that regulation of HGP is the result of the interaction between both neural and hormonal stimuli, although hormonal stimulation likely predominates under moderate exercise conditions.[10,30]

Animal studies have suggested that liver nerves are not essential for the increased hepatic glucose output during moderate exercise.[31,32,33] In rats there was no change in HGP following surgical or chemical denervation of the liver,[31,32] and in dogs the exercise-induced increase in liver glycogenolysis and gluconeogenesis was not influenced by hepatic denervation.[33] In humans, the exercise-induced enhancement of sympathetic nervous activity and the increase in hepatic glucose output occur much more rapidly than the release of hormones. This indicates that liver nerves may play a key regulatory role in the early exercise-induced increase in HGP in humans. However, α- and β-blockade experiments,[22,34,35] sympathetic coeliac ganglionic blockade experiments,[22] and studies in liver transplant patients,[36–38] all showing maintenance of the exercise-induced increase in HGP, indicate that neural stimulation is not essential for the occurrence of this response, although it does play a role in the modulation of hepatic glycogenolysis and glycogenesis.[30]

Much of the research that has examined the role of hormones other than insulin and glucagon in HGP has focused on the role of the catecholamines. Considerable evidence exists to support a correlation between plasma catecholamine concentration and glucose output during exercise and hypoxia.[22,38–40] The degree of predominance of catecholamine regulation is difficult to ascertain since removal of the adrenal medulla is accompanied by an increase in plasma insulin, which disfavors liver glycogenolysis and diminishes the effect of epinephrine.[41–44] Moreover, it is possible that the primary role of epinephrine is on glycogenolysis at the level of the muscle, thereby enabling the provision of gluconeogenic precursors for the liver to increase HGP.[45,46] This is particularly important during long-duration exercise.[47] In the insulin deficient state, however, a small increase in plasma epinephrine production that stimulates both gluconeogenesis and glycogenolysis may, in fact, worsen a preexisting state of hyperglycemia.[48]

The role of cortisol and growth hormone during exercise is likely to be minor. The stimulation of gluconoegenic enzymes by corticosterone injections in exercising rats can delay the onset of fatigue, likely through greater provision of gluconoegenic substrates to the liver.[49] Cortisol promotes glucose cycling through glycogen, greatly inhibits nonhepatic glucose utilization, increases hepatic gluconeogenesis in vivo through enhanced substrate delivery, and raises plasma insulin levels, which limits intrahepatic gluconeogenesis.[50]

Regulation of Muscle Carbohydrate Metabolism. We have previously described factors that regulate glucose production. Plasma glucose levels are maintained throughout steady-state exercise despite the increase in HGP due to the matching increase in muscle glucose uptake that occurs in response to the energy demands of the contracting tissue(s).

The uptake of glucose is closely regulated by both hormonal and nonhormonal factors (Fig. 17–4). Kinetic analyses of glucose uptake, conducted in vivo [51] and in vitro,[52–55] generally indicate that the maximal velocity (Vmax) for glucose uptake is increased by exercise without affecting the Michaelis-Menton constant (Km) (Fig. 17–6). The Km for glucose oxidation by the working limb is the same as that for glucose uptake, implying that both processes are characterized by the same rate-limiting step. It is likely that except for perhaps at the onset of exercise[56] or during heavy exercise,[57] when there is a large accumulation of intracellular glucose, the transport of glucose across the plasma membrane is

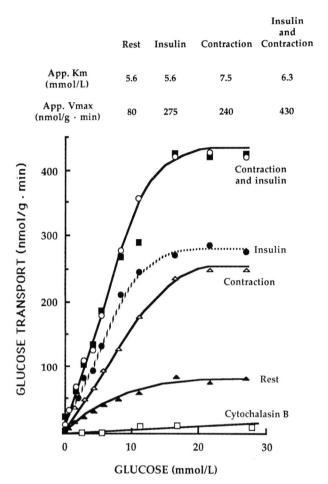

	Rest	Insulin	Contraction	Insulin and Contraction
App. Km (mmol/L)	5.6	5.6	7.5	6.3
App. Vmax (nmol/g · min)	80	275	240	430

Figure 17–6. Dose-response relationship between glucose concentration and glucose transport in epitrochlearis muscle at rest, during contractions (48 twitches/min), and incubated in the presence and absence of insulin (10 mU/mL). Also shown are the rates of nonfacilitated glucose diffusion obtained by incubating the muscle in the presence of cytochalasin B (50 uM). Note that both insulin and contractile activity increase the apparent Vmax without significantly changing the apparent Km (5–8 mmol). (From Ref. 54)

the rate limiting step in glucose uptake. Saturation kinetic data indicate that plasma glucose uptake occurs by the process of facilitated diffusion.[58] These *"glucose transporters"* have subsequently been identified as transmembrane proteins (GLUT 1–GLUT 7). In muscle, GLUT 4 is the dominant transporter with GLUT 1 (and GLUT 3) also present, but at a significantly lower concentration.[58–62] GLUT 4 has a Km of 5 mM,[63] which makes it suitable for the transport of glucose into the muscle after eating and during periods of enhanced glucose production when plasma glucose is elevated. It is predominantly located in tissues that are insulin sensitive, e.g., heart, skeletal muscle, and adipose tissue (insulin-responsive glucose transporter). GLUT 1 is most important in facilitating basal glucose uptake. During the basal state GLUT 4 is located in intracellular vesicles while GLUT 1 is located mainly within the plasma membrane. The increase in Vmax for glucose uptake, without a change in Km, suggests that exercise increases predominantly the number, turnover, and availability of active glucose transporters without changing the affinity of the transporter for glucose. Indeed, during periods of muscle contraction and/or insulin stimulation GLUT 4 vesicles are translocated to the surface membrane of the cell. The transporters then fuse with and are inserted within the cell membrane, and glucose uptake can be increased.[64] The increase in the plasma membrane transporters is associated with a decrease in transporter content in the intracellular microsomal fraction.[65] In addition to the actual transporters it is believed that other proteins, such as Rab4, various vesicle-associated membrane proteins (VAMPs), and secretory carrier membrane proteins, are also involved in the translocation process.[58,66–68] It is currently believed that the GLUT 4 translocation system is recycled between the intracellular tubulovesicular endosomes and the cell-surface membrane.[58,66–71] The majority of glucose transporters in the muscle are concentrated within the transverse tubular membranes, an anatomically favorable site since it enables glucose to be moved rapidly and transported to the myofibrillar area where it is most needed for energy. Both insulin and muscle contraction cause translocation of transporters to the t-tubule membranes. However, it is still unknown whether muscle contraction alone is responsible for translocating glucose transporters to the sarcolemmal membrane.[65,72–81]

Muscle glucose uptake can be increased both in the presence and the absence of insulin. The stimulation of glucose uptake by contraction alone has been demonstrated in situ using perfused rat hindlimb preparations,[82–85] in vitro with the epitrochlearis muscle,[54,86] and in vivo in pancreatectomized dogs.[87] Studies in the isolated perfused rat hindlimb also indicate that contraction per se can also stimulate muscle glycogenolysis in the absence of catecholamines. Insulin modulates steps during the endocytotic and exocytotic phases of the GLUT 4 translocation process. This occurs primarily through the activation of PI-3 kinase, which increases highly acidic lipid products near the endosomal membranes. This interaction affects important regulatory steps of vesicle movement.

Separate mechanisms of contraction versus insulin-induced glucose uptake come primarily from studies in the rat epitrochlearis muscle incubated at various glucose concentrations. Muscle contraction and insulin both stimulate glucose transport with an apparent Km for glucose ranging between 5.6 and 7.5 mM. The combination of contraction with insulin increases the Vmax in an additive fashion, without altering the Km. This suggests that contractile activity can increase glucose uptake independently of insulin and further supports the notion of separate pools of glucose transporters.[74,88]

However, the fact that cytochalasin B inhibits the stimulatory effects of both muscle contraction and insulin indicates that both processes are mediated by facilitated diffusion. Thus, these two effects are additive and the stimulation of transporter translocation is different, but the endpoint of transporter translocation must be common. Indeed, polymyxin B inhibited the stimulation of glucose transport by both insulin and muscle contraction.[89] Similarly, studies involving alterations in the concentration of calcium or the release of calcium have suggested that effects of both insulin and contraction require an increase in calcium.[90–93]

It is evident that the signaling pathways for the effects of insulin and muscle contraction are different. Muscle contraction can increase glucose uptake independently of changes in tyrosine phosphorylation of IRS-1 or the activation of PI-3 kinase while insulin, but not exercise, causes an increase in insulin receptor kinase activity.[94] Wortmannin, an inhibitor of PI-3 kinase activity, inhibits glucose uptake with insulin but not by muscle contraction.[95,96] A differential role of Rab proteins and MAP kinase enzymes for contraction and insulin-induced glucose uptake has also been demonstrated. Insulin, but not exercise, translocates Rab4 from the microsomal fraction of muscle,[66] while exercise, not insulin, increased the c-jun NH2-terminus kinase (JNK) in muscle.[97] Finally, experiments with insulin-resistant animals also support two separate signaling pathways. In such studies muscle contraction results in a normal glucose uptake,[98–101] despite significant insulin resistance, emphasizing that glucose transport can occur without insulin. Collectively, it appears that there are differences between muscle contraction and insulin in the pathways, or points within the pathway which they act upon, that result in the stimulation of glucose transport. The endpoint, however, is likely to be common.

It appears that exercise stimulates insulin-independent glucose uptake, increases insulin action, or both. In addition, increased blood flow during exercise can counterbalance the decrease in plasma insulin concentration. Studies in vitro show that contraction can stimulate glucose uptake in the absence of insulin[83] without affecting structure or function of the insulin receptor.[94] In streptozotocin-diabetic rats deprived of insulin injection for 3 days, nuclear magnetic resonance imaging and biochemical studies indicate that all bioenergetic changes (force of contraction, energy-rich phosphorus-containing compounds, intracellular pH [Fig. 17–7], and the activity of pyruvate dehydrogenase) were not different from normal or insulin-treated subjects, but glycogen resynthesis was decreased during the recovery period. The exercise-induced increase in glucose uptake and oxidation in normal dogs with somatostatin-induced insulinopenia and normal FFA and glucose levels occurs primarily by insulin-independent processes.[102] Thus it would appear that exercise can

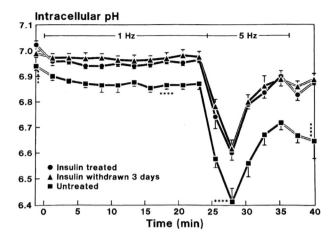

Figure 17–7. Changes in intracellular pH in gastrocnemius muscle during stimulation at 1 and 5 Hz and during the initial recovery period for insulin-treated diabetic (●), untreated diabetic (■), and diabetic animals from which insulin therapy was withdrawn for 72 hr prior to study (▲). Values are shown as means ±SE for six experiments in each study group.

stimulate both insulin-independent glucose uptake and insulin action.

Finally, there is a strong correlation between contraction stimulation of myofibrillar ATPase activity and muscular glucose uptake. Both in man and in laboratory animals glucose uptake is related to the ATP-ADP ratio and to the Phosphocreatine (PCr) content of the muscle before, during, and after exercise.[39,57,103–106] In addition, glucose transport is linearly related to the force expended during isometric contraction of the epitrochlearis muscle. Thus, factors that affect an increase in ATP turnover and stimulate oxidative and nonoxidative carbohydrate metabolism would also enhance extracellular glucose uptake.

Other Factors Affecting Muscle Carbohydrate Metabolism. In addition to muscle contraction, other factors such as glycemia, the abundance of noncarbohydrate fuels such as fat, blood flow, catecholamine level, and hypoxia can influence glucose uptake and metabolism. Hyperglycemia decreases glucose clearance but enhances glucose uptake by its mass effect. For example, acute hyperglycemia (10 mmol) in healthy humans induces a substantial increase in carbohydrate oxidation during 2 hr of intense cycling, while muscle glycogenolysis in unaltered.[107] In resting type 2 subjects, acute hyperglycemia fully compensated for the defects in the fasting and insulin-stimulated oxidative and nonoxidative glucose disposal.[108] The mechanisms whereby glycemia regulates muscle glucose uptake may be complex, but involve at least modulation of the quantity, and probably also the activity, of GLUT 4 on the plasma membrane of the muscle.[109–112] Suppression of lipolysis in partially insulin-deficient (alloxan-induced) diabetic dogs enhanced the exercise-induced

increment in glucose uptake largely by decreasing glucose production and improving hyperglycemia.[113,114]

Muscle metabolism is affected by chronic hyperinsulinemia.[115,116] More recently it has been shown that there is a sensitization to the presence of the low levels of insulin present during exercise.[117] Thus, in addition to an increase in insulin-independent glucose uptake, an added stimulus may be provided by an increase in the sensitivity of working muscles to insulin. The mechanism by which exercise enhances insulin action may be related to an increase in blood flow, increased transendothelial transport of insulin, indirect effects mediated by insulin-induced suppression of (FFA) levels, or some as-yet undefined insulin receptor or postinsulin receptor modification.

Regulation by Hypoxia and Metabolic State. The notion of the role of the "energy-state" of the muscle in affecting glucose uptake has been previously introduced. This is particularly evident under conditions of limited oxygen availability such as hypoxia,[39] anemia,[28] or during severe exercise.[57,103–106] The high rate of glucose uptake in anemic dogs[28] or in human subjects[39] breathing a hypoxic gas mixture occurs even though insulin levels are normally maintained and catecholamines, often antagonistic to glucose uptake, are elevated. The mechanism by which muscle metabolism may be linked to glucose uptake remains to be determined. However, the energy state of the muscle, as determined by the muscle PCr levels, correlates strongly to glucose uptake in the exercising limb.[57] The effect of hypoxia and the muscle metabolic state in increasing glucose uptake may be important in the individual with diabetes that has cardiovascular impairments.

Regulation by Increased Blood Flow. The exercise-induced increase in skeletal muscle blood flow increases the exposure of this insulin-sensitive tissue to circulating insulin and glucose. A strong positive correlation exists between insulin delivery to the working muscle and insulin's action.[115] Furthermore, insulin action in specific muscles correlates to the resting blood flow of those muscles. Nevertheless, re-creating the exercise-induced increase in glucose and insulin loads to the hindlimb of resting, conscious dogs results in an increase in limb glucose uptake and oxidation that are only a small fraction of the rates obtained during exercise.[118] Studies examining insulin action following exercise, when basal hemodynamic changes have been restored, still show an increase in insulin action. An increase in the Km and Vmax of insulin action is clearly evident for 2 days after just 1 hr of cycle exercise.[119] Thus, factors aside from muscle blood flow must be important.

Regulation by Catecholamines. The β-adrenergic metabolic effects of the catecholamines can antagonize insulin-mediated glucose uptake in skeletal muscle.[120] This is evident by the ability of propranolol to stimulate glucose uptake during exercise.[106,121] This effect is probably related to the ability of the β-adrenergic blocker to limit muscle glycogen and fat oxidation, which then increases the reliance of the working muscle on blood glucose. Data from diabetic dogs indicate that catecholamines may regulate glucose uptake during exercise only when some insulin is available to prevent markedly elevated FFA levels.[87,113] β-Adrenergic blockade does not increase metabolic clearance in exercising depancreatized dogs with excessive FFA levels. Instead, there is a threshold of FFA (about 1.1 mmol) above which changes in FFA do not affect glucose clearance, but below which a fall in this variable increases clearance.

Fat as a Source of Fuel.   Fat is by far the most abundant potential energy source. On average, our body fat stores can provide us with enough energy to sustain low-intensity exercise for more than 24 hr. In most instances, 10–25% of total body weight is made up of adipose tissue. Although the capacity of this energy system is large, the rate at which energy is supplied by this system is considerably slower than that of the immediate energy sources or from carbohydrate metabolism. Hence, fat is used in those instances when a large amount of energy is required, but the rate at which it is required is moderate to low.

The utilization of fat as a source of energy involves several different processes; lipolysis, mobilization, transportation, uptake, activation, translocation, and B-oxidation/electron transport system. Hormone-sensitive lipase (HSL) regulates the breakdown of stored adipose triglyceride (TG) molecules to glycerol and the individual fatty acid(s).[122,123] This process is stimulated by several hormones, the most potent of which are the catecholamines, which regulate the phosphorylation state of HSL.[124–128] The rate of adipose tissue *lipolysis* is increased with moderate exercise[9] and depends on the intensity and duration of exercise.[9] Once *mobilized* from the adipose tissue into the bloodstream the FFA binds with albumin so it can be *transported* to the muscle. In addition to neuroendocrine factors, FFA mobilization and subsequent transportation are determined by the availability of blood albumin, the arterial FFA/albumin molar ratio, and the perfusion rate through the adipose tissue. During exercise the FFA/albumin ratio is increased due to the exercise-induced increase in FFA concentration. However, because FFA binding to albumin results in a decrease in the binding affinity, unbound FFA concentration increases, favoring an increase in the reesterification of FFA, a factor that could ultimately decrease FFA mobilization. However, net mobilization is maintained by the increase in adipose tissue blood flow that occurs during prolonged

exercise.[9] At the muscle membrane the albumin and fatty acid dissociate and the free fatty acid moves into the muscle via a carrier-mediated process involving a fatty acid binding protein (FABP). Support for this carrier-mediated uptake has been demonstrated in human muscle through net uptake or tracer studies that have shown that saturation occurs with an increase in plasma unbound FFA concentration.[129–133] Isolated adipocyte data has demonstrated that this permeation and mobilization into the cell are enhanced by epinephrine[129,134,135] and suppressed by physiologic concentrations of insulin.[136] However, the role of these hormones in regulating FFA mobilization into skeletal muscle has yet to be elucidated. Once inside the cell the FFA is either stored (as TG for later breakdown by the hormone lipoprotein lipase) or oxidized. Fatty acid molecules to be oxidized are activated and then translocated into the mitochondria where the actual oxidation of the FFA and the generation of ATP occurs. The relative contribution of each individual fat as a fuel is dependent upon the carbon chain length of the fat and its saturation, with additional energy being produced by the breakdown of the glycerol backbone through gluconeogenesis. The rate of oxidation is dependent upon the intensity and the duration of the exercise bout and highly correlated to plasma FFA concentration.[137–139] Plasma FFA concentration increases during light to moderate intensity exercise, and an increase in total lipid utilization is evident until exercise intensity reaches between 60 and 70% of maximal oxygen uptake. The energy contribution by fat similarly increases as the duration of the exercise increases. Unlike most other processes associated with lipid metabolism, FFA utilization does not appear to be hormonally regulated. In contrast, factors such as FFA availability,[140–142] the oxidative potential of the muscle (B-oxidative and Krebs cycle enzymes),[143–145] malonyl-CoA levels,[146,147] and carbohydrate availability[148–150] are important factors in the regulation of FFA utilization.

The onset of exercise is characterized by a decrease in plasma arterial FFA levels emphasizing that, in contrast to glucose regulation, plasma FFA levels are not as well matched to the energy demands of the exercising tissue(s).[9] This decrease occurs as a result of the inability of FFA mobilization to be immediately upregulated at the onset of exercise. As a result, the increased muscle FFA uptake induced by the enhanced flow of blood to the working muscles is not compensated for by a comparable increase in FFA mobilization and plasma FFA decline. As exercise continues, FFA mobilization is enhanced and plasma FFA increases. The linear relationship between FFA concentration and muscle utilization emphasizes the importance of enhanced mobilization in the utilization of FFA by the exercising tissue. As has been previously mentioned the release of FFA is determined by HSL. Thus, the availability of

FFA for oxidation is also determined by the balance between insulin's inhibitory effect on HSL and the stimulatory effects of the catecholamines and blood flow through the adipose tissue. Upon completion of exercise plasma FFA levels continue to increase during the recovery phase until clearance of regulatory hormones has been completed.

In addition to the energy provided by FFA and glycerol, it is important to emphasize the contributions of intramuscular and plasma TGs and ketone bodies to the lipid energy pool. Intramuscular TGs are important contributors of energy during prolonged exercise periods. Both human and dog experiments demonstrate that in the postabsorptive state only a little more than 50% of the lipids that are oxidized are represented by the plasma FFA concentration. Utilization of intramuscular TG stores also depends on the predominant muscle fiber type. The greatest utilization is usually evident in fast-oxidative glycolytic (FOG) fibers, then slow-oxidative (SO). Most data suggest the intramuscular TG utilization in fast-glycolytic (FG) fibers is nonexistent. Since fiber recruitment is dictated by the intensity and the nature of the exercise the differing quantitative contribution of intramuscular TGs may often be a function of the exercise type and intensity. Moreover, the mode and intensity also determine hormonal contribution, a factor that might also contribute to the degree of intramuscular TG utilization. Ketone body production during exercise is limited to the incomplete breakdown of fats to acetoacetate and/or B-hydroxybutyrate. Blood ketone body levels have been shown to increase with increasing exercise duration[7] and during the postexercise recovery period. Exercise training enhances the ability of muscle to utilize ketone bodies; however, their energy contribution remains limited to between 2 and 5%.

Training enhances ketone body utilization and utilization of FFA for energy, primarily through adaptations in lipase and other oxidative enzymes, improved blood flow, and a more favorable hormonal response. Red skeletal muscle is well suited for fat utilization since it has a high myoglobin content and is well capillarized and its mitochondrial content is well adapted to utilize fats as fuel. Mitochondrial capacity can as much as double with endurance training, a factor that raises the apparent Vmax of fat oxidation such that in trained individuals the absolute utilization of fat is greater at any given fat concentration.[151]

In addition to acting as an abundant source of energy, FFA levels also affect carbohydrate (CHO) utilization. By preferentially utilizing FFA for energy the body is able to preserve its carbohydrate stores for more intense periods of exercise and to ensure adequate glucose supply to the brain. Since glycogen depletion is directly associated with muscle fatigue, utilizing fat to preserve glycogen can postpone fatigue.

This relationship is called the glucose-fatty acid cycle, which describes how elevated levels of FFA oxidation can decrease muscle glucose oxidation and/or glucose uptake.[152] When FFA oxidation is increased, the byproducts of the oxidation process act to decrease carbohydrate utilization, thus preserving carbohydrate stores until the energy demand of the working muscles can no longer be met by FFA oxidation. While this interaction has been convincingly demonstrated in heart and diaphragm muscle its significance in skeletal muscle has generated considerable controversy. Studies in the rat hindquarter have, for the most part, failed to demonstrate an inhibitory effect of FFAs on glucose utilization.[153–156] In contrast, FFAs[156,157] and ketone bodies[156] inhibit glucose uptake in slow-twitch muscles. This may be due to a greater capacity of slow-twitch muscle to metabolize fats coupled with a greater reliance on glucose. Recent investigations[158–160] highlighted the importance of the duration of FFA elevation. Much of the failure to demonstrate the glucose-fatty acid cycle in whole body studies is due to limited duration of exposure to elevated FFA. Changes in glucose uptake were not evident until 3–4 hr of elevated FFA exposure, while a decrease in glucose oxidation occurred as early as 2 hr.[161]

During exercise, when energy metabolism is accelerated, FFAs may influence carbohydrate metabolism to a greater extent.[157,162,163] In the rat hindquarter the inhibitory effect of oleate on glucose uptake and glycogen breakdown was much greater when the muscle was stimulated to contract.[157] Increments in glucose uptake in the working limb of the dog are unaffected by a nicotinic acid infusion that suppresses circulating FFA levels, while the increments in the rate of glucose and lactate oxidation are augmented under these conditions.[163] FFA replacement normalized the accelerated oxidation evident during nicotinic acid infusion. When FFA levels were elevated with heparin infusion in the rat, liver and muscle glycogen breakdown and lactate levels were reduced in red but not white skeletal muscle fibers during exercise, but not at rest.[162] More recently, there has been increased interest in the impact of high-fat diets on carbohydrate metabolism. Several studies[164] have demonstrated that a high-fat diet (with augmented blood FFA) in the rat significantly impairs carbohydrate metabolism, as evident by a decrease in Vmax and intrinsic activity (Vmax/cytochalasin binding rate) of GLUT 4 in hindlimb muscles in response to both exercise and insulin stimulation.[164] Studies in humans also demonstrated a sparing effect of elevated FFA levels on muscle glycogen and a reduced rate of total carbohydrate oxidation over 30 min of moderate-intensity exercise.[163] The FFA-glucose cycle was also shown to be operative in humans at the levels of both whole-body glucose disposal and muscle glucose metabolism under both high and low insulin conditions.[165] Thus, it would appear that the role of FFA availability has a carbohydrate-sparing effect that is most evident in slow-twitch muscle, particularly as exercise duration is prolonged. The carbohydrate-sparing effect of FFAs during exercise may be due to an attenuation of muscle glycogen breakdown as well as muscle glucose uptake. Because the apparent rate of glucose uptake does not reflect the intracellular fate of glucose, it would be important to track the intracellular glucose along both oxidative and nonoxidative pathways under the influence of the glucose-fatty acid cycle.

Protein as a Source of Fuel. The contribution of amino acids to energy metabolism during exercise is limited (5–18%).[7,166] However, it is important that during intense prolonged exercise even a small additional source of energy is extremely valuable to an otherwise failing energy system. Moreover, amino acids contribute significantly to the substrate pool for hepatic gluconeogenesis, they are important in the synthesis and/or repair of muscle proteins, and, since they act as common intermediary compounds of both carbohydrate and fat metabolism, they are essential to metabolic integration. Thus, while the actual energy contribution of proteins may be limited, their overall value to the exercising system is emphasized.

Proteins, like other energy fuels, can be either synthesized or degraded during exercise. The amount of protein that is actually available for breakdown to energy or as substrate for liver gluconeogenesis is therefore dependent upon the balance between synthesis and degradation. During endurance exercise protein degradation is the "favored" process in both skeletal muscle and the liver.[166–170] However, although the degradation of noncontractile proteins is increased, the breakdown of contractile proteins is, in fact, suppressed.[166,171,172] The magnitude of breakdown is exercise intensity and duration dependent.[173,174] Protein degradation is also enhanced by fasting and an increase in the level of glucocorticoids.[175,176] Increases in dietary protein intake and enhanced levels (infusion) of medium chain triglycerides and leucine decrease the rate of degradation.[177–179]

The amount of protein degradation can be determined through the measurement of the levels of (1) protein in liver and muscle following exercise; (2) essential amino acids postexercise, since levels of these amino acids would only increase in the plasma following dietary consumption or via tissue breakdown; (3) tyrosine and phenylalanine, as markers of noncontractile protein breakdown; or (4) 3-methylhistidine (3-MH), which is a measure of contractile muscle protein breakdown. Of these four potential measures the most commonly used is the measurement of plasma and/or urinary 3-MH. Data from these studies have revealed a biphasic response of 3-MH excretion to exer-

cise and indicate that 3-MH excretion is decreased during exercise but increased during recovery from exercise. In addition to being intensity and duration dependent,[173,174] it has also been shown that 3-MH excretion is dependent on the type of exercise, specifically whether the exercise involves eccentric (muscle lengthening—e.g., downhill running) or concentric (muscle shortening—e.g., lifting a bag) contractions. In animal studies eccentric exercise appears to enhance 3-MH excretion.[83]

As might be expected, protein synthesis during exercise is decreased.[171,172,174,180–182] This decrease has been documented in muscle and liver and in whole-body studies.[172,183,184] The magnitude of this decrease is dependent upon exercise intensity and duration, with duration the more critical factor. Insulin, growth hormone, and leucine have all been shown to increase synthesis.[185–187] Factors that cause a decrease in synthesis are associated with the cell's energy status, for instance, reduced energy intake, and exercise decrease protein synthesis.[171,174,177] Protein synthesis and protein degradation are closely linked, and glucocorticoids are the most important regulators. During exercise glucocorticoids increase and promote net protein breakdown.

Once the proteins themselves have been degraded into amino acids they become part of the amino acid pool available for energy metabolism. Endogenous protein is the greatest contributor to this pool,[168] with the tissue free amino acid pools and dietary protein being complimentary additional sources.[169,188] Of the amino acids available in the total pool, six have been identified, to date, as being oxidizable by skeletal muscle. These are the three branch-chain amino acids (BCAA—leucine, isoleucine, valine) and glutamate, aspartate, and alanine. Of these six, the BCAA are the most often utilized. Unlike fat and carbohydrate, amino acids are broken down by numerous complex pathways, the nature of which are dependent upon the specific amino acid being oxidized. What is common is the initial removal of the α-amino group by either transamination or oxidative deamination and ultimately the conversion of the resulting carbon skeleton to a metabolite that is part of the fat and carbohydrate pathway. Collectively these amino acid sources or their resultant metabolites are either processed as gluconeogenic precursors for the liver or oxidized by the muscle. Although the ability of the skeletal muscle to actually use amino acids as an energy source is limited, during prolonged exercise amino acids may contribute from 3% to 18%.[7,189,190] Individual amino acids such as valine, leucine, and isoleucine may generate between 32 and 43 moles of ATP/mole of amino acid.[189,190] The activity of rate-limiting enzymes of amino acid breakdown increases in linear relation to the intensity and duration of the exercise. BCAA release from the liver is increased with exercise, although there is not a corresponding net accumulation in the plasma or in the muscle, thereby suggesting that active muscle participates in both the removal and oxidation of these amino acids. The ability of muscle to oxidize the BCAA is facilitated by an appropriate enzyme distribution in the skeletal muscle. Exercise stimulates the activation of the rate-limiting enzyme (BCOADH complex) and, together with the energy provided by gluconeogenesis, can be supported during prolonged periods by energy provided through protein metabolism.

Intense Exercise

Exercise at and above 80% of maximum VO_2 imposes energy requirements that are different from those of lesser intensities and has regulatory mechanisms that are correspondingly different. This type of exercise is typically engaged in by athletes, for example, in short sprints or during repeated short shifts on the ice or court, as in hockey and basketball. The very nature of the activity is such as to require near-maximal or maximal performance over periods measured in minutes, as compared to less that 3–4 hr for moderate intensity and longer for endurance activities of lower relative intensity. Another important difference between intense and other levels of exercise is that exercise induces hyperglycemia and the early recovery phase continues and intensifies the hyperglycemia, which may last an hour or more. The regulation of the response in this phase is not merely a return to the preexercise hormone-substrate milieu. Importantly, it appears to immediately favor repletion of some part of the muscle glycogen mobilized during the bout, whether or not exogenous carbohydrate has been consumed. Therefore, the physiology will be reviewed under the same headings used for the more general case of exercise to highlight the ways in which it is different.

Intense exercise is almost entirely dependent upon glycogen and circulating glucose as fuel for the muscles involved, so the whole-body response is dominated by the need to produce glucose as fuel and use it at the maximal rates found in any physiologic state. Although the majority of the fuel, especially at the onset, is from glycogenolysis, there is a massive and extremely rapid increase in hepatic glucose release into the circulation that increases progressively throughout the bout or, in the case of repeated bouts, increases stepwise. The anaerobic threshold is exceeded within minutes of onset, and huge increases in blood lactate and corresponding decreases in bicarbonate levels occur. There is a loss of the elegant matching of the increase in production to that of muscle uptake, such that a progressive rise in the circulating glucose occurs, usually of no more than 2 mmol/L (36 mg/dL) by exhaustion, in a single bout, but may be more with repeated bouts. This increases further for the first min-

utes of recovery, then gradually returns to the preexercise baseline over the succeeding hour (Fig. 17–8A–C).

The hormonal responses are qualitatively similar to those described earlier, but quantitatively radically different. We and others have postulated that the main regulators of the increase in glucose production are no longer the small decline in insulin and either no change or a small rise in glucagon. There is a rise in the glucagon-insulin ratio, but insufficient when compared to responses in lesser intensity to be the main regulator. In contrast, there is a comparable rise in both norepinephrine and epinephrine that is about the largest known in physiology (14 to 18-fold). Given that norepinephrine release directly into the liver by sympathetic nerve endings could produce even higher levels in proximity to the hepatocytes, this sympathetic adrenergic response is a prime candidate as regulator of the glucose production response (reviewed in Ref. 191). It is likely a main regulator of the cardiovascular responses as well, which include a 5 to 6-fold increase in cardiac output, up to a 40-fold increase in blood flow to the exercising regions, and either a decrease or a relatively small increase in splanchnic blood flow. In the latter case, there may be enough diminution of flow to the main organs that clear the regulatory peptide hormones to be a more important factor in determining their circulating levels than in lesser intensities of exercise. Indeed, in pancreatic clamp experiments with a somatostatin analog (octreotide) infusion and replacement of insulin, glucagon, and growth hormone at basal levels, if the infusion rates were not decreased during intense exercise, levels of these regulatory hormones rose considerably.[192] Similarly, in subjects with type 1 diabetes, a constant insulin infusion led to increases in levels with such exercise.[193] The catecholamine response in lesser intensities of exercise have been postulated by Galbo and colleagues to be a feedback response to peripheral signals indicating the need for the increases, whereas they propose that in intense exercise it is an anticipatory, feed-forward response to mobilize and deliver the requisite glucose. This notion is based in part on the overshoot of production in excess of uptake that is responsible for the hyperglycemic response.[194]

The hormonal responses during recovery after mild to moderate intensity exercise consist of a return (at rates related to the intensity) to their respective values prior to the exercise. In contrast, there is a marked rise in insulin to 1.5 to 2-fold preexercise levels that takes 40–60 min to decline, in a pattern that follows glycemia. Glucagon remains constant, and the catecholamines decline within 20–30 min to preexercise concentrations. This hyperglycemic-hyperinsulinemic response maintains the glucose uptake at higher levels than production as both decline progressively. This is an adaptation consistent with endogenous circulating glucose being

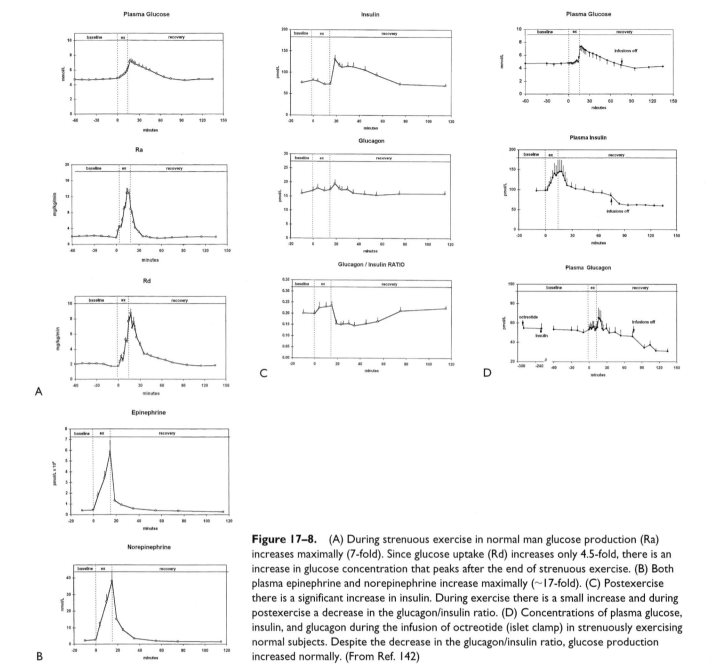

Figure 17–8. (A) During strenuous exercise in normal man glucose production (Ra) increases maximally (7-fold). Since glucose uptake (Rd) increases only 4.5-fold, there is an increase in glucose concentration that peaks after the end of strenuous exercise. (B) Both plasma epinephrine and norepinephrine increase maximally (~17-fold). (C) Postexercise there is a significant increase in insulin. During exercise there is a small increase and during postexercise a decrease in the glucagon/insulin ratio. (D) Concentrations of plasma glucose, insulin, and glucagon during the infusion of octreotide (islet clamp) in strenuously exercising normal subjects. Despite the decrease in the glucagon/insulin ratio, glucose production increased normally. (From Ref. 142)

made available for partial repletion of muscle glycogen. If a second identical bout of intense exercise follows 1 hr after the first, the responses are almost identical, although with somewhat more circulating glucose contributing to energy requirements.[105]

Glucose uptake by intensely exercising muscle is controlled in the manner described above, with differences largely accounted for by the magnitude of the catecholamine responses. As noted, the stimulation of muscle glycogenolysis increases the intracellular glucose-6-phosphate, which in intense exercise is likely to be sufficient to restrain the uptake of circulating glucose and account for the hyperglycemia. Consistent with this explanation is the effect of β-adrenergic receptor blockade in both dogs[113] and intensely exercised normal and type 1 diabetic human subjects[106,195] in whom β-blockade increases the uptake of glucose.

There is compelling evidence that the up to 8-fold increase in hepatic glucose production is mainly mediated by the catecholamine response. In many different protocols (reviewed in Ref. 191), there is an extraordinarily tight correlation between rates of glucose production and the individual catecholamines from the beginning of exercise until both reach their preexisting levels. While this does not establish a regulatory relationship, the levels reached are consistent with this. In

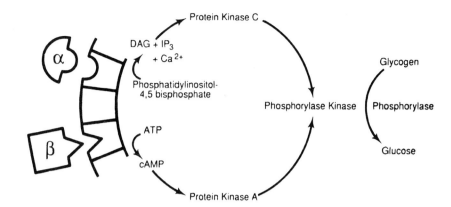

Figure 17–9. Catecholamines can increase glucose production either through α or β receptors, which can act as back-up systems. (From Ref. 398, with permission.)

the dog, epinephrine infusion during a pancreatic clamp induced a maximal 4-fold increase of glucose production. The additional increment observed during strenuous exercise in man reflects either the additional effect of norepinephrine or other unknown factors released during this type of exercise.[196] In contrast, there is no situation in which the magnitude of the glucagon-insulin ratio changes observed were shown to produce such a huge increase in production. The change in the ratio could have contributed to the responses. But this contribution is not even necessary, as in the islet cell clamp experiments,[192] the same magnitudes of increment in production and catecholamines occurred as in control experiments (Fig. 17–8D), yet there either was no increase or even a decrease in glucagon-insulin ratio. If catecholamines were the main mediators, the adrenergic blockade should provide not only support for this notion, but also inferences as to the receptor mechanism(s) involved (that is not certain in the human). In our β-blocker experiments,[106,195] there was an enhanced increment in glucose production at VO_2 levels matching to control nonblocked subjects. This suggests an α-receptor-mediated component to the stimulation. Such in vivo experiments are complex to interpret, as there are effects in secretion of other regulatory hormones—in the case of β-blocker infusion, a greater fall in insulin. This was still insufficient in itself to result in such a glucagon-insulin ratio to be responsible for the magnitude of increase in glucose production. Experiments with α-blockade were even more complex, in that the catecholamine responses were markedly increased and insulin increased during exercise, yet the increase in glucose production was as great as in unblocked persons. This also argues for an α-adrenergic component to augmented glucose production, as there might otherwise have been an even greater increase in relation to the catecholamine levels. The critical experiments would require local α and β hepatic blockade without systemic or other hormonal effects to find out whether the increment of glucose production would be attenuated or abolished. It is possible that α- and β-adrenergic stimulation of glucose

production reflect two back-up systems signaling through kinases C and A, respectively. Thus, the effect of blocking one receptor is compensated by the effect of the other receptor, particularly because such blockades induce marked increase of catecholamines in blood (Fig. 17–9).

Arguments against catecholamines being the primary mediators have included the demonstration of no apparent effect of denervation (liver transplantation) or of coeliac ganglion blockade.[22,38] Here, although the subjects exercised at high relative workloads, their absolute workload was so low that it could not really be considered to be intense. Thus the mechanisms of stimulation of glucose production that are more applicable are those of moderate exercise, where catecholamines play only a minimal role. Holloszy and Kohrt in their recent review emphasize that the metabolic requirements of exercise are imposed as much by absolute level as by level relative to the individual's maximum.[196]

If catecholamines or additional unknown factors were the important mediators of the glucose production response, they should be able to overcome the postprandial suppression of hepatic glucose output by the insulin response to the meal. This has been tested in the glucose-infused state, both with constant glucose before and during exercise and by providing all the glucose increment required by increasing the infusion rates during intense exercise. In both cases there was still a marked increase in endogenous glucose production, despite the exogenous glucose supply and the hyperinsulinemia it induced. The catecholamine responses were unaffected, and there was again a tight correlation of their levels with the rates of endogenous glucose production.[197] Of interest is that the rates of glucose uptake were elevated prior to exercise, as expected with the insulin response, and increased more rapidly during exercise and greater uptake persisted for the first hour of recovery. Thus prior hyperinsulinemia does enhance muscle glucose uptake with exercise, and the effect persists into the recovery period. The latter would further enhance glycogen repletion in preparation for the next challenge. Very analogous results were obtained with intense exercise 3 hr following a mixed meal. The hyperglycemic response was shorter in duration, yet the endogenous glucose production response was preserved and was associated with the same magnitude of catecholamine response.[198]

In both of the settings in which exercise was performed during or not long after exogenous carbohydrate, the plasma free fatty acid concentrations were suppressed, presumably by the insulin response. In the setting of intense exercise, this likely had little effect on fuel homeostasis, except to enhance the insulin effect on glucose uptake, at least into muscle. Of interest is that with the sum of all the potent lipolytic stimuli of intense exercise in the postabsorptive state, fatty acid levels actually decline during exercise, return partially early in recovery, then fall again as a consequence of the postexercise hyperinsulinemia. The fall during exercise is a contrast with lesser intensities, in which there is a progressive rise. This is explained in part by a decrease in FFA release from adipose tissue, perhaps because of decreased blood flow[22] and/or a greater rate of uptake in the muscles exercising at a lower intensity such as the arms and chest when the legs are intensively exercising on an upright cycle ergometer. The respiratory exchange ratio rises to or even above unity during intense exercise, suggesting that there is relatively little energy derived from fat oxidation (though the interpretation of Respiratory exchange ratio is complex in this situation).

Exercise in Diabetes Mellitus

Considering the complexity of fuel fluxes during exercise and the important regulatory role played by many hormones, it is not surprising that individuals with diabetes respond to exercise differently than do nondiabetic individuals. This is most evident in those receiving exogenous insulin, since the delivery of insulin in these subjects is subcutaneous and they cannot respond to changes in minute-to-minute regulation as the β-cell does. Varying states of insulin deficiency or excess and different time intervals between subcutaneous insulin injection and onset of exercise occur. These factors together with the type of insulin administered subcutaneously all influence the metabolic response to exercise in diabetes. Thus, interest is focused mainly on the effects of insulin deficiency and different states of insulin treatment during exercise.[199] Although exercise physiology in type 2 diabetes has been the subject of less study, it is the insulin *resistance* characteristic of this state that influences fuel homeostasis.

Type 1 Diabetes. The inability of type 1 diabetic subjects to regulate insulin access to the circulation is a problem when trying to meet the metabolic requirements of muscular work. While, in general, the diabetic person is able to meet the energy needs of exercise, it is often with less than the optimal balance of substrate usage that create undesirable swings in blood glucose. Both insulin sensitivity (SI) and glucose effectiveness (SG) (glucose uptake independent of a change in insulin) are impaired in type 1 diabetes, even when glycemia is under satisfactory control.[200] Exercise, as a form of stress, stimulates release of catecholamines, among other counterregulatory factors, and has been shown to decrease SI in type 1 diabetes.[201] The metabolic response to exercise in the diabetic individual will vary with type of exercise and diet. An important variable is the degree of metabolic control and insulinization, portal and peripheral, achieved with therapy.[202] The effect of exercise on glucose homeostasis in diabetes is characterized by three different phenomena as illustrated in the scheme in Figure 17–10: (1) During constant intravenous infusion of insulin, which generates normoglycemia, glucose homeostasis may be preserved because glucose production and utilization can be balanced. (2) In insulin–deficient states, increments in glucose fluxes can be normal, but fuel homeostasis is abnormal. When insulin deficiency is substantial, exercise fails to stimulate glucose utilization. Hence, the exercise–induced increase in hepatic glucose production leads to a rise in blood glucose levels. (3) If exercise is performed following the subcutaneous injection of insulin, the continuous absorption of exogenous insulin into the circulation is maintained or may even be accelerated, causing elevated plasma insulin levels. Glucose

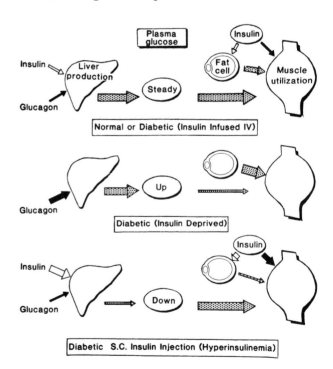

Figure 17–10. Scheme indicating changes in glucose fluxes during exercise in insulin-treated diabetics.

production rates are inhibited (or prevented from rising) during exercise because of hyperinsulinemia and hence, increased peripheral glucose utilization leads to a fall in blood glucose levels (Fig. 17–11). Hypoglycemia can also occur several hours after exercise in type 1 diabetes because of overinsulinization at the time of the exercise-induced increase in insulin sensitivity.

The metabolic response to exercise has been investigated in each of three conditions: normal, hypoinsulinization, and hyperinsulinization.

Normoinsulinization.   Although a fall in insulin is essential for normal metabolic responses to exercise, it is not clear whether this is the case in subjects with type 1 diabetes receiving a peripheral insulin infusion (Fig. 17–11). When type 1 diabetic subjects were exercising during a constant insulin infusion that maintained normoglycemia, the response of glucose production was either insufficient[203] or just adequate[204,205] to prevent a fall in

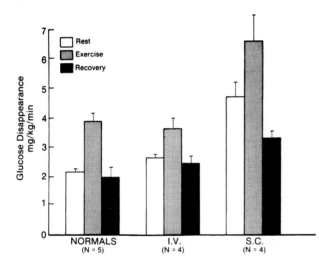

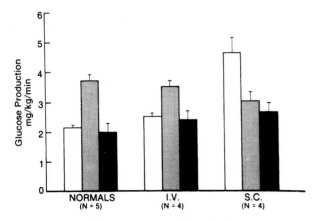

Figure 17–11. Glucose turnover: (upper) glucose disappearance and (lower) glucose production at rest, at 45 min of exercise, and at 60 min recovery for the normal controls. Insulin-infused (IV) and subcutaneous (SC) insulin-treated diabetics. (From Ref. 204)

glycemia. It is likely that with peripheral insulin infusion, a smaller decrease in insulin is required during exercise than with portal insulin administration. This could relate to portal hyperinsulinemia, which inhibits the actions of neural inputs and the counterregulatory hormones that serve to increase glucose production during exercise. Responses of glucose production and utilization to exercise could be completely normalized only when peripheral insulin infusion in persons with type 1 diabetes fully normalized glycemia. Thus plasma glucose levels as well as adequate insulinization are critical regulators during exercise in insulin-dependent diabetes mellitus (IDDM).[202]

Hypoinsulinization.

Moderate Insulin Deficiency   Twenty-four hr after the injection of intermediate insulin in type 1 diabetic subjects, increments in glucose fluxes are often normal during exercise. The mechanisms for the increase in glucose fluxes, however, are very different from those in nondiabetic subjects. For example, although the increase in glucose production is quantitatively similar, hyperglycemic diabetic subjects rely more heavily on glucose derived from gluconeogenesis.[206] Total gluconeogenic precursor uptake by the splanchnic bed could account for up to 30% of the splanchnic glucose output after 40 min of exercise compared to just 11% in normal subjects, due to a greater delivery and fractional extraction of gluconeogenic substrate by the splanchnic bed in diabetic subjects.[206]

Generally, glucose utilization also increases similarly in both diabetic and nondiabetic subjects, but whereas in the latter this increase is due to an increase in glucose clearance, in inadequately controlled diabetic subjects it is a result of an increased mass action related to hyperglycemia, coupled with a smaller increment in glucose clearance.[87,11,103] In addition, a smaller percentage of the glucose utilized is completely oxidized in diabetic subjects,[207] probably due to decreased pyruvate dehydrogenase activity. Increased utilization of FFAs is likely the cause of and appears to compensate, at least in part, for the reduction in energy production that results from the diminished capacity to oxidize glucose. From the data of Wahren et al.[206] it can be estimated that during 40 min of moderate exercise FFA uptake can account for 27% of the energy needs of the working limb in normal subjects, but as much as 33% and 56% in nonketotic and ketotic diabetic subjects, respectively. Poorly controlled type 1 diabetes is also associated with a greater availability of ketone bodies for energy metabolism.[103,208]

Splanchnic ketone body production is elevated during exercise due to an increased splanchnic fractional extraction and a greater intrahepatic conversion of FFA to ketone bodies as assessed by ^{14}C-oleic acid infusion.[209] The effects of insulin on muscle glucose uptake can be partly mediated by insulin's effects on fat metabolism.[114,209]

Individuals with diabetes may also exhibit differences in intramuscular substrate metabolism in response to exercise. Diabetic subjects deprived of insulin for 24 hr have decreased intramuscular glycogen storage and increased intramuscular fat storage. This shift in substrate stores leads to a greater metabolism of intramuscular fat and a diminished breakdown of glycogen.[210] By using radioactive palmitate and glucose in combination with gas exchange measurements, it was calculated that in the insulin-deficient depancreatized dog over twice as much intramuscular fat, but only about 60% of the muscle glycogen, is utilized during exercise of moderate intensity.[211] Thus, individuals with type 1 diabetes in poor control rely on fat metabolism to a greater extent in exercise of low-moderate intensity.

Severe Insulin Deficiency Severe insulin deficiency, manifested by substantial hyperglycemia and ketosis, can result in a deterioration of glycemic control during exercise,[208,212] and ketone bodies rose substantially. It was shown in depancreatized dogs that this rise in glucose with severe insulin-deficiency is due to an attenuated increase in glucose utilization, accompanied by an increase in glucose production that is generally similar to that in nondiabetic animals.[11,213] The attenuated increment in glucose utilization is due to the lack of a direct effect of insulin on glucose transport and/or to an indirect effect to restrain catecholamine-induced lipolysis and/or glycogenolysis. The stimulatory role of hypoinsulinemia on glucose production can be counteracted by the suppressive effect of hyperglycemia.[214] Underinsulinization also leads to further increases in FFA and ketone body levels with exercise. Thus, exercise in the poorly-controlled diabetic subjects may contribute to the existing hyperglycemia and hyperlipidemia and lead to ketoacidosis. The extent to which exercise may worsen control in the individual with diabetes is affected by the work intensity. Heavy exercise can be more deleterious to diabetic control than moderate exercise of similar duration.[215,216] Even subjects in good metabolic control may develop a progressive increase in glycemia and FFA levels after intense exercise to exhaustion.[217]

The deleterious effects of underinsulinization in individuals with diabetes during exercise is not exclusively due to the diminished insulin levels per se, as exercise in these subjects or animals is characterized by excessive increases in glucagon,[113,206,208,214,218] the catecholamines,[113,214,219] growth hormone,[208,220] and cortisol levels,[113,208] all of which aggravate the diabetic state. An excessive increase in glucagon is also seen in resting diabetic dogs during physiologic infusion of epinephrine.[221] Therefore excessive glucagon response

to exercise is due to catecholamine release as well as hypoinsulinemia. Insulin therapy that improves metabolic control can normalize the excessive counterregulatory response to exercise in subjects with type 1 diabetes.[208,219] It is unknown whether excessive counterregulation can be due to brain hyperglycemia. If this is the case, it would indicate that hypo- and hyperglycemia can have similar effects on efferent signals from the autonomic nervous system. It is interesting not only that excessive counterregulation in poorly controlled diabetes occurs during exercise, but also that it is a general characteristic of the metabolic responses to stress. Chronic stimulation of counterregulatory mechanisms by hyperglycemia may be one of the factors that interferes with acute counterregulation to hypoglycemia in type 1 diabetes (see the section on "Stress" later in this chapter).

The mechanism of accelerated gluconeogenesis in the insulin-deficient state was studied in depancreatized dogs. It was concluded that gluconeogenesis from alanine, lactate, and glycerol is exaggerated at rest due to an increased capacity of hepatic lactate extraction, increased hepatic precursor loads and a greater gluconeogenic efficiency. In addition, it is accelerated by exercise due to added increments in hepatic precursor loads and because of a greater net gut alanine and lactate output.[222]

Role of Counterregulatory Hormones Studies in the alloxan-diabetic dog deprived of exogenous insulin for 24 hr demonstrate that, as in normal dogs, the presence of glucagon is a major determinant of hepatic glucose production during exercise.[218] In this model of poorly controlled type 1 diabetes, glucagon suppression with somatostatin prevented the rise of hepatic glucose production during exercise. Despite the substantial role of glucagon in poorly controlled diabetes, it was somewhat less important to the rise in glucose production than it was in normal dogs,[113,218,223] although insulin deficiency was present, which sensitizes the liver to glucagon. This might be related to suppression of hepatic glucose production by hyperglycemia. Elevated glucagon also plays a role in increasing ketogenesis in the liver and in diabetes, and it was demonstrated that physiologically, the exercise-induced rise in glucagon is an important regulator of ketogenesis.[224]

The role of the catecholamines in moderate intensity exercise has been studied using adrenergic blockade in well-controlled type 1 diabetes,[203] alloxan-diabetic dogs with residual insulin secretion,[113] and totally insulin-deprived depancreatized dogs.[87] In well-maintained, insulin-infused diabetic subjects (basal plasma glucose of 144 mg/dL) with normal increments in counterregulatory hormones, β-adrenergic blockade did not affect hepatic glucose output.[203] However, this finding is difficult to interpret because even in the absence of β-blockade the subjects did not have an appreciable increase in glucose output in response to exercise. Nevertheless, glucose production during exercise in alloxan-diabetic dogs in poor metabolic control and with excessive counterregulatory hormone levels was also unaffected by β-blockade.[113] In contrast, in depancreatized dogs that were totally insulin-deprived, β-blockade markedly decreased increments in glucose production during exercise.[87] Extrapancreatic glucagon fails to rise during exercise in these dogs. It therefore appears that in the total absence of insulin and in the presence of basal levels of glucagon, the control of glucose production is shifted to the catecholamines.

The role of catecholamines in stimulating hepatic glucose production in intense exercise has been reviewed earlier. Type 1 diabetic subjects rendered euglycemic prior to intense exercise by intravenous insulin infusion show the same effects upon glucose production as normal control subjects when infused with the β-blocker propranolol. Their increment in production was greater than in unblocked subjects, again suggesting an α-receptor component to stimulation.[106] To our knowledge, neither α-blocker studies of euglycemia nor studies with either α- or β-blockers plus hyperglycemia have been done with intense exercise in diabetic subjects. The adrenergic receptor mechanisms involved may be different across species and may even be influenced by chronic hyperglycemia within the same species.

Although the role of the catecholamines in regulating glucose release from the liver during exercise in type 1 diabetes still remains to be fully defined, they clearly have potent peripheral effects. Plasma epinephrine increments during insulin deficiency can significantly worsen the resulting hyperglycemia through stimulation of both glycogenolysis and gluconeogenesis.[48] In moderate-intensity exercise β-blockade markedly decreased FFA levels during exercise in alloxan-diabetic[113] and depancreatized dogs[87] deprived of exogenous insulin and also prevented the exercise-induced increment in FFA concentration in insulin-infused diabetic humans.[203] On the other hand, α-blockade in insulin-infused diabetic subjects caused a twofold increase in the FFA increment during exercise.[203] β-Blockade prevented the rise in lactate in alloxan-diabetic dogs,[113] offering indirect evidence that muscle glycogenolysis may have been stimulated by β-adrenergic mechanisms. As previously mentioned, in alloxan-diabetic dogs but not in depancreatized dogs, β-blockade increased glucose uptake and clearance during exercise. Also in well-maintained, insulin-infused diabetic subjects, β-blockade induced a marked rise in glucose utilization.

In intense exercise, the same occurred and to the same extent as in control subjects and in euglycemic diabetic subjects during propranolol infusion. The pro-

pranolol markedly decreased FFA levels, and they remained suppressed during and after exercise.[106,194] These observations are consistent with the β-blocker attenuating lipolysis and muscle glycogenolysis. The latter allowed for greater uptake of circulating glucose both during and after intense exercise, to the extent that in the diabetic subjects, euglycemia was restored soon into recovery *without* the usual need for sustained hyperinsulinemia.[106]

The response to adrenergic blockade in moderate exercise in type 1 diabetes is, in a qualitative manner, similar to the response of adrenergic blockade seen in normal subjects. However, in a quantitative sense the activity of the catecholamines appears enhanced in poorly controlled diabetes.[203] It is not clear whether this difference is due to a change in sensitivity to the catecholamines or to other abnormalities in diabetes. Regardless of the mechanism involved, the previous studies indicate that propranolol, a common drug used for treatment of hypertension or angina, may increase the risk of exercise-induced hypoglycemia in insulin-treated diabetic subjects.

Cardiovascular function and plasma catecholamine response was examined in diabetic patients with or without autonomic neuropathy. While VO$_2$max was not different among the diabetic groups, it was much less than in control subjects. During exercise, the heart rate, systolic blood pressure, and norepinephrine and epinephrine increments were significantly blunted when autonomic neuropathy was associated with parasympathetic and sympathetic defects.[225]

Hyperinsulinization It is evident that adequate insulin is important to avoid aggravating the diabetic state during exercise. However, the more common problem in type 1 diabetes is hypoglycemia resulting from overinsulinization during and after exercise. It has been demonstrated in man, in the dog, and in the rat that exercise can accelerate the absorption of subcutaneous insulin injection.[204,226–228] However, hypoglycemia may occur during exercise in type 1 diabetes even when insulin mobilization from its injection site is not accelerated.[229,230] The crucial factor seems to be ongoing insulin absorption, which results in hyperinsulinemia during exercise and may be excessive after exercise when the exercise-induced increase in insulin sensitivity occurs.

The hypoglycemia that may ensue during exercise in type 1 diabetes or diabetic animals is mainly due to deficient release of glucose from the liver.[204,227] A subcutaneous injection of long-acting insulin 8 hr prior to exercise in depancreatized dogs resulted in a substantial rise in circulating insulin levels and led to a 100 mg/dL fall in plasma glucose after 60 min of exercise, due to a failure of hepatic glucose production to rise normally.[227] These findings in the depancreatized dog are consistent with those obtained in the type 1 subjects treated subcutaneously with intermediate-acting insulin 1 hr prior to exercise (Fig. 17–11).[204] These results contrast to subjects rendered euglycemic overnight by intravenous insulin, whose glycemic glucose turnover responses during and after exercise were normalized. The actions and mechanisms of peripheral insulin infusion on hepatic glucose production in these patients during exercise are not clear. It should be noted that, at least during rest, insulin exerts its inhibition of hepatic glucose production primarily through the peripheral mechanism.[231–234] In man and dog, peripheral signals due to hyperinsulinemia are suppression of FFA and glucagon.[234–238]

The three panels of Figure 17–10 summarize the interactions of insulin and glucagon in regulating glucose turnover in exercising patients with type 1[239] and in depancreatized dogs.[87,114,240] During constant intravenous infusion of insulin, glucose homeostasis is preserved because glucose production and use are balanced as in nondiabetic subjects. Due to the direct or indirect (FFA-glucose cycle) effects of insulin deficiency,[87,240,241] exercise does not stimulate glucose use adequately, and hence the exercise-induced increase in hepatic glucose production leads to or enhances hyperglycemia, a key factor restraining metabolic glucose clearance during exercise.[240] Absolute or relative overinsulinization, due to absorption of subcutaneous insulin injected before exercise, results in inhibition of hepatic glucose production, enhanced peripheral glucose uptake, and a fall in blood glucose levels.

The mechanism of the delayed hypoglycemia has been poorly investigated. Peripheral mechanisms related to increased glucose uptake for glycogen repletion in previously depleted muscles may be more important. The non-physiological route of administration of insulin and consequent peripheral hyperinsulinemia could be particularly disadvantageous for this type of hypoglycemia. Of course, extent and timing of overinsulinization depend on the modality of insulin treatment. Therefore, the problem of exercise-induced hypoglycemia in insulin-treated diabetic subjects has to be evaluated in conjunction with the individual diet

and insulin regimen. Specific problems arising in subjects on conventional or intensive insulin treatment are dealt with, together with practical recommendations, in the section on "Clinical Considerations."

Type 2 Diabetes.   Despite the high prevalence of type 2 diabetes, in comparison to type 1 diabetes there have been fewer studies examining the effects of acute exercise on glucose kinetics in type 2 diabetes. To understand the effects of exercise in type 2 diabetes one must take into account the specific treatment modality. Obese type 2 diabetic subjects maintained on diet or diet plus sulfonylurea (chlorpropamide) with postabsorptive hyperglycemia (above 200 mg/dL) and normal basal insulin showed a fall in glycemia of about 50 mg/dL during a 45-min moderate intensity exercise period (Fig. 17–12).[242] The fall in glucose was due to an attenuation of the rise in hepatic glucose production while glucose utilization increased normally. In another study, however, the rise in glucose utilization was variable among lean type 2 diabetic subjects with mild hyperglycemia (8 mM).[243] This led to inconsistent changes in plasma glucose levels, which decreased, remained unchanged, or even increased. This emphasizes the heterogeneity in pathophysiology of non-insulin-dependent diabetes mellitus (NIDDM), that affects glucoregulation differently in both the exercised and rested states. Interestingly, however, in both studies the rise in glucose production was attenuated. This could relate to hyperglycemia or to a defect in a proposed feedback mechanism that couples the increase in glucose production to glucose utilization during exercise.[244] However, the main factor is probably the fact that in type 2 diabetes insulin secretion is not inhibited.[242] Thus type 2 diabetic subjects have a defect in insulin secretion both when challenged with glucose (inadequate or uncoordinated increase) and when challenged with exercise (inadequate or uncoordinated decrease). The latter could be a consequence of hyperglycemia prevailing over adrenergic stimulation or of reduced sympathetic activity due to autonomic neuropathy. Alternatively, it might reflect an intrinsic abnormality of β-cell function. It was not due to the

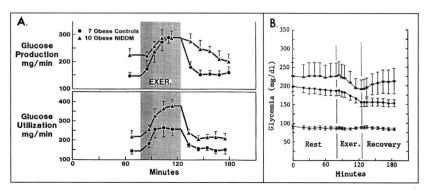

Figure 17–12.   (A) Glucose production and utilization in seven obese controls and ten obese NIDDM subjects during rest, exercise (60% VO_2 max), and recovery. (B) Glycemia in seven obese controls (X), four obese diabetic subjects treated by diet (C), and five diabetic subjects treated with sulfonylureas (●). EXER signifies the 45 min exercise period. Mean and SE are shown. (From Ref. 242)

effect of sulfonylureas in the studies cited, as it was present without such treatment. The failure of β-cell secretion to decrease seems to also depend on the duration of exercise. Obese women with type 2 diabetes and mild hyperglycemia (approx. 160 mg/dL) showed a decrease in plasma glucose during 20–40 min moderate exercise, with no change in plasma insulin. Using different techniques, one study did show an increase in splanchnic glucose output as well as a decline in plasma insulin in postabsorptive exercise.[245] Also, during 3 hr of moderate-intensity exercise in type 2 diabetic subjects with borderline fasting hyperglycemia (140 mg/dL) and hyperinsulinemia (23 uU/mL), plasma glucose fell by about 40 mg/dL[246] and there was some decrease in plasma insulin. It is likely that with increased duration of exercise the falling glycemia reduces stimulation of the β-cell. This could explain why the fall in glucose during such exercise in type 2 diabetic subjects tends not to lead to hypoglycemia. These data demonstrate that acute exercise might have beneficial glucose-lowering effect in type 2 diabetes, which is of great importance clinically. Even more interesting is the effect of acute exercise to enhance insulin sensitivity in the postexercise period. Twelve to sixteen hr after a single bout of glycogen-depleting exercise, hepatic and peripheral insulin sensitivity increased in type 2 diabetes.[247] The increased peripheral insulin sensitivity is due to an enhanced rate of nonoxidative glucose disposal.[247]

A well-designed recent study assessed for the first time the responses to postprandial moderate exercise of obese NIDDM subjects treated with diet alone.[248] Forty-five min of 50% VO$_2$max exercise beginning 45 min after a standardized breakfast markedly attenuated the glycemic response to the same breakfast without exercise. However, the values reached the same mildly hyperglycemic level of 8mmol/L (144mg/dL) by 4 hr after breakfast with or without exercise. Of special note is that there was no effect on the glycemic excursion following a standardized *lunch* with or without exercise after breakfast. The decrease in postprandial glycemia during exercise was associated with a correspondingly lowered insulin response, both of which rose immediately following exercise toward the levels in the control nonexercised experiment (Fig. 17–13). Reduction of breakfast caloric intake has the same effect on postprandial glycemia and insulin secretion as an equivalent exercise-induced increase in caloric expenditure. This is very reminiscent of the response in lean, normal subjects, although this occurred at higher glucose and insulin concentrations in diabetic subjects.[249] As in certain postabsorptive NIDDM subjects,[242] in these postprandial diabetic studies there was no increase in isotopically estimated glucose appearance (i.e., the sum of meal plus endogenous glucose production) during exercise, the rates being the same as in the absence of exercise. It seems improbable that there was a decrease

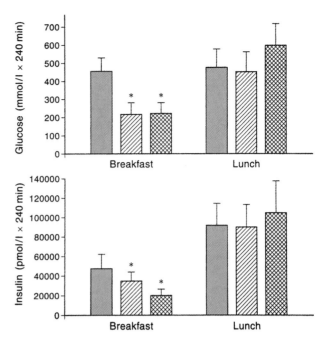

Figure 17–13. Area under curve (AUC) for glucose and insulin in NIDDM patients studied on three occasions: control day (CD) (■) (n = 9), exercise day (ED) (▨) (n = 9), and diet day (DD) (⧆) (n = 7). Breakfast AUC (B-AUC) was calculated from time 0 min to time 240 min, lunch AUC was calculated from time 240 min $p < 0.05$, difference in comparison to CD. (From Ref. 248.)

in glucose absorption from the intestine.[250] The attenuation of the postprandial hyperglycemic response could thus be explained by the increased glucose uptake during exercise, occurring during a *dip* in the postprandial hyperinsulinemic response. Of interest is that the authors included experiments with a smaller breakfast that produced a comparable decrease in glycemic and insulin excursions as with the larger meal plus exercise, although with a different time course. These findings are especially relevant to clinical management, as most patients will exercise postprandially rather than in the overnight-fasted state.

Subjects with type 2 diabetes who are on diet therapy alone should be able to exercise like normal subjects, provided there are no major vascular complications. However, when oral hypoglycemic drugs are used, there may be a tendency for hypoglycemia during prolonged exercise. Type 2 diabetic subjects on insulin treatment are at similar risk for hypoglycemia as those with IDDM, so caution is advisable in matching diet and insulin treatment to meet the glucose requirements of physical activity.

Effect of Hyperglycemia: Possible Protection of Muscle Against Excessive Glucose. Decreased metabolic glucose clearance in hyperglycemia may reflect a protective mechanism against excessive glucose in the muscle.

It is tempting to speculate that this is the reason that muscle doesn't have diabetic complications seen in so many other tissues. It is particularly important that the determination of Metabolic Clearance Rate (MCR) in vivo corresponds to some changes seen in muscle glucose transporters. Indeed, chronic hyperglycemia decreases the concentration of glucose transporters in both plasma and internal membranes. This was shown by cytochalasin binding and by measurements of specific glucose transporters GLUT 4 and GLUT 1. It is only the insulin-sensitive GLUT 4 that is downregulated. It is notable that in streptozotocin-diabetic rats this effect occurs even when fasting insulin levels are normal. Restoration of normal glycemia by phlorizin treatment normalizes glucose transporters in plasma membrane. Importantly, this effect of normalization of plasma glucose occurs without any changes of plasma insulin. In the same experiments, hyperglycemia also suppressed mRNA of GLUT 4 and normoglycemia brought about partial restoration. The conclusion is that hyperglycemia itself suppresses both gene expression and translocation of the GLUT 4 protein (Fig. 17–14).[109,110,112,251,252]

Similarly, normalization of glycemia with phlorizin in alloxan-diabetic dogs increases MCR, while glucose uptake is unchanged. This applies both to resting conditions[253,254] and to exercise (Fig. 17–15).[255] Regulation of glucose uptake and metabolism during rest and exercise is normal because hyperglycemia maintains glucose use through its mass effect, and excessive metabolism of glucose is prevented as metabolic glucose clearance is suppressed. This mechanism works in the presence of very small amounts of insulin, and a defect in glucose use is noted only in depancreatized dogs that are totally insulin deficient.[114,240] On the cellular level, the efficiency of glucose uptake is related to the number of glucose transporters in the plasma membrane.[109] The observation that hyperglycemia decreases the number of glucose transporters in plasma membrane also supports the notion of the adaptive effect of hyperglycemia.[109,251] Interestingly, glucose uptake and clearance during exercise may not be affected by levels of FFA. Higher levels of FFA, however, decreased glucose oxidation, a reflection of lactate release. This is in concordance with the notion that the FFA/glucose cycle initially affects only glucose oxidation, and only after 3–4 hr does it also decrease glucose uptake.[157] Figure 17–16 compares responses of glycemia, glucose utilization (Rd), and glucose metabolic clearance (MCR) in lean nondiabetic and lean IDDM subjects. IDDMs were maintained at moderate hyperglycemia on constant insulin infusion during the preceding night and through the experimental protocols. In both groups, exercise induced an equivalent increase in plasma glucose, but in IDDMs, glucose did not decline during exercise. MCR was decreased in IDDM during rest and exercise, but glucose utilization was the same as in nor-

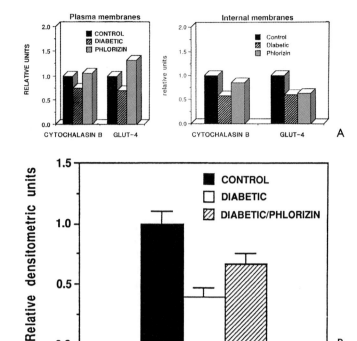

Figure 17–14. (Top) Effect of normalization of glycemia on cytochalasin B binding and GLUT4 glucose transporters in hyperglycemic normoinsulinemic diabetic rats. The isolated fractions were isolated for protein and 5-nucleotidase activity. Forth micrograms of protein-isolated membrane fractions were analyzed by Western blot using an anti-GLUT4 antibody. The blots were quantified by laser densitometry and the results were plotted in arbitrary units relative to the values in the plasma membrane of control animals. Plasma membrane glucose transporters were suppressed by diabetes and restored by normalization of glucose with phlorizin. Normalization of glucose with phlorizin restores cytochalasin B binding but not the GLUT4 transporters in internal membranes. (Bottom) GLUT4 mRNA is suppressed by diabetes and partially restored by normalization of glucose with phlorizin. (Reprinted from Ref. 10.)

mal controls. This indicates that adaptation of glucose utilization also occurs in diabetic man.[193] This mechanism of self-regulation also explains observations in streptozotocin-diabetic rats where endogenous pH and energy stores measured with Nuclear Magnetic Resonance (NMR) techniques and the activity of pyruvate dehydrogenase during rest and muscular contraction were normal, not only in insulin-treated rats but also in rats with insulin treatment discontinued for 3 days (Fig. 17–7).[256] However, there was a defect in glycogen resynthesis following contractions. A severe defect was noted only when the diabetic rats did not receive insulin for 3 weeks.

Physical Training

Effects on Insulin Sensitivity, Glucose Tolerance, and Glycemic Control.

Nondiabetic Subjects. Athletes or endurance-trained subjects have normal or even increased glucose toler-

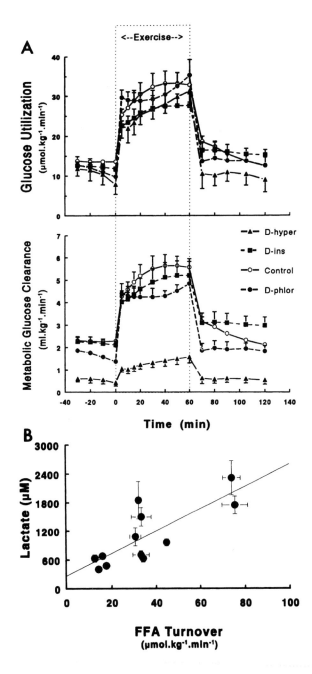

Figure 17–15. (A) Glucose utilization and metabolic clearance rates of plasma glucose in dogs before, during, and after 60 min treadmill exercise (100 m/min, 5% slope). Experiments were conducted in four dog protocols consisting of one protocol with normal control dogs (C, O) and three protocols with alloxan-diabetic dogs studied under conditions of hyperglycemia (DH, ⅄), and during acutely induced normoglycemia ($<$160 min) with either insulin (2.6 ± 0.6 pmol.kg^{-1}/min^{-1}, DI, ■) or phlorizin (50 ìg/kg^{-1}/min^{-1}, DP, ⊠). Values are presented as mean $\pm$ SE from six experiments in each protocol. During hyperglycemia metabolic clearance of glucose was markedly suppressed during rest and exercise. It was normalized with normoglycemia and independently of insulin or FFA levels—glucose utilization was only slightly decreased in hyperglycemic dogs, reflecting the balance between mass effect of hyperglycemia and suppressed clearance. (B) Correlation between rates of FFA turnover and lactate concentrations in all four dog protocols consisting of normal control dogs and alloxan-diabetic dogs studied under conditions of hyperglycemia and during acutely induced normoglycemia ($<$160 min) with either insulin or phlorizin. Plotted data indicate the mean $\pm$ SE during the basal period, exercise period, and recovery period for each protocol ($r = 0.72$, $P < 0.001$). Increased FFA turnover did not affect glucose uptake but it decreased glucose oxidation—a reflection of lactate release. (From Ref. 255.)

ance, while fasting and glucose-stimulated insulin levels are lower.[257,258] Considered under *usual* daily conditions of meals and activity, Dela et al. showed that despite athletes' ingesting considerably more energy (and expending correspondingly more as well), their 24 hr integrated glucose responses and insulin secretion were the *same* as in sedentary subjects.[259] This translates into greater efficiency in disposing that part of the dietary intake that is dependent upon insulin's effects. In testing for maximal insulin responses, hyperinsulinemic, euglycemic clamp experiments have demonstrated that submaximal insulin-stimulated glucose disposal is increased in aerobically trained athletes.[258,260] In a comprehensive study, it was demonstrated that insulin action in trained distance runners

was enhanced in muscle, liver, and adipose tissue (Figure 17–17).[258] This was demonstrated by combining tracer methods with regional catheterization and by taking biopsies of fat depots. The sensitivity to physiologic insulin levels was assessed in trained distance runners using a euglycemic clamp with insulin infusions that maintained levels of 10 and 50 uU/mL. At the low and high insulin concentrations, respectively, trained subjects had glucose uptakes that were 25% and 38% increased, while glucose production was 47% and 70% below that in controls. Furthermore, insulin-stimulated glucose uptake was 43% higher than in controls. Thus, at physiologic insulin levels, trained subjects have both increased peripheral and hepatic sensitivity to insulin. These effects of training are probably specific

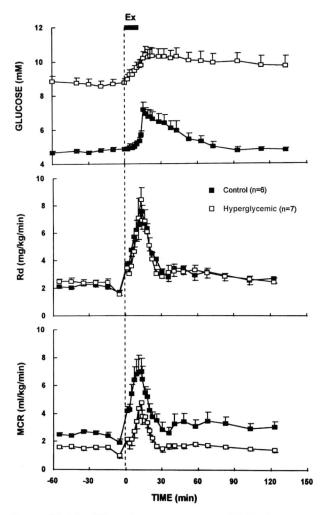

Figure 17–16. Effect of intense exercise in IDDM subjects whose glycemia was normalized (■) or kept moderately elevated (□) by constant insulin infusions maintained overnight and during the experiment. (Modified from Ref. 193.)

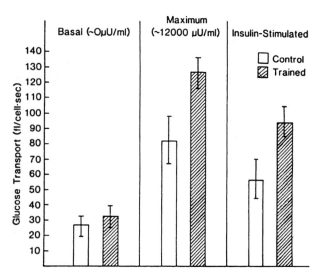

Figure 17–17. Mean ± SE values for basal, maximal, and insulin-stimulated glucose transport in adipocytes isolated from control (open bars) and trained (hatched bars) individuals. (From Ref. 258)

for aerobic exercise. Although strength training results in a net increase in submaximal insulin-stimulated glucose disposal[260] and glucose tolerance,[261] this increase is proportional to the increased muscle mass and probably does not represent an increase in insulin sensitivity per se.

Considering the fundamental role of skeletal muscle during exercise and that it represents the bulk of insulin-sensitive tissue, it is likely that muscle is the major site of the increase in insulin action that occurs with training. In trained rats, skeletal muscle is more insulin sensitive than that from sedentary controls due mainly to increased glucose oxidation.[262–264] Hyperinsulinemic, euglycemic clamps combined with the 2-deoxyglucose technique demonstrated an increase in insulin sensitivity or responsiveness in several muscles from exercise-trained rats compared to sedentary controls.[264,265] Exercise alone does not appear to normalize insulin sensitivity in muscle in insulin-resistant rats.[262,266] However, diet and exercise together may correct this situation.[266,267]

In the rat, the increase in insulin action in skeletal muscle was associated with an increase in insulin binding to its skeletal muscle receptor.[268,269]

The advancement of molecular technology has made it possible to frequently relate changes in tissue glucose uptake to the synthesis and translocation of glucose transporters.[79,110,270–273] It is well documented that both insulin and exercise translocate GLUT 4 from internal sites to the plasma membrane. The effect of insulin is more pronounced in red muscle than in white.[270] The translocation from internal membranes to the muscle transverse tubules is at least as important as the transfer to plasma membrane[79] because the area of transverse tubules that penetrates the various muscle structures is much larger than that of plasma membrane. Swimming or free-wheel running induces rapid increases in the expression of the insulin-sensitive GLUT 4 protein and enhancement of glucose transport capacity in insulin-induced glycogen storage in the muscle in the normal rat.[274,275] In nine male type 1 patients, acute exercise (3 hr of cycling) decreased cellular GLUT 4 mRNA content while GLUT 4 protein content remained unchanged in the quadriceps femoris. The authors concluded that there is abnormal GLUT 4 mRNA production or degradation or both in patients with type 1 diabetes.[276] In contrast, in type 2 patients physical training increased both muscle GLUT 4 protein and mRNA.[277] In most human studies, only total GLUT 4 content was measured, and that does not indicate the membrane abundance of this protein. In nine male healthy athletes, both muscle blood flow and glucose uptake were increased. The cellular mechanisms of glucose uptake are increased GLUT 4 protein content, glycogen synthase activity, and glucose storage as glycogen. A correlation between glycogen synthase fractional activity and blood flow suggested that they are causally related in promoting glucose disposal.[278] The signaling whereby insulin can increase translocation of GLUT 4 protein has been in part characterized. It requires an intact actin network[279] and activation of phosphatidylonositol 3-kinase (PI-3).[280] In contrast, PI-3 kinase and the actin network are not required for the stimulation of glucose transport caused by uncoupling the oxidative chain. Muscle contraction does not affect the insulin receptor autophosphorylation or IRS-1 tyrosine phosphorylation,[281] and it does not lead to stimulation of muscle PI-3 kinase. Such data indicate different signaling pathways[57,65] of translocation of GLUT 4 by insulin and exercise and explain their additive effects on glucose uptake.

Skeletal muscle adapts to aerobic exercise training so that it more readily uses fuels and oxygen. To enhance its metabolic capacity, mitochondrial enzyme concentrations and capillary density increases in muscle in response to habitual training, and the improved insulin sensitivity in diabetic subjects may be due to these adaptations.

In addition to skeletal muscle, adipose tissue represents another site of adaptation to training. Regular physical activity increases insulin-stimulated glucose uptake,[264,282–284] oxidation,[264,284] and incorporation into fatty acids[264,284] in rat adipocytes. This is consistent with the demonstration that trained rats have a greater number of glucose transporters in fat cell membranes.[283] The improvement of insulin action may also relate to the reduced fat cell size after physical training. The increase in insulin action in adipocytes of trained rats occurs in the absence of any changes in insulin binding,[284] indicating a modification in a postbinding event.

In the rat, the marked increase of glucose uptake in the resting muscle was only observed up to 2 days after the last bout of exercise.[285] The effect of training on adipose tissue was also short-lived.[286] Such transience of the effects of training has also been reported in humans. As rapidly as 14 days after cessation of exercise training the insulin response increased, as demonstrated during a hyperglycemic clamp technique. However, rates of whole body glucose disposal were not different between exercising and inactive states, indicating a large magnitude of the physiologic range of modulation of the action of insulin due to level of activity.[287,288] These observations suggest that the improvement in insulin action in trained subjects could be due to the cumulative action of single bouts of exercise rather than to long-term adaptations from exercise training. An acute bout of exercise and training share some similar effect, and the effects of training on insulin action can be reversed by inactivity. However, some studies[289,290] show that an increase in insulin action can also be related to the trained state itself. It therefore appears that the improvement in insulin action induced by training is mainly related to acute processes, such as depletion of glycogen stores. However, it is also feasible that training might also increase the capacity of the muscle to utilize glucose through chronic processes, such as increased content of oxidative enzymes and number, intrinsic activity, and regulation of transporters. The question is whether some of these effects persist for a prolonged period of time up to cessation of training. It is interesting that exercise adds to the effect of maximal insulin on whole body glucose uptake. Training increases contraction-induced glucose tranport in vitro but not glucose utilization in human muscle exercising during normal insulinemia. This effect is in part due to the increased blood flow due to insulin. However, training increases the effect of acute exercise but without influencing blood flow.[291]

Type 1 Diabetic Subjects. Insulin sensitivity as assessed by the euglycemic clamp technique can be increased following training in type 1 diabetic subjects that are on conventional[86,291] or insulin pump therapy.[292] Studies in streptozotocin-diabetic rats indicate that the ability to adapt to chronic exercise in insulin-deficient states may depend on the severity of the condition. Mildly diabetic rats increase insulin sensitivity in response to exercise training,[293] whereas severely diabetic rats do not show this change.[294,295] Streptozotocin-diabetic rats have deficits in cytoplasmic and mitochondrial enzyme in their muscle fibers, and these enzymes are increased by training.[296] In type 1 diabetic subjects, training programs can lead to increases in skeletal muscle citrate synthase and succinate dehydrogenase that parallel the increase in insulin sensitivity.[86] The evidence available so far indicates that training sufficient to increase insulin sensitivity in persons with both type 1 and 2 diabetes is not accompanied by an increase in muscle capillary density.[297,298] However, it should be pointed out that in older nondiabetic and diabetic adults habitual exercise prevented the thickening of the skeletal muscle capillary basement membrane that is characteristic of advancing age. Moreover, the thickening of the capillary basement membrane appears to be readily reversed as a result of exercise training, even in older individuals.[299] Although insulin sensitivity is improved and insulin requirements may be reduced in some subjects, there is no evidence that glycemic control is effectively improved in trained IDDM individuals. Indeed, there was no improvement in glycosylated hemoglobin levels, glycosuria, or fasting plasma glucose following training programs, which resulted in significant increments in maximum oxidative capacity.[86,291,300,301] Concomitant increase in food intake may explain these findings,[301] indicating that more sophisticated strategies for managing insulin and diet in training and in athletic persons are required.

Type 2 Diabetic Subjects. Studies in NIDDM have shown that an exercise training program that is feasible for most individuals can cause an increase in glucose tolerance[302–307] and lower basal[246,305,308] and glucose-stimulated insulin levels.[302] Insulin sensitivity, as assessed by glucose disposal during hyperinsulinemic, euglycemic clamps, improves with exercise training (Fig. 17–14).[246,302,305,308] Studies on whether hepatic as well as peripheral sensitivity increase in both type 1 and II diabetic subjects are lacking.

Since insulin resistance is one of the main features of type 2 diabetes, exercise training might be particularly beneficial for these subjects. A combined exercise training and diet program increased the total glucose disposal rate during an insulin clamp by approximately 27%, due primarily to an accelerated rate of nonoxidative carbohydrate disposal (storage).[308] In contrast, diet alone did not affect glucose storage (Figure 17–18). Thus, it appears that the combination of diet and exercise has a more physiologic metabolic effect than diet alone. Basal and insulin-suppressed hepatic glucose output was also reduced by diet and training, but no more than the diet program alone.[308] Training program lead to an improvement in insulin sensitivity in obese subjects even without concurrent weight loss or change in body composition.[304] Nevertheless, since weight reduction by itself can

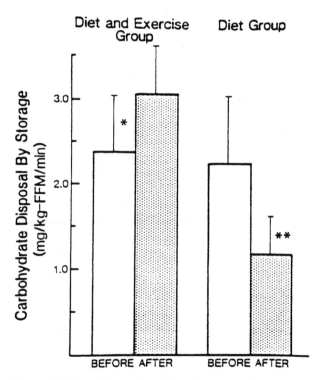

Figure 17–18. Carbohydrate disposal by nonoxidative processes, "storage." The single asterisk indicates the significant increase in estimated storage within the group in the dietary therapy plus physical training group (*P* < 0.05), and the double asterisk shows the significant reduction in the group given dietary therapy alone. (From Ref. 308)

also improve insulin sensitivity,[309] it is likely that exercise training as part of a program that results in loss of body fat will yield maximal effectiveness.

Training has been shown to decrease basal and glucose-stimulated insulin secretion in most,[310,311] but not all,[312] nondiabetic individuals. Following exercise, endogenous insulin secretion in healthy man is reduced and insulin clearance is enhanced both in healthy man and in individuals with type 1 diabetes. This indicates that there are two mechanisms for decreased insulin availability, both of which may allow enhanced muscle lipid utilization and spare glucose after long-term exercise. This has been generally interpreted as a consequence of enhancement in insulin sensitivity. Studies on type 2 diabetic subjects have shown a reduction or no change[246,305–308] in fasting and glucose-stimulated insulin levels following physical training. However, an increase in first-phase insulin secretion has also been reported.[303,308] Fasting and glucose-stimulated C-peptide increased after training in obese diabetic subjects with low C-peptide levels, while it decreased in both diabetic and control subjects with moderately elevated C-peptide concentrations. Insulin levels after training did not change.[302] Such a beneficial effect on β-cell function, selective for individuals with type 2 diabetes, was positively correlated with an improvement in glucose tolerance.

In contrast to type 1 diabetes, training does seem to improve glycemic control in type 2 diabetes.[303–305,308] Training programs that induced a 10–20% increase in maximum oxygen uptake caused significant reductions in glycosylated hemoglobin and fasting plasma glucose.[303–305] However, the improvement in fasting glucose and in glucose tolerance seems to be rapidly reversible with inactivity.[304] Increased insulin action in skeletal muscle due to training in some individuals with type 2 diabetes can even normalize glycemic control. However, the increase in trained muscle cannot fully account for the increase in whole body glucose clearance. Improvement in glucose clearance involves enhancement of insulin-mediated increase in muscle blood flow and the ability to extract glucose. They are accompanied by enhanced, nonoxidative glucose disposal and increases in glycogen synthase mRNA. The improvements in insulin action were short lived.[313] It is important to note that physical training in type 2 patients increased muscle GLUT 4 protein and mRNA.[314] In contrast to other reports in the literature, it appeared that in type 2 diabetes insulin can stimulate leg blood flow normally.[315] Therefore, exercise seems to be helpful in improving glycemic control in type 2 diabetes, but has to be maintained and, for the best effect, combined with diet or pharmacologic intervention.

Effects on the Atherogenic Complications of Diabetes. A recent review has concluded that quantitative estimates indicate that a sedentary lifestyle is responsible for about one-third of deaths due to coronary heart disease, colon cancer, and diabetes—three diseases for which physical inactivity is an established causal factor: "Presumably, if everyone were highly active, the death rate from these three diseases would be only two-thirds of the current rate."[316]

Atherosclerotic vascular disease, affecting arteries in the heart, brain, and extremities, is accelerated in subjects with all forms of diabetes. Retrospective epidemiologic data and animal studies indicate that physical training might retard cardiovascular disease (CVD) in the general population. Epidemiologic studies concerning exercise and CVD, however, are exceedingly difficult because of the selection of less healthy people in the lower activity category and the difficulty in quantifying levels of habitual physical activity.[317] Longitudinal population studies have given mixed results. For example, in a frequently quoted prospective study,[318] 10-year follow-up showed that the incidence of fatal myocardial infarction among Harvard alumni with a weekly recreational energy expenditure over 2,000 Kcal was one-half of that of their less active classmates, independent of other known risk factors, including hypertension, cigarette smoking, and hypercholesterolemia. In Framingham, an inverse relationship between the index of overall job and leisure time activity and 14-yr mortality for coronary heart disease was found in men but not in women.

Available epidemiologic data suggest that physical inactivity is probably not as potent an individual risk factor as elevated serum cholesterol, hypertension, or cigarette smoking. On the other hand, there is some evidence that exercise may attenuate other risk factors both directly and through associated weight reduction. Physical inactivity has been inversely associated with obesity, hypertension, and blood lipid abnormalities in some population studies. Although the association between total cholesterol and physical inactivity is inconclusive, physically inactive people usually have higher LDL and lower HDL cholesterol levels than active people. The atherogenic potential of triglyceride, uncertain in the general population, has been established in diabetes. Regarding associated risk factors for CVD, some data are available on lipid metabolism and lipid profiles in diabetes. Recent studies in type 1 diabetes[86,292,300] have shown that exercise training increases the ratio of HDL cholesterol to total cholesterol. One study in type 2 diabetes did not observe these changes.[319] Other studies have revealed a tendency for training to reduce circulating triglyceride levels in type 2 diabetics,[304,306] an effect that appears to be readily reversed by inactivity.[304] Training has been shown to improve glucose intolerance and hyperinsulinemia, ascertained and suspected risk factors for CVD. Therefore, it is likely that the atherogenic risk of

diabetes might be lessened by regular training programs. For this potential effect and for the beneficial effect on glycemic control, exercise training is being increasingly considered as part of the treatment strategy for type 2 diabetes.

Exercise in Prevention and Treatment of Diabetes Mellitus. The 1998 position statement of the American Diabetes Association (ADA)[320] and the recent Surgeon General's report on physical activity and health[321] underscore the pivotal role that physical activity plays in health promotion and disease prevention. It is becoming increasingly clear that the epidemic of type 2 diabetes sweeping the globe is associated with decreasing levels of activity and an increasing prevalence of obesity. Promoting exercise as a vital component of prevention as well as management of type 2 diabetes is viewed as a high priority. The benefit is the greatest when it is used early in its progression from insulin resistance to impaired glucose tolerance to overt hyperglycemia. The benefits with respect to glycemic control are prevention of cardiovascular disease, improvement of hyperlipidemia and hypertension, and weight maintenance control. People with type 1 diabetes should have the opportunity to benefit from all valuable effects of exercise, although the evidence of its effect on glycemic control is less conclusive. It appears that in the elderly, the progressive decrease in fitness, muscle mass, strength, and insulin sensitivity is in part preventable. It is likely that better levels of fitness will lead to less chronic vascular disease and improved quality of life. The recommendations of the ADA are based in part on two technical reviews.[322,323]

Physical inactivity is significantly associated with type 2 diabetes (for a review, see Ref. 321), and there is considerable evidence to support the relationship between physical inactivity and the incidence of type 2 diabetes.[318–327] Early suggestions emerged from the observation that societies that had discontinued their traditional lifestyles experienced major increases in the prevalence of type 2 diabetes.[328] Groups who migrated to a more technologically advanced environment had a higher prevalence of type 2 diabetes than those who remained in their native land,[329–331] and rural dwellers had a lower prevalence than their urban counterparts.[332–335] Most importantly, prospective cohort studies of college alumnae, female registered nurses, and male physicians have demonstrated that physical activity protects against the development of type 2 diabetes.[336] Each 5 Kcal of additional leisure time physical activity/week was associated with a 6% decrease in the risk of developing type 2 diabetes (independent of other risk factors) (Fig. 17–19). Similar observations were reported, in a different study on female registered nurses;[317–319] in a feasibility study in Malmo, Sweden;[338] and in a study in Daqing, China.[339] The lack of random

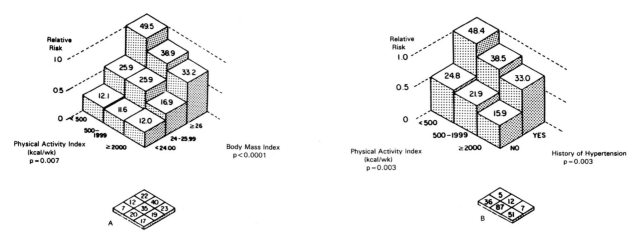

Figure 17–19. Age-adjusted incidence rates and relative risks of NIDDM among 5,990 men, based on (A) 1962 data for the physical activity index in relation to the body mass index and (B) any history of hypertension. Each block represents the relative risk based on the rate of NIDDM per 10,000 person-years of follow-up, with the risk for the tallest block set at 1.0. The numbers on the blocks are the incidence rates of NIDDM, and the numbers of patients with NIDDM are shown below in the corresponding grid. (Modified from Ref. 336.)

assignment of participants in many studies limits the generalization of these findings.

In explaining some of the beneficial effects of exercise, the report of the Surgeon General also reviews the short and long-term effects of physical activity on carbohydrate metabolism and glucose tolerance. It is indicated that the effect of muscular contraction is related to both increased blood flow in the muscle and enhanced glucose transport in the muscle cell. It appears that physical activity is primarily beneficial when abnormalities are caused by insulin resistance than when they are caused be deficient amounts of circulating insulin (for review, see Ref. 321).

Most interestingly, exercise training also has a significant effect in lean, insulin resistant offspring of type 2 diabetic parents. These individuals are characterized by (1) trimodal distribution of insulin sensitivity, (2) high fasting FFA concentrations, (3) an inverse correlation between insulin sensitivity and FFA concentration, (4) low plasma gluconeogenic amino acid concentrations, and (5) defective insulin secretion when related to insulin sensitivity in the subgroup of very resistant offspring.[340] Following exercise, NMR studies have shown that glycogen synthesis is normal during the insulin-independent phase of recovery but is severely diminished during the late recovery period, 2–5 hr which is insulin dependent.[341] Since insulin resistance in these individuals is the best predictor of development of the disease it was determined whether training improves insulin sensitivity in these subjects. Indeed, insulin sensitivity was increased because of a twofold increase in insulin-stimulated glycogen synthesis in muscle due to an increase in insulin-stimulated glucose transport-phosphorylation.[342]

Clinical Considerations

Exercise has been recommended as an adjuvant therapy for diabetes mellitus for many decades. With the discovery of insulin, Joslin recommended that diet, insulin, and exercise represent the management triad in insulin-treated diabetic subjects. In the last 20 years, the importance of exercise in the management of both type 1 and type 2 diabetes has been extensively reexamined in humans and tested in animals as well as nondiabetic persons. Unquestionably, it is important for both diabetic and nondiabetic individuals to optimize cardiovascular and pulmonary parameters. In addition, improved fitness can improve one's sense of well-being and ability to cope with the physical and psychological stresses that can be aggravated in diabetes. There have been a number of studies, reviewed earlier, indicating that the risk of cardiovascular disease may decrease in trained individuals, an observation of particular importance to individuals with diabetes, who are already at high risk.

Type 1 Diabetes. From the point of view of intermediate and long-term glycemic control, individuals with type 1 diabetes do not seem clearly to benefit from training programs. Due to the present modalities of insulin treatment, exercise is clearly associated with the risk of hypoglycemia in type 1 diabetes. In poorly controlled subjects, exercise may also aggravate hyperglycemia. However, these subjects do exercise as part of a more active population than type 2. They should not be restricted from sport, recreational activities, or even organized athletics or most occupations on the basis of their insulin dependency. On the contrary, diet and insulin therapy should be optimized and, most importantly, combined with self blood glucose monitoring (SBGM) to allow them to cope with the increased metabolic demands of physical activity. Patient and health professional education is fundamental in this respect. Also, it should be remembered that specific types of exercise may be contraindicated when complications of diabetes occur, so that subjects need to be evaluated before engaging in strenuous exercise or vigorous training. Specific guidelines vary according to type, intensity, duration of exercise, timing and type of diet and insulin therapy, and glycemic control. In general, metabolic control during and after exercise is more easily achieved and the risk of hypoglycemia is lessened if exercise can be planned.

Certain general considerations apply to all persons with diabetes who are treated with insulin, whether the physical activity is related to work, training, or leisure: (1) Supervisors, trainers, and team members should be aware that the person has diabetes and should be able to deal with symptoms suggesting hypoglycemia. (2) Very dangerous activities or those that require physical isolation are probably better not undertaken by such persons. One such activity that has elicited significant controversy is scuba diving; another might be working as a telephone lineman. (3) Where endurance-type or prolonged activity is undertaken the person must be accompanied by an informed partner. (4) A readily absorbable source of glucose should be available and at hand at all times. (5) Finally, in the case of a person demonstrably prone to severe hypoglycemia, injectable glucagon and a qualified person to administer it should be in proximity.

Diabetic subjects should not exercise when under- or overinsulinized, so that SBGM is mandatory. It is thus a prerequisite to have all the SBGM equipment on hand before and after exercise and to adjust carbohydrate intake accordingly. If exercise is prolonged and vigorous, frequent carbohydrate feedings (approximately every 30 min) should be taken, and food intake should be increased after exercise to avoid postexercise hypoglycemia. If hypoglycemia tends to occur during exercise, glucose requirements for activity at 50% VO_2max (moderate exercise) are calculated to be 1.25 g/min. Therefore, a 35–40 g carbohydrate snack every 30 min is suitable.

Although not considered a safeguard against hypoglycemia, it is often helpful to avoid injecting insulin 60–90 min before exercise and to use an injection site that is not in the area being exercised to avoid the rapid mobilization of insulin from an exercising extremity. Persons treated with conventional insulin therapy (one or two daily injections of intermediate insulin with short-acting insulin) should not exercise at the peak of action of the intermediate insulin. If exercise is planned, a 30–50% reduction of both short- and intermediate-acting insulin, according to blood glucose, is advisable.

Postprandial exercise has actually been proposed as a means of improving postprandial hyperglycemia, which results from the inadequate matching of depot insulin absorption with the absorption of carbohydrate from the gastrointestinal tract. However, the glycemic response to postprandial exercise has been found to be quite variable, and the risk of delayed hypoglycemic events, which are the most unpredictable and dangerous, is considerable. In practice, since exercise is often spontaneous and unplanned, it is extremely difficult to match insulin administration to insulin need with standard depot insulin. Since the risk of hypoglycemia is substantial, criteria of control are often loosened. This type of insulin treatment lacks flexibility so that SBGM is helpful to anticipate the need for carbohydrate snacks and to help adjust the insulin dose in subsequent exercising days, but does not allow readjustment of the insulin dose immediately after exercise.

Presently, more persons are being treated with intensive insulin therapy, including continuous subcutaneous insulin infusion (CSII) and multiple daily injections (MDI), including ultrarapidly acting insulin prior to meals with either one injection of ultra Lente insulin before supper or two intermediate insulins. The risk of hypoglycemia with these modalities is greater overall than with conventional insulin treatment. However, in the specific context of exercise these modalities provide a distinctive advantage over standard therapy because of their flexibility. Timely adjustment of insulin dose according to SBGM makes it possible to achieve relative normalization of the glycemic and metabolic response to exercise with less risk of hypoglycemia. The ability to readjust each pre-meal insulin bolus provides the opportunity to modify the insulin requirement both in anticipation of and following postprandial exercise. Depending on prior experience with the same exercise, timing and duration of exercise and on initial blood glucose concentration, the pre-meal bolus of insulin might be reduced by up to one-half the usual amount. In healthy subjects, postprandial exercise reduced insulin requirements from the artificial pancreas by 30%.[217] There is often a long-term effect from one bout of exercise on the glycemic excursion that extends well beyond the exercise period.[343] It is desirable in some patients to improve control, but in others it can be the cause of late, postexercise hypoglycemia. Again, SBGM makes it possible to adjust subsequent insulin boluses, or in the case of CSII, the basal rate of insulin.

Exercise studies in subjects with intensified insulin treatment have been carried out almost exclusively in subjects on CSII. Published information about exercise in multiple injection regimens is scanty. For postprandial exercise, extrapolation of the results obtained with CSII is justifiable. Subjects treated with CSII can safely exercise in both the postabsorptive and postprandial state, since free insulin levels in these subjects are lower postabsorptively than postprandially. For postabsorptive exercise, adjustment of the basal infusion rate will not usually be required, although for prolonged exercise it is probably prudent to reduce the basal rate by 30% to 50%. However, this has not been substantiated by detailed studies.

Multiple Daily Injection regimens regimens have fewer practical problems than insulin pumps. Diabetic subjects on CSII often have to remove their pumps before engaging in water sports and vigorous exercise, due to vulnerability of the subcutaneous infusion site to trauma and disruption. In these cases, SBGM and familiarity of the subjects with switching from CSII to multiple injection regimens are essential. For people engaged regularly in such kinds of physical activity, multiple injection regimens are probably advisable.

Type 2 Diabetes. Type 2 diabetes is characterized by insulin resistance and impaired insulin secretion. Fasting hyperinsulinemia is often present. Obesity, hyperlipidemia, and hypertension, all of which increase the risk for cardiovascular disease, are commonly associated with type 2 diabetes. As reviewed earlier, exercise has been shown to increase insulin sensitivity, reduce fasting hyperinsulinemia, and possibly improve insulin secretion. In contrast to type 1 diabetes, glycemic control has also been found to be improved by exercise. Increased energy expenditure by physical activity helps in weight-reducing, and hyperlipidemia and hypertension may also be ameliorated. There is some evidence that the risk for cardiovascular disease may be lessened by exercise through an indirect effect on risk factors and possibly also through direct effects on glycemic control. For all of these reasons, exercise training is being increasingly considered as part of the treatment of type 2 diabetes in association with diet regimens. Type 2 diabetic subjects on diet are not under risk of hypoglycemia, and in those diabetic subjects on sulphonylureas, the risk is minimal. This makes exercise programs easier for such subjects. In insulin-treated individuals with type 2 diabetes, however, exercise-induced hypoglycemia can occur. Clinically, the risk of hypoglycemia is often deemed to be less than in type 1 diabetes due to insulin resistance. However, despite the fact that insulin-treated type 2 diabetics make up the majority of diabetic subjects on insulin treatment, no studies have been carried out concerning the responses to acute exercise. These subjects are generally treated with standard insulin therapy, which may make normalization of the glycemic response to exercise quite difficult and increase the risk of hypoglycemia. At present, the same practical recommendations apply to these subjects as to type 1 subjects on conventional insulin treatment.

Individuals with type 2 diabetes under any type of treatment should not exercise when in poor metabolic control (glycemia >250 mg/dL). However, the most important risk is precipitating cardiovascular events related to unsuspected coronary heart disease. Therefore, subjects with type 2 diabetes should undergo a complete physical examination and stress electrocardiogram (ECG) testing before embarking on training programs. Furthermore, strenuous, anaerobic, isometric activities (i.e., weight lifting) are contraindicated in these subjects. Training programs should be gradual in onset in sedentary individuals. Aerobic, dynamic types of exercise, such as swimming, bicycling, and, for subjects free of peripheral neuropathy or known vascular disease, brisk walking, jogging, and running are ideal types of activity. Training sessions should be preceded and followed by 5–15 min warm-up or slow-down stretching or other gentle exercises. Expenditure of at least 500 calories/week by moderate activity exercise appears to be required to achieve any reduction in risk for coronary heart disease. An additional reduction in risk is provided by an expenditure up to 2,000 calories/week, but still further activity does not appear to provide any additional protection.[318] It is unknown how much exercise is required for the metabolic benefits. Such benefits have been shown after at least 6 weeks of exercise regimens, which increased VO_2 more than 10%. Presently, 20 to 40-min training sessions three to five times weekly are recommended.

Inasmuch as the majority of type 2 diabetic subjects are overweight, diet and exercise regimens are almost always instituted together. Exercise alone does not usually result in significant weight loss, and even its addition to a low-calorie regimen may not add significantly to the rate of weight loss. However, it will serve to improve insulin sensitivity, result in increased level of physical conditioning, and perhaps, limit the loss in lean body mass. Regular exercise has been associated with improvement in mood and relief of symptoms of depression, when present. A number of practical considerations enter into the prescription of exercise to obese persons with NIDDM. Since 80% of all persons with diabetes are in this category, it has enormous potential impact. Like with diet prescription, the assessment of the individual readiness to make durable behavioral changes is critical. Most patients will recognize the desirability to make changes, but when confronted with the challenge not only to eat fewer calories but also to perform unaccustomed physical activity, many will find the latter a deterrent to even start controlling eating behavior. Thus the strategy must be individualized and must often be approached stepwise, with eating behavior first and activity next. Emphasis needs to be placed on the overwhelming evidence that changes in eating and a consequent *small* decrease in weight can have substantial influence first on diabetes medication dose reduction, then eventual discontinuation, and the glycemic improvement that drives this. Several studies have confirmed that 3–8 kg weight reduction can induce marked improvement in glycemic control.

The concept of *activity* versus *exercise* needs then to be introduced to prevent discouragement at the mere concept of having to do what for many is daunting, even at the conditions mentioned two paragraphs earlier. Increase in *activity* is possible for almost all such patients, and this consists of walking, taking stairs rather than escalators, parking the car at the far end of the lot, and other such components of daily life that can be performed without a special exercise time. Those who succeed will be more willing to then take the next step. One *cannot overemphasize* the need for obese diabetic persons to enroll in programs that include persons like themselves. The mere act of enrolling in an *inappropriate* program will lead to premature discontinuation, either because of being physically overextended too early or because of explicit or implied competition with others who may be younger and leaner to begin with.

The reasons for including systemic activity/exercise in prescription for NIDDM therapy are not only for cardiovascular risk reduction and improvement of metabolic control, but also because those who both exercise and control diet are more likely to achieve sustained weight reduction. In addition to earlier studies on small cohorts (e.g., Refs. 344, 345), one recent study of a registry of almost 800 subjects who lost on average 30 kg and maintained a 13.6 kg loss for a mean duration of 5.5 years documented that 89% did so by combining decreased dietary intake with increased physical activity.[346] Only 10% used diet modification alone, whereas only 1% used modification of activity level only. This is to be contrasted with the more typical published work that tends to come from university centers and emphasizes recidivism, especially in persons with NIDDM. Although it was not reported how many of the registrants had type 2 diabetes, it seems reasonable to presume that the results are relevant to obese persons with NIDDM. The calculable savings in lessened comorbid factors in such successful maintainers both in direct and indirect costs, as well as sustained quality of life improvement, justifies that intensive efforts be made to encourage obese NIDDM patients to follow this route.

Diets under 400 calories have been associated with the risk of cardiac arrhythmias and sudden death,[347] suggesting that physical exercise may carry an increased risk under these conditions. Very low calorie (<800 calories), carbohydrate-restricted diets (<36%) result in impaired capacity for high-intensity exercise.[348] Otherwise, exercise programs are safe in subjects on caloric restriction.[349–351]

It should be indicated that in addition to endurance training, resistance training may provide physiologic benefits to the individual with diabetes that may equal or exceed those gained through aerobic training. These benefits include improved blood lipid profiles, increased absolute left ventricular wall contractility, decreased resting blood pressure, improved insulin sensitivity and glucose tolerance, improved glycemic control, improved muscular strength and endurance, and increased bone and connective tissue strength. The combination of aerobic and resistance training is a more comprehensive exercise that also increases the number of exercise modalities.[225]

Exercise and Its Risks in Subjects with Complications of Diabetes. All potential risks can be attenuated in frequency and severity by *gradual* introduction of *activity* (such as walking or climbing stairs) followed by structured *exercise* programs. If the exercise program is directed by a qualified professional, it need not necessarily be preceded by an unsupervised increase in activity. Both the physician and the health professional involved must be sensitive to this issue and must recommend a return to a level of activity/exercise below that which induces symptoms, then progress slowly only if clearly safe. It is interesting that in older persons and postmenopausal females, bone mass may be maintained better in active persons, thus *protecting* them to a certain extent from bone injury. This is important because the musculoskeletal system is at greatest risk of complications of exercise. There are no data to indicate whether persons with diabetes who do *not* have complications or concurrent musculoskeletal disorders are at a *greater* risk of injury from exercise. The frequency of exercise-related injuries is highest in the lower limb involving foot, knee, and hip. In the presence of preexisting arthritis in these joints, consultation with a rheumatologist or orthopedic surgeon may be indicated prior to starting exercise programs. Although the prevalence of osteoarthritis of weight-bearing joints is not increased in obesity per se, when present it tends to be more severe. This can be limiting in terms of the effectiveness of an activity/exercise program. Nonetheless, most persons can engage in at least some forms of increased activity or special exercises to strengthen the muscles around the affected joints. This has benefits directly for the arthritis and indirectly as it may enable greater mobility.

Exercise is clearly associated with some risk in both type 1 and type 2 patients with diabetic complications. In subjects with underlying coronary heart disease, exercise may precipitate angina pectoris, myocardial infarction, cardiac arrhythmias, or sudden death. Diabetic subjects with coronary heart disease are often asymptomatic, so that screening prior to exercise prescription is essential. As for all cardiac subjects, exercise is absolutely contraindicated in the 6 weeks postinfarct period and in the presence of heart failure or unstable or intractable angina. Currently, however, in stable coronary heart disease, increased rather than decreased physical activity is recommended for secondary prevention. Judicious and supervised exercise training programs are also included in postinfarct rehabilitation. The benefit seems to be related to improved work tolerance with consequently reduced sympathetic activity. No studies on physical activity in diabetic subjects with coronary heart disease are available. However, since in these subjects cardiac damage is generally more extensive than in nondiabetic subjects and small vessel disease and cardiomyopathy may be present, more caution than in nondiabetics is probably advised.

Peripheral vascular disease is often more extensive than in otherwise comparable persons, but is asymptomatic in diabetic subjects until ischemic lesions occur. Exercise that may traumatize the foot (e.g., jogging, running) is contraindicated in subjects with peripheral vascular disease because healing of traumatic lesions is impaired. When other kinds of exercise can be performed, increased rather than decreased physical activity is advised. In subjects with transient ischemic attacks (TIA) blood perfusion may be jeopardized in ischemic areas by the lowering of systemic vascular resistance that occurs during exercise. Appropriate footwear can allow persons with mild to moderate neuropathy to perform activity beyond walking as long as the feet are inspected after each session and all routine aspects of diabetic footwear are respected. Activity, and perhaps even supervised exercise by experts, may even improve effort tolerance and symptoms in persons with leg claudication.

Subjects with peripheral neuropathy should avoid pounding movements of the lower extremities, such as jogging and running, which may cause soft tissue and bone injury of the insensitive foot.

Exercise is also contraindicated in proliferative retinopathy because it is associated with increased risk for developing retinal or vitreous hemorrhages and retinal detachment. High-intensity exercise, such as isometric weight lifting, head down positions, and jarring of the head, are particularly dangerous. Exercise tolerance is reduced in autonomic neuropathy and the response to dehydration is reduced. On the other hand, metabolic responses such as the fall in glycemia and the increase in lactate levels are similar to normal or type 1 diabetes without autonomic neuropathy, but the counterregulatory hormone responses (catecholamines, cortisol and growth hormones) are impaired.[201] When cardiovascular symptoms are present (e.g., orthostatic hypotension), exercise is best avoided for the risk of syncope and cardiac arrhythmia. Diabetic nephropathy per se does not contraindicate exercise. Proteinuria may be aggravated by vigorous exercise,[202,203] which results in decreased renal perfusion. However, it is unlikely that exercise interferes with the course of the disease. Fluid and electrolyte imbalance contraindicate exercise, which is poorly tolerated in chronic renal failure. In addition, proliferative retinopathy is usually present.

Problem Statement and Research Directions

This section summarizes data that have been described in detail in the preceding sections and therefore reference will not be made again to original contributions of various research groups. There has been considerable progress in analyzing the effects of various metabolic hormones on glucoregulation and fat metabolism during moderate exercise. Combination of tracer methodology with balance techniques across the liver, kidney, and leg provided valuable data, and it was also possible to quantify the rates of gluconeogenesis and glycogenolysis across the liver. A major advance in tracer technique was to adjust the tracer infusion rate to minimize fluctuations of specific activity. This new technique yields much more reliable data of glucose turnover. There has been considerable advance in characterizing the metabolic responses to strenuous exercise. It was concluded that the main regulators of hepatic glucose production are the changes of glucagon and insulin, whereas in strenuous exercise it seems that the catecholamines take over. However, it is not established whether the increment of glucose production in strenuous exercise can be attenuated by combined α- and β-blockade. It is possible that there are other regulators (perhaps back-up systems) that safeguard against attenuation of glucose production during strenuous exercise. Application of techniques of NMR has yielded new insights into the regulation of glycogenolysis and gluconeogenesis in the liver and metabolic events in the muscle.

In the last decade, there has been a major advance in our knowledge of how insulin regulates glucose uptake in muscle and fat cells. Clearly, the effect of insulin and of muscular contraction yields different signaling cascades, and this is why the effects of insulin and exercise can be synergistic. Presently, a very important task is to unravel the signaling cascades initiated by muscle contraction. Deficient glucose uptake results from insulin resistance. The question is what is defective and what are the differences in insulin- and exercise-induced signaling.

It is remarkable that the liver, under normal conditions, can precisely match the increased fuel needs of the muscle during moderate exercise. Further research is needed to determine whether there are functional signals transmitted from the muscle to the liver and vice versa and what is the role of the nervous system in this coordination.

Methods to assess lactate turnover and its relationship to glucose, FFA, and turnover of amino acids still need to be developed.

There have been large, epidemiologic studies delineating the importance of exercise in treatment and prevention of diabetes. Although there has been considerable evidence for the importance of physical training and fitness both in treatment of both types of diabetes and prevention of type 2, it is still not possible to generalize because epidemiologic studies frequently target selective groups of people.

Prescribing and Planning the Exercise

Guidelines for Activity Behavior Modification. In making the distinction between activity and exercise, a number of issues are important. In general, the type 1 diabetic patient without complications, being younger, generally lean, and in a better state of fitness than the typical type 2 patient, should engage in regular, programmed exercise as described herein. If the patient is neither fit nor sufficiently motivated to enter such a program directly, then starting with increases in daily life activities may be the appropriate way to initiate such changes, as in type 2 patients. Secondly, from the point of view of weight and glycemic control, eating correctly has quantitatively much greater effects and should receive greater emphasis in new patients and those in need of improved control. Third, if the obese type 2 patient is *required* to make changes to eating *and* activity patterns that are beyond her or his current state of motivation, neither will be addressed. Fourth, in the case of both eating and activity behaviors, changes should be encouraged to be stepwise. Approaches such as those promoted in formal behavior modification programs for both the stages of weight control and maintenance have considerable merit (e.g., that of Brownell[352]). (See Chapters 15 and 16).

Approaches to increase activity may include the following suggestions. To increase walking, clearly it is desirable to find an *extra* time during the day and week when one does this as a specific activity: the evening after supper, weekend mornings, etc. If this is not possible (or is resisted), then the suggestions of getting off public transit one stop before destinations may be accepted and can be done on regular daily trips, e.g., to and from work, as well as others. It can be escalated, if feasible, to two stops and more. A similar approach applies to replacing escalators and elevators progressively by stairs. If one works or lives in an upper floor of a tall building, one can get off the first week one floor below the destination, the next week two floors below, and progress accordingly. One should park as far away from the destination in the parking lot as feasible. (The argument can be made that this will actually *save* time, since everyone else is circulating *near* the door of the shopping center and it takes longer to find a spot there.) If one has a job in which there are materials to be delivered to different persons or locations within the workplace, deliver each item individually rather than collecting several and making one trip. Needless to say, the stairs should be taken as much as possible. Break and lunch times at work should be used

as opportunities to walk (and shorten the eating/sitting times concurrently).

In most patients' routines there can be ways like these that can be adapted to each individual. Positive feedback for *any* such changes on the part of the supervisory health professionals is an exceedingly important part of reinforcing these behavioral changes.

Problem　　What guidelines should the primary physician follow when giving an exercise prescription for an individual with type 2 or with type 1 diabetes?

1. *Subjective:* Is the patient less than or more than 35 years of age? Is she or he already physically active (regular exercise) or physically sedentary (little, erratic, or no exercise)? If the individual is more than 35 years of age, is there any history of CVD or pulmonary, neurologic, or joint disease? Does the individual have type 2 or type 1 diabetes? Is weight acceptable or excessive? What is the level of metabolic control? Are there any chronic complications of diabetes (retinopathy, nephropathy, neuropathy, or vascular disease)?

2. *Objective:* Complete physical examination, laboratory studies.

3. *Assessment:* If an individual is asymptomatic, less than 35 years of age, has no subjective or objective findings or risk factors for CVD (myocardial infarction [MI], arrhythmia, congestive heart failure, ECG abnormalities, hypertension, hyperlipidemia, cigarette smoking, intermittent claudication, TIAs with or without neurologic findings on physical examination, autonomic or peripheral neuropathy, diabetic nephropathy, or diabetic retinopathy), no *medical clearance* is necessary before the *physician* gives a prescription to increase the level of physical activity.

All others should have a *complete medical evaluation* and exercise stress test prior to a significant increase in the physical activity level.[353,354] A complete report of the exercise stress test must include all of the following: (1) heart (pulse) rate and blood pressure preexercise (every minute for 9 min); (2) energy cost of the maximum work load (exercise level) achieved; (3) symptoms and the test stage at which they appeared; (4) ECG abnormalities noted at any stage; (5) reason for termination of the test; target achieved (at least 90% of age-predicted pulse rate, with maximum predicted being $220 -$ age in years, e.g., $220 - 60$ years $= 160 \times 90\% = 144$ heartbeat/min; volitional exhaustion; symptoms; ECG abnormalities; and interpretation of the stress test as positive or negative for cardiac ischemia).

Initial Plan　　The energy costs of exercise during the stress test may be quantified in a number of ways: (1) the cost in "calories" (Kcalories) or in kilojoules in SI units (1 Kcal $= 4.189$ kjoules); (2) the oxygen cost in liters/min; (3) the oxygen cost in mL/kg/min.[354]

The oxygen cost of each exercise level may be represented as multiples of the cost of sitting at rest, designated as metabolic equivalents (METs). One MET (sitting at rest) equals about 3.5 mL oxygen consumed/kg body weight/min (about 1.6 mL/pound/min). Multiples of this value are used to represent the energy (calorie or oxygen) cost of higher levels of work. For example, oxygen consumption of 35 mL/kg/min equals 10 METs.[353–355]) The energy cost of treadmill work varies with body size, and MET values reflect the energy cost/unit of body size. Thus, the treadmill work will be the same for all body weights. For example, walking 3 miles/hr up a 5% grade will cost the 100 kg person about 1,890 mL/min but will cost the 50 kg person only 945 mL/min. The rate in mL/kg/min will be the same in both individuals (18.9 mL/kg/min, or 5.4 METs).

If the stress test is performed by cycle ergometry, the work rate is measured as kilopond meters/min (kPM/min) or in watts (joules/min). Cycle ergometry involves external work only (moving the wheel a given distance against a resistance load over time) and does not involve moving the whole body. Thus, the relative energy cost (METs) must be corrected for body size. For example, the absolute oxygen cost of bicycle work at 300 kPM/min is approximately 900 mL (600 mL to do the external work plus the 300 mL due to sitting). Thus, the oxygen cost is 18 mL/kg/min (or 5.1 METs) for the 50 kg person, but only 9 mL/kg/min (2.6 METs) for the 100 kg person.

A comparison of the heart rate response plotted against the cost in METs of graded exercise (rest, average intensity, peak intensity) as shown in Fig. 17–20,[353] and the approximate cost of various physical activities is shown in Exhibit 17–1.[354]

The Exercise Prescription   Four factors should be considered: type, frequency, duration, and intensity of exercise that is appropriate for the individual. Program characteristics for preventive, interventive, and cardiac rehabilitation exercise programs are outlined in Exhibit 17–2.[354] Since there is no risk of hypoglycemia in those with ty<pe 2 diabetes who are not being treated with insulin or a sulfonylurea, an interventive exercise program can be initiated if metabolic control is adequate (plasma glucose consistently less than 200 mg/dL, 11 mmol/L, fasting) and provided there are no contraindications to such a program. Since there is always risk of hypoglycemia in those who are being treated with insulin and there is always risk of intensifying hyperglycemia (and perhaps inducing diabetic ketoacidosis) in those whose metabolic control is unsatisfactory, the insulin administration routine (see Chapter 18) and food intake routine (see Chapters 15 and 16) should be carefully adjusted to the prescribed exercise routine to minimize the risks of hypoglycemia and of significant hyperglycemia.

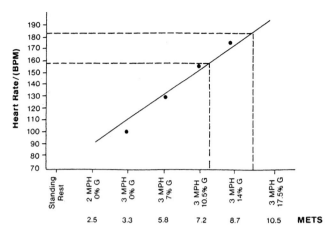

Figure 17–20. Heart rate response in beats per minute (BPM) plotted against the MET costs of a treadmill exercise stress test. Functional capacity = 10.5 METs. Average intensity = 7.4 METs, heart rate = 158 BPM, peak intensity = 9.5 METs, heart rate 182 BPM. (*Source:* Paolone AM: Prescribing exercise programs. *In* Bore AA, Lowenthal DT (eds): Exercise Medicine: Physiologica Principles and Clinical Application. New York: Academic Press, 1993, pp 361–381. With permission.)

The type of exercise recommended would depend on the age, health status (symptoms and risk factors), current state of physical conditioning, functional capacity (as determined by the stress test), and physical activity interests and skills of the individual.

The intensity of the exercise (prescribed METs) should be controlled by the heart rate response to the prescribed work level of the activity.

The frequency of the exercise (prescribed times for exercising) is important in those with diabetes. Exercise shortly after each of the three meals, 7 days/week is ideal in terms of minimizing hypoglycemia in insulin-treated patients (less likely to occur immediately after food intake) and hyperglycemia (more likely to occur after food intake). Such regularity facilitates standardizing insulin doses and diet that otherwise have to be changed for the nonexercising days. On the other hand, it is a minority of patients who can actually achieve this, for practical reasons. In those with tipe 2 diabetes who are being treated with diet and exercise therapy alone, exercise sessions should be scheduled at least four times/week, more frequently if possible.[356,357]

The duration of exercise sessions may vary from 30 to 38 min, with warm-up (stretching and rhythmic large muscle group isotonic activities) occupying 5–8 min, training (elevate the heart rate to the desired training level) occupying 20 min, and cool-down (tapering-off period to allow body systems to return to the preexercise state) occupying 5–10 min.[354–357]

Absolute contraindications to a training exercise program include: (1) proliferative retinopathy: avoid high-intensity exercises such as isometrics, weight lifting, and

EXHIBIT 17–1 Approximate Metabolic Cost of Activities[a]

Metabolic Equivalents (Mets)	Occupational	Recreational
1.5 to 2 METS[b] 4 to 7 mL O_2/min/kg 2 to 2.5 cal[d]/min (70 kg person)	Desk work Automobile driving[c] Typing Operating electric calculating machine	Standing Walking (strolling 1.6 km/hr or 1 mile/hr) Flying airplane, motorcycling[c] Playing cards[c] Sewing, knitting
2 to 3 METS 7 to 11 mL O_2/min/kg 2.5 to 4 cal[d]/min (70 kg person)	Auto repair Radio, television repair Janitorial work Typing, manual Bartending	Level walking (3.2 km/hr or 2 miles/hr) Level bicycling (8.0 km/hr or 5 miles/hr) Riding lawn mower Billiards, bowling Skeet,[c] shuffleboard Woodworking (light) Powerboat driving[c] Golf (power cart) Canoeing (4 km/hr or 2.5 miles/hr) Horseback riding (walk) Playing piano and many musical instruments
3 to 4 METS 11 to 14 mL O_2/min/kg 4 to 5 cal[d]/min (70 kg person)	Bricklaying, plastering Pushing wheelbarrow (45.4 kg or 100 pound load) Machine assembly Trailer-truck traffic Welding (moderate load) Cleaning windows	Walking (4.8 km/hr or 3 miles/hr) Cycling (9.7 km/hr or 6 miles/hr) Horseshoe pitching Volleyball (6-person noncompetitive) Golf (pulling bag cart) Archery Sailing (handling small boat) Fly fishing (standing with waders) Horseback (sitting to trot) Badminton (social doubles) Pushing light power mower Playing musical instrument energetically
4 to 5 METS 14 to 18 mL O_2/min/kg 5 to 6 cal[d]/min (70 kg person)	Painting, masonry Paperhanging Light carpentry	Walking (5.6 km/hr or 3.5 miles/hr) Bicycling (12.9 km/hr or 8 miles/hr) Table tennis Golf (carrying clubs) Dancing (fox-trot) Badminton (singles) Tennis (doubles) Raking leaves Hoeing Many calisthenics
5 to 6 METS 18 to 21 mL O_2/min/kg 6 to 7 cal[d] (70 kg person)	Digging garden Shoveling light earth	Walking (6.4 km/hr or 4 miles/hr) Cycling (16.1 km/hr or 10 miles/hr) Canoeing (6.4 km/hr or 4 miles/hr) Horseback riding ("posting" to trot) Stream fishing (walking in light current in waders) Ice or roller skating (14.5 km/hr or 9 miles/hr)
6 to 7 METS 21 to 25 mL O_2/min/kg 7 to 8 cal[d]/min (70 kg person)	Shoveling 10/min (4.5 kg or 10 pounds)	Walking (8.0 km/hr or 5 miles/hr) Cycling (17.7 km/hr or 11 miles/hr) Badminton (competitive) Tennis (singles) Splitting wood Snow shoveling Hand lawn mowing Folk (square) dancing Light downhill skiing Ski touring (4.0 km/hr or 2.5 miles/hr) (loose snow) Water skiing

(continued)

EXHIBIT 17–1 (continued) Approximate Metabolic Cost of Activities

Metabolic Equivalents (Mets)	Occupational	Recreational
7 to 8 METS 25 to 28 mL O_2/min/kg 8 to 10 cal[d]/min (70 kg person)	Digging ditches Carrying 36.3 kg or 80 pounds Sawing hardwood	Jogging (8.0 km/hr or 5 miles/hr) Bicycling (19.3 km/hr or 12 miles/hr) Horseback (gallop) Vigorous downhill skiing Basketball Mountain climbing Ice hockey Canoeing (8.0 km/hr or 5 miles/hr) Touch football Paddleball
8 to 9 METS 28 to 32 mL O_2/min/kg 10 to 11 cal[d]/min (70 kg person)	Shoveling 10/min (6.4 kg or 14 pounds)	Running (8.9 km/hr or 5.5 miles/hr) Bicycling (20.9 km/hr or 13 miles/hr) Ski touring (6.4 km/hr or 4 miles/hr) (loose snow) Squash racquets (social) Handball (social) Fencing Basketball (vigorous)
10 + METS 32 plus mL O_2/min/kg 11 + cal[d]/min (70 kg person)	Shoveling 10/min (7.3 kg or 16 pounds)	Running 6 mph = 10 METS 7 mph = 11.5 METS 8 mph = 13.5 METS 9 mph = 15 METS

[a] Reprinted from Fox SM, Naughton JP, and Gorman PA: Physical activity and cardiovascular health. III. The exercise prescription; frequency and and type of activity. Mod Concepts Cardiovasc Dis 41:6, 1972. Includes resting metabolic needs.

[b] 1 MET is the energy expenditure at rest, equivalent to approximately 3.5 ml O_2/kg body weight/min.

[c] A major excess metabolic increase may occur due to excitement, anxiety, or impatience in some of these activities, and a physician must assess his patient's psychologic reactivity.

[d] A calorie is defined in this book as the energy equivalent of a kilocalorie.

[Source: Paolone AM: Prescribing exercise programs. In Bove AA, Lowenthal DT (eds): Exercise Medicine: Physiological Principles and Clinical Applications. New York: Academic Press, 1983, pp 361–381. With permission.]

so on, head-low positions, and excessive jarring of the head; (2) MI in last 6 weeks, congestive heart failure, unstable or intractable angina, severe intermittent claudication, TIAs with symptoms and signs; (3) autonomic neuropathy with symptomatic postural hypotension, peripheral neuropathy with insensitive feet that are easily traumatized (including stress fractures) by running (cycling and swimming are better).

Relative contraindications to a formal training exercise program include: (1) diabetic nephropathy with renal failure; (2) poor metabolic control (individuals with type 2 and type 1 diabetes who have persistently elevated plasma glucose levels); (3) individuals on insulin or sulfonylurea therapy are always at risk of developing hypoglycemia, especially if they are on high-dose salicylate therapy, β-adrenergic blocking agents, phenylbutazone, sulfonamides, monoamine oxidase inhibitors, or dicumarol.

For those on either insulin or sulfonylureas, care should be taken to avoid hypoglycemia by scheduling the activity immediately after meals or after a supplementary carbohydrate-containing snack and by carrying a readily absorbable form of carbohydrate to consume during exercise to prevent hypoglycemia or on stopping the exercise, should hypoglycemia occur.

Three Examples of Exercise Program Prescriptions. An exercise program prescribed for a 35-year-old man who has IDDM of 8 years duration but who has no complications and is at acceptable body weight and is under good control on home blood glucose monitoring (mean fasting blood glucose level 108 mg/dL, 6 mmol/L, Hb A_{1c} 7.1%, mean postprandial blood glucose 154 mg/dL, 8.6 mmol/L), on 20 U (units) NPH (Neutral Protamine Hagedorn), and 6 U regular insulin at 8:00 A.M. and 8 U NPH insulin at 8:00 P.M.) is shown in Exhibit 17–3.

An exercise program prescribed for a 45-year-old man whose weight is 220 pounds (100 kg) and body mass index (BMI) is 28.5 kg/m², who had no complications after 4 years of type 2 diabetes and who was under good control on diet therapy alone (mean postprandial blood glucose 148 mg/dL, 8.2 mmol/L, Hb A_{1c} 7.4%), is shown in Exhibit 17–4.

An exercise program prescribed for a 55-year-old man whose weight is 167 pounds (76 kg) and BMI is

EXHIBIT 17–2   Preventive, Interventive, and Cardiac Rehabilitation Exercise Programs

Preventive Exercise Program

1. For asymptomatic, clinically normal adults with no significant risk factors
2. Can be relatively unstructured and utilize a wide variety of activities, including recreational sports and games
3. Can be individually undertaken and relatively unsupervised.
4. Reevaluation and assessment can be infrequent
5. Can have a greater cosmetic emphasis and include resistive exercise, isometrics, and other muscle toning activities
6. Conducted by community recreation agencies, YMCAs, YMHAs, health spas, company recreation personnel.

Interventive Exercise Program

1. Serves asymptomatic persons with significant risk factors for coronary heart disease (no one with documented coronary heart disease or positive stress test)
2. Must be structured to provide for strict control of work intensity
3. Must be designed for individual limitations and modifications of risk factors such as obesity, high blood pressure, diabetes, smoking, emotional stress
4. Sessions should be supervised at least in the early phase
5. Participants must be trained in monitoring techniques
6. Less emphasis on cosmetic effects
7. Frequent assessment and reevaluation
8. Participants should be under a physician's care

9. Detailed emergency procedures must be defined and rehearsed
10. Conducted by hospitals, commercial rehabilitation clinics, YMCA groups, health spas with specially trained personnel, college and university physical education departments, certain companies for employees

Cardiac Rehabilitation Program

1. Serves postmyocardial infarction, documented coronary heart disease, symptomatic angina pectoris, and postcoronary bypass surgery patients, and patients with positive stress tests
2. Must be structured to provide strict control of work intensity, which is checked frequently and in some cases monitored continuously
3. All sessions supervised by trained exercise leaders and medical personnel are present on site
4. Frequent assessment and reevaluation
5. Patients must be referred by a physician
6. Exercise prescription reviewed and endorsed by a physician
7. Competition should be avoided
8. Emergency equipment must be on site and detailed procedures must be defined and rehearsed
9. Conducted by hospitals, commercial rehabilitation clinics, YMCA groups, health spas with specially trained personnel, college and university physical education departments

(*Source*: Paolone AM: Prescribing exercise programs: *In* Bove AA, Lowenthal DT (eds): Exercise Medicine: Physiological Principles and Clinical Applications. New York: Academic Press, 1983, pp. 361–381. With permission.)

26 kg/m^2, with a history of type 2 diabetes for 2 years, under good control on diet therapy alone (mean postprandial blood glucose 142 mg/dL, 7.9 mmol/L, Hb A$_{1c}$ 6.7%), who had a family history of coronary heart disease, an abnormal treadmill exercise stress test (test terminated because of dyspnea and ECG evidence of ischemia manifested by premature ventricular contractions and ST-segment depression), and a coronary angiogram revealing single vessel coronary disease, is shown in Exhibit 17–5.

Follow-up Plan.   The initial exercise prescription should be adjusted to the progress of the individual's program during follow-up and to the objectives that have been set for the program, as illustrated in Exhibits 17–3 to 17–5.

Stress

Introduction

All stress situations are characterized by increased activity of all counterregulatory hormones, such as epinephrine, norepinephrine, glucagon, adrenocorti-

cotropin (ACTH), and cortisol. There may also be multiple insults to the individual such as infection supervening upon injury. Pain and anxiety can also contribute to hormonal and metabolic derangements. In the case of severe injury involving shock—hypovolemic, cardiac, or endotoxic—the survival of the individual may ultimately depend upon the ability of the glucoregulatory system to increase arterial glucose concentrations to compensate for decreased blood flow to the brain and to provide substrate for wound healing.

Recognition of the importance of neuropeptides in regulating stress responses is well established. It is interesting that corticotrophin-releasing hormone (CRH) can stimulate not only ACTH, but also epinephrine and norepinephrine release.[358–361] This would imply that CRH can control the autonomic nervous system and adrenomedullary secretion, as well as adrenocorticol responses to stress.[362,363] Vasopressin could have a similar function to CRH, thus generating a supporting regulatory system during stress. CRH-induced hyperglycemia, secondary to the multiple hormonal and neural responses, could provide glucose for the brain under conditions of stress. With respect to glucoregulation, it is interesting that insulin secretion in

EXHIBIT 17–3 Exercise Prescription for a 35-Year-Old Man with type 1 diabetes of 8 Years' Duration, with No Complications, at Ideal Body Weight, Under Satisfactory Metabolic Control

Treadmill Exercise Stress Test					
Treadmill Speed/Grade	Mets	Heart Rate (Beats/min)	Blood Pressure (mmHg)	Symptoms	ECG
Standing, at rest	1 (estimated)	80	126/78	None	Normal
2 mph/0% grade	2.5	90	120/80	None	No change
3 mph/0% grade	3.3	100	120/80	None	No change
3 mph/7% grade	5.8	130	140/70	None	No change
3 mph/10.5% grade	7.2	155	160/65	None	No change
3 mph/14.0% grade	8.7	175	180/60	None	No change
3 mph/17.5% grade	10.5	190	200/60	Volitional exhaustion	No change

Test was terminated because of volitional exhaustion.
Functional capacity = 10.5 METS at a heart rate of 190 beats/min
ECG negative for ischemia.

Exercise Prescription

Intensity
Peak   = 9.5 METS, heart rate 182 beats/min
Average = 7.4 METS, heart rate 158 beats/min
The prescribed intensity was calculated as follows:
Peak   = 90% of functional capacity (0.90 of 10.5
    METS = 9.5 METS)
Heart rate corresponding to 9.5 METS is calculated by
    interpolation between the rates of 8.7 METS and 10.5
    METS using the following formula:
$$\frac{9.5 - 8.7}{10.5 - 8.7} = 0.44$$
    $0.44 (190 - 175) = 7 + 175 = 182$
Average = 70% of functional capacity (0.70 × 10.5
    METS = 7.41 METS)
Heart rate corresponding to 7.4 METS is calculated as
    follows:
$$\frac{7.4 - 7.2}{8.7 - 7.2} = 0.13$$
    $0.13 (175 - 155) = 3 + 155 = 158$

Duration (training stimulus phase only)
    15 to 30 min
Frequency
    7 days/week, immediately after a meal
Type
    Isotonic rhythmic large muscle group activities such as
        fast walking (120 steps/min), jogging, running,
        stationary cycling, outdoor cycling, and so forth
    Work late: jogging 5 miles/hr, cycling 600 KPM/min,
        outdoor cycling 12 miles/hr
Follow-up progression
    After 4 to 6 weeks of uneventful activity, recreational
        games may be incorporated, e.g., singles tennis,
        soccer, basketball, and so on. The MET cost of the
        work should be increased to maintain average initial
        heart rate.
Objective
    To increase functional capacity

stress can be inhibited, enhanced, or unchanged. When it is inhibited it provides increased FFA to tissues that use them, further sparing glucose. This enhances the glucose supply from the central nervous system and other obligatory glycolytic tissues.

To gain understanding of hormonal interactions in glucoregulation under conditions of stress, several experimental stress models have been used:

(1) *Pyrogen* induces fever and stress hormones are released.[364]

(2) *Hypoglycemia* provides a model for moderate to severe stress. Both glucagon and the catecholamines play a major role in the recovery from hypo-glycemia.[19,365-375] The relative importance of these hormones relates to the rapidity of the fall in plasma glucose and the degree and duration of hypoglycemia. Also, insulin levels during hypoglycemia can affect pancreatic hormone release and the sensitivity of the liver to the their effects. When phlorizin infusion was used to decrease plasma glucose without hyperinsulinemia, there was a small decrease in plasma glucose followed by a rise in glucose production (Ra), which was mediated by an increase in plasma glucagon. The decrease in plasma insulin that accompanied the drop in plasma glucose increased hepatic sensitivity to glucagon. On the other hand, during insulin–induced hypoglycemia,[369] plasma glucose fell precipitously and profoundly, and although glucagon rose together with Ra, the importance of the catecholamines became apparent. ACTH, cortisol, and β-endorphin are also released in response to the hypoglycemia.[376,377] It is interesting that naloxone (opiate antagonist), injected into a peripheral vein, accelerated the release of epinephrine, glucagon, β-endorphin, ACTH, and cortisol.[376] The greater compensatory increase in glucose production lessened the hypoglycemic excursion. In contrast, when naloxone was given centrally (into the third ventricle of the brain), during insulin infusion[377]

EXHIBIT 17–4 Exercise Prescription for a 45-Year-Old Man with type 2 diabetes of 4 Years Duration, No Complications, 122% of Ideal Body Weight, Under Satisfactory Metabolic Control

Treadmill Speed/Grade	Mets	Heart Rate (Beats/min)	Blood Pressure (mmHg)	Symptoms	ECG
Standing, at rest	1 (estimated)	88	160/90	None	Normal
2 mph/0% grade	2.5	95	160/90	None	Normal
3 mph/2.5% grade	4.3	110	165/96	None	Normal
3 mph/5% grade	5.4	135	180/100	None	Normal
3 mph/7.5% grade	6.4	155	250/110	None	0.05 mV ST-segment depression

Treadmill Exercise Stress Test

Test was terminated because of systolic blood pressure 250 mmHg
Functional capacity = 6.4 METS at a heart rate of 155 beats/min
ECG negative for ischemia.

Exercise Prescription

Intensity Peak = 5.8 METS, heart rate 143 beats/min
 Average = 4.2 METS, heart rate 109 beats/min
 (See Exhibit 17–3 for formulas that were used to calculate the prescribed peak and average intensity.)
Duration
 30 to 45 min
Frequency
 5 to 7 days/week
Type
 Rhythmic large muscle group activities, preferably controlled on treadmill or cycle ergometer
 Work rate: 3 mph/2.5% grade on treadmill, 600 kPM/min on cycle ergometer

Follow-up progression
 After 4 to 6 weeks of uneventful activity, the duration should be increased to maintain the initial average training heart rate.
Objectives
 1. To increase caloric expenditure for weight reduction
 2. To increase functional capacity
 3. To reduce resting blood pressure
 4. To reduce plasma glucose and hemoglobin A_{1c} levels, and possibly to return the response to a glucose load (glucose tolerance test) to normal

the increase in glucagon and cortisol was unaffected, but catecholamine release was diminished.

In addition to stimulating release of counterregulatory hormones, hypoglycemia induces other responses that increase Ra, such as hepatic autoregulation,[378,379] a change in the autonomic nervous system inputs to the liver,[380,381] and increased hepatic sensitivity to counterregulatory hormones.[382] The role of the brain in regulating counterregulatory responses has been studied in great detail.[383] More recently, Bergman et al. discovered a specific sensor for hypoglycemia in the portal vein. It appears that the glycemic threshold for the portal receptor is 3.6 mM, identical to the glucose level for counterregulatory response; the threshold for the central receptor is 3.1 mM, identical to the value of glucose where behavioral responses are detected (sweating, nervousness, etc.). They argued that the portal vein glucose sensor with a higher receptor threshold can protect the brain from hypoglycemic awareness and behavioral changes.[384,385]

(3) *Epinephrine* infusion simulates some of the hormonal changes that occur in response to stress, and has been used to provide a partial model of moderate to severe stress.[386] As described in the previous section, it appears that in the liver, β and α effects can represent back-up additive systems to increase hepatic glucose production. In contrast, β and α effects are antagonistic in control of peripheral glucose utilization. Epinephrine infusion transiently increases plasma glucagon (IRG) and insulin (IRI) in normal dogs. However, epinephrine's effect on hepatic glucose production is independent of glucagon release. This was demonstrated by concomitant epinephrine and somatostatin infusions that suppressed plasma glucagon but did not attenuate insulin release.[387] This was also demonstrated in man.[385,388] The combined infusion of epinephrine, glucagon, and cortisol increases Ra to a greater extent than the additive effect of the individual hormones, suggesting a synergism among the stress-related hormones.[389,390]

Many stress situations involve repeated insults, for example, infection supervening upon trauma, therefore repeated epinephrine infusions have been used as a model by which to study responses to multiple stresses.[391] Although there were equivalent increases in plasma glucagon and hepatic glucose production in response to two successive epinephrine infusions, there was a diminished insulin response and a much greater decrease in glucose MCR in response to the second epinephrine infusion, which was associated

EXHIBIT 17–5   Exercise Prescription for a 55-Year-Old Man with type 2 diabetes of 2 Years' Duration, Evidence of Coronary Artery Disease, 112% of Ideal Body Weight, Under Satisfactory Metabolic Control

Treadmill Exercise Stress Test					
Treadmill Speed/Grade	Mets	Heart Rate (Beats/min)	Blood Pressure (mmHg)	Symptoms	ECG
Standing, at rest	1 (estimated)	75	140/100	None	Normal
2 mph/0% grade	2.5	80	135/90	None	Normal
3 mph/0% grade	3.3	88	135/90	None	Normal
3 mph/7% grade	5.8	120	140/90	Slight dyspnea	0.1 mV ST-segment depression
3 mph/10.5% grade	7.2	150	185/100	Severe dyspnea	0.15 mV, ST-segment depression, PVCs

Test was terminated because of dyspnea and PVCs.
Functional capacity = 7.2 METS at a heart rate of 150 beats/min.
ECG positive for ischemia. Follow-up coronary angiogram revealed single-vessel disease.

Exercise Prescription

Intensity
  Peak   = 6.5 METS, heart rate 135 beats/min
  Average = 4.8 METS, heart rate 107 beats/min
  (See Exhibit 17–3 for formulas that were used to calculate
    the prescribed peak and average intensity.)
Duration
  15 to 20 min
Frequency
  Four to five times per week
Type
  Rhythmic large muscle group activities, controlled on
    treadmill or cycle ergometer
  Work rate: walking on treadmill at 3.5 mph 2.5% grade,
    or 450 kPM/min on a cycle ergometer

Follow-up progression
  After 4 to 6 weeks of uneventful activity, the duration
    should be increased to 25 to 35 min and the work rate
    increased to maintain the initial average training heart
    rate.
Objectives
  1. To increase functional capacity so that a greater
     work capacity will be achieved before symptoms
     appear
  2. To increase caloric expenditure for weight reduction
  3. To reduce resting blood pressure
  4. To reduce plasma glucose and hemoglobin A_{1c} levels,
     and possibly to return the response to a glucose load
     (glucose tolerance test) to normal

Abbreviations: PVC, premature ventricular contractions, others as in text.

---

with exaggerated hyperglycemia. This indicates that the stress regulatory systems may have a "memory" that sensitizes and augments the responses.

(4) *Intracerebroventricular (ICV) injection of substances* such as neuropeptides, hormones and neurotransmitters such as carbachol, an acetylcholine analogue has given rise to hormonal and metabolic responses similar to those seen in clinical stress states (Fig. 17–21). This has provided a very useful experimental stress model. Brain or gut peptides that have shown hyperglycemic effects when injected ICV include CRH, β-endorphin, neurotensin, thyrotropin-releasing hormone, bombesin, gastrin-releasing peptide, growth hormone-releasing factor, glucagon, angiotensin II, substance P, and cholecystokinin.[392] For example, in the rat ICV injection of CRH resulted in increased plasma concentrations of ACTH, epinephrine, norepinephrine, and glucagon[362,363] with resultant hyperglycemia. Neither hypophysectomy nor adrenalectomy prevented this CRH-induced hyperglycemia. Pretreatment with the ganglionic

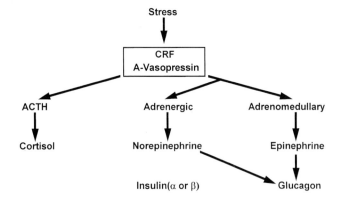

Figure 17–21. Scheme of release of counterregulatory hormones during stress.

blocker chorisondamine prevented the CRH-induced increase in plasma epinephrine, norepinephrine, and glucose. Such studies lend credence to the hypothesis that CRH may be physiologically involved in integrating neuroendocrine, autonomic, cardiovascular, and metabolic responses to stressful stimuli.[362,363] We examined tracer-determined glucose fluxes during ICV carbachol injection.[393,394] Epinephrine, norepinephrine, and cortisol were released. This was associated with a substantial increase in glucose production, which was offset by a concomitant rise in glucose MCR. Thus, there was only a 5% increase in glycemia (Fig. 17–22). Carbachol injection not only mobilized glucose, but also increased lipolysis as evidenced by increases in plasma glycerol and FFA. It is interesting that when somatostatin octapeptide (ST-8) was given together with carbachol, the epinephrine and cortisol responses were virtually abolished, but ST-8 only partially inhibited carbachol-induced norepinephrine release. ST-8

prevented the carbachol-induced increase in glucose production and utilization. It also enhanced the increase in FFA seven-fold but decreased the carbachol-induced rise in glycerol, indicating inhibition of FFA reesterification in the adipocytes due to decreased glucose uptake (Fig. 17–23). It is possible that analogs of somatostatin that are present in the brain are antagonists of CRH in control of counterregulatory responses to stress. The fact that carbachol prevented the increase of catecholamines can imply, as will be described later, that catecholamines are in part responsible for the increased glucose production during stress. However, inhibition of glucose uptake is not related to inhibition of catecholamine release, as such inhibition actually increases glucose uptake.

To assess the role of adrenergic activation on the ICV carbachol stress-induced increase in glucose clearance and production, selective or combined α- and β-adrenoceptor blockade was applied using infusions of phentolamine (α-blocker, 5 mg/kg/min) and/or propranolol (β-blocker, 7 mg/kg/min). Simultaneously, the effects of catacholamines on pancreatic hormone release were circumvented by means of a

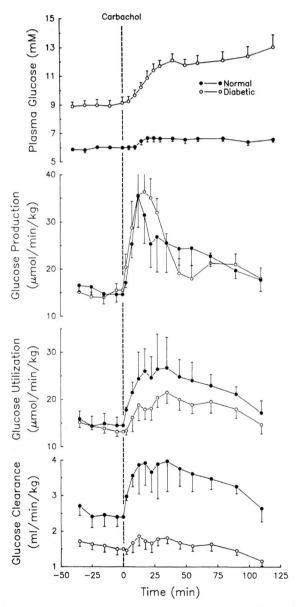

Figure 17–22. The effect of carbachol (27 nmol per 50 μl of water) injected into the third ventricle ($t = 1$ min) of normal (●) and moderately controlled diabetic (○) dogs ($n = 7$) (mean ± SEM). (From Ref. 393.)

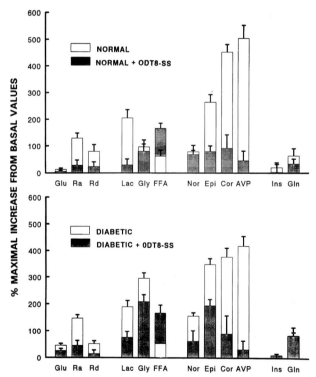

Figure 17–23. The percent above basal levels of the maximal stress-induced increase in glucose, glucose production (Ra), glucose utilization (Rd), lactate, glycerol, FFA, norepinephrine, epinephrine, cortisol, arginine vasopressin (AVP), insulin, and glucagon in response to carbachol (27 nmol/50 mL water) injection into the third ventricle of the brain in normal (top) and alloxan-diabetic (bottom) dogs either with (shaded boxes) or without (open boxes) prior to intracerebroventricular injection of a somatostatin analog, octapeptide ODT8-SS (20 nmol/200 mL water). (From Ref. 395.)

pancreatic clamp (PC group) to maintain basal insulinemia and glucagonemia. The stress-induced increase in MCR was augmented above that observed in the PC group with PC + α and β (two-fold) and PC + β-blockade (three-fold). Thus our data suggest a role for β-adrenoceptor mechanisms in restraining the increment in MCR during stress. Both α + β- and β-blockade unmask the inhibitory effects of adrenergic activity on glucose clearance. The increase in glucose clearance observed in all groups was independent of increments in insulin and not mediated by the mass action effect of glycemia. The augmented glucose clearance observed under both β- and α + β-blockade conditions is consistent with the inhibition of muscle glycogenolysis. β-Blockade also resulted in inhibition of lipolysis with a 33% fall in FFA levels. A fall in lipolysis, resulting in increased reliance on glucose as a fuel, could have further contributed to the enhanced glucose uptake and clearance in the β-blockade group. Stress resulted in an increase in glucose production that was 50% reduced because of the glucagon clamp. However, α + β-blockade largely abolished the acute increase in glucose production during stress. Catecholamines therefore accounted for most of the remaining 50% of the PC group increment in glucose production during stress. We observed that both α- and β-adrenoceptors are capable of increasing glucose production during stress in the dog.[395]

To mimic stress the effect of chronic administration (70 hr) of counterregulatory hormones (glucagon, cortisol, epinephrine, and norepinephrine) was examined in fasted, conscious dogs. The infusion of these hormones doubled plasma glucose and tripled plasma insulin. Glucose production increased by 80% from both the liver and the kidney, with gluconeogenesis accounting for 70% of the response. Glucose clearance did not change, presumably because hyperinsulinemia counteracted the effects of the catecholamines. These experiments would indicate that chronically, these hormones do not increase glucose clearance directly. This could indicate that the increase in glucose clearance observed during ICV carbachol injections is mediated by other neuroendocrine mechanisms.[396]

In summary, ICV injection of carbachol in the dog represents an acute model of moderate stress encompassing the increased neuroendocrine activity characteristic of stress. The stress-induced increase in glucose uptake and clearance demonstrates a new neuroendocrine pathway that increases availability of glucose for muscle and fat during stress. This pathway is insulin independent. β-Adrenoceptor blockade unmasks the inhibitory effects of catecholamines on glucose clearance through inhibition of muscle glycogenolysis and lipolysis. Thus, the full impact of the novel neuroendocrine pathway is revealed during such a blockade. Moreover, the combined effects of catecholamines and glucagon are responsible for increasing glucose production during stress (Fig. 17–9).[395]

Fuel Sources During Stress

Stress can greatly affect carbohydrate, fat, and protein metabolism. Their effects are mediated through changes in circulating hormones, particularly the increase in catecholamines and glucagon and the relative contribution of or decreased sensitivity to insulin.

Carbohydrates as a Source of Fuel. The catecholamines induce hyperglycemia by increasing glucose production and sustaining impairment in glucose clearance.[387,397] It seems that catecholamines can increase hepatic glucose production by both α- and β-adrenergic mechanisms. β-receptors stimulate the activity of protein kinase A, while α-receptors stimulate protein kinase C. The evidence of two signaling systems implies two backup systems (Fig. 17–9).[398] We have shown, for example, that during strenuous exercise in healthy subjects, complete blockade of β-receptors does not decrease but actually enhances hepatic glucose production. β-Blockade resulted in excessive concentration of plasma catecholamines. Our interpretation was that the maximum increase of catecholamines induced a maximal stimulation of α-receptors, thus overcompensating for the inhibitory effects of the β-receptors.[399]

Catecholamines can also accelerate glycogenolysis in muscle and decrease muscle uptake of glucose.[400] Increased glucagon levels during stress can increase hepatic glycogenolysis, through activation of cAMP–dependent protein kinase.[401] Cortisol can also increase gluconeogenesis and impair insulin sensitivity, but these effects are delayed for several hours after cortisol levels increase.[402] With respect to all of these observations, species differences may alter the relative importance of the above mechanisms.

Fat as a Source of Fuel. Catecholamine excess, via β–adrenergic receptors in adipose tissue,[403] together with insulin lack or insulin resistance can stimulate lipolysis, resulting in increased release of FFA and glycerol to the liver, thus increasing ketogenesis under the appropriate hormonal milieu.[365,404] Hyperglucagonemia and hypoinsulinemia can also activate hepatic carnityl transferase, which stimulates ketogenesis.[405] In shock, an extreme form of stress, there is a decreased ability to oxidize FFA.[406]

Protein as a Source of Fuel. Short infusions of norepinephrine can decrease circulatory alanine in man,[407] but epinephrine does not decrease alanine, glutamate, or glutamine.[365,408] However, prolonged infusions of epinephrine, which simulate stress, can decrease amino acids. In shock, massive protein breakdown can occur.[406] It should be pointed out that the effect of stress on protein breakdown will greatly vary depending on the type of stress applied. Also, there would be a big difference between short experiments versus prolonged clinical "shock" situations.

Glucoregulation During Stress

Elevated epinephrine and norepinephrine levels occur in stress situations such as major surgery,[409,410] burns,[411,412] severe infection,[413] myocardial infarction,[410,414] head injury,[415] severe hypoglycemia,[365,366,416–420] ketoacidosis,[412] and in emotional stress in normal man[421] and diabetic children.[422]

The increased catecholamine levels of stress may be associated with changes in insulin secretion. Normal[381] or elevated[413,414] circulating insulin levels have been reported, but in some situations these levels are inappropriately low relative to the prevailing hyperglycemia. This indicates at least a relative suppression of insulin secretion,[423–425] which represents a balance between α–adrenergic suppression and β–adrenergic stimulation of insulin release,[426–428] as well as the effects of catecholamine-induced hyperglycemia on pancreatic β-cell function. The predominance of one of these effects depends upon the circulating catecholamine levels and also on temporal factors.[375]

Glucocorticoids have been shown to stimulate catecholamine biosynthesis, and conversely, the catecholamines may stimulate ACTH release[361] through β adrenoreceptors in the pituitary. Afferent neurogenic stimuli from the area of injury are also of major importance in the endocrine–metabolic response to injury.[429,430] Tracer–determined glucose turnover has been studied in experimental animals and injured subjects, under several severe stress states, associated with catecholamine and glucagon release and a relative insulin deficiency. In burn injury, the rates of both glucose production and metabolic clearance of glucose (MCR) increased.[431,432] This appeared to involve both α- and β-adrenoreceptor mechanisms, and insulin resistance was also reported.[432] In sepsis, however, both Ra and MCR decreased,[432] and gluconeogenesis could not be suppressed by glucose administration.[433,434] Gluconeogenesis was also increased after major trauma, and this was suppressible by glucose administration.[435]

Stress in Diabetes Mellitus

Introduction Counterregulatory hormone release has been well documented, but few studies have examined counterregulatory hormone release or glucoregulation in diabetic subjects subjected to stress conditions. It is widely perceived, however, that acute ketoacidosis can develop rapidly under conditions of stress, and one or more of the stress hormones have been implicated.[436–439] The major stress hormones, epinephrine, norepinephrine, cortisol, glucagon, and growth hormone, were measured close to the onset of illness in a large group of young insulin-dependent diabetic subjects.[422] A history of severe infections or physical or emotional stress was reported in the majority of these subjects. Despite receiving their usual dose of insulin, hyperglycemia, dehydration, and ketoacidosis developed within a few hours of their experiencing the stress stimulus, and the metabolic derangements were associated with increased release of at least three of the counterregulatory hormones. Cortisol and the catecholamines were the most consistently released.

All of the counterregulatory hormones could act to overwhelm the actions of insulin on one or more of its target tissues and bring about an increase in glycogenolysis, gluconeogenesis, or lipolysis with a resultant deterioration in metabolic control. Thus, under conditions of stress, the usual insulin dose may be insufficient to offset the actions of the counterregulatory hormones, and ketoacidosis may ensue.[440]

Emotionally stressful events have been shown to result in increased sympathetic activity and hyperglycemia in diabetic subjects[441] and the relationship between stress and impaired glucoregulation is thought of as unidirectional. However, one study has raised the possibility of a reciprocal interactive model in which hyperglycemia-induced nervous system arousal may make an individual more susceptible to environmental stress,[442] explaining some of the psychiatric symptoms associated with poor metabolic control.

In summary, it is well recognized in the clinical setting that much greater doses of insulin are required in acute and severe stress states in type 1 and type 2 diabetic subjects. This is especially apparent in states in which total parenteral nutrition is required using hypertonic glucose. If intravenous insulin at 5–10 U/hr are insufficient to control glycemia, the glucose infusion rates have to be dropped, sometimes considerably.

Experimental Stress Models in Diabetes Mellitus As the hormonal and metabolic responses to various types of stress have not been well characterized in diabetic subjects, some understanding may be gained by studying experimental stress models.

The effects of pyrogen, which simulate mild stress, have been studied in well controlled insulin-dependent diabetic subjects during basal insulin infusion.[443] The rise in plasma glucose was preceded by the rise in plasma glucagon. The rise in FFA and ketone bodies, heralding the deterioration of the metabolic state in these subjects, was preceded by a rise in the catecholamines, cortisol, and growth hormone. Thus the stress hormones can initiate the metabolic deterioration in stressed diabetic subjects.

Insulin-induced hypoglycemia provides a model for moderate to severe stress. Type 1 diabetic subjects have diminished glucagon secretory responses to hypoglycemia,[444-447] which is related to the duration of the disease but can occur independently of autonomic neuropathy.[448] With respect to glucoregulation, these subjects are more dependent on epinephrine-induced β-adrenergic mechanisms than nondiabetic subjects.[449,450] However, with the development of autonomic neuropathy, there is a progressive blunting of epinephrine[447,451] and further blunting of glucagon responses. This correlates with a progressive deterioration in glucose recovery from hypoglycemia. Thus, it has been suggested that despite a markedly reduced glucagon secretory response to hypoglycemia, type 1 diabetic subjects may not be subjected to severe prolonged hypoglycemic episodes as long as epinephrine responses remain adequate.[452] However, if epinephrine secretory responses are deficient or the effects of epinephrine are blocked, for example, by propranolol, recurrent and profound hypoglycemia would occur as reported in one well-documented case history.[452] In type 1 diabetic subjects in whom gluconeogenesis is proportionately greater than in normal subjects, nonselective β-adrenoreceptor blockade attenuated glucose recovery from hypoglycemia by reducing the availability of gluconeogenic precursors such as lactate and glycerol.[453] The impairment in glucagon responsiveness may involve at least a defect in glucose sensing mechanism of the pancreatic α-cell.[454,455] The α-cell defect appears to be selective, since the glucagon response to arginine was maintained when its response to hypoglycemia was impaired.[456] We have indicated that chronic hyperglycemia plays an important role in desensitizing the α-cell response to hypoglycemia. In streptozotocin-diabetic rats the impaired glucagon responsiveness to hypoglycemia was significantly improved by insulin-independent correction of hyperglycemia, achieved by phlorizin treatment. Normalization of glycemia with insulin did not improve responsiveness of α-cells, which is presumably due to the inhibitory effect of exogenous insulin on the islet α-cells (Fig. 17–24).[457,458] An intriguing aspect of the pancreatic hormonal response to changes in circulating glucose is the somatostatin/glucagon ratio in the pancreas and circulation. We reported increased total pancreatic somatostatin content with no change in glucagon in hyperglycemic alloxan diabetic dogs.[459,460] However, acute normalization of glycemia using insulin in these dogs resulted in a marked decrease (five-fold) in total pancreatic glucagon content, with a relatively smaller decrease in the somatostatin content. We hypothesized that the relative abundance of the somatostatin/glucagon combined with the decreased total pancreatic glucagon content in normoglycemia could explain, at least in part, the impaired glucagon response to hypoglycemia in diabetic dogs.

Epinephrine infusions in diabetes provide a partial model for moderate stress since epinephrine infusion

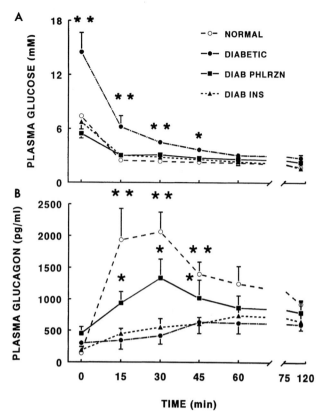

Figure 17–24.   (A) Plasma glucose and (B) glucagon levels during acute hypoglycemia experiments. Insulin was injected immediately after 0 min blood sampling. Hypoglycemia was attained between 75–120 min, when the animals were killed. Plasma glucagon levels in the NC and DP groups are significantly higher than those in the DU group, as indicated (**, $P < 0.01$; $P < 0.05$). (Reprinted from Ref. 457.)

simulates some of the hormonal and metabolic responses to stress. In type 1 diabetic subjects, epinephrine-stimulated glucagon release accounted for approximately 50% of epinephrine's effect on hepatic glucose production.[426] The response to epinephrine was also more prolonged in juvenile-onset diabetic subjects than in normal subjects.[389]

We have studied the effects of epinephrine in alloxan diabetic dogs that have a small residual amount of plasma insulin. In contrast to normal dogs in which the main effect of epinephrine on hepatic glucose production was direct, in diabetic dogs the response of plasma glucagon was excessive. Therefore, glucagon played a major role in enhancing glucose production during infusion of epinephrine. In addition, hypoinsulinemia sensitizes the liver to both glucagon and epinephrine. In depancreatized dogs glucagon is secreted from the fundus of the stomach[461,462] and is released in response to some glucagonotropic stimuli. The dogs were studied under normoglycemic and hyperglycemic conditions by infusing insulin. Under both conditions epinephrine induced only a modest and equivalent increase in glucagon. Glucagon was a mediator of epinephrine's effect only in poor diabetic control. This was attributed to increased sensitivity of the liver during hypoinsulinemia. These experiments clearly demonstrated that glucagon is an important mediator of epinephrine's effect either when glucagon release is excessive or when liver sensitivity to glucagon is enhanced.[463] Thus glucagon suppression would be effective in countering the diabetic instability of stress only when the patient is in poor diabetic control.[463–465] It is interesting that with repeated epinephrine infusions the hyperglycemic responses were intensified. β-Endorphins that decreased glucose production in response to epinephrine in normal dogs did not effect hyperglycemic and hepatic responses to epinephrine in diabetic dogs. β-Endorphins induced a markedly exaggerated decrease in glucose clearance during stress in normal dogs but not in diabetic dogs. Thus the action of β-endorphins during stress requires intact pancreatic endocrine function.[466,467]

Intracerebroventricular injection of carbachol in alloxan-diabetic dogs[393] induced a ten-fold greater increase in glycemia than in normal dogs. This was not due to enhanced hepatic glucose production, but rather to the failure of glucose MCR to increase. A physiologic amount of insulin was infused and the plasma glucose levels were moderately hyperglycemic. Therefore, these dogs were not insulin deficient, but were insulin resistant. The epinephrine and cortisol levels were not exaggerated in the diabetic animals, but norepinephrine release was markedly enhanced, suggesting that the sympathetic nervous system may play a greater role in diabetic than in normal subjects under conditions of stress (Fig. 17–22).

As in normal dogs, somatostatin octapeptide greatly attenuated the release of epinephrine, norepinephrine, and cortisol. There was improvement in glycemia relating solely to suppression of glucose production. ICV carbachol had a greater lipolytic effect in the diabetic animals as compared to normal controls (Fig. 17–23). We were interested to find out why stress in diabetic animals did not increase metabolic glucose clearance resulting in excessive hyperglycemia.[468] In our previous experiments alloxan diabetic dogs were maintained hyperglycemic with insulin infusions. In the recent experiments we maintained alloxan diabetic dogs either normoglycemic with an adequate amount of insulin or infused excessive insulin during glucose clamps. These two experiments were designed to answer the question whether acute normalization of glucose or excessive insulin can normalize resistance to stress. In both cases clearance was not improved. When the normoglycemic diabetic dogs were treated with a β-blocker stress did not induce hyperglycemia and the response to clearance of stress was near normal. That indicated that, perhaps under certain conditions of acute stress in diabetic subjects, β-blockade, in addition to insulin treatment, could help normalize glucose responses.[468]

Problem Statement and Research Directions

Basic mechanisms that regulate various glucoregulatory responses to stress, particularly those in diabetes, have not been studied as extensively as exercise. Part of the reason is that there is a spectrum of stress stimuli that involve a variety of different responses. It is not known, for example, what is the mechanism that increases glucose uptake independently of insulin in physiology but not in the diabetic condition. This altered response to stress is different than the responses to exercise. For example, in alloxan diabetic dogs normalization of glucose for only 2 hr fully normalized the response of glucose metabolic clearance to exercise but not to stress.[468] In exercise the main reason for abnormal glucose clearance was hyperglycemia and not insulin deficiency.[255] On the other hand, β-blockade could normalize the response of clearance to both exercise[113] and stress.[468] The question is whether β-blockade could be a useful adjunct to the treatment of diabetes during acute stress. Outline of neural pathways that control glucose uptake during stress could lead to new pharmacologic modalities that could be useful during some stress conditions. Methods of molecular biology could be used in experimental animals to delineate the importance of the genetic expression of a number of stress hormones in the brain. Of special importance in diabetes is are he stress response during insulin-induced hypoglycemia. The Diabetes Control and Complication Trial[469] has demonstrated the importance of optimal control of glucose concentration in individuals with diabetes to prevent diabetic complications. Optimal control requires insulin treatment, which increases the threat of hypoglycemia. It is also indicated that the threat of hypoglycemia is enhanced by antecedent episodes (repeated episodes of hypoglycemia). In view of the fact that glucose uptake by the muscle is regulated by adaptive physiological mechanisms,[111,255,470] the question is what adaptations occur in the pancreatic α-cells in muscle and in the genetic expression of hormones that regulate stress mechanisms of the brain in diabetes, and whether such adaptive processes are affected transiently or more permanently by antecedent hypoglycemia.

Practical Considerations for the Management of Subjects with Diabetes Mellitus in Stress Situations

It should be helpful to consider the practical management of the diabetic patient in certain stress situations. These include (1) elective surgery; (2) emergency surgery for uncontrolled bleeding and for serious injury and its complications, such as hypovolemic shock or hypoxemia due to chest trauma; and (3) supervening infections and spinal cord or head injury, which can impair the transmission of neural stimuli that initiate the neuroendocrine responses.[470–473] (See Exhibit 17–6).

Preparation of Diabetic Subjects for Elective Surgery.

1. Collection preoperatively of a complete database (see Appendix VII) must be done and assessment made of metabolic control (Hb A_{1c}, SMBG).

2. If metabolic control is not optimal (>75% of SMBG between 80 and 150 mg/dL without significant hypoglycemia), adjust diet or insulin therapy, or both, so that control is optimal for at least 2 weeks before surgery.

3. Evaluate and treat appropriately any complications of diabetes and of any associated diseases.

4. To maintain optimal blood glucose control during and after surgery requires work by a team (surgeon, anesthesiologist, internist, nurses).

5. Consider local or regional anesthesia (such as epidural or spinal), with concomitant general anesthesia if needed, to decrease the exaggerated neuroendocrine response to the surgical stress.

6. Do not forget to prepare the patient both mentally (by education) and emotionally, as well as metabolically and physically, for the surgery.

Preparation of Subjects with Diabetes Mellitus for Emergency Surgery.

1. Minimal workup consistent with need for immediate surgery is essential. In some situations, such as acute appendicitis and simple mechanical bowel obstruction, one can afford to spend 2 or 3 hr assessing the status of the diabetes and implementing insulin therapy if needed and therapy to repair fluid and electrolyte (especially potassium and sodium) deficits (see Exhibit 17–6).

2. A frequent problem is the undiagnosed diabetic patient presenting for emergency surgery. For this reason, all subjects must have a preoperative urinalysis and preferably a random plasma glucose to rule out undiagnosed diabetes (see Chapters 11 and 12). Infections, especially an abscess, may be the harbinger of diabetes. Surgical drainage of abscesses and appropriate antibiotic therapy results in more rapid control of the diabetes.

Management of Severely Injured Subjects Who Are Known to Have or Who Develop Overt Diabetes Mellitus in the Course of Their Illness. Assessment should be similar to that noted under "Emergency Surgery." Blood, fluid, electrolyte, and insulin deficits should be replaced and metabolic control attained and maintained,[474–480] as previously noted.

For management in the presence of major trauma, the normal physiologic responses are integrated and directed at restoring cardiovascular stability, correcting hypoxia, and mobilizing fuels, particularly glucose for use by the brain and for wounded healing. In diabetes, the neuroendocrine responses can be exaggerated, and although there is hyperglycemia, this can be deleterious rather than beneficial because of the development of insulin resistance. In addition, the enhanced glucocorticoid release can impair the inflammatory response to trauma and increase the risk of the development of infection and impair would healing. The situation may be made worse by factors such as advanced age, ethanol intake, certain preexisting medical conditions, and medications that have been administered, such as β-blockers, systemic steroids, and drugs used to treat hypertension.

In the severely injured diabetic patient, it is of even greater importance than in nondiabetic subjects to restore homeostasis as quickly as possible. Release of vasopressin, the catecholamines, and aldosterone and activation of the renin-angiotensin system may support the circulation for some time, depending on the severity of the injury and related factors, such as the extent of blood loss. However, careful attention must be paid not only to restoring normal circulating blood volume, but also to replacing total body fluid and electrolyte losses and insulin deficits. Also in the diabetic, appropriate hemodynamic monitoring is vital because there is frequently coexistent arteriosclerotic vascular disease and defective autonomic nervous system function.

Hypoxia must be treated by appropriate use of oxygen and prompt treatment of any life-threatening thoracic injuries, such as pneumothorax, tension pneumothorax, and hemothorax. Appropriate chest tube drainage and chest wall stabilization must be carried out when indicated. Again, blood gas monitoring assumes more importance in the diabetic patient because diabetic control can deteriorate deceptively and quickly, and ketoacidosis can ensue (see Exhibit 17–6).

Quick recognition of infection is also crucial in the diabetic, in whom the inflammatory response may be blunted, and prompt treatment with appropriate antibiotics and/or surgical drainage when indicated must be done. When stabilization has been achieved, the nutritional needs (calories, protein, vitamins, minerals) aimed at restoring positive nitrogen balance and providing optimal substrate and insulin (if needed) for excellent blood glucose control to promote wound healing must be met (see Chapters 15 and 16).

Finally, in the rush to take care of life-threatening emergencies, the surgeon must not forget that the psychological overlay of pain and emotional arousal may have profound neuroendocrine and autonomic nervous system effects. Endogenous opiate release either can play a beneficial role or, conversely, can increase insulin resistance. Attention must be given to provid-

EXHIBIT 17–6 Therapy of IDDM (Type 1) and of NIDDM (Type 2) During Elective Surgery and During Emergency Surgery.

I. Therapy for IDDM and NIDDM during *elective* surgery

A. *For IDDM*

1. The anesthesiologist, internist, surgeon, and nurses should coordinate and plan for the patient's care before, during, and after the surgical procedure (see Chapter 43). Plasma glucose (PG) control should have been satisfactory for at least 2 weeks before surgery, and the fasting PG level should be in the 100 to 150 mg/dL range at the beginning of the procedure.

   (a) If the PG is 100 to 150 mg/dL, 5% dextrose in 0.45% NaCl or in D/W may be infused intravenously (IV) at a rate of 100 to 200 ml/hr (5 to 10 g glucose/hr) with piggyback regular human insulin being infused intravenously at an initial rate of 2 U/hr. The insulin infusion rate is increased if the PG increases to >150 mg/dL, and decreased if the PG decreases to <100 mg/dL.

   (b) If the plasma glucose is >250 mg/dL, an insulin bolus of 10 U/hr should be given IV at hourly intervals (in addition to 0.45% NaCl without glucose) until the PG is <150 mg/dL. Then 5% dextrose in D/W or in 0.45% NaCl can be substituted and the insulin infusion rate reduced to 2 U/hr, with the infusion rate being adjusted to keep the PG in the 100 to 150 mg/L range.

   (c) Postoperatively, the infusion rates should continue as above with hourly monitoring and adjustments being made by the nurses, surgeon, internist, or anesthesiologist to maintain the PG level between 100 and 180 mg/dL without hypoglycemia until oral feedings are resumed.

B. *For NIDDM*

1. Same as I.A.1 above

   (a) If the PG is <150 mg/d before, during, and after the procedure, insulin therapy is not needed; 0.45% saline should be infused at a rate of 100 ml/hr.

   (b) If the PG is >150 mg/dL at the beginning of the procedure, or if during the procedure the hourly monitored PG rises to ≥180 mg/dL, the infusion should be changed to piggybacked human insulin infusion (2 U/hr) and 100 to 200 ml/h of 5% dextrose (5 to 10 g glucose/hr), with the insulin and dextrose infusion rates being adjusted to maintain the PG (monitored hourly) at the 100 to 150 mg/dL level during and after the procedure until oral feedings are resumed.

II. Therapy for IDDM and for NIDDM during *emergency* surgery

A. *For IDDM*

1. The surgeon, anesthesiologist, internist, and nurses should coordinate the plan for the patient's care before, during, and after the surgical procedure (see Chapter 43). In some situations, such as acute appendicitis and simple mechanical bowel obstruction, one may have 2 or 3 hr to assess the status of the diabetes and to implement insulin therapy to attain optimal PG control and to replace water and electrolyte deficits (potassium and sodium) before the surgical procedure begins.

2. In the presence of *major trauma* (head, chest, other) or *uncontrolled bleeding*, immediate surgery may be necessary even though the patient may be in diabetic ketoacidosis. In this situation, surgery should be accompanied *in parallel* by replacement of blood, water, electrolyte, and insulin therapy to maintain life and restore metabolic homeostasis as soon as possible (see Chapter 24 for details).

3. Careful monitoring of vital signs (respirations, pulse, blood pressure) and blood gases, with maintenance of an open airway (intubation, if necessary) and use of oxygen therapy if hypoxia occurs.

4. Prompt treatment of life-threatening thoracic (lung, cardiac, other) injuries (pneumothorax, tension pneumothorax, hemothorax, hemopericardium, and so forth) with appropriate chest tube drainage or chest wall stabilization or other procedure being carried out promptly.

5. Quick recognition of infection with appropriate antibiotic therapy and surgical drainage when indicated.

6. Insulin, water, and electrolyte therapy.

   (a) if the plasma glucose is >250 mg/dL, the initial dose of regular human insulin should be an IV bolus of 10 to 20 U, followed by an IV infusion of 10 U/hr (more if the PG does not fall at a rate of about 100 mg/dL/hr) until the PG decreases to <200 mg/dL. In *insulin-resistant individuals* [many with serious injury, obesity, and major brain injury with hypothalamic and pituitary dysfunction secondary to cerebral edema similar to the effects of injuries in the region of the fourth ventricle (or the *piqure diabetique* of Claude Bernard)] the insulin dose requirement may be much higher, and the insulin infusion rate must be adjusted to meet those requirements (rarely up to 50 to 100 U/hr). PG monitoring should continue at hourly intervals during recovery with the insulin infusion rate being adjusted downward to the level that sustains the PG at the 100 to 200 mg/dL level until oral feedings are resumed.

   (b) Careful monitoring at hourly intervals of serum sodium and potassium should continue with levels being kept in or near the normal range (serum sodium 140 ± mmol/L, serum potassium 4.8 ± 0.3 mmol/L.) Both *hypo- and hypernatremia* and *hypo- and hyperkalemia* should be avoided because all can terminate fatally.

   (c) Careful monitoring of fluid infusion so that underhydration and overhydration and their consequences are avoided.

B. *For NIDDM*

1. If initial PG is <150 mg/dL, same as I.B.1 (a).

2. If initial PG is 150-249 mg/dL, same as I.B.1 (b).

3. If initial PG is ≥250 mg/dL, or if patient is in DKA (see Chapter 24), same as II.A.1.2.3.4.5.6.(a) (b) and (c).

ing, when safe, appropriate pain relief and sedation, and emotional support should be provided routinely for the patient and the family.

Acknowledgements

The authors would like to thank Dr. Lavina Lickley and Dr. Adria Giacca, whose important contributions to previous editions of this chapter have helped to shape the present version. Special thanks are due to Linda Vranic for editing and revising the chapter and to Debbie Bilinski for additional administrative help. Some of the work reported here has been supported by the Medical Research Council of Canada (M. Vranic and E. Marliss) and by a Canadian Diabetes Association Grant (M. Vranic).

References

1. Toates F: Stress: Conceptual and Biological Aspects. West Sussex, England: Wiley, 1995

2. Stockvis BJ: Zur Pathologie und Therapie des Diabetes Mellitus. Verhandlungen des Kongresses fur innere Medizin:126, 1886.

3. Trousseau A: Glycosuria: Saccharine diabetes. Lectures Delivered at the Hotel Dieu, Paris. Philadelphia: P. Blakiston, 1882.

4. Allen FM, Stillman E, Fitz R: Total dietary regulation in the treatment of diabetes. In Allan FM, Stillman E, Fitz R (eds.): Exercise. New York: Rockefeller Institute, 1919.

5. Joslin EP, Root HF, White P, et al: The Treatment of Diabetes Mellitus. Philadelphia: Lea & Febiger, 1935.

6. Lawrence RH: The effects of exercise on insulin action in diabetes. Br Med J 1:648, 1926.

7. Brooks GA, Fahey TD, White TP: Exercise Physiology: Human Bioenergetics and Its Applications. Mountain View, CA. Mayfield Publishing Co., 1996.

8. Brooks GA, Mercier J: The balance of carbohydrate and lipid utilization during exercise: the "crossover" concept. J Appl Physiol Respirat Environ Exercise Physiol 49: 1057–1069, 1994.

9. Brooks GA: Importance of the "crossover" concept in exercise metabolism. Clin Exp Pharm Physiol 24: 889–895, 1997.

10. Shi ZQ, Wasserman D, Vranic M: Metabolic implications of exercise and physical fitness in physiology and diabetes. In Porte D, Sherwin R, (eds.): Ellenberg and Rifkin's Diabetes Mellitus, Ed. 5 Norwalk, Appleton and Lange, 1997, pp. 653–687.

11. Vranic M, Kawamori R, Pek S, et al.: The essentiality of insulin and the role of glucagon in regulating glucose utilization and production during strenuous exercise in dogs. J Clin Invest 57:245–256, 1976.

12. Wasserman DH, Cherrington AD: Hepatic fuel metabolism during exercise: Role and regulation. Am J Physiol 260:E811, 1991.

13. Zinker BA, Mohr T, Kelly P, et al.: Exercise-induced fall in insulin: Mechanism of action at the liver and effects on muscle glucose metabolism. Am J Physiol 265(5pt 1): E683–689, 1994.

14. Wasserman DH, O'Doherty RM, Zinker BA: Role of the endocrine pancreas in control of fuel metabolism by the liver during exercise. Intern J Obesity Rel Metab Dis 19 (Suppl. 4:)S22–30, 1995.

15. Wasserman DH, Williams PE, Lacy DB, et al.: Importance of intrahepatic mechanisms to gluconeogenesis from alanine during prolonged exercise and recovery. Am J Physiol 254:E518, 1988.

16. Wasserman DH, Lacy DB, Bracy DP: Relationship between arterial and portal vein immunoreactive glucagon during exercise. J Appl Physiol 75(2):724–729, 1993.

17. Wasserman DH, Lickley HLA, Vranic M: Interactions between glucagon and other counterregulatory hormones during normoglycemic and hypoglycemic exercise. J Clin Invest 74:1404–1413, 1984.

18. Issekutz B, Vranic M: Role of glucagon in regulation of glucose production in exercising dogs. Am J Physiol 238:E13, 1980.

19. Cherrington AD, Liljenquist JE, Shulman GI, et al.: Importance of hypoglycemia-induced glucose production during isolated glucagon deficiency. Am J Physiol 236:E263, 1979.

20. Liljenquist JE, Mueller GL, Cherrington AD, et al.: Evidence for an important role of glucagon in the regulation of hepatic glucose production in normal man. J Clin Invest 59:369, 1977.

21. Hirsch IB, Marker JC, Smith LJ, et al.: Insulin and glucagon in prevention of hypoglycemia during exercise in humans. Am J Physiol 260:E695, 1991.

22. Kjaer M, Engfred K, Fernandez A, et al.: Regulation of hepatic glucose production during exercise in humans; role of sympathoadrenergic activity. Am J Physiol 265: E275, 1993.

23. Wolfe RR, Nadel ER, Shaw JHF, et al.: Role of changes in insulin and glucagon in glucose homeostasis in exercise. J Clin Invest 77:900, 1986.

24. Wasserman DH, Williams PE, Lacy DB, et al.: Exercise-induced fall in insulin and hepatic carbohydrate metabolism during muscular work. Am J Physiol 256:E500, 1989.

25. Wasserman DH, Spalding JS, Lacy DB, et al.: Glucagon is a primary controller of hepatic glycogenolysis and gluconeogenesis during muscular work. Am J Physiol 257: E108, 1989.

26. Issekutz B Jr: The role of hypoinsulinemia in exercise metabolism. Diabetes 29:629, 1980.

27. Wasserman DH, Lacy DB, Colburn CA, et al.: Efficiency of compensation for the absence of the fall in insulin during exercise. Am J Physiol 261:E587, 1991.

28. Wasserman DR, Lickley HLA, Vranic M: Effect of hematocrit reduction on hormonal and metabolic responses to exercise. J Appl Physiol 58:1257, 1985.

29. Wasserman DH, Cherrington AD: Regulation of hepatic glucose production during exercise. In Kawamori R, Hoshi M (eds.): Proceedings of the First International Symposium on Exercise for Diabetes. Osaka: Doubenshoin 33, 1989.

30. Moore MC, Pagliassotti MJ, Wasserman DH, et al.: Hepatic denervation alters the transition from the fed to the food deprived state in conscious dogs. J Nutr 123(10):1729–1746, 1993.

31. Richter EA, Galbo H, Sonne B, et al.: Adrenal medullary control of muscular and hepatic glycogenolysis and of pancreatic hormonal secretion in exercising rats. Acta Physiol Scand 108:253–242, 1980.

32. Sonne B, Mikines KL, Richter EA, et al.: Role of liver nerves and adrenal medulla in glucose turnover in running rats. J Appl Physiol 59:1640, 1985.

33. Wasserman DH, Williams PE, Lacy DB, et al.: Hepatic nerves are not essential to the increase in hepatic glucose production during muscular exercise. Am J Physiol 259:E195, 1990.

34. Hoelzer DR, Dalsky GP, Clutter WE, et al.: Glucoregulation during exercise: Hypoglycemia is prevented by redundant glucoregulatory systems, sympathochromaffin activation, and changes in islet hormone secretion. J Clin Invest 77:212–221, 1986.

35. Hoelzer DR, Dalsky GP, Schwartz NS, et al.: Epinephrine is not critical to prevention of hypoglycemia during exercise in humans. Am J Physiol 251:E104, 1986.

36. Kjaer M, Engfred K, Galbo H, et al.: Hepatic glucose production during exercise in liver-transplanted subjects. Scand J Gastroenterol 26 (Suppl):Abstract 183, 1991.

37. Kjaer M, Jurlander J, Keiding S, et al.: No reinnervation of hepatic sympathetic nerves after liver transplantation in human subjects. J Hepatol 20:97-100,1994.

38. Kjaer M, Keiding S, Engfred K, et al.: Glucose homeostasis during exercise in humans with a liver or kidney transplant. Am J Physiol 268:E636, 1995.

39. Cooper DM, Wasserman DH, Vranic M, et al.: Glucose turnover in response to exercise during high- and low-FiO2 in humans. Am J Physiol 14:E209–E214, 1986.

40. Kjaer M, Kiens B, Hargreaves M, Richter EA: Influence of active muscle mass on glucose homeostasis during exercise in humans. J Appl Physiol 71:552–557, 1991.

41. Arnall DA, Marker JC, Conlee RK, Winder WW: Effect of infusing epinephrine on liver and muscle glycogenolysis during exercise in rats. Am J Physiol 250:E641–E649, 1986.

42. Carlson KI, Marker JC, Arnall DA, et al.: Epinephrine is unessential for stimulation of liver glycogenolysis during exercise. J Appl Physiol 58:544–548, 1985.

43. Marker JC, Arnall DA, Conlee RK, et al.: Effect of adrenodemedullation on metabolic responses to high-intensity exercise. Am J Physiol 251:R552, 1986.

44. Winder WW, Terry ML, Mitchell VM, et al.: Role of plasma epinephrine in fasted exercising rats. Am J Physiol 248:R302, 1985.

45. Richter EA, Galbo H, Christensen NJ: Control of exercise-induced muscular glycogenolysis by adrenal medullary hormones in rats. J Appl Physiol 58:544–548, 1985.

46. Winder WW, Yang HT, Jaussi AW, et al.: Epinephrine, glucose and lactate infusion in exercising adrenomedullated rats. J Appl Physiol 62:1442, 1997.

47. Moates JM, Lacy DB, Goldstein RE, et al.: The metabolic role of exercise-induced increment in epinephrine in the dog. Am J Physiol 255:E428–E436, 1988.

48. Goldstein RE, Abumrad NN, Lacy DB, et al.: Effects of an acute increase in epinephrine and cortisol on carbohydrate metabolism during insulin deficiency. Diabetes 44(6):672–681, 1995.

49. Sellers TL, Jaussi AW, Yang HT, et al.: Effect of the exercise-induced in glucocorticoids on endurance in the rat. J Appl Physiol 58:544–548, 1985.

50. Goldstein RE, Wasserman DH, McGuinness OP, et al.: Effects of chronic elevation in plasma cortisol on hepatic carbohydrate metabolism. Am J Physiol 264(1 Pt 1): E119–E127, 1993.

51. Zinker BA, Bracy D, Lacy DB, et al.: Regulation of glucose uptake and metabolism during exercise: an in vivo analysis. Diabetes 42:956, 1993.

52. Goodyear LJ, King PA, Hirshman MF, et al.: Contractile activity increases plasma membrane glucose transporters in absence of insulin. Am J Physiol 258:E667–E672, 1990.

53. Holloszy JO, Narahara HT: Studies of tissue permeability, 10: Changes in permeability to 3-methylglucose associated with contraction of isolated frog muscle. J Biol Chem 240:3493, 1965.

54. Nesher R, Karl IE, Kipnis KM: Dissociation of the effect(s) of insulin and contraction on glucose transport in rat epitrochlearis muscle. Am J Physiol 249:C226–C232, 1985.

55. Sternlicht E, Barnard RJ, Grimditch GK: Exercise and insulin stimulate skeletal muscle glucose transport through different mechanisms. Am J Physiol 256:E227, 1989.

56. Katz A, Sahlin K, Broberg S: Regulation of glucose utilization in human skeletal muscle during moderate dynamic exercise. Am J Physiol 260:E411, 1991.

57. Katz A, Brobert S, Sahlin K, et al.: Leg glucose uptake during maximal dynamic exercise in humans. Am J Physiol 251:E65–E70, 1986.

58. Cortright RN, Dohm GL: Mechanism by which insulin and muscle contraction stimulate glucose transport. Can J Appl Physiol 22(6):519–530, 1997.

59. Thorens B, Sarkar HK, Kaback HR, Lodish HF: Cloning and function expression bacteria of a novel glucose transporter present in liver, intestine, kidney, and B-pancreatic islet cells. Cell 55:281–290, 1988.

60. Fukumoto H, Kayano T, Buse JB, et al.: Cloning and characterization of the major insulin-responsive glucose transporter express in human skeletal muscle and other insulin-responsive tissues. J Biol Chem 264:7776–7779, 1989.

61. James DE, Strube M, Mueckler M: Molecular cloning and characterization of an insulin-regulatable glucose transporter. Nature (London) 338:83–87, 1989.

62. Flier JS, Mueckler M, McCall AL, Lodish HF: Distribution of glucose transporter messenger RNA transcripts in tissues of rat and man. J Clin Invest 79:657–661, 1987.

63. Bell GI, Kayano T, Buse JB, et al.: Molecular biology of mammalian glucose transporters. Diabetes Care 13(3): 198-208, 1990.

64. Stephens J, Pilch P: The metabolic regulation and vesicular transport of GLUT4, the major insulin responsive glucose transporter. Endocrine Rev 26:529–546, 1995.

65. Goodyear LJ, Hirshman, MF, Horton ES: Exercise-induced translocation of skeletal muscle glucose transporters. Am J Physiol 261:E795–E799, 1991.

66. Sherman L, Hirshman M, Cormont M, et al.: Differential effects of insulin and exercise on rab4 distribution in rat skeletal muscle. Endocrinology 137:266–273, 1996.

67. Kristiansen S, Hargraves M, Richter E: Exercise-induced increase in glucose transport, GLUT-4, and vamp-2 in plasma membrane from human muscle. Am J Physiol 270:E197–E201, 1996.

68. Del Vecchio RL, Pilch PF: Phosphatidylinositol 4–kinase is a component of glucose transporter (GLUT4)-containing vesicles. J Biol Chem 266:13278–13283, 1991.

69. Czech MP: Molecular actions of insulin on glucose transport. Ann Rev Nutr 15:441–471, 1995.

70. Kelly KL, Ruderman, NB: Insulin-stimulated phosphatidylinositol 3-kinase. J Biol Chem 268:4391–4398, 1993.

71. Mueckler M: Facilitative glucose transporters. Eur J Biochem 219:713–725, 1994.

72. Fushiki T, Wells JA, Tapscott EB, et al.: Changes in glucose transporters in muscle in response to exercise. Am J Physiol 256:E580, 1989.

73. Brozinick JT Jr, Etgen GJ Jr, Yaspelkis BB III, Ivy JL: The effects of muscle contraction and insulin on glucose-transporter translocation in rat skeletal muscle. Biochem J 297:539–545, 1994.

74. Douen AG, Ramlal T, Klip A, et al.: Exercise-induced increase in glucose transporters in plasma membrane of rat skeletal muscle. Endocrinology 124:449, 1989.

75. Ploug T, Galbo H, Ohkuwa T, Tranum-Jensen J, Vinten J: Kinetics of glucose transport in rat skeletal muscle membrane vesicles: Effects of insulin and contractions. Am J Physiol 262(Endocrinol. Metab.) 253(16):E12–E20, 1987.

76. Lund S, Holman G, Schmitz O, Petersen O: Contraction stimulates translocations of glucose transporter GLUT4 in skeletal muscle through a mechanism distinct from that of insulin. Proc Natl Acad Sci USA 92:5817–5821, 1995.

77. Ploug T, Wojtaszewski J, Kristiansen S, et al.: Glucose transport and transporter in muscle giant vesicles: Differential effects of insulin and contractions. Am J Physiol 264:E270–E278, 1993.

78. Friedman J, Dudek R, Whitehead D, et al.: Immunolocalization of glucose transporter GLUT4 within human skeletal muscle. Diabetes 40:150–154, 1991.

79. Marette A, Burdett E, Douten A, et al.: Insulin induces the translocation of GLUT4 glucose transporters from a unique intracellular organelle to transverse tubules in rat skeletal muscle. Diabetes 41:1562, 1992.

80. Dohm G, Dolan P, Frisell W, Dudek R: Role of transverse tubules in insulin stimulated muscle glucose transport. J Cell Biochem 52:1–7, 1993.

81. Roy D, Marette A: Exercise induces the translocation of GLUT4 to transverse tubes from an intracellular pool in ratskeletal muscle. Biochem Biophys Res Commun 223:147–152, 1996.

82. Wallberg-Henriksson H, Holloszy JO: Contractile activity increases glucose uptake in muscle of severely diabetic rats. J Appl Physiol 57:1045–1049, 1984.

83. Ploug T, Galbo H, Vinten J, et al.: Increased muscle glucose uptake during contraction: No need for insulin. Am J Physiol 247:E726–E731, 1984.

84. Richter EA, Ploug T, Galbo H: Increased muscle glucose uptake after exercise. Diabetes 34:1041–1048, 1985.

85. Idstrom JP, Rennie MJ, Schersten T, et al.: Membrane transport in relation with net glucose uptake in the perfused rat hinlimb. Biochem J 233:131–137, 1986.

86. Wallberg-Henriksson H, Gunnarsson R, Henriksson J, et al.: Increased peripheral insulin sensitivity and muscle mitochondrial enzymes but unchanged blood glucose control in type 1 diabetics after physical training. Diabetes 31:1044, 1982.

87. Bjorkman O, Miles P, Wasserman D, et al.: Regulation of glucose turnover in pancreatectomized, totally insulin deficient dogs: Effects of beta-adrenergic blockade. J Clin Invest 81:1759–1767, 1988.

88. Coderre L, Kandron K, Vallega G, Pilch P: Identification and characterization of an exercise-sensitive pool of glucose transporters in skeletal muscle. J Biol Chem 46: 27584–27588, 1995.

89. Henriksen E, Sleeper M, Zierath J, Holloszy J: Activation of glucose transport in skeletal muscle by phospholipase c and phorbol ester. J Biol Chem 264:21536–21543, 1989.

90. Westfall M, Sayeed M: Effect of Ca2+-channel agonists and antagonists on skeletal muscle sugar transport. Am J Physiol 258: R462–R468, 1990.

91. Youn J, Gulve E, Holloszy J: Calcium stimulates glucose transport in skeletal muscle by a pathway independent of contraction. Am J Physiol 260:C555–C561, 1991.

92. Youn J, Gulve E, Henriksen E, Holloszy J: Interactions between effects o W-7, insulin, and hypoxia on glucose transport in skeletal muscle. Am J Physiol 267: R888–R894, 1994.

93. Cartee G, Briggs-Tung C, Holloszy J: Diverse effects of calcium channel blockers on skeletal muscle glucose transport. Am J Physiol 263:R70–R75, 1992.

94. Treadway JL, James DE, Burcel E, et al.: Effect of exercise on insulin receptor binding and kinase activity in skeletal muscle. Am J Physiol 256:E138, 1989.

95. Yeh J, Culves E, Rameh L, Birnbaum M: The effects of Wortmannin on rat skeletal muscle. J Biol Chem 270: 2107–2111, 1995.

96. Lee AD, Hansen A, Holloszy JO: Wortmannin inhibits insulin-stimulated but not contraction-stimulated glucose transport activity in skeletal muscle. FEBS Lett 361: 51–54, 1995.

97. Goodyear L, Chang P, Sherwood D, Dufresne S, Moller D: Effects of exercise and insulin on mitogen-activated protein kinase signaling pathways in rat skeletal muscle. Am J Physiol 271:E403–E408, 1996.

98. Dolan P, Tapscott E, Dorton P, Dohm G: Contractile activity restores insulin responsiveness in skeletal muscle of obese zucker rats. Biochem J 289:423–426, 1993.

99. Brozinick JT Jr, Etgen GJ Jr, Yaspelkis BB III, Ivy JL: Contraction-activated glucose uptake is normal in insulin-resistant muscle of obese Zucker rat. J Appl Physiol 73: 382–387, 1992.

100. King PA, Betts JJ, Horton ED, Horton ES: Exercise, unlike insulin, promotes glucose transporter transloca-tion in obese zucker rat muscle. Am J Physiol 265: R447–R452, 1993.

101. Kusunoki M, Storlien L, MacDessi J, et al.: Muscle glucose uptake during and after exercise is normal in insulin-resistant rats. Am J Physiol 264:E167–E172, 1993.

102. Wasserman DH, Bupp JL, Johnson JL, et al.: Impact of insulin deficiency on glucose fluxes and muscle glucose metabolism during exercise. Diabetes 41:1229, 1992.

103. Wahren J, Felig P, Ahlborg G, et al.: Glucose metabo-lism during leg exercise in man. J Clin Invest 50: 2715–2725, 1971.

104. Calles J, Cunningham JJ, Nelson L, et al.: Glucose turnover during recovery from intense exercise. Diabetes 32:734, 1983.

105. Marliss EB, Simantirakis E, Miles PDG, et al.: Glucoreg-ulatory and hormonal responses to repeated bouts of intense exercise in normal male subjects. J Appl Physiol 71(3):924–933, 1991.

106. Sigal RJ, Purdon C, Vranic M, et al.: Glucoregulation during and after intense exercise: Effect of beta block-ade. J Clin Endocrinol Metab 78:359–366, 1994.

107. Coyle EF, Hamilton MT, Alonso JG, et al.: Carbohydrate metabolism during intense exercise when hyper-glycemic. J Appl Physiol 70:834, 1991.

108. Vaag A, Damsbo P, Hother-Nielsen O, et al.: Hypergly-caemia compensates for the defects in insulin-mediated glucose metabolism and in the activation of glycogen synthase in the skeletal muscle of patients with type 2 (non-insulin-dependent) diabetes mellitus. Diabetologia 35:80, 1992.

109. Dimitrakoudis D, Ramlal T, Rastogi S, et al.: Glycemia regulates the glucose transporter number in the plasma membrane of rat skeletal muscle. Biochem J 284:341, 1992.

110. Klip A, Marette A: Acute and chronic signals control-ling glucose transport in skeletal muscle. J Cell Biochem 48:51, 1992.

111. Klip A, Marette A, Dimitrakoudis D, et al.: Effect of dia-betes on glucoregulation. From glucose transporters to glucose metabolism in vivo. Diabetes Care 15: 1747–1766, 1992.

112. Dimitrakoudis D, Vranic M, Klip A: Effects of hyper-glycemia on glucose transporters of the muscle: Use of the renal glucose reabsorption inhibitor phlorizin to control glycemia. J Am Soc Nephrol 3:1078, 1992.

113. Wasserman DH, Lickley HLA, Vranic M: Role of beta-adrenergic mechanisms during exercise in poorly-con-trolled insulin deficient diabetes. J Appl Physiol 59:1282–1289, 1985.

114. Yamatani K, Shi Z, Giacca A, et al.: Role of FFA-glucose cycle in glucoregulation during exercise in total absence of insulin. Am J Physiol 263:E646, 1992.

115. DeFronzo RA, Ferrannini E, Sato Y, et al.: Synergistic interaction between exercise and insulin on peripheral glucose uptake. J Clin Invest 68:1468–1474, 1981.

116. Wasserman DH, Geer RJ, Rice DE, et al.: Interaction of exercise and insulin action in humans. Am J Physiol 260:E37, 1991.

117. Wasserman DH, Bupp JL, Johnson JL, et al.: Glucoregu-lation during rest and exercise in depancreatized dogs: Role of the acute presence of insulin. Am J Physiol 262:E574, 1992.

118. Zinker BA, Lacy DB, Bracy D et al.: Role of glucose and insulin loads to the exercising limb in increasing glucose uptake and metabolism J Appl Physiol 74:2915, 1993.

119. Mikines KJ, Sonne B, Farrell PA et al.: Effect of physical exercise on sensitivity and responsiveness to insulin in man. Am J Physiol 254:E248, 1988.

120. Chiasson JL, Shikama H, Chu DTW, et al.: Inhibitory effect of epinephrine on insulin-stimulated glucose uptake by rat skeletal muscle. J Clin Invest 68:706–713, 1981.

121. Issekutz B: Role of beta-adrenergic receptors in mobi-lization of energy sources in exercising dogs. J Appl Physiol 44:869, 1978.

122. Fredrikson G, Tornqvist H, Belfrage P: Hormone-sensi-tive lipase and monoacylglycerol lipase are both required for complete degradation of adipocyte triacyl-glycerol. Biochim Biophys Acta 876:288–293, 1986.

123. Yeaman SJ: Hormone sensitive-lipase—a multipurpose enzyme in lipid metabolism. Biochim Biophys Acta 1052:128–132, 1990.

124. Fredrikson G, Stralfors P, Nilsson NO, Belfrage P: Hor-mone-sensitive lipase of rat adipose tissue. Purification and some properties. J Biol Chem 256(12):6311–6320, 1981.

125. Nilsson NO, Stralfors P, Fredrikson G, Belfrage P: Regu-lation of adipose tissue lipolysis: Effects of noradrenaline and insulin on phosphorylation of hormone-sensitive lipase and on lipolysis in intact rat adipocytes. FEBS Lett 111(1):125–130, 1980.

126. Stralfors P, Belfrage P: Phosphorylation of hormone-sensitive lipase by cyclic AMP-dependent protein kinase. J Biol Chem 258(24):15146–15152, 1983.

127. Stralfors P, Bjorgell P, Belfrage P: Hormonal regulation of hormone-sensitive lipase in intact adipocytes: Iden-tification of phosphorylated sites and effects on the phosphorylation by lipolytic hormones and insulin. Proc Natl Acad Sci USA 81:3317–3321, 1984.

128. Stralfors P, Honnor RC: Insulin-induced dephosphory-lation of hormone-sensitive lipase. Correlation with lipolysis and cAMP-dependent protein kinase activity. Eur J Biochem 182:379–385, 1989.

129. Abumrad NA, Perkins RC, Park JH, Park CR: Mechanisms of long chain fatty acid permeation in the isolated adipocyte. J Biol Chem 256(17):9183–9191, 1981.

130. Sorrentino D, Robinson RB, Kiang, C-L, Berk PD: At physiologic albumin/oleate concentrations oleate uptake by isolated hepatocytes, cardiac myocytes, and adipocytes is a saturable function of the unbound oleate concentration. Uptake kinetics are consistent with the conventional theory. J Clin Invest 84:1325–1333, 1989.

131. Stremmel W, Strohmeyer G, Berk PD: Hepatocellular uptake of oleate is energy dependent, sodium linked, and inhibited by an antibody to a hepatocyte plasma membrane fatty acid binding protein. Proc Natl Acad Sci USA 83:3584–3588, 1986.

132. Turcotte LP, Richter EA, Srivastava AK, Chiasson J-L: First evidence for the existence of a fatty acid binding protein in the plasma membrane of skeletal muscle. Diabetes 41(Suppl 1):172A, 1992.

133. Kiens B, Essen-Gustavsson B, Christensen NJ, Saltin B: Skeletal muscle substrate utilization during submaximal exercise in man: effect of endurance training. J Physiol (London) 469:459–478, 1993.

134. Brauer RW, Pessotti RL: The removal of bromosulphthalein from blood plasma by the liver of the rat. J Pharmacol Exp Ther 97:358–370, 1949.

135. Abumrad NA, Park JH, Park CR: Permeation of long-chain fatty acid into adipocytes. Kinetics, specificity, and evidence for involvement of a membrane protein. J Biol Chem 259(14):8945–8953, 1984.

136. Abumrad NA, Harmon CM, Barnela US, Whitesell RR: Insulin antagonism of catecholamine stimulation of fatty acid transport in the adipocyte. Studies on its mechanism of action. J Biol Chem 263(29):14678–14683, 1988.

137. Christensen EH, Hansen O: Respiratorischer quotient und Os-aufnahme. Scan Arch Physiol 81:180–189, 1939.

138. Paul P: FFA metabolism of normal dogs during steady-state exercise at different work loads. J Appl Physiol 28(2):127–132, 1970.

139. Pruett EDR: FFA mobilization during and after prolonged severe muscular work in men. J Appl Physiol 29(6):809–815, 1970.

140. Armstrong DT, Steele R, Altszuler N, et al.: Regulation of plasma free fatty acid turnover. Am J Physiol 210:9–15, 1961.

141. Hagenfeldt L, Wahren J, Pernow B, Raf L: Uptake of individual free fatty acids by skeletal muscle and liver in man. J Clin Invest 51:2324–23330, 1972.

142. Essen-Gustavsson B, Tesch P: Glycogen and triglyceride utilization in relation to muscle metabolic characteristics in men performing heavy resistance exercise. Eur J Appl Physiol 61:5–10, 1990.

143. Gollnick PD, Saltin B: Significance of skeletal muscle oxidative enzyme enhancement with endurance training: hypothesis. Clin Physiol 2:1–12, 1992.

144. Holloszy HO, Coyle EF: Adaptations of skeletal muscle to endurance exercise and their metabolic consequences. J Appl Physiol 56(4):831–838, 1984.

145. McGarry JD, Mills SE, Long CS, Foster DW: Observations on the affinity for carnitine, and malonyl-CoA sensitivity, of carnitine palmitoyltransferase I in animal and human tissues. Biochem J 214:21–28, 1983.

146. Winder WW, Arogyasami J, Barton RJ, Elayan IM, Vehrs PR: Muscle malonyl-CoA decreases during exercise. J Appl Physiol 67(6):2230–2233, 1989.

147. Hopp JF, Palmer WK: Effect of electrical stimulation on intracellular triacylglycerol in isolated skeletal muscle. J Appl Physiol 68(1):348–354, 1990.

148. Richter EA, Sonne B, Mikines KJ, Ploug T, Galbo H: Muscle and liver glycogen, protein and triglyceride in the rat. Effect of exercise and of the sympatho-adrenal system. Eur J Physiol 52:346–350, 1984.

149. Turcotte LP, Hespel PJL, Graham TE, Richter EA: Impaired plasma FFA oxidation imposed by extreme CHO deficiency in contracting rat skeletal muscle. J Appl Physiol 77:517–525, 1994.

150. Randle PJ, Garland PB, Hales CN, et al.: The glucose-fatty acid cycle: Its role in insulin sensitivity and the metabolic disturbances of diabetes mellitus. Lancet 1:785, 1963.

151. Berger M, Hagg SA, Goodman MN, et al.: Glucose metabolism in perfused skeletal muscle. Biochem J 158:191, 1976.

152. Goodman MN, Berger M, Ruderman NB: Glucose metabolism in rat skeletal muscle at rest: Effect of starvation, diabetes, ketone bodies and free fatty acids. Diabetes 23:881, 1974.

153. Jefferson LS, Koehler JO, Morgan HE: Effect of insulin on protein synthesis in skeletal muscle of an isolated perfused preparation of rat hemicorpus. Proc Natl Acad Sci USA 69:816, 1972.

154. Maizels EZ, Ruderman NB, Goodman MN, et al.: Effects of acetoacetate on glucose metabolism in the soleus and extensor digitorum longus muscles of the rat. Biochem J 162:557, 1977.

155. Rennie MJ, Holloszy JO: Inhibition of glucose uptake and glycogenolysis by availability of oleate in well-oxygenated perfused skeletal muscle. Biochem J 68:161–170, 1977.

156. Boden G: Fatty acids and insulin resistance. Diabetes Care 19:394–395, 1996.

157. Boden G, Chen X, Ruiz J, White JV, Rossetti L: Mechanisms of fatty acid-induced inhibition of glucose uptake. J Clin Invest 93:2438–2446, 1994.

158. Boden G, Jadali F, White J, et al.: Effects of fat on insulin-stimulated carbohydrate metabolism in normal men. J Clin Invest 88:960–966, 1991.

159. Bonadonna RC, Zych K, Boni C, Ferrannini E, DeFronzo RA: Time dependence of interaction between lipid and glucose in humans. Am J Physiol 257:E49–E56, 1989.

160. Rennie MJ, Winder WW, Holloszy JO: A sparing effect of increased plasma fatty acids on muscle and liver glycogen content in the exercising rat. Biochem J 156:647–655, 1976.

161. Bracy DP, Zinker BA, Jacobs JC, et al.: Carbohydrate metabolism during exercise: Influence of circulating fat availability. J Appl Physiol 79:506, 1995.

162 . Rosholt MN, King PA, Horton ES: High-fat diet reduces glucose transporter responses to both insulin and exercise. Am J Physiol 35:R95, 1994.

163. Vaag AA, Handberg A, Skott P, et al.: Glucose-fatty acid cycle operates in humans at the levels of both whole body and skeletal muscle during low and high physiological plasma insulin concentrations. Eur J Endocrinol 130:70, 1994.

164. Graham TE, Rush JWE, MacLean DA: Skeletal muscle amino acid metabolism and ammonia production during exercise. In Hargreaves M (ed.): Exercise Metabolism. Champaign, IL: Human Kinetics. 1995, pp. 131–176.

165. Dohm GL, Beecher GR, Warren RQ, Williams RT: The influence of exercise on amino acid concentrations in rat tissues. J Appl Physiol 50:41–44, 1981.

166. Dohm GL, Kasperek GJ, Tapscott EB, Barakat HA: Protein metabolism during endurance exercise. Fed Proc 44:348–352, 1985.

167. Dohm GL: Protein as a fuel for endurance exercise. Exer Sport Sci Rev 14:143–173, 1986.

168. Haralambie G, Berg A: Serum urea and amino nitrogen changes with exercise duration. Eur J Appl Physiol 36:39–48, 1976.

169. Bylund-Fellenius AC, Ojamaa KM, Flaim KE, et al.: Protein synthesis versus energy state in contracting muscle of perfused rat hindlimb. Am J Physiol 246:E297–305, 1984.

170. Rennie MJ, Edwards RHT, Krywawych S, et al.: Effect of exercise on protein turnover in man. Clin Sci 61:627–639, 1981.

171. Calles-Escandon J, Cunningham JJ, Snyder P, et al.: Influence of exercise on urea, creatinine, and 3-methyl-histidine excretion in normal human subjects. Am J Physiol 246:E334–E338, 1984.

172. Dohm GL, Tapscott EB, Kasperek GJ: Protein degradation during endurance exercise and recovery. Med Sci Sports Exerc 19:S166–S171, 1987.

173. Fryburg DA, Barrett EJ, Louard RJ, Gelfand RA: Effect of starvation on human muscle protein metabolism and its response to insulin. Am J Physiol 259:E477–E482, 1990.

174. Beaufrere B, Tessari P, Cattalini M, Miles J, Haymond W: Apparent decreased oxidation and turnover of leucine during infusion of medium-chain triglycerides. Am J Physiol 249:E175–E182, 1985.

175. Nair KS, Schwartz RG, Welle S: Leucine as a regulator of whole body and skeletal muscle protein metabolism in humans. Am J Physiol 263:E928–E934, 1992.

176. Tawa NE Jr, Goldberg AL: Suppression of muscle protein turnover and amino acid degradation by dietary protein deficiency. Am J Physiol 263:E317–E325, 1992.

177. Kasperek GJ, Snider RD: Increased protein degradation after eccentric exercise. Eur J Appl Physiol 54:30–34, 1985.

178. Booth FW, Watson PA: Control of adaptations in protein levels in response to exercise. Fed Proc 44:2293–2300, 1985.

179. Dohm GL, Hecker AL, Brown WE, et al.: Adaptation of protein metabolism to endurance training. Biochem J 164:705–708, 1977.

180. Dohm GL, Kasperek GJ, Tapscott EB, Beecher GR: Effect of exercise on synthesis and degradation of muscle protein. Biochem J 188:255–262, 1980.

181. Haag SA, Morse EL, Adibi SA: Effect of exercise on rates of oxidation turnover, and plasma clearance of leucine in human subjects. Am J Physiol 242:E407–E410, 1982.

182. Wolfe RR, Goodenough RD, Wolfe MH, Royle GT, Nadel ER: Isotopic analysis of leucine and urea metabolism in exercising humans. J Appl Physiol 52:458–466, 1992.

183. Marshal S, Monzon R: Amino acid regulation of insulin action in isolated adipocytes. J Biol Chem 264:2037–2042, 1989.

184. Fryburg DA, Gelfand RA, Barrett EJ: Growth hormone acutely stimulates forearm muscle protein synthesis in normal humans. Am J Physiol 260:E499–E504, 1991.

185. Watt PE, Corbett ME, Rennie MJ: Stimulation of protein synthesis in pig skeletal muscle by infusion of amino acids during constant insulin availability. Am J Physiol 263:E453–460, 1992.

186. Smith K, Rennie MJ: Protein turnover and amino acid metabolism in human skeletal muscle. Clin Endocrin Metab 4:461–498, 1990.

187. Brooks GA: Amino acid and protein metabolism during exercise and recovery. Med Sci Sports Exerc 19: S150–S156, 1987.

188. Poortmans JR: Protein turnover and amino acid oxidation during and after exercise. Med Sports Sci 17: 130–147, 1984.

189. Khatra BS, Chawla RK, Sewell CW, Ruderman D: Distribution of branched chain amino alpha-keto acid dehydrogenase in primate tissues. J Clin Invest 59: 558–564, 1977.

190. Wagenmakers AJM, Brookes JH, Coakley JH, Reilly T, Edwards RHT: Exercise-induced activation of the branched-chain-2-oxo acid dehydrogenase in human muscle. Eur J Appl Physiol 59:159–67, 1989.

191. Marliss EB, Sigal RJ, Miles PDG, et al.: Glucoregulation in intense exercise and its implications for persons with diabetes mellitus. In Kawamori R, Vranic M, Horton ES, Kubota M (eds.): Proceedings of IDF Satellite Symposium on Glucose, Fluxes, Exercise and Diabetes. London: Smith-Gordon and Company Ltd. 1996, pp. 55–66.

192. Sigal RJ, Fisher S, Vranic M, Halter JB, Marliss EB: The roles of catecholamines in glucoregulation in intense exercise as defined by the islet cell clamp technique. Diabetes 45:148–56, 1996.

193. Sigal R, Purdon C, Fisher SJ, et al.: Hyperinsulinemia prevents prolonged hyperglycemia following intense exercise in insulin-dependent diabetic subjects. J Clin Endocrinol Metab 79:1049–1057, 1994.

194. Kjaer M, Farrell PA, Christensen NJ, Galbo H: Increased epinephrine response and inaccurate glucoregulation in exercising subjects. J Appl Physiol 61:1693–1700, 1986.

195. Sigal RJ, Fisher SJ, Vranic M, et al.: Glucoregulation during and after intense exercise: Effect of b-adrenergic

blockade in subjects with type 1 diabetes mellitus. 1998 (Submitted)

196. Holloszy JO, Kohrt WM: Regulation of carbohydrate and fat metabolism during and after exercise. Annu Rev Nutr 16:121–38, 1996.

197. Manzon A, Fisher SJ, Morais JA, et al.: Glucose infusion partially attenuates glucose production and increases glucose uptake during intense exercise. J Appl Physiol 85(2):514-524, 1998.

198. Marliss EB, Manzon A, Nessim S, et al.: Glucoregulation Responses to Intense Exercise (IE) in the Postprandial (PP) State. American Diabetes Association, Boston; MA, June 21–24, 1997. Diabetes 46 (Suppl 1):253A, 1997.

199. Wasserman DH, Vranic M: Exercise and diabetes. In Alberti KGMM, Krall LP (eds): The Diabetes Annual/4. Amsterdam: Elsevier Science Publishers, 1988, pp.116–142.

200. Ward GM, Weber KM, Walters JM: A modified minimal model analysis of insulin sensitivity and glucose-mediated glucose disposal in insulin-dependent diabetes. Metabolism 40:4, 1991.

201. Walters JM, Ward GM, Kalfas A, et al.: The effect of epinehprine on glucose-mediated and insulin-mediated glucose disposal in insulin-dependent diabetes. Metabolism 41:671, 1992.

202. Zinman B, Marliss EB, Hanna AK, et al.: Exercise in diabetic man: glucose turnover and free insulin responses after glycemic normalization with intravenous insulin. Can J Physiol Pharmacol 60(10):1236–1240, 1982.

203. Simonson DC, Koivisto V, Sherwin RS, et al.: Adrenergic blockade alters glucose kinetics during exercise in insulin-dependent diabetics. J Clin Invest 73:1648–1658, 1984.

204. Zinman B, Murray FT, Vranic M, et al.: Glucoregulation during moderate exercise in insulin treated diabetics. J Clin Endocrinol Metab 45:641–652,1977.

205. Tuttle K, Marker J, Dalsky G, et al.: Glucagon, not insulin, may play a secondary role in defense against hypoglycemia during exercise. Am J Physiol 17:E713–E719, 1988.

206. Wahren J, Hagenfeldt L, Felig P: Splanchic and leg exchange of glucose, amino acids and free fatty acids and ketones in insulin-dependent diabetics during exercise. J Clin Invest 55:1303–1314, 1975.

207. Krzentowski G, Pirnay F, Pallikarakis N, et al.: Glucose utilization in normal and diabetic subjects. The role of insulin. Diabetes 30:983–989, 1981.

208. Berger M, Berchtold P, Cuppers HJ: Metabolic and hormonal effects of muscular exercise in juvenile type diabetics. Diabetologia 13:355–365, 1977.

209. Wahren J, Sato Y, Ostman J, et al.: Turnover and splanchnic metabolism of FFA and ketones in insulin-dependent diabetics during exercise. J Clin Invest 73: 1367–1376, 1984.

210. Standl E, Lotz N, Dexel TH, et al.: Muscle triglycerides in diabetic subjects. Diabetologia 18:463–469, 1980.

211. Issekutz B, Paul P: Intramuscular energy sources in exercising normal and pancreatectomized dogs. Am J Physiol 215:197–204, 1968.

212. Zander E, Burns W, Wulfert P, et al.: Muscular exercise in type 1 diabetics. I. Different metabolic reactions during heavy muscular work is dependent on actual insulin availability. Exp Clin Endocrinol 82:78–90, 1983.

213. Vranic M, Wrenshall GA: Exercise, insulin and glucose turnover in dogs. Endocrinology 85:165–171, 1969.

214. Walker PM, Idstrom JP, Schersten T, et al.: Glucose uptake in relation to metabolic state in perfused rat hindlimb at rest and during exercise. Eur J Appl Physiol 48:163–176, 1982.

215. Hubinger A, Ridderskamp I, Lehmann E: Metabolic response to different forms of physical exercise in type 1 diabetics and the duration of the glucose lowering effect. Eur J Clin Invest 15:197–205, 1985.

216. Zander E, Schulz B, Chlup R, et al.: Muscular exercise in type 1 diabetics. II. Hormonal and metabolic responses to moderate exercise. Exp Clin Endocrinol 85:95–104, 1985.

217. Mitchell T, Abraham G, Schiffrin A, et al.: Hyperglycemia after intense exercise in IDDM subjects during continuous subcutaneous insulin infusion. Diabetes Care 11:311–317, 1988.

218. Wasserman DH, Lickley HLA, Vranic M: Important role of glucagon during exercise and diabetes. J Appl Physiol 59(4):1272–1281, 1985.

219. Tamborlane WV, Sherwin RS, Koivisto V, et al.: Normalization of the growth hormone and catecholamine response to exercise in juvenile-onset diabetic subjects treated with a portable insulin infusion pump. Diabetes 28:785–788, 1979.

220. Hansen AP: Abnormal serum growth hormone response to exercise in juvenile diabetics. J Clin Invest 49:1467–1478, 1970.

221. Perez G, Kemmer FW, Lickley L, et al.: Importance of glucagon in mediating epinephrine-induced hyperglycemia in alloxan-diabetic dogs. Am J Physiol 241(4): E328–E335, 1981.

222. Wasserman DH, Johnson JL, Bupp JL, et al.: Regulation of gluconeogenesis during rest and exercise in the depancreatized dog. Am J Physiol 265:E51–E60, 1993.

223. Wasserman DH, Vranic M: Interaction between insulin and counterregulatory hormones in control of substrate utilization in health and diabetes during exercise. Diabetes/Metabol Rev 1:359–384, 1986.

224. Wasserman DH, Spalding JS, Bracy D, et al.: Exercise-induced rise in glucagon and ketogenesis during prolonged muscular work. Diabetes 38:799, 1989.

225. Soukup JT, Kovaleski JE: A review of the effects of resistance training for individuals with diabetes mellitus. Diabetes Educator 19(4):307–312, 1993.

226. Berger M, Halban PA, Muller WA, et al.: Mobilization of subcutaneously injected tritiated insulin in rats: Effect of muscular exercise. Diabetologia 15:113–140, 1978.

227. Kawamori R, Vranic M: Mechanism of exercise-induced hypoglycemia in depancreatized dogs maintained on long-acting insulin. J Clin Invest 59:331–337, 1977.

228. Koivisto V, Felig P: Effects of leg exercise on insulin absorption in diabetic subjects. New Engl J Med 298: 77–83, 1978.

229. Kemmer FW, Berchtold P, Berger M, et al.: Exercise-induced fall of blood glucose in insulin treated diabetics unrelated to alteration of insulin mobilization. Diabetes 28:1131–1137, 1979.

230. Susstrunk H, Morell B, Ziegler WH, et al.: Insulin absorption from the abdomen and the thigh in healthy subjects during rest and exercise: blood glucose, plasma insulin, growth hormone, adrenaline, and noradrenaline levels. Diabetologia 22:171–174, 1982.

231. Ader M, Bergman RN: Peripheral effects of insulin dominate suppression of fasting hepatic glucose production. Am J Physiol 245:E1020, 1990.

232. Giacca A, Fisher S, Shi ZQ, et al.: Importance of peripheral insulin levels for insulin-induced suppression of glucose production in depancreatized dogs. J Clin Invest 90:1769, 1992.

233. Lewis G, Zinman B, Groenwould Y, et al.: Hepatic glucose production is regulated both by direct hepatic and extrahepatic effects of insulin in humans. Diabetes 45: 454–462, 1996.

234. Giacca A, Fisher S, McCall RH, et al.: Direct and indirect effects of insulin in suppressing glucose production in depancreatized dogs: Role of glucagon. Endocrinology 138:999–1007, 1997.

235. Lewis GF, Vranic M, Harley P, Giacca A: Fatty acids mediate the acute extrahepatic effects of insulin on hepatic glucose production in humans. Diabetes 46: 1111–1119, 1997.

236. Sindelar DK, Balcom JH, Chu CA, Neal DW, Cherrington AD: A comparison of the effects of selective increases in peripheral or portal insulin on hepatic glucose production in the conscious dog. Diabetes 45: 1594–1604, 1996.

237. Rebrin K, Steil GM, Getty L, Bergman RN: Free fatty acid as a link in the regulation of hepatic glucose output by peripheral insulin. Diabetes 44:1038–1045, 1995.

238. Rebrin K, Steil GM, Mittelman SD, Bergman RM: Causal linkage between insulin suppression of lipolysis and suppression of liver glucose output in dogs. J Clin Invest 98:741–749, 1996.

239. Zinman B, Murray FT, Vranic M, et al.: Glucoregulation during moderate exercise in insulin treated diabetics. J Clin Endocrinol Metabol 45:641, 1977.

240. Shi ZQ, Giacca A, Yamatani K, et al.: Effects of subbasal insulin infusion on resting and exercise-induced glucose uptake in depancreatized dogs. Am J Physiol 264: E334, 1993.

241. Shi ZQ, Giacca A, Fisher S, et al.: Indirect effects of insulin in regulating glucose production in postabsorptive state and glucose fluxes during exercise. In Efendic S, Ostenson C, Vranic M (eds.): New Concepts in the Pathogenesis of NIDDM. New York: Plenum, 1993, p. 151.

242. Minuk HL, Vranic M, Marliss EB, et al.: Glucoregulatory and metabolic response to exercise in obese noninsulin-dependent diabetes. Am J Physiol 240:E458–E464, 1981.

243. Issekutz B Jr, Miller HI, Paul P et al.: Aerobic work capacity and plasma FFA turnover. J Appl Physiol 20: 293–296, 1965.

244. Jenkins AB, Furler SM, Bruce DG, et al.: Regulation of hepatic glucose output during moderate exercise in non-insulin dependent diabetes. Metabolism 37: 966–969, 1988.

245. Martin IK, Katz A, Wahren J: Splanchnic and muscle metabolism during exercise in NIDDM patients. Am J Physiol 269:E583–590, 1995.

246. Koivisto V, DeFronzo R: Exercise in the treatment of type 2 diabetes. Acta Endocrinol 262(Suppl.):107–116, 1984.

247. Devlin JT, Hirshman M, Horton ED, et al.: Enhanced peripheral and splanchnic insulin sensitivity in NIDDM men after single bout of exercise. Diabetes 36: 434–439, 1987.

248. Larsen JJS, Dela F, Kjaer M, Galbo H: The effect of moderate exercise on postprandial glucose homeostasis in NIDDM patients. Diabetologia 40:447–453, 1997.

249. Nelson JD, Poussier P, Marliss EB, et al.: Metabolic response of normal man and insulin-infused diabetics to postprandial exercise. Am J Physiol 242:E309–E316, 1982.

250. Fordtran JS, Saltin B: Gastric emptying and intestinal absorption during prolonged severe exercise. J Appl Physiol 23:331–335, 1967.

251. Klip A, Marette A, Dimitrakoudis D, et al.: Effect of diabetes on glucoregulation. From glucose transporters to glucose metabolism in vivo. Diabetes Care 15:1747, 1992.

252. Ramlal T, Rastogi S, Vranic M, et al.: Decrease in glucose transporter number in skeletal muscle of mild diabetic (streptozotocin-treated) rats. Endocrinology 125: 890, 1989.

253. Hetenyi G Jr, Gautier C, Byers M et al.: Phlorizin induced normoglycemia partially restores glucoregulation in diabetic dogs. Am J Physiol 256:E277, 1989.

254. Lussier B, Vranic M, et al.: Glucoregulation in alloxandiabetic dogs. Metabolism 35:18, 1986.

255. Fisher SJ, Lekas M, Shi ZQ, et al.: Glycemia acutely regulates glucose clearance during exercise in diabetic dogs. Diabetes 46:1805–1812, 1997.

256. Challis RAJ, Vranic M, Radda GK: Bioenergetic changes during contraction and recovery in diabetic rat skeletal muscle. Am J Physiol 256:E129, 1989.

257. Mikines KJ, Sonne B, Farrell PA, et al.: Effect of physical exercise on sensitivity and responsiveness to insulin in man. Am J Physiol 254:E248–259, 1988.

258. Rodnick KJ, Haskell WL, Swislocki ALM, et al.: Improved insulin action in muscle, liver and adipose tissue in physically trained human subjects. Am J Physiol 253:E489, 1987.

259. Dela F, Mikines KJ, Von Linstow M, Galbo H: Twenty-four-hour profile of glucose and glucoregulatory hormones during normal living conditions in trained and untrained men. J Clin Endocrinol Metab 73:982–989, 1991.

260. Yki-Jarvinen H, Koivisto V: Effects of body composition on insulin sensitivity. Diabetes 32:965–969, 1983.

261. Miller WJ, Sherman WM, Ivy JL: Effect of strength training on glucose tolerance and post-glucose insulin response. Med Sci Sport Exer 16:539, 1984.

262. Crettaz M, Horton ES, Warzala LJ, et al.: Physical training of Zucker rats: Lack of alleviation of muscle insulin resistance. Am J Physiol 244:E414–E420, 1983.

263. Davis TA, Klahr S, Tegtmayer ED, et al.: Glucose metabolism in epitrochlearis muscle of acutely exercised and trained rats. Am J Physiol 250:E137–E143, 1986.

264. James DE, Kraegen EW, Chisholm DJ: Effects of exercise training on in vivo insulin action in individual tissues of the rat. J Clin Invest 76:657–666, 1985.

265. Bouchard C, Shepard RJ, Stephens T, et al.: Exercise, Fitness and Health Champaign, IL: Human Kinetic Publishers, 1989.

266. Ivy JL, Sherman WM, Cutler CL, et al.: Exercise and diet reduce muscle insulin resistance in obese Zucker rat. Am J Physiol 251:E299–E305, 1986.

267. Vallerand AL, Lupien J, Bukowiecki LJ: Synergistic improvement of glucose tolerance by sucrose feeding and exercise training. Am J Physiol 250:E607–E614, 1986.

268. Bonen A, Clune PA, Tan MH: Chronic exercise increases insulin binding in muscles but not liver. Am J Physiol 251:E196–203, 1986.

269. Dohm GL, Sinha MK, Caro JF: Insulin receptor binding and protein kinase activity in muscles of trained rats. Am J Physiol 252:E170–E175, 1987.

270. Marette A, Richardson JM, Ramlal T, et al.: Abundance, localization and insulin-induced translocation of glucose transporters in red and white muscle of the rat hindlimb. Am J Physiol 263:C443, 1992.

271. Douen AG, Burdett E, Ramlal T, et al.: Characterization of glucose transporters enriched membranes from rat skeletal muscle: Assessment of endothelial cell contamination, and of presence of sarcoplasmic reticulum and transverse tubules. Endocrinology 128:611, 1991.

272. Klip A, Ramlal T, Bilan PJ, et al.: Recruitment of GLUT4 glucose transporter by insulin in diabetic rat skeletal muscle. Biochem Biophys Res Comm 172:728, 1990.

273. Hirshman MF, Goodyear LJ, Wardzala LJ et al.: Identification of an intracellular pool of glucose transporters from basal and insulin-stimulated rat skeletal muscle. J Biol Chem 265:987, 1990.

274. Ren JM, Semenkovich CF, Gulve EA, et al.: Exercise induces rapid increases in GLUT4 expression, glucose transport capacity, and insulin-stimulated glycogen storage in muscle. J Biol Chem 269:14396, 1994.

275. Rodnick KJ, Henriksen EJ, James DE, et al.: Exercise training, glucose transporters and glucose transport in rat skeletal muscles. Am J Physiol 262:C9, 1992.

276. Koivisto VA, Bourey RE, Vuorinen-Markkola H et al.: Exercise reduces muscle glucose transport protein (GLUT4) mRNA in type I diabetic patients. J Appl Physiol 74:1755, 1993.

277. Dela F, Ploug T, Handberg A, et al.: Physical training increases muscle GLUT4 protein and mRNA in patients with NIDDM. Diabetes 43:862, 1994.

278. Ebeling P, Bourey R, Koranyi L, et al.: Mechanism of enhanced insulin sensitivity in athletes. Increased blood flow, muscle glucose transport protein (GLUT-4) concentration, and glycogen synthase activity. J Clin Invest 92(4):1623–1631, 1993.

279. Tsakiridis T, Vranic M, Klip A: Disassembly of the actin network inhibits insulin-dependent stimulation of glucose transport and prevents recruitment of glucose transporters in plasma membrane. J Biol Chem 269:29934–29942, 1994.

280. Tsakiridis T, McDowell HW, Walker T, et al.: Multiple roles of phosphatidylinositol 3–kinase in the regulation of glucose transport, amino acid transport and glucose transporters in L-6 skeletal muscle cells. Endocrinology 136:4315–4322, 1995.

281. Goodyear LJ, Giorgino F, Balon TW, et al.: Effects of contractile activity on tyrosine phosphoproteins and PI 3-kinase activity in rat skeletal muscle. Am J Physiol 268:E987–E995, 1995.

282. Craig BW, Garthwaite SM, Holloszy JO: Adipocyte insulin resistance: Effects of aging, obesity exercise and food restriction. J Appl Physiol 62:95-100, 1987.

283. Vinten J, Norgaard-Peterson L, Sonne B, et al.: Effect of physical training on glucose transporters in fat cell fractions. Biochem Biophys Act 841:223, 1985.

284. Wardzala LJ, Horton ES, Crettaz M, et al.: Physical training of lean and genetically obese Zucker rats: Effect on fat cell metabolism. Am J Physiol 243:E418–E426, 1982.

285. Craig BW, Thompson K, Holloszy JO: Effects of stopping training on size and response to insulin of fat cells in female rats. J Appl Physiol 54(2):571–575, 1983.

286. Ivy JL, Young JC, McLane JA, et al.: Exercise training and glucose uptake by skeletal muscle in rats. J Appl Physiol 55(5):1393–1396, 1983.

287. King DS, Dalsky GP, Clutter WE, et al.: Effects of exercise and lack of exercise on insulin sensitivity and responsiveness. J Appl Physiol 64(5):1942–1946, 1988.

288. King DS, Dalsky GP, Clutter WE, et al.: Effects of lack of exercise on insulin secretion and action in trained subjects. Am J Physiol 254(17):E537–E542, 1988.

289. Mikines KJ, Sonne B, Farrell PA, et al.: Insulin action in man. Effects of different levels of physical activity. Diabetologia 31(7):522A (abstract), 1988.

290. Skor D, et al.: Diabetes 25(Suppl. 2):64A (abstract), 1983.

291. Landt KW, Campaigne BN, James FW, et al.: Effects of exercise training on insulin sensitivity in adolescents with type 1 diabetes. Diabetes Care 8:461–465, 1985.

292. Yki-Jarvinen H, DeFronzo R, Koivisto V: Normalization of insulin sensitivity in type 1 diabetic subjects by physical training during insulin pump therapy. Diabetes Care 7:520, 1984.

293. Tancrede G, Rousseau-Migneron S, Nadeau A: Beneficial effects of physical training in rats with a mild streptozotocin-induced diabetes mellitus. Diabetes 31:406, 1982.

294. Vallerand AL, Lupien J, Deshaies Y, et al.: Intensive exercise training does not improve intravenous glucose tolerance in severely diabetic rats. Horm Metab Res 18:79, 1986.

295. Goodyear LJ, Hirshman MF, Knutson SM, et al.: Effect of exercise training on glucose homeostasis in normal and insulin-deficient diabetic rats. J Appl Physiol 65(2):844–851, 1988.

296. Noble EG, Ianuzzo CD: Influence of training on skeletal muscle enzymatic adaptations in normal and diabetic rats. Am J Physiol 249:E360–E365, 1985.

297. Lithell H, Krotkiewski M, Kiens B: Non-response of muscle capillary density and lipoprotein-lipase activity to regular training in diabetic subjects. Diabetes Res 2: 17, 1985.

298. Wallberg-Henriksson H, Gunnarsson R, Henriksson J, et al.: Influence of physical training on formation of muscle capillaries in type 1 diabetes. Diabetes 34: 412–414, 1984.

299. Williamson JR, Hoffmann PL, Kohrt WM, et al.: Endurance exercise training decreases capillary basement membrane width in older non-diabetic and diabetic adults. J Appl Physiol 80(3):747–753, 1996.

300. Wallberg-Henriksson H, Gunnarsson R, Rossner S, et al.: Long-term physical training in female type 1 (insulin dependent) diabetic subjects: Absence of significant effect on glycemic control and lipoprotein levels. Diabetologia 29:53–65, 1986.

301. Zinman B, Zuniga-Guajardo S, Kelly D: Comparison of the acute and long-term effects of exercise on glucose control in type 1 diabetes. Diabetes Care 7:515–519, 1984.

302. Krotkiewski M, Lonnroth P, Mandroukas K, et al.: The effects of physical training on insulin secretion and effectiveness and on glucose metabolism in obesity and type 2 (non-insulin dependent) diabetes mellitus. Diabetologia 28:881–890, 1985.

303. Reitman JS, Vasquez B, Klimes I, et al.: Improvement of glucose homeostasis after exercise training in non-insulin dependent diabetes. Diabetes Care 7:434–441, 1984.

304. Schneider SH, Amorosa LF, Khachadurian AK, et al.: Studies on the mechanism of improved glucose control during regular exercise in type 2 (non-insulin dependent) diabetes. Diabetologia 26:355–360, 1984.

305. Trovati M, Carta Q, Cavalot F, et al.: Influence of physical training on blood glucose control, glucose tolerance, insulin secretion, and insulin action in non-insulin dependent diabetic subjects. Diabetes Care 7:416–420, 1984.

306. Ruderman NB, Ganda OP, Johansen K: Effects of physical training on glucose tolerance and plasma lipids in maturity onset diabetes mellitus. Diabetes 28(Suppl.):89, 1979.

307. Saltin B, et al.: Physical training and glucose tolerance in middle-aged men with chemical diabetes. Preceedings of a Conference on Diabetes and Exercise (Vranic M, Horuath S and Wahner J, editors). Diabetes 28(Suppl.1): 30-32, 1979.

308. Bogardus C, Ravussin E, Robbins DC, et al.: Effects of physical training and diet therapy on carbohydrate metabolism in subjects with glucose intolerance and non-insulin dependent diabetes mellitus. Diabetes 33: 311–318, 1984.

309. Bjorntorp P, Fahlen M, Grimby G, et al.: Carbohydrate and lipid metabolism in middle aged physically well-trained men. Metabolism 21:631, 1972.

310. Bjornthorp P, et al.: The effect of physical training on insulin production in obesity. Metabolism 19:631-638, 1970.

311. Krotkiewski M, et al.: Effects of physical training insulin, correcting peptide (c-peptide), gastric inhibitory polypeptide (GIP) and pancreatic polypetide (PP) levels in obese subjects. Int J Obesity 8:193-199, 1984.

312. LeBlanc J, Nadeau A, Richard D, et al.: Effect of physical training and adiposity on glucose metabolism and 125I-insulin binding. J Appl Physiol 46:235–239, 1979.

313. Dela F, Larsen JJ, Mikines KJ, et al.: Insulin-stimulated muscle glucose clearance in patients with NIDDM. Effects of one-legged physical training. Diabetes 44(9): 1010–1020, 1995.

314. Dela F, Ploug T, Handberg A, et al.: Physical training increases muscle GLUT4 protein and mRNA in patients with NIDDM. Diabetes 43(7):862–865, 1994.

315. Dela F, Larsen JJ, Mikines KJ, Galbo H: Normal effect of insulin to stimulate leg blood flow in NIDDM. Diabetes 44(2):221–226, 1995.

316. Powell KE, Blair SN: The public health burdens of sedentary living habits: Theoretical but realistic estimates. Med Sci Sports Exercise 26(7):851–856, 1994.

317. Schneider SH, Vitug A, Ruderman NB: Atherosclerosis and physical activity. Diabetes/Metabol Rev 1: 513–553, 1986.

318. Paffenbarger RS, Wing AL, Hyde RT, et al.: Physical activity as an index of heart attack risk in college alumni. Am J Epidemiol 108:161–175, 1978.

319. Kaplan RM, Wilson DK, Hartwell SL, et al.: Prospective evaluation of HDL cholesterol changes after diet and physical conditioning programs for subjects with type 2 diabetes mellitus. Diabetes Care 8:343, 1985.

320. American Diabetes Association: Diabetes mellitus and exercise: Position statement. Diabetes Care 21(Suppl. 1): S40–S44, 1998.

321. U.S. Department of Health and Human Services: The effects of physical activity on health and disease. Surgeon General's Report on Physical Activity and Health. U.S. Department of Health and Human Services, Centers for Disease Control and Prevention, National Center for Chronic Disease Prevention and Health Promotion. Atlanta, GA pp. 81–172, 1996.

322. Schneider SH, Ruderman NB: Exercise and NIDDM (technical review). Diabetes Care 13:785–789, 1990.

323. Wasserman DH, Zinman B: Exercise in individuals with IDDM (technical review). Diabetes Care 17: 924–937, 1994.

324. Kriska AM, Blair SN, Pereira MA: The potential role of physical activity in the prevention of noninsulin-dependent diabetes mellitus: the epidemiological evidence. Exercise Sport Sci Rev 22:121–143, 1994.

325. Zimmet PZ: Kelly West Lecture 1991 challenges in diabetes epidemiology—from West to the rest. Diabetes Care 15:232–252, 1992.

326. King H, Kriska AM: Prevention of type 2 diabetes by physical training: Epidemiology considerations and study methods. Diabetes Care 15:1794–1799, 1992.

327. Kriska, AM, Bennett PH: An epidemiological perspective of the relationship between physical activity and NIDDM: From activity assessment to intervention. Diabetes/Metabol Rev 8:355–372, 1992.

328. Bennett PH, Rewers MJ and Knowler WC: Epidemiology of Diabetes Mellitus. In Ellenberg and Rifkin's Diabetes Mellitus, 5th edition (D. Porte and RS. Sherwing editors). Appleton and Lange. Stamford, Conn 1997.

329. Hara H, Kawase T, Yamakido M, Nishimoto Y: Comparative observation of micro- and macroangiopathies in Japanese diabetics in Japan and U.S.A. In Abe H, Hoshi M (eds.): Diabetic Microangiopathy. Basel: Karger, 1983.

330. Kawate R, Yamakido M, Nishimoto Y, et al.: Diabetes mellitus and its vascular complications in Japanese migrants on the island of Hawaii. Diabetes Care 2: 161–170, 1979.

331. Ravussin E, Bennett PH, Valencia ME, et al.: Effects of a traditional lifestyle on obesity in Pima Indians. Diabetes Care 17:1067–1074, 1994.

332. Cruz-Vidal M, Costas R Jr, Garcia-Palmiere MR, et al.: Factors related to diabetes mellitus in Puerto Rican men. Diabetes 28:300–307, 1979.

333. Zimmet P, Faaiuso S, Ainuu J, et al.: The prevalence of diabetes in the rural and urban Polynesian populations of Western Samoa. Diabetes 30:45–51, 1981.

334. Taylor RJ, Bennett PH, LeGonidec G, et al.: The prevalence of diabetes mellitus in a traditional-living Polynesian population: The Wallis Island survey. Am J Public Health 6:334–340, 1983.

335. King H, Taylor R, Zimmet P, et al.: Non-insulin-dependent diabetes mellitus (NIDDM) in a newly independent Pacific nation: The Republic of Kiribati. Diabetes Care 7:409–415, 1984.

336. Helmrich SP, Ragland DR, Leung RW, Paffenbarger RS Jr: Physical activity and reduced occurrence of non-insulin-dependent diabetes mellitus. New Engl J Med 325:147–152, 1991.

337. Manson JE, Rimm EB, Stampfer MJ, et al.: Physical activity and incidence of non-insulin-dependent diabetes mellitus in women. Lancet 338:774–778, 1991.

338. Eriksson K-F, Lindgarde F: Prevention of type 2 (non-insulin-dependent) diabetes mellitus by diet and physical exercise. Diabetologia 34:891–898, 1991.

339. Pan X, Li G, Hu Y: Effect of dietary and/or exercise intervention on incidence of diabetes in 530 subjects with impaired glucose tolerance from 1986–1992. Chinese J Internal Med 34–108–112, 1995.

340. Persheghin G, Ghosh S, Gerow K, Shulman GI: Metabolic defects in lean nondiabetic offspring of NIDDM parents: a cross-sectional study. Diabetes 46:1001–1009, 1997.

341. Price TB, Persheghin G, Duleba A, et al.: NMR studies of muscle glycogen synthesis in insulin-resistant offspring of parents with non-insulin-dependent diabetes mellitus immediately after glycogen-depleting exercise. Proc Natl Acad Sci USA 93:5329–5334, 1996.

342. Perseghin G, Price TB, Petersen KF, et al.: Increased glucose transport-phosphorylation and muscle glycogen synthesis after exercise training in insulin-resistant subjects. New Engl J Med 335:1357–1362, 1996.

343. Caron D, Pousseir P, Marliss EB: The effect of postprandial exercise on meal-related glucose intolerance in insulin-dependent diabetic individuals. Diabetes Care 5(4):364–369, 1982.

344. Colvin RH, Olson, SB: A descriptive analysis of men and women who have lost significant weight and are highly successful at maintaining the loss. Addict Behav 8:287–295, 1983.

345. Kayman S, Bruvold W, Stern JS: Maintenance and relapse after weight loss in women: behavioral aspects. Am J Clin Nutr 52:800–807, 1990.

346. Klem ML, Wing RR, McGuire MT, et al.: A descriptive study of individuals successful at long-term maintenance of substantial weight loss. Am J Clin Nutr 66: 239–246, 1997.

347. Lantigua RA, Amatruda JM, Biddle TL, et al.: Cardiac arrhythmias associated with a liquid protein diet for the treatment of obesity. New Engl J Med 303:735–738, 1980.

348. Bogardus C, LaGrange CM, Horton ES, et al.: Comparison of carbohydrate-containing and carbohydrate-restricted hypocaloric diets in the treatment of obesity: Endurance and metabolic fuel homeostasis during strenuous exercise. J Clin Invest 68:399–404, 1981.

349. Phinney SD, Horton ES, Sims EAH, et al.: Capacity for moderate exercise in obese subjects after adaptation to a hypocaloric ketogenic diet. J Clin Invest 66:1152–1161, 1980.

350. Horton ES: Effects of low energy diets on work performance. Am J Clin Nutr 35:1228–1233, 1982.

351. Horton ES: Role and management of exercise in diabetes mellitus. Diabetes Care 11(2):201, 1988.

352. Brownell KD: The Learn Program for Weight Control, Ed. 7. Dallas, TX: American Health Publishing Company, 1997.

353. American College of Sports Medicine: Guidelines for Graded Exercise Testing and Exercise Prescription, Ed. 2. Philadelphia: Lea & Febiger, 1980.

354. Paolone AM: Prescribing exercise programs. In Bove AA, Lowenthal DT (eds.): Exercise Medicine: Physiological Principles and Clinical Applications. New York: Academic Press, 1983, pp. 361–481.

355. Whitehouse FW: Get wise, exercise. Diabetes Forecast, March–April 1978.

356. Flood TM: Ten steps to a successful exercise program. Med Times 108:67–71, 1980.

357. Beeken RK: Initiating exercise programs for patients with non-insulin dependent diabetes. Diabetes Care 3: 627–628, 1980.

358. Orth DN, Jackson RV, DeCherney GS, et al.: Effect of synthetic ovine corticotropin-releasing factor. J Clin Invest 71:587–589, 1983.

359. Grossman A, Neiuwenhuyzen-Kruseman AC, Perry L, et al.: New hypothalamic hormone, corticotropin-releasing factor, specifically stimulates the release of adreno-corticotropin hormone and cortisol in man. Lancet 1: 921–922, 1982.

360. Linton EA, Tilders FJH, Hodgkinson, et al.: Stress-induced secretion of adrenocorticotropin in rats is inhibited by administration of antisera to ovine corticotropin-releasing factor and vasopressin. Endocrinology 116:966–970, 1985.

361. Axelrod J, Reisine TD: Stress hormones: Their interaction and regulation. Science 224:452–459, 1984.

362. Brown MR, Fisher L, Spiess J, et al.: Corticotropin-releasing factor: Actions on the sympathetic nervous system and metabolism. Endocrinology 111:928–931, 1982.

363. Brown M, Fisher L: Corticotropin-releasing factor: Effects on the autonomic nervous system and visceral systems. Fed Proc 44:243–248, 1985.

364. Wexler BC, Dolgin DE, Tryczynski EW: Effects of bacterial polysaccharide (Piromen R) on the pituitary-adrenal axis, adrenal ascorbic acid, cholesterol and histologic alterations. Endocrinology 61:300–308, 1957.

365. Christensen NJ, Alberti KGMM, Brandsborg O: Plasma catecholamines and blood substrate concentrations: Studies in insulin-induced hypoglycemia and after adrenaline infusions. Eur J Clin Invest 5:415–423, 1975.

366. Gerich J, Davis J, Lorenzi M, et al.: Hormonal mechanisms of recovery from insulin-induced hypoglycemia in man. Am J Physiol 236:E380–E385, 1979.

367. Sacca L, Perez G, Carteni G, et al.: Evaluation of the role of the sympathetic nervous system in the glucoregulatory response to insulin-induced hypoglycemia in the rat. Endocrinology 101:1016–1022, 1977.

368. Rizza RA, Cryer PE, Gerich JE: Role of glucagon, catecholamines and growth hormone in human glucose counterregulation. Effects of somatostatin and combined alpha- and beta-adrenergic blockade in plasma glucose recovery and glucose flux rate after insulin-induced hypoglycemia. J Clin Invest 64:62–70, 1979.

369. Gauthier C, Vranic M, Hetenyi G Jr: Importance of glucagon in regulatory rather than emergency responses to hypoglycemia. Am J Physiol 238:E131–E140, 1980.

370. Garber AJ, Karl IE, Kipnis DM: Alanine and glutanine synthesis and release from skeletal muscle. IV. Beta-adrenergic inhibition of amino acid release. J Biol Chem 251:1851–1857, 1976.

371. Goldfien A, Zileli S, Despointes RH, Bethune JE: The effect of hypoglycemia on the adrenal secretion of epinephrine and norepinephrine in the dog. Endocrinology 62:749–757, 1958.

372. Garber AJ, Cryer PE Santiago JV, et al.: The role of adrenergic mechanisms in the substrate and hormonal response to insulin-induced hypoglycemia in man J Clin Invest 8:7–15, 1976.

373. Cryer PE: Glucose counterregulation in man. Diabetes 30:261–264, 1981.

374. Frizzell RT, Hendrick GK, Brown LL, et al.: Stimulation of glucose production through hormone secretion and other mechanisms during insulin-induced hypoglycemia. Diabetes 37:1531–41, 1988.

375. Cryer PE, Tse TF, Clutter WE, Shah SSD: Roles of glucagon and epinephrine in hypoglycemic and nonhy-poglycemic glucose counterregulation in humans. Am J Physiol 247(10):E198–E205, 1984.

376. El-Tayeb K, Brubaker P, Lickley L, et al.: Effects of naloxone on hormonal and metabolic responses to insulin-induced hypoglycemia. Am J Physiol 250: E236–E242, 1986.

377. Nash JA, Radosevich PM, Lacy DB, et al.: Effects of naloxone on glucose homeostasis during insulin-induced hypoglycemia. Am J Physiol 257(20): E367–E373, 1989.

378. Soskin S, Essex H, Herrick J, Mann F: The mechanism of regulation of the blood sugar by the liver. Am J Physiol 124:558–567, 1938.

379. Bolli G, DeFeo P, DeCosmo G, et al.: Role of hepatic autoregulation in defense against hypoglycemia in man. J Clin Invest, 75:1623–1631, 1985.

380. Gardemann A, Jungermann K: Control of glucose balance in the perfused rat liver by the parasympathetic innervation. J Biol Chem, 367:559–566, 1986.

381. Fagius J, Niklassen F, Berne C: Sympathetic outflow in human muscle nerves increases during hypoglycemia. Diabetes, 35:1124–1129, 1986.

382. Sacca L, Cryer PE, Sherwin RS: Blood glucose regulates the effects of insulin and counterregulatory hormones on glucose production in vivo. Diabetes 28: 533–536, 1979.

383. Biggars DW, Myers SR, Neal D, et al.: Role of brain in counterregulatlion of insulin-induced hypoglycemia in dogs. Diabetes, 37:7–16, 1989.

384. Hamilton-Wessler M, Donovan CM, Bergman RN: Role of the liver as a glucose sensor in the integrated response to hypoglycemia (R. Kawamori, E. Horton, M. Vranic editors). In Glucose Fluxes, Exercise and Diabetes (IDF Satellite/Nara), London: Smith-Gordon, 1996, pp. 131–141.

385. Hevener AL, Bergman RN, Donovan CM: Novel glucosensor for hypoglycemic detection localized to the portal vein in the rat. Diabetes 46:1521–1525, 1997.

386. Rizza RA, Haymond MW, Miles JM, et al.: Effect of alpha-adrenergic stimulation and its blockade on glucose turnover in man. Am J Physiol 238:E467–E472, 1980.

387. Gray D, Lickley HLA, Vranic M: Physiologic effects of epinephrine on glucose turnover and plasma FFA concentrations mediated independently of glucagon. Diabetes 29:600–609, 1980.

388. Rizza RA, Verdonk C, Miles J, et al.: Effect of intermittent endogenous hyperglucagonemia on glucose homeostatis in normal and diabetic man. J Clin Invest 63:1119–1123, 1979.

389. Shamoon H, Hendler R, Sherwin R: Altered responsiveness to cortisol, epinephrine and glucagon in insulin-infused juvenile onset diabetics: a mechanism for diabetic instability. Diabetes 29:284–291, 1980.

390. Exton HH, Assimocopoulos-Jeannet FD, Blackmore PF, et al.: Mechanisms of catecholamine action on liver carbohydrate metabolism. Adv Nucleotide Res 9:441–452, 1978.

391. El-Tayeb KMA, Brubaker PL, Vranic M, et al.: Beta-endorphin modulation of the glucoregulatory effects of repeated epinephrine infusion in normal dogs. Diabetes 34:1293–1300, 1985.

392. Sasaki H, Marubashi S, Yawata Y, et al.: Neuropeptides and glucose metabolism. In Cohen MP, Foa PP (eds.): The Brain as an Endocrine Organ, Endocrinology and Metabolism III, Progress in Research and Clinical Practice. New York: Springer-Verlag, 1988, pp.150–192.

393. Miles P, Yamatani K, Lickley HLA, et al.: Mechanism of glucoregulatory responses to stress and their deficiency. Proc Natl Acad Sci USA 88(4):1296–1300, 1991.

394. Miles PDG, Yamatani K, Brown MP, Lickley A, Vranic M: Intracerebroventricular administration of somatostatin octapeptide counteracts the hormonal and metabolic responses to stress in normal and diabetic dogs. Metabolism 43:1134–1143, 1994.

395. Fisher S, Lekas MD, McCall RH, et al.: Determinants of glucose turnover in pathophysiology and diabetes: An in vivo analysis in diabetic dogs. Diabetes Metabol 22: 111–121, 1996.

396. McGuinness OP, Fugiwara T, Murrell S, et al.: Impact of chronic stress hormone infusion on hepatic carbohydrate metabolism in the conscious dog. Am J Physiol (Endocrinol Metab 28) 265:E314–E322, 1993.

397. Rizza RA, Haymond M, Cryer P, et al.: Differential effects of epinephrine on glucose production and disposal in man. Am J Physiol 237:E356–E362, 1979.

398. Goodman, HM: Basic Endocrinology, Ed. 2. Raven Press, New York, 1994.

399. Sigal R, Purdon C, Bilinski D, et al.: Glucoregulation during and after intense exercise: Effects of beta-blockade. J Clin Endocr Metab 78:359–366, 1994.

400. Walaas O, Walaas E: Effect of epinephrine on rat diaphragm. J Biol Chem 187:769–775, 1950.

401. Cherrington AD, Exton JH: Studies on the role of cAMP-dependent protein kinase in the action of glucagon and catecholamines on liver glycogen metabolism. Metabolism 23:729–744, 1976.

402. McPartland RP: Metabolic and pharmacologic actions of glucocorticoids. In Mulrow PJ (ed): The Adrenal Gland, Current Endocrinology: Basic & Clinical Aspects. New York: Elsevier, 1986, pp. 85–116.

403. Himms-Hagen J: Adrenergic receptors for metabolic responses in adipose tissue. Fed Proc 29:1388–1401, 1970.

404. Muller WA, Aoki TT, Egdahl RH, et al.: Effects of exogenous glucagon and epinephrine in physiological amounts on the blood levels of free fatty acids and glycerol in dogs. Diabetologia 13:55–58, 1977.

405. McGarry JD, Foster DW: Hormonal control of ketogenesis. Arch Intern Med 137:485–501, 1977.

406. Liddel MJ, MacLean LD, Shizgal HM: The role of stress hormones in the catabolic metabolism of shock. Surg Gynecol Obstet 149:822–830, 1979.

407. Silverberg AB, Shah SD, Haymond MW, et al.: Norepinephrine: Hormone and neurotransmitter in man. Am J Physiol 234:E252–E256, 1978.

408. Clutter N, Bier D, Shah S, et al.: Epinephrine plasma metabolic clearance rate and physiologic thresholds for metabolic and hemodynamic actions in man. J Clin Invest 66:94–101, 1980.

409. Halter JB, Pflug AE, Porte D Jr: Mechanism of plasma catecholamine increases during surgical stress in man. J Clin Endocrinol Metab 45:936–944, 1977.

410. Cryer PE: Physiology and pathophysiology of the human sympathoadrenal neuroendocrine system. New Engl J Med 303:436–444, 1980.

411. Wilmore DW, Long JM, Mason AD: Catecholamines: mediator of the hypermetabolic response to thermal injury. Ann Surg 180:653–669, 1974.

412. Wolfe RR, Durkot MJ, Allsop JR, et al.: Glucose metabolism in severe burned subjects. Metabolism 28:1031–1039, 1979.

413. Rocha DM, Santeusanio F, Faloona GR, et al.: Abnormal pancreatic alpha-cell function in bacterial infection. New Engl J Med 288:700–703, 1973.

414. Christensen NJ, Videbaek J: Plasma catecholamines and carbohydrate metabolism in subjects with acute myocardial infarction. J Clin Invest 54:278–286, 1974.

415. Clifton GL, Ziegler MG, Grossman RG: Circulating catecholamines and sympathetic activity after head injury. Neurosurgery 8:10–14, 1981.

416. Cannon WB, McIver MA, Bliss SW: Studies on the conditions of activity in endocrine glands. XIII. A sympathetic and adrenal mechanism for mobilizing sugar in hypoglycemia. Am J Physiol 69:46–66, 1924.

417. Houssay BA, Lewis JT, Molinelli EA: Role de la secretion d'adrenaline pendant l'hypoglycemie produite par l'insuline. CR Soc Biol (Paris) 91:1011–1013, 1924.

418. Garber AJ, Cryer PE, Santiago JV, et al.: The role of adrenergic mechanisms in the substrate and hormonal responses to insuin-induced hypoglycemia. J Clin Invest 58:7–15, 1976.

419. Sacca L, Sherwin R, Hendler R, et al.: Influence of continuous physiologic hyperinsulinemia on glucose kinetics and counterregulatory hormones in normal and diabetic humans. J Clin Invest 63:849–857, 1979.

420. Frier BM, Corrall RJM, Ratcliffe JG, et al.: Autonomic neural control mechanisms of substrate and hormonal responses to acute hypoglycemia in man. Clin Endocrinol (Oxford) 14:425–433, 1981.

421. Kemmer FW, Bisbing R, Steingruber J, et al.: Psychological stress and metabolic control in subjects with type 1 diabetes mellitus. New Engl J Med 314:1078–1084, 1986.

422. MacGillivray MH, Bruk E, Voorkess ML: Acute diabetic ketoacidosis in children: Role of the stress hormones. Pediatr Res 15:99–106, 1981.

423. Iversen J: Adrenergic receptors and the secretion of glucagon and insulin from the isolated perfused canine pancreas. J Clin Invest 52:2102–2116, 1973.

424. Samols E, Weir GC: Adrenergic modulation of pancreatic A, B and D cells. J Clin Invest 63:230–238, 1979.

425. Porte D, Graber A, Kuzuya T, et al.: The effects of epinephrine on IRI levels in man. J Clin Invest 45: 228–236, 1966.

426. Gerich JE, Lorenzi M, Tsalikian E, et al.: Studies on the mechanism of epinephrine-induced hyperglycemia in man. Diabetes 25:67–71, 1976.

427. Nakhooda AF, Sole MJ, et al.: Adrenergic regulation of glucagon and insulin secretion during immobilization stress in normal and spontaneously diabetic BB rats. Am J Physiol 240:E373–E378, 1981.

428. Atkinson RL, Kahms WT, Bray GA, et al.: Adrenergic modulation of glucagon and insulin secretion in obese and lean humans. Horm Metab Res 13:249–253, 1981.

429. Kehlet H, Brnadt MR, Rem J: Role of neurologic factors in mediating the endocrine-metabolic response to surgery. J Parent Ent Nutr 4:152–156, 1980.

430. Engquist A, Fog-Moller F, Christiansen C, et al.: Influences of epidural analgesia on the catecholamine and cyclic AMP responses to surgery. Acta Anaesthesiol Scand 24:17–21, 1980.

431. Allsop JR, Wolfe RR, Burke JF: Glucose kinetics and responsiveness to insulin in the rat injured by burn. Surg Gynecol Obstet 147:565–573, 1978.

432. Durkot MJ, Wolfe RR: Effects of adrenergic blockade on glucose kinetics in septic and burned guinea pigs. Am J Physiol 241:R222–R227, 1981.

433. Wolfe RR, Allsop JR, Burke JF: Experimental sepsis and glucose metabolism: Time course of response. Surg Forum 28:42–43, 1977.

434. Long CL, Schiller WR, Geiger JW, et al.: Gluconeogenic response during glucose infusion in subjects following skeletal trauma or during sepsis. J Parent Ent Nutr 2:619–626, 1978.

435. Elwyn DH, Kinney JH, Jeevanandam M, et al.: Influence of increasing carbohydrate intake on glucose kinetics in injured subjects. Am Surg 190:117–127, 1979.

436. Alberti KGMM, Christensen NJ, Iversen J, et al.: Role of glucagon and other hormones in the development of diabetes. Lancet 1:1307–1311, 1975.

437. Garces LY, Kenny FM, Drask A: Cortisol secretion rate in acidotic and non-acidotic juvenile diabetes mellitus. J Pediatr 74:517, 1969.

438. Unger RH, Aquilar-Parado E, Muller WA, et al.: Studies on pancreatic alpha-cell function in normal and diabetic subjects. J Clin Invest 49:837–848, 1970.

439. Waldhausl W, Kleinberger G, Korn A, et al.: Severe hyperglycemia: Effects of rehydration on endocrine derangement and blood glucose concentration. Diabetes 28:577–584, 1979.

440. Schade DS, Eaton RP: The controversy concerning counterregulatory hormone secretion. A hypothesis for the prevention of diabetic ketoacidosis. Diabetes 26:596–599, 1977.

441. Lustman P, Carney R, Amado H: Acute stress and metabolism in diabetes. Diabetes Care 4:568–569, 1981.

442. Lustman PJ, Skor DA, Carney RM, et al.: Stress and diabetic control (letter). Lancet (8324): 588, 1983.

443. Schade DS, Eaton RP: The temporal relationship between endogenously secreted stress hormones and metabolic decompensation in diabetic man. J Clin Endocrinol Metab 50:131–136, 1980.

444. Gerich JE, Langlois M, Noacco C, et al.: Lack of glucagon response to hypoglycemia in diabetes: Evidence for an intrinsic pancreatic alpha-cell defect. Science 182:171–173, 1973.

445. Benson JW Jr, Johnson DG, Palmer JP, et al.: Glucagon and catecholamine secretion during hypoglycemia in normal and diabetic man. J Clin Endocrinol Metab 44:459–464, 1977.

446. Maher TD, Tanenberg RJ, Greenberg BZ, et al.: Lack of glucagon response to hypoglycemia in diabetic autonomic neuropathy. Diabetes 26:196–200, 1977.

447. Bolli G, De Feo P, Campagnucci P, et al.: Abnormal glucose counterregulation in insulin dependant diabetes mellitus: Interaction of anti-insulin antibodies and impaired glucagon and epinephrine secretion. Diabetes 32:134–141, 1983.

448. Cryer PE: Hypoglycemic glucose counterregulation in subjects with insulin dependent diabetes mellitus. J Clin Lab Med 99:451–456, 1982.

449. Papp DA, Shah SD, Cryer PE: The rate of epinephrine mediated beta-adrenergic mechanisms in hypoglycemic glucose counterregulation and posthypoglycemic hyperglycemia in insulin dependent diabetes mellitus. J Clin Invest 69:315–326, 1982.

450. Bolli G, De Feo P, Campagnucci P, et al.: Important role of adrenergic mechanisms in acute glucose counterregulation following insulin-induced hypoglycemia in type 1 diabetes: Evidence for an effect mediated by beta-adrenoreceptors. Diabetes 31:641–647, 1982.

451. Hilstead J, Madsbad S, Krarup T, et al.: Hormonal, metabolic and cardiovascular responses to hypoglycemia in diabetic autonomic neuropathy. Diabetes 30:626–633, 1981.

452. Cryer PE, Gerich JG: Relevance of glucose counterregulatory system to subjects with diabetes. Diabetes Care 6:95, 1983.

453. Lager I, Smith U: Beta-adrenoreceptor blockade and recovery from hypoglycemia in diabetic subjects: Normalization after lactate and glycerol infusions. Clin Sci 62:131–136, 1982.

454. Ganda O, Srikanta S, Gleason, RE, et al.: Diminished A-cell secretion in the early phase of type 1 diabetes mellitus. 35:1074–1077, 1986.

455. Stark AS, Grundy JD, McGarry JD, Unger RH: Correction of hyperglycemia with phlorizon restores the glucagon response to glucose in insulin deficient dogs: implications for human diabetes. Proc Natl Acad Sci USA, 82:1544–1546, 1985.

456. Gerich JE, Lanlois M, Noacco C, et al.: Lack of glucagon response to hypoglycemia in diabetes: Evidence for an intrinsic pancreatic alpha cell defect. Science 182:171–173, 1973.

457. Shi ZQ, Rastogi KS, Lekas M, et al.: Glucagon response to hypoglycemia is improved by insulin-independent restoration of normoglycemia in diabetic rats. Endocrinology 137:3193–3199, 1996.

458. Rastogi KS, Cooper RL, Shi ZQ, Vranic M: Quantitative measurement of islet glucagon response to hyperglycemia by confocal fluorescence imaging in diabetic

rats: Effect of phlorizin treatment. Endocrine 7:367-375, 1997.

459. Rastogi KS, Lickley L, Jokay M, et al.: Paradoxical reduction in pancreatic glucagon with normalization of somatostatin, decrease in insulin in normoglycemic alloxan diabetic dogs: a putative mechanism of glucagon irresponsiveness to hypoglycemia. Endocrinology 126:1096–1104, 1990.

460. Rastogi KS, Brubaker PL, Kawasaki A, et al.: Increase in somatostatin to glucagon ratio in islet of alloxan-diabetic dogs. Can J Physiol Pharmacol 71:512–517, 1993.

461. Vranic M, Pek S, Kawamori B: Increased "glucagon immunoreativity" in plasma of totally depancreatized dogs. Diabetes 23:905–912, 1974.

462. Doi K, Prentki M, Yip C, et al.: Identical biological effects of pancreatic glucagon and a purified moiety of canine gastric glucagon. J Clin Invest 63:525–531, 1979.

463. Perez G, Kemmer FW, Lickley HLA, Vranic M: Importance of glucagon in mediating epinephrine-induced hyperglycemia in alloxan-diabetic dogs. Am J Physiol 241:E328–E335, 1981.

464. Kemmer FW, Lickley HLA, Gray DE, et al.: The state of metabolic control determines the role of epinephrine-glucagon interactions of glucoregulation in diabetes. Am J Physiol 242:E428–E436, 1982.

465. Lickley HLA, Kemmer FW, Doi K, Vranic M: Glucagon suppression improves glucoregulation in moderate but not chronic severe diabetes. Am J Physiol 245: E424–E429, 1983.

466. El-Tayeb KMA, Brubaker PL, Vranic M, Lickley HLA: Beta endorphin modulation of the glucoregulatory effects of repeated epinephrine infusion in normal dogs. Diabetes, 34:1293–1300, 1985.

467. El-Tayeb KMA, Vranic M, Brubaker PL, et al.: Beta-endorphin modulation of the glucoregulatory effects of epinephrine infusion in alloxan diabetic and normal dogs. Diabetologia 30:745–754, 1987.

468. Rashid S, Niwa M, Van Delangeryt M, et al.: Improvement of impaired glucose clearance during stress in diabetes with hyperinsulinemia or beta-blockade. Diabetes 46(Suppl. 1): 230A(Abstract) #0881, 1997.

469. The DTCC Research Group: The Diabetes Control and Complications Trial (DCTT): Design and methodologic considerations for the feasibility phase. Diabetes 35: 530–545, 1986.

470. Vranic M: Glucose turnover: a key to understanding the pathogenesis of diabetes. Indirect effects of insulin. The Banting Lecture. Diabetes 41:1188–1206, 1992.

471. Gann DS, Amaral JF: Endocrine and metabolic responses to injury. In Schwartz DS (ed.): Principles of Surgery, Ed. 5. New York: McGraw-Hill, 1989, pp. 3–68.

472. Hume DM, Egdahl RH: The importance of the brain in the neuroendocrine response to surgery. Ann Surg 150:697, 1959.

473. Hume DM, Bell CL, Bartter FC: Direct measurement of adrenal secretion during operative trauma and convalescence. Surgery 52:174, 1962.

474. Galloway JA, Shuman CR: Diabetes and surgery. Am J Med 34:177–191, 1963.

475. Husband DV, Thai AC, Alberti KGMM: Management of diabetes during surgery with glucose-insulin-potassium solution. Diabetic Med 3:69–74, 1986.

476. Page MMB, Watkins, PJ: Cardiorespiratory arrest with diabetic autonomic neuropathy. Lancet 1:14, 1978.

477. Axelrod J, Reisine TD: Stress hormones: Their interaction and regulation. Science 224:452–459, 1984.

478. Watson BG, Elliott MJ, Pay DA, Williamson M: Diabetes mellitus and open heart surgery. Anaesthesia 41: 250–257, 1986.

479. Crock PA, Ley CJ, Martin IK, et al.: Hormonal and metabolic changes during hypothermic coronary artery bypass surgery in diabetic and non-diabetic subjects. Diabetic Med 5:47–52, 1987.

480. Fraser CL, Arieff AI: Fatal central diabetes mellitus and insipidus resulting from untreated hyponatremia: a new syndrome. Ann Intern Med 112:113–119, 1990.

18

Insulin Therapy

John K. Davidson, James H.J. Anderson Jr., and Ronald E. Chance

Historical Perspective

De Mayer coined the French word *insuline* in 1909 and Sharpey-Schafer the English word *insulin* in 1916. The dramatic events of 1921–1922 in Toronto are described by Dr. Barbara Hazlett in Chapter 1. The discovery (Fig. 18–1)[1] and clinical use of the hormone saved the lives of many with type 1 diabetes mellitus (IDDM) and converted them from almost moribund children to healthy young individuals (Figs. 18–2 and 18–3).[2–9] This initiated a series of clinical, physiologic, pharmacologic, and pathologic research programs that have intensified during the last three decades. Since its discovery, over 200,000 scientific papers have been published on insulin and related matters, and eleven persons have received Nobel prizes for insulin-related research (Table 18–1). Although the precise number of individuals with diabetes is not known, it is estimated from available data[10] that worldwide at least 25 million individuals with IDDM depend for their lives on the continuing availability of insulin.

In an article that was published shortly after his sudden death on July 8, 1998, Dr. Geza Hetenyi reflected on the continuing controversies and changes in published beliefs of some contemporary historians about who deserves credit for the discovery of insulin. He concluded that *the discoverers* were obviously Banting and Best, while Collip and MacLeod in the early days after the discovery played significant roles in the development and production of insulin for *clinical use*. (Figure 18–3). Fred Banting in his lecture accepting the Cameron Prize of 1928 from the University of Edinburgh stated "I am fully aware that this award is also meant to include the group of workers who were closely associated with the development of insulin, and without whose whole-hearted assistance the work could not have been done. The chief among these was Dr. Charles Herbert Best." Thus almost from the beginning in 1921, the *discovery* and *clinical use* of insulin was a *team effort*. Progressively increasing numbers of individuals contributed knowledge as time passed. By 1999

thousands of scientists are involved in research on the nature and treatment of diabetes mellitus with insulin.

The discovery of insulin made it necessary to devise methods for assessing its activity. Banting, Best, Collip, Macleod, and Noble (1922)[11] found that insulin-induced convulsions in rabbits were associated with a blood

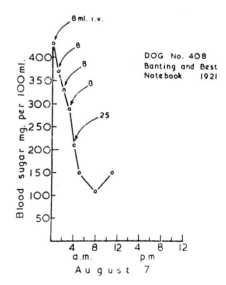

EFFECT OF INJECTION OF EXTRACT OF PANCREAS ON BLOOD SUGAR OF DEPANCREATIZED DOG

SALINE EXTRACT OF DEGENERATED PANCREAS

DOG No. 408
Banting and Best
Notebook 1921

Figure 18–1. Early graph of the effect of injection of a cold saline extract made from dog pancreas removed after the pancreatic duct had been ligated and the pancreas had degenerated. The dog into which the injections were made was rendered diabetic by removal of its pancreas. Its blood sugar when injections began, 430 mg/dL, was greatly above normal. The moment of each injection is indicated by an arrow. The time scale is along the bottom line. The blood sugar fell to normal within 8 hr. [*Source:* Wrenshall GA, Hetenyi G, Feasby WR (eds): The Story of Insulin: Forty Years of Success Against Diabetes. Toronto: Max Reinhardt, 1962. With permission.]

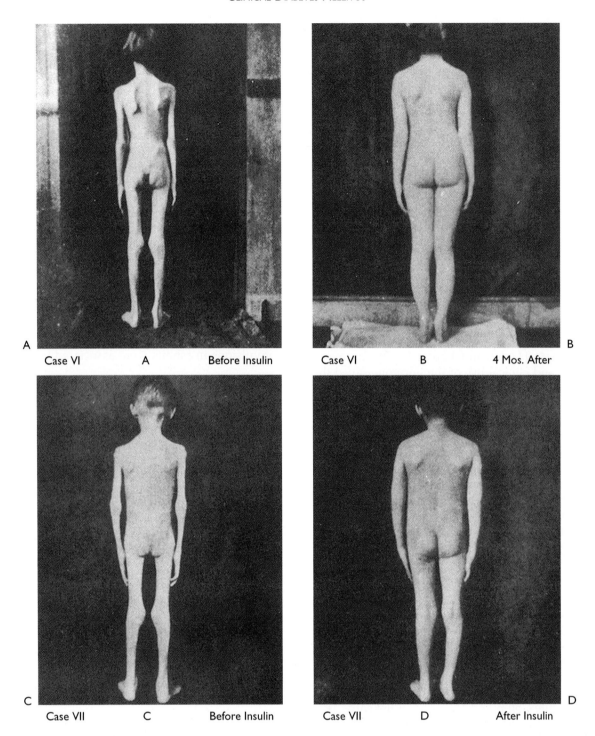

Case VI   A   Before Insulin   Case VI   B   4 Mos. After

Case VII   C   Before Insulin   Case VII   D   After Insulin

Figure 18–2. A,B. A diabetic girl (top) before and 4 months after initiation of insulin therapy in 1922. C,D. A diabetic boy (bottom) before and after initiation of insulin therapy in 1922. [*Sources:* Geyelin HK, Harrop G, Murray MF, et al.: The use of insulin in juvenile diabetes. J Metab Res, November 1922, pp. 767–792; Wrenshall GA, Hetenyi G, Feasby WR (eds): The Story of Insulin: Forty Years of Success Against Diabetes. Toronto: Max Reinhardt, 1962. With permission.]

sugar concentration of 45 mg/dL or less. The amount of insulin that lowered the blood sugar to this level in 2 to 4 hr was used as a unit of activity (the rabbit unit). Later (League of Nations, 1926),[12] the *unit* was defined as *one-third the amount of insulin required to lower the blood sugar in a rabbit starved for 24 hr to 45 mg/dL within 5 hr after injection.* The first international standard for insulin con-

tained 8 U of insulin activity per milligram of dry powder. Since 1925 all preparations of insulin have been assayed directly or indirectly in terms of the first international standard. The second international standard (1935) contained 22 U/mg, the third international standard (1952) contained 24.5 U/mg, and the fourth international standard (1958) contained 24.0 U/mg

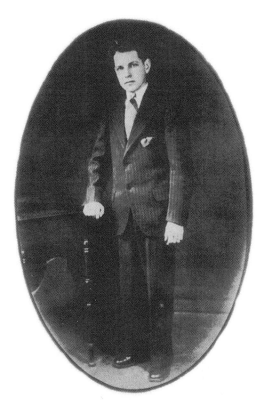

Figure 18–3. Leonard Thompson, who received his first insulin injection (preparation of Banting and Best) on January 11, 1922, and a more potent pancreatic extract (preparation of Collip) on January 23, 1922. The second extract lowered the blood sugar from 520 to 120 mg/dL by the next day and ketonuria disappeared. This picture was taken some years later and is reproduced from the cover of the *University of Toronto Medical Journal.*[4] Thompson died of pneumonia complicated by severe diabetic ketoacidosis on April 20, 1935, age 27 years. (*Sources:* Bliss M: The Discovery of Insulin, Toronto: McClelland and Stewart, 1982, pp. 112–113, 120–121, 242–243; Burrow GN, Hazlett BE, Phillips MS: A case of diabetes mellitus. N Engl J Med 306:340–343, 1982. With permission.)

(52% beef insulin, 48% pork insulin). The first three standards were dry powder, the fourth contained 5.56% water. The fourth international standard contained 25.36 U/mg when completely dry.

The international standard became a reference material for assaying the potency of unknown materials until 1985. Either the international standard, or a local standard carefully calibrated against it, were used in four-point parallel slope assays [blood sugar lowering in rabbits or convulsions in mice to measure the potency, which the United States Pharmacopeia (USP) required be within 95 to 105% of the potency stated on the labels of the marketed products].[12,13]

In 1985, an agreement was reached between the Food and Drug Administration (FDA), the USP, and insulin manufacturers to supply bulk quantities of purified standards to the USP. In 1999, beef, pork, and human insulin standards are supplied by Eli Lilly to all companies marketing insulin in the United States. This

permits all companies marketing insulin in the United States to establish the *bioidentity* of their master lots of insulin according to the *USP method* [USP 23 NF 18, the United States Pharmacopeia, the National Formulary, (121) insulin assay, second supplement United States Pharmacopeial Convention, Inc., Rockville, MD, 1999]. In addition, these insulin standards are used to determine the *actual potency* of batches of insulin by *high-performance* liquid chromatography.[13]

Since 1991, the potency of human and animal (pork, beef) insulins have been determined by chemical identity and weight based on high-pressure liquid chromatography (HPLC) measurement. In 1999 one-milligram human insulin RDNA contains 28.7 units.[13]

In the 1950s, attempts to measure insulin activity in blood serum were begun using mice with endocrine alterations (in vivo) and tissues surgically removed from animals and incubated in vitro. Hypophysectomized alloxan-diabetic mice (Anderson, 1957) and adrenalectomized alloxan-diabetic mice (Baird, 1959) were used, but the difficulty of preparing and maintaining the animals made studies of this sort impractical. In vitro bioassay techniques used various metabolic responses to insulin by muscle (diaphragm of rats and mice) and by adipose tissue (epididymal fat pad and isolated fat cells of rats) to estimate the level of insulin activity in serum. These metabolic parameters included glucose uptake by rat diaphragm (Groen, 1952; Vallance-Owen, 1954), and mouse diaphragm (Oyama, 1960), incorporation of ^{14}C glycine into diaphragm protein (Manchester, 1959), and glycogen synthesis by mouse diaphragm (Wardlaw, 1961). Glycogen synthesis in muscle (mouse diaphragm) was shown to be the in vitro assay with the highest specificity for insulin in serum. Glycogen synthesis is also stimulated by non-suppressible insulinlike activity, [NSILA, subsequently designated somatomedins C and A, or insulinlike growth factors 1 and 2 (IGF-1, IGF-2), respectively] and by an increase in the glucose level in the medium, but it is not affected by normal levels of other serum factors.[14]

The raising of insulin-binding antibodies in the serum of immunized guinea pigs (beef insulin in Freund's complete adjuvant)[15] and the labeling of insulin with the gamma-emitting tracer[131] I led to the development of the first radioimmunoassay (RIA) for insulin.[16,17] This procedure made it possible to measure as little as 2 to 3 µU insulin per milliliter of serum (12 to 18 pM—Exhibit 18–1), and to measure changes in endogenous insulin levels after stimulants or depressants to endogenous insulin secretion had been applied. Insulin assays and other procedures designed to evaluate metabolic perturbations in humans and in experimental animals have been responsible for greatly expanding knowledge of the pathophysiology of IDDM, non-insulin-dependent diabetes mellitus (NIDDM), insulinomas, and other related problems during the last 40 years.

TABLE 18–1   Nobel Prize Winners for Insulin-Related Research

Name	Country	Year	Category of Award	Nature of Research
		Prizes related directly to insulin		
Banting, Frederick G.	Canada	1923	Physiology-medicine	Discovery of insulin
Macleod, John J.R.	Canada	1923	Physiology-medicine	Discovery of insulin
Sanger, Frederick	Great Britain	1958	Chemistry	Amino acid sequence of insulin
Hodgkin, Dorothy C.	Great Britain	1964	Chemistry	X-ray crystallographic analysis of insulin and other biologically active molecules
Yalow, Rosalyn S.	United States	1977	Physiology-medicine	Radioimmunoassay of insulin and other hormones
		Prizes related to metabolic activities influenced by insulin		
Cori, Carl F.	United States	1947	Physiology-medicine	How glycogen is catalytically converted
Cori, Gerty T.	United States	1947	Physiology-medicine	How glycogen is catalytically converted
Houssay, Bernardo A.	Argentina	1947	Physiology-medicine	Role of pituitary hormones in sugar metabolism
Leloir, Luis F.	Argentina	1970	Chemistry	Mechanisms of glycogen formation
Sutherland, Earl W	United States	1971	Physiology-medicine	Discovery of cyclic adenosine monophosphate and its function in sugar metabolism
Rodbell, Martin	United States	1994	Physiology-medicine	Discovery of G-proteins and their relationships to intracellular cascading actions of insulin

Until 1983, the main sources of insulin were the cow (about 70%) and the pig (about 30%). Cow insulin is also designated as beef, bovine, and ox insulin, and pig insulin is designated as porcine insulin. Sheep, fish (bonito), and whale have provided small amounts of insulin from time to time in the past. Insulin was crystallized in 1926 by Abel[18] and shown to be protein in nature. Until the early 1970s commercial insulin was prepared by repeated crystallization. It is now known that these preparations contained up to 5% proinsulin, as well as proinsulin-insulin conversion intermediates, connecting peptide (C-peptide), glucagon, vasoactive intestinal polypeptide (VIP), pancreatic polypeptide (PP), and somatostatin, all of which contaminated conventionally crystallized insulin (Fig. 18–4).[19]

The use of sophisticated protein separation techniques [Sephadex and diethylaminoethyl (DEAE) cellulose columns, high-performance liquid chromatography (HPLC), and so forth] permitted the removal of contaminants and the preparation of highly purified animal insulins that contained less than 0.001% proinsulin.

Sanger described the primary structure of insulin from the cow in 1953.[20] The structure of human insulin (Fig. 18–5) was reported by Nichol and Smith in 1960,[21] and the structures of more than 80 other insulins became known from then until now (Table 18–2).[22–24]

In 1963–1965, three groups (Zahn's group in Aachen, Germany, the Shanghai Insulin Research Group, and the group of Katsoyannis at the University of Pittsburgh) reported the organic chemical synthesis of insulin.[25] Although this approach was cumbersome and expensive, and provided yields that were too low to be of commercial importance,[26] it provided techniques that led to the ability to modify chemically and synthesize insulin and its analogs and derivatives. It then became possible to determine the biologic and immunologic activities of these peptides.[27]

The structure of connecting peptides (Table 18–3), proinsulins (Fig. 18–5), and preproinsulins (Table 18–4)[28–31] from a number of animal species are now known. Using human insulin as the reference standard, only 21 of 51 amino acids in insulin (41%) are invariant (11 of 21 in the A chain and 10 of 30 in the B chain). None of the 31 in the C-peptide (0%) and only 4 of 24 in the proinsulin prepeptide (17%) are invariant.

Structural differences largely account for the antigenicity of one animal's insulin when it is injected into an animal of a different species.[32] Also, the immune response to insulin is under genetic control.[33] Other potential antigens in commercial animal insulins include insulin derivatives, proinsulin and its intermediates, glucagon, somatostatin, PP, VIP, protamine, and other contaminants[19] (See Fig. 18–4). It has been shown that regular crystalline insulin is less immunogenic in a subcutaneous repository form than are neutral protamine Hagedorn (NPH) and lente insulins,[34,35] and that sulfated beef insulin (no longer available) is less immunogenic than lente beef insulin.[36] It is possible that noninsulin substances in insulin preparations increase the antigenicity of insulin by an adjuvant effect.

EXHIBIT 18–1 Diagnostic Applications for Assays for Insulin, Insulin Receptor, Connecting Peptide (C-Peptide), Proinsulin, Glucagon, Insulin-Like-Growth Factors (IGF-1, IGF-2), and Somatostatin and Other Gastroenteropancreatic Hormones

I. Insulin Assays

The fourth international standard for insulin (52% beef, 48% pork) contains 25.36 U/mg dry powder, or 1 U/0.04167 mg (1 mU = 0.04167 μg, 1 μU = 0.04167 ng. rDNA human insulin contains 28.7 mg, or 1 U/0.0348 mg (1 mU = 0.0348 μg, 1 μU = 0.0348 ng).

Peripheral serum insulin in the fasting state usually ranges in nondiabetics from 4 to 24 μU/ml serum (24–144 pM), but varies with the specificity of the assay (in some assays up to 30% of the immunoreactive "insulin" measured is actually proinsulin). Insulin levels in portal venous blood serum and pancreatic venous blood serum are much higher in nondiabetic animals.

Insulin in peripheral serum in easily measured (in those who have not been treated with exogenous insulin) by a radioimmunoassay technique, preferably utilizing monoiodinated A-14 tyrosine species-specific insulin (i.e., ^{125}I-labeled plus unlabeled rDNA human insulin plus antibodies to human insulin when human serum samples are being assayed).

Radioimmuno assays (RIAs) are based on the principles of competitive protein-binding in which fixed amounts of tracer (such as I^{125}-labeled insulin) and antiserum to insulin are added simultaneously to tubes containing standard amounts of insulin or serum containing unknown amounts of insulin and other materials. Immunometric assays [immunoradiometric assays (IRMAs) and immunochemiluminometric assays (ICMAs)] utilize two or more antisera that recognize epitopes (different segments of proteins) that are present in the anylate. *IRMA* reporters are labeled with radioactive iodine, and *ICMAs* detect a particular wavelength of light. ICMAs avoid radioactive exposure and disposal, are less costly, more precise, and easy to perform (results can be available in 20 minutes if necessary).[91]

In those who have been treated with exogenous insulin, antibody-bound insulin may be precipitated by polyethylene glycol (PEG)[90] and "free" insulin measured in the supernate by radioimmunoassay (RIA). The antibody-bound insulin may be liberated by acid-alcohol extraction,[92] and the "total" insulin measured by RIA. Antibody-bound insulin may be calculated by subtracting "free" from "total" insulin. Alternatively, serum may be treated with hydrochloric acid to free antibody-bound insulin, antibody precipitated with PEG, and supernatant insulin measured, with *bound insulin* being the difference between "free" and "total" insulin corrected for recovery and assay variability.[74]

Similar measurements may be done using glycogen content of mouse hemidiaphragm as the in vitro indicator of insulin action,[14] but this in vitro bioassay is more expensive and cumbersome. Now it is seldom used unless one wishes to measure insulin's biologic activity rather than its immunologic activity.

The clinical utility of insulin assays is now essentially limited to evaluating fasting hypoglycemic states, especially insulinomas (see Fig. 18–11). Insulin assays in those not treated with insulin have some utility in differentiating those with IDDM (serum insulin absent or low) from those with NIDDM (serum insulin low, normal, or high). See Fig. 18–12. C-peptide assays have essentially replaced the insulin assay in evaluating insulin secretion levels fasting, after stimulation (Sustacal, glucagon, glucose, protein meal, leucine, and so on) and after suppression (0.1 U insulin/kg IV with hypoglycemia maintained for 1 hr with serial C-peptide measurements). Diagnosis of insulinoma requires demonstration of: (1) hypoglycemic attacks during fasting of up to 72 hr [measure immunoreactive insulin (IRI), C-peptide, and plasma glucose (PG) levels every 6 hr]; (2) PG <2.5 mM (<45 mg/dL) during attack; and (3) prompt relief of symptoms by administration of glucose. These three phenomena are known as *Whipple's triad.*

In normal individuals, serum insulin falls to undetectable levels during a 72-hour fast, but they remain above the 36 to 60 pM (6 to 10 μU/mL of serum) range (depending on the assay used) in those with an insulinoma when the venous PG falls below 2.2 mM (40 mg/dL). C-peptide and proinsulin assays are also of value in diagnosis of insulinoma (C-peptide increased, ratio of proinsulin to insulin may be increased). The presence and location of an insulinoma can be confirmed prior to surgical removal in 80% of patients by selective celiac angiography. Computed tomography scan may be helpful.

Since stimulation-of-insulin-secretion tests (glucagon, tolbutamide, leucine) produce many false-positive and many false-negative in those with insulinomas, and may be dangerous because of induced severe hypoglycemia, they are no longer used.

II. *Radio Receptor Assays (RRAs)* measure the interaction of a ligand (such as insulin) with biological receptors (such as the cellular insulin receptor), that mediates the actions of the hormone. Target tissues or clonal cell lines are widely used to characterize the properties of receptors. RRAs have been used to measure autoantibodies to cell receptors. Autoantibodies to the insulin receptor can mimic the effects of insulin and cause hypoglycemia, or block the effects of insulin and cause hyperglycemia.[93,94]

III. Connecting Peptide (C-Peptide) Assays

C-peptide is produced in equimolar concentrations with insulin during conversion of proinsulin to insulin. When insulin antibodies in the circulation prevent accurate assessment of insulin levels by the standard insulin immunoassay (as in IDDMs who have been treated with beef or pork insulin), C-peptide levels are clinically useful in assessing pancreatic islet beta cell secretory activity (fasting and after stimulation with Sustacal, IV glucose, or 1 mg glucagon subcutaneously). C-peptide in IDDMs may be

(continued next page)

EXHIBIT 18–1 *(continued)*　Diagnostic Applications for Assays for Insulin, Insulin Receptor, Connecting Peptide (C-Peptide), Proinsulin, Glucagon, Insulin-Like-Growth Factors (IGF-1, IGF-2), and Somatostatin and Other Gastroenteropancreatic Hormones

undetectable but also may overlap levels in normals and in NIDDMs. A fasting value below 0.33 pmol/mL (1.00 ng/mL) and a glucagon-stimulated value below 0.49 pmol/mL (1.48 ng/mL) has been suggested as the highest levels to be accepted for those to be classified as IDDMs, with those who have higher C-peptide levels in the presence of diabetes being classified as NIDDMs (fasting greater than 0.33 pmol/mL or 1.0 ng/mL, stimulated greater than 0.49 pmol/mL or 1.48 ng/mL). The Diabetes Control and Complications Trial (DCCT) required a fasting level of less than 0.2 pmol/mL (<0.6 ng/mL) and a 90-minute Sustacal-stimulated level less than 0.5 pmol/mL (<1.5 ng/mL) to distinguish IDDM from NIDDM. Levels in nondiabetic normal individuals vary, *fasting* from 0.4 to 1.6 pmol/mL (1.2 to 4.8 ng/mL). *Sustacal-stimulated* from 0.4 to 12 pmol/mL (1.2 to 36 ng/mL).[113] Many NIDDMs have high normal levels fasting, especially in the presence of modest hyperglycemia and obesity, but nearly all have a subnormal C-peptide response to Sustacal, 30 g IV glucose, and 1 mg glucagon subcutaneously.

In normals, insulin-induced hypoglycemia (0.1 U/kg body weight IV) for 1 hr results in suppression of C-peptide levels to less than 0.4 pmol/mL (1.2 ng/mL) serum.[91] Some insulinoma patients have undetectable or low C-peptide levels initially, whereas some other insulinoma patients do not suppress their C-peptide levels below 0.63 pmol/mL (1.9 ng/mL). In other words, despite 1 hr of insulin-induced hypoglycemia which suppresses C-peptide levels to <0.4 pmol/mL (<1.2 ng/mL in normals), in some insulinoma patients serum C-peptide levels remain ≤0.66 pmol/mL (≤2.0 ng/mL).

Also, the C-peptide assay may be of value in assessing the level of insulin secretion[113] in diabetic ketoacidosis (absent or decreased) stable IDDM (usually decreased but not absent), unstable IDDM (usually absent or decreased), and NIDDM (usually normal or increased fasting, decreased stimulated). it is of value in follow-up of a patient after *complete pancreatectomy* (absent), *partial pancreatectomy* (normal or decreased), the remission or "honeymoon" phase of IDDM (near-normal or normal fasting, decreased stimulated), hypoglycemia with spontaneously developed insulin antibodies (decreased), and in detecting individuals who are surreptitiously (factitiously) injecting insulin (absent with elevated insulin levels plus hypoglycemia).[113]

Reported mean 24-hr urine C-peptide levels in normal individuals have ranged from 36 to 65 μg (11.9 to 21 nmol).[95] There is a good correlation between normal and low serum and urine C-peptide levels. Urine C-peptide levels may be determined noninvasively and may be monitored sequentially over time during various physiologic states, such as after fasting and after stimulation with carbohydrate, protein, a mixed meal, or Sustacal (usually 12 oz

containing 350 calories, 48 g carbohydrate, 21 g protein, and 8 g fat). B-cell reserve mg be evaluated after stimulation with oral prednisone.[95]

IV. Proinsulin Assays

Older proinsulin assays (column chromatography plus enzyme degradation) have been replaced by new methods utilizing antibodies that measure human proinsulin specifically and monoclonal antibodies that are directed either at the antigenic site connecting the B-chain and C-peptide or at the antigenic site connecting the A-chain and C-peptide. Mean normal levels (in fmol/mL) are: *fasting*, lean 2.7, obese 4.7; *after glucose*, lean 10.7, obese 23. The mean level in a group of insulinoma patients was 151 (range, 17 to 600). There is a disproportionate increase in the proinsulin level in NIDDM and after glucocorticoid administration. Depending on the method of analysis, 10 to 30% of the insulin immunoreactive material fasting is proinsulin, but the percent decreases in the fed state.[113]

Human proinsulin has about 10% of the biologic activity of insulin, but clinical research on its effects was put on hold because an increased incidence of myocardial infarction that occurred in one study group.[102] Six mutations have been reported in the structural gene for proinsulin. Three consist of alterations in the alpha and the beta chains that impair binding of the peptide to its receptor; the other mutations affect the processing of proinsulin. All subjects had hyperinsulinemia but little impairment of glucose homeostasis.

V. Glucagon Assays

Plasma glucagon is heterogenous and consists of four fractions: (1) immunoreactive glucagon (IRG), the physiologically important molecule secreted by the pancreatic islet alpha cells, 3,500 daltons, which for accurate measurement requires a specific antibody that reacts only with the C-terminal part of the glucagon molecule, since nonspecific antibodies react with both N-terminal and C-terminal ends of IRG; (2) glucagon-like immunoactivity (GLI) is gut-derived and reacts with antibody directed toward the N-terminal part of glucagon. The four fractions of glucagon in the serum weigh 160,000, 9,000, 3,500, and 2,000 daltons.[97,98]

The IRG level in serum of healthy fasting individuals is 50 to 150 ng/L (50 to 150 pg/ml) serum (46%, 3,500 daltons; 54%, 160,000 daltons). In normal individuals during hypoglycemia there is a two- to threefold rise; during hyperglycemia there is a fall to about half the fasting level. In renal failure the 9,000-dalton fraction increases fivefold. In alpha cell tumors (glucagonoma), which are characterized by a migrating necrotizing skin rash, stomatitis, glossitis, and anemia (two-thirds of which have metastasized at time of diagnosis), the IRG level is 700 to 7,800 pg/ml serum [700 to 7,800 ng/L (700 to 7,800 pg/ml.)] (See Chapter 46.)

Familial (autosomal-dominant) hyperglucagonemia (9,000-dalton component) has been described.

EXHIBIT 18–1 *(continued)* Diagnostic Applications for Assays for Insulin, Insulin Receptor, Connecting Peptide (C-Peptide), Proinsulin, Glucagon, Insulin-Like-Growth Factors (IGF-1, IGF-2), and Somatostatin and Other Gastroenteropancreatic Hormones

In satisfactorily controlled IDDM, the IRG level is within the normal range, but in uncontrolled hyperglycemia and in diabetic ketoacidosis the IRG does not decrease appropriately in response to the hyperglycemia as it does in normal subjects. There is also an exaggerated response of IRG to stimuli such as protein loading in those with diabetes. After 5 years or more of IDDM, IRG does not rise appropriately in response to insulin-induced hypoglycemia.

VI. Insulin-like Growth Factors (IGF-1, IGF-2)
Normal levels of insulin-like growth factor-1 (IGF-1 or somatomedin-C) are: adult women 0.45–2.2KU/L, adult men, 0.34–1.9KU/L. At puberty, levels are 2–3 times as high as adult levels. IGF-1 is a basic peptide of 70 amino acids and IGF-2 is a slightly acidic peptide of 67 amino acids. The two peptides share 45 of 75 possible amino acid positions and have approximately 50% amino acid homology to insulin. This structural similarity explains the ability of IGF-1 and IGF-2 to bind to the insulin receptor, and of insulin to bind to the IGF-1 receptor. Conversely, the structural differences explain why insulin *does not bind* to IGF-binding proteins (IGFBPs), of which there are six. There are several variants of the IGF-peptides. *BIG IGF-2* may be produced by Mesenchymal Tumors that may produce hypoglycemia that disappears when the tumor is removed.[97b]

VII. Somatostatin
This tetradecapeptide is produced by the delta cells of the pancreatic islets, the hypothalamus, gastric mucosa, and intestine, but it cannot be detected in circulating blood. When injected IV it has a half-life of only 1 min. It acts on endocrine tissue as a local modulator in suppressing insulin, glucagon, growth hormone, thyrotropin, gastrin, secretin, and vasointestinal peptide secretion, and on nonendocrine tissue by suppressing gastric acid secretion and gastric emptying, gallbladder contraction, pancreatic bicarbonate and pancreatic enzyme release, and acetylcholine release from peripheral nerve endings.

A few somatostatin-producing delta cell pancreatic tumors have been described (malabsorption, achlorhydria, hyperglycemia, hypoglucagonemia). Somatostatin in these tumors is measured by RIA.

The hypothalamus and the pituitary gland are central to an understanding of the regulation of growth. The pulsatile pattern characteristic of growth hormone (GH) secretions reflects the interplay of two hypothalamic regulatory peptides [GH-releasing hormone (GHRH) and somatostatin]. The pulsatile secretion of GH results from a simultaneous reduction in hypothalamic somatostatin release and increase in GHRH. The synthesis and secretion of GH are regulated also by insulin-like growth factors (IGFs).

The somatostatin analogue SMS 201-995 inhibits gastrointestinal secretion [serotonin, vasoactive intestinal peptide (VIP), pancreatic polypeptide (PP), gastrin, glucagon, insulin, secretin, motilin]. It has been used to treat acromegaly, carcinoid syndrome, glucagonoma, insulin-secreting tumors, VIPomas, and Zollinger-Ellison syndrome. Experiments have shown that the secretion of islet amyloid polypeptide (amylin), which has been proposed as a hormone related to beta cell function and possibly to the pathogenesis of NIDDM, is inhibited by SMS 201-995.

VIII. Non-insulin-secreting tumors of the gastroentropancreatic system
The gastroentropancreatic system of clear cells produce more than 30 known hormones or hormone-like peptides. These presumably neuroendocrine cells have many physiologic functions. They rarely produce tumors [examples: Gastrinomas (Zollinger-Ellison Syndrome) 1 per 2 million persons per year, VI Pomas 1 per 10 million per year, Glucagonomas 1 per 20 million per year, somatostatinomas 1 per 40 million per year.] Pancreatic endocrine tumors, can be a part of the syndrome of multiple endocrine neoplasia type 1 (men 1). Other tumors that may originate from clear cells are: Pancreatic polypeptide secreting-tumor (PPOMA), Neurotensinoma, Parathyroid hormone-related protein (PTHRP) tumor, corticotropinoma, growth hormone releasing hormone (GHRH)-secreting tumors. Immuno Assays are available to measure serum and extractable hormone levels in these tumors.[97a,97b]

[*Sources:* Davidson JK, Haist RE, Best CH: Studies employing a new method for recovery of biologically active insulin from acid alcoholic extracts of pancreas and blood serum. Diabetes 12:448–453,1963; Desbuquois B, Arbach GD: Use of polyethylene glycol to separate free and antibody-bound hormones in radloimmunoassay. J Clin Endocrinol Metab 33:732–738, 1971; Hoogwerf BJ, Goetz FC: Urinary C-peptide: a simple measure of integrated insulin production with emphasis on the effects of body size, diet, and corticosteroids. J Clin Endocrinol Metab 56:60–67, 1983; Howanitz PJ, Howanitz JH; Carbohydrates: pancreatic hormones, insulinoma. *In* Henry JB (ed): Todd-Sanford-Davidsohn's Clinical Diagnosis and Management by Laboratory Methods, Ed. 17. Philadelphia: W. B. Saunders, 1984. pp. 165–172; Kuzuya H, Blix PM, Horwitz DL, et al.: Determination of free and total insulin and C-peptide in insulin-treated diabetics. Diabetes 26:22–29, 1977; Lehmann HP, Henry JB: SI units (International System of Units). *In* Henry JB (ed): Todd-Sanford-Davidsohn's Clinical Diagnosis and Management by Laboratory Methods, Ed. 17. Philadelphia: W. B. Saunders, 1984, pp. 1429, 1434; Perry-Keene DA, Alford FP, Chisholm DJ, et al.: Glucagon and diabetes. Clin Endocrinol 6:417–423, 1977; Service FJ, Horwitz DL, Rubenstein AH, et al.: C-peptide suppression test for insulinoma. J Lab Clin Med 90:180–186, 1977; Sperling MA.. Insulin biosynthesis and C-peptide. Am J Dis Child 134:1119–1121, 1980; Unger RH, Orci L: The role of glucagon in diabetes. Diabetes 8:53–68,1982; Yalow RS, Berson SA: Dynamics of insulin secretion in hypoglycemia. Diabetes 14:341–349,1965. Mitsukawa T, Takemura J, Asai J, Nakazato M, Kangawa K, Matsou H, Matsukura S: Islet amyloid polypeptide response to glucose, insulin, and somatostatin analogue administration. Diabetes 39:639–642, 1990. With permission.] Krejs GR: Non-insulin secreting tumors of the gastroenteropancreatic system in Williams textbook of Endocrinology, 9th Ed: Wilson J, Foster D, Kronenberg H, Larsen R (eds), pp 1663–1673, WB Saunders CO, Philadelphia, 1998.[97a] Edwards R. Immuno Assays in Rickwood D, Hames BD, Series Eds. Essential Data Series. John Wiley and Sons, New York, 1996.[91] Taylor SI, Grunberger G, Marcus-Samuels B, et al: Hypoglycemia Associated with Antibodies to the Insulin Receptor." N Engl J Med 307:1422–1426, 1982.[93] Dons RF, Havlik R, Taylor SI, et al: Clinical Disorders Associated with Autoantibodies to the Insulin Receptor." J Clinical Invest 72:1072–1080, 1983.[94] Leroith D: Tumor-Induced Hypoglycemia. N Engl J Med 241:757–758, 1999.[97b]

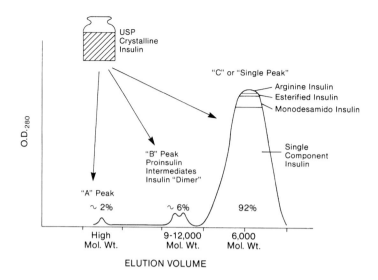

Figure 18–4. Gel filtration pattern of an older animal USP grade insulin on Sephadex G-50. Many recrystallized insulins contained up to 5% proinsulin and were contaminated with glucagon, pancreatic polypeptide, vasoactive intestinal peptide, and somatostatin. [*Source:* Kahn CR: Antibodies to insulin and insulin receptors: mechanisms of insulin resistance. *In* Gupta S (ed): Immunology of Clinical and Experimental Diabetes. New York: Plenum, 1984, pp. 249–327. With permission.]

TABLE 18–2   Primary Structures of Insulins from 26 Different Species[a]

A-Chain[a]	1	2	3	4	5	6	7	8	9	10	11	12
Human	Gly	Ile	Val	Glu	Gln	Cys	Cys	Thr	Ser	Ile	Cys	Ser
Abnormal (1)[b]												
Abnormal (2)[c]												
Abnormal (3)[d]			Leu									
Pig												
Dog												
Cow								Ala		Val		
Sheep								Ala	Gly	Val		
Rabbit												
Horse									Gly			
Sperm whale												
Sei whale								Ala		Thr		
Elephant									Gly	Val		
Rat (1)				Asp								
Rat (2)				Asp								
Mouse (1)				Asp								
Mouse (2)				Asp								
Guinea pig				Asp					Gly	Thr		Thr
Coypu				Asp					Asn			
Chinchilla				Asp								Thr
Casiragua				Asp					Asn			
Porcupine				Asp					Gly	Val		
Cod				Asp				His	Arg	Pro		Asp
Angler fish								His	Arg	Pro		Asn
Hagfish								His	Lys	Arg		
Toadfish (1)								His	Arg	Pro		Asp
Toadfish (2)								His	Arg	Pro		Asp
Tuna (2)								His	Lys	Pro		Asn
Chicken								His	Asn	Thr		
Turkey								His	Asn	Thr		
Duck								Glu	Asn	Pro		
Rattlesnake								Glu	Asn	Thr		

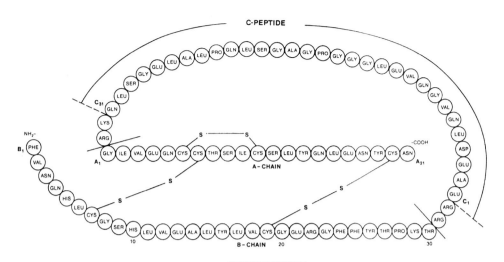

HUMAN PROINSULIN

Figure 18–5. The primary structure of human proinsulin consists of 86 amino acid residues. Of these, 51 are in insulin (21 in the A chain, 30 in the B chain), 35 are in the connecting peptide; two (LYS-ARG) join C_{31} to A_1, and two (ARG-ARG) join C_1 to B_{30}.[29] These 4 amino acids are enzymatically removed resulting in insulin and the 31 amino acid C-peptide. The structure of insulin, proinsulin, and the preregion of preproinsulin differ according to the species of animal, and some animals produce two different insulins. (See Tables 18–2 through 18–4). Abbreviations for amino acids (in this figure and in Tables 18–2 through 18–4) are as follows: ALA, alanine; ARG, arginine; ASN, asparagine; ASP, aspartic acid; CYS, cysteine; GLN, glutamine; GLU, glutamic acid; GLY, glycine; HIS, histidine; ILE, isoleucine; LEU, leucine; LYS, lysine; MET, methionine; PHE, phenylalanine; PRO, proline; SER, serine; THR, threonine; TYR, tyrosine. (*Sources:* Adapted from Nicol DSHW, Smith LF: Amino-acid sequence of human insulin. Nature 187:483–485, 1960; Chance RE: Amino-acid sequences of proinsulins and intermediates. Diabetes 21:462–467, 1972; Kitabchi AE: Proinsulin and C-peptide: a review. Metabolism 26:547–587, 1977. With permission.)

13	14	15	16	17	18	19	20	21	22	No. of Amino Acids Different from Human Insulin
Leu	Tyr	Gln	Leu	Glu	Asn	Tyr	Cys	Asn		
										0
										0
										1
										0
										0
										2
										3
										0
										1
										0
										2
										2
										1
										1
										1
										1
Arg	His			Gln	Ser					8
Arg	Asn			Met	Ser				Asp	7
										2
Arg	Asn			Leu	Thr					6
					Gln					4
Ile	Phe	Asp		Gln						9
Ile	Phe	Asp		Gln						8
Ile		Asp								5
Ile	Phe	Asp		Gln	Ser					9
Lys	Phe	Asp		Gln	Ser					9
Ile	Phe	Asp		Gln						8
										3
										3
										3
										3

(continued next page)

TABLE 18–2　*(continued)*　Primary Structures of Insulins from 26 Different Species[a]

B-Chain	−1	1	2	3	4	5	6	7	8	9	10	11	12	13	14	15	16
Human		Phe	Val	Asn	Gln	His	Leu	Cys	Gly	Ser	His	Leu	Val	Glu	Ala	Leu	Tyr
Abnormal (1)[b]																	
Abnormal (2)[c]																	
Abnormal (3)[d]																	
Pig																	
Dog																	
Cow																	
Sheep																	
Rabbit																	
Horse																	
Sperm whale																	
Sei whale																	
Elephant																	
Rat (1)				Lys						Pro							
Rat (2)				Lys													
Mouse (1)				Lys						Pro							
Mouse (2)				Lys													
Guinea pig				Ser	Arg						Asn				Thr		
Coypu		Tyr		Ser		Arg					Gln			Asp	Thr		
Chinchilla					Lys									Asp			
Casiragua		Tyr		Gly		Arg					Gln			Asp	Thr		
Porcupine																	
Cod	Met	Ala	Pro	Pro										Asp			
Angler fish	Val	Ala	Pro	Ala										Asp			
Hagfish		Arg	Thr	Thr	Gly					Lys	Asp			Asn			
Toadfish (1)	Met	Ala	Pro	Pro										Asp			
Toadfish (2)	Met	Ala	Pro	Pro										Asp			
Tuna (2)	Val	Ala	Pro	Pro										Asp			
Chicken		Ala	Ala														
Turkey		Ala	Ala														
Duck		Ala	Ala														
Rattlesnake		Ala	Pro			Arg										Phe	

[a] Blank spaces indicate residues identical with human sequence. A dash (—) indicates an amino acid deletion at that position.

(*Sources:* Blundell TL, Wood SP: Is the evolution of insulin Darwinian or due to selectively neutral mutation? Nature 257:197–203, 1975; Chance RE: Personal communication, 1985; Cutfield JF, Cutfield SM, Dodson EJ, et al.: Structure and biological activity of hagfish insulin. J Mol Biol 132:85–100, 1979; Nicol DSHW, Smith LF: Amino-acid sequence of human insulin. Nature 187:483–485, 1960. Chan ST, Emdin SO, Kwok SCM: Messenger mRNA sequence and primary structure of preproinsulin in a primitive vertebrate, the Atlantic hagfish. J Biol Chem 256:7595–7602, 1981. See reference 23. With permission.)

[b] insulin Chicago

[c] insulin Los Angeles

[d] insulin Wakayama

Abbreviations: Ala, alanine; Arg, arginine; Asn, asparagine; Asp, aspartic acid; Cys, cysteine; Gln, glutamine; Glu, glutamic acid; Gly, glycine; His, histidine; Ile, isoleucine; Leu, leucine; Lys, lysine; Met, methionine; Phe, phenylalanine; Pro, proline; Ser, serine; Thr, threonine; Tyr, tyrosine; Val, valine.

The tertiary structure of insulin was determined by x-ray crystallography by Hodgkin and colleagues.[38] Since that time, continuing crystallographic studies have provided a detailed understanding of the variable residues in the insulin monomer that are involved in antibody binding and receptor binding, as well as various areas involved in activation from proinsulin and self-association in intermonomer and interdimer contacts.[39–41] (Fig. 18–6). The presence of zinc permits insulin self-association and the formation of hexamers and higher aggregates with crystallization of insulin in B-cell storage granules.[38,40] The residues on the surface of hexamers of different species vary. Some rodents (guinea pig, coypu, casiragua) cannot dimerize their insulin because of amino acid differences at A-21, B-20, B-22, and/or B-26,[39] and such insulins exist as monomers only.[41,42]

17	18	19	20	21	22	23	24	25	26	27	28	29	30	31	No. of Amino Acids Different from Human Insulin
Leu	Val	Cys	Gly	Glu	Arg	Gly	Phe	Phe	Tyr	Thr	Pro	Lys	Thr		
							Leu								1
							Ser								1
															0
													Ala		1
													Ala		1
													Ala		1
													Ala		1
													Ser		1
													Ala		1
													Ala		1
													Ala		1
															0
													Ser		3
												Met	Ser		3
													Ser		3
												Met	Ser		3
Ser			Gin	Asp	Asp					Ile			Asp		10
Ser			Arg	His				—		Arg		Asn	Asp		13
				Asp								Met	Ala		5
Ser			Lys	His				—		Arg		Ser	Glu		13
			Asn	Asp						Arg			Ala		4
			Asp							Asn			—		8
			Asp							Asn			—		8
Ile	Ala		Val							Asp		Thr	Lys	Met	14
			Asp							Asn			—		8
			Asp							Asn	Ser	—	—		10
			Asp							Asn			—		8
										Ser			Ala		4
										Ser			Ala		4
										Ser					3
	Ile								Tyr	Ser		Arg	Ser		9

X-ray analysis of rhombohedral porcine two-zinc insulin crystals has permitted model-building and proposed conformations for proinsulin, IGF-1 (also known as somatomedin C), IGF-2 (also known as somatomedin A), and porcine relaxin (Fig. 18–7).[43–45]

IGFs are produced in the liver and some other tissues and are growth hormone dependent. Target cells include bone, liver, adipocytes, and muscle cells and fibroblasts, all of which produce different insulin-growth factor-binding proteins (IGFBPs 1, 2, 3, 4, 5, and 6) which modulate the various biologic effects of IGFs.[46]

The amino terminal 29 amino acids of IGF-1 are homologous to the B-chain of insulin (B-domain), and the next 12 amino acids (C-domain) link the B-domain with the A-domain (residues 42-62) which is homologous to the A-chain of insulin. The carboxyl terminus of IGF-1 is extended by eight amino acids to form the D-domain.[47] Both polyclonal and neutralizing monoclonal antibodies to IGF-1 are available.[48] It appears that the major antigenic epitopes of IGF-1 are residues 15 and 16 in the B-domain and residues 49-51 and 55, 56 in the A-domain.[47]

IGFs bind to specific receptors on the cell surface, and the IGF-1 receptor is similar in structure to the insulin receptor.[49] See Chapter 8.

There is a decrease in circulating IGF-1 levels and a concomitant decrease in growth in laboratory rats with experimental diabetes,[50] which can be corrected by administration of IGF-1.[51] Also, insulin therapy can restore normal IGF-1 levels in animals with uncontrolled diabetes, whereas growth hormone cannot.[52]

In evolutionary terms, insulin is related to the group of gastroenteropancreatic hormones found in many prostomian and deuterostomian lines, including the alimentary tract of mollusks.[53] In cyclostomes, including hagfish, the B cells have been relocated from the gut to the primitive islet organ. In holocephalan and elasmobranchian, cartilaginous fish a distinct pancreatic organ, which empties with the bile duct into the

TABLE 18–3 Amino Acid Sequences of Proinsulin C-Peptides from 15 Species[a,b,c]

Species	BC -2'	BC -1	C 1	2	3	4	5	6	7	8	9	10	11	12	13	14	15	16	17	18	19
Human	Arg	Arg	Glu	Ala	Glu	Asp	Leu	Gln	Val	Gly	Gln	Val	Glu	Leu	Gly	Gly	Gly	Pro	Gly	Ala	Gly
Monkey							Pro											Leu			
Guinea pig				Leu						Glu		Thr				Met	Val		Glu		
Chinchilla				Leu								Ala	Asp	Pro		Val			Glu		
Rat (1)				Val						Pro		Leu									
Rat (2)				Val						Ala		Leu									
Horse											Glu									Leu	
Pig				Ala		Asn			Ala		Ala							Leu		—	
Cow				Val		Gly					Ala	Leu		Ala	Ala						
Sheep				Val		Gly					Ala	Leu		Ala	Ala						
Dog				Val		Glu			Arg		Asp			Ala	Ala		Ala			Glu	
Rabbit				Val								Ala									
Duck			Asp	Val		Gln	Pro	Leu		Asn	Gly	Pro	—		His		Glu	Val		Glu	
Chicken			Asp	Val		Gln	Pro	Leu		Ser	Ser	Pro	—		Arg		Glu	Ala		Val	
Angler fish			Asp	Val	Asp	Gln		Leu	Gly	Phe	Leu	Pro	Pro	Lys	Ser	Ala	Glu	Ala	Ala	Ala	
Hagfish			Asp	Thr	Gly	Ala		Ala	Ala	Phe	Leu	Pro	Leu	Ala	Tyr			Asp	Asn	Ser	

Species	20	21	22	23	24	25	26	27	28	29	30	31	32	33	34	35	36	37	38	C 31	CA -1	CA -2
Human	Ser	Leu	Gln	Pro	Leu	Ala	Leu	Glu	Gly	Ser	Leu	Gln									Lys	Arg
Monkey																						
Guinea pig	Gly							Gln		Ala												
Chinchilla	Arg								Met	Thr												
Rat (1)	Asp			Thr					Val	Ala	Arg											
Rat (2)	Asp			Thr					Val	Ala	Arg											
Horse	Gly							Ala		Pro	Gln											
Pig	—			Ala						Pro												
Cow	Gly				—	—	—			Pro	Pro											
Sheep	Gly				—	—	—			Pro	Pro											
Dog	Gly									Ala	Pro											
Rabbit	Gly			Ser						Ala												
Duck	—		Pro	Phe	Gln	His	Glu		—	—	Tyr	Val										
Chicken	—		Pro	Phe	Gln	Gln	Glu		—	Glu	Lys	Glu										
Angler fish	Gly		Asp	Asn	Glu	Val	Ala		Phe	Ala	Phe	Lys	Asp	Gln	Met	Glu	Met	Met	Val			
Hagfish	Gln		Asp	Glu	Ser	Ile	Gly		Asn	Glu	Val	Leu	Lys	Ser	Met	Met	Met	Val				

[a] If an amino acid position is blank the amino acid residue in that position is identical to the amino acid residue in human C-peptide. If the amino acid in a position is different from the amino acid at that position in human C-peptide, the different amino acid is indicated. If an amino acid is not present at a position, the deletion is indicated by —.

[b] See Figure 18–5.

Abbreviations: Ala, alanine; Arg, arginine; Asn, asparagine; Asp, aspartic acid; BC = the 2 amino acids (Arg-Arg) that connect B-30 to C-1; C = the 31 amino acids of the C-peptide; CA = the 2 amino acids (Lys-Arg) that connect C-31 to A-1; Gln, glutamine; Glu, glutamic acid; Gly, glycine; His, histidine; Ile, isoleucine; Leu, leucine; Lys, lysine; Met, methionine; Phe, phenylalanine; Pro, proline; Ser, serine; Thr, threonine; Tyr, Tyrosine; Val, valine.

[*Sources:* Chance RE: Personal communication, 1985; Chance RE: Amino acid sequences of proinsulins and intermediates. Diabetes 21:461–467, 1971. Kwok SCM, Chan SJ, Steiner DF: Cloning and nucleotide sequence analysis of the dog insulin gene. J Biol Chem 258:2357–2363, 1983. See References 23, 24, 26. With permission.]

TABLE 18–4 Comparison of Amino Acid Sequences of Proinsulin Prepeptides from Six Species[a]

	−20[b]	−15[b]	−10[b]	−5[b]	−1[b]	+1[b]
Human	Met Ala Leu Trp Met Arg Leu Leu Pro	Leu Leu Ala Leu Leu	Ala Leu Trp Gly Pro	Asp Pro Ala Ala	Ala	Phe
Dog	Met Ala Leu	Leu	Ala	Ala Ala	Thr	Arg
Rat (1)	Met Ala Leu	Phe	Val Glu	Lys Gln		
Rat (2)	Met Ala Leu	Phe	Ile Glu	Arg Gln		
Chicken	Met Ala Leu	Ser	Val Phe Ser	Gly Thr Ser	Tyr	Ala
Angler fish	Met Ala Ala Leu	Ser Phe Ser	Val Val Trp	Gly Ser —	Gln	Val
Hagfish	Met Ala Leu Ser Pro Phe Leu	Ala Val Ile Pro	Leu Ser Arg Ala	Pro Ser Ser Asp	Thr	Arg

[a] Comparison of amino acid sequence of human proinsulin prepeptide with those of dog, rat 1 and 2, chicken, angler fish, and hagfish proinsulin prepeptides. Blank spaces indicate residues identical with human sequence. Arrow denotes position of cleavage by the signal peptidase. A — is introduced at position −3 in the angler fish sequence to maximize homology. The highly conserved NH_2-terminal Met-Ala-Leu sequence is underlined.

[b] +1 represents the first (N-terminal) amino acid in the B chain of proinsulin. −1 represents the —COOH terminal amino acid of the proinsulin prepeptide. Hagfish prepeptide contains 26 amino acids, and the N-terminal Met is numbered −26.

Abbreviations: As in Table 18–2; Trp, tryptophane.

[*Sources:* Chance RE: Personal communication, 1985; Kwok SCM, Chan SJ, Steiner DF: Cloning and nucleotide sequence analysis of the dog insulin gene. J Biol Chem 258:2357–2363, 1983. See References 23, 24, 26, and 28. With permission.]

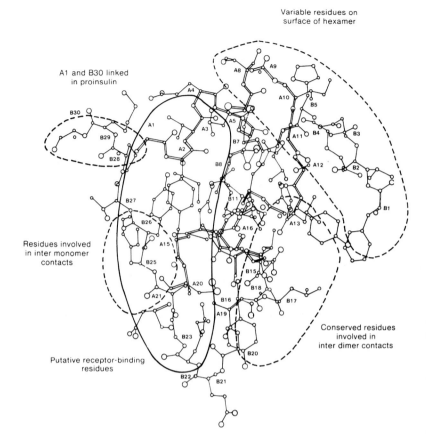

Variable residues on
surface of hexamer

A1 and B30 linked
in proinsulin

Residues involved
in inter monomer
contacts

Putative receptor-binding
residues

Conserved residues
involved in
inter dimer contacts

Figure 18–6. View of the insulin monomer indicating how the surface may be described in terms of various areas involved in activation from the prohormone, variable residues involved in antibody binding, binding to the receptor, and self-association. (*Source:* Blundell TL, Wood SP: Is the evolution of insulin Darwinian or due to selectively neutral mutation? Nature 257:197–203, 1975. With permission.)

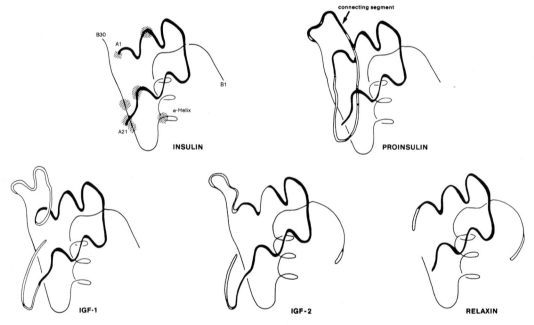

INSULIN

PROINSULIN

IGF-1

IGF-2

RELAXIN

Figure 18–7. Schematic presentation of the three-dimensional structure of insulin based on an x-ray analysis of rhombohedral two-zinc insulin crystals, and proposed conformations based on model-building for proinsulin, IGF-1, IGF-2, and relaxin, showing the close structural homology. The B chain is designated by the lines with a helix structure, the A chain by heavy dark lines, and connecting segments by double lines. The shaded areas on the insulin molecule depict the biologically active sites. The first four share similar biologic actions (insulin > proinsulin > IGF-1 and IGF-2), but relaxin does not share any biologic actions with insulin. (*Source:* Blundell TL, Humbel RE: Hormone families: pancreatic hormones and homologous growth factors. Nature 287:781–787, 1980. With permission.)

gut cavity, is present, and this represents the final link in the evolution of insulin-producing cells from very primitive life forms to mammals.[54]

Steiner and Oyer (1967)[55] elucidated the mechanism of insulin synthesis in human insulinoma tissue by showing that it was preceded by biosynthesis of an insulin-containing peptide (proinsulin) about 1.5 times the size of insulin (Fig. 18–5).[21,29] Later it was shown that an even larger molecule (preproinsulin)[30,31] was synthesized prior to the production of proinsulin (see Table 18–4).

There has been a rapid increase in the knowledge of genetic structure deoxyribonucleic acid (DNA) and control of intracellular metabolism during the last 25 years.

The human insulin gene is located within the short arm of chromosome 11 and contains 1,789 base pairs. The B-cell response to physiologic stimuli is controlled by the insulin gene and the intranuclear events that regulate its expression (Fig. 18–8).[56]

Rarely, mutation of the human insulin gene produces a structurally abnormal gene that produces an abnormal insulin with lower than normal biologic activity[57,58] or a proinsulin that is not normally converted to insulin and that has lower than normal biological activity. (Exhibit 18–1).

B-25 leucine (for phenylalanine) insulin (insulin Chicago) has 1 to 4% of the biologic and receptor-binding activities of normal insulin; B-24 serine (for phenylalanine) insulin (insulin Los Angeles) has 0.5 to 1.0% of the activities of normal insulin; A-3 leucine (for valine) insulin (insulin Wakayama) has 0.14% of the biologic activity of normal insulin.[59]

These three mutant insulins are referred to in Table 18–3 as abnormal insulins (1), (2), and (3), respectively.

These individuals have an abnormality in the insulin gene. The reduced affinity of these abnormal insulins for binding to the insulin receptor results in a markedly prolonged half-life in the circulation, decreased clearance from the plasma, and high immunoreactive insulin levels. Clinically, these individuals may present with overt diabetes or with mild glucose intolerance and high immunoreactive insulin and C-peptide levels.

Another group of patients has been identified who have defects in the conversion of proinsulin to insulin. Two families have a histidine substituting for arginine at the 65th position in the proinsulin molecule (which is attached to the glycine at A1). The loss of arginine at this position prevents enzymatic splitting of histidine from the glycine and this results in a circulating proinsulin intermediate that has only been split at the B32, 33 positions but not at the 65 position. Another defect was noted in which B10 histidine was replaced by aspartic acid with a three-dimensional change in the folding of proinsulin with a resultant failure of conversion of the mutant proinsulin to insulin.[59]

Similarly, another family with a proline at B65 which also cannot be enzymatically processed has been reported.

Patients with familial hyperproinsulinemia (either partially cleaved or intact) may present nonstressed as normoglycemic, or stressed as glucose intolerant or hyperglycemic. Typically, immunoreactive insulin levels are high, but levels depend on cross-reactivity of the antiserum used with proinsulin and split proinsulin. On *molecular sieve chromatography*, there is an increase in the 9,000 molecular weight range. With HPLC, using standards of human proinsulin and its intermediate, the component that is increased can be identified.

Substitution of aspartic acid for histidine at B-10 produces an insulin with increased biologic activity.[60,61] There is considerable continuing research interest in insulins and proinsulins with increased or decreased biologic activity, and in the chemical changes in the molecules that are responsible.

The first important clinical application of genetic engineering involved the production of recombinant DNA (rDNA) human insulin.[63–75] Synthetic genes for the human A chain of insulin and for the human B chain of insulin were inserted into separate batches of the K12 strain of *Escherichia coli*. The synthetic genes were placed adjacent to the promoter regions of the betagalactosidase or tryptophan synthetase in the bacterial plasmid. Bacteria, thus modified, produced proteins from which the A and B chains were cleaved by cyanogen bromide. The chains were purified, then combined through chemical procedures that resulted in appropriate disulfide bond formation and the production of biosynthetic human insulin (human insulin rDNA) whose chemical, physical, and biologic properties were equivalent to those of insulin produced by the human pancreatic B cell.[73]

Since 1986 human insulin (from Lilly) has been produced via the recombinant human proinsulin process as outlined in Figure 18–9.[62,75]

The first dose of rDNA human insulin was administered to an individual in the United Kingdom in June, 1980.[63–69] It became available for use in the United States in 1983, at which time beef insulin accounted for over two thirds of insulin usage. Since then, the majority of those being treated with beef or pork insulins have been transferred to rDNA human insulin.[70–75]

Semisynthetic (SS) human insulin has been produced by an enzymatic transpeptidation process in which the B-30 alanine in pork insulin is replaced by the B-30 threonine of human insulin.[76,77]

It is important to note that the amino acid sequence of human connecting peptide varies from cow connecting peptide at 16 positions and from pig connecting peptide at 10 positions (Table 18–3 and Fig. 18–5), thus accounting for antigenicity of cow and pig connecting

Molecular events   **Cellular events**

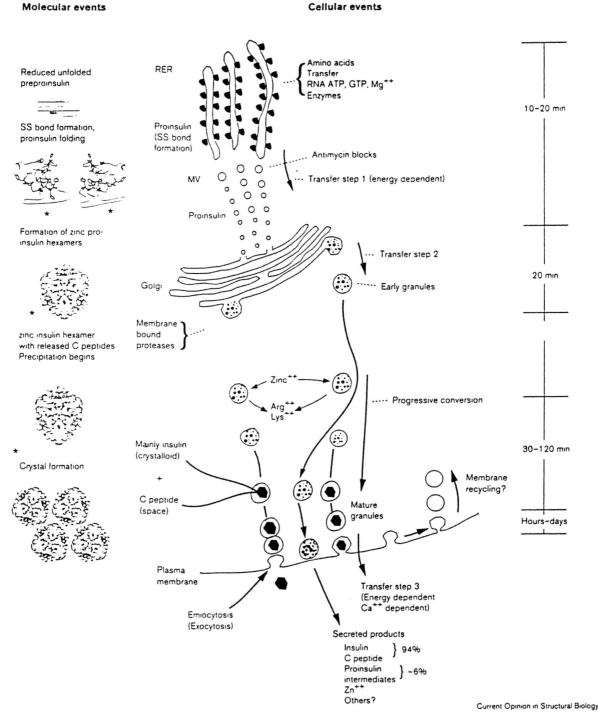

Figure 18–8. A schematic representation of the molecular events (left) and cellular events (right) that occur in insulin's biosynthesis the asterisk indicates the bound (or C peptide) free connecting peptide. RER, rough endoplasmic reticulum. Reproduced with permission from Dodson G and Steiner D: The role of assembly in insulin's biosynthesis. Current Opinion in Structural Biology 8:189–194, 1998.[104]

peptides (and part of the antigenicity of cow and pig proinsulins) in the human.

Human insulin is less immunogenic and also more hydrophilic than purified beef and purified pork insulins,[74] and this probably accounts, at least in part, for the slightly earlier onset and peak of action and slightly shorter duration of action compared with that of animal insulins in some individuals.

Highly purified animal insulins[78] (<0.0003% proinsulin content) were introduced at about the same time as were rDNA human insulin,[69,72] and SS human insulin.[77] It was predicted that the insulin marketplace would be thrown into turbulence by these advances.[79] Although there is no question that competition between insulin producers has intensified, the overall effect has been very positive in that both clinical research and

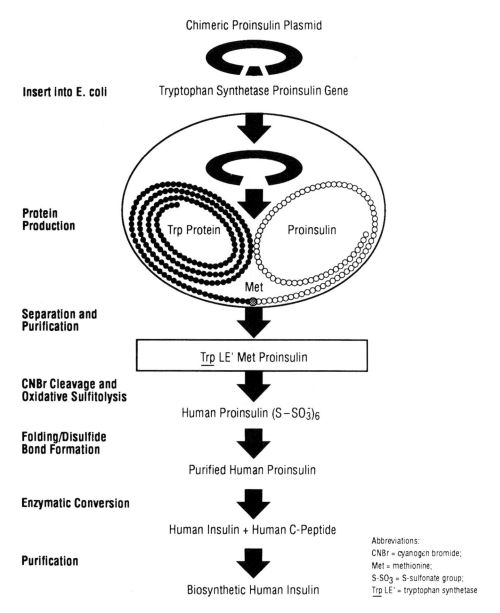

Chimeric Proinsulin Plasmid

Insert into E. coli   Tryptophan Synthetase Proinsulin Gene

**Protein
Production**   Trp Protein   Proinsulin

Met

**Separation and
Purification**

Trp LE' Met Proinsulin

**CNBr Cleavage and
Oxidative Sulfitolysis**

Human Proinsulin $(S-SO_3^-)_6$

**Folding/Disulfide
Bond Formation**

Purified Human Proinsulin

Enzymatic Conversion

Human Insulin + Human C-Peptide

Abbreviations:
CNBr = cyanogen bromide;
Met = methionine;
$S-SO_3$ = S-sulfonate group;
Trp LE' = tryptophan synthetase

Purification

Biosynthetic Human Insulin

Figure 18–9.   General scheme for producing biosynthetic insulin via the proinsulin route. (*Source:* Adapted from Frank BH, Chance RE: The preparation and characterization of human insulin of recombinant DNA origin. Therapeutic agents produced by genetic engineering. *Quo Vadis?* Symposium, Sanofi Group, Toulouse-Labège, France, May 29–30, 1985. With permission.)

basic research on insulin have intensified. Also, the cost to the patient of human insulin is lower in 1999 than is the cost of highly purified pork insulin.

Until 1936, because of the relatively short duration of action of regular insulin (4 to 8 hr; Fig. 18–10)[80] it was necessary to inject the hormone subcutaneously three or four times per day. It was natural that attempts would be made to produce longer-acting insulins so that the needed number of daily injections could be reduced. Early attempts to do so involved combining insulin with epinephrine and similar substances that altered local blood flow in order to delay absorption. A major break through came with physical and chemical modifications of the molecule. Hagedorn[81] found that insulin's time action could be prolonged by combina-

tion with basic proteins of which fish (trout, salmon) protamine was the most successful. Scott and Fisher (1936)[82] showed that the addition of increasing amounts of heavy metals such as zinc would lengthen the period of action of protamine insulin for up to 3 days.

For about 10 years, protamine zinc insulin (PZI) was used extensively in North America and the United Kingdom, whereas protamine insulin (isophane or NPH) gained popularity in Europe. Use of NPH insulin in the United States started in 1950. PZI contains approximately 0.15 to 0.25 mg zinc and 1.2 mg protamine/100 U insulin, whereas isophane (NPH) insulin contains only 0.016 to 0.04 mg zinc and 0.4 mg protamine/100 U insulin (Table 18–5). It should be noted, however, that protamine added to zinc-free

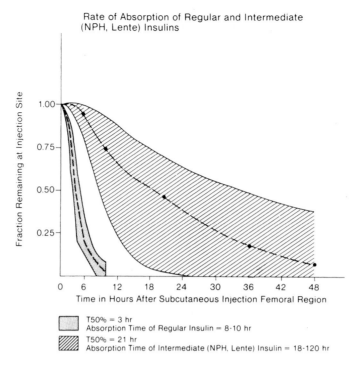

Figure 18–10. Absorption rates (means and ranges) of regular and intermediate (NPH, Lente) insulins from subcutaneous tissue. T50% = the mean time at which 50% of the insulin had been absorbed. Absorption time is the range in hours required for essentially complete absorption of the injected insulin. Note the wide range of absorption time of intermediate insulins in different individuals. It is estimated that variability in rates of absorption of intermediate-acting insulin in the same individual accounts for 80% of the variations in the amplitude of glucose excursion from day to day. (See Exhibits 18–2 and 18–3. (*Source*: Binder C: Insulin pharmacokinetics. Diabetes Care 7:188–199, 1984. With permission.)

insulin (protamine sodium insulin) does prolong its action.[83,84] Neither PZI or PSI is available in the United States.

Globin insulin was introduced by Burroughs Wellcome Company in 1939. In the case of globin insulin, zinc plus the protein present in hemoglobin was used. Globin had a less-marked effect on prolonging the duration of action of insulin than did protamine, and its time of action did not extend beyond 24 hr. It is no longer available in the United States.

PZI had the twin disadvantages of insufficient hypoglycemic action during the day and too much hypoglycemic action during the night. For that reason, a combination of various amounts of PZI and regular insulin (with ratios ranging from 1:1 to 1:4, usually 1 U PZI and 2 U regular) were commonly used and were adjusted to the individual's need. PZI insulin contains an excess of protamine which converts some regular insulin that is mixed with it to the longer-acting protamine insulin. NPH insulin can be mixed with neutral regular insulin and essentially all of the regular insulin remains short-acting.[84,108] NPH-regular insulin mixtures (usually freshly made and immediately injected) have been used instead of PZI-regular insulin mixtures since the mid-1950s. Extemporaneous mixtures containing NPH (10 to 90%) and regular (10 to 90%) may be prepared and injected, without changing the time-

action curves of either of the two insulins. Stable premixed NPH (70%)/R (30%) and NPH(50%)/R (50%) preparations are now available (Humulin 70/30, Humulin 50/50, and Novolin 70/30) (see Table 18–5).

Lente insulin was introduced in 1952 by Hallas-Moller.[85] Lente insulin contains no foreign protein. The time of insulin action depended on whether the insulin was amorphous (short-acting Semilente whose action is slightly longer than that of regular insulin) or microcrystalline (long-acting Ultralente). Lente insulin is a mixture of three parts of Semilente insulin and seven parts of Ultralente insulin. The time action of the Lente insulins can be modified by preparing extemporaneous mixtures containing more Semilente (more early effect) or more Ultralente (more late effect). Regular insulin remains fast acting when added to NPH, but not when added to Lente because excess zinc in the Lente binds the regular insulin and blunts its quick effect.[62]

Insulin lispro (Humalog®, Eli Lilly and Company) is a marketed analog of human insulin created by reversing the amino acids on the B-chain of the insulin molecule from $Pro^{B28}Lys^{B29}$ to $Lys^{B28}Pro^{B29}$. The pharmacokinetic profile of insulin lispro with its more rapid absorption over a shorter duration of time produces a more physiologic profile characteristic of mealtime endogenous insulin secretion.[247] This allows insulin lispro to be administered just before the meal, and in some cases after the meal,[288] in contrast to regular insulin, which should be administered 30 to 45 minutes before the meal. In clinical use it has been associated with improvements in the postprandial control, overall control and less frequent hypoglycemia.[251,254]

The pharmacokinetics of insulin lispro offer unique advantages over traditional regular insulins. With regular human insulin administered subcutaneously, as one increases the dose both the time to peak activity and the total duration of action are increased. In contrast, with insulin lispro, as the dose increases the time to peak activity and the total duration of action remain relatively constant providing much greater predictability of response as the patient adjusts their dose to manage changes in food consumption and/or physical activity.[264] Another study demonstrates that the differences in absorption rates due to anatomic site of injection are significantly reduced using insulin lispro compared to regular human insulin.[245]

Insulin lispro, with its peak of activity at about 60 minutes after injection, consistently reduces the postprandial rise in blood glucose compared to regular human insulin in patients with type 1 or type 2 diabetes.[251,254] This improved postprandial control leads to a 0.3 to 0.4 percentage point drop in hemoglobin A1c in studies in which basal insulin therapy is adjusted to provide adequate premeal and nocturnal coverage.[289,290] Studies demonstrate that best control is achieved when basal insulin requirements are supplied by subcutaneous insulin infusion pumps or, in the majority of patients, when 2 injections of human NPH insulin are used.[265,266] Some European studies demonstrate additional improvements in control when NPH is used 3 or 4 times per day.[266] It is important to note that 20 to 40% of the activity of regular human insulin occurs during the time period normally associated with basal insulin activity. Thus it is not surprising that in many studies there are slight decreases in the amount of insulin lispro (mealtime insulin) used and an increase in the proportion as well as total dose of basal insulin administered.

The shorter duration of activity of insulin lispro has resulted in a decrease in hypoglycemia. Clinical studies in patients with type 1 diabetes have demonstrated an 11% reduction in the number of hypoglycemic episodes in patients treated with insulin lispro compared to regular human insulin with the largest difference observed at night.[254] Although patients with type 2 disease have less hypoglycemia overall, a reduction was seen in nocturnal hypoglycemia.[251] A cumulative meta-analysis of over 2327 patients using insulin lispro and 2339 patients using regular human insulin demonstrated that insulin lispro reduces severe hypoglycemia by 30% compared to regular human insulin.[267]

The hormonal counterregulatory response and cognitive function were studied in patients with type 1 diabetes after hypoglycemia induced by injection of insulin lispro or regular human insulin. The glucagon, epinephrine, norepinephrine, growth hormone and cortisol responses as well as the cognitive function changes after each insulin were superimposable. The blood glucose rebound was faster and the posthypoglycemia hyperglycemia was slightly greater following insulin lispro.[268]

The immunogenic potential of insulin lispro is minimized because of its structural similarity to human insulin and the extremely short residence time at the site of injection in the subcutaneous tissue. Measurements of lispro specific, human insulin specific, and cross-reactive antibodies during one year studies have demonstrated that there were no differences in the immunogenicity of insulin lispro compared to regular human insulin in type 1 or type 2 patients previously treated with insulin therapy[271] or new, insulin-naïve type 1 or type 2 patients.[272] Studies have also demonstrated no significant change from baseline to endpoint in insulin antibodies over 50 months of therapy.[273]

Interestingly, two recent papers have described patients with severe, antibody mediated insulin resistance that developed 3 to 9 years after their onset of diabetes. Both of these patients responded to insulin lispro delivered by CSII with significant decreases in insulin requirements and greatly improved glucose profiles.[274,275]

Recent studies have also evaluated the use of insulin lispro in pediatric populations. Prepubertal and adolescent studies have demonstrated that insulin lispro improved postprandial glucose control with the convenience of injection at mealtime.[276,277] The adolescent patients also had a significantly reduced rate of hypoglycemia.[278] A third study in patients under the age of 5 compared insulin lispro given immediately before the meal to (1) regular human insulin given up to 30 minutes before the meal, and (2) insulin lispro given after the meal. Results indicated that insulin lispro given after the meal produced blood glucose results as good as or better than regular insulin given before the meal.[279] This offers the advantage of being able to assess the amount of food consumed by the child, and then administer the appropriate dose of insulin lispro thus reducing the potential risk of hypoglycemia.

Endogenous Insulin, Proinsulin, and C-Peptide

Ogilvie (1937)[86] showed that pancreatic islet cell volume was markedly reduced in young diabetics and moderately reduced in adult diabetics. Wrenshall (1952)[87] reported that the total extractable insulin of the pancreata from seven of nine individuals dying in diabetic ketoacidosis was less than 4 U in each pancreas. The amount extractable from the pancreas of those with onset of diabetes between 0 and 20 years of age was less than 2% of normal, whereas the amount extractable

TABLE 18–5

Manufacturer	Type and Brand of Insulin	Species	Strength
	Rapid Acting		
Lilly	Humalog (Insulin lispro) 10 mL vial[1]	Analog (rDNA)	U-100
	Humalog 1.5 mL cartridges[1]	Analog (rDNA)	U-100
	Humalog 3.0 mL prefilled pen[1]	Analog (rDNA)	U-100
	Short Acting		
Lilly	Humulin R (human insulin injection) 10 mL vial	Human (rDNA)	U-100
	Humulin R 1.5 mL cartridges	Human (rDNA)	U-100
	Humulin R (U-500) 20 mL vial[1]	Human (rDNA)	U-500
	Iletin II Regular (Purified Pork) 10 ml vial	Pork	U-100
Novo-Nordisk	Novolin R (human insulin injection) 10 mL vial	Human (rDNA)	U-100
	Novolin R 1.5 mL cartridges	Human (rDNA)	U-100
	Novolin R 3.0 mL cartridges	Human (rDNA)	U-100
	NovoPen 1.5 (regular) prefilled pen	Human (rDNA)	U-100
	Velosulin BR (buffered regular) 10 mL vial	Human (semi-synthetic)	U-100
	Purified Pork Regular 10 mL vial	Pork	U-100

(continued next page)

TABLE 18-5 Insulins avaiable in the United States (1999)

Manufacturer	Type and Brand of Insulin	Species	Onset (hours)	Peak (hours)	Duration (hours)	Preservative	Buffer/pH	Zinc (mg/100 U)	Protamine (mg/100 U)
Lilly	**Rapid Acting**								
	Humalog (Insulin lispro) 10 mL vial *2	Analog (rDNA)	0.1–0.25	0.5–1.5	3–5	metacresol	phosphate/neutral	0.019	
	Humalog 1.5 mL cartridges *2	Analog (rDNA)	0.1–0.25	0.5–1.5	3–5	metacresol	phosphate/neutral	0.019	
	Humalog 3.0 mL prefilled pen *2	Analog (rDNA)	0.1–0.25	0.5–1.5	3–5	metacresol	phosphate/neutral	0.019	
Lilly	**Short Acting**								
	Humulin R (human insulin injection) 10 mL vial	Human (rDNA)	0.5–1.5	2–4	6–8	metacresol	none/neutral	0.01–0.04	
	Humulin R 1.5 mL cartridges	Human (rDNA)	0.5–1.5	2–4	6–8	metacresol	none/neutral	0.01–0.04	
	Humulin R (U 500)[3] 20 mL vial *2	Human (rDNA)	0.5–3	3–8	8–20	metacresol	none/neutral	0.01–0.04	
	Iletin II Regular (Purified Pork) 10 mL vial	Pork	0.5–1.5	2–4	6–8	metacresol	none/neutral	0.01–0.04	
Novo-Nordisk	Novolin R (human insulin injection) 10 mL vial	Human (rDNA)	0.5–1.5	2–4	6–8	metacresol	none/neutral	trace	
	Novolin R 1.5 mL cartridges	Human (rDNA)	0.5–1.5	2–4	6–8	metacresol	none/neutral	trace	
	Novolin R 3.0 mL cartridges	Human (rDNA)	0.5–1.5	2–4	6–8	metacresol	none/neutral	trace	
	NovoPen 1.5 (regular) prefilled pen	Human (rDNA)	0.5–1.5	2–4	6–8	metacresol	none/neutral	trace	
	Velosulin BR (buffered regular) 10 mL vial	Human (semi-synthetic)	0.5–1.5	2–4	6–8	metacresol	phosphate/neutral	trace	
	Purified Pork Regular 10 mL vial	Pork	0.5–1.5	2–4	6–8	metacresol	none/neutral	0.01–0.04	

(continued next page)

TABLE 18-5 *(continued)*

Manufacturer	Type and Brand of Insulin	Species	Strength
	Intermediate Acting		
Lilly	Humulin L (Lente®2 Human Insulin Zinc Suspension) 10 mL vial	Human (rDNA)	U-100
	Humulin N (NPH Human Insulin Isophane Suspension) 10 mL vial	Human (rDNA)	U-100
	Humulin N (NPH Human Insulin Isophane Suspension) 1.5 mL cartridges	Human (rDNA)	U-100
	Humulin N (NPH Human Insulin Isophane Suspension) 3.0 mL prefilled pen	Human (rDNA)	U-100
	Iletin II Lente® (Zinc Suspension, Purified Pork) 10 ml vial	Pork	U-100
	Iletin II NPH (Isophane Suspension, Purified Pork) 10 ml vial	Pork	U-100
Novo-Nordisk	Novolin L (Lente® Human Insulin Zinc Suspension) 10 mL vial	Human (rDNA)	U-100
	Novolin N (NPH Human Insulin Isophane Suspension) 10 mL vial	Human (rDNA)	U-100
	Novolin N 1.5 mL cartridges	Human (rDNA)	U-100
	Novolin N 3.0 mL cartridges	Human (rDNA)	U-100
	NovoPen 1.5 (NPH Human Insulin Isophane Suspension) prefilled pen	Human (rDNA)	U-100
	NovoPen 3.0 (NPH Human Insulin Isophane Suspension) prefilled pen	Human (rDNA)	U-100
	Lente® (Zinc Suspension, Purified Pork) 10 ml vial	Pork	U-100
	NPH (Isophane Suspension Purified Pork) 10 ml vial	Pork	U-100

(continued next page)

TABLE 18-5 Insulins avaiable in the United States (1999)

Manufacturer	Type and Brand of Insulin	Species	Onset (hours)	Peak (hours)	Duration (hours)	Preservative	Buffer/pH	Zinc (mg/100 U)	Protamine (mg/100 U)
	Intermediate Acting								
Lilly	Humulin L (Lente® Human Insulin Zinc Suspension) 10 mL vial	Human (rDNA)	1-3	8-14	18-24	methil-paraben	acetate/neutral	0.12-0.25	
	Humulin N (NPH Human Insulin Isophane Suspension) 10 mL vial	Human (rDNA)	1-3	6-12	18-24	phenol/metacresol	phosphate/neutral	0.01-0.04	0.32-0.44
	Humulin N (NPH Human Insulin Isophane Suspension) 1.5 mL cartridges	Human (rDNA)	1-3	6-12	18-24	phenol/metacresol	phosphate/neutral	0.01-0.04	0.32-0.44
	Humulin N (NPH Human Insulin Isophane Suspension) 3.0 mL prefilled pen	Human (rDNA)	1-3	6-12	18-24	phenol/metacresol	phosphate/neutral	0.01-0.04	0.32-0.44
	Iletin II Lente® [4] (Zinc Suspension, Purified Pork) 10 mL vial	Pork	1-3	8-14	18-24	methil-paraben	acetate/neutral	0.12-0.25	
	Iletin II NPH (Isophane Suspension Purified Pork) 10 mL vial	Pork	1-3	6-12	18-24	phenol/metacresol	phosphate/neutral	0.01-0.04	0.32-0.44
Novo-Nordisk	Novolin L (Lente® Human Insulin Zinc Suspension) 10 mL vial	Human (rDNA)	2.5	7-15	22	methil-paraben	acetate/neutral	0.15 (approx)	
	Novolin N (NPH Human Insulin Isophane Suspension) 10 mL vial	Human (rDNA)	1.5	4-12	24	phenol/metacresol	phosphate/neutral	trace	0.35 (approx)
	Novolin N 1.5 mL cartridges	Human (rDNA)	1.5	4-12	24	phenol/metacresol	phosphate/neutral	trace	0.35 (approx)
	Novolin N 3.0 mL cartridges	Human (rDNA)	1.5	4-12	24	phenol/metacresol	phosphate/neutral	trace	0.35 (approx)
	NovoPen 1.5 (NPH Human Insulin Isophane Suspension prefilled pen	Human (rDNA)	1.5	4-12	24	phenol/metacresol	phosphate/neutral	trace	0.35 (approx)
	NovoPen 3.0 (NPH Human Insulin Isophane Suspension prefilled pen	Human (rDNA)	1.5	4-12	24	phenol/metacresol	phosphate/neutral	trace	0.35 (approx)
	Lente® (Zinc Suspension, Purified Pork) 10 mL vial	Pork	2.5	7-15	22	methil-paraben	acetate/neutral	0.15 (approx)	
	NPH (Isophane Suspension, Purified Pork) 10 mL vial prefilled pen	Pork	1.5	4-12	24	phenol/metacresol	phosphate/neutral	trace	0.35 (approx)

(continued next page)

351

TABLE 18–5 *(continued)*

Manufacturer	Type and Brand of Insulin	Species	Strength
	Long Acting		
Lilly	Humulin U (Ultralente®[2] Human Insulin Extended Zinc Suspension) 10 mL vial[3]	Human (rDNA)	U-100
	Fixed Mixtures (Intermediate/short-acting)		
Lilly	Humulin 70/30 (70% human insulin isophane suspension/30% human insulin injection) 10 mL vial	Human (rDNA)	U-100
	Humulin 70/30 (70% human insulin isophane suspension/30% human insulin injection) 1.5 mL cartridges	Human (rDNA)	U-100
	Humulin 70/30 (70% human insulin isophane suspension/30% human insulin injection) 3.0 mL prefilled pen	Human (rDNA)	U-100
	Humulin 50/50 (50% human insulin isophane suspension/50% human insulin injection) 10 mL vial	Human (rDNA)	U-100
Novo-Nordisk	Novolin 70/30 (70% human insulin isophane suspension/30% human insulin injection) 10 mL vial	Human (rDNA)	U-100
	Novolin 70/30 (70% human insulin isophane suspension/30% human insulin injection) 3.0 mL cartridges	Human (rDNA)	U-100
	Novolin 70/30 (70% human insulin isophane suspension/30% human insulin injection) 1.5 mL prefilled pen	Human (rDNA)	U-100

[1] Available by prescription only.
[2] Lente® and Ultralente® are registered trademarks of Novo-Nordisk A/S.
[3] Because the duration of human Ultralente® is less than that of beef Ultralente, some clinicians group human Ultralente with the Intermediate-acting insulins.

TABLE 18–5 Insulins avaiable in the United States (1999)

Manufacturer	Type and Brand of Insulin	Species	Onset (hours)	Peak (hours)	Duration (hours)	Preservative	Buffer/pH	Zinc (mg/100 U)	Protamine (mg/100 U)
	Rapid Acting								
Lilly	Humulin U[3] (Ultralente®[4] Human Insulin Extended Zinc Suspension) 10 mL vial	Human (rDNA)	4–6	8–20	24-28	methil-paraben	acetate/neutral	0.12–0.25	
	Fixed Mixtures (Intermediate/short-acting)								
Lilly	Humulin 70/30 (70 % human insulin isophane suspension/30% human insulin injection) 10 mL vial	Human (rDNA)	0.5–1	2–12	up to 24	phenol/metacresol	phosphate/neutral	0.01–0.04	0.22–0.26
	Humulin 70/30 (70 % human insulin isophane suspension/30% human insulin injection) 1.5 mL cartridges	Human (rDNA)	0.5–1	2–12	up to 24	phenol/metacresol	phosphate/neutral	0.01–0.04	0.22–0.26
	Humulin 70/30 (70 % human insulin isophane suspension/30% human insulin injection) 3.0 mL prefilled pen	Human (rDNA)	0.5–1	2–12	up to 24	phenol/metacresol	phosphate/neutral	0.01–0.04	0.22–0.26
	Humulin 50/50 (50 % human insulin isophane suspension/50% human insulin injection) 10 mL vial	Human (rDNA)	0.5–1	2–12	up to 24	phenol/metacresol	phosphate/neutral	0.01–0.04	0.22–0.26
Novo-Nordisk	Novolin 70/30 (70 % human insulin isophane suspension/30% human insulin injection) 10 mL vial	Human (rDNA)	0.5	2–12	24	phenol/metacresol	phosphate/neutral	trace	0.25 (approx)
	Novolin 70/30 (70 % human insulin isophane suspension/30% human insulin injection) 3.0 mL cartridges	Human (rDNA)	0.5	2–12	24	phenol/metacresol	phosphate/neutral	trace	0.25 (approx)
	Novolin 70/30 (70 % human insulin isophane suspension/30% human insulin injection) 1.5 mL prefilled pen	Human (rDNA)	0.5	2–12	24	phenol/metacresol	phosphate/neutral	trace	0.25 (approx)

[1] All insulins shown are U-100 (100 units/mL) except for Humulin R® U-500 (500 units/mL).

[2] Available by prescription only.

[3] Because of the high concentration of U-500 insulin the time-action profile is markedly extended.

[4] Lente® and Ultralente® are registered trademarks of Novo-Nordisk A/S.

[5] Because the duration of human Ultralente® is less than that of beef Ultralente® , some clinicians group human Ultralente® with the Intermediate-acting insulins.®

Source: Adapted from American Diabetes Association Forecast Resource Guide (1999) and American Pharmaceutical Association Formulations and Feature '98-99.

from the pancreas of those with onset of diabetes between 20 and 80 years of age averaged about 50% of the amount extractable from the pancreas of nondiabetics of comparable age. The normal human pancreas contains about 4 U of extractable insulin/g of pancreas (i.e., about 320 U extractable insulin/80 g pancreas).

Since 1960, it has been shown by many investigators that individuals with IDDM at time of diagnosis have undetectable or low-fasting and stimulated serum insulin levels.[88,89] After 5 years of IDDM, most individuals have undetectable serum C-peptide levels. Antibodies generated to exogenous insulin invalidate insulin assays in most of these individuals. (See Exhibit 18–1.)

Fasting serum insulin and C-peptide levels in those with NIDDM are usually normal or elevated, but stimulated levels are usually lower than those in age- and weight-matched nondiabetic control subjects. First-phase glucose-stimulated insulin release (first 10 min) in NIDDM is usually reduced or lost. Obese individuals who lose excess body weight may have their insulin secretion pattern and glucose tolerance test return to normal. Others may progress to insulinopenic diabetes (IDDM) despite therapeutically induced weight loss. (See Fig. 2–2).

Clinical indications for insulin, proinsulin, C-peptide, and glucagon assays are listed in Exhibit 18–1,[88–98] and the results of a series of insulin assays for insulinomas are illustrated in Figure 18–11.[96]

It has been estimated that the average lean nondiabetic adult secretes 33 to 60 U insulin/day and this maintains normoglycemia (Fig. 18–12).[99] Normal pancreatic B-cell insulin-secretion reserve permits the markedly obese nondiabetic individual to secrete up to 120 to 130 U/day to maintain normoglycemia. An abnormal glucose tolerance test followed by fasting hyperglycemia will develop in a majority of these individuals despite continuing excess insulin secretion (when compared with insulin secretion levels in lean, nondiabetic, age-and sex-matched control subjects).

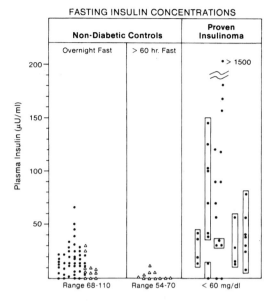

Figure 18–11. Fasting insulin concentrations in normal subjects after an overnight fast (left) and after more than 60 hr fasting (center). The open triangles represent the patients studied under both conditions. Right: fasting insulin concentrations in hypoglycemic patients with proven insulinoma. The solid circles in the rectangles represent multiple samples in the same subjects. (*Source:* Yalow RS, Berson A: Dynamics of insulin secretion in hypoglycemia. Diabetes 14:341–349, 1965. With permission.)

Insulin secretion gradually decreases in those who develop NIDDM when compared with insulin secretion in equally obese nondiabetic, age- and sex-matched control subjects. Individuals with NIDDM are at increased risk of progressing to IDDM for reasons that are as yet largely shrouded in mystery. It is estimated that more than 90% of those who are being treated with insulin in North America had NIDDM when diabetes was diagnosed. It is not known whether these individuals have a diminished genetic B-cell insulin secretion capacity, "B-cell exhaustion"[100] because of sustained hyperglycemia, immunologic B-cell destruction, or a

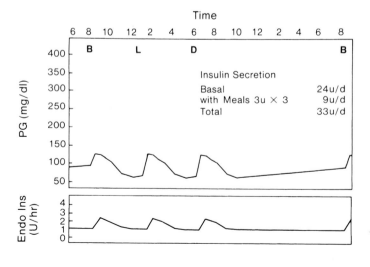

Figure 18–12. This graph represents insulin secretion and plasma glucose patterns in a hypothetical 176 pound (80 kg) adult at ideal body weight. The pancreatic B-cell mass is normal (0.64 g), and the insulin receptor number is normal. *Abbreviations:* B, breakfast, D, dinner, L, lunch. [*Source:* Davidson JK: Diabetes mellitus and its treatment with diet, exercise, insulin and sulfonylureas. *In* Wang RIH (ed): Practical Drug Therapy. Philadelphia: J. B. Lippincott, 1979, pp. 417–444. With permission.]

combination of these and other causes. Methodology currently available will permit detailed study of the various possibilities (see Chapters 2 through 9).

About 40 to 50% of secreted endogenous insulin is removed on its first pass through the liver.[101–106] In the systemic plasma compartment, the half-life of endogenous insulin is about 4.3 min. About 5% of secreted endogenous proinsulin is removed on its first pass through the liver. The half-life of endogenous proinsulin is about 26 min.[106–111] Only negligible amounts of endogenous C-peptide are removed by the liver.

It is estimated that about 70% of the C-peptide secreted by the B cell is extracted by the kidney.[112] Normal subjects excrete 36 to 65 μg C-peptide/24 hr in the urine.[95] A good estimate of maximal B-cell secretory capacity is provided by the 24-hr urine C-peptide level after oral prednisone. Serum fasting C-peptide levels in normal subjects are 0.4 to 1.6 pmol/mL (1.2 to 4.8 ng/mL); these levels rise two- to threefold after stimulation by glucose or food.

Peripheral fasting serum insulin levels in normal subjects range from 24 to 144 pmol/L (0.14–0.84 ng/mL, or 4 to 24 μU/mL); these levels rise severalfold after stimulation by glucose, food, and other stimuli.

From 30 to 80% of the insulin entering the peripheral circulation is removed by the kidney.

Because of its longer half-life (six times as long as the half-life of insulin), the molar concentration of C-peptide in the peripheral plasma compartment is 5 to 15 times that of insulin.

Also, because of its longer half-life (five times as long as the half-life of insulin), even though proinsulin and its conversion intermediates account for only 3 to 4% of the B-cell secretion products, proinsulin may account for up to 30% of the insulin immunoreactivity in peripheral serum. About 50% of the proinsulin entering the peripheral circulation is removed by the kidney.

When an insulinoma or familial hyperproinsulinemia is suspected, the proinsulin level should be measured (see Exhibit 18–1).

The body distribution space of insulin in normals approximates that of the extracellular compartment (see Fig. 18–28). The metabolic clearance rate of insulin is 11.3 mL/min/kg, of C-peptide is 4.4 mL/min/kg, and of proinsulin is 2.1 to 3.7 mL/min/kg.[113] The half-life of insulin is about 4.3 to 4.8 min, of C-peptide is about 33.5 ± 3 min, and of proinsulin is about 25.6 min.[113]

The kidney metabolizes a larger fraction of exogenous insulin (which is absorbed directly into the venous systemic circulation) than of endogenous insulin (about half of which is removed on its first pass through the liver before it reaches the systemic circulation).

The glomerular filtration rate (GFR) of insulin is about 90% of the GFR of the freely filtered (100%) fructose-polymer inulin. C-peptide's GFR is probably 100%, and proinsulin's GFR is probably less than insulin's GFR.

Normally, 99% of the filtered insulin is reabsorbed and enzymatically degraded in the proximal tubule. Less than 1% of the filtered insulin appears in the urine.

Thirty to 80% of the insulin and 50% of the proinsulin in the peripheral circulation are removed by the kidney (two thirds by luminal clearance via glomerular filtration, one third by the postglomerular peritubular circulation). Contraluminal insulin receptors are distributed throughout the nephron, especially along the medullary thick ascending limb of Henle's loop and along the distal convoluted tubule. It is thought that the peritubular clearance of insulin delivers it to its major sites of action on the kidney (reabsorption of sodium, phosphate, and glucose).[112]

Fifty percent of the secreted C-peptide is removed by the kidney, with 10% being excreted in the urine. The metabolic clearance rate of C-peptide is about 300 mL/min. Urinary C-peptide excretion is about 20% of the renal excretion rate, resulting in a urinary elimination rate of about 50 pmol/min. The fate of the remaining secreted C-peptide is not known.

When renal clearance of insulin is impaired, the half-life of insulin is longer than normal. The dose of exogenous insulin needed to maintain near normoglycemia may fall dramatically, frequently to none in those who can still secrete some endogenous insulin.

Much more knowledge is needed of the manner in which diabetic nephropathy and renal failure affect insulin, proinsulin, C-peptide, and substrate metabolism.[112,113]

C-peptide has generally been considered not to possess biological activity. Studies during the last five years have demonstrated that administration of C-peptide in physiological amounts in Type 1 (IDDM) patients on a short-term basis (1–3 hr) results in decreased glomerular hyperfiltration, augmented glucose utilization, and improved autonomic nerve function.[118] More prolonged administration (1–3 months) of C-peptide to IDDM patients is accompanied by improvements in renal function (diminished microalbuminuria) and autonomic and sensory nerve function. Both in vitro and in vivo data indicate that C-peptide may have a role in insulin secretion. C-peptide's mechanism of action is not known, but it may be related to its ability to stimulate Na, K(+)-ATPase activity, probably by activating a receptor coupled to a pertussis toxin-sensitive G protein with subsequent activation of $Ca_2(+)$-dependent intracellular signaling pathways. These findings indicate that C-peptide is a biologically active hormone. The possibility that C-peptide therapy in IDDM patients may be beneficial is being explored.

When endogenous insulin levels are not adequate to maintain near normoglycemia with diet and exercise therapy alone in those who are near or below ideal body weight (Fig. 18–13), glucosuria and hyperglycemia become more marked and diabetic

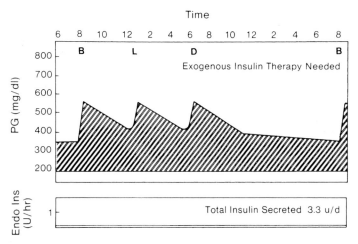

Figure 18–13. This graph represents the abnormal insulin secretion, plasma glucose, and urine glucose patterns in a hypothetical 176 pound (80 kg) adult at ideal body weight who has IDDM. His pancreatic B-cell mass is markedly reduced (0.05 g), and is secreting only 3.3 U of insulin per day. The plasma glucose ranges from 350 to 575 mg/dL, and glucosuria is persistent (represented by cross-hatching on plasma glucose graph). Exogenous insulin therapy is needed. *Abbreviations:* B, breakfast; D, dinner; L, lunch. [*Source:* Davidson JK: Diabetes mellitus and its treatment with diet, exercise, insulin and sulfonylureas. *In* Wang RIH (ed): Practical Drug Therapy. Philadelphia: J. B. Lippincott, 1979, pp. 417–444. With permission.]

ketoacidosis (DKA) may develop.[114] To maintain life and health, exogenous insulin therapy then becomes mandatory (Fig. 18–14).

Pharmacokinetics of Exogenous (Injected) Insulin

The introduction of highly purified animal (beef, pork) insulin[78] in the late 1970s and of human insulin (rDNA),[69,72] and of human insulin SS in the early 1980s[77] made available to physicians a large number of commercial insulin preparations (see Table 18–5).

The hope of the 1950s that most individuals with diabetes could be controlled by intermediate-acting or long-acting insulin administered once daily was not realized.[81,82,85] Also the hope of the 1970s and 1980s that individuals could be perfectly controlled by intensive conventional insulin therapy (ICIT) or by (open-loop) continuous subcutaneous insulin infusion (CSII)

was not realized.[115–117] Some individuals absorb insulin (intermediate and/or rapid-acting) quickly, and some absorb it slowly (see Fig. 18–10 and Figs. 18–15 through 18–19). Most individuals absorb it at different rates on different days. Thus, because the pharmacokinetics and bioavailability of injected insulin varies between individuals, and from day to day in the same individual, all persons with IDDM require an initially tailored treatment routine (insulin, diet, exercise), and appropriate adjustments by the responsible professional and the patient during follow-up (see Exhibits 18–4 and 18–5).

Regular insulin may be administered by bolus either subcutaneously, intramuscularly IV, or intraperitoneally, or continuously by insulin infusion devices. In some individuals, programmed continuous subcutaneous insulin infusion may provide excellent continuing control of the plasma glucose level (Fig. 18–20), but the open-loop devices in use from 1985 to 1998 have not been uniformly safe and effective and there

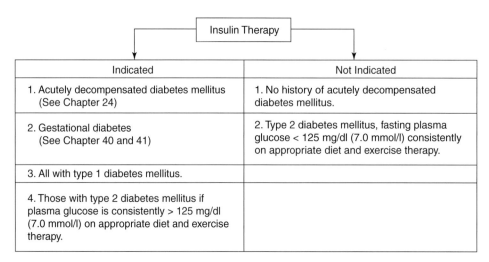

Figure 18–14. A list of the problems for which insulin therapy is indicated and for which insulin therapy is not indicated. [*Sources:* Davidson JK: (Topic 203) Diabetes Mellitus. *In* Hurst JW (ed): Medicine for the Practicing Physician, Butterworth, Woburn, MA. Pp 435–448, 1988.

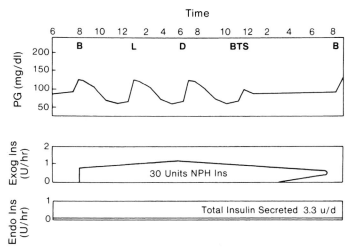

Figure 18–15. This graph represents a hypothetical individual with IDDM who absorbed NPH insulin administered once daily (before breakfast) at a rate (24 hr) that permitted him to maintain his plasma glucose range (AGEs) between 70 and 130 mg/dL without hypoglycemia. Only a small fraction of those with IDDM attain and maintain this level of control with one injection of intermediate-acting insulin per day. Those who do are usually secreting a significant amount of endogenous insulin, and are on a consistent diet and exercise pattern.[114–131] *Abbreviations:* B, breakfast; BTS, bedtime snack; D, dinner; L, lunch. [*Source:* Davidson JK: Diabetes mellitus and its treatment with diet, exercise, insulin and sulfonylureas. *In* Wang RIH (ed): Practical Drug Therapy. Philadelphia J. B. Lippincott, 1979, pp. 417–444. With permission. See also: Bretcher C, Malmquist J: Insulin requiring diabetes mellitus of sixty years duration without significant late manifestations. Acta Med Scand 210:239–240, 1981; Cochran HA, Jr, Alexander M, Galloway JA: Factors in the survival of patients with insulin-requiring diabetes for 50 years. Diabetes Care 2:363–368, 1979; Deckert T: The influence of supervision and endogenous insulin secretion on the course of insulin-dependent diabetes mellitus. Acta Endocrinol 94 (Suppl 238):31–38, 1980.]

may be a slightly increased risk of DKA and of hypoglicemia for those using CSII.

One fairly common problem that has been encountered in attempts to implement successful CSII programs has been the tendency of regular insulin to aggregate as larger crystals and to plug the infusion devices.[119] Buffered insulins, which are prepared to prevent aggregation, are an improvement compared with conventional regular insulin when CSII programs are being used (Table 18–5).

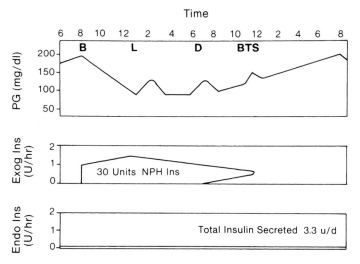

Figure 18–16. This graph represents a hypothetical individual with IDDM who absorbed NPH insulin administered before breakfast rapidly (16 hr) so that the plasma glucose level was normal in the afternoon, but elevated before and after breakfast. More NPH insulin before breakfast would have made him hypoglycemic in the afternoon, and hyperglycemia before and after breakfast would have persisted because of the waning of insulin action. Also, hyperglycemia in the morning may have been intensified by posthypoglycemic hyperglycemia (Somogyi phenomenon). See Figs. 18–24, 18–25, Exhibit 18–12, and Table 18–8. *Abbreviations:* B, breakfast; BTS, bedtime snack; D, dinner; Endo Ins, endogenous insulin; Exog Ins, exogenous insulin; L, lunch, PG, plasma glucose. [*Source:* Davidson JK: Diabetes mellitus and its treatment with diet, exercise, insulin and sulfonylureas. *In* Wang RIH (ed): Practical Drug Therapy. Philadelphia; J. B. Lippincott, 1979, pp. 417–444. With permission.]

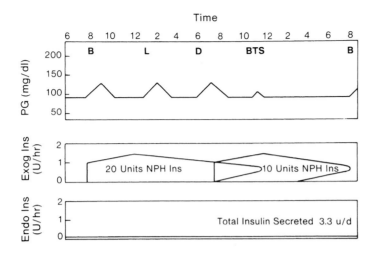

Figure 18–17. This graph represents the hypothetical individual depicted in Figure 18–16 and the decrease in the AGEs that occurred when a single dose of 30 U NPH insulin was split into two doses (20 U at 8 a.m., 10 U at 8 p.m.). See Figs. 18–24, 18–25, Exhibit 18–12, and Table 18–7. Abbreviations as in Figure 18–15. [*Source:* Davidson JK: Diabetes mellitus and its treatment with diet, exercise, insulin and sulfonylureas. *In* Wang RIH (ed): Practical Drug Therapy. Philadelphia: J. B. Lippincott, 1979, pp. 417–444. With permission.]

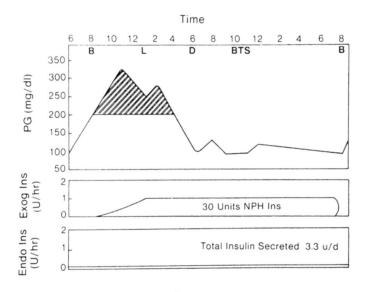

Figure 18–18. This graph represents a hypothetical individual with IDDM who absorbed NPH insulin administered before breakfast slowly in the morning so that the plasma glucose was elevated in the morning and early afternoon and there was morning glucosuria, but the plasma glucose was within the normal range from 6 p.m. to 8 a.m. See Table 18–8. Abbreviations as in Figure 18–15. [*Source:* Davidson JK: Diabetes mellitus and its treatment with diet, exercise, insulin and sulfonylureas. *In* Wang RIH (ed): Practical Drug Therapy. Philadelphia, J. B. Lippincott, 1979, pp. 417–444. With permission.]

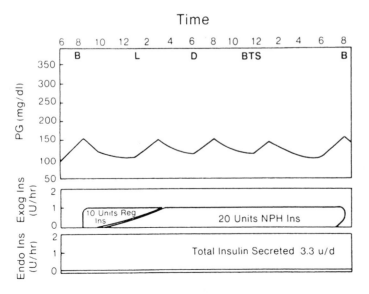

Figure 18–19. This graph represents the hypothetical individual depicted in Figure 18–17 and the decrease in the amplitude of glucose excursions that occurred when he was given 20 U NPH insulin mixed with 10 U regular insulin at 8 a.m. rather than 30 U NPH insulin at 8 a.m. See Table 18–8. Abbreviations as in Figure 18–15. [*Source:* Davidson JK: Diabetes mellitus and its treatment with drug, exercise, insulin and sulfonylureas. *In* Wang RIH (ed): Practical Drug Therapy. Philadelphia: J. B. Lippincott, 1979, pp. 417–444. With permission.]

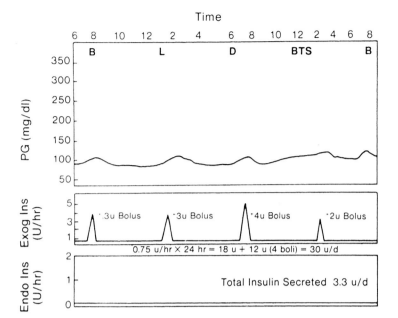

Figure 18–20. This graph represents a hypothetical individual with IDDM on continuous subcutaneous insulin infusion (CSII) or open-loop pump therapy. See Table 18–12. A basal infusion of 0.75 U/hr (18 U/24 hr) plus three boluses at mealtimes and one bolus at snack time (total 12 U) maintains near normoglycemia.

It should be noted that aggregation of NPH insulin in the vial was a problem encountered rather frequently in 1986 through 1988 (see Fig. 18–39), but it has been noted only rarely since then, because adjustments in the pH and reformulation of commercially available insulin solutions since that time decreased the risk of aggregation. Yet, it can still occur in vials of insulin subjected to vigorous or prolonged *shaking* (as it occurs in a pocket when walking for a week or longer) or to *high temperatures* (above 100°F). Thus, all individuals should routinely inspect the insulin in the vial that they are using to be certain that it is not aggregated, because aggregation can reduce the potency to 25% or less than the designated potency on the label, and this can lead to poor metabolic control and diabetic ketoacidosis.

The availability of radioactively labeled insulin (^{131}I, ^{125}I, ^{123}I, ^{3}H, ^{14}C) not only has made it possible to measure serum insulin levels in vitro, but also has made it possible to measure in vivo the metabolic clearance rate (milliliters of plasma cleared of insulin per minute), the half-life $(T_{1/2})$, the body DS of insulin (percent of body weight or volume of distribution in liters) after IV administration of labeled insulin (see Fig. 18–28), and the 50% absorption time of insulin from a subcutaneous depot (see Fig. 18–10).[120–124] It has been shown that A-14 monoiodinated ^{125}I insulin retains essentially 100% of its biologic and immunologic reactivity, whereas A-19 monoiodinated insulin retains only about 50% of its biologic and immunologic activity. Thus, it is important to use a labeled insulin whose biologic and immunologic activities are similar or identical to those of unlabeled insulin. Similar parameters have been measured by injecting unlabeled insulin IV and measuring sequential insulin levels over appropriately timed intervals.

Insulin absorption rates from subcutaneous and intramuscular depots have been measured and these rates have been correlated with the biologic effects of the injected insulin. As a result, knowledge of the factors that influence the pharmacokinetics of injected (exogenous) insulin have expanded greatly in recent years (Exhibits 18–2 and 18–3; see also Exhibit 18–5). Similar studies have been done with proinsulin and with C-peptide.

The attempts that have been made to administer insulin in a format that will mimic the metabolic control provided by normal pancreatic B-cell insulin secretion include: (1) conventional insulin therapy (CIT) (three versions including split doses of intermediate-acting insulin and mixtures of intermediate-acting and regular (or lispro) insulin), (2) ICIT (several visions), (3) open-loop CSII, and (4) closed-loop intravenous insulin infusion (Biostator) (Exhibit 18–4; Fig. 18–21). Only the closed-loop IV insulin infusion system (Biostator), which continuously monitors the plasma glucose level and infuses insulin to attain and to maintain sustained normoglycemia (without hypoglycemia or hyperglycemia), has succeeded, and an individual can be treated with this device for only a few days. (See Chapter 19.)

Although self blood glucose monitoring (see Chapter 22) has been of assistance in minimizing the amplitude of glucose excursions (AGEs) in those with IDDM, and at least partially "closing the loop," variations in the pharmacokinetics of injected insulin are now known to be the most important uncontrollable variables (see Exhibit 18–2). Controllable and uncontrollable factors that influence AGE and that influence the pharmacokinetics, bioavailability, and biologic actions of exogenous insulins are summarized in

EXHIBIT 18–2   Factors That Influence the Pharmacokinetics, Bioavailability, and Biologic Action of Exogenous Insulin

I. Factors that can be controlled
A. Insulin formulations

1. Rapid-acting	(a) Insulin lispro
2. Short-acting	(b) Regular
3. Intermediate-acting	(c) NPH
	(d) Lente
4. Long-acting	(e) Ultralente
5. Future insulin analogs	A variety of rapid-and longer-acting insulin analogs are anticipated in the near future

B. Mixtures of different types of insulin
   1. Self-mixed
      (a) NPH and regular insulin
      (b) NPH and insulin lispro
      (c) Lente and regular insulin*
      (d) Lente and insulin lispro
      (e) Ultralente and regular insulin*
      (f) Ultralente and insulin lispro
   2. Fixed mixtures*
      (a) 70/30 (70% NPH/30% Regular)
      (b) 50/50 (50% NPH/50% Regular)
C. Insulin source
   1. Human
      (a) rDNA (from genetically programmed *Escherichia coli* or *Saccharomyces cerevisiae*)
      (b) Semisynthetic (from pork)
   2. Pig (pork, porcine)
   3. Cow (beef, bovine)
   4. Other-sheep, fish, whale, and so forth
D. Insulin concentration and volume injected
E. Site of injection
   1. Intravenously
   2. Intramuscularly
   3. Subcutaneously
      (a) Abdomen
      (b) Deltoid
      (c) Gluteal
      (d) Femoral
      (e) other
F. Subcutaneous injection technique
   1. Depth
   2. Needle
   3. Syringe
   4. The rete cutis is about 2 mm thick. A needle, equal to or greater than 12 mm in length (8 mm needles are used by many pediatric or thin adult patients), should be inserted to the hilt at a 90° angle so that the insulin will be deposited by the injection at a depth of at least 10 mm in the subcutaneous tissue. The injection site should be massaged gently as the needle is being removed to prevent insulin from escaping through the needle tract.
G. Exercise
H. Ambient temperature
I. Diet

II. Factors that cannot be controlled
A. Rate of absorption of exogenous insulin
   1. Interperson variation of up to 50% (see Fig. 18–10)
   2. Intraperson variation from day to day up to 25%
   3. The rate of absorption from a subcutaneous site is influenced primarily by rate of blood flow, which in turn is influenced by depth of injection, site of injection, massaging the injection site, exercise, ambient temperature, physical state of the insulin, and concentration and volume of insulin injected
B. Rate of insulin degradation
   1. Subcutaneous
   2. Liver
   3. Kidney
   4. Insulin-sensitive cells
C. Numbers and affinity of insulin receptors and dynamics of the receptor-insulin interaction. See Chapters 8 and 9
D. Insulin antibodies
   Antibodies can combine with and hold in the plasma compartment exogenous insulin (and endogenous insulin as well). This prolongs the action of the insulin, and can result in the wastage of up to 95% of the injected insulin as a result of sequestration by the reticuloendothelial system.[133–137] Beef insulin is more antigenic than human or pork insulin. Insulin antibodies injected in sufficient amounts into nondiabetic experimental animals can produce an acute endogenous insulin deficit, diabetic coma, and death[15]
   See chapter section entitled "Immunologic Insulin Resistance"

---

* Self-made mixtures of Lente or Ultralente and regular insulin should be administered within 15 minutes of mixing to avoid loss of the faster acting effect of the regular insulin due to interaction with the zinc.

* *Footnote:* The United States uses the Intermediate Short-acting ratio in naming fixed mixtures while the majority of the world uses the Short (or Insulin lispro) Intermediate ratio for the naming convention.

[*Sources:* Binder C: Insulin pharmacokinetics. Diabetes Care 7:188–199, 1984; Galloway JA, Wentworth SM: A short review of the factors that affect the absorption and disposal of insulin. *In* Peterson CM (ed): Diabetes Management in the 80s. New York: Praeger, 1980, pp. 100–108; Galloway JA, deShazo RD: The clinical use of insulin and the complications of insulin therapy. *In* Ellenberg M, Rifkin H (eds): Diabetes Mellitus—Theory and Practice. New Hyde Park, NY: Medical Examination Publishing, 1983, pp. 519–538; Galloway JA, Root MA, Bergstrom R, et al.: Clinical pharmacologic studies with human insulin (recombinant DNA). Diabetes Care 5 (suppl 2):13–22, 1982; Galloway JA, Spradlin CT, Jackson RL, et al.: Mixtures of Intermediate-Acting Insulin (NPH and Lente) with Regular insulin: An Update. *In* Skyler JS (ed.) Proceedings of a symposium, "Insulin update 1982," December 1981, Key Biscayne, Fla. Amsterdam: Excerpta Medica, pp. 111–119; Galloway JA, Spradlin CT, Nelson RL, et al.: Factors influencing the absorption, serum insulin concentration, and blood glucose responses after injections of regular insulin and various insulin mixtures. Diabetes Care 4:366–376, 1981; Kobayashi T, Sawano S, Itoh K, et al.: The pharmacokinetics of insulin after continuous subcutaneous infusion or bolus subcutaneous injection in diabetic patients. Diabetes 32:331–336, 1983. With permission.]

EXHIBIT 18–3   Evaluation of Timing of Insulin Action

I. Indirect methods
   A. Time course of its effect on plasma glucose levels after injection
      1. Time to plasma glucose minimum = time to peak insulin effect
      2. Time for return of plasma glucose to fasting level = duration of insulin action
   B. Plasma glucose clamping techniques (Biostator) in which plasma glucose level is kept at a constant level. The amount of glucose infused and the time course reflect the magnitude and duration of insulin action. When this technique is combined with measurement of free insulin, plasma C-peptide, and a direct measurement of local clearance of subcutaneously injected insulin (see "Direct Methods," below), one has a complete picture of pharmacokinetics, bioavailability, and biologic action of exogenous subcutaneously injected insulin

II. Direct methods
   A. Time course of ^{125}I insulin remaining at injection site (measured by gamma-counter). (See Fig. 18–10.)
   B. B1-[^{3}H]phenylalanine insulin has been used to study the time course of insulin absorption as affected by exercise, the rate of insulin degradation at the injection site, and the in vitro rate of insulin degradation by insulin protease
   C. During conventional insulin therapy (CIT) or intensive conventional insulin therapy (ICIT), variation in the absorption rate of intermediate insulin (NPH or Lente) *accounts for up to 80% of the day-to-day fluctuations in the plasma glucose level* [amplitude of glucose excursions (AGE)]. *A major part of the variation is related to changes in blood flow at the injection site.* Coefficients of variation for the half-time of insulin absorption (T_{50}) are approximately 25% from day-to-day within the same individual, and up to 50% between individuals. See Figure 18–10
   D. The T_{50} for subcutaneously injected regular insulin (12 U) varied significantly by region of injection. The mean T_{50}s $\pm$ the standard error of the means were: *subcutaneous* (1) abdomen 87 $\pm$ 12 min, (2) deltoid 141 $\pm$ 23 min, (3) gluteal 155 $\pm$ 28 min, (4) femoral 164 $\pm$ 15 min; *intramuscular* (1) deltoid 69 $\pm$ 12 min, (2) femoral 89 $\pm$ 31 min
   E. The *relative absorption rate* rises during the first hours after injection, then remains constant. The initial absorption delay disappears when the concentration of injected insulin is reduced from 40 U/ml to 4 U/ml, and when the volume injected is increased from 0.01 to 1 mL. The absorption rate increases with increasing blood flow, but plateaus at high flow rates. This supports the hypothesis that available capillary surface area is the rate-limiting factor that determines the maximum absorption rate. Smoking-induced vasoconstriction slows the absorption rate
   F. Presumably zinc insulins (Semilente, Lente, Ultralente) are dissolved in situ and protamine insulins (NPH, PZI) are split before absorption takes place. Yet there is evidence that some NPH may enter the plasma compartments without being split
   G. Mixtures: See Exhibit 18–2, Section 1.B.
   H. Regional differences in the absorption rates of intermediate (NPH, Lente) and long-acting (Ultralente, PZI) insulins are probably great enough so that random rotation of injection sites between regions should be avoided
   I. The larger the dose of insulin, the longer its biologic action

(*Sources:* Same works as listed in footnote to Exhibit 18–2. With permission.)

Exhibit 18–2. The indirect and direct methods that are used in evaluating the timing of exogenous insulin actions are listed in Exhibit 18–3. The different subcutaneous insulin therapy routines in current use are listed in Exhibit 18–4. The effects of different insulin administration routines on the size of the exogenous *insulin depot* are described in Exhibit 18–5.

Molnar and associates[127–129] have described three methods for quantitating blood (or plasma) glucose changes over time: (1) *mean amplitude of glucose excursions (MAGE)*, a within-day blood glucose variability index; (2) *mean (diurnal) blood glucose (MBG)*, an index of overall glycemia; and (3) *mean of daily differences (MODD)* (referring to paired blood glucose values on successive days), an index of between-day blood glucose variability. Figure 18–22 illustrates each of the three methods of quantitating these changes in *normals*, in those with *stable diabetes*, and in those with *unstable diabetes*.

The enormous intrasubject coefficient of variation of insulin absorption rates and plasma glucose responses in normal test subjects prompted Galloway and coworkers[131] to state: "Considering the magnitude of the coefficient of variation in response to injected insulin of normal subjects, the phenomenon of diabetic instability as quantified by Molnar et al.[127–129] is more easily explained. These variations emphasize the shortcomings of conventional insulin therapy (CIT) in the management of IDDM." It is estimated that about 80% of the day-to-day variation in plasma glucose levels in the same individual are related to the day-to-day variation in rates of insulin absorption (Exhibit 18–2).

Simple ways to estimate the amplitude and causes of glucose excursions is shown in Figures 18–23 to 18–25. Frequent monitoring of the blood (plasma) glucose in the hospital or at home can provide the information needed to make appropriate adjustments in insulin, diet, and exercise routines to optimize

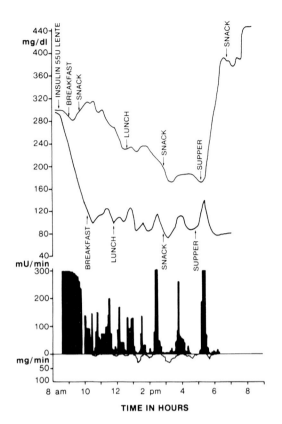

Figure 18–21. Continuous records of blood sugar profiles in subject S.M. sustained by subcutaneous insulin (top curve) and regulated by artificial pancreas (center curve). Minute-by-minute infusion patterns (lower curve) of insulin (black) and dextrose (white). Note dextrose infusion scale is inverted with respect to the insulin infusion scale. Total insulin infused was 53.1 U. (*Source:* Albisser AM, Leibel BS, Ewart TG, et al.: Chemical control of diabetes by the artificial pancreas. Diabetes 23:397–404, 1974. With permission.)

metabolic control, and to attain the *goal target zone* more than 75% of the time.

Figures 18–15 through 18–20 illustrate hypothetical examples of the effects of different types of insulin therapy (a.m. NPH, a.m. and p.m. NPH, a.m. NPH plus regular, and open-loop pump CSII).

Six examples of unsatisfactory blood glucose control on one insulin routine that improved on a subsequent routine are shown in Tables 18–6 through 18–12.

Molnar and associates[129] have characterized levels of control as (1) *ideal*, (2) *adequate*, and (3) *inadequate* for plasma glucose levels fasting and 2 hr postprandial. The recommended levels were for those with *mild diabetes*: (1) *ideal*, fasting <110 mg/dL (<6.1 mM) and 2 hr postprandial; (2) *adequate* <130 mg/dL (<7.2 mM) fasting, <170 mg/dL (<9.4 mM) 2 hr post prandial; (3) *inadequate*, >130 mg/dL (>7.2 mM) fasting, >170 mg/dL (>9.4 mM) 2 hr postprandial. The recommended levels were for those with severe *diabetes*: (1) ideal, < 110 mg/dL (<6.1 mM) fasting and 2 hr postprandial; (2) *adequate*, ≤170 mg/dL (≤9.4 mM) fasting and ≤170 mg/dL (<9.4 mM) 2 hr postprandial; (3) inadequate >170 mg/dL (>9.4 mM) fasting and/or 2 hr postprandial. See Table Intro-I.

Undesirable fluctuations of plasma glucose levels resulting in hypoglycemia and/or hyperglycemia despite the prescription by the physician of the best available therapeutic modalities (diet, insulin, exercise) and conscientious self-monitoring of blood glucose by the patient has long been a source of frustration. Studies have shown that those with the greatest fluctuations, those with so-called "unstable", "labile," or "brittle" diabetes, have no beta cell insulinogenic reserve. Those who are stable usually have more beta cell insulinogenic reserve than those who are unstable.[126,127] (See Fig. 18–22.)

EXHIBIT 18–4   Subcutaneous Insulin Therapy Routines (See Figs. 18–15 to 18–21 and Tables 18–6 to 18–12)

I. Conventional Insulin Therapy (CIT)
  A. Intermediate-acting insulin (NPH or Lente) before breakfast (See Fig. 18–15)
  B. For those on CIT format (I.A.) whose fasting plasma glucose is consistently >120 mg/dL (see Fig. 18–16): Intermediate-acting insulin (NPH or Lente) before breakfast and 12 hr later (some give the second dose before supper or at bedtime). (See Figure 18–17)
  C. For those on CIT format (I.A.) whose postbreakfast and prelunch plasma glucose is >150 mg/dL (see Fig. 18–18): Intermediate-acting (NPH or Lente) plus regular or lispro insulin before breakfast. (See Fig. 18–19)
II. Intensive Conventional Insulin Therapy (ICIT)
  A. Intermediate-acting insulin plus regular insulin twice daily (every 12 hr, or before breakfast and before supper, or before breakfast and at bedtime)

  B. Regular insulin before meals plus intermediate-acting insulin before supper or at bedtime
  C. Regular insulin every 6 or 8 hr
  D. Insulin lispro before each meal with a basal insulin (NPH or Lente or Ultralente) at bedtime or twice a day.
III. For those not satisfactorily controlled on any of the above routines
  A. (Open-loop) continuous subcutaneous insulin infusion (CSII): Basal rate, and bolus before meals (see Fig. 18–20). Doses determined on individual basis. Careful home monitoring is essential. Minicomputer dose planning adjustment may be helpful. See Chapter 19
  B. Closed-loop IV insulin infusion (Biostator)—can be used only for a few days. (See Fig. 18–21.) Has been used during surgery, delivery of baby, treatment of DKA, and to estimate 24-hr insulin requirement prior to initiating CSII or ICIT. See Chapter 19

EXHIBIT 18–5   The Effects of Different Insulin Administration Routines on the Size of the Exogenous Insulin Depot

For one taking 40 U insulin/day, *the size of the body tissue depot of insulin* will vary depending on how insulin is administered. For example, for 32 U NPH SC at 8:00 a.m. and 8 U NPH SC at 6:00 p.m. and an insulin T_{50} of 15 hr, the size of the depot varies from 26 to 52 U. A T_{50} variation of 30% in either direction from 4:00 to 6:00 a.m. can result in a range of insulin absorption of 2 to 4.2 U. See Figure 18–10. For regular insulin three times daily (8 U at 8:00 a.m. and 12 noon, 12 U at 6:00 p.m., and 12 U NPH at 11:00 p.m.), the depot varies from 12 to 21 U. A T_{50} variation of 30% in either direction from 4:00 to 6:00 a.m. can result in a range of insulin absorption of 1 to 1.9 U. For CSII (continuous subcutaneous insulin infusion) at a basal rate of 0.5 U/hr plus three boluses of 9.33 U each (containing a total of 28 U insulin) administered at 8:00 a.m., 12:00 noon, and 6:00 p.m., the depot varies from 1 to 14 U. A T_{50} variation of 30% in either direction from 4:00 to 6:00 a.m. can result in a range of insulin absorption from 0.7 to 1.8 U.

Large fluctuations in insulin absorption rates with conventional insulin therapy (CIT) is the most significant cause of unpredictably large swings in plasma glucose levels (with intermittent episodes of hypoglycemia and hyperglycemia). The amplitudes of glucose excursion (AGE) may decrease during CSII if the insulin dose is properly designed to meet the patient's needs. Since the insulin depot with CSII is very small, diabetic ketoacidosis may develop rapidly if insulin infusion is interrupted by a break, or by an obstruction that develops in the insulin infusion system.

Another reason for large variations in plasma glucose levels is that some individuals may be five times as sensitive to small changes in circulating free insulin as are others who are less sensitive.

Some individuals whose plasma glucose levels cannot be regulated satisfactorily with large doses of insulin may have one or more of the problems listed in Exhibit 18–15 (items A through J). If appropriate, these ten problems should be considered.

(*Source:* Binder C: Insulin pharmacokinetics. Diabetes Care 7:188–189, 1984. With permission.)

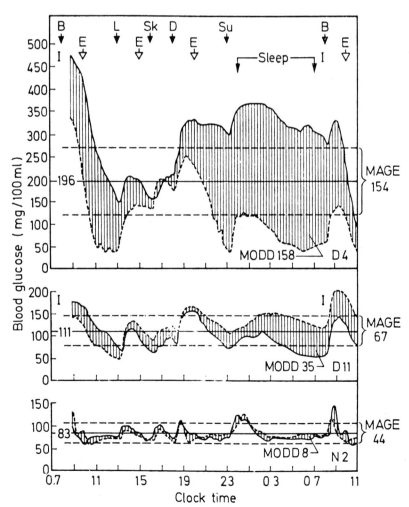

Figure 18–22.   Continuously sampled and analyzed blood glucose patterns over two successive 24 hr periods in a normal subject (bottom), a stable diabetic (middle), and an unstable diabetic (top). The first 24 hr is plotted as a solid line and the second 24 hr, as a broken line. The 48 hr mean blood glucose (MBG) is shown by the horizontal line transecting each panel; its numerical value is at the left. Mean of daily differences of paired blood glucose values (MODD) is shown by the hatched area (absolute difference between the first and second 24 hr); its numerical value is below. Mean amplitude of glycemic excursions (MAGE) is shown by interrupted lines bracketing the MBG; its numerical value is at the right. *Abbreviations:* B, breakfast; L, lunch; Sk, snack; D, dinner; Su, supper; E, 1 hr of exercise; I, insulin. (*Source:* Molnar GD, Taylor WF, Langworthy A: On measuring the adequacy of diabetes regulation: comparison of continuously monitored blood glucose patterns with values at selected time points. Diabetologia 10:139–143, 1974.[128]

Blood Glucose mg/dl (mM)

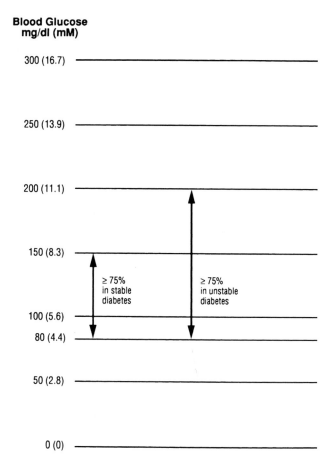

Figure 18–23. Target zone goals for blood glucose control in those with stable diabetes mellitus and in those with unstable diabetes mellitus.

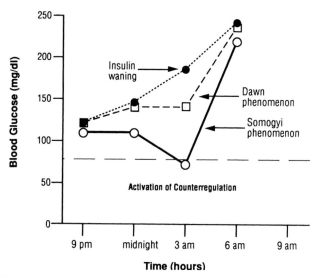

Figure 18–24. Distinguishing between insulin waning and dawn and Somogyi phenomena using overnight blood glucose profiles. (*Source:* Distinguishing between dawn, Somogyi phenomena called critical for proper patient management. Diabetes Outlook 22:3, 1987. With permission.)

In a study of 148 type 1 patients who had never received insulin and were then treated with insulin for 1 year, only 12% had normal hemoglobin A_{1c} levels, and over two thirds had levels indicative of significant, probably sustained, hyperglycemia.[131] It was believed that these unsatisfactory therapeutic results were due primarily to two factors: (1) the erratic pharmacokinetics of insulin, mainly due to variable absorption rates from day-to-day (see Fig. 18–10), and poor patient adherence to prescribed diet, exercise, and insulin therapy.

Harris[132] compiled fasting and nonfasting plasma glucose levels in normals, IDDMs, and NIDDMs from a variety of sources in the United States. In normals,

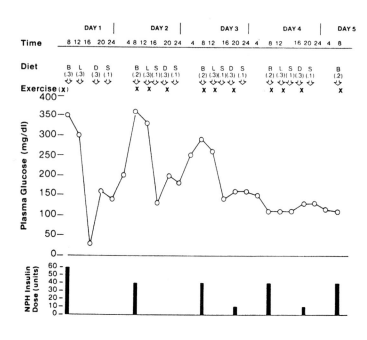

Figure 18–25. An example of posthypoglycemic hyperglycemia plus the waning of insulin effect which resulted in a wide amplitude of glycemic excursions. The amplitude of glycemic excursions was decreased significantly by splitting the dose of NPH insulin, and by stabilizing the diet and exercise routine. See text for detailed description of the patient's clinical course. *Abbreviations:* B, breakfast; D, dinner; L, lunch; S, snack.

mean fasting plasma glucose was 91 mg/dL (5.1 mM) and nonfasting was 97 mg/dL (5.4 mM). In patients with established diabetes (IDDMs and NIDDMs) in three university diabetes clinics, mean fasting plasma glucoses [mg/dL (mM)] were: 199 (11.1), 217 (12.1), 224 (12.4). In the WHO multinational study, mean fasting plasma glucose in those using insulin was 221 mg/dL (12.3 mM). Mean fasting plasma glucose levels in those with diabetes who were under treatment were more than twice as high as those in normals. Thus, *ideal control* and *adequate control*, as described by Molnar, have been attained and maintained in only a small percent of those with IDDM up to 1999. More studies are needed.

Because of varying day-to-day rates of exogenous insulin absorption, it is not surprising that it has not been possible to maintain the amplitude of glycemic excursions in those who are being treated with insulin within the range that is characteristic of those who have normally responsive pancreatic B cells.[115–117,126–129] (see Fig. 18–10). In 1999, it seems that the only possible solution to this problem will be the eventual development of a completely reliable closed-loop insulin infusion system that monitors the plasma glucose level and that infuses insulin as needed to keep the AGE normal.[115] (See Chapter 19)

The controversy[138–140] concerning whether or not optimal plasma glucose control can be attained and maintained has not been resolved. Some regard the goal of persistent "good control" of the plasma glucose level in IDDM with insulin delivery devices available in 1999 as a "mass delusion,"[139] and some question whether good control" is "achievable or desirable."[140]

Others have shown that many patients with insulin-requiring diabetes can survive for 50 years or more,[141] and some, after 65 years of IDDM, have no significant complications.[142] It appears that the ability to secrete some endogenous insulin, and continuing supervision by a diabetologist, contribute to an increased duration of survival and to an improved quality of life.[143]

Short-term amelioration of hypercalcuria,[144] improvement in nerve conduction velocity,[145] correction of lipid and lipoprotein abnormalities,[146] correction of exercise-induced microalbuminuria,[147] and marked improvement in plasma glucose control during short-term CSII have been reported. However, very "tight" control risks severe (sometimes fatal) hypoglycemia,[148] and other undesirable side effects.[149,150] CSII is expensive, and it requires an intensive time commitment by both the patient and physician or diabetes nurse.

A study to assess the relationship between metabolic control and development and/or progression of complications of IDDM was initiated in 1982 by the National Institute of Arthritis, Diabetes, Digestive and Kidney Disease (NIADDKD) in 27 centers in the United States and Canada. This study, known as the DCCT, was conducted in four sequential phases. Its goal was to assess the relationship between metabolic control and the clinical course of early vascular complications in persons with IDDM. Diabetic retinopathy was the primary outcome assessed. Secondary outcomes included neuropathy, nephropathy, and neurobehavioral and cardiovascular complications.[151–155]

1441 individuals with IDDM participated in the diabetes control and complications trial (DCCT).[151–155] On entry 726 had no retinopathy and 715 had mild retinopathy. They were randomly assigned to conventional therapy (one or two insulin injections per day) or intensive therapy (three or more insulin injections per day or insulin administered continuously by an external pump).

The mean plasma glucose in the conventional therapy group was 232 mg/dl, mean hemoglobin A_{1c} was 9.0%. Mean plasma glucose in the intensive therapy group was 151 mg/dl (81 mg/dl less), mean hemoglobin A_{1c} was 7.1% (1.9% less).

After a mean of 6.5 years follow up, in the intensive therapy group, the appearance of retinopathy in retinopathy-free individuals was reduced by 76% and progression of mild retinopathy by 54%, the occurrence of microalbuminuria by 54% and clinical neuropathy was decreased by 60%.

In the intensive therapy group, the frequency of severe hypoglycemia was much more common, with a disproportionate number occurring during sleep. One-third of the daytime episodes were not accompanied by warning symptoms. One intensive therapy study participant who was driving a car, killed two other individuals, but survived.

At the conclusion of the study, 33.6% in the intensive study group were significantly overweight, whereas only 17.5% in the conventionally treated group were. Thus in 1999, it is clear that utilizing currently available knowledge, medications, and devices will not produce continuous near-normoglycemia (see Figure 18–22) that most professionals and individuals with IDDM desire. Those who attempt such levels of control must pay a high price (hypoglycemic coma, weight gain, money and time) for the effort. We do not yet know whether the rewards are worth the price that must be paid.

A follow-up study of those who participated in the DCCT is underway (the EDIC). The EDIC (Epidemiology of Diabetes Interventions and Complications Research Group)[156, 157] could over the next several decades answer some of the long-term effects on morbidity and mortality in tightly controlled versus conventionally controlled individuals who participated in the DCCT.

The suggestion that hyperinsulinemia might contribute to the development of atherosclerosis was first reported in 1969, and the evidence since accumulated that such may be the case has been recently reviewed.[158]

It has been known for more than 20 years that peripheral arteries of both NIDDMs and IDDMs are exposed for prolonged periods to higher than normal insulin levels. Endogenous hyperinsulinemia is closely associated with a cluster of cardiovascular risk factors: hypertriglyceridemia, low HDL, levels, upper body obesity, hypertension, and hyperglycemia. Insulin stimulates proliferation of arterial smooth muscle cells and stimulates cholesterol synthesis and low density lipoprotein binding to smooth muscle cells and monocyte macrophages (to form foam cells). Stout[158] has recommended that hyperinsulinemia be avoided insofar as possible in normals and in NIDDMs (diet to attain and maintain ideal body weight, exercise) and in IDDMs by maintaining good metabolic control with the lowest possible circulating insulin levels in order to minimize the putative, yet unproved, atherogenic effects of elevated circulating insulin levels.

Epidemiology and Pathophysiology of IDDM

See Chapters 3 and 6.

Problem Statement

When is insulin therapy indicated? What insulin therapy routines are available? When and how should they be used?[261]

Berger and colleagues[210] have suggested that it may be best to initiate insulin therapy in type 2 diabetes if fasting plasma glucose consistently exceeds 125 mg/dl (7 mmol/l) and HbA1c 7%. Thus the dangers and expense of oral agent therapy can be avoided.[261] See Chapters 20 and 54.

The International Diabetes Federation (IDF) reported recently on its survey of patient access to insulin, particularly in economically deprived populations. The IDF is leading efforts to make insulin available to all who need it.[260] See Appendix II.

Subjective

See Chapters 3 and 6.

Objective

See Chapters 3 and 6.

Assessment

Before insulin therapy is initiated, it should be determined that the individual has IDDM, or gestational diabetes that requires insulin therapy to protect the fetus, or NIDDM that requires insulin therapy (possibly transiently) because of DKA, hyperglycemic hyperosmolar state (HHS), or a fasting plasma glucose level persistently >125 mg/dL in those who are within 10% of ideal body weight.[114,159–161] See Figure 18–14.

Plan

Initial Available insulin preparations and their characteristics are shown in Table 18–5, and subcutaneous insulin therapy routines in common use at the present time are listed in Exhibit 18–4.

If the patient when initially seen is in DKA or a HHS, regular insulin therapy should be used until metabolic homeostasis has been restored (see Chapter 24). Then an intermediate (NPH or Lente) insulin should be started promptly to prevent recurrence of DKA. Later, an intermediate-acting insulin (NPH or Lente) should be administered once per day to determine whether one injection per day is sufficient to sustain a near-normal amplitude of glucose excursion (hospital- or home-monitored) (see Fig. 18–15), or whether two doses of intermediate-acting insulin (so-called *split dose*) are needed (see Figs. 18–16 and 18–17), or whether intermediate-acting insulin mixed with regular insulin or insulin lispro (so-called *mixed dose*) is needed (see Figs. 18–18 and 18–19). In some individuals it will be appropriate to try another insulin administration routine or to try CSII (see Fig. 18–20). Most physicians aim for the hypothetical near-normoglycemia depicted in Figures 18–15, 18–17, 18–19, and 18–20, but they recognize that the continuing risk of hypoglycemia makes it unattainable in many individuals with IDDM. See Tables 18–6 to 18–12 for examples of patients with unsatisfactory blood glucose control which improved when the prescribed insulin routine was changed.

Follow-up

A number of algorithms for prescribing insulin and adjusting the dose have been described.[116, 117] None of them are successful in some individuals with IDDM, especially in those with unstable diabetes and/or autonomic neuropathy. Exhibit 18–4 lists in order the routines used by one of the authors (J.K.D.) in trying to attain optimal plasma glucose control in as many individuals with IDDM as possible. (See Tables 18–6 to 18–12 and Figs. 18–15 to 18–20.)

The size of the exogenous insulin depot varies with different insulin administration routines, as noted in Exhibit 18–5. Variables that determine the plasma concentration of exogenous insulin are listed in Exhibit 18–6. *For each individual, the dose(s) and type(s) of insulin must be adjusted to their needs (determined by AGE), and must be coordinated with prescribed diet and exercise routine to maximize the likelihood of success* in attaining and maintaining optimal metabolic control. (See Chapters 3, 15, 16, and 17.)

Patient Education Supplies that may be needed to treat individuals on insulin therapy are: (1) Syringes (Table 18–13), (2) injection aids (Table 18–15), (3) insulin pumps (Table 18–16), (4) aids for individuals who are visually impaired (Table 18–17), insulin pump supplies (Table 18-I) and insulin jet injectors (Table 18-II).[291]

Instructions on insulin measurement, on preparation of extemporaneous mixtures of NPH and regular (or Lispro) insulins, on skin sterilization and injection routines, and on the technique of rotating insulin injection

TABLE 18–6 Example of Unsatisfactory Blood Glucose (mg/dL) Control on 8 a.m. NPH Insulin Which Improved on 8 a.m. NPH Insulin Plus 8 p.m. NPH Insulin

Day	Insulin: 24 N + 4 R am. B	L	S	BT	3 a.m.	Insulin: 20 N + 4 R a.m., 6 N p.m. B	L	S	BT	3 a.m.
1	186	156	144	161		131	102	96	115	
2	211	142	130	138	148	114	108	105	102	113
3	191	118	102	128	136	127	118	113	98	108
4	176	126	131	141	149	98	90	92	78	121
5	203	134	126	160		117	115	104	88	
6	208	104	100	120		122	107	93	103	
7	198	113	98	114		116	120	111	128	
Mean	196	128	119	142	144	118	109	102	102	114
SD	12.6	17.9	18.4	15.2	7.2	10.7	10.4	8.5	16.5	6.6
SEM	4.8	6.7	6.9	5.7	4.2	4.0	3.9	3.2	6.2	2.5

Abbreviations: B, before breakfast; L, before lunch; S, before supper; BT, at bedtime; SD, standard deviation; SEM, standard error of the mean; N, NPH insulin; R, regular insulin.

TABLE 18–7 Example of Unsatisfactory Blood Glucose (mg/dL) Control on 8 a.m. NPH and 8 p.m. NPH Insulin Which Improved on 8 a.m. NPH Plus Regular and 8 p.m. NPH Insulin

Day	Insulin: 18 N 8:00 a.m., 10 N 8:00 p.m. B	L	S	BT	3 a.m.	Insulin: 14 N + 6 R 8 a.m., 10 N 8:00 p.m. B	L	S	BT	3 a.m.
1	118	189	143	121		93	142	121	131	
2	103	194	127	103	104	114	138	116	96	
3	85	217	134	117	113	91	114	137	121	
4	98	183	141	138	119	116	132	98	117	
5	115	163	98	100		121	127	117	87	
6	137	228	151	116		97	158	126	136	
7	94	204	141	123		119	148	123	101	
Mean	107	197	134	117	112	107	137	120	113	
SD	17.5	21.7	17.4	12.8	7.5	13.0	14.4	11.9	17.1	
SEM	6.6	8.2	6.6	4.8	4.3	4.9	5.4	4.5	6.5	

Abbreviations: Same as in Table 18–6.

TABLE 18–8 Example of Unsatisfactory Blood Glucose (mg/dL) Control on 8 a.m. and 8 p.m. NPH Insulin Which Became More Unsatisfactory on Supplementary Regular Insulin and Improved When Supplementary Regular Insulin Was Discontinued and 8 p.m. NPH Insulin Dose Was Decreased: An Example of Hypoglycemia-Induced Reactive Hyperglycemia (the Somogyi Phenomenon)

Day	Insulin: 24 N a.m., 16 N 8 p.m. B	L	S	BT	3 a.m.	Insulin: 24 8 a.m., 16 N 8 p.m., + Suppl R[b] B	L	S	BT	3 a.m.	Insulin: 14 N 8 a.m., 8 N 8 p.m. B	L	S	BT	3 a.m.
1	330	286	142	120		286	178	118	72		148	102	110	133	
2	415	314	185	132	51[a]	381	312	40[a]	317	31[a]	156	153	93	96	86
3	295	320	161	144	38[a]	510	172	316	215	26[a]	123	98	127	116	110
4	362	220	114	115	23[a]	480	230	216	90	16[a]	176	123	104	121	104
5	420	380	232	192		310	35[a]	196	362		131	146	137	148	
6	274	190	178	117		460	32[a]	232	294		96	109	88	84	
7	385	261	153	89		340	410	248	156		168	141	149	113	
Mean	354	282	166	130	37	395	196	195	215	24	143	125	115	116	100
SD	57.1	64.3	37.3	32.2	14.0	88.5	137.9	90.6	113.9	7.6	27.9	22.4	21.3	21.5	12.5
SEM	21.5	24.3	14.1	12.2	8.1	33.4	52.0	34.2	43.0	4.4	10.5	8.5	8.0	8.1	7.2

[a] Symptomatic hypoglycemia.

[b] Suppl R = Supplementary regular insulin according to the following algorithm: when blood glucose >300, give 5 U; >250, give 3 U; >200, give 2 U.

Abbreviations: Same as in Table 18–6.

TABLE 18–9   Example of Waning of Insulin Action Before Breakfast: Improved by Moving Evening NPH Insulin Dose from 6 to 11 p.m.

| Day | Insulin: 20 N + 6 R 8 a.m., 8 N 6 p.m. | | | | | | | Insulin: 20 N + 6 R 8 am., 8 N 11 p.m. | | | | | | |
	B	L	S	BT	2 a.m.	4 a.m.	6 a.m.	B	L	BT	S	2 a.m,	4 a.m.	6 a.m.
1	210	111	104	122	136	148	161	141	136	117	131	115	102	108
2	180	125	116	141				115	104	134	126			
3	230	132	138	118	116	142	138	161	128	86	94	96	107	83
4	165	103	81	98				92	88	80	80			
5	214	142	133	131	151	165	198	113	141	151	118	121	124	132
6	243	118	136	114	121	164	174	137	129	104	138	118	98	117
7	178	116	114	102				124	114	126	142			
Mean	203	121	117	118	131	155	169	126	108	114	118	113	108	110
SD	29.1	13.1	20.5	15.2	15.8	11.5	24.7	22.4	44.6	25.7	23.2	11.3	11.4	20.5
SEM	11.0	4.9	7.7	5.7	7.9	5.8	12.4	8.5	16.8	9.7	8.8	5.7	5.7	10.3

Abbreviations: Same as in Table 18–6.

TABLE 18–10   Example of the Dawm Phenomenon Improved by Moving Evening NPH Insulin Dose from 8 to 11 p.m. and Increasing the Dose Modestly

| Day | Insulin: 35 N + 10 R 8 a.m., 15 N 8 p.m. | | | | | | | Insulin: 35 N + 10 R 8 a.m., 18 N 11 p.m. | | | | | | |
	B	L	S	BT	2 a.m.	4 a.m.	6 a.m.	B	L	S	BT	2 a.m,	4 a.m.	6 a.m.
1	201	181	131	86				131	116	110	114			
2	216	143	98	141	119	114	182	101	123	93	103	108	114	118
3	198	124	123	116				124	127	134	131			
4	171	98	114	127	126	118	214	116	143	116	127	131	108	134
5	256	178	142	111				141	112	84	104			
6	212	153	78	98	106	132	198	132	128	96	118	117	101	119
7	243	114	116	123				116	91	131	98			
Mean	214	142	100	115	117	121	198	123	120	109	114	119	108	124
SD	28.5	31.6	42.8	18.4	10.1	9.5	16.0	13.2	16.2	19.2	12.6	11.6	6.5	9.0
SEM	10.8	11.9	16.2	6.9	5.8	5.5	9.2	5.0	6.1	7.2	4.8	6.7	3.8	5.2

Abbreviations: Same as in Table 18–6.

TABLE 18–11   Example of an Unstable Type 1 with Unsatisfactory Blood Glucose (mg/dL) Control and Hypoglycemia on 8 a.m. NPH + R and 8 p.m. NPH Insulin Which Improved on 8 a.m. Lispro and NPH, 12 noon Lispro, 6 p.m. Lispro and 11 p.m. Lispro and NPH Insulin

| Day | Insulin | | | | | | | |
| | 19N + 6R 8 a.m. | | 12 N 8 p.m. | | 22 N + 6 IL 8 a.m. | 4 IL 12 noon | 6 IL 6 p.m. | 14 N + 2 IL 11 p.m. |
	B	L	S	BT	B	L	S	BT
1	143	110	121	148	110	86	106	84
2	105	48*	143	178	88	94	118	82
3	159	123	92	137	107	88	98	76
4	82	37*	94	143	120	104	116	94
5	162	101	136	156	106	100	110	106
6	131	78	42*	171	108	82	92	87
7	146	108	157	131	114	93	120	104
Mean	133	72	112	138	108	92	109	90
SD	29.4	42.1	39.3	49.3	9.9	7.8	10.6	11.3
SEM	11.1	15.8	14.8	18.6	3.74	2.94	4.0	4.26

* Symptomatic hypoglycemia.

Abbreviations: Same as in Table 18–6.

TABLE 18–12 Example of an Unstable IDDM with Unsatisfactory Blood Glucose (mg/dL) Control on NPH + R Insulin 8 a.m. and 6 p.m. Which Improved on Continuous Subcutaneous Regular Insulin Infusion (CS11)

Day	Insulin: 20 N + 4 R 8 a.m., 14 N 8 p.m.					R Insulin CS11: Basal/IU/hr Boluses: 5,2,5,2 U				
	B	L	S	BT	3 a.m.	B	L	S	BT	3 a.m.
1	121	78	94	142		104	84	113	106	
2	112	132	143	158	142	96	117	87	102	116
3	98	116	118	126		114	103	121	141	
4	117	84	121	113	126	118	106	114	101	104
5	82	52[a]	168	178		102	100	104	93	
6	141	68	114	112	119	126	93	98	115	105
7	101	121	133	111		103	118	103	121	
Mean	110	79	113	135	129	109	103	106	111	108
SD	18.9	37.5	42.4	26.0	11.8	10.6	12.2	11.4	16.0	6.7
SEM	7.1	14.2	16.0	9.8	6.8					

[a] Symptomatic hypoglycemia.

Abbreviations: Same as in Table 18–6.

EXHIBIT 18–6 Variables that Determine the Plasma Concentration of Insulin

The plasma concentration of insulin is a product of four variables[a]:
1. Secretion rate of endogenous insulin
2. Absorption rate of exogenous insulin
3. Volume of distribution (similar to extracellular fluid volume or about 18 ± 3% of body volume)
4. Metabolic clearance rate or "catabolism" of insulin in the liver, kidney, and other insulin-sensitive cells which internalize and degrade it after it has combined with the insulin receptor. The half-life of ^{125}I monoiodinated A-14 (tyrosine) insulin (which retains essentially 100% of its biologic and immunologic activities) in the plasma compartment is about 4.5 min, and the half-life of proinsulin in the plasma compartment is about 26 min.

[a] A fifth variable, i.e., circulating insulin-binding and insulin-neutralizing antibodies can affect 2, 3, and 4. When antibodies are present in high titer (>30 mU/mL serum or >0.216 nM) the volume of distribution is similar to or only slightly greater than that of the plasma compartment, or 5 to 8% of the body volume. Endogenous insulin may also be neutralized by the antibody. The metabolic clearance rate of insulin is slowed. If the antibody titer and affinity constant are high, there may be a very low level of circulating "free insulin," or none at all. Up to 95% of the antibody-bound insulin can be sequestered (presumably in the reticuloendothelial system) without ever having interacted with the insulin receptors on insulin-sensitive cells. See text, section entitled "Immunologic Insulin Resistance."

(*Sources*: Binder C: Insulin pharmacokinetics. Diabetes Care 7:188–199, 1984; Galloway JA, Spradlin CT, Nelson RL, et al.: Factors influencing the absorption, serum insulin concentration, and blood glucose responses after injections of regular insulin and various insulin mixtures. Diabetes Care 4:366–376, 1981; Kobayashi T, Sawamo S, Itoh K, et al.: The pharmacokinetics of insulin after continuous subcutaneous infusion or bolus subcutaneous injection in diabetic patients. Diabetes 32:331–336, 1983; Davidson JK, Fineberg SE, De Meyts P, et al.: Immunologic and metabolic responses of patients with a history of antibody-induced-beef-insulin-resistance to treatment with beef, pork, human (rDNA), and sulfated beef insulin. Diabetes Care 15:702–704, 1992; Davidson JK: Transferring patients with insulin-dependent diabetic mellitus from animal-source insulins to recombinant DNA human insulin: clinical experience. Clin Ther 11:319–330, 1989; Sodoyez JC, Sodoyez-Goffaux F, Guillaume M, et al.: (^{123}I) Insulin metabolism in normal rats and humans: external detection by a scintillation camera. Science 219:865–867, 1983. With permission.)

sites (Figure 18–26) should be given. Feedback by patient demonstration to a professional should be observed and confirmed (Exhibit 18–2).

It has been shown (Davidson, Grunberger) that it is safe for the same individual to reuse disposable insulin syringes with needles as many as ten times if aseptic precautions are observed. Pen injection devices (Table 18–15) have become increasingly popular and effective especially in adolescents. Occasionally it is necessary to utilize aids for insulin measurement and injection for the visually impaired (Table 18–17).

The patient should become proficient in home blood glucose and urine glucose and ketone monitoring (See Chapter 22), and should be taught how to make modest adjustments in insulin doses, diet, and exercise to min-imize hyperglycemia and to avoid hypoglycemia. Any symptoms or signs of acutely decompensated diabetes mellitus (see Chapter 24) should be reported promptly to the physician or nurse (see Chapter 14).

Adherence and Audit

See Chapters 14 and 22.

Adverse Effects of Insulin Therapy

Hypoglycemia

Historical Perspective The effects in dogs of insulin-induced hypoglycemia and their reversal with IV

TABLE 18–13 Syringes

Manufacturer/Distributor and Name	Insulin	Needle Gauge	Needle Size	Packaging
1-cc syringes				
Aimsco Ultra Thin II	U-100	29G	$\frac{1}{2}''$	100 (10 packs of 10 individually wrapped)
Aimsco Maxi Comfort	U-100	28G	$\frac{1}{2}''$	100 (10 packs of 10 individually wrapped)
Aimsco Uni Body Ultra II	U-100	29G	$\frac{1}{2}''$	100 (10 packs of 10)
Aimsco Uni Body Ultra II	U-100	28G	$\frac{1}{2}''$	100 (10 packs of 10)
B-D Ultra-Fine	U-100	29G	$\frac{1}{2}''$	100 (10 packs of 10)
B-D Ultra-Fine II Short	U-100	30G	$\frac{5}{16}''$	100 (10 packs of 10)
B-D Micro-Fine IV	U-100	28G	$\frac{1}{2}''$	100 (10 packs of 10)
Can-Am Care				
Monoject Ultra Comfort 28	U-100	28G	$\frac{1}{2}''$	100 (individually sterile wrapped)
Monoject Ultra Comfort 29	U-100	29G	$\frac{1}{2}''$	100 (individually sterile wrapped)
Various store brands	U-100	29G	$\frac{1}{2}''$	100 (individually sterile wrapped)
Various store brands	U-100	28G	$\frac{1}{2}''$	100 (individually sterile wrapped)
MediSense				
Precision Sure-Dose Plus	U-100	29G	$\frac{1}{2}''$	100 (individually sterile wrapped)
Precision Sure-Dose	U-100	28G	$\frac{1}{2}''$	100 (individually sterile wrapped)
$\frac{1}{2}$-cc syringes				
Aimsco Ultra Thin II	U-100	29G	$\frac{1}{2}''$	100 (10 packs of 10 individually wrapped)
Aimsco Maxi Comfort	U-100	28G	$\frac{1}{2}''$	100 (10 packs of 10 individually wrapped)
Aimsco Uni Body Ultra II	U-100	29G	$\frac{1}{2}''$	100 (10 packs of 10)
Aimsco Uni Body Ultra II	U-100	28G	$\frac{1}{2}''$	100 (10 packs of 10)
B-D Ultra-Fine	U-100	29G	$\frac{1}{2}''$	100 (10 packs of 10)
B-D Ultra-Fine II Short	U-100	30G	$\frac{5}{16}''$	100 (10 packs of 10)
B-D Micro-Fine IV	U-100	28G	$\frac{1}{2}''$	100 (10 packs of 10)
Can-Am Care				
Monoject Ultra Comfort 28	U-100	28G	$\frac{1}{2}''$	100 (individually sterile wrapped)
Monoject Ultra Comfort 29	U-100	29G	$\frac{1}{2}''$	100 (individually sterile wrapped)
Various store brands	U-100	29G	$\frac{1}{2}''$	100 (individually sterile wrapped)
Various store brands	U-100	28G	$\frac{1}{2}''$	100 (individually sterile wrapped)
MediSense				
Precision Sure-Dose Plus	U-100	29G	$\frac{1}{2}''$	100 (individually sterile wrapped)
Precision Sure-Dose	U-100	28G	$\frac{1}{2}''$	100 (individually sterile wrapped)
$\frac{3}{10}$-cc syringes				
B-D Ultra-Fine	U-100	29G	$\frac{1}{2}''$	100 (10 packs of 10)
B-D Ultra-Fine II Short	U-100	30G	$\frac{5}{16}''$	100 (10 packs of 10)
B-D Micro-Fine IV	U-100	28G	$\frac{1}{2}''$	100 (10 packs of 10)
Can-Am Care				
Monoject Ultra Comfort 29	U-100	29G	$\frac{1}{2}''$	100 (individually sterile wrapped)
Various store brands	U-100	29G	$\frac{1}{2}''$	100 (individually sterile wrapped)
MediSense				
Precision Sure-Dose	U-100	29G	$\frac{1}{2}''$	100 (Individually sterile wrapped)

* Adapted from *American Diabetes Association's Forecast Buyers Guide 1999* [291] with permission.

glucose were known in 1921[164] and were reported in the *British Medical Journal* on January 6, 1922, 5 days prior to the first clinical use of insulin in the treatment of Leonard Thompson on January 11, 1922. Less than 2 years later, several deaths from hypoglycemia had been observed. In 1924, Campbell and Macleod[3] stated: "It is important to remember that with insulin we are dealing with a most powerful drug, many times as toxic as strychnine. Its toxic action arises from the fact that when present in excess, it inhibits the utilization of, or fixes in an unavailable form, the soluble carbohydrate of the body." Seventy-five years later (1999), deaths and permanent brain damage from hypoglycemia[124,125,165–173] still occur (Table 18–14).

TABLE 18–14 Audit of Causes of 240 Consecutive Cases of Hypoglycemia in Patients Known to Have Diabetes Mellitus[a] (Grady Memorial Hospital Emergency Clinic, 1973–1975)

Inadequate food (carbohydrate) intake	66%
Excess insulin dose	12%
Sulfonylurea therapy	12%
Strenuous exercise	4%
Ethanol intake	4%
Other (kidney failure, liver failure, decrease in corticosteroid dose)	2%

[a] Eight cases (3.3%) terminated fatally. Four of these patients were on insulin therapy, and four were on sulfonylurea therapy.

[*Source:* Davidson JK: Hypoglycemia. *In* Schwartz GR, Wagner D (eds): Principles and Practice of Emergency Medicine. Philadelphia: W.B. Saunders, 1978, pp. 1075–1078; Davidson JK: Hypoglycemia. *In* Conn RB (ed): Current Diagnosis, Ed. 7. Philadelphia: W.B. Saunders, 1985, pp. 749–752. With permission.]

As Cryer has emphasized, hypoglycemia is the limiting factor in the management of diabetes.[124] The devastating effects of hypoglycemia on the brain, which results in death of 4% or more of IDDMs, also are responsible for much physical and psychosocial morbidity. Physicians should always be on guard to help patients minimize its frequency and severity.

Although the incidence, prevalence, and severity of hypoglycemia in different groups and in individuals with diabetes remains unknown, some measurements and estimates are available. For instance, it is estimated that among IDDMs, *mild symptomatic episodes* that can be treated by the patient occur at least 30 times each year, and that *severe episodes with coma and/or convulsions* that require hospitalization or treatment by professionals occur at a minimal rate of 0.09 episodes per patient per year and a maximal rate of 0.28 episodes per patient per year. About 10% of the individuals who have hypoglycemia experience repeated episodes.

It is estimated that one third of the children with IDDM have experienced episodes of severe hypoglycemia. During the feasibility phase of the DCCT,[151] severe hypoglycemia occurred in 26% of the intensively treated ("tight control") group, but only in 9.8% of the "conventionally controlled" group. Severe hypoglycemia was associated with young age, a history of prior severe hypoglycemia, a long duration of IDDM, autonomic neuropathy, and defective glucose counterregulation (deficient glucagon or epinephrine secretion, or both). During intensive therapy for IDDM, glucose counterregulation is initiated at a lower glucose level than is the case with conventional therapy during which mean glucose levels are higher.

Hypoglycemic unawareness is common in those with IDDM. Of the severe hypoglycemic episodes that occurred in the feasibility phase of the DCCT during hours when patients were awake, 80% were associated with hypoglycemic unawareness. Two-thirds of the total number of episodes of severe hypoglycemia that developed occurred during sleep.

Studies of hospitalized IDDMs have shown that 30 to 55% had blood glucose levels during the night from 40 to 54 mg/dL (2.2 to 3.0 mM), and that more than 50% had levels below 50 mg/dL (below 2.8 mM) during 24 hours of continuous blood glucose monitoring. (See Fig. 18–22.) Three to 5% of deaths in those with IDDM are hypoglycemia related (Table 18–14). It is estimated that 10% of the deaths in sulfonylurea-treated NIDDMs are secondary to sulfonylurea-induced hypoglycemia.[124]

Although more than 95% of cases of hypoglycemia occur in those with diabetes who are being treated with insulin or a sulfonylurea,[174] a number of other uncommon or rare causes of hypoglycemia (both exogenous and endogenous) have been described[166] (see Exhibit 18–10, Assessment). Since 1980, as aggressive attempts to maintain normoglycemia have increased, in those with IDDM,[117,152–156] the risks of hypoglycemia also have increased. The incidence of morbidity and mortality (especially in those with unstable diabetes and in those with autonomic neuropathy) may continue to increase in the 21st century if the use of ICIT and CSII becomes widespread (see Fig. 18–24 and 18–25, Table 18–8, Exhibit 18–12). (See Chapter 20 for description of the hypoglycemic effects of the sulfonylureas.)

Epidemiology Two hundred forty cases of severe hypoglycemia in those being treated for diabetes were observed in the Grady Memorial Hospital Medical Emergency Clinic over a 2-year period (1973–1975) and eight (3.3%) of the affected individuals died (see Table 18–14). Four of the fatal cases were on insulin therapy and four were on sulfonylurea therapy. It was judged that two thirds of the severe cases of hypoglycemia were secondary to inadequate carbohydrate intake prior to the episode.[165]

Pathophysiology (Exhibit 18–7) The mean plasma glucose level in normal humans fasted overnight is 92 mg/dL (range, 78 to 115 mg/dL). In such individuals, the glucose level fluctuates over a remarkably narrow range, rising modestly after feeding and falling modestly during fasting. When *glucose production* (primarily from glucose absorbed from the gastrointestinal tract after feeding and from liver gluconeogenesis during fasting) lags behind *glucose utilization* (primarily to provide substrate for energy production during exercise, or to be stored as glycogen when insulin levels are elevated) for a significant period of time, hypoglycemia results.

The lowest level of plasma glucose that can be regarded as normal varies from person to person. Some patients are symptomatic when the plasma glucose falls

TABLE 18–15   Injection AIDS

Product Name (Manufacturer/Distributor)	Description	Syringe Used	Needle Visible	Adjustable Depth of Skin Penetration	Comments
Insertion					
Autoject Autoject 2 (Owen Mumford, Inc.)	Spring-loaded plastic syringe holder positioned over skin. Press device against site, push button to insert needle and deliver insulin simultaneously.	Autoject: Most 1-cc, $\frac{1}{2}$-cc. $\frac{3}{10}$-cc, and $\frac{1}{4}$-cc plastic syringes Autoject 2: MediSense 1-cc, $\frac{1}{2}$-cc; B-D 1-cc, $\frac{1}{2}$-cc	no	yes	Increases injection-site alternatives.
Automatic Injector (Becton Dickinson)	Spring-loaded plastic syringe holder positioned over skin. To insert needle, press button.	B-D 1-cc, $\frac{1}{2}$-cc, and $\frac{3}{10}$-cc syringes	no	yes (2 adjustments)	Increases injection-site alternatives.
Instaject (Jordan Medical)	Combination syringe injector and blood lancet device. Button-activated.	Most 1-cc, $\frac{1}{2}$-cc, and $\frac{3}{10}$-cc syringes	no	yes	Self-contained as injector. Lancet adapter only.
Inject-Ease (Palco)	Spring-loaded plastic syringe holder positioned over skin. To insert needle, press button.	Most 1-cc, $\frac{1}{2}$-cc. and $\frac{3}{10}$-cc syringes	no	yes (2 adjustments)	Includes plunger cap to pre-load syringes.
Monoject Injectomatic (Can-Am Care)	Spring-loaded metal syringe holder positioned over skin. Press device against selected site to insert needle.	Monoject 1-cc, $\frac{1}{2}$cc, and $\frac{3}{10}$-cc syringes	no	no	Increases injection-site alternatives.
Subcutaneous Infusion Sets					
Insuflon (Chronimed)	A flexible Teflon catheter that remains beneath the skin for several days. Insulin is injected through a discreet external port.	Any syringe or insulin pen			Give injections into Insuflon instead of through skin. Minimizes needle punctures.

Insulin Pens and Pen Needles	**Comments**
Autopen (Owen Mumford, Inc.)	For use with pre-filled 1.5-ml insulin cartridges; dial-a-dose selector offers both visual and audio indication of setting. Two models: 2 to 32 units in 2-unit dose increments and 1 to 16 units in 1-unit dose increments; side-mounted activation button for easy one-hand delivery.
B-D Pen (Becton Dickinson)	For use with all brands of 150-ml insulin cartridges; delivers 1 to 30 units in 1-unit increments; dose dial has black numbers on white background; reset groove for correction of dialing error; free magnifier accessory available by calling Becton Dickinson. Works with B-D Ultra-Fine Original (29G $\times$ $\frac{1}{2}$″) or B-D Ultra fine II Short (30G $\times$ $\frac{5}{16}$″) pen needles.
NovoPen 1.5 (Novo Nordisk)	Will deliver insulin in 1-unit increments up to 40 units; designed for use with Novolin PenFill 1.5-ml cartridge and NovoFine 30 disposable needle.
Novolin Prefilled (Novo Nordisk)	Prefilled; will deliver insulin in 2-unit increments up to 58 units; use only with Novofine 30 disposable needles.
NovoPen 3 (Novo Nordisk)	Delivers insulin in single-unit increments from 2 to 70 units. Designed for use with (Novo Nordisk) Novolin Penfill 3-ml cartridges and NovoFine 30 disposable needle. Each Novolin Penfill 3-ml cartridge contains 300 units and is available in Regular, NPH, and 70/30.
Unifine Pentips (Owen Mumford, Inc.)	Comfortable pen needles fit all 1.5- and 3.0-ml insulin pens; available in 29-gauge original length (12 mm) or short (8mm).

* Adapted from *American Diabetes Association's Forecast Buyer's Guide 1999* [291] with permission.

as low as 75 mg/dL (4.2 mmol/L), whereas some are asymptomatic when the plasma glucose falls as low as 30 mg/dL (1.7 mM). Thus, the level from 3 to 5 hr after a glucose load may fall as low as 35 mg/dL (1.9 mM) in some asymptomatic individuals, and during fasting the level may fall as low as 30 mg/dL (1.7 mM) in some asymptomatic individuals. See Table 12–7.

Since prolonged or repeated hypoglycemic episodes can result in permanent brain damage and death,[167] it is prudent, as a general rule, to regard all patients with measured plasma glucose levels <50 mg/dL (<2.8 mM) as having hypoglycemia until proved otherwise. Individuals who have a plasma glucose level of 30 to 50 mg/dL (1.7 to 2.8 mM) and who are asymptomatic when initially seen should be classified as *hypoglycemia suspects*. They should be carefully studied to determine whether or not they develop symptomatic hypoglycemia after fasting (for up to 3 days), or whether or not they develop symptomatic reactive hypoglycemia 3 to 6 hr after a glucose load (see Table 12–7), or whether or not there is some other cause of fasting or reactive hypoglycemia (see Exhibit 18–10, Assessment).[97b]

Symptoms of hypoglycemia result from overactivity of the adrenal medulla with hyperepinephrinemia and neurologic dysfunction due to glucopenia. The subjective and objective findings of hyperepinephrinemia and neurologic dysfunction are listed in Exhibit 18–7.

Causes of hypoglycemia in patients being treated for diabetes are listed in Exhibit 18–8, and some drugs that can lower the plasma glucose level and abolish or diminish the subjective and objective findings characteristic of hypoglycemia are listed in Exhibit 18–9.

Symptoms and signs similar to those of hypoglycemia frequently occur in emotionally disturbed patients. Thus, *a diagnosis of symptomatic hypoglycemia cannot be confirmed unless the timing of symptoms and signs coincides with the lowest plasma glucose levels.* One should avoid an erroneous diagnosis of hypoglycemia because of improper blood specimen collection, preservation, or analysis ("desk-top hypoglycemia"). It is important not to confuse *asymptomatic* and *unrecognized* hypoglycemia. Many diabetics, especially those with autonomic neuropathy, have severe hypoglycemic episodes which neither they (*hypoglycemic unawareness*) nor their peers recognize. Many patients with insulinomas have been confined to mental institutions because hypoglycemia was not suspected.

Hypoglycemia of brief duration may cause cerebral malfunction which can result in accidental injury or jail confinement (suspected ethanol intoxication). Prolonged hypoglycemia (usually 4 or more hr) may result in irreversible brain damage (with paralysis and/or imbecility) or death. Pathologic findings secondary to prolonged hypoglycemia have varied from slight loss of cortical neurones with secondary gliosis to extensive necrotizing injury of the cortex (preponderantly temporal) and gliosis. Also, lesions may occur in the amygdala, hippocampus, putamen, caudate nucleus, globus pallidus, and thalamus.[167]

Electroencephalography has been reported as showing suppression of the alpha rhythm, generalized theta activity, and a moderate number of delta waves without asymmetry.[167] Since the amount of brain damage varies from patient to patient, it seems reasonable to assume that the electroencephalogram (EEG) abnormalities will vary between individuals and over time.

Problem: Hypoglycemia (Subsets: Exogenous, Endogenous Reactive, Endogenous Fasting) See Exhibit 18–10.

All cases of drug-induced (insulin or sulfonylurea) hypoglycemia should be regarded as *true medial emergencies* that require prompt confirmation by a stat plasma glucose measurement and immediate treatment with oral or IV glucose or glucagon administered subcutaneously or intramuscularly (Exhibit 18–11). If a Beckman glucose analyzer (see Chapters 11, 12, 13) is not immediately available, a glucose oxidase test strip blood glucose meter reading, either visually or meter-read (see Chapter 22) can, when appropriately used, provide an estimate of the capillary blood glucose level in a few minutes.

Nocturnal hypoglycemia[176] may be missed. Hypoglycemia occurring in drivers of private or public transportation vehicles and in those working in a dangerous environment is particularly dangerous,[177] as is hypoglycemic coma that occurs during CSII therapy.[178] *Factitious hypoglycemia* may occur in emotionally disturbed diabetics individuals (see Exhibit 18–15), or in a suicide or homicide attempt.[179–181]

Plan

Initial   See Exhibit 18–11.

Follow-up   See Exhibit 18–11.

Reactive Hyperglycemia Induced by Hypoglycemia

Historical Perspective   The hyperglycemic response to hypoglycemia was noted less than 15 years after the first clinical use of insulin (Somogyi, 1938.)[182,183] It was designated the Somogyi phenomenon" in deference to the scientist (a Ph.D., not an M.D.) who originally reported that hyperglycemia and ketoacidosis may occur in the wake of hypoglycemia.

Epidemiology   Although the prevalence and incidence of posthypoglycemic hyperglycemia are not precisely known, it seems likely that the phenomenon is very common and that it has occurred on multiple

TABLE 18–16   Insulin Pumps

Pump Model (Manufacturer)	Size (inches)	Wt.	Battery Type/Life	Infusion Set	Basals	
					#	Range
MiniMed 507C (MiniMed)	3.4 × 1.9 × 0.8	<3.5 ounces <100 grams	Three 1.5-volt silver oxide (2–3 mo. life, available in drug and camera stores).	24″ and 42″ Sof-set and Sof-set QR (disconnectable) soft catheter sets: 23″ and 43″ Silhouette, angled, soft catheter complete and combo sets (disconnected at the site). 24″ and 42″ Polyfin. Polyfin QR, and Polyfin QR with wings, with bent or straight needle sets. Sot-set designed for use with Sof-serter automatic insertion tool.	48 profiles plus an advanced temporary basal rate gives users the ability to finetune their insulin delivery; both the basal and temporary rates can begin on the hour or half hour; temporary rate can be increased or decreased for up to 24 hours.	0.0–35.0 U/hr
H-TRONplus (Disetronic Medical Systems)	3.36 × 2.16 × 0.75	<3.5 ounces	Two 3-volt silver oxide (2-4 mo. life).	21″ and 43″ polyolefin bent needle sets; 21″, 31″, and 43″ soft cannula set with disconnect/ reconnect mechanism; 21″, 31″, and 43″ metal needle set with 90-degree bend and adhesive disk with 3 needle lengths.	24 profiles so a different rate can be set each hour for a patient-specific insulin delivery profile plus advanced temporary basal rate, which can be increased or decreased in 10-percent increments.	0.0–99.0 U/hr

* Adapted from *American Diabetes Association's Forecast Buyer's Guide 1999* [291] with permission.

occasions in many individuals who have unstable IDDM and in some insulin-treated individuals who have NIDDM.

Pathophysiology[98,168,169,184–190]   Counterregulatory hormones (glucagon, epinephrine, norepinephrine, cortisol, growth hormone), which defend the brain against glucopenia, produce transient hyperglycemia in nondiabetics. It is quickly corrected by increased insulin secretion by normal B cells. In diabetics, the plasma concentration of counterregulatory hormones increases in response to the stress of emotional upsets, infections, surgery, trauma, unplanned erratic and vigorous exercise, and diabetic ketoacidosis. This increase in counterregulatory hormones causes a prolonged increase in glucose production by the liver.[189] Modest deficiency of insulin in the posthypoglycemia state in individuals with IDDM accentuates the hyperglycemic effects of the counterregulatory hormones.[190] Also, the islets of some individuals with IDDM have not only lost the ability to secrete insulin in response to hyperglycemia, they have lost at least a part of their ability to respond to hypoglycemia by secreting glucagon appropriately. Some individuals, especially those with autonomic neuropathy, release not only less glucagon, but also release less epinephrine.[190] These individuals are at greatly increased risk of severe hypoglycemia on intensive insulin therapy treatment programs (ICIT and CSII). See Exhibit 18–12.

Glucagon,[262] through its stimulatory effect on glucose production, is the key hormone responsible for recovery from hypoglycemia; epinephrine is not nor-

Smallest Bolus	Alarms			Warranty	Features
	Occlusion	Over-Delivery	Near Empty		
0.1 unit	yes, within 2 to 3 units	Patented solenoid motor can't over-deliver insulin. Watchdog system monitors programming. 30.000+ software safety checks are performed every hour.	Empty Reservoir Alert (yes): Near empty (no)	4 yr. plus lifetime motor warranty.	Multipte bolus options include: normal for immediate delivery: square-wave bolus for delivery over a timed duration dual wave combines a normal bolus with a square wave, and audio bolus for setting a bolus without looking at display; mini-glo backlight and self-test; Com Station memory includes approximately 90 days delivery history that can be downloaded from 507 or 507 C to a PC; pump accessible memory includes last 24 boluses and 7 combined daily totals; PC software included (compatible with Mellitus Manager from MetaMedix); water tight without any additional plugs or cases: user-defined safety limits; 24-hour, toll-free clinical services help line staffed by RNs; free videos and educational materials; insurance assistance.
0.1 unit	yes	Patented system incapable of hardware or software over-delivery. Dual microprocessor control.		4 yr. with free safety inspection every 2 yrs.	Patient receives two pumps; three minute insulin delivery system; audible bolus delivery; pump is waterproof without additional case; glass and plastic cartridges available; free video; 24-hour, toll-free telephone support; insurance assistance; color choice, durable clip case, and other accessories available.

mally critical but becomes important when glucagon is deficient. Growth hormone, cortisol, neural mechanisms, and hepatic glucose autoregulation do not play critical roles, and are not sufficient to promote recovery from hypoglycemia when both glucagon and epinephrine secretion are deficient.

It is important to distinguish between *nocturnal posthypoglycemic hyperglycemia* and the *dawn phenomenon* in a person with early morning hyperglycemia, since treatment of the *dawn phenomenon* usually requires an increase in the insulin dose.[191] See Fig. 18–24 and Tables 18–8 to 18–10.

Example of Posthypoglycemic Hyperglycemia Plus the Waning of Insulin Action (see Fig. 18–25) A 20-year-old white male was referred for evaluation and treatment of unstable diabetes diagnosed 3 years earlier by his family physician. He had been on an unmeasured diet, an erratic exercise pattern, and 60 U NPH insulin subcutaneously each morning before breakfast. He frequently had rather severe hypoglycemic episodes between 3:00 and 6:00 p.m., and usually spilled 5% glucose and occasionally acetone in the urine the next morning. He was moderately active physically, was 69 in. tall and of medium frame, and weighed 160 pounds.

He was hospitalized and his plasma glucose was monitored every 4 hr on 60 U NPH insulin before breakfast, a 2,400-calorie diet divided 0.3, 0.3, 0.3, 0.1, and an unregulated exercise pattern (Fig. 18–25). On the first hospital day, the fasting plasma glucose was 360 mg/dL. It fell to 28 mg/dL at 4:00 p.m.

TABLE 18–17　AIDS for People Who Are Visually Impaired

Product	Description/Use
Syringe Magnifiers	
HypOview Brilliant Syringe Viewer	Magnifies and lights a loaded syringe against a dark background, enabling user to see calibrations and entrapped air bubbles (similar to lava lamp). Five element optic system. Size of a small flashlight.
Insul-eze (Palco)	Holds syringe and insulin bottle while dosage is drawn. Magnifies syringe calibration. Allows device to sit on any flat surface. Works with all types of insulin bottles.
Magni-Guide (Becton Dickinson)	Syringe is slipped into curved channel of Magni-Guide. At opposite end insulin vial is snapped into collar. Guide maunifies entire scale 2 times.
Syringe Magnifier (Apothecary Products)	Clips to syringe barrel.
Tru-Hand (Whittier Medical)	Insulin bottle holder-syringe guide-magnifier. Locks in syringes with direct guide into vial stopper. Magnifier entire scale. Insulin bottles can be changed without removing syringe from device.
Non-Visual Insulin Measurement	
Count-a-Dose	Syringe-filling device. Empty syringe secured in easy-to-locate platform; slide moves syringe plunger to control insulin intake. Click wheel activates slide to ensure accurate dosage in 1-unit increments. Click heard and felt as wheel is rotated. Holds 1 or 2 bottles of insulin for mixed doses.
Insulgage	Permanent, pre-calibrated device, purchased according to dose (from 2 to 85 units). Dose marked in Inkprint, raised numbers, Braille and raised numbers, or Braille. Two gauges can be used for mixed dosages.
Load-Matic (Palco)	Allows person to load syringes by touch alone. Aligns needle with bottle top; loads syringe by separate 10 or single-unit increments. Holds any size insulin bottle. After setting the desired dosage, it can be used repeatedly without further adjustment.
Needle Guides and Vial Stabilizers	
Holdease	Needle guide and syringe/vial holder. Unit holds syringe and insulin together in easy-to-handle unit while user fills syringe.
Insulin Needle Guide	Guide fits over vial cap; funnel-shaped opening guides needle into rubber seal of vial.
Blood Glucose Meters and Attachments	
Diascan Partner	Same features as the Diascan-S (see Blood Glucose Meters). Compact, all-in-one, battery powered with built-in voice module. Voice instructions guide user through entire procedure; error codes announced. Minimal cleaning required. Available in English, Spanish, and German.
Digi-Voice Deluxe, Mini-DV	Speech module plugs into data jack on One Touch II and One Touch Profile. Talks user through self-test procedure. Repeat feature. Earphone, cassette instructions. Mini-DV is a smaller version of the Digi-Voice. Other languages available.
Touch-n-Talk Profile	Voice synthesizer connects to One Touch Profile. Annunciates all messages that appear on the meter's display. Jacks and controls are labeled in Braille. Includes one data cable, earphone, and large-print and cassette instructions. Available in other languages.
Voice Touch, Voice Touch Pro	Voice synthesizer attaches to the One Touch II or One Touch Profile. Annunciates all messages. Includes earphone, and large-print and cassette instructions. Any language with minimum order or choice of two languages. Optional accessories.

* Adapted from the *American Diabetes Association Forecast Buyer's Guide 1999* [291] with permission.

(AGE = 360 − 28 = 332 mg/dL) and the patient was symptomatically hypoglycemic. On the second hospital day, the fasting plasma glucose was 355 mg/dL. The NPH insulin dose was dropped to 40 U, and one third of the breakfast calories were moved to a 3:30 p.m. snack. Twenty minutes of walking at a rate of 100 steps/min after each meal was prescribed. The plasma glucose at 4:00 p.m. that day was 130 mg/dL, and there were no hypoglycemic symptoms during the 24 hr period. The next day, the fasting plasma glucose was 290 mg/dL,

and the 4:00 p.m. plasma glucose level was 140 mg/dL (AGE = 290 − 150 mg/dL). At 8:00 p.m., 10 U NPH insulin was given. The following day, the plasma glucose ranged from 110 to 130 mg/dL (AGE = 130 − 110 = 20 mg/dL) and there were no hypoglycemic episodes.

Comment　This individual was having posthypoglycemic hyperglycemia (Somogyi's phenomenon). Also, the effect of his morning NPH insulin waned in

Syringe Used	Source (see resource list)
Any syringe up to $\frac{1}{2}''$ in diameter	HypOview
Holds 25-, 30-, 50-, and 100-unit syringes by most manufacturers	Local pharmacies; home health centers; Science Products
B-D 1-cc, $\frac{1}{2}$-cc, or $\frac{3}{10}$-cc syringe	B-D Consumer Products; local pharmacies: Lighthouse Catalog
Any standard-size syringe	Local pharmacies
B-D, MediSense, and Monoject (all sizes)	Local pharmacies
Use with B-D U-100, $\frac{1}{2}$-cc Lo-Dose syringe	Jordan Medical; Science Products; local pharmacies: Lighthouse Catalog
For B-D 1-cc or B-D $\frac{1}{2}$-cc Lo-Dose syringe and Monoject 1-cc; every size available from 2 through 45	Meditec, Inc.
B-D 100-unit syringe	Local pharmacies; home health centers; Science Products; Lighthouse Catalog
none	Meditec, Inc.
none	Lighthouse Catalog
none	Home Diagnostics
none	Science Products
none	Lighthouse Catalog
none	Myna Corporation

less than 24 hr (rapid absorption). Thus, he needed less 8:00 a.m. NPH insulin and some 8:00 p.m. NPH insulin. A stable diet and exercise routine helped decrease the AGE during the 24-hr period.

Problem Reactive hyperglycemia induced by hypoglycemia.

Subjective and Objective Findings are those noted under hypoglycemia above. Occasionally, very subtle subjective and objective findings of unrecognized hypoglycemia may suggest reactive hyperglycemia: nocturnal sweating, hypothermia, and so on.

Assessment It is important to maintain a high index of suspicion in all unstable IDDM patients. Around-the-clock home blood glucose monitoring or hospital plasma glucose monitoring to detect plasma glucose levels <65 mg/dL is sufficient to diagnose all patients. Some individuals have reactive hyperglycemia only, others have reactive hyperglycemia plus a waning

TABLE 18-I Insulin Pump Supplies

Product Name (Manufacturer)	Type of Product	Features
PureLine Basic (Chronimed)	Infusion set	Needle is pre-bent at a 30-degree angle. Available with or without butterfly. Tubing available in 43″ and 23″.
PureLine Comfort (Chronimed)	Infusion set	Soft Teflon catheter in all that remains in place after insertion. Allows user to disconnect from the pump for bathing, etc. Tubing available in 43″ and 23″.
PureLine Contact (Chronimed)	Infusion set	Needle is pre-bent at a 90-degree angle. Tubing available in 43″ and 23″.
Sof-serter (Minimed)	Automatic insertion device	For use with Sof-set infusion sets: provides placements at optimal depth for insulin absorption.

* Adapted from the *American Diabetes Association Forecast Buyer's Guide 1999* [291] with permission.

TABLE 18-II Jet Injectors

Product Name (Manufacturer)	Size/Weight	Features
Advanta Jet (Activa Brand Products, Inc.)	Size: 6″ × 1″ Weight: 5.6 oz	Standard model Activa injector for the average skin type. Delivers from $\frac{1}{2}$ to 50 units in $\frac{1}{2}$-unit increments; accepts all types and mixes of U-100 insulin; 14 comfort settings; tactile detents for visually impaired; video included; toll-free help line; immediate service.
Gentle Jet (Activa Brand Products, Inc.)	Size: 6″ × 1″ Weight: 5.6 oz	A lower power model Activa Jet specifically designed for children and those with low levels of subcutaneous tissue; two-year warranty; same features as Advanta Jet.
Advanta Jet ES (Activa Brand Products, Inc.)	Size: 6″ × 1″ Weight: 5.6 oz	An extra strength Activa Jet for those whose skin conditions require additional power from an injector, same features as Advanta Jet.
Medi-Jector Choice (Medi-Ject Corp.)	Size: 7.75″ × 1.2″ Weight: 6.4 oz	Disposable drug chamber (Needle-Free Insulin Syringe) eliminates cleaning or maintenance and allows for viewing of insulin dose; delivers single or mixed doses from 2 to 50 units in $\frac{1}{2}$-unit increments with 14 comfort settings; includes manual, video, carrying case, and toll-free help line. Full one-year warranty and 30-day trial period.
Vitajet 3 (Bioject Corp.)	Size: 6″ × 1″ Weight: 5.6 oz	No cleaning or maintenance required; disposable nozzles allow visual verification of entire dose; adjustable pressure and choice of two nozzle sizes; delivers 2 to 50 units of single or mixed insulin; training video included; 2-year warranty and 30-day money-back guarantee.

* Adapted from the *American Diabetes Association Forecast Buyer's Guide 1999* [291] with permission.

action of insulin due to rapid absorption of a single daily dose of intermediate-acting insulin (see Fig. 18–16, 18–17, 18–24, and 18–25).

Plan Revise insulin dose until hypoglycemia (blood glucose <75 mg/dL) no longer occurs. Then reactive hyperglycemia will disappear.

Insulin-Induced Hypovolemia

Historical Perspective The circulatory response to IV insulin therapy was first noted in 1968.[192] Later it was shown that in diabetics with autonomic neuropathy, IV insulin can cause profound hypotension and fainting in the upright position.[193–195]

Epidemiology Although prevalence and incidence of an insulin-induced decrease in plasma volume is not known, it has been observed with increasing frequency in recent years.

Pathophysiology Intravenous insulin causes a decrease of about 6% in plasma volume (mean, 190 mL; range, 75 to 425 mL) in those with uncomplicated diabetes. This in turn causes an increase in plasma norepinephrine and an increase in heart rate.[195] In diabetics with severe autonomic neuropathy who had smaller than normal initial plasma volumes intravenous insulin produced no further decrease in the plasma volume.[195] Yet it produced profound hypotension 5 to 10 min after injection, particularly in the upright position. These individuals have impaired renin responses. An insulin effect on blood vessel tone with transfer of fluid and albumin out of the vascular system may contribute. If the

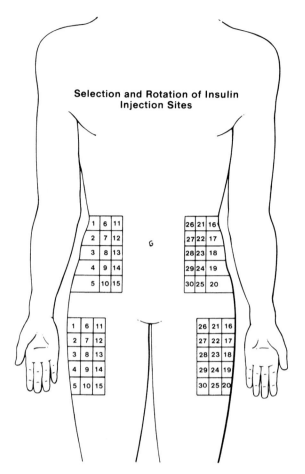

Selection and Rotation of Insulin Injection Sites

Figure 18–26. Insulin injection sites should be selected in the same area and sites should be rotated on a preplanned grid so that no site is injected more than once each month. If an individual makes one injection daily, sites on the abdomen or thighs may be used; if two or more injections are made, the grid should be expanded and the same area should be used to minimize the variation in day-to-day insulin absorption rates. The first injection on the first day of each month should be at position number 1. See Exhibits 18–2 and 18–3.

plasma glucose is high initially and drops abruptly after IV insulin, the transfer of water from the plasma compartment to the intracellular compartment (to maintain the Donnan equilibrium across cell membranes; see Chapter 24) also could contribute to the hypotension. A drop of plasma glucose from 500 to 100 mg/dL would decrease the plasma osmolality by 22 mOsm, and this could result in the transfer of a significant amount of water (estimated 300 to 800 mL) from the plasma compartment into the intracellular compartment with a concomitant decrease in the plasma volume.

Problem Statement Insulin-induced hypovolemia.

Subjective and Objective Fainting, hypotension especially in the erect position, and tachycardia after IV insulin therapy: more common and more severe in those with autonomic neuropathy.

Assessment Rule out hypoglycemia, autonomic neuropathy with orthostatic (postural) hypotension, and cardiovascular and other problems that may result in hypotension, fainting, and so on.

Plan

Initial When giving IV insulin therapy, prevent insulin-induced contraction of plasma volume by giving IV 0.9% saline to replace prospectively or concurrently the estimated intravascular fluid deficit plus the additional deficit that may result from the use of IV insulin therapy with a rapid marked decrease in the plasma glucose level and plasma osmolality.

Follow-up Control plasma glucose as carefully as possible and treat autonomic neuropathy as indicated (see Chapter 36).

Research Considerations Further studies are needed to elucidate completely the mechanics and optimal

EXHIBIT 18–7 Pathophysiology of Symptomatic Hypoglycemia

Adrenal medulla overactivity with hyperepinephrinemia
Subjective: Anxiety, palpitation, occasionally angina pectoris
Objective: Perspiration, pallor, hypothermia, tachycardia, hypertension, cardiac arrhythmias, dilated pupils
Neurologic dysfunction: Initially the higher cortical centers malfunction because the glucose supply is insufficient to maintain normal metabolic activity; oxygen utilization decreases; later, centers in the midbrain and medulla are similarly affected. In fatal reactions there is cerebral edema, multiple petechial hemorrhages, and widespread necrosis of cortical ganglion cells.

Prolongation of hypoglycemia (usually 4 or more hr), not depth to which plasma glucose falls, is responsible for irreparable brain damage.
Subjective: Headache, blurring of vision, transient diplopia, paresthesias, hunger, nausea, fatigue, drowsiness, irritability, vertigo
Objective: Mental confusion, bizarre behavior, speech difficulties, irrational agitation, combativeness, delirium, vomiting, lethargy, somnolence, aphasia, tremor, ataxia, nystagmus, paralysis, seizures, coma. Babinski reflexes, shallow respiration, bradycardia

[*Sources:* Davidson JK: Hypoglycemia. *In* Schwartz GR, Wagner D (eds): Principles and Practice of Emergency Medicine. Philadelphia: W. B. Saunders, 1978, pp. 1075–1078; Davidson JK: Hypoglycemia. *In* Corn RB (ed): Current Diagnosis, Ed. 7. Philadelphia: W. B. Saunders, 1985, pp. 749–752. With permission.]

EXHIBIT 18–8   Causes of Hypoglycemia in Patients Being Treated for Diabetes Mellitus

I. Inadequate carbohydrate intake
II. Vigorous exercise
III. Insulin therapy
   A. Excess insulin dose
      1. Erroneously prescribed
      2. Failure to match insulin potency with correct syringe (i.e., each U-100)
      3. Visual failure with inability to measure correct dose
      4. Attempted suicide or homicide
   B. Failure to reduce insulin dose when need for insulin decreases
      1. During reduction of body weight
      2. Endocrine deficiency
         (a) Hypopituitarism

         (b) Adrenal cortical insufficiency
      3. Reduction in dose of corticosteroid
      4. Decreased rate of insulin degradation due to kidney failure or liver failure
      5. After recovery from stressful situations
         (a) Infection
         (b) Pancreatitis
         (c) Acutely decompensated diabetes
         (d) Surgery
      6. At termination of pregnancy
IV. Sulfonylurea therapy (tolbutamide, tolazamide, chlorpropamide, acetohexamide, glyburide, glipizide). See Chapter 20.
V. Ethanol, drugs, and toxins that lower plasma glucose level

[*Sources:* Davidson JK: Hypoglycemia. *In* Schwartz GR, Wagner D (eds): Principles and Practice of Emergency Medicine. Philadelphia: W. B Saunders, 1978, pp. 1075–1078; Davidson JK: Hypoglycemia. *In* Conn RB (ed): Current Diagnosis, Ed. 7. Philadelphia: W. B. Saunders, 1985, pp. 749–752. With permission.]

EXHIBIT 18–9   Some Drugs that Lower the Plasma Glucose Level in Patients Being Treated for Diabetes Mellitus

I. Potentiation of sulfonylureas
   A. Barbiturates
   B. Dicumarol
   C. Chloramphenicol
   D. Monoamine oxidase inhibitors
   E. Phenylbutazone
   F. Salicylates
   G. Sulfonamides
   H. Thiazides
II. Increased insulin production
   A. Alpha-adrenergic blockers
   B. Beta-adrenergic stimulators
   C. Monoamine oxidase inhibitors

III. Decreased hepatic glycogenolysis
   A. Propranolol[175]
IV. Mechanism unknown
   A. Antihistamines
      1. Antazoline phosphate
      2. Tripelennamine hydrochloride
   B. Morphine
   C. Probenecid
   D. Propylthiouracil
   E. Tuberculostatic drugs
      1. Isoniazid
      2. Aminosalicylic acid

[*Sources:* Davidson JK: Hypoglycemia. *In* Schwartz GR, Wagner D (eds): Principles and Practice of Emergency Medicine. Philadelphia: W. B. Saunders, 1978, pp. 1075–1078; Davidson JK: Hypoglycemia. *In* Conn RB (ed): Current Diagnosis, Ed. 7. Philadelphia: W. B. Saunders, 1985, pp. 749–752. With permission.]

treatment of insulin-induced hypovolemia, of the pathophysiology of the reduced plasma volume in autonomic neuropathy, and of the clinical consequences for these individuals of IV insulin therapy.

Insulin Allergy

Historical Perspective   Campbell and MacLeod reported in 1924[3] that "when our first patient returned to us in a state of severe acidosis bordering on coma, considerable care was taken to avoid an anaphylactic reaction. Desensitization precautions (Besredka method) were used. Fortunately no evidence of sensitization has appeared in this patient, though it is now 2 years since pancreas extract was first given, and insulin has been given daily during the last 16 months." Until that time, "the large majority of patients" showed no sensitization phenomena. Occasionally mild local urticaria, and rarely swelling, itching, pain, and generalized urticaria had occurred. It was their impression

that these reactions had steadily decreased in number as the purity of the insulin preparations increased. In persistent cases of allergy, they recommended using insulin from a source other than beef pancreas, or desensitization as was the custom in treating hay fever. These recommendations of 1924 are still valid today (1999).

In 1942, Lowell[196] demonstrated the presence of two antibodies in the sera of two patients with dermal hypersensitivity to insulin and insulin resistance [one antibody associated with generalized urticaria which could be passively transferred to normal skin, the Prausnitz-Küstner (P-K) reaction; one antibody that neutralized the biologic effect of commercial crystalline beef insulin but not of human insulin].

For many years after the discovery of insulin, it was assumed that antigenic impurities, not insulin itself, were responsible for immunologic reactions. By 1950, 50 cases of resistance to insulin had been reported,[197] and 15 of these patients (30%) had a history of an aller-

EXHIBIT 18–10   Problem: Hypoglycemia (Subsets: Exogenous, Endogenous Reactive, Endogenous Fasting)

Recognition (defined data base)
  Subjective
    Neurologic dysfunction: headache, blurring of vision, transient diplopia, paresthesias, hunger, nausea, fatigue, drowsiness, irritability, vertigo
    Hyperepinephrinemia: anxiety, palpitation, occasionally angina pectoris
    Known diabetes mellitus
    Insulin therapy: type, dose, time
    Sulfonylurea therapy: type, dose
    Diet prescription: calories, grams of protein, carbohydrate, and fat, division
    Missed food: time
    Vigorous exercise: time
    Level of control of diabetes
    Previous hypoglycemia
    Weight loss
    Duration of symptoms (minutes)
    Drugs: salicylates, steroids, other
    Ethanol
    Toxins
    Gastrectomy
  Objective
    Neurologic dysfunction: mental confusion, bizarre behavior, speech difilculties, irrational agitation, combativeness, delirium, vomiting, lethargy, somnolence, aphasia, tremor, ataxia, nystagmus, paralysis, seizures, coma, Babinski reflexes, shallow respiration, bradycardia
    Hyperepinephrinemia: perspiration, pallor, hypothermia, tachycardia, hypertension, cardiac arrhythmias, dilated pupils
    Venous plasma glucose <50 mg/dL (absolute requirement)
Assessment
  Exogenous hypoglycemia?
    Insulin
    Sulfonylurea
    Insulin or sulfonylurea plus missed meal and/or strenuous exercise
    Ethanol
    Drugs (See Exhibit 18–9)
    Toxins (such as hypoglycin in Jamaican vomiting sickness)
  Endogenous reactive hypoglycemia?
    Alimentary hypoglycemia

Physiologic postmeal or postglucose load (rule out anxiety, depression, psychosis)
Hereditary fructose intolerance (postfructose load) (see Chapter 22)
Galactosemia (after infant ingests lactose or galactose) (see Chapter 22)
Endogenous fasting hypoglycemia?
  Malnutrition
  Hyperinsulinemia (benign adenoma—single or multiple, microadenomatosis, carcinoma, nesidioblastosis)
  Nonpancreatic tumors (mesenchymal retroperitoneal or mediastinal, hepatoma, adrenocortical carcinoma, lymphoma, gastrointestinal, other)
  Severe liver disease (e.g., cirrhosis, congestive heart failure, viral destruction)
  Severe kidney disease (renal failure)
  Endocrine abnormalities (hypopituitarism, adrenal cortical insufficiency, congenital adrenal hyperplasia, epinephrine deficiency, hypothyroidism, cretinism)
  Hypothalamic disease
  Liver glycogenosis due to deficiency of liver enzymes that produce glucose from liver glycogen stores (types I, II, VI, IX) and other hereditary enzyme deficiencies (glycogen synthetase, fructose 1–6 diphosphatase, pyruvate-carboxylase, phosphoenol pyruvate, carboxykinase)
  Glycerol intolerance
  Hereditary defects in amino acid metabolism (maple syrup urine disease, propionic acidemia, methylmalonic acidemia, tyrosinosis, phenylketonuria, type 2 glutaric acidemia, hydroxymethylglutaric acidemia)
  Ketotic hypoglycemia (due to hepatic glycogen depletion in 30 to 50% of patients secondary to inadequate amino acid precursors for gluconeogenesis, especially alanine; cause of 50 to 70% of cases unknown)
  Reye's syndrome
  Insulin-like growth factor one (IGF-1) deficiency (Laron dwarf)
  Transient neonatal hyperinsulinemia in infant of diabetic mother (usually when mother's diabetes has been poorly controlled)
  Idiopathic in neonate

[*Sources:* Davidson JK: Hypoglycemia. *In* Schwartz GR, Wagner D (eds): Principles and Practice of Emergency Medicine. Philadelphia: W. B. Saunders, 1978, pp. 1075–1078; Davidson JK: Hypoglycemia. *In* Conn RB (ed): Current Diagnosis, Ed. 7. Philadelphia: W. B. Saunders, 1985, pp. 749–752. With permission.]

gic response to insulin (nine generalized urticaria, four local urticaria, and two eosinophilia; four had positive P-K transfer tests).

In 1955, Moloney and Coval[15] produced antibodies to beef insulin in guinea pigs. In 1959, Berson and Yalow[16] demonstrated that the serum of nearly all humans who had been injected with commercial (beef or pork) insulin for as long as 3 months contained antibodies, usually of

low titer, that bound ^{131}I insulin. When the chemical structures of insulin became known, it was apparent that the greater the structural differences between the donor and recipient animals' insulins, the greater the antigenic response of the recipient.

Patterson et al.[198] demonstrated that immunoglobulin E (IgE) and P-K titers fall slowly (1 to 4 years) when insulin therapy is discontinued, and that the IgE titer

EXHIBIT 18–11   Treatment Plan

Initial (in Emergency Department):
  Initiate immediately after capillary blood glucose (visually or meter-read Chemstrip bG, Visidex, or Dextrostix) and after drawing stat venous plasma glucose (central laboratory measurement).
    If able to swallow: oral glucose, candy, orange juice or food, or sugar-containing soft drinks (not diet soft drinks).
    If unable to swallow: administer IV glucose (25 g) or subcutaneous (SC) or intramuscular (IM) glucagon (1 mg).
    Observe until complete recovery, repeat plasma glucose, and give additional food.
    Patient and family education: if prompt recovery, reinstruct on and/or revise as indicated: diet, insulin, and/or exercise. Omit ethanol, drugs, toxins. See Follow-up (in hospital and after discharge), below.
    Additional diagnostic data: if delayed recovery, neurologic damage, or uncertain etiology of hypoglycemia, hospitalize.
Follow-up (in hospital and after discharge):
  If fasting hypoglycemia: up to 72-hr fast with plasma glucose and serum insulin assay every 6 hr (see Exhibit 18–1 and Fig. 18–11). Terminate test if hypoglycemia occurs. If reactive hypoglycemia: do 6-hr oral GTT (after 300 g C/d for 3 days prior to test), and IV GTT if indicated. See Exhibits 22–3 and 22–4 if fructose or galactose intolerance suspected. See Exhibit 18–10, Assessment, for other causes of endogenous fasting and endogenous reactive hypoglycemia.
  Complications: evaluate residual neurologic damage: EEG, motor, sensory, cerebellar, judgment, memory, IQ, cranial nerves; evaluate electrocardiogram and cardiac status.
  Predischarge examination: were precipitating factors identified and appropriately treated, and precautions taken to avoid recurrence?
  Management after hospital discharge: if indicated, revise diet and/or insulin therapy and/or exercise pattern. Carry Lifesavers or another conveniently packaged and transported sugar source at all times; prescribe snack 60 min before hypoglycemia is prone to occur; prescription for and instruction of relatives on use of glucagon if recurrence of hypoglycemia and unable to swallow; give diabetes identification card, bracelet, and/or necklace; caution patient about driving motor vehicles and working around dangerous machinery and in unprotected high places; arrange continuing follow-up in ambulatory care facility such as diabetes clinic or physician's office.

Abbreviations: GTT, glucose tolerance test; C/d, carbohydrate per day.
[*Sources:* Davidson JK: Hypoglycemia. *In* Schwartz GR, Wagner D (eds): Principles and Practice of Emergency Medicine. Philadelphia: W. B. Saunders, 1978, pp. 1075–1078; Davidson JK: Hypoglycemia. *In* Conn RB (ed): Current Diagnosis, Ed. 7. Philadelphia: W. B. Saunders, 1985, pp. 749–752. With permission.]

EXHIBIT 18–12   Glucagon, Epinephrine, Norepinephrine, Cortisol, and Growth Hormone Secretion During Hypoglycemia

The body's first defense against hypoglycemia is epinephrine (and norepinephrine) and glucagon secretion, and then adrenocorticotropic hormone (ACTH), cortisol, and growth hormone secretion. When glucagon secretion is suppressed (somatostatin), epinephrine becomes the primary defense hormone, but when both glucagon and epinephrine are suppressed, the body cannot recover from insulin-induced hypoglycemia with cortisol, norepinephrine, and growth hormone combined.

In a majority of those who have had IDDM for at least 5 years, glucagon responsiveness to hypoglycemia is blunted.

After 10 to 20 years of IDDM, about one third of patients have not only impairment of glucagon release, but impairment of epinephrine release as well (possibly secondary to autonomic neuropathy).

These patients are at 20-fold greater risk of developing severe hypoglycemia on intensive conventional insulin therapy (ICIT) or continuous subcutaneous insulin infusion (CSII) than those who have had IDDM for less than 5 years. They should be identified prospectively and excluded from intensive insulin therapy programs. See Table 18–9 and Fig. 18–25.

Sources: Bolli GB, Dimitriadis GD, Pehling GB, et al.: Abnormal glucose counterregulation after subcutaneous insulin in insulin-dependent diabetes mellitus. N Engl J Med 310:1706–1711, 1984; Bolli GB, Gotterman IS, Campbell PJ et al.: Glucose counterregulation and waning of insulin in the Somogyi phenomenon (posthypoglycemic hyperglycemia). N EnglJ Med 311:1214–1218, 1984; Bright GM, Melton TW, Rogol AD, et al.: Failure of cortisol blockade to inhibit early morning increases in basal insulin requirements in fasting insulin-dependent diabetics. Diabetes 29:662–664, 1980; Rizza R, Cryer P, Gerich J: Role of glucagon, catecholamines and growth hormone in human glucose counterregulation: effect of somatostatin and combined A and B adrenergic blockade on plasma glucose recovery and glucose flux rates after insulin-induced hypoglycemia. J Clin invest 64:62–71, 1979; Shamoon H, Hendler R, Sherwin RS: Altered responsiveness to cortisol, epinephrine, and glucagon in insulin-infused juvenile-onset diabetics. Diabetes 29:289–291, 1980; Shima K, Tanaka P, Morishita S, et al.: Studies on the etiology of "brittle diabetes." Diabetes 26:717–725, 1977; White NH, Skor DA, Cryer PE, et al.: Identification of Type I diabetic patients at increased risk for hypoglycemia during intensive therapy. N Engl J Med 308:485–491, 1983. Cryer PE: Hypoglycemia: The Limiting Factor in the Management of IDDM. Diabetes 43:1378–1389, 1994;[124] Hypoglycemic Disorders. F. John Service (ed.), W. B. Saunders Co., Philadelphia, 1999.[125] With permission.)

falls rapidly (within 2 to 3 days) during desensitization. They suggested that IgE antibodies are neutralized by insulin desensitization, that continued IgE antibody production does not occur, and that these two phenomena combined result in disappearance of the local and/or general allergic reactions. Others have suggested that since immunologic insulin resistance (IgG-mediated) may follow insulin allergy, the IgG antibodies may serve to protect desensitized patients by acting as "blocking antibodies" and preventing the combination of insulin with IgE antibodies and the allergic reactions that follow (see Fig. 18–27).

IgE antibodies may be measured by the in vitro radioallergosorbent test (RAST), by an indirect immunofluorescence technique using fluorescein-labeled anti-IgE, and by a quantitative insulin-specific IgE (IgE$_I$) assay.[199,200] It is not appropriate, as of 1999, to use the in vivo P-K assay because of the possibility of

transferring the hepatitis or AIDS viruses (or other infections) to the recipient.

Prior to the 1970's, USP crystalline insulin contained a number of impurities that were themselves antigenic (see Fig. 18–4), and that may have acted as adjuvants in increasing the antigenicity of insulin when it was injected subcutaneously into certain individuals. Yet, the primary antigenicity of insulin resides in the insulin molecule itself, with beef (three amino acids different) being more antigenic than pork (one amino acid different) which in turn is more antigenic than rDNA human insulin (no amino acids different).[133]

It has been suggested that "insulin" allergy may be due to zinc,[201] but the evidence for this claim is not convincing. Protamine, preservatives (0.25% m-cresol, and so forth), and rubber stopper allergies have been described, but are extremely rare. One of us (J.K.D.), over a period of 50 years, has not observed or been

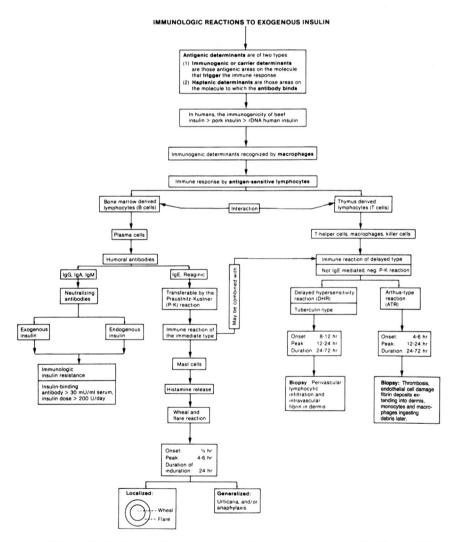

Figure 18–27.   A summary of the pathophysiology of immunologic reactions to exogenous insulin. (*Sources:* Davidson JK: Insulin allergy and immunologic insulin resistance. Comp Ther 8:46–52, 1982; deShazo RD, Boehm TM, Kumar D, et al.: Dermal hypersensitivity to insulin: correlations of three patterns to their histopathology. Allergy Clin Immunol 69:229–237, 1982. With permission.)

shown a single case of subsequently confirmed zinc, protamine, preservative, or rubber stopper allergy.[201]

A number of cases of local and or general allergy occurring after transfer from conventional to highly purified animal insulins have been reported.[197–200] Some patients previously allergic to beef-pork insulin have developed general urticaria when transferred to semisynthetic human insulin[206] or to rDNA human insulin.[207] Animals immunized with one compound eventually develop antibodies that react with related compounds. Thus, it is not surprising that those with diabetes and an allergic diathesis who have been chronically exposed to insulin from one species eventually develop antibodies that cross-react with insulins from other species, including human insulin.[208]

While reports of generalized allergy in patients treated only with rDNA human insulin are exceedingly rare,[207] cases of local insulin allergy have been reported at lower rates than with animal insulins. Whether or not intermittent treatment with exogenous human insulin will result in an amnestic antigenic response is yet to be determined. Very low-level antibody responses to human insulin, lower than those with purified pork insulin, have been observed.[209]

Epidemiology The prevalence and incidence of insulin allergy is not precisely known. Insulin anaphylaxis is rare. Galloway observed four cases of anaphylaxis to animal insulins, but was not aware of any deaths due to insulin anaphylaxis.[62,122] It is estimated that wheal-and-flare reactions (WFR) occurred in the 1980s in less than 5% of the individuals being treated with insulin and that most of the reactions were so mild that less than one in five was observed by a physician. Many individuals who have been treated with beef or pork insulins have desensitized themselves after mild local WFR by continuing daily insulin injections for 30 to 60 days. As previously noted, local allergy to the human insulins is rare, and general allergy to human insulin has been observed only in a few individuals who were previously allergic to animal insulins.

Intermittent insulin therapy and an atopic or allergic background predispose a patient to have immunologic reactions to insulin. Whether racial or other genetic factors predispose one to these reactions, is not known, but it seems possible that they do. Since life-threatening anaphylactic reactions are very rare and there have been no confirmed reported deaths,[62,122] and it is estimated that about 600 billion injections of insulin from animal sources have been administered to humans during the last 78 years, it seems safe to assume that fatal anaphylactic reactions to beef and/or pork insulins have not occurred.

Pathophysiology The sequence of events that occurs during immunologic reactions to insulin are summa-

rized in Figure 18-27.[202,211] When exogenous insulin is administered to humans, the immunogenicity of beef insulin is greater than that of pork insulin, which in turn is greater than that of rDNA and semisynthetic human insulins. Studies of patients transferred from combined beef-pork and from pork to human insulin have revealed that the serum IgG antibody response to human insulin is smaller, and about one half of patients with severe animal insulin allergy have not been allergic to rDNA human insulin. Conventional animal insulin therapy may induce the formation of species-specific IgE insulin antibodies that decrease on transfer to human insulin.[199,200] Studies of patients who have been treated with human insulin only have shown that IgG antibody production is less than that of control subjects treated with purified pork insulin.[208]

Problem Statement

Insulin allergy: Subsets: (1) local immediate WFR; (2) local delayed allergy (LDA) due to either delayed hypersensitivity reaction (DHR) or to Arthus-type reaction (ATR): (3) combination of WFR and LDA; (4) generalized urticaria; (5) anaphylaxis.

Subjective Is there a history of penicillin, food, pollen, dander, or physical (freezing temperature, skin trauma, and so forth) allergies? Any history of urticaria, hay fever, asthma, or dermatographia? Any history of intermittent insulin therapy, lipoatrophy, or immunologic insulin resistance? Is the patient overweight? See Table 18–19 for profiles of 591 patients with beef-pork insulin allergy reported by Galloway.[62,122,209]

Objective Erythematous, indurated, cutaneous, and subcutaneous nodules, varying from small, invisible, palpable-only, subcutaneous lesions to large, indurated, urticarial lesions at insulin injection sites.[211]

Observe insulin injection techniques to be certain that they are correct and that the patient is not injecting insulin intradermally (see Exhibit 18–2, Section I.F.). Evaluate for local infection, especially in those using CSII.

Assessment In the individual with IDDM who has local allergy to beef or pork insulin (Exhibit 18–13),[62,122] presence or absence of local allergy to human insulin should be determined first by intradermal skin tests (saline control, and rDNA human insulin). Measure WFR at 20 to 30 min and 1 hr, and induration at 6 to 72 hr at each site after injection of 0.001 U (0.1 mL of a 0.01 U/mL solution). If no WFR to human insulin occurs after 30 min, serially increase the human insulin dose tenfold (to 0.01 U, 0. 1 U, and 1 U intradermally, then 10 U subcutaneously). If there is still no reaction, therapy with human insulin may be continued without desensitization. If a WFR to human insulin occurs, desensitization to human insulin should be carried out. If suspected, skin tests for pro-

TABLE 18-19 Frequency of Subjective and Objective Findings in 591 Patients with Beef-Pork Insulin Allergy

Observation	Local Allergy (%) (n = 295)	Systemic Allergy[a] (%) (n = 296)
History of penicillin allergy	28	36
Other allergies	40	35
Total	68	71
Intermittent insulin therapy	29	59
Insulin resistance	14	20
Lipoatrophy	17	5
Overweight (>120% IBW)	30	30

[a] Alone or in combination with local allergy.
Abbreviation: IBW, ideal body weight.
[*Source:* Galloway JA, de Shazo RD: insulin chemistry, pharmacology, dosage algorithms, and complications of insulin treatment. *In* Rifkin H, Porte D (eds): Diabetes Mellitus: Theory and Practice. Amsterdam: Elsevier, 1990, pp. 497–513. With permission.]

tamine, preservative(s), rubber stopper, and zinc allergies may be carried out.

Skin tests for general allergy may be done in the same way (Exhibit 18–14),[62,122] but should be carried out in an intensive care unit that is prepared to deal with an anaphylactic reaction.

Plan

Initial (1) If the patient has either local or general allergy and NIDDM, and is not in DKA or HHS, and is not pregnant, discontinue insulin therapy and treat with aggressive low-calorie diet and exercise therapy (including an initial 1-week fast). (2) If the patient has IDDM, is in DKA or HHS, or is pregnant, and has either local or general allergy to human insulin, it will not be possible to institute treatment with human insulin without first desensitizing the individual. *Quick desensitization* to human insulin should be done in an intensive care unit that is prepared to deal with an anaphylactic reaction. Observation should be continuous.

After skin testing, administer every 20 to 30 min human insulin (start with 0.001 U and double the dose sequentially to 0.002, 0.004, 0.008, 0.016, and so on) until an intradermal dose of 1 U has been attained, or until a WFR develops. if no reaction at 1 U intradermally occurs, shift to subcutaneous administration of 2 U and continue to double the dose until plasma glucose is under satisfactory control. *Quick desensitization* can be accomplished within 6 hr. If a WFR occurs, drop the next dose to one-fourth the level that produced the reaction, and again start doubling the dose every 20 min. If desensitization is not possible, add dexamethasone (4 μg/U of insulin) to the injected insulin,[212] or give an antihistamine drug, such as diphenhydramine (25 to 50 mg orally every 4 to 6 hr) or oral prednisone until plasma glucose is under satisfactory control (see Exhibit 18–13).

If the antigenic response is local only (a WFR and/or LDA) and the patient is not in DKA or HHS, *slow desensitization* may be accomplished by giving four to six doses of insulin/day at 1 to 2 hr intervals, beginning with 0.001 U intradermally, then switching to the subcutaneous route of administration using 2 U initially and continuing to double the dose until the therapeutic level of insulin has been attained without an allergic reaction (2 to 3 days required).

Follow-up Over 90% of patients with local allergy to beef or pork insulins have improved within 2 months, and half of the remainder have improved within 6 to 12 months.[62,122] Once desensitized, insulin therapy should continue daily, since interruption of therapy and resumption at a later time is known to lead to an amnestic response with local or general allergy or anaphylaxis. Some individuals, to maintain desensitization to animal insulins, have required two doses of insulin daily. Immunologic insulin resistance may develop in some individuals who are allergic to animal insulins.

Once satisfactorily transferred to human insulin therapy, patients should *not* be given beef or pork insulin subsequently because of the significant risk of an amnestic reaction with recurrent allergy or resistance.

EXHIBIT 18–13 Assessment and Treatment Plan(s) for Local Insulin Allergy in Those with Insulin-Dependent Diabetes Mellitus (IDDM)

1. Rule out poor injection technique (failure to inject insulin under the skin), infection, and impurities in cleansing alcohol.
2. Evaluate with skin tests for wheal-and-flare reaction (WFR) to human insulin. If no WFR, treat with human insulin. If WFR to human insulin, desensitize to human insulin.
3. If local allergy persists, the possibility of allergy to protamine, preservative(s), rubber stopper, or zinc should be considered and ruled out by appropriate skin testing.
4. If desensitization is not possible, add dexamethasone [1 μg/U of insulin (1 mg/10 ml of U-100 insulin)]. Oral antihistamines (such as diphenhydramine, 25 to 50 mg every 4 to 6 hours) may be administered orally as therapy with regular insulin from the least antigenic source continues. Rarely, oral prednisone therapy may be needed. In some individuals, desensitization may require weeks or months.

[*Source:* Galloway JA, de Shazo RD: Insulin chemistry, pharmacology, dosage algorithms, and complications of insulin treatment. *In* Rifkin H, Porte D (eds): Diabetes Mellitus: Theory and Practice. Amsterdam: Elsevier, 1990, pp. 497–513. With permission.]

EXHIBIT 18–14   Treatment Plan(s) for Systemic Insulin Allergy

I. A. If the patient has NIDDM (and is above ideal body weight, is not pregnant, and has no history of DKA), reduce patient's body weight and attempt to control plasma glucose level with aggressive diet therapy, including 1-week total fast initially. (See Chapter 16.)

    B. If diet and exercise therapy alone or in conjunction with an oral agent (in the case of those with NIDDM) fails, then consider desensitization.

II. A. If the patient has IDDM, perform intradermal testing using rDNA, human insulin 0.001 and 0.01 U. If these are negative, test with 0.1 U.

    B. Unless the results in II.A. indicate a wheal-and-flare reaction (WFR) to rDNA human insulin, initiate therapy with human insulin without desensitization.

C. If the patient has a generalized allergic reaction (including anaphylaxis) to human insulin, desensitization to human insulin should be done in a carefully monitored setting where personnel knowledgeable in the treatment of anaphylactic reactions are available.

III. The authors are unaware of any reports of fatal anaphylactic reactions to rDNA human insulin.

IV. In fact, in 78 years of insulin use and reports of a number of cases of anaphylaxis thereunto related, there are no clearly confirmed cases of death related to insulin allergy after an estimated 600 billion injections of animal insulin into humans.

[*Source:* Galloway JA, de Shazo RD: Insulin chemistry, pharmacology, dosage algorithms, and complications of insulin treatment. *In* Rifkin H, Porte D (eds): Diabetes Mellitus: Theory and Practice. Amsterdam: Elsevier, 1990, pp. 497–513. With permission.]

Research Considerations

It seems reasonable to hypothesize that the complete replacement of animal (beef, pork) insulin therapy by human insulin therapy will result in a continuing decrease, and possibly eventual disappearance, of allergic reactions to insulin. In the last 15 years, primarily because of the low immunogenicity of human insulin,[122,134] the incidence and prevalence of allergy and resistance have dropped remarkably, especially in hospitals where human insulin therapy has been used exclusively.

Immunologic Insulin Resistance

Historical Perspective   Five years after the initial clinical use of insulin, the first case of resistance to the hormone was reported in an individual who required 1,100 U/day and who had both local and general allergy, but no insulin-neutralizing antibodies detected by mouse convulsion tests.[213] Root (1929)[214] defined insulin resistance as a "metabolic state that required 200 units or more for metabolic regulation," and that definition is still in use. Root thought that the normal human pancreas secreted 200 U/day, and that any diabetic who required more was "resistant" to the metabolic effects of the injected hormone. The first case in which the patient's serum was shown to contain a substance that neutralized the convulsant effects of insulin in mice was reported in 1938.[215] This individual required 1,050 U/day for 3 years and had no evidence of local allergy. By 1950,[197] 50 cases of insulin resistance had been reported, and the sera of eight of the individuals contained a substance that protected mice from insulin-induced convulsions. Moloney and Coval[15] (1955) produced insulin-neutralizing antibodies to beef insulin in guinea pigs, and in 1964 Moloney et al.[216]

reported that sulfated beef insulin (which contained an average of six sulfate groups) retained only one fifth of its ability to bind antibodies to unmodified beef insulin but retained one half of its biologic activity. It was shown that sulfated insulin, which in solution was a monomer and did not dimerize, was less antigenic than Lente beef insulin.[36]

In 1959 Berson and Yalow[16] reported that, after 3 months of insulin therapy, the sera of a majority of insulin-treated individuals contained insulin-binding antibodies, usually of low titer and that a small number who had high antibody titers required large doses of insulin (>200 U/day) for metabolic control. Shipp and coworkers[217] reported on 34 cases of insulin resistance observed at the Joslin Clinic. Seven required more than 2,000 U/day, but only one required more than 3,300 U/day (5,700 U/day). It is likely that some of these individuals had a disorder other than immunologic insulin resistance (see Exhibit 18–15). Of the 34 cases of immunologic insulin resistance reported by Davidson and DeBra,[218] none required more than 2,000 U regular beef insulin/day (mean dose, 550 U regular beef insulin/day). All responded to sulfated beef insulin, the initial dose being 89 U/day or 16% as much sulfated beef as regular beef insulin.

By 1990, the less immunogenic highly purified pork insulins and rDNA human insulins had been shown to be comparably effective in the treatment of immunologic insulin resistance.[133,134]

In 1978 Davidson and DeBra reported 34 cases of immunologic insulin resistance (IIR) that had been successfully treated with sulfated insulin imported to the USA from Toronto, Canada.[218] Eventually over 100 Americans were treated with sulfated insulin.

Between 1985–1988, Davidson started newly-diagnosed IDDMs on rDNA human insulin and transferred many from animal to human insulin therapy.[134]

EXHIBIT 18–15   Assessment (Differential Diagnosis) of Insulin-Resistant States

I. Common
  A. Obesity (see Chapter 9)
  B. Significant infection (see Chapter 45)
II. Uncommon
  C. Diabetic ketoacidosis (see Chapter 24)
  D. Immunologic insulin resistance (prevalence 0.1 to 1.0% of animal insulin-treated individuals)
    Maximum insulin-binding capacity ≥ 30 mU/mL (>0.216 nM) serum, ^{125}I insulin half-life in vivo >200 min, insulin dose ≥ 200 U/day
    Immunologic insulin resistance of less magnitude

may be present in those whose insulin dose is less than 200 U/day[133]
III. Rare
  E. Lipoatrophic diabetes
  F. Insulin receptor absence (see Chapter 9)
  G. Insulin receptor antibodies (see Chapter 9)
  H. Proteolytic degradation of subcutaneously injected insulin
  I. Significant complicating endocrine disease(s)
  J. Factitious insulin resistance in emotionally disturbed individuals

[*Source:* Davidson JK, DeBra DW: Immunologic insulin resistance. Diabetes 27:307–318, 1978. With permission.)

Sulfated insulin therapy was continued on IIRs until a study[133] comparing immunological and metabolic responses of patients with a history of antibody-induced beef insulin resistance to treatment with beef, pork, human, and sulfated beef insulin was initiated.

26 patients started the study; 21 completed it. 8 had been on sulfated insulin for >1 year, 11 for 1–5 wk., 2 for less than 1 wk. While on beef, 12 of 21 required an increased dose, 6 developed recurrent IIR (>200 U/d), plasma glucose and HbA$_{1c}$ increased. Recurrent resistance did not occur in any patient during 2 months on each of the other three insulins (sulfated beef, human, pork).

Sulfated insulin therapy for >1 year but *not* for <6 weeks reduced the risk of recurrent IIR on subsequent beef insulin therapy.[133]

In 1989, Naquet et al. had reported that sulfated beef insulin treatment elicits CD8$^+$T cells which might abrogate IIR in Type I diabetes.[219]

In 1997, Carpentier et al. reported that all remaining Canadians who had been on sulfated insulin therapy had been successfully transferred to human insulin therapy, and that the production of sulfated beef insulin had been terminated by its manufacturer[220] thus the availability and low immunigenicity of rDNA human insulin has obviated the need for sulfated beef insulin in preventing and treating IIR.

Recent papers have reported patients in whom severe insulin resistance to human insulin caused by insulin antibodies was ameliorated by *continuous insulin lispro infusion therapy*. While not successful in all cases, several patients have been able to maintain normal insulin doses at this point for up to 4 years.[221,222]

Epidemiology   With beef-pork insulin therapy, the prevalence of immunologic insulin resistance was estimated to be from 0.1 to 1.0%, with the greatest prevalence occurring in those who had been treated intermittently with insulin and in blacks.[133] The incidence has decreased significantly since the introduction of rDNA human, SS human, and highly purified pork insulins.

Pathophysiology   Insulin binding (neutralizing) antibodies, when present in a titer ≥ 30 mU/mL (0.216 nM) serum, may result in an increase in the insulin requirement to ≥ 200 U/day for metabolic regulation. The in vivo insulin half-life is prolonged and the space of insulin distribution in the body is reduced (compare Fig. 18–28 and Fig. 18–29). When the antibody titer is ≥ 30 mU/mL serum, the in vivo half-life of ^{125}I insulin is usually ≥ 200 min. The resistant state may wax (as the insulin-binding antibody titer reaches or exceeds ≥ 100 mU/mL serum) and wane (as the insulin-binding antibody titer falls as low as 10 mU/mL serum). See Figure 18–30. There was a good correlation between the maximum binding capacity (MBC) and the mouse hemidiaphragm assay (MHD) insulin antibody titers (Fig. 18–31).[218] Although there was a good correlation between the half-life ($T_{1/2}$) of ^{125}I beef insulin in vivo and the MBC of serum in vitro, there was an overlap of MBC titers (in the range of 30 to 90 mU/mL) in those who were classified as nonresistant (<200 U/day) and resistant (>200 U/day) (Fig. 18–32).[218] However, the insulin dose can increase significantly in some individuals without reaching >200 U/day when they are being treated with the most immunogenic (i.e., beef) insulin, presumably as a result of the increase in the titer and/or avidity of circulating insulin antibodies.[133] This can lead in turn to significant *insulin waste* from the plasma compartment by sequestration of insulin-antibody complexes by the reticuloendothelial system.[135-137]

In immunologic insulin resistance, insulin-binding antibodies are predominantly of the IgG type (see Fig. 18–27). The relative immunogenicity of purified beef, pork, sulfated, and rDNA human insulins was studied in a group of 21 patients with a documented history of immunologic insulin resistance.[133] Beef insulin was clearly more immunogenic than the other insulins, and metabolic control with beef insulin was less satisfactory. Yet some individuals with very high antibody titers did not require an increase in the dose of beef insulin. Thus, an insulin-binding antibody titer

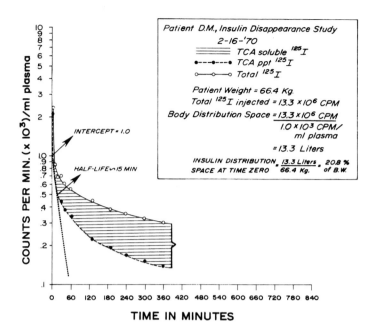

Figure 18–28. Calculation of the half-life and body distribution space of IV injected ^{125}I insulin. Plasma samples were collected at the indicated time intervals, and total ^{125}I and trichloroacetic acid (TCA; 10%)-precipitable ^{125}I measured. The shaded area represents TCA-soluble ^{125}I, or degraded insulin. The body distribution space was 20.8%, the estimated half life of the undegraded insulin was about 15 min. This individual had not been treated with insulin, and his serum contained no insulin-binding antibodies. The mean $T_{1/2}$ in ten non-insulin-treated humans was 13.9 min (range, 11.8 to 16.5 min), which is longer than the half-life of unlabeled insulin because the older ^{125}I insulins did not retain all of their biologic and immunologic activity. The mean $T_{1/2}$ for monoiodinated A14 tyrosine insulin, which retains essentially 100% of its biologic and immunologic activity, is about 4.5 min. (See Figure 18–29.)

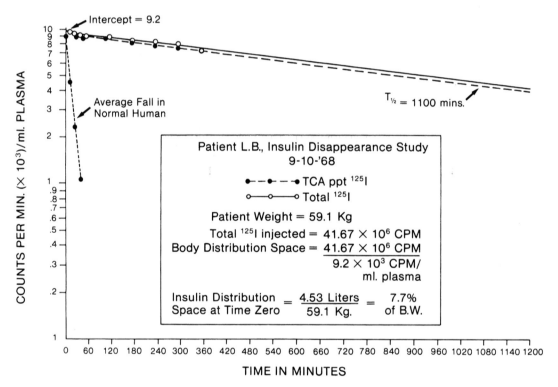

Figure 18–29. The body distribution space (7.7%) and $T_{1/2}$ (1,100 min) for ^{125}I beef insulin were both markedly abnormal. (See Fig. 18–28.) This individual required 2,000 U regular beef insulin per day for metabolic regulation and had a very high serum insulin antibody binding titer (1,000 mU/mL serum), and there was essentially no degraded insulin (TCA-soluble ^{125}I) in the serum 6 hr after the injection of ^{125}I beef insulin. (*Source:* Davidson JK, DeBra DW: Immunologic insulin resistance. Diabetes 27:307–318, 1978. With permission.)

of ≥30 mU/mL cannot be taken alone as being diagnostic of immunologic insulin resistance.

Treatment of immunologic insulin resistance to beef insulin for more than 1 year with sulfated beef insulin prevents recurrence of immunologic resistance on subsequent beef insulin therapy, presumably because the appearance of insulin-specific CD8+ T cells inhibits the response of A-loop-specific CD4+T cells.[133,219]

IMMUNOLOGIC INSULIN RESISTANCE

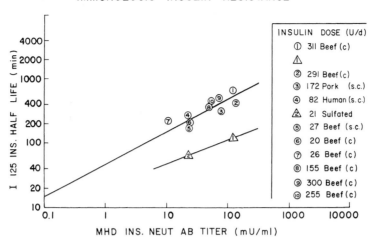

Figure 18–30. This 50-year-old black woman with IDDM had a high insulin antibody titer (>100 mU serum) and a markedly prolonged in vivo ^{125}I beef insulin $T_{1/2}$ (400 to 600 min) while on USP regular beef insulin therapy [beef (C) = beef (commerial)] or USP beef regular insulin), and required 291 to 311 U/day for metabolic control. The initial in vivo ^{35}S-sulfated beef insulin half-life was 100 min. The patient was then treated for 1 week on single-component pork [pork (SC)], then human [human (SC)], then sulfated, then beef [beef (SC)] insulins. The immunologic resistance started remitting on pork insulin (several hypoglycemic reactions) and continued on human insulin (several hypoglycemic reactions). During this period the ^{125}I beef insulin $T_{1/2}$ dropped (to about 200 min) and the insulin antibody titer dropped (to about 30 mU/mL serum). The patient's immunologic insulin resistance remained in remission on sulfated beef [sulfated, beef (SC)] and commercial beef insulin until the antibody titer started rising. When the $T_{1/2}$ reached about 400 min and the antibody titer exceeded about 60 mU/mL serum, recurrent immunologic resistance (dose of commercial beef insulin 255 to 300 U/day) was again evident.

MAXIMUM INSULIN BINDING CAPACITY (MBC) VS. MOUSE
HEMI-DIAPHRAGM (MHD) NEUTRALIZING ANTIBODY TITER

Figure 18–31. Comparison of insulin antibody titers measured in the same serum samples (numbers refer to individual patients) by the maximum ^{125}I insulin binding capacity (MBC) by the Berson-Yalow method[16] and by the mouse hemidiaphragm (MHD) method.[14] In the hemidiaphragm method, free insulin activity is measured in native serum and total insulin is measured after insulin is extracted by an acid alcoholic dialysis method.[92] The total insulin minus the free insulin represents the insulin bound to antibody in native serum. The two techniques provided very similar results with a correlation coefficient of 0.98. (*Source:* Davidson JK, DeBra DW: Immunologic insulin resistance. Diabetes 27:307–318, 1978. With permission.)

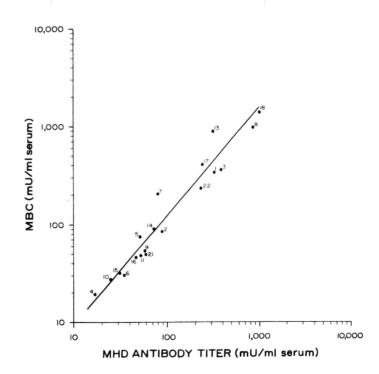

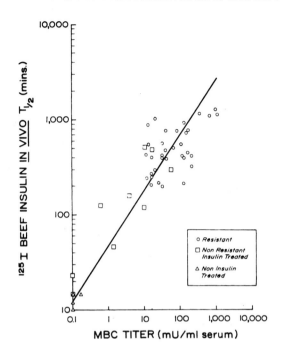

RELATIONSHIP BETWEEN IN VIVO T$_{1/2}$ OF ^{125}I BEEF INSULIN
AND MAXIMUM INSULIN BINDING CAPACITY (MBC)

Figure 18–32. Comparison of the in vivo T$_{1/2}$ of ^{125}I beef insulin and the maximum binding capacity (MBC) of serum in vitro. Patients who had never been treated with insulin had a short T$_{1/2}$ and bound essentially no insulin, whereas patients with immunologic insulin resistance had a high MBC (generally >30 mU/niL serum) and a long T$_{1/2}$ (>200 min). Insulin-treated nonresistant patients (i.e., dose <200 U/day) fell into an intermediate group, with some overlap. (*Source:* Davidson JK, DeBra DW: Immunologic insulin resistance. Diabetes 27:307–318, 1978. With permission.)

Problem Statement   Immunologic insulin resistance.

Subjective   History of intermittent animal insulin therapy, rapidly increasing dose without satisfactory metabolic control, possibly DKA, possibly history of insulin allergy.

Objective   Insulin dose >200 U/day, possibly greater prevalence in blacks.

Assessment   Rule out problems listed in Exhibit 18–15.

If insulin dose is >200 U/day and the serum insulin-binding antibody titer $\geq$30 mU/mL ($\geq$0.216 nM), a diagnosis of immunologic insulin resistance is almost certain. If the antibody titer is greater than 10 mU/mL (>0.072 nM) and the insulin dose has risen significantly (i.e., to greater than 50 U/day) in those who are not overweight, who are not rapidly growing juveniles with IDDM, and who do not have any of the other problems noted in Exhibit 18–15, the possibility of emerging immunologic insulin resistance should be considered.

Plan

Initial   An insulin-binding antibody titer should be measured. If it is >30 mU/mL (>0.216 nM) serum, and the patient is on animal insulin, the patient should be transferred to rDNA human insulin.

Follow-up   If the patient is currently receiving human insulin, a trial of insulin lispro (using CSII) is indi-

cated.[221,222] The insulin dose and the level of metabolic control should be assessed at frequent intervals initially, since the dose needed may fall dramatically during the first few weeks and severe hypoglycemia may result.[218]

Insulin Lipoatrophy

Historical Perspective   Insulin lipoatrophy, which consists of loss of subcutaneous fat at insulin injection sites, was first noted in 1926.[223,224] Lipoatrophy in response to immunogenic growth hormone and narcotic injections and jellyfish stings have also been reported.[122]

Epidemiology   Although the precise prevalence and incidence are not known, Renold et al.[225] reported a 24% prevalence of lipoatrophy in 1957. It is estimated that prior to the use of highly purified animal and human insulins, from 1 to 5% of individuals treated with USP conventional animal insulins developed clinically significant lipoatrophy[62,122] (Figs. 18–33 and 18–34). It has become less common in the last 10 years, probably due to the use of human insulin and highly purified animal insulins.[212,226,227]

Pathophysiology   In the past, most cases were thought to have been due to lipolytic impurities (not identified) in the insulin preparations. About 5% had evidence of local insulin allergy. In rare individuals, lipoatrophy recurred in previously filled-in lipoatrophic sites when insulin was injected into another part of the body. Such cases were thought to be due to an ill-defined immunogenic response to exogenous animal insulins.[212]

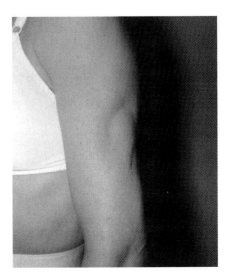

Figure 18–33. Insulin lipoatrophy of the arm in a 31-year old woman who had IDDM for 5 years and who had been treated with USP mixed beef-pork NPH and regular insulins. Disfiguring lipoatrophy of arms, buttocks (see Fig. 18–34), and thighs had been present for 3 years. Insulin therapy was changed to highly purified pork NPH and regular insulins, and one atrophic site was selected for injection daily, starting peripherally and moving centrally, until the atrophic site was filled with fat. It required over 700 injections over a period of 2 years to fill all atrophic sites.

Problem Insulin lipoatrophy.

Subjective, Objective, Assessment See Figures 18–33 through 18–35. Rule out causes of lipoatrophy other than insulin. Lipoatrophy and lipohypertrophy may coexist in the same person.

Plan

Initial Human insulin may be injected into the atrophic site(s) beginning at the edge of the atrophy and moving centrally until the site is filled.[62,122,226] If atrophic sites are multiple, one site should be filled before moving to another.

Follow-up About 95% of atrophic sites will fill when treatment with human insulin is carried out, as noted before.[62,122] Periodic injection of the previously atrophic sites may be needed in some individuals to keep the sites filled. Some individuals who excavate sites distal to the insulin-injection site may benefit from insulin desensitization. Some individuals benefit from dexamethasone (4 μg/U of insulin) injected with the insulin.[212]

The incidence of lipoatrophy has decreased on human insulin therapy.[224–229] Lipoatrophy has been reported in patients receiving human insulin. Injection site rotation and local administration of steroids has been helpful in some of these cases.

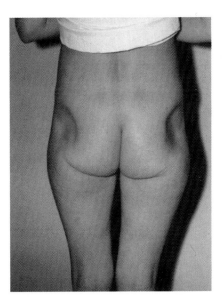

Figure 18–34. Insulin lipoatrophy of the buttocks in the same individual described in legend of Figure 18–33.

Insulin Lipohypertrophy

Historical Perspective That insulin repeatedly injected into the same subcutaneous site could produce unsightly accumulations of fat has been known since the 1930s, but it was not until 1950 that Renold et al.[228, 263]

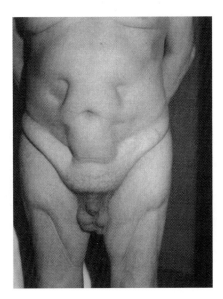

Figure 18–35. Insulin lipoatrophy in a 59-year-old man who had had IDDM for 15 years and had been treated with USP mixed beef-pork NPH and regular insulins. Disfiguring lipoatrophy of arms, buttocks, abdomen, and thighs had been present for 12 years. He had no history of local or general insulin allergy. Insulin therapy was changed to highly purified pork NPH and regular insulins. One abdominal atrophic site was injected daily during a 3-year period (over 1,000 injections), but the atrophic site did not fill completely. The other sites remained atrophic.

showed fat accumulation in experimental animals at insulin injection sites.

Epidemiology   Modest fat tissue hypertrophy probably occurs in a large number of individuals who do not rotate insulin injection sites appropriately. The prevalence and incidence of slight or modest lipohypertrophy is unknown. Five of 148 patients (3.4%) developed insulin hypertrophy after 1 year of insulin therapy.[229] Marked hypertrophy rarely develops, and then only in those who do not rotate injection sites within a specific area (abdomen, thigh, and so on) so that no site is injected more than once each month (see Fig. 18–26).

Pathophysiology   The lipogenic effect of insulin produces triglyceride accumulation and fat cell hypertrophy in areas exposed repeatedly to high insulin concentrations (Figs. 18–36 and 18–37).

Plan

Initial and Follow-up   Select insulin injection sites where lipohypertrophy has not occurred. Plan a grid in the *same* region [(abdomen, thigh, and so forth (Fig. 18–26)] so that 30 injections can be placed at 1 inch intervals during a 1-month period (60 injection sites at 1 inch intervals if two injections per day are used). Start on the first day of each month at position 1. This approach will establish an injection routine and will minimize the subsequent development of lipohypertrophic areas.

Insulin Edema

Historical Perspective   It has been known for more than 40 years that insulin therapy promotes sodium retention by the kidney.[230,231]

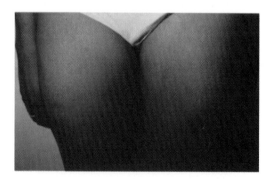

Figure 18–36.   Insulin lipohypertrophy of the thighs in a 33-year-old man who had had IDDM for 12 years and who had been treated with USP mixed beef-pork NPH insulin. He had injected insulin at the same site of each thigh on alternate days. He said that injections at the hypertrophic sites were less painful. He had not been instructed to rotate injection sites so that no site was injected more than once every 30 days. After the injection area was shifted to the abdomen and sites were rotated as illustrated in Figure 18–26, lipohypertrophy did not occur at the new injection sites. The lipohypertrophy of the thighs decreased markedly over a 2-year follow-up period.

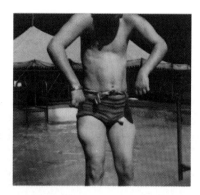

Figure 18–37.   Insulin lipohypertrophy of the thighs in a 17-year-old man who had had IDDM for 14 years and who had been treated with USP mixed beef-pork NPH and regular insulins for 14 years. He had not been instructed to rotate injection sites and had injected the lipohypertrophic sites on each thigh on alternating days because injections in those sites were less painful.

Epidemiology and Pathophysiology   Although modest sodium retention occurs in almost everyone treated with exogenous insulin because of increased sodium reabsorption by the ascending loop of Henle and the distal convoluted tubule,[112,113] it rarely becomes pronounced enough to be of clinical significance. It usually occurs in those who have been poorly controlled and is more likely to develop in those who are prone to congestive heart failure and in those who have kidney or liver disease, or significant peripheral neuropathy.

Problem   Edema induced by insulin therapy (Fig. 18–38).

Plan

Initial and Follow-up   The edema will clear with diuretic therapy (furosemide 40 to 80 mg/day preferred). After the edema has subsided, diuretic therapy may be used thereafter on an as-needed basis. Dietary sodium intake should be limited (usually 2 g daily) until the edema clears.

An Overview of Research Considerations Related to Insulin Therapy

Human insulin rDNA assures an unlimited supply of insulin for future use. It is significantly less immunogenic than beef insulin.[133,134] Insulin aggregation shown in Figure 18–39 may occur with all types of insulin when vials are subjected to vigorous agitation or high environmental temperatures. Each vial should be inspected to be sure that this has not occurred.

Research continues related to the development of closed-loop insulin delivery systems that can measure glucose and concomitantly infuse insulin at a rate that

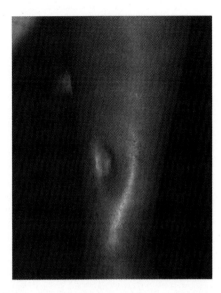

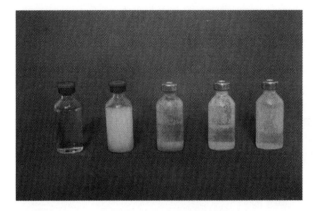

Figure 18–39. Insulin vials containing from left to right: (1) Normal regular insulin, (2) normal NPH insulin, (3), (4), and (5) NPH insulin that has clumped, settled, and stuck to the inside of the vial.

Figure 18–38. Insulin edema in a 62-year-old woman who had been started on insulin therapy 1 month earlier during an episode of severe diabetic ketoacidosis. Marked pitting edema to the knees developed, and she gained 20 pounds. The edema disappeared within 2 weeks after sodium intake was restricted to 2 g/day and 80 mg furosemide/day was given orally. Metabolic control remained satisfactory during the next month, and edema did not recur despite the omission of furosemide therapy.

will maintain normoglycemia. No such device is available in 1999.

A great deal is yet to be learned about the nature of insulin action on cells and about the etiology and pathogenesis of IDDM and NIDDM. (See Chapters 3 through 9.)

Human Proinsulin

Because limited studies in animals and man suggested that porcine proinsulin had pharmacologic properties that could have clinical utility,[232–234] the rDNA technology that was first used to produce human insulin was utilized to manufacture human proinsulin (HPI).[232–235] Initial pharmacologic studies demonstrated that, like porcine proinsulin, HPI was a soluble intermediate-acting insulin agonist that was relatively hepatospecific. Moreover, early studies indicated that the intrasubject variation in response of patients receiving repeated doses of HPI was significantly less than that observed with NPH insulin. However, since metabolic control observed in patients treated with HPI was not better than that observed with insulin, these advantages apparently were not translatable into clinical benefit. Furthermore, in one multicenter clinical trial in which insulin-naive patients were randomized to treatment with HPI or human insulin, six patients on HPI, all of whom had been treated for 1 year or more, developed acute myocardial infarctions (MIs), two of which resulted in death. There were no MIs in the human insulin group.[102] This finding and the facts that on a

molar basis serum hormone concentrations of HPI were several hundred times those found in normal individuals and that hyperinsulinemia was alleged to be a risk factor for atherogenesis,[236,237] combined with a failure to demonstrate unique efficacy, led to the suspension of the clinical development of HPI.[102]

Insulin Analogues

The focus in recent years on intensification of metabolic control in order to forestall the chronic complications of the disease has heightened the awareness of physicians and patients of the extraordinary difficulty encountered in attempting to normalize the blood glucose, a phenomenon that increasingly is being ascribed to the failure to simulate the serum insulin profile of normal individuals during feeding and fasting. Substitution of aspartic acid for histidine at B-10 was shown to produce an insulin with increased biologic activity. This stimulated considerable continuing research interest into insulins and proinsulins with increased or decreased biologic activity, and in the chemical changes in the molecule that are responsible.

Insulin lispro, created by reversing the amino acids on the B-chain of the insulin molecule from $Pro^{B28}Lys^{B29}$ to $Lys^{B28}Pro^{B29}$, produced a molecule with the same amino acid composition and molecular weight, but with a decreased propensity for self-association into dimers resulting in an insulin with a more rapid onset of action and shorter duration of action than regular human insulin[282, 283] (Fig. 18–40). In contrast to true monomeric insulin analogs, both regular human insulin and insulin lispro, in their respective formulations, exist as hexamers that are stabilized with zinc ions and phenolic preservatives. The insulin lispro hexamer complex, however, dissociates into monomers immediately upon injection producing a rapid absorption pattern that is indistinguishable from true monomeric insulins.[249] Insulin lispro became the first

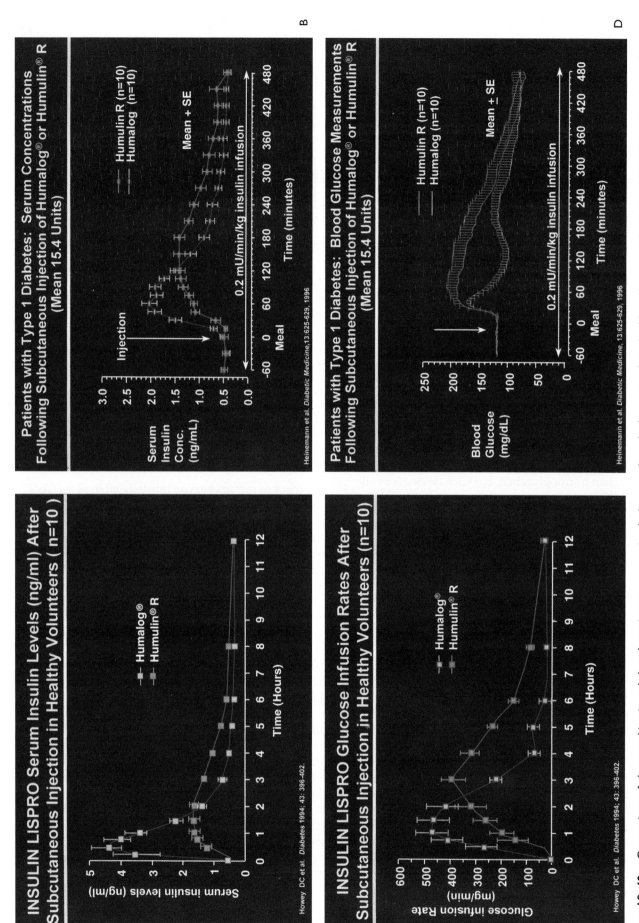

Figure 18–40. Comparison of pharmacokinetic and glucodynamic responses to insulin lispro and regular human insulin in healthy volunteers (18–40-A and 18–40-C) and patients with type I diabetes mellitus (18–40-B and 18–40-D) demonstrating the more rapid onset, earlier peak and shorter duration of activity of insulin lispro compared to regular human insulin. The healthy volunteer study was conducted using a glucose clamp technique and the type I patient study was a high carbohydrate, high lipid meal challenge study.

insulin analog commercially available and offered a more physiologic approach to insulin therapy, by providing improved postprandial glucose control, the potential for improved overall glucose control, and reductions in hypoglycemia (especially nocturnal hypoglycemia) and in severe hypoglycemia, while also providing the convenience of injection just before (or even after) mealtime.[251, 254, 288, 291] Thus, the role for insulin analogs was established in providing more physiologic control of diabetes.

Other insulin analogs are currently in development for addressing both mealtime and basal therapy. Insulin aspart (Asp^{B28}-human insulin, NovoRapid^{TM}, Novo-Nordisk, AS) is being studied as a mealtime insulin with an activity profile in terms of time of injection and improved postprandial control similar to Insulin lispro.[285] Although proinsulin could be considered the first longer acting insulin analog to be studied clinically, insulin glargine (Gly^{A21} L-Arg^{Ba30} L-Arg^{Bb30}-human insulin, Hoechst Marion Roussel) is a designed, longer-acting insulin analog currently being evaluated.

This analog is formulated in an acidic solution and forms microprecipitates upon injection into physiologically neutral pH subcutaneous tissue resulting in a prolonged absorption from the site. Characterized by a more prolonged duration with a less pronounced peak activity, clinical trials have focused on comparisons with once or twice daily NPH insulin with better fasting plasma glucose and lower or equivalent hypoglycemia.[286] Another approach to basal analog development has been the fatty acid acylated insulins. Lys^{B29} tetradecanoyl-des^{B30}-human insulin (NN304, Novo-Nordisk, AS)[286] and N$^{\varepsilon}$-palmitoyl Lys^{B29}-human insulin (C16-HI, Eli Lilly and Company)[281, 287] are two examples of analogs that have been evaluated which use binding to circulating proteins (albumin) as the basis for prolongation of activity.[287] Extensive biochemical and pharmacological work remains to determine the effectiveness of this approach. It does remain quite evident that the future of insulin therapy is moving in the direction of insulin analogs that can contribute additional advantages over human insulin.

References

1. Banting FG, Best CH: The internal secretion of the pancreas. J Lab Clin Med 7:251–266, 1922.

2. Geyelin HR, Harrop G, Murray MF, et al.: The use of insulin in juvenile diabetes. J Metab Res, November 1922, pp. 767–792.

3. Campbell WR, Macleod JJR: Insulin. Medicine 3:195–308, 1924.

4. Campbell WR: Anabasis: a lecture on the fortieth anniversary of the discovery of insulin. Univ Toronto Med J 39:189–194, 1962.

5a. Wrenshall GA, Hetenyi G, Feasby WR (eds): The Story of Insulin: Forty Years of Success Against Diabetes. Toronto: Max Reinhardt, 1962.

5b. Hetenyi G.: "Why Can't we Get it Right? Notes on the Discovery of Insulin." Annals Royal Canadian Physiological Society 31:237–239, August 1998.

5c. Banting FG: "The History of Insulin." *Edinburgh Medical Journal*, Jan, 1929, p. 1–18.

6. Burrow GN, Hazlett BE, Phillips MJ: A case of diabetes mellitus. N Engl J Med 306:340–343, 1982.

7. Proceedings: Fiftieth Anniversary Insulin Symposium. Diabetes 21 (Suppl 2)385–714, 1972.

8. Bliss M: The Discovery of Insulin. Toronto: McClelland and Stewart, 1982, pp. 112–113, 120–121, 242–243.

9. Bliss M: Banting, A Biography. Toronto: McClelland and Stewart, 1984.

10. West KM: Epidemiology of Diabetes and Its Vascular Lesions. New York: Elsevier, 1978, pp. 127–158, 289–321.

11. Banting FG, Best CH, Collip JB, et al.: The effect of pancreatic extract (insulin) on normal rabbits. Am J Physiol 43:162–176, 1922.

12. Stewart GA: Methods of insulin assay. Br Med Bull 16:196–201, 1960.

13. Volund A, Brange J, Drejer K, et al.: In vitro and in vivo potency of insulin analogs designed for clinical use. Diabet Med 8:839–847, 1991.

14. Davidson JK: Islet cell function. Ph.D. thesis in physiology. University of Toronto, 1965.

15. Moloney PJ, Coval M: Antigenicity of insulin: diabetes induced by specific antibodies. Biochem J 59:179–185, 1955.

16. Berson SA, Yalow RS: Quantitative aspects of the reaction between insulin and insulin binding antibody. J Clin Invest 38:1996–2016, 1959.

17. Yalow RS, Berson SA: Immunoassay of endogenous plasma insulin in man. J Clin Invest 39:1157–1175, 1960.

18. Abel JJ, et al.: Crystalline insulin. J Pharmacol Exp Ther 31:65–85, 1927.

19. Kahn CR: Antibodies to insulin and insulin receptors: mechanisms of insulin resistance. *In* Gupta S (ed): Immunology of Clinical and Experimental Diabetes. New York: Plenum, 1984, pp. 249–327.

20. Sanger F: Chemistry of insulin. Br Med Bull 16:183–187, 1960.

21. Nicol DSHW, Smith LF: Amino-acid sequence of human insulin. Nature 187:483–485, 1960.

22. Smith LF: Amino acid sequences of insulins. Diabetes 21 (Suppl 2):457–460, 1972.

23. Derewenda U and Dodson GG: The structure and sequence of insulin, in molecular structures in biology. Eds. Diamond R, Koetzle TF, Prout K, Richardson JS. Chapter 9, pp. 260–277, Oxford University Press, NY, 1993.

24. Shuldiner AR, Bennett C, Robinson EA, Androth J: Isolation and characterization of two different insulins from an amphibian, Xenopus Laevis, Endocrinology 125:469–477, 1989.

25. Katsoyannis PG, Trakatellis AC, Johnson S, et al.: Studies on the synthesis of insulin from natural and synthetic A and B chains. II. Isolation of insulin from recombination mixtures of natural A and B chains. Biochemistry 6:2642–2654, 1967.

26. Warren-Perry MG, Manley SE, Ostrega D, et al.: A novel point mutation in the insulin gene giving rise to hyperproinsulinemia. Jour Clin Endo Metab 82:1629–1631, 1997.

27. Brandenburg D, Wollmer A (eds): insulin: Chemistry, Structure and Function of Insulin and Related Hormones. Berlin: Walter de Gruyter, 1980.

28. Rachman J, Levy Jc, Barrow BA: Relative hyperproinsulinemia of NIDDM persists despite the reduction of hyperglycemia with insulin or sulfonylurea therapy. Diabetes 46:1557–1562, 1997.

29. Chance RE: Amino acid sequences of proinsulins and intermediates. Diabetes 21:462–467, 1972.

30. Perler F, Efstratiadis A, Gilbert W, et al.: The evolution of genes: the chicken preproinsulin gene. Cell 20:555–566, 1980.

31. Kwok SCM, Chan SJ, Steiner DF: Cloning and nucleotide sequence analysis of the dog insulin gene. J Biol Chem 258:2357–2363, 1983.

32. Pitts JE, Bajaj M: Structure and function of insulin. In Gupta S (ed): Immunology of Clinical and Experimental Diabetes. New York: Plenum, 1984, pp. 3–50.

33. Rosenthal AS, Mann D, Kahn CR: Genetic control of the immune response to insulin in man. In Gupta S (ed): Immunology of Clinical and Experimental Diabetes. New York: Plenum, 1984, pp. 51–72.

34. Galloway JA, Bressler R: Insulin treatment in diabetes. Med Clin North Am 62:663–680, 1978.

35. Chance RE, Root MA, Galloway JA: The immunogenicity of insulin preparations. Acta Endocrinol 83:185–197, 1976.

36. Little JA, Lee R, Sebriakova M, et al.: Insulin antibodies and clinical complications in diabetes treated for five years with lente or sulfated insulin. Diabetes 26:980–988, 1977.

37. Young CWT, Moule ML, Yip CC: Functional role of the N-terminal region of the B-chain of insulin. In Brandenburg, D, Wollmer A (eds): Insulin: Chemistry, Structure and Function of Insulin and Related Hormones. Berlin: Waiter de Gruyter, 1980, pp. 417–423.

38. Blundell TL, Cutfield JF, Cutfield SM, et al.: Atomic positions in rhombohedral 2-zinc insulin crystals. Nature 231:506–511, 1971.

39. Blundell TL, Dodson GG, Hodgkin D, et al.: Insulin: the structure in the crystal and its reflection in chemistry and biology. Adv Protein Chem 26:279–402, 1972.

40. Blundell TL, Wood SP: Is the evolution of insulin Darwinian or due to selectively neutral mutation? Nature 257:197–203, 1975.

41. Dodson EJ, Dodson GG, Hubbard RE, Reynolds CD: Insulin molecular structure and molecular behavior. In Besser GM, Bodansky HJ, Cudworth AG (eds): Clinical Diabetes—An Illustrated Text. London: Gower Medical Publishers, 1988, pp. 4.1–4.8.

42. Blundell TL, Hawk R: A monomeric insulin from the casiragua: model building using computer graphics. Hoppe Seylers Z Physiol Chem 362:727–737, 1981.

43. Rinderknecht E, Humbel RE: The amino acid sequence of human insulin-like growth factor 1 and its structural homology with proinsulin. J Biol Chem 253:2769–2776, 1978.

44. Rinderknecht E, Humbel RE: Primary structure of human insulin-like growth factor 2. FEBS Lett 89:283–286, 1978.

45. Blundell TL, Humbel RE: Hormone families: pancreatic hormones and homologous growth factors. Nature 287:781–787, 1980.

46. Conover CA: Regulation of insulin-like growth factor (IGF)-binding protein synthesis by insulin and IGF-1 in bovine fibroblasts. Endocrinology 126:3139–3145, 1990.

47. Cascieri MA, Bayne ML, Ber E, et al.: Identification of the insulin-like growth factor I (IGF I) epitopes recognized by monoclonal and polyclonal antibodies to IGF I. Endocrinology 126:2773–2777, 1990.

48. Yancey GG, Van Wyk JJ, Underwood LE, Svoboda ME: Derivation of monoclonal antibodies to human somatomedin C/insulin-like growth factor I. Methods Enzymol 146:207–216, 1987.

49. Czech MP: Signal transmission by the insulin-like growth factors. Cell 59:235, 1989.

50. Goldstein S, Sertich GJ, Levan KR, Phillips LS: Nutrition and somatomedin. XIX. Molecular regulation of insulin-like growth factor-1 in streptozotocin-diabetic rats. Mol Endocrinol 2:1093–1100, 1988.

51. Scheiwiller E, Guler HP, Merryweather J, et al.: Growth restoration of insulin-deficient diabetic rats by recombinant human insulin-like growth factor I. Nature 11:169–171, 1986.

52. Leaman DW, Simmer FA, Ramsay TG, White ME: Insulin-like growth factor-I and -II: messenger RNA expression in muscle, heart, and liver of streptozotocin-diabetic swine. Endocrinology 126:2850–2857, 1990.

53. Davidson JK, Falkmer S, Mehrotra BK, et al.: Insulin assays and light microscopical studies of digestive organs. Gen Comp Endocrinol 17:388–401, 1971.

54. Van Noorden S, Falkmer S: Gut-islet endocrinology—some evolutionary aspects. Invest Cell Pathol 3:21–35, 1980.

55. Steiner DE, Oyer PE: Biosynthesis of insulin and a probable precursor of insulin by a human islet cell adenoma. Proc Natl Acad Sci USA 57:473–480, 1967.

56. Robbins DC, Tager HS, Rubenstein AH: Biologic and clinical importance of proinsulin. N Engl J Med 310:1165–1175, 1984.

57. Ullrich A, Dull TJ, Gray A: Genetic variation in the human insulin gene. Science 209:612–615, 1980.

58. Tager HS: Abnormal products of the human insulin gene. Diabetes 33:693–699, 1984.

59. Steiner DF, Tager HS, Chan SJ, et al.: Lessons learned from molecular biology of insulin-gene mutations. Diabetes Care 13:600–609, 1990.

60. Schwartz GP, Burke GT, Katsoyannis PG: A superactive insulin: [B-10 aspartic acid] insulin (human). Proc Natl Acad Sci USA 84:6408–6411, 1987.

61. Schwartz GP, Burke GT, Katsoyannis PG: A highly potent insulin: (DES B26-B30)-[ASP B10, TYR B25-NH$_2$] insulin (human). Proc Nad Acad Sci USA 86:458–461, 1989.

62. Galloway JA: Chemistry and clinical use of insulin. *In* Galloway JA, Potvin JH, Shuman CR (eds): Diabetes Mellitus. Indianapolis: Eli Lilly, 1988, pp. 105–138.

63. Goeddel DV, Kleid DG, Bolivar F, et al.: Expression in Escherichia coli of chemically synthesized genes for human insulin. Proc Natl Acad Sci USA 76:106–110, 1979.

64. Riggs AD, Itakura K, Crea R, et al.: Synthesis, cloning, and expression of hormone genes in Escherichia coli. Rec Prog Horm Res 36:261–276, 1980.

65. Riggs AD: Bacterial production of human insulin. Diabetes Care 4:64–68, 1981.

66. Galloway JA, Marsden JH: Clinical trials with biosynthetic human insulin. Diabetes Care 4:260–261, 1981.

67. Galloway JA, Peck FB, Fineberg SE, et al.: The U.S. "new patient" and "transfer" studies. Diabetes Care 5 (Suppl 2): 135–139, 1982.

68. Johnson IS, Human insulin from recombinant DNA technology. Science 219:632–637, 1983.

69. Keen H, Glymme A, Pickup JC, et al.: Human insulin produced by recombinant DNA technology: safety and hypoglycemic potency in healthy men. Lancet ii (8191): 398–401, 1980.

70. NIH: Insulin and human growth hormone: triumphs in genetic engineering. JAMA 245:1724–1725, 1981.

71. Galloway JA: Insulin treatment for the early 80s: facts and questions about old and new insulins and their usage. Diabetes Care 3:615–622, 1980.

72. Skyler JS (ed): Symposium on human insulin of recombinant DNA origin. Diabetes Care 5 (Suppl 2)1–186, 1982.

73. Chance RE, Kroeff EP, Hoffmann JA et al.: Chemical, physical and biologic properties of biosynthetic human insulin. Diabetes Care 4:147–154, 1981.

74. Fineberg SE, Galloway JA, Fineberg NS, et al.: Immunogenicity of recombinant DNA human insulin. Diabetologia 25:465–469, 1983.

75. Frank BH, Pettee JM, Zimmerman RE, et al.: The production of human proinsulin and its transformation to human insulin and C-peptide. *In* Peptides: Synthesis-Structure-Function. Proceedings of the Seventh American Peptide Symposium. Rockford: Pierce Chemical Company, 729–783, 1981.

76. Inouye K, Watanabe K, Morihara K, et al.: Enzyme-assisted semisynthesis of human insulin. J Am Chem Soc 101:751–752, 1979.

77. Karam JH, Etzwiler DD: International symposium on human insulin. Diabetes Care 6 (Suppl 1):1–68, 1983.

78. Abramowics M (ed): Purified insulin preparations. Med Lett Drugs Ther 23(12)53–56, 1981.

79. Sun M: Insulin wars: new advances may throw market into turbulence. Science 210:1225–1228, 1980.

80. Galloway JA, Root MA, Radimacher RP, et al.: A comparison of acid regular and neutral regular insulin. Diabetes 22:471–479, 1973.

81. Hagedorn HC: Modification of insulin. Phys Bull 12:26–33, 1947.

82. Scott DA, Fisher AL: Studies on insulin with protamine. J Pharmacol Exp Ther 58:78–92, 1936.

83. Galloway JA, Spradlin CT, Nelson RL, et al.: Factors influencing the absorption, serum insulin concentration, and blood glucose responses after injections of regular insulin and various insulin mixtures. Diabetes Care 4:366–376, 1981.

84. Galloway JA, Spradlin CT, Jackson RL, et al.: Mixtures of intermediate-acting insulin (NPH and Lente) with regular insulin. *In* Insulin Update, 1982, Amsterdam: Excerpta Medica, 1982, pp. 111–119.

85. Hallas-Moller K, Petersen K, Schlichtkrull J: Crystalline and amorphous insulin-zinc compounds with prolonged action. Science 116:394–398, 1952.

86. Ogilvie R: A quantitative estimation of the pancreatic islet tissue. Q J Med 6:287–300, 1937.

87. Wrenshall GA, Bogoch A, Ritchie RC: Extractable insulin of pancreas. Diabetes 1:87–107, 1952.

88. Howanitz PJ, Howanitz JH: Carbohydrates: pancreatic hormones, insulinoma. *In* Henry JB (ed): Todd-Sanford-Davidsohn's Clinical Diagnosis and Management by Laboratory Methods, Ed. 17. Philadelphia: W. B. Saunders, 1984, pp. 165–172.

89. Lehmann HP, Henry JB: SI Units (International System of Units). *In* Henry JB (ed): Todd-Sanford-Davidsohn's Clinical Diagnosis and Management by Laboratory Methods, Ed. 17. Philadelphia: W. B. Saunders, 1984, pp. 1429–1434.

90. Desbuquois B, Arbach GD: Use of polyethylene glycol to separate free and antibody-bound hormones in radioimmunoassay. J Clin Endocrinol Metab 33:732–738, 1971.

91. Edwards R. Immuno Assays in Rickwood D, Hames BD, Series Eds. Essential Data Series. John Wiley and Sons, New York, 1996.

92. Davidson JK, Haist RE, Best CH: Studies employing a new method for recovery of biologically active insulin from acid alcoholic extracts of pancreas and blood serum. Diabetes 12:448–453, 1963.

93. Taylor SI, Grunberger G, Marcus-Samuels B, et al: Hypoglycemia Associated with Antibodies to the Insulin Receptor." N Engl J Med 307:1422–1426, 1982.

94. Dons RF, Havlik R, Taylor SI, et al: Clinical Disorders Associated with Autoantibodies to the Insulin Receptor." J Clinical Invest 72:1072–1080, 1983.

95. Hoogwerf BJ, Goetz FC: Urinary C-peptide: a simple measure of integrated insulin production with emphasis on the effects of body size, diet, and corticosteroids. J Clin Endocrinol Metab 56:60–67, 1983.

96. Yalow RS, Berson SA: Dynamics of insulin secretion in hypoglycemia. Diabetes 14:341–349, 1965.

97a. Krejs GF: Non-insulin secreting tumors of the gastroen-teropancreatic system in Williams textbook of Endo-crinology, 9th Ed: Wilson J, Foster D, Kronenberg H, Larsen R (eds), pp 1663–1673, WB Saunders CO, Philadelphia, 1998.

97b. Leroith D: Tumor-induced hypoglycemia. N Engl J Med: 241:757–758, 1999.

98. Unger RH, Orci L: The role of glucagon in diabetes. Diabetes 8:53–68, 1982.

99. Cohn C, Berger S, Norton M: Relationships between meal size and frequency and plasma insulin response in man. Diabetes 17:72–75, 1968.

100. Logothetopoulos J, Jain K: In vivo incorporation of (^{3}H) leucine and (^{3}H) tryptophan into proinsulin-insulin and other islet cell proteins in normoglycemic, hyperglycemic, and hypoglycemic rats. Diabetes 29:801–805, 1980.

101. Madison LL, Kaplan L: The hepatic binding of I^{131} labeled insulin in human subjects during a single tran-shepatic circulation. J Lab Med 52:927–932, 1948.

102. Galloway JA, Hooper SA, Spradlin CT, Howey DC, Frank BH, Bowsher RR, and Anderson JH: Biosynthetic Human Proinsulin: Review of chemistry, in vitro and in vivo receptor binding, animal and human pharmacol-ogy studies, and clinical trial experience. Diabetes Care 15:666–692, 1992.

103. Steiner, DF: The Proprotein Convertases. Curr Opin Chem Biol 2(1):31–39, 1998.

104. Dodson G and Steiner DF: The role of assembly in insulins's biosynthesis. Current opinion in structural biology 8:189–194, 1998.

105. Rubenstein AH, Pottenger LA, Mako M, et al.: The metabolism of proinsulin and insulin by the liver. J Clin Invest 51:912–921, 1975.

106. Misbin RI, Merimee JJ, Lowenstein J: Insulin removal by the isolated perfused rat liver. Am J Physiol 230: 171–177, 1976.

107. Rubenstein AH, Clark JL, Melani F, et al.: Secretion of proinsulin, C-peptide by pancreatic beta cells and its cir-culation in blood. Nature (Lond) 224:697–699, 1969.

108. Anderson JH, Campbell RK: Mixing Insulins in 1990. Diabetes Educator 16(5)380–387.

109. Stoll RW, Toubert JL, Menahan LA, et al.: Clearance of porcine insulin, proinsulin and connecting peptide by the isolated rat liver. Proc Soc Exp Biol Med 133: 894–896, 1970.

110. Block M, Mako M, Steiner D, et al.: Circulating C-peptide immunoreactivity studies in normals and diabetic patients. Diabetes 21:1013–1024, 1972.

111. Faber OK, Hagen C, Binder C, et al.: Kinetics of human connecting peptide in normal and diabetic subjects. J Clin Invest 62:197–203, 1979.

112. Rabkin R, Ryan MP, Duckworth WC: The renal metab-olism of insulin. Diabetologia 27:351–357, 1984.

113. Kitabchi AE, Duckworth WC, Steutz FB: Insulin synthe-sis, proinsulin and C-peptides. In Rifkin H, Porte D (eds): Diabetes Mellitus: Theory and Practice, Amster-dam: Elsevier, 1990, pp. 71–88.

114. Davidson JK: Diabetes mellitus and its treatment with diet, exercise, insulin and sulfonylureas. In Wang RIH (ed): Practical Drug Therapy. Philadelphia: J. B. Lippin-cott, 1979, pp. 417–444.

115. Albisser AM, Leibel BS, Ewart TG, et al.: Chemical con-trol of diabetes by the artificial pancreas. Diabetes 23:397–404, 1974.

116. Rizza RA, Gerich JE, Haymond MW, et al.: Control of blood sugar in insulin-dependent diabetes: comparison of an artificial endocrine pancreas, continuous subcuta-neous insulin infusion, and intensified conventional insulin therapy. N Engl J Med 303:1313–1318, 1980.

117. Skyler JS, Skyler DL, Seigler DE, et al.: Algorithms for adjustment of insulin dosage by patients who monitor blood glucose. Diabetes Care 4:311–318, 1981.

118. Wahren J, Johansson BL: New aspects of C-peptide physiology. The Ernst-Friedrich-Pfeiffer Memorial Lec-ture. Horm Metab Res 30:A2-5(1) Jan, 1998.

119. Loughweed WD, Woulfe-Flanagan H, Clement JR, et al.: Insulin aggregation in artificial delivery systems. Dia-betologia 19:1–9, 1980.

120. Galloway JA, Wentworth SM: A short review of factors that affect the absorption and disposal of insulin. In Peterson CM (ed): Diabetes Management in the 80s. New York: Praeger, 1980, pp. 100–108.

121. Galloway JA, Root MA, Berstrom R, et al: Clinical phar-macologic studies with human insulin (recombinant DNA). Diabetes Care 5 (suppl 2):13–22, 1982.

122. Galloway JA, de Shazo RD: Insulin chemistry, pharma-cology, dosage algorithms, and the complications of insulin treatment. In Rifkin H, Porte D (eds): Diabetes Mellitus: Theory and Practice, Amsterdam: Elsevier 1990, pp. 497–513.

123. Binder C: Insulin pharmacokinetics. Diabetes Care 7:188–199, 1984.

124. Cryer PE: Hypoglycemia: The Limiting Factor in the Management of IDDM. Diabetes 43:1378–1389, 1994.

125. Hypoglycemic Disorders. F. John Service (ed). W.B. Saunders Co., Philadelphia, 1999.

126. Cremer GM, Molnar GD, Taylor WF, et al.: Studies of diabetic instability. Il. Tests of insulinogenic reserve. Metabolism 20:1083–1098, 1971.

127. Molnar GD, Taylor WF, Ho MM: Day-to-day variation of continuously monitored glycemia: a further measure of diabetic instability. Diabetologia 8:342–348, 1972.

128. Molnar GD, Taylor WF, Langworthy A: On measuring the adequacy of diabetes regulation: comparison of con-tinuously monitored blood glucose patterns with values at selected time points. Diabetologia 10: 139–143, 1974.

129. Molnar GD, Marien GJ, Hunter AN, et al.: Methods of assessing diabetic control. Diabetologia 17:5–16, 1979.

130. Galloway JA: Chemistry and Clinical use of insulin. In Galloway JA, Potvin JH, Shuman CR (eds): Diabetes Mellitus. Eli Lilly Co, Indianapolis, 1988, pp. 105–137.

131. Galloway JA, Jackson RL, Bechtel LD: Factors affecting the bioavailability of insulin. Diabetes Care 3:366–376, 1981.

132. Harris MI: Screening for undiagnosed non-insulin-dependent diabetes mellitus. *In* Albert KGMM, Mazze RS (eds): Frontiers of Diabetes Research: Current Trends in Non-Insulin-Dependent Diabetes Mellitus. Amsterdam: Excerpta Medica, International Congress Series 859, 1989, pp. 119–131.

133. Davidson JK, Fineberg SE, De Meyts P, et al.: Immunologic and metabolic responses of patients with a history of antibody-induced-beef-insulin-resistance to treatment with beef, pork, human (rDNA), and sulfated beef insulin. Diabetes Care 15:702–704, 1992.

134. Davidson JK: Transferring patients with insulin-dependent diabetes mellitus from animal-source insulins to recombinant DNA human insulin: clinical experience. Clin Ther 11:319–330, 1989.

135. Sodoyez JC, Sodoyez-Goffaux F, Guillaume M, et al.: (^{123}I) Insulin metabolism in normal rats and humans: external detection by a scintillation camera. Science 219:865–867, 1983.

136. Sodoyez JC, Sodoyez-Goffaux F: Effects of insulin antibodies on bioavailability of insulin: preliminary studies using ^{123}I-insulin in patients with insulin-dependent diabetes. Diabetologia 27:143–145, 1984.

137. Sodoyez JC, Sodoyez-Goffaux F, Von Frenchell R, et al.: Differing effects of antiinsulin serum and antiinsulin receptor serum on ^{123}I-insulin metabolism in rats. J Clin Invest 75:1452–1455, 1985.

138. Ingelfinger FJ: Debates on diabetes. N Engl J Med 296:1228–1230, 1977.

139. Malone JI, Hellrung JM, Malphus EW, et al.: Good diabetic control—a study in mass delusion. J Pediatr 88:943, 1976.

140. Drash A: The control of diabetes mellitus: is it achievable? Is it desirable? J Pediatr 88:1074, 1976.

141. Cochran HA Jr, Marble A, Galloway JA: Factors in the survival of patients with insulin-requiring diabetes for 50 years. Diabetes Care 2:363–368, 1979.

142. Bretcher C, Malmquist J: Insulin-requiring diabetes mellitus of sixty years duration without significant late manifestations. Acta Med Scand 210:239–240, 1981.

143. Deckert T: The influence of supervision and endogenous insulin secretion on the course of insulin-dependent diabetes mellitus. Acta Endocrinol 94(Suppl 238)31–38, 1980.

144. Raskin P, Stevenson MRM, Barilla DE, et al.: The hypercalcuria of diabetes mellitus: its amelioration with insulin. Clin Endocrinol 9:329–335, 1978.

145. Pietri A, Ehle AL, Raskin P: Changes in nerve conduction velocity after six weeks of glucoregulation with portable insulin infusion pumps. Diabetes 29:668–671, 1980.

146. Pietri A, Dunn FL, Raskin P: The effect of improved diabetic control on plasma lipid and lipoprotein levels. Diabetes 29:1001–1005, 1980.

147. Viberti G, Pickup JC, Bilous RW, et al.: Correction of exercise-induced microalbuminuria in insulin-dependent diabetics after 3 weeks of subcutaneous insulin infusion. Diabetes 30:818–823, 1981.

148. Macek C: Diabetics' deaths: insulin pump connection? JAMA 247:1918–1919, 1982.

149. Christiansen JS, Svendsen PA, Mathiesen E, et al.: Comparison of 24-hour insulin requirements in IDDM patients during control by an artificial beta cell and during conventional therapy. Horm Metab Res 13:537–541, 1981.

150. Pietri A, Raskin P: Cutaneous complications of chronic continuous subcutaneous insulin infusion therapy. Diabetes Care 4:624–626, 1981.

151. The Diabetes Control and Complications Trial Research Group: The effect of intensive treatment of diabetes on the development and progression of long-term complications in insulin-dependent diabetes mellitus. N Engl J Med 329:977–986, 1993.

152. DCCT Research Group: Prevention of neuropathy: the effect of intensive diabetes therapy on the development and progression of neuropathy in the DCCT. Ann Intern Med 122:564–568, 1995.

153. DCCT Research Group: Effect of intensive therapy on the development of diabetic nephropathy in the DCCT. Kidney Int 47:1703–1720, 1995.

154. DCCT Research Group: The effect of intensive diabetes management on macrovascular events and risk factors in the DCCT. Am J Cardiol 75:894–903, 1995.

155. Diabetes Control and Complications Trial Research Group: Effect of intensive diabetes management on macrovascular events and risk factors in the Diabetes Control and Complications Trial. Am J Cardiol 75:894–903, 1995.

156. Epidemiology of Diabetes Interventions and Complications (EDIC) Research Group. Design, implementation, and preliminary results of a long-term follow-up of the Diabetes Control and Complications Trial cohort. Diabetes Care. 1999 Jan; 22(1):99–111.

157. Epidemiology of Diabetes Interventions and Complications (EDIC) Research Group. Effect of intensive diabetes treatment of carotid artery wall thickness in the epidemiology of diabetes interventions and complications. Diabetes, 1999 Feb; 48(2):383–90.

158. Stout RW: Insulin and atheroma: 20 year perspective. Diabetes Care 13:631–654, 1990.

159. Kromann H, Borch E, Gale EAM: Unnecessary insulin treatment for diabetes. Br Med J 283:1386–1388, 1981.

160. Galloway JA, Davidson JK: Clinical use of insulin. *In* Rifkin H, Raskin P (eds): Diabetes Mellitus, Vol. 5. pp. 117–127. Bowie, MD: R.J. Brady, 1981.

161. Davidson JK: (Topic 203) Diabetes Mellitus. In Hurst JW (ed): Medicine for the Practicing Physician. Woburn, MA: Butterworth, 1988, pp. 435–448.

162. Borders LA, Bingham PR, Riddle MC: Traditional insulin-use practices and the incidence of bacterial contamination and infection. Diabetes Care 7:121–127, 1984.

163. Products for People with Vision Problems (catalogue). New York: American Foundation for the Blind, Consumer Products Department.

164. Fletcher AA, Campbell WR: The blood sugar following insulin administration and the symptom complex-hypoglycemia. J Metab Res 2:637–649, 1922.

165. Davidson JK: Hypoglycemia. *In* Schwartz GR, Wagner D (eds): Principles and Practice of Emergency Medicine. Philadelphia: W.B. Saunders, 1978, pp. 1075–1078.

166. Davidson JK: Hypoglycemia. *In* Conn RB (ed): Current Diagnosis, Ed. 7. Philadelphia: W.B. Saunders, 1985, pp. 749–752.

167. Kalimo H, Olsson Y: Effects of severe hypoglycemia on the human brain. Acta Neurol Scand 62:345–356, 1980.

168. Alberti KGMM: Diabetic emergencies. *In* Galloway JA, Potvin JH, Shuman CR (eds): Diabetes Mellitus. Indianapolis: Eli Lilly, 1988, pp. 254–257.

169. Cryer PE, Gerich JE: Hypoglycemia in insulin dependent diabetes mellitus: insulin excess and defective glucose counterregulation. *In* Rifkin H, Porte D, (eds): Diabetes Mellitus: Theory and Practice. Amsterdam: Elsevier, 1990, pp. 526–546.

170. Potter J, Clark P, Gale EAM, et al.: Insulin induced hypoglycaemia in an accident and emergency department: the tip of an iceberg. Br Med J 285:1180–1182, 1982.

171. Goldgewicht C, Slama G, Papoz L, Tchobrutsky G: Hypoglycaemic reactions in 172 Type 1 insulin-dependent diabetic patients. Diabetologia 24:95–99, 1983.

172. Eeg-Olofsson O: Hypoglycemia and neurological disturbances in children with diabetes mellitus. Acta Paediatr Scand 270 (Suppl):91–95, 1977.

173. Muhlhauser I, Berger M, Sonnenberg G, et al.: Incidence and management of severe hypoglycemia in 434 adults with insulin-dependent diabetes mellitus. Diabetes Care 8:268–273, 1985.

174. Asplund K, Wilholm BE, Lithner F: Glibenclamide-associated hypoglycemia: a report of 57 cases. Diabetologia 24:412–417, 1983.

175. Barnett AH, Leslie D, Watkins PH: Can insulin-treated diabetics be given beta-adrenergic blocking drugs? Br Med J 280:976–978, 1980.

176. Asplin CM, Hockaday TD, Smith RF, et al.: Detection of unrecognized nocturnal hypoglycemia in insulin treated diabetes. Br Med J 280:357–360, 1980.

177. Clark BC, Ward JD, Enoch BA: Hypoglycemia in insulin-dependent diabetic drivers. Br Med J 281:586, 1980.

178. Lock DR, Rigg IA: Hypoglycemic coma associated with subcutaneous insulin infusion by portable pump. Diabetes Care 4:389–391, 1981.

179. Rynearson EH: Hyperinsulinism among malingerers. Med Clin N Am 31:477–480, 1947.

180. Mayefsky JH, Sarnaik AP, Postellon DC: Factitious hypoglycemia. Pediatrics 69:804–805, 1982.

181. Grunberger G, Weiner JL, Silverman R, et al.: Factitious hypoglycemia due to surreptitious administration of insulin. Diagnosis, treatment, and long-term follow-up. Ann Intern Med 108:252–257, 1988.

182. Somogyi M: Hyperglycemic response to hypoglycemia in diabetic and in healthy individuals. Proc Soc Exp Biol Med 38:51–55, 1938.

183. Somogyi M: Exacerbation of diabetes by excess insulin action. Am J Med 26:169–191, 1959.

184. Shima K, Tanaka R, Morishita S, et al.: Studies on the etiology of "brittle diabetes." Diabetes 26:717–725, 1977.

185. Rizza R, Cryer P, Gerich J: Role of glucagon, catecholamines and growth hormone in human glucose counterregulation: effect of somatostatin and combined A and B adrenergic blockage on plasma glucose recovery and glucose flux rates after insulin-induced hypoglycemia. J Clin Invest 64:62–71, 1979.

186. Shamoon H, Hendler R, Sherwin RS: Altered responsiveness to cortisol, epinephrine, and glucagon in insulin-infused juvenile-onset diabetics. Diabetes 29:289–291, 1980.

187. Bright GM, Melton TW, Rogol AD, et al.: Failure of cortisol blockage to inhibit early morning increases in basal insulin requirements in fasting insulin-dependent diabetics. Diabetes 29:662–664, 1980.

188. White NH, Skor DA, Cryer PE, et al.: Identification of Type I diabetic patients at increased risk for hypoglycemia during intensive therapy. N Engl J Med 308:485–491, 1983.

189. Bolli GB, Dimitriadis GD, Pehling GB, et al.: Abnormal glucose counterregulation after subcutaneous insulin in insulin-dependent diabetes mellitus. N Engl J Med 310:1706–1711, 1984.

190. Bolli GB, Gottesman IS, Campbell PJ, et al.: Glucose counterregulation and waning of insulin in the Somogyi phenomenon (posthypoglycemia hyperglycemia). N Engl J Med 311:1214–1218, 1984.

191. Bolli GB, Gerich JE: The "dawn phenomenon"—a common occurrence in both non-insulin-dependent and insulin—dependent diabetes mellitus. N Engl J Med 310:746–750, 1984.

192. Miles DW, Hayter CT: The effect of intravenous insulin on the circulatory responses to tilting in normal and diabetic subjects with special references to baroreceptor block and atypical hypoglycemic reactions. Clin Sci Mol Med 34:419–430, 1968.

193. Page MM, Watkins PJ: Provocation of postural hypotension by insulin in diabetic autonomic neuropathy. Diabetes 25:90–95, 1976.

194. Gundersen HJG, Christensen NJ: Intravenous insulin causing loss of intravascular water and albumin and increased adrenergic nervous activity in diabetics. Diabetes 26:551–557, 1977.

195. Mackay JD, Hayakawa H, Watkins PJ: Cardiovascular effects of insulin: plasma volume changes in diabetics. Diabetologia 15:453–457, 1978.

196. Lowell FC: Evidence for the existence of two antibodies for crystalline insulin. Proc Soc Exp Biol Med 50:167–172, 1942.

197. Davidson JK, Eddelman EE: Insulin resistance: review of the literature and report of a case associated with carcinoma of the pancreas. Arch Intern Med 86:727–742, 1950.

198. Patterson R, Grammer LC, Chen PY: Insulin hypersensitivity: pathogenesis, diagnosis and management. *In* Gupta S (ed): Immunology of Clinical and Experimental Diabetes. New York: Plenum, 1984, pp. 401–414.

199. Falholt K: Determination of insulin-specific IgE in serum of diabetic patients by solid-phase radioimmunology. Diabetologia 22:254–257, 1982.

200. Falholt K, Hoskian JAM, Karamanos BG, et al.: Insulin specific IgE in serum of 67 diabetic patients against human insulin (NOVO), porcine insulin, and bovine insulin. Four case reports. Diabetes Care 6:61–65, 1983.

201. Feinglos MN, Jegaam RW, Russell RO, et al.: Insulin resistance: clinical features, natural course, and effects of adrenal steroid treatment. Medicine (Baltimore) 44:165–186, 1965.

202. Davidson JK: Insulin allergy and immunologic insulin resistance. Comp Ther 8:46–52, 1982.

203. Reisner C, Moul DJ, Cudworth AG: Generalized urticaria precipitated by change to highly purified porcine insulin. Br Med J 56, 1978.

204. Simmonds JP, Russel GI, Coweley, et al.: Generalized allergy to porcine and bovine monocomponent insulins. Br Med J 355–356, 1980.

205. Galloway JA, Fineberg SE, Fineberg NS, et al.: Effect of purity and beef content on complications of insulin therapy in Hormone Drugs (Proceedings of the Food and Drug Administration—United States Pharmacopeia Workshop on Drug and Reference Standards for Insulins, Somatotropins, and Thyroid-axis Hormones). Rockville, MD: United States Pharmacopeial Convention, 1983, p. 244.

206. Carveth-Johnson AO, Mylvaganam K, Child DF: Generalized allergic reaction with synthetic human insulin. Lancet 2:1287, 1982.

207. Galloway JA, Fireman P, Fineberg SE: Complications of insulin therapy—a brief overview of four years of experience with human insulin (rDNA). Diabetes Symposium, Athens, March 1984.

208. Galloway JA, Peck FB, Jr, Fineberg SE, et al.: The U.S. "new patient" and "transfer" studies. Diabetes Care 5 (Suppl 2):135–139, 1982.

209. Fineberg SE, Galloway JA, Fineberg NS, et al.: Immunologic improvement resulting from the transfer of animal insulin-treated diabetic subjects to human insulin (recombinant DNA). Diabetes Care 5 (Suppl 2):107–113, 1982.

210. Berger M, Jorgens V, Mülhauser I: Rational for the use of insulin therapy alone as the pharmacological treatment of type 2 diabetes. Diabetes Care 22(Suppl 3):671–675, 1999.

211. deShazo RD, Boehm TM, Kumar D, et al.: Dermal hypersensitivity reactions to insulin: correlations of three patterns to their histopathology. J Allergy Clin Immunol 69:229–237, 1982.

212. Kumar D, Miller LV, Mehtalia SD: Use of dexamethasone in treatment of insulin lipoatrophy. Diabetes 26:296–299,1977.

213. Glassberg BY, Somogyi M, Taussig AE: Diabetes mellitus: report of a case refractory to insulin. Arch Intern Med 40:676–685, 1927.

214. Root HF: Insulin resistance and bronze diabetes. N Engl J Med 201:201–206, 1929.

215. Glen A, Eaton JC: Insulin antagonism. Q J Med 7: 272–291, 1938.

216. Moloney PJ, Aprile MA, Wilson S: Sulfated insulin for treatment of insulin resistant diabetes. J New Drugs 4:258–263, 1964.

217. Shipp JC, Cunningham RW, Russel RO, et al.: Insulin resistance: clinical features, natural course, and effects of adrenal steroid treatment. Medicine (Baltimore) 44:165–186, 1965.

218. Davidson JK, DeBra DW: Immunologic insulin resistance. Diabetes 27:307–318, 1978.

219. Naquet P, Ellis J, Kenshole A, et al.: Delovitch TL: Sulfated beef insulin treatment elicits CD8$^+$ T cells that may abrogate immunologic insulin resistance in Type I diabetes. J Clin Invest 84:1479–1487, 1989.

220. Carpentier A, Wither J, Vukusic B, Lawday K, Boss AH, Lewis GF: An epitaph for sulfated insulin. Diabetes Care 21:1571–1572, 1998.

221. Lahtela JT, Knip M, Paul R, Antonen J, and Salmi J: Severe antibody mediated human insulin resistance. Successful treatment with the insulin analog lispro: A case report. Diabetes Care 20:71–73, 1997.

222. Henrichs FIR, Unger H, Trautmann ME, Pfutzner A: Severe insulin resistance treated with insulin lispro. Lancet 348:1248, 1996.

223. Depisch F: Uber lokale-lipodystrophie bie lange zeit mit insulin behandelten fällen von diabetes. Klin Wochenschr 5:1965–1966, 1926.

224. Barborka CJ: Fatty atrophy from injections of insulin. JAMA 87:1646–1647, 1926.

225. Renold AE, Winegrad AI, Martin DB: Diabète sucré et tissu adipeux. Helv Med Acta 24:322–327, 1957.

226. Wentworth SM, Galloway JA, Haunz EA; et al.: The use of purified insulins in the treatment of patients with insulin lipoatrophy. Diabetes 22 (suppl 1):290, 1973.

227. Watson BM, Calder JS: A treatment for insulin-induced fat atrophy. Diabetes 20:628–632, 1971.

228. Renold AE, Marble A, Fawcett DW: Action of insulin on deposition of glycogen and storage of fat in adipose tissue. Endocrinology 46:55–56, 1950.

229. Galloway JA: Insulin treatment for the early 80s: facts and questions about old and new insulins and their usage. Diabetes Care 3:615–622, 1980.

230. Saudek CD, Boulter PR, Knopp RH, et al.: Sodium retention accompanying insulin treatment of diabetes mellitus. Diabetes 23:240–246, 1974.

231. Bleach NR, Dunn PJ, Khalafalla ME, et al.: Insulin oedema. Br Med J 177–178, 1979.

232. Galloway JA, Anderson JH, Spradlin CT: Clinical experiences with human proinsulin. *In* Larkins RG, Zimmet PZ, Chisholm DJ (eds): Diabetes 1988. Proceedings of the 13th Congress of the International Diabetes Federation, Sydney, November 20–25, 1988. Amsterdam: Excerpta Medica, 1989, pp. 85–88.

233. Galloway JA: Treatment of NIDDM with insulin agonists or substitutes. Diabetes Care 13:1209–1239, 1990.

234. Galloway JA, Chance RE: Insulin agonist therapy: the challenge for the 1990's. Clin Ther 12:460–472, 1990.

235. Frank BH, Pettee JM, Zimmerman RE, Burck PJ: The production of human proinsulin and its transformation to human insulin and C-peptide. *In* Peptides: Synthesis-Structure-Function. Proceedings of the Seventh American Peptide Symposium. Rockford: Pierce Chemical Company, 1981, pp. 729–738.

236. Stout RW: Diabetes and atherosclerosis—the role of insulin, Diabetologia 16:141–150, 1979.

237. Pyorala K, Laakso M, Uusitupa M: Diabetes and atherosclerosis: an epidemiologic view. Diabetes Metab Rev 3:463–524, 1987.

238. Brange J, Owens DR, Kang S, Volund A: Monomeric insulins and their experimental and clinical implications, Diabetes Care 13:923–954, 1990.

239. Galloway JA, Chance RE, Su KSE: Human insulin and its modifications. Proceedings of the Esteve Foundation Symposium, Mallorca, Spain, October 7–11, 1990.

240. Bruce DG, Chisholm DJ, Storlien LH, Kraegen EW: Physiological importance of deficiency in early prandial insulin secretion in non-insulin-dependent diabetes, Diabetes 37:736–744, 1988.

241. Stolar MW: Atherosclerosis in diabetes: the role of hyperinsulinemia. Metabolism 37(Suppl 1):1–9, 1988.

242. Jorgensen S, Vaag A, Langkjaer L, Hougaard P, Markussen J: NovoSol Basal: Pharmacokinetics of a novel soluble long acting soluble insulin analogue. Br. Med J 299:415–419, 1989.

243. Prescriber's Letter (March 15, 1999) of the Therapeutic Research Center: Mixing Humalog (Insulin Lispro) with Long-acting Insulins (NPH, Lente, Ultralente).

244. Mohn A, Matyka KA, Harris DA, Ross KM, Edge JA, Dunger DB: Lispro or regular insulin for multiple injection therapy in adolescence-differences in free insulin and glucose levels overnight. Diabetes Care 22:27–32, 1999.

245. ter Braak EW, Woodworth JR, Bianchi R, et al., Injection site effects on the pharmacokinetics and glucodynamics of insulin lispro and regular insulin. Diabetes Care 1996, 19:1437–40.

246. Howey DC, Bowsher RR, Brunelle RL, Woodworth JR: [Lys(B28), Pro(B29)] B human insulin: a rapidly absorbed analog of human insulin. Diabetes 43:396–402, 1994.

247. Wilde MI, McTavish D: Insulin lispro: a review of its pharmacological properties and therapeutic use in the management of diabetes mellitus. Drugs 54:597–614, 1997.

248. Campbell RK, Campbell LK, White JR: Insulin lispro: its role in the treatment of diabetes mellitus. Ann Pharmacother 30:1263–1271, 1996.

249. Howey DC, Bowsher RR, Brunelle RL, Rowe HM, Santa PF, Downing-Shelton J, Woodworth JR: [Lys(B28), Pro(B29)] - human insulin: effect of injection time on postprandial glycemia. Clin Pharmacol Ther 58:459–469, 1995.

250. Vignati L, Anderson JH Jr, Iversen PW: Efficacy of insulin lispro in combination with NPH human insulin twice per day in patients with insulin-dependent, or non-insulin-dependent diabetes mellitus: Multicenter Insulin Lispro Study Group. Clin Ther 19:1408–1421, 1997.

251. Anderson JH Jr, Brunelle RL, Keohane P, Koivisto VA, Trautmann ME, Vignati L, DiMarchi R: Mealtime treatment with insulin analog improves postprandial hyperglycemia and hypoglycemia in patients with non-insulin-dependent diabetes mellitus: Multicenter Insulin Lispro Study Group. Arch Intern Med 157:1249–1255, 1997.

252. Burge MR, Castillo KR, Schade DS: Meal composition is a determinant of lispro induced hypoglycemia in IDDM. Diabetes Care 20:152–155, 1997.

253. Heinemann L, Heise T, Wahl LC, Trautmann ME, Ampudia J, Starke AA, Berger M: Prandial glycemia after a carbohydraterich meal in type 1 diabetic patients: using the rapid acting insulin analogue [Lys(B28), Pro(B29)] human insulin. Diabet Med 13:625–629, 1996

254. Anderson JH, Brunelle RL, Koivisto VA, Pfützner A, Trautman ME, Vignati L, DiMarchi R, the Multicentre Insulin Lispro Study Group: Reduction of postprandial hyperglycemia in type 1 diabetic patients on insulin-analog treatment. Diabetes 46:265–270, 1997.

255. Ebeling P, Jansson PA, Smith U, Lalli C, Bolli GB, Kohisto V: Strategies toward improved control during insulin lispro therapy in IDDM, importance of basal insulin. Diabetes Care 20:1287–1289, 1997.

256. Tubiana-Rufi N, Munz-Licha G: Lispro analog and quality of life. Diabetes Metab 3 (Suppl. 1):58–62, 1997.

257. Anderson JH Jr, Brunelle RL, Koivisto VA, Trautmann ME, Vignati L, DiMarchi R: Improved mealtime treatment of diabetes mellitus using an insulin analogue: Multicenter Insulin Lispro Study Group. Clin Ther 19:62–72, 1997.

258. Zinman B, Ross S, Campus RV, Stack T, The Canadian Lispro Study Group: Effectiveness of human ultralente versus NPH insulin in providing basal insulin replacement for an insulin lispro multiple daily injection regimen: a double-blind randomized prospective trial. Diabetes Care 22:603–608, 1999.

259. Bell DSH, Clements RS, Perentesis G: Hypoglycemia in children with insulin-dependent diabetes mellitus. J Pediatr 340–341, 1990.

260. Tan MH, Jervell J, of the IDF Task Force on Insulin. Results of global IDF survey: access to insulin. IDF Bulletin 43, Dec. 1998, pp. 12–16.

261. Functional Insulin Treatment: Principles, Teaching Approach, and Practice. K Howrka (ed), Second Edition, 1996. Springer Verlag, Berlin, ISBN 3-540-60352-2.

262. Glucagon: I, II, III. P Lefèbvre (ed), 1998. Springer Verlag, Berlin. ISBN 3-540-60989-X.

263. Contributions of physiology to the understanding of diabetes: ten essays in memory of Albert E. Renold, Grzahnd and Wollheim (eds.), 1997. Springer Verlag, Berlin. ISBN 3-540-61385-4.

264. Woodworth J, Howey D, Lutz S, Santa P, Brady P, Bowsher R, [Lys(B28), Pro(B29)] human insulin (K): Dose-

ranging versus Humulin R (H). Diabetologia 1993, 36 (Suppl. 1)A155.

265. Zinman B, Tildesley H, Chiasson J.-L, Tsui E, Strack T: Insulin lispro in CSII: Results of a double-blind crossover study. Diabetes 1997, 46:440–3.

266. Ebeling P, Jansson P.-A, Smith U, Lalli C, Bolli G. B, Koivisto V. A: Strategies toward improved control during insulin lispro therapy in IDDM. Importance of basal insulin. Diabetes Care 1997, 20:1287–9.

267. Brunelle RL, Llewelyn J, Anderson JH, Gale EAM, Koivisto VA. Meta-Analysis of the Effect of Insulin Lispro on Severe Hypoglycemia in Patients with Type I Diabetes. Diabetes Care 1998; 21:1726–1731.

268. Torlone, E, Fanelli C, Rambotti AM, et al. Pharmacokinetics, pharmacodynamics and glucose counterregulation following subcutaneous injection of the monomeric insulin analogue [Lys(B28), Pro(B29)] in IDDM. Diabetologia 1994, 37:713–20.

269. Heinermann L, Kapitza C, Strake AAR, Heise T (1996) Time-action profile of the insulin analogue B28 Asp. Diabet Med 13:683–684.

270. Home PD, Lindholm A, Hylleberg B. Round P, for the UK Insulin Aspart Study Group (1998) Improved glycaemic control with Insulin Aspart—a multicentre randomized, double-blind cross-over trial in type 1 diabetic patients. Diabetes Care 21:1904–1909.

271. Fineberg NS, Fineberg SE, Anderson JH, Birkett MA, Gibson RG, Hufferd S. Immumologic effects of insulin lispro [Lys(B28), Pro(B29)-human insulin] in IDDM and NIDDM patients previously treated with insulin. Diabetes 1996, 45:1750–4.

272. Fineberg SE, Fineberg NS, Anderson JH, Birkett M. Insulin immune response to lispro human insulin therapy in insulin naive type 1 and type 2 patients. Diabetologia 1995, 38 (Suppl. 1): A4.

273. Huang J, Brunelle R, Fineberg E, and Anderson JH. Long Term Monitoring of Insulin Antibody Responses in Patients Treated with Insulin Lispro (Humalog) Diabetes 1999; 48 (Suppl. 1): A94.

274. Lahtela JT, Knip M, Paul R, Antonen J, and Salmi J. Severe antibody mediated human insulin resistance. Successful treatment with the insulin analog lispro: A case report. Diabetes Care 1997, 20:71–3.

275. Henrichs HR, Unger H, Trautmann ME, Pfutzner A. Severe insulin resistance treated with insulin lispro. Lancet 1996, 348:1248.

276. Holcombe J, Zalani S, Arora V. Comparative study of insulin lispro and regular insulin in 481 adolescents with type 1 diabetes. Diabetologia 1997, 40(Suppl. 1):A344.

277. Holcombe J, Zalani S, Arora V, at al. Patient preference for insulin lispro versus Humulin® in adolescents with type 1 diabetes. Diabetologia 1997, 40(Suppl. 1):A343.

278. Halcombe J, Zalani S, Arora V, et al. Insulin lispro (LP) results in less nocturnal hypoglycemia compared with regular human insudn in adolescents with type 1 diabetes. Diabetes 1997, 46 (Suppl. 1):103A.

279. Rutledge KS, Chase HP, Klingensmith GJ, Walravens PA, Slover RH, Garg SK. Effectiveness of postprandial Humalog in toddlers with diabetes. Pediatrics 1997, 100:958–72.

280. Heinemann L, Sinha K, Weyer C, et al. (1999) Time-action profile of the soluble, fatty acid acylated long-acting insulin analogue NN304. Diabet Med 16:332–338.

281. Radziuk J, Pye S, Bradley B et al. (1998) Basal activity profiles of NPH and [N$^{\epsilon}$–palmitoyl Lys (B29)] human insulins in subjects with IDDM. Diabetologia 41: 116–120.

282. Howey DC, Bowsher RR, Brunelle RL, Woodworth JR: [Lys(B28), Pro(B29)]-human insulin: A Rapidly absorbed analogue of human insulin. Diabetes 43(3):396–402, 1994.

283. Heinemann L, Heise T, Wahl LC, Trautmann ME, Ampudia J, Starke AAR, Berger M: Prandial glycaemia after a carbohydrate-rich meal in type I diabetic patients: Using the rapid acting insulin analogue [Lys(B28), Pro(B29)]-human insulin. Diabet Med 13(7):625–629, 1996.

284. Anderson JH and Koivisto VA: Clinical studies on insulin lispro. Drugs Today; 34(Suppl. C): 37–50,1998.

285. Home PD, Barriocanal L, Lindholm A: Comparative pharmacokinetics and pharmacodynamics of the novel rapid-acting insulin analogue, insulin aspart, in healthy volunteers. Eur J Clin Pharmacol 55(3):199–203, 1999.

286. Rosskamp RH, Park G. Long-acting insulin analogs. Diabetes Care 22(Suppl 2):B109–13, 1999.

287. Hamilton-Wessler M, Ader M, Dea M, Moore D, Jorgensen PN, Markussen J, Bergman RN: Mechanism of protracted metabolic effects of fatty acid acylated insulin, NN304, in dogs: retention of NN304 by albumin. Diabetologia 42(10):1254–63, 1999.

288. Schernthaner G, Wein W, Sandholzer K, Equiluz-Bruck S, Bates PC, Birkett MA. Postprandial insulin lispro. A new therapeutic option for type 1 diabetic patients. Diabetes Care 21(4):570–3, 1998.

289. Koivisto VA: The human insulin analogue insulin lispro. Ann Med 30(3):260–6, 1998.

290. Anderson J, Garg S, MacKenzie T, Shephard M, Peery B, Chase H. The Impact of DCCT and Humalog® treatment on glycohaemoglobin and hypoglycaemia in type 1 diabetes. Diabetologia 42(Suppl. 1): A210, 1999.

291. American Diabetes Association Forecast Buyers Guide, 1999.

19

Computer-Assisted Diabetes Care

A.M. Albisser, S. Sakkal, R.I. Harris, S.C. En Chao,
and I.D. Parson

Historical Perspective

Is an insulin pump really necessary? A study comparing diabetes control in patients receiving either insulin infusions from the open-loop pump or simply just multiple daily injections found an essential equivalence of the two methods of treatment.[1] Obviously, continuously pumped insulin has the same limitations as frequently but intermittently injected insulin: both develop a depot.[2] Pumps therefore add much to the complexity of management but little to enhancing the delivery of insulin subcutaneously.

In spite of its complications, the pump, however, promises absolute freedom to the diabetic in regard to meal size and timing because administration of the interprandial basal infusion is independent of the meal bolus. To a select population of patients, this may be of major importance, and thus the open-loop pump for them may be the treatment modality of choice. However, its benefits are rapidly lost if the regularity and intensity of self-blood glucose measurement are relaxed from the minimum four to seven times/day.

In practice, the effect of the meal bolus is also not entirely independent of the basal rate, so that identical results in terms of near normalization of metabolic control are also achieved by *intensified* conventional therapy.[1] This process utilizes the same high frequency of self-measurement and provides detailed, individualized scales for insulin dosage selection.

Today, for those patients prepared to make the required ongoing commitment to self-care, to measure their capillary blood glucose, to carry a pump, or to perform multiple daily injections and bear the added costs, such intensified therapy has much to offer.[3] Interestingly, teaching each patient is no minor commitment, requiring in the first instance some 30 hours of instruction coupled with weekly follow-up with the patient in person by health professionals: either the nurse practitioner, diabetes educator, or the diabetologist. This system is obviously demanding and questions of its practicality arise from the patient as well as the health provider points of view.

There is clearly a need right now for a more practical diabetes care system that can bring convenience rather than complexity to insulin delivery for those many patients who must nonetheless take the hormone on a daily basis. Recently, two approaches have been suggested that are more practical than the open- and closed-loop systems. These approaches place major emphasis on the functional characteristics of the real clinical situation with the intent of optimizing performance with due reference to the many limitations inherent in a truly practical system. Interestingly, one common approach involves educating the patient. The other harnesses modern technology, information theory, artificial intelligence, and microcomputer devices.[4] Both complement existing clinical methods by providing *expert* intervention for the patient not just once a month, but at each injection in regard to insulin dosage adjustment. In effect, the latter is a new yet practical closed-loop system that seeks to control diabetes within acceptable limits by exploiting conventional methods with once, twice, or (when necessary) multiple daily insulin injection therapy. It turns out to be more easily implemented than educating the patient about diabetes. In many respects it is just like power steering on an automobile. Although strictly unnecessary, it does make the vehicle easier to drive. However, it does appear to need the support of a designated center of expertise.

Problem Statement

Modern medicine's thrust is to provide the best possible care. In diabetes this has been formalized in the St. Vincent Declaration.[5] Furthermore, newly derived knowledge[6] now suggests substantial increases in effort for diabetes care, possibly beyond what was previously accepted as "conventional care." As a consequence, expanding patient care services to achieve these ends may be inescapable. However, rising costs are projected.[7] Computers will most likely play a role in this approach.

Accordingly, we describe a new computer system for outpatient care in diabetes mellitus. The system is designed to include the patient as an on-line participant in the care process and assists the health professional in providing intervention at a distance. This work extends previous effort with a bed-side, computer-assisted, closed-loop control system[8,9] and experience with a hand-held device for daily self-management.[10–12] We also outline the characteristics of the system and summarize initial experiences from a β-testing phase. These document safety and efficacy. Formal, randomized, and controlled studies are beginning.

Computer-Assisted Diabetes Care

The drawing in Figure 19–1 illustrates the various components of the computer-assisted care system. Patients electronically access the computer remotely via any convenient touch-tone telephone. At the computer site, the diabetes nurse educator (or case manager) has direct control over the system through its keyboard and monitor. Reports are dispatched to the clinic and physician(s). Medical interventions can be routed to the patient conveniently via the nurse or case manager and thence through the voice messaging features of the computer system to the patient. Although this appears circuitous, it carries the technical advantage of being asynchronous: The patient and the doctor need not be on the phone at the same time, yet the message is transmitted and received at each party's convenience.

Computational Platform

The personal computer is the platform on which the design of the system is based. Two user interfaces are provided: one for the nurse or case manager and one for the patient. The former allows data storage while the latter interface accepts diabetes self-management information from patients.

Health Professional Interface. The health professional user interface permits an on-screen review of

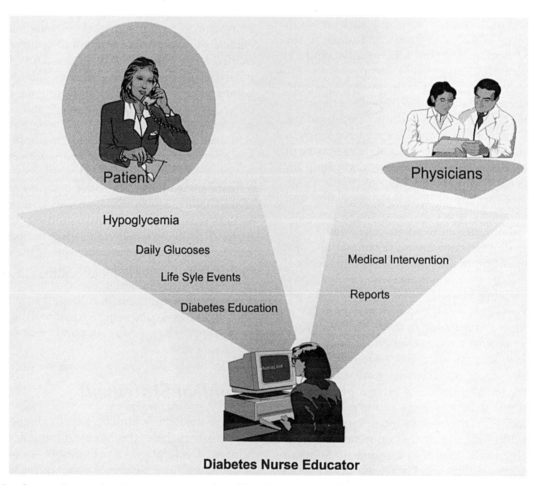

Figure 19–1. System diagram showing remote patient (possibly at home or elsewhere) using a telephone to access the on-line computer system for daily diabetes care. Diabetes nurse (or case manager) provides education and physician-directed interventions in response to reported blood glucose readings, hypoglycemia, lifestyle events (diet, exercise, stress, ketonemia, illness, etc.) entered daily or, preferably, at each measurement. The computer system can help the patient manage his or her blood glucose levels automatically.

patient-entered daily blood glucose measurements, lifestyle events (such as changes in diet, exercise, stress, etc.), and other indices (such as intercurrent illness, fever, loss of appetite, vomiting, ketonuria, etc.). Besides receiving the information from the patient, the system serves as a database not just for storing the results but also for processing the information in order to coordinate and format the patient-entered data. This database is used by the system for subsequent daily, weekly, or monthly report generation in the doctor's office. All reports are standardized in format but customized to accommodate each center's specific details, such as physician names, addresses, and telephone numbers. Furthermore, the diabetes nurse educator can activate a virtual recorder and, using a microphone, leave voice messages for the patient regarding specific instructions. All interactions by the health professional are documented in electronic, medical chart, and "on-line" notes with facilities to enter time spent and briefly describe actual effort or medical management activities as may be required. These become part of the legal medical record as well as the basis for evaluation and management claims against the patient's health insurance.

A facility is included to forward courtesy reports automatically by fax to referring physicians. Daily, weekly, or monthly summary reports of each patient's data are generated as ordered by the physician. When prescheduled, these are printed overnight, typically at 3:00 AM. Otherwise they can be printed immediately.

Patient Interface. The patient user interface is separate hardware, realized through a voice-interactive hardware link to an analog telephone line. Patients may use any available touch-tone telephone as a data-entry terminal through which each glucose measurement, crisis event, lifestyle factor, and self-administered medication is entered (directly by the patient) in response to supportive prompts and verbal instructions given by the system. The system talks to relay instructions and messages over the telephone when the patient calls. However, it only deciphers key-press tones interpreted as digits (0–9) and symbols (* and #) on the telephone keypad. With experience, the transaction time for a patient to report a single blood glucose measurement and associated lifestyle event is less than 30 sec.

Data Storage

Every number entered by the patient using a touch-tone telephone is verified before being accepted. Only the physician (or the authorized diabetes nurse educator or case manager) can make changes in medication and direct instructions and messages to patients. The physician can request confirmation that the information has been delivered. Patient access to the system is via a personal identification number (PIN).

The system accumulates the number of telephone calls made, the number of blood glucose readings entered, the number of crises (which includes the number of hyperglycemic and hypoglycemic events), and the number of days used over the month. Every month the system summarizes use by each patient.

Automatic Control Algorithms

The patient interface includes algorithms. These computer routines, if enabled by the physician, must be programmed for each particular patient. Thereafter, using the physician's specified medications, dosages, trigger points, target levels, rates, limits, guidelines, and verbal instructions, it acts on behalf of the physician immediately when a blood glucose is entered or a crisis is reported. In all cases, the physician uses his or her own algorithms for each patient. As a consequence, treatment outcome directly reflects the physician's goals or targets for the particular patient and indirectly reflects the patient and physician's combined skills in managing diabetes. Assistance for the patient in self-managing his or her blood glucose levels is also provided, as presented previously.[13,14] When the automatic control features are disabled, the system supports patient-directed control. With patient-directed control, the health professional only receives data from the patient, who may utilize manual methods[15] for blood glucose control. In the automatic mode, predetermined adjustments for hypoglycemia are provided.

Safety Considerations

Safety issues are fundamental and of concern during β-testing. The Food and Drug Administration, Center for Devices and Radiological Health, determined that this technology is a medical device.[16] It conforms to the definitions under Section 201(h) of the Federal Food, Drug and Cosmetic Act.[17]

Professional User Instruction and Training

Teaching and supporting the health professional was necessary. Teaching focused on how to exploit daily machine-mediated information exchanges to facilitate medication review and how to provide remote interventions for many patients. None of the health professionals offered the opportunity to test this new technology for diabetes care were prepared for it. Much about the process, however, is intuitive and supported by the system design.

β-Test Methods

System evaluation was done in the two centers. Patients were included under broad criteria and participated in the use of the system following a simple registration procedure and brief user instructions. Using the system is similar to many telephone banking or credit card systems.

β-Study Centers

Two clinic sites agreed to collaborate in a β-testing phase of this new system: a diabetes clinic in a managed care organization in a medium sized urban area and a private practice office in a rural area. Each site included about 100 patients. Utilization statistics were assessed after the first 12 months while the metabolic outcomes were compared after 9 months of specific use in each patient. Parenthetically, use continues and patient registration expands in each center.[18,19]

The β-study was designed as an open and ongoing (prospective) case study. Patients who were registered but did not (of their own accord) access the system were also followed, as a "reference" group.

Inclusion Criteria

Entrance criteria were unrestricted with respect to gender, age, socioeconomic class, type of diabetes, method of treatment, type(s) of medication, method of glucose self-measurement, and so on. No additional laboratory tests were done for the purposes of the β-studies beyond those usually ordered. The physicians recommended mainly difficult-to-manage diabetic patients to participate solely on a judgment of the patient's need for increased intervention specifically (1) to improve blood glucose control, (2) to lower glycated hemoglobin, (3) to stabilize diabetes, (4) to reduce frequent hypoglycemia and/or hyperglycemia, or (5) to make medication adjustments safely. In this way a cross-section of patients representative of such clinical practice sites was included. The mix of patients included both types 1 and 2 diabetic patients.

Crisis Ranges

Hyperglycemia in the crisis range was defined as any blood glucose entry greater than 400mg/dL or moderate to strong ketones. Hypoglycemia in the crisis range was defined as either symptoms of hypoglycemia (without measurement) or any reported blood glucose less than 50mg/dL.

Registration and Patient Instruction

Patients directed by their physicians to use the system were registered into the computer database. Registration and instruction involved about 10 min and was usually done by nurses or case managers. If the automatic control subsystem was to be activated, additional parameters, as mentioned earlier, must be defined by the physician for the patient. Advanced user features allow the patient to provide information about lifestyle and other events or planned actions. Specifically, they can annotate symptomatic hypoglycemia as being mild, typical, or strong and coarsely classify changes in carbohydrates, activity/exercise, stress, fever, monthly cycles, steroid medication, appetite, nausea, and urinary ketones. Patients can also declare supplemental medication doses taken at any time. Each category has associated with it a three-level grading scale: less, typical, or more. All of these lifestyle factors are coded by adding a suffix to the glucose reading when it is entered or when confirming a medication dosage.

Most patients experienced minimal difficulties using the system. Patients usually began phoning results the same day. A few (generally the older patients) required some additional time, typically in the form of direct telephone support on one or more occasions, before they "got the skill" of doing the task. In all cases, the system allowed the patient to make his or her own decisions regarding medication dosages but captured and documented everything for the health professional to monitor and review.

Training and Follow-up

Initial training and subsequent ongoing support in the interests of follow-up for the professional users in each center was done. In each center, the daily use of the system (through the professional user interface) was carried out by a specially trained diabetes nurse educator or case manager who registered the patients and then provided most of the actions and responses (interventions) to support the registered patients using the system. The physicians generally reviewed the patients' data from the printed reports on a weekly basis and noted treatment plans, which the nurse or case manager would implement. Most patients received at least a voice message each week or so along with whatever physician-directed interventions in their diabetes treatment plan were deemed necessary. Medication interventions were infrequent, ranging from small increments in insulin or tablet dosages to revisions of treatment plans and changes in type or timing of medications. These occurred until desired targets were reached.

Weekly reports were generated for each active user. Monthly reports were generated for all registered users whether or not they used the system. An example and lower excerpt of the weekly report provided to the patient's own doctor is presented in Figure 19–2. All data entered by the patient are assembled into a notebook format with columns for pre-breakfast, pre-lunch, pre-dinner, and pre-bedtime readings. The time of the glucose entry is included automatically and inserted in brackets next to the blood glucose value. Between-meal values, when entered by the patient, appear above the pre-meal values shown in the figure. As illustrated, the pre-meal averages realized over the week and the ranges in the blood glucose levels reported are computed. The parameters of the particular physician's programming are also shown (as the physician set tar-

Health Professional: Dr. Sakkal MR# 1234567

Patient: Ms. Grace Hyden phone: 555-1212

	DATA: Glucose (time)	MEDICATION: Prescribed / Taken		
Day	pre-Breakfast	pre-Lunch	pre-Dinner	pre-Bedtime
Mon Aug-5 -	**217 (08:29)** R 2 / 2 NPH 29 / 29	**123 (11:48)**	**285 (17:45)** R 4 / 4 NPH 11 / 11	**142 (22:19)** **Doctor reviewed data: glucose averages, medication timing and approved alterations. SS**

(A)

Mon Aug-12 - -	**127 (07:55)** R 0 / 0 NPH 31 / 31	**112 (12:12)**	**104 (18:03)** R 3 / 3 NPH 12 / 12	**132 (22:45)**
min-max	**127 - 217**	**123 - 246**	**104 - 285**	**142 - 216**
Averages (7)	**166**	**191**	**168**	**167**
Physician Set	**140**	**140**	**140**	**140**
Slope +/-	**1 / 1**	**1 / 1**	**1 / 1**	**1 / 1**
Dosecure	**R 1 / 1 < 4 >** V ^	- V ^	**R 3 / 3 < 10>** V ^	- V ^
Total = 44 / 44	**NPH 31 / 31** V ^	- V ^	**NPH 12 / 12** V ^	- V ^
Crib	**pre-Breakfast**	**pre-Lunch**	**pre-Dinner**	**pre-Bedtime Snack**

Medications last revised *on* *Mon Aug 5, 1996* *by* *Dr. Sakkal*

Print Graph | Print Logbook

Chart Note | Recorder | Crib Note | E&M

(B)

Figure 19–2. Example of weekly report generated by computer system. (a) Header section showing physician's name, with patient's name, telephone number, and medical record number above columns for the day; pre-meal glucose readings; and medication doses prescribed by the doctor and confirmed by patient. (b) Footer section showing computed values (pre-meal glucose averages and ranges over previous week or month, physician-set blood glucose targets, and mode of prescribing medications. Buttons with arrows (↑↓) allow health professional to immediately modify any dosage during on-screen review of displayed patient's data. From Ref. 20 with permission.

gets and the gradient or slope of the relationship between the actual medication dosage changes and the blood glucose levels reported by the patient). The maximum permissible medication levels set by the physician are also shown. With these settings the system helps the individual patient manage his or her own blood glucose levels.

All parameters used by the system for a given patient must be set for each patient by the physician, who also defines the types, mixtures, and times of administration of each medication, i.e., the particular patient's prescription. Changes in any dosage can be made by clicking on the ↑↓ buttons displayed during on-screen review of the weekly or monthly data. Other changes in types of medication and/or times of administration can also be made using a dialog box (not shown in the figure) specifically for this purpose. Typed notes for medico-legal and billing purposes can be entered on-line during review under "Chart Notes." On-line "Crib Notes" relate to details about medication, sites of injection, exercise, and diet. These can be redisplayed immediately during review without resorting to the medical chart. Finally, voice messages can be left for the patient, using a Recorder button to activate a virtual recorder (also not shown). Other buttons allow the physician or case manager to print the displayed logbook or a bar graph of the week's data. The E&M button is for documenting time spent for evaluation and management.

Metabolic Considerations

Each center undertook a retrospective review of metabolic data in patients registered in the system. Registrants failing to use the system in the two centers were similarly reviewed to serve as a control or reference group. In the former group, we recorded the number of blood glucose measurements and lifestyle events entered into the system, and in both groups we calculated the changes from their baseline in subsequently measured glycated hemoglobin A_{1c} fractions and body weights.

β-Test Results

As illustrated in Table 19–1, total system usage among the two centers was summarized over the first 12 months. Registered users totaled 204 in the two centers. Active users were a majority, representing 62% of registrants. Active users generated 60,707 calls to the system. Total calls reporting hyperglycemia were 613; total calls reporting hypoglycemia were 1,319.

As shown in Table 19–2, the accumulating β-testing experience reached 888 patient-months in the first year.

Specific usage on average was greatest in the managed care center, at 72 ± 36 calls/patient/month. The corresponding mean rate in the private practice office (48 ± 32) was significantly less ($p < 0.001$).

A diabetic crisis was noted when a call reported a blood glucose level either over 400mg/dL or under 50mg/dL or symptoms of hypoglycemia without measurement. The average rate of such crises was 2.9 ± 4.8/patient/month in the managed care setting. Corresponding rates in the private office (0.8 ± 1.7) were significantly less ($p < 0.001$). Among the crises, the mean rate of hypoglycemia was 1.9 ± 3.1 events/patient/month in the managed care center with 0.7 ± 1.7 in the private office center. Clinic visits were unchanged at 4.4 visits/patient/year in the managed care center and rose from 2.6 to 4.4 physician visits/patient/year in the private practice office ($p < 0.001$).

Metabolic outcomes are shown in Figure 19–3. Glycated hemoglobin fell significantly in both centers. Changes from baseline values prevailing at the start dropped by 1.0–1.3% ($p < 0.01$ or $p < 0.001$). There was no change in this index in the control group followed at the managed care center. In the private practice office, the parallel reference group showed a slight rise in glycated hemoglobin ($p = 0.009$). Also, there were no significant changes in body weight among the patients in either group in either of the centers (data not shown).

Specific rates of hyperglycemia were followed in each center. Nonlinear regression lines fitted to the data revealed no change with time in the managed care center, where it remained at about 1% of calls. Notably very low rates of hyperglycemia (0.2% of calls throughout the period of observation) were reported in the private practice office.

Hypoglycemia represented as much as 4% of calls in month 1, as shown in Figure 19–4. By month 12, 1

TABLE 19–1   Computer System Usage in Two Centers[a]

Period in each center	1 year
Registered users	204
Active users	124 (62%)
Nonusers	80 (38%)
Total calls accessing system	60,707
Total calls reporting hyperglycemia	613
Total calls reporting hypoglycemia	1,319

[a] Adapted from Ref. 20 with permission.

TABLE 19–2   Specific Usage and Rates of Diabetic Crises (50mg/dL > Blood Glucose > 400mg/dL), Symptomatic Hypoglycemia, and Physician Visits in each Center[a]

	Managed Care Organization	Private Practice Office
Usage (patient-months)	531	357
Rate of calls made	72 ± 36	48 ± 32[b]
Rate of days used (max = 31)	25 ± 7	14 ± 10[b]
Rate of crises reported	2.9 ± 4.8	0.8 ± 1.7[b]
Rate of mild hypoglycemia	1.9 ± 3.1	0.7 ± 1.7[b]
Rate of severe hypoglycemia	0	0
Physician visits per year before[c]	4.4 ± 2.6 (N = 17)	2.6 ± 1.2 (N = 21)
Physician visits per year after[c]	4.4 ± 2.2 (N = 17)	4.4 ± 1.2 (N = 21)

[a] From Ref. 20 with permission; all rates mean ± SD in units of per patient/month.

[b] Statistical comparisons: $p < 0.001$ vs. managed care organization.

[c] N = subset of patients whose clinic records extended back 1 or more years before and after starting on the system.

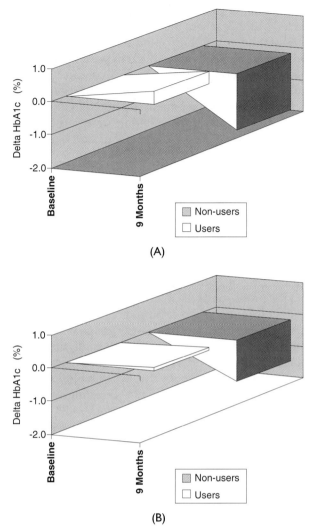

Figure 19–3. Metabolic issues: Mean glycated hemoglobin changes (%) from baseline to 9 months in system users versus nonusers at managed care center (A) $N = 58$ and at private practitioner office (B) $N = 54$. Nonusers are a reference group, registered but not using the system. Changes in users at 9 months vs. baseline ($p < 0.001$) and nonusers ($p < 0.01$).

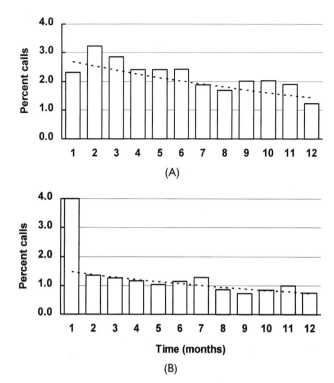

Figure 19–4. Percent of total calls to computer system each month reporting hypoglycemia (blood glucose $< 50mg/dL$ or symptoms) at managed care center (A) $N = 57$ and at private practitioner office (B) $N = 43$. Nonlinear regression lines shown (—). From Ref. 20 with permission.

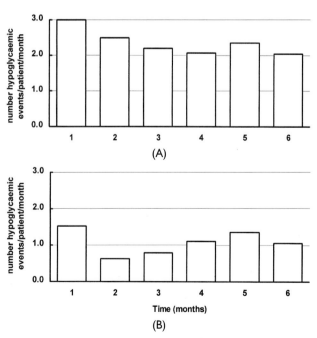

Figure 19–5. Average number of hypoglycemic events (blood glucose $< 50mg/dL$ or symptoms)/month in patients reporting recurrent hypoglycemia at managed care center (A) $N = 30$, decreasing to 22 and at private practice office (B) $N = 11$, not changing. Only patients reporting hypoglycemia are included, while followed prospectively from starting use of the system in month 1. (From Ref. 20 with permission.)

year later, the fraction of calls reporting hypoglycemia was down to an average rate of about 1% month. The nonlinear regression lines fitted to the data indicate that the falls were statistically significant ($p < 0.05$) in both centers.

To explore the mechanisms for the observed fall in reports of hypoglycemia, the data were examined by specific patient reporting of one or more episodes of hypoglycemia/month. As can be seen in Figure 19–5, these specific rates of recurrent hypoglycemia on average fell in the managed care center, where the number of reports of hypoglycemia at month 6 was less ($p < 0.02$) than those reported at month 1. Recurrent rates of hypoglycemia in patients in the private practice office were low initially and, except for a transient fall, did not change significantly with time.

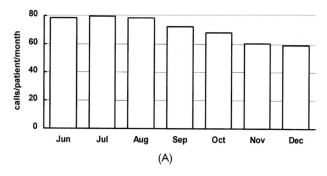

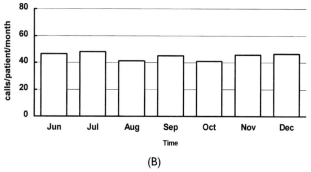

Figure 19–6. Average number of calls/patient/month (adherence) at managed care center (A) and at private practice office (B).

The average number of phone calls (by specific patient by month) is shown in Figure 19–6. In the managed care center, seven gestational diabetes patients were included among those followed while using the system. Each stopped using the system at the conclusion of pregnancy over the months of September through December. This accounted in large part for the fall in average number of calls from 79 ± 42 in June to 59 ± 29 in December. Eight others showed a significant reduction, while the remainder showed either an increase ($N = 1$) or no change ($N = 40$). In the private practice office, the number of calls/patient/month averaged 45 ± 32, reflecting the use of the system to enter blood glucose profiles as instructed "on no less than 2 days per week."

Conclusions and Indications for the Future

Frequent, appropriate intervention improves metabolic control in diabetes,[2] but face-to-face intervention is costly.[7] It is possible to facilitate intervention manually by using a telephone, a modem, or a fax machine.[20–23] In such manual methods, patients are instructed to measure their blood glucose each day and to call, modem, or fax a report of their results to the clinic or office, in

some cases several times a day. A case manager (nurse or clerk) receives these transmissions and passes a written note thereof to the patient's doctor, who reviews the new data in reference to the patient's medical history of previous results, activity level, diet patterns, and so on. A decision regarding medication dosing, diet, or exercise is then made and noted in the medical chart, and pertinent instructions are returned to the nurse or case manager for transmission back to the patient, usually by phone. This manual method achieves the goal of frequent intervention. However, because it also is time intensive, the manual method is usually not attractive to the health care administrator, managed care organization, or health insurance company. As a consequence, it is difficult to offer this approach to many patients or even to practice it for long periods of time with any given patient.

Recognizing both the need for frequent intervention and the problems of the manual methods, we see a role for a voice-interactive computer assistant capable of linking patients directly to their care providers. Such systems must be automatic to reduce the time/effort inherent in such interactions. Several are being developed.[20,24] With the American system, a representative initial experience (also known as β-testing) was accumulated. This testing included some 888 patient-months of prospective follow-up in a cross-section of patients from two independent health care settings. Positive findings on acceptance, safety, efficacy, and fiscal and administrative aspects (results not shown) as well as favorable preliminary metabolic outcomes resulted with the use of the computer technology.

Physician and health professional acceptance was binary. The β-site participants obviously represented an enthusiastic professional user group. Their acceptance of the technology was high, and they were willing to work diligently to acquire the necessary new skills in information technology and to participate in a β-test thereof. The role of the engineer/computer experts was to design and adapt the system to the physician's and patient's needs, teach the fundamentals of information technology to the health professionals, and train them in its use for diabetes care.

The fraction of all health professionals who may effectively work with such information technology is not large. Most fear computers and what these devices may do to their job security. This points to the need for a new generation of "computer-tolerant" health professionals to assume this task. We foresee these new information-age care providers as being required in large numbers. Among their numbers, some may possibly be located in managed care organizations, in hospital clinics, or in private practice offices. Most are likely to be located outside, independently contracting to provide diabetes management services as consultants to health care organizations and to support individual practitioners not equipped or personally motivated to acquire these skills. Cost-recovery issues are now becoming favorable for this form of care.

The present evaluation involved β-testing in a heterogeneous population broadly representative of diabetes patients in subspecialty medical practices. This β-testing is preliminary. It should not be considered a randomized, controlled clinical trial either of a particular clinician's treatment method or of the response thereto of a specific subset of his or her patients. As this information system does not of itself provide medical management or independent medication decision making, the evaluation in β-testing was mainly on safety and efficacy of a telecommunication link. Notwithstanding, preliminary reports[17–19] have shown improvements in mean blood glucose concentrations, glycated hemoglobin A_{1c}, fructosamine, and lipid levels in patients using the system. Contrary to expectations,[25] body weight did not increase (data not shown), and hypoglycemia, as shown herein, was reduced. We attribute this favorable outcome to the effects of the daily (albeit machine) and weekly (human) intervention that this system fosters. Others[26] using patient-directed, manual methods reported no change in metabolic control after one year but noted a reduction in nurse task time with a modem system for receiving blood glucose readings transmitted every 2 weeks from memory meters. Parenthetically, this interval may be too long for effective closed-loop control.[8,9,27]

The design of the present system and the selection of the particular hardware, operating systems, and supporting software were satisfactory. Together, this computational platform maintained safety, confidentiality, data security, redundancy, and prompt turn-around of patient data and individual reports. We found that one telephone line can serve some 200 users. This obviously depends on how frequently each patient accesses the system.

Notwithstanding, we are seeing this service expand each year as more patients in each clinic are registered. Eventually all patients should be offered the opportunity to participate in the on-line care of their diabetes. With the help of such systems, physicians will realize interactive control over the well-being of their patients, and their patients will receive the direct benefit of continuous medical supervision. Depriving patients or not informing them of these opportunities may make such practitioners liable for future outcomes, particularly if they are adverse.[6]

A key question was whether patients would abandon this method of care following an initial enthusiasm. The data suggest an adherence to the process. Although they range widely, the specific number of telephone calls remained constant month by month in the majority of patients. An approximately 10% turnover was noted, with some falling away from and others returning to more active use. Strikingly, about one-quarter of patients willing to be registered into the system dropped out because their insurance companies would not pay for the medical services they were receiving. The remainder never made a single call. Why this occurs and what ought be done to change these treatment failures is not obvious. The psychological underpinnings, possible machine aversions, and personality traits contributing to the various behaviors clearly require further study.

Although successful for hospital use, earlier bedside[8,9] instruments have not been suitably miniaturized through further development, and a unique, hand-held device[10] for outpatient use was too expensive for wide-scale application. In the present design[18–20] there are no communication or computer devices needed by the patient and therefore no device costs to the patient, who is only responsible for the medical fees associated with the increased intervention and case management or care plan oversight services he or she may require. Where third-party insurance exists, the costs of providing service may be adequately covered.[28] Physician visits tended toward accepted average rates of 3–4/year in all centers.

Evaluation[29] and cost-benefit analyses[30] of intensive treatment and teaching programs for type 1 (insulin-dependent) diabetes mellitus can be found in the literature. Metabolically, the present early results using the information technology appear similar. As computers can provide ongoing follow-up by convenient telecommunication, we hope the benefits so far gained will persist rather than dissipate with time in the longer term. It remains to be seen in our model in the United States whether urine glucose self-monitoring can be substituted. This wonderful observation[30] could represent major savings in the immense cost of blood glucose test strips if improved diabetes care is to be implemented on a wider scale.

The limitations of the present open β-study are numerous, and the results must be cautiously interpreted in this context. In particular, the observed improvements in glycated hemoglobin and reductions in incidences of hyperglycemia and hypoglycemia may represent a placebo effect or a case selection effect. Further clinical studies with larger numbers of patients, randomized to treatment regimens with longer follow-up, are obviously required to confirm and extend the current findings.

In summary, an information technology approach has been developed, applied, and tested in two centers motivated to increase intervention, in a computer-assisted, ostensibly time-effective way. Early clinical experience indicates that this computer technology is safe and that it may empower physicians, nurse educators, and case managers to improve metabolic outcome in diabetes in their constituency (see also chapter 48).

References

1. Schiffrin A, Belmonte MM: Comparison between continuous subcutaneous insulin infusion and multiple injections of insulin. A one-year prospective study. Diabetes 31:255–264, 1982.

2. Berger M: Subcutaneous Insulin Therapy. Heidelberg: Springer-Verlag, 1985.

3. Howorka K: Feasibility of long-term near-normoglycemic insulin substitution (NIS) by multiple injections. In Brunetti P, Waldhausl WK (eds): Advanced Models for the Therapy of Insulin-Dependent Diabetes. Serono Symposium. New York: Raven Press, 1987, pp. 147–152.

4. Albisser AM: Insulin therapy: closing the loop with a microprocessor. *In* Clarke WL, Larner J, Pohl S (eds): Methods in Diabetes Research, vol. II: Clinical Methods. New York: John Wiley & Sons, 1986, pp. 329–345.

5. WHO/IDF EUROPE Diabetes Care and Research in Europe: The Saint Vincent Declaration. Diabetic Medicine 7:360, 1990.

6. The Diabetes Control and Complications Trial Research Group. The effect of intensive treatment of diabetes on the development and progression of long-term complications in insulin-dependent diabetes mellitus. [New England Journal of Medicine 329:977–986, 1993.

7. 2 ed. National Institutes of Diabetes, Digestive and Kidney Diseases, National Institutes of Health: Diabetes in America, (Pub no. 95-1468). NIH, Bethesda, MD, 1995.

8. Albisser, A.M., Leibel, B.S., Ewart, T.G., Davidovac, Z., Botz, C.K. and Zingg, W. (1974) An artificial endocrine pancreas. *Diabetes*, 23, 389–396.

9. Albisser AM, Leibel BS, Ewart TG, et al.: Clinical control of diabetes by the artificial pancreas. Diabetes 23:397–404, 1974.

10. Schiffrin A, Mihic M, Leibel BS, Albisser AM: Computer assisted insulin dosage adjustment. Diabetes Care 8:545–552, 1985.

11. Peters A, Rubsamen M, Jacob U, et al.: Clinical evaluation of decision support system for insulin dose adjustment in IDDM. Diabetes Care 14:875–880, 1991.

12. Albisser AM: Intelligent instrumentation in diabetic management. CRC Critical Review in Biomedical Engineering 17:1–24, 1989.

13. Schiffrin A, Albisser AM: Evaluating a computer algorithm for exercise in type I diabetic subjects. Diabetes Nutrition and Metabolism 1:29–35, 1988.

14. Sakkal S: Brittle diabetes treated with intensified therapy and a pocket insulin dosage computer. Diabetes Nutrition and Metabolism 6:97–101, 1993.

15. Skyler J, Skyler D, Seigler D, Sullivan MO: Algorithms for adjustment of insulin dosage by patients who monitor blood glucose. Diabetes Care 4:311–318, 1981.

16. Kessler DA, Pape SM, Sundwall DN: The federal regulation of medical devices. New England Journal of Medicine 317:357–366, 1987.

17. Federal Register sept. of Health and Human Services, Food and Drug Administration. Pub L No. 94-295, 90 Stat 539 (1976), codified at 21CFR 807.65(d), 1991.

18. Albisser AM, Meneghini LM, Mintz DH: New on-line computer system for daily diabetes intervention: First year experience. Diabetes 46(Suppl 2):P256(abstract), 1996.

19. Sakkal S, Wright C: Cost effectiveness of the use of telecommunication in diabetes management for daily diabetes control. Proceedings, 77th Annual Meeting of the Endocrine Society, Washington DC: June 14–17, P3-295(abstract), 1995.

20. Albisser AM, Harris RI, Sakkal S, et al.: Diabetes intervention in the information age. Med Inform 21:297–316, 1996.

21. Shultz EK, Bauman A, Hayward M, Holzman R: Improved care of patients with diabetes through telecommunications. Ann. NY Acad Sci 670:141–145, 1992.

22. Billiard A, Rohmer V, Roques MA, et al.: Telematic transmission of computerised blood glucose profiles for IDDM patients. Diabetes Care 14:130–134, 1991.

23. Del Pozo F, Gomez, E, Arrendo MT: A telemedicine approach to diabetes management. Diabetes Nutrition and Metabolism 4 (Suppl 1): 149–153, 1991.

24. Albisser AM, Sperlich M: Adjusting insulins. Diabetes Educator 18:211–219, 1992.

25. The Diabetes Control and Complications Trial Research Group: Epidemiology of severe hypoglycemia in the Diabetes Control and Complications Trial. Am J Med 90: 450–459, 1991.

26. Marrero DG, Vandagriff JL, Kronz K, et al.: Using telecommunication technology to manage children with diabetes: The computer-linked outpatient clinic (CLOC) study. Diabetes Educator 21:313–319, 1995.

27. Franklin GF, Powell JD, Workman ML: Digital Control of Dynamic Systems, 2 ed. Reading, MA: Addison-Wesley, 1990.

28. Kirschner CG, Frankel LM, Jackson JA: Physician's current procedural terminology CPT96. Prolonged evaluation and management service (without direct face-to-face patient contact) CPT99358. Chicago, IL: Amercian Medical Association, 1996.

29. Muhlhauser I, Bruckner I, Berger M, et al.: Evaluation of an intensified insulin treatment and teaching programme as routine management of type 1 (insulin-dependent) diabetes. The Bucharest-Dusseldorf Study. Diabetologia 30:681–690, 1987.

30. Starostina EG, Antsiferov M, Galstyan GR, et al.: Effectiveness and cost-benefit analysis of intensive treatment and teaching programmes for type 1 (insulin-dependent) diabetes mellitus in Moscow—blood glucose versus urine glucose self-monitoring. Diabetologia 37:170–176, 1994.

20

Oral Agents in the Treatment of Diabetes Mellitus

Michael Berger and Bernd Richter

The story of oral antidiabetic agents reflects in many ways the forces that govern clinical and pharmaceutical investigations as well as the treatment of chronic diseases that afflict a sizable proportion of the world's population.

The drive to investigate potentially useful oral pharmacotherapies for patients with diabetes mellitus (beginning in 1926 with the guanides) has always been, and remains, a powerful motivator. Discovery of an effective and safe oral hypoglycemic agent that could replace insulin injection therapy and/or render diet treatment unnecessary is greatly desired by both professionals and patients who suffer from a *relative* insulin deficiency only, i.e., those defined as having type 2 or non-insulin-dependent diabetes mellitus (NIDDM).

In industrialized societies, NIDDM represents approximately 95% of all patients with diabetes mellitus. A drug treatment for these patients could be successful by stimulation of insulin secretion or by increasing the body's sensitivity to insulin. Furthermore, the possibilities of decreasing hyperglycemia by inhibiting gastrointestinal glucose absorption or hepatic glucose production, or by increasing the peripheral disposal of glucose, have been explored. In fact, all of these potential approaches to decreasing hyperglycemia in NIDDM have been and are being investigated with enormous investments by the pharmaceutical industry and by other research funding organizations throughout the world. These efforts are stimulated by the rapidly growing prevalence of NIDDM, which now afflicts 4–8% of industrialized populations.

The leading oral hypoglycemic agents, however, were discovered by chance in the early 1940s in the south of France.[1] Mainly due to the occupation of France by the German army, Dr. Loubatières' clinical studies of the new hypoglycemic agents did not continue. Ironically, *German* scientists introduced sulfonylurea drugs for clinical use some 10 years later, and in the 1980s Germany topped the list of countries that used these drugs excessively.

Since 1970, the sulfonylureas have become the center of one of the most heated controversies in modern medicine.[2] Because of the enormous medical and financial implications of policy decisions regarding the prescription and utilization of these drugs, relevant discussions increasingly have been taken away from the medical profession by pharmaceutical manufacturers, politicians, health care economists, lawyers, consumer advocates, and the like. The principal multicenter clinical trials in this field, carried out with an unprecedented amount of planning and biometric expertise, i.e., the University Group Diabetes Program (UGDP)[3] study and the very recent United Kingdom Prospective Diabetes Study (UKPDS)[4], in some respects have been difficult to interpret. In any case, the heated controversies that erupted, as overshadowed as they may have been by commercial and political powers, have alerted the medical profession and the public to the potential risks of chronic drug therapy for NIDDM.[2] In some countries, the steady increase in use of sulfonylurea drugs had been stopped temporarily because of concern over possible side effects of sulfonylureas on the part of physicians and the public. Even though major issues of effectivity and safety of oral antidiabetic drug treatment are still unresolved to date, sulfonylurea drugs have remained by far the most popular treatment for type 2 diabetes throughout the world.

More recently, a number of additional pharmaceutical strategies are being propagated. The use of the biguanide metformin has experienced a worldwide renaissance after phenformin (and buformin) had been banned in the late 1970s. Glucosidase-blocking agents such as acarbose or miglitol, introduced in the early 1990s, aim at decreasing postprandial hyperglycemia. In recent years, the thiazolidinediones, a group of drugs described as "insulin sensitizers," have been developed and marketed with the particular objective to improve insulin sensitivity in patients with type 2 diabetes.

In line with the aforementioned powerful drive to market oral antidiabetic agents, these drugs have been the focus of *unparalleled marketing campaigns* throughout the world. In fact, the vast majority of type 2 diabetic patients is presently treated with one or more of these drugs, frequently in combination with insulin therapy.

It needs to be pointed out that the efficacy and safety of oral antidiabetic therapy remain an open issue to date. The main health problem of the type 2 diabetic patient is his or her excess cardiovascular morbidity and mortality. For none of the available oral antidiabetic drugs, there has never been any proof that they lower type 2 diabetic patients' excessive rates of cardiovascular morbidity and mortality, with the possible exception of metformin monotherapy in younger overweight type 2 diabetic patients.[4] Rather, for tolbutamide and phenformin the UGDP study provided evidence that these drugs were unsafe, as they led to increased cardiovascular mortality. It remains difficult to understand why oral antidiabetic drugs have been approved by national licensing authorities and most successfully marketed worldwide based upon their effectivity on surrogate markers only (such as glycemia, HbA$_{Ic}$ levels, body weight), whereas data on the clinically relevant endpoints, such as cardiovascular morbidity and mortality or incidence rates for microangiopathic complications of diabetes, have only recently become available.[4]

Comprehensive reviews on the clinical pharmacology and clinical use of oral antidiabetic drugs have been published in the recent past. This chapter will summarize the clinically relevant aspects of these drugs for the practicing physician.

Historical Perspective

The search for oral agents to treat hyperglycemia and glycosuria and other signs and symptoms of diabetes mellitus is as old as the disease itself. In the desperate times of the preinsulin era, every available drug was tried—without success. Even following the introduction of insulin treatment, research and trials on orally administered pharmaceuticals (including insulin[5]) continued.

Despite intensive efforts to develop blood sugar–lowering drugs, the discovery of the first hypoglycemic agent was made by chance. In 1941 observant physicians in Montpellier, France, diagnosed hypoglycemia following the administration of sulfonamides being used to treat a patient for pneumonia. Dr. A. Loubatières and colleagues between 1942 and 1946 described the hypo-

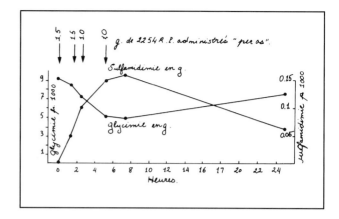

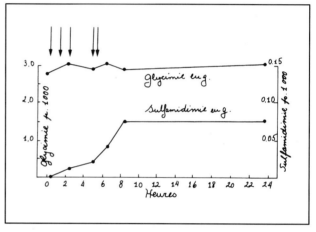

Figure 20–1. (Upper panel) First experimental demonstration of the hypoglycemic action of the sulfonamide 2254 RP in the normal dog. (Lower panel) First demonstration of the absence of the hypoglycemic action of the sulfonamide 2254 RP in the totally depancreatectomized dog. [*Source:* Ref. 1, with permission.]

glycemic action of a sulfonamide [p-amino-benzene-sulfamido-isopropyl-thiodiazole (2254 RP)] in a series of sophisticated animal experiments (Fig. 20–1).[1] Loubatières was able to demonstrate that in dogs the hypoglycemic effect of sulfonamide compounds was dependent on intact pancreatic tissue; i.e., in totally depancreatectomized animals, the drug failed to lower blood glucose levels (see Fig. 20–1). Loubatières concluded that these drugs exerted their blood glucose–lowering effects via stimulation of insulin secretion, and, consequently, he called them "beta-cytotropic agents." Due to the sequelae of World War II, Loubatières and colleagues were unable to continue their pharmacologic studies on the hypoglycemic effects of sulfonamides. It was not until the mid-1950s that a number of German investigators described the use of another sulfonamide derivative, 1-butyl-3-sulfonylurea (carbutamide), for the treatment of certain diabetic patients. In these early publications it was noted that carbutamide was effective only in nondiabetic individuals and in moderately severe maturity-onset diabetic patients, but it was not effective in patients who had what now is classified as type 1 or insulin-dependent diabetes mellitus (IDDM).

In 1956 the first report of experimental and clinical data on the sulfonamide derivative N-(4-methyl-benzoyl-sulphonyl)-N'-butyl-carbamide (tolbutamide), a substance virtually free of bacteriostatic, but possessing unequivocal hypoglycemic properties, was published.[6] Since then, uncounted reports on an ever-increasing number of sulfonylurea drugs have appeared in the literature. In fact, sulfonylurea drugs are being marketed *as generations*, with tolbutamide, chlorpropamide, tolazamide, and acetohexamide being coined as first-generation sulfonylureas. By now, these drugs have been almost completely replaced by the second-generation sulfonylureas, namely glibenclamide, glibornuride, gliclazide, and glipizide, which are much more potent on an effect-to-weight basis. Most recently, a third-generation sulfonylurea, glimepiride, and the benzoic acid derivative repaglinide have been introduced into various international markets—in an attempt to decrease the risks of iatrogenic hypoglycemia. Interestingly, the respective marketing concepts are aimed in opposite directions: Glimepiride is advocated because a once-daily dose suffices; repaglinide is praised because it is to be given several times daily, i.e., before each main meal ("one meal, one dose—no meal, no dose"). Unknown is the number of congresses, symposia, and monographs on the pharmacology, mechanism of action, and clinical use of sulfonylurea drugs. Some observers maintain that the sulfonylureas stimulated the investigators more than the (ailing) β cells, as Rachmiel Levine stated some 40 years ago.[7] In fact, a Medline search covering 1966–1997 has identified 8824 publications devoted to sulfonylurea drugs, whereas only two studies (UGDP,[3] UKPDS[4]) were actually directed to document long-term endpoint-related effectivity and safety as the basis for a rational use of these drugs in type 2 diabetic patients.

Still, some opinion leaders praise the discovery of the sulfonylurea drugs as a hallmark of modern medicine. The opinions of diabetologists with respect to their clinical usefulness are equally divided. Some diabetologists stopped prescribing them 25 years ago, such as Dr. J.K. Davidson in his memorandum to the House Staff of Grady Memorial Hospital at Emory University, Atlanta, dated November 20, 1970 (Exhibit 20–1). Yet as of today, in most countries, notably Germany, the vast majority of NIDDM patients are treated with sulfonylurea drugs (Table 20–3).

EXHIBIT 20–1. Memorandum of Dr. J. K. Davidson
To: Faculty and House Staff of Department of Medicine
   Chiefs of other services

Oral Anti-Diabetic Agents

The University Group Diabetes Program (UGDP) findings (published in a supplement to the November, 1970 issue of *Diabetes*) have recently been reviewed by an Ad Hoc Committee of the American Diabetes Association, the Council on Drugs of the American Medical Association and the Food and Drug Administration of the Department of Health, Education, and Welfare. Since there was a significantly higher death rate from cardiovascular disease in the tolbutamide-treated group than in the placebo-treated group, the three agencies named above have made the following recommendations: (1) the use of tolbutamide, chlorpropamide, acetohexamide, and tolazamide should be *limited to those patients with symptomatic adult-onset nonketotic diabetes mellitus which cannot be adequately controlled by diet or weight loss alone and in whom the addition of insulin is impractical or unacceptable (to the patient)*, and (2) oral hypoglycemic agents are not recommended in the treatment of chemical or latent diabetes, in suspected diabetes, or in prediabetes, and are contraindicated in patients with ketoacidosis.

Dr. Preedy and I have carefully studied and taken into account all available information and have concluded that we have no alternative but to follow for the present the recommendations of the above national agencies in the management of diabetes mellitus at Grady Memorial Hospital.

House Staff in the Department of Medicine are accordingly advised to discontinue *all* oral anti-diabetic agents as soon as practicable and to control the diabetes by diet alone or diet plus insulin. It is anticipated that the majority of cases now taking oral anti-diabetic agents will be controlled by diet alone, and only a minority will need small amounts of insulin.

Clearly close adherence to diet will be essential particularly in the obese subject. The greatest emphasis must be given to this form of treatment during patient interviews.

Additional facilities for the management of clinic diabetics are planned.

Yours sincerely,
John K. Davidson, M.D., Ph. D.
Director of the Diabetes Unit

JKD:mm

Thus it is not surprising that the use of sulfony-lureas in NIDDM treatment became the central issue in a major controversy of contemporary clinical pharmacology; the welcome publication of the final results from the UKPDS[4] is unlikely to end this debate.

The history of the development of biguanides dates back as far as 1918, when a blood glucose–lowering effect of guanidine was described in rabbits. During the 1920s, the diguanides synthaline A and B (Exhibit 20–2) were tested for their hypoglycemic potencies in clinical studies, without success. Almost in parallel with the sulfonylureas, three biguanides, i.e., phenformin, buformin, and metformin (see Exhibit 20–2) were introduced into the treatment of diabetic patients. However, despite their increasing popularity with physicians and patients and apparent overuse in the 1960s and 1970s, the mechanism of action of these drugs remains obscure. Due to the frequent association between the therapeutic use of biguanides and the occurrence of fatal lactic acidosis (and possibly hypertension), the prescription of biguanides was severely restricted in most countries and banned in the United States in 1977. However, in many European countries, notably Italy, France, and Great Britain, metformin has always been used to an appreciable amount during the treatment of overweight type 2 diabetic patients, both as monotherapy and in combination with sulfonylureas or insulin treatment. Toward the late 1980s, a revival of biguanide treatment was initiated in Europe in the context of a marketing campaign that was widely referred to as the "renaissance of metformin." It was felt that metformin was useful in its antihyperglycemic action, which was not associated with increasing levels of circulating insulin, and that the incidence of lactic acidosis could be kept at a minimum when certain contraindications were observed. Even though no further evidence on efficacy and safety of the drug was put forward, metformin was introduced into the market of the United States effective 1995—where it subsequently became a remarkable marketing success. Most recently, the UKPDS documented metformin's endpoint-related efficacy and safety when used as monotherapy in younger, newly diagnosed overweight type 2 diabetic patients—whereas when given in combination with sulfonylureas it was associated with increased mortality.[4]

Further efforts to develop oral antidiabetic drugs were directed at improvements of insulin sensitivity, with the aim of avoiding hyperinsulinemia, which was considered—by some investigators at times—to be a potential independent risk factor for macroangiopathy.

EXHIBIT 20–2.   Biguanide Drugs and Acarbose

Synthaline A (diguanide)	$H_2N-CNH-CH-(CH_2)_{10}-NH-CNH-NH_2$
Synthaline B (diguanide)	$H_2N-CNH-NH-(CH_2)_{12}-NH-CNH-NH_2$
Phenformin	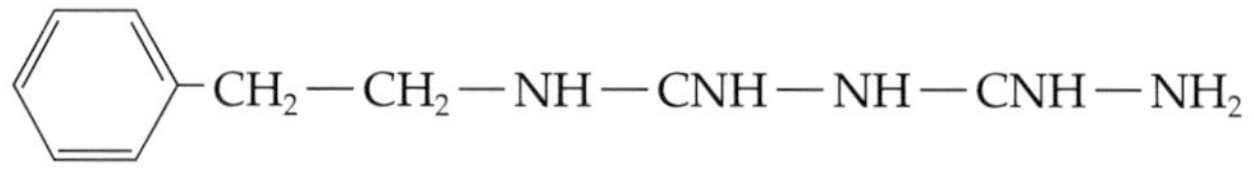 $-CH_2-CH_2-NH-CNH-NH-CNH-NH_2$
Buformin	$H_3C-CH_2-CH_2-CH_2-NH-CNH-NH-CNH-NH_2$
Metformin	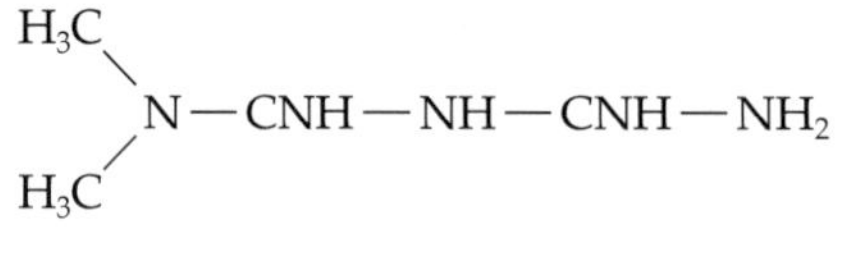 $H_3C,\ H_3C > N-CNH-NH-CNH-NH_2$
Acarbose	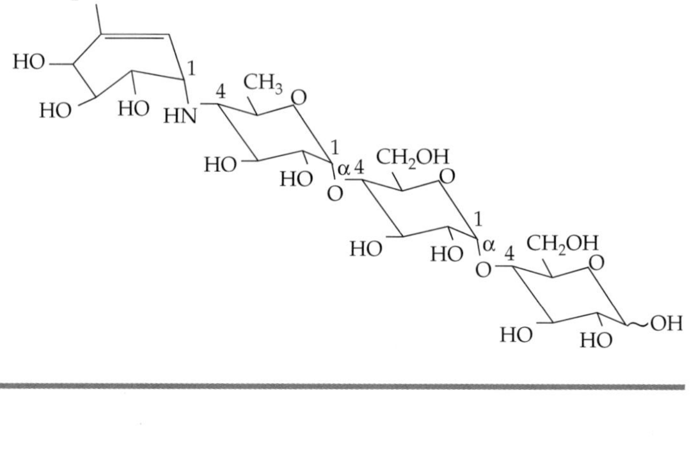

First attempts were made to delay the absorption of carbohydrates with the aim to decrease postprandial hyperglycemia. Whereas the administration of guar substances in various galenic preparations and formulas never became popular among physicians and their patients, the use of disaccharidase inhibitors, such as the α-glucosidase inhibitor acarbose (see Exhibit 20–2), has rapidly become widespread after these drugs first were marketed in the early 1990s. Finally, a group of drugs called thiazolidinediones (Exhibit 20–3) have been explored as antidiabetic agents since they seem to increase insulin sensitivity, in particular at the level of the muscular cell. These drugs are agonists for the peroxisome proliferator-activated nuclear receptor (PPAR-γ); their mechanism of action remains incompletely understood. As of 1997, troglitazone has been marketed in Japan and in the United States; following reports of hepatotoxicity, the attempts to market the drug in Europe have been suspended.

Among the reasons for the plethora of development and marketing of oral antidiabetic drugs, many of similar or even doubtful effectiveness, may be their commercial profitability. However, it also seems that patients' attitudes have not changed profoundly since Dr. John Rollo stated 200 years ago:

> We have to lament that our mode of cure is so contrary to the inclinations of the sick. Though perfectly aware of the efficacy of the [diet] regimen, and the impropriety of devi-

ations, yet they commonly trespass, concealing what they feel as a transgression on themselves. They express a regret that a medicine could not be discovered, however nauseous or distasteful, which would suppress the necessity of any restriction of diet.[8]

Sulfonylurea Drugs

Mechanism of Action

The mechanism of action by which sulfonylurea drugs (Table 20–1) exert their hypoglycemic effects has been known since the initial investigation of Loubatières and colleagues. Thus, these compounds have always been referred to as "beta-cytotropic agents," indicating that their primary and probably only mechanism of action is the stimulation of the pancreatic β-cell. A beneficial effect of sulfonylurea treatment of IDDM has never been shown.

The stimulation of insulin secretion by sulfonylurea drugs has been extensively studied in a variety of experimental models, such as the isolated perfused pancreas and perfused islets and islets cells in culture. It has been shown repeatedly that the insulinotropic effect of sulfonylureas is dependent, at least in large part, on the presence of glucose. Some authors have rephrased these findings by stating that the sulfonylureas increase the sensitivity of the β-cell to glucose.

EXHIBIT 20–3. Thiazolidinediones, structural formulas

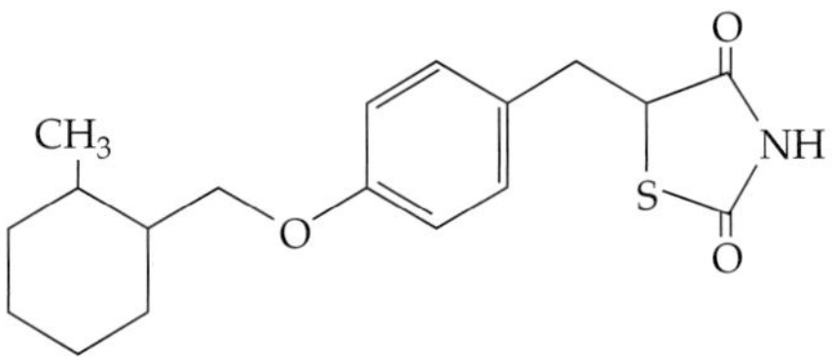

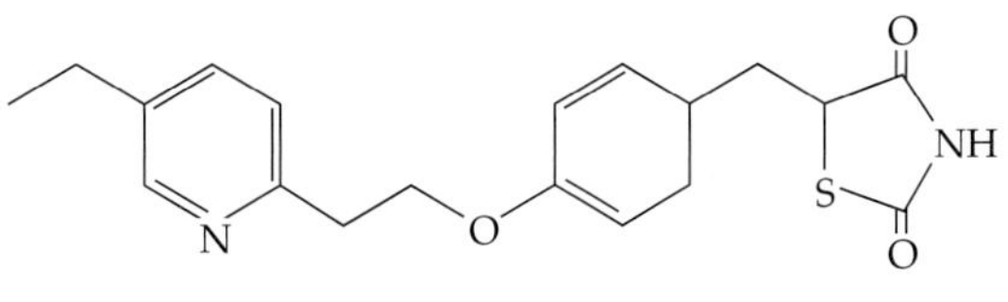

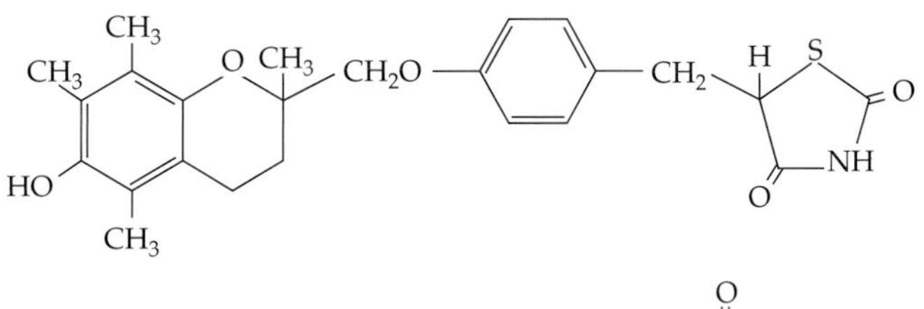

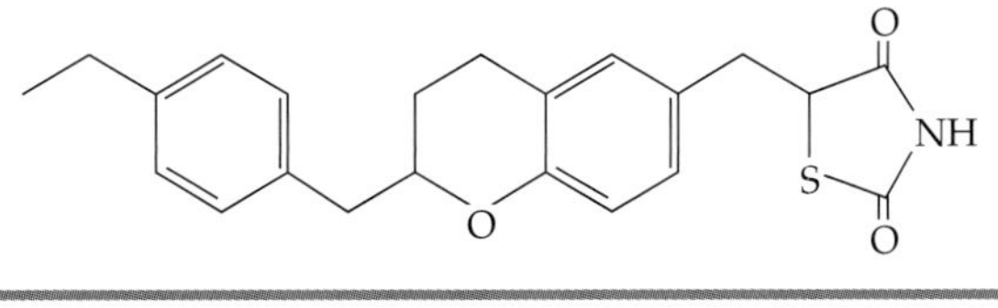

TABLE 20–1   Sulfonylurea Drugs R_1—⟨phenyl⟩—$SO_2NHCONH$—R_2 and Repaglinide

Name of Drug	R_1	R_2	Metabolism	Elimination of the Drug		
				Half-Life Range (hr)	Duration of Action (hr)	Daily Dose Range (mg)
First-generation sulfonylurea drugs						
Tolbutamide	CH_3—	—$(CH_2)_3CH_3$	Hepatic metabolism, renal excretion of less active metabolites	7 (4–25)	6–10	500–3,000
Chlorpropamide	Cl—	—$(CH_2)_2CH_3$	80% hepatic metabolism, renal excretion of drug and less active metabolites	35 (25–60)	24–72	100–500
Second-generation sulfonylurea drugs						
Glibenclamide (glyburide)			Hepatic metabolism, renal excretion of less active metabolite	5 (low compartment) 10 (deep compartment)	16+	1.25–15
Glipzide			Hepatic metabolism, renal excretion of inactive metabolites	6	8–12	2.5–40
Gliclazide	CH_3—		Hepatic metabolism, renal excretion of inactive metabolites	10–12	8–16	80–240
Third-generation sulfonylurea drugs						
Glimepiride			Hepatic metabolism, renal (60%) and biliary excretion of inactive metabolites	5–8	24	1–6
Benzoic acid derivatives						
Repaglinide			Hepatic metabolism, biliary excretion	1	?	1.5–16

The fact that they can be quite potent stimulators of insulin secretion in their own right is evident from the repeated reports of *severe and prolonged (sometimes fatal) hypoglycemia* due to administration of excessive doses of sulfonylureas.

The cellular biochemical events that are responsible for the stimulatory action of sulfonylurea drugs on insulin secretion by the β-cells have recently been described. Presently, it is assumed that sulfonylurea drugs exert their β-cytotropic action by blocking ATP-dependent potassium channels (K_{ATP}-channels),[9] the subsequent inhibition of the potassium ion efflux leading to an increased influx of calcium ions and, hence, to the calmodulin-triggered activation of kinases that stimulate the exocytosis of insulin-loaded secretory granules[10] (Fig. 20–2). All of this appears to be initiated by an interaction between the sulfonylurea with high-affinity sulfonylurea receptors at the surface of the pancreatic β-cell, whereas the binding affinity of the different sulfonylurea compounds to these receptors seems to be correlated to their respective potencies in stimulating insulin secretion. Likewise, a new group of hypoglycemic agents, the benzoic derivatives, namely repaglinide, exhibit their β-cytotropic action via a blockage of K_{ATP} channels (even though their molecular structure does not coincide with that of sulfonylurea drugs; see Table 20–1).

Early claims that sulfonylureas might inhibit glucagon secretion by the pancreatic α-cells have not been supported by recent investigations. Despite the general assumption that these drugs exert their blood glucose-lowering effect via the stimulation of insulin secretory processes, in some studies, but not all, long-term treatment with these compounds resulted in relatively low levels of circulating insulin despite an improvement of glycemic control. The initial amelioration of hyperglycemia in sulfonylurea-treated patients with NIDDM is associated with an increase of insulinemia. However, in many patients successfully managed on oral sulfonylureas, serum insulin levels have reverted to or fallen below initial concentrations on long-term follow-up. It thus appears that in a sizable percentage of sulfonylurea-treated NIDDM patients improved glycemic control can be maintained *á la longue* in association with rather low serum insulin levels when compared with the initial phases of drug therapy. This phenomenon might have a number of explanations. The improvement of metabolic control as such is expected to result in an increase in the body's insulin sensitivity. Alternatively, extrapancreatic effects of sulfonylureas on long-term use have always been discussed. However, in vivo evidence for a causal relationship between sulfonylurea effects on glycemia and insulin sensitivity of the organism and the action of sulfonylurea drugs on insulin receptor numbers or insulin-receptor interaction has not been documented. Quite often authors have been tempted to draw premature conclusions from in vitro studies. In conclusion, any claims of hypothetical extrapancreatic effects of sulfonylureas on glucose metabolism remain to be substantiated. If such an effect were present, one would have to presume that the addition of sulfonylurea treatment would be beneficial to diabetic patients with IDDM, at least to those in suboptimal metabolic control with decreased insulin sensitivity. However, numerous attempts to demonstrate such a beneficial effect by combination sulfonylurea-insulin therapy in IDDM have unanimously failed.

On the other hand, sulfonylurea drugs (and the aforementioned benzoic acid derivatives) do block K_{ATP} channels far beyond the endocrine pancreas.[9,11] Particular attention centers on their effects on the heart. Whereas ischemic preconditioning is based upon the opening of K_{ATP} channels, sulfonylurea drugs prevent this phenomenon of autoprotection of the heart against ischemia; in fact, during experimental coronary occlusion, ischemic damage to the myocardium is enhanced during sulfonylurea treatment.[11] This observation may differ between various sulfonylurea drugs; it may represent the pathophysiologic plausibility for earlier observations of increased cardiovascular mortality in patients with type 2 diabetes (and coronary artery disease) on tolbutamide therapy.

Description of Individual Sulfonylurea Drugs

During the past 40 years a number of different sulfonylurea drugs have been introduced. Despite enormous efforts made in investigating and promoting the growing number of sulfonylurea drugs, few relevant differences

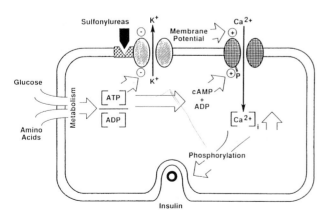

Figure 20–2. Mechanism of action of sulfonylureas (adapted from Ref. 10).

are demonstrable on comparison of the currently available preparations (Table 20–1). The sulfonylureas are classified into first-generation compounds (discovered before 1970) such as tolbutamide and chlorpropamide and second-generation compounds (discovered after 1970) such as glibenclamide (glyburide), glipizide, glisoxepide, and gliclazide. Despite this seemingly fundamental differentiation according to *generations*, few basic differences are demonstrable with the exception of the increased potency on an effect-to-weight basis for the second-generation sulfonylurea drugs. There is, however, no unequivocal difference with respect to the *efficacy* and *safety* of the drugs, and most diabetologists support the idea not to try a second sulfonylurea in case the first one has ceased to be effective in a patient with NIDDM. Glyburide and glipizide were introduced in the United States as late as 1984. The Food and Drug Administration (FDA) required that the package insert for these drugs contain a warning of possible increased risk of cardiovascular death based on the results of the UGDP studies.[12] Nevertheless, they have rapidly gained a large market share in the United States.[13]

More recently, glimepiride has been introduced as a *third-generation* sulfonylurea. As its duration of action is rather long, it needs to be given only once daily. Suggestive research might indicate that the risk of iatrogenic hypoglycemia is decreased and the potentially harmful side effects of other sulfonylureas on the (ischemic) myocardium are avoided. Also most recently, the benzoic acid derivative repaglinide that exerts its β-cytotropic action via the same mechanism as sulfonylurea drugs has been marketed in a number of countries. Its action is deliberately short, which should predispose the drug to preprandial use aiming at selectively increasing prandial insulinemia.

The main characteristics of the leading sulfonylurea drugs are listed in Table 20–1. In contrast to their widespread use, only a limited amount of information is available with regard to their pharmacokinetics and bioavailability after oral administration. Most of the current knowledge related to pharmacokinetics and dose–response relationships of sulfonylurea drugs has been critically reviewed by Jackson and Bressler[14] and by Gerich.[15]

Absorption

It appears that all sulfonylureas are completely absorbed from the intestinal tract into the bloodstream. As with other drugs, the absorption process may be delayed by fiber-rich nutrition. In the circulation, sulfonylureas are 75–95%, protein bound, as a result of which their bioavailability may be influenced by dysproteinemias and by various other drugs competing for the same albumin-binding sites. The binding to serum albumin is different for tolbutamide and chlorpropamide, which are connected to the protein through ionic forces, and for glibenclamide and other drugs of the second-generation sulfonylureas, which bind by nonionic forces. Consequently, these groups of sulfonylureas differ also in their interaction with other drugs.

While there is no evident alteration of absorption rates for glibenclamide by food, to obtain maximal effectiveness the drug should be given (30 min) before meals.[16] The absorption of oral sulfonylurea drugs is substantially inhibited during hyperglycemia.[17]

Metabolism and Elimination

Sulfonylureas are metabolized by the liver, mostly resulting in compounds of less hypoglycemic potency. The sulfonylurea metabolites are mainly excreted by tubular secretion in the kidney. In patients with liver and kidney disease the pharmacokinetics of sulfonylureas are changed. The drugs and/or their metabolites may accumulate in the blood and increase the risk of severe prolonged hypoglycemia. Thus, sulfonylurea treatment should not be considered in patients with liver or renal disease. Furthermore, the elimination of sulfonylurea drugs extensively metabolized by hepatic enzymes may be subjected to enzyme activation and/or inhibition by other drugs, giving rise to potential drug interference problems.

The main differences between various sulfonylurea compounds are related to their rates of inactivation and elimination. Sartor et al.[18] found a surprisingly weak relationship between the dosage of oral glibenclamide and the resulting levels of serum glibenclamide in a group of 37 NIDDM patients who had been treated for at least 1 year with the drug. The authors stated that the lack of correlation between prescribed dosage and blood levels of the drug cannot be explained on the basis of poor patient compliance only. Rather, interindividual differences in the elimination rates of the glibenclamide must be assumed in order to explain this disturbing observation. Systemic investigations of elimination rates for sulfonylureas have been carried out for tolbutamide. Scott and Poffenbarger[19] reported tolbutamide elimination rates after IV administration of the drug in 50 normal volunteers. In accordance with other investigators, they found a mean half-life for the elimination process (disappearance from the blood) of approximately 7 hr for the entire cohort of probands. However, in a more detailed analysis of their data, these authors were able to identify three distinct subpopulations with tolbutamide elimination half-lives of 4, 6, and 10.5 hr, respectively. Scott and Poffenbarger have demonstrated that the tolbutamide disappearance rate appears to be a constant characteristic of an individual and that the elimination of tolbutamide by a given individual appears to be under strong genetic influence. Similar to findings on the other drugs, Scott and Poffenbarger have introduced the term of *pharmacogenetics* of tolbutamide metabolism. These observations appear to be of considerable relevance for the clinical use of sulfonylurea drugs. If, as suggested by the data from Scott and Poffenbarger on tolbutamide metabolism, one-third of the population are slow eliminators of sulfonylurea drugs, it might be likely that it is this subpopulation of patients that tends to develop side effects of sulfonylurea treatment. It might also be that patients who are fast eliminators of sulfonylurea drugs represent a majority of the cases of primary or secondary drug failure(s) because on standard dosage much lower circulating drug levels are achieved than in medium or slow eliminators. However, in contrast to the observations of Scott and Poffenbarger[19] with regard to tolbutamide, the elimination of glibenclamide seems to follow a uniform elimination pattern, at least on the basis of a study in healthy white males.[20] For decades, tolbutamide was the most widely used sulfonylurea drug in the United States. Its relatively short half-life necessitates several daily doses to maintain effective circulating drug levels in most patients. Chlorpropamide has a much longer half-life before disappearance from the blood. It is believed to remain effective for up to 2 to 3 days. A once daily dose is the prescription of choice. On the other hand, many physicians have become concerned about chlorpropamide's excessively long half-life, its risk of drug accumulation, the problems of accurate dosing, and its untoward side effect on blood pressure.[4] In most European countries, the use of chloropropamide has practically been discontinued during the 1980s, while as of 1986 chlorpropamide was still the most frequently used oral antidiabetic in the United States.[13]

Worldwide, the most widely used and studied sulfonylurea drug is presently glibenclamide (glyburide), a comparably potent hypoglycemic agent on an effect-to-weight basis. In its prolonged action, it appears to resemble chlorpropamide. In fact, several pharmacologic and clinical studies have reported very prolonged elimination rates for glibenclamide, possibly due to a hypothetical, slowly equilibrating "deep" compartment of distribution of the drug in vivo. It follows from these data that the risks of drug accumulation have to be taken into account; dose increases should not be made more often than once every 3 or 4 days. Particular emphasis must be placed on the warning not to use glibenclamide in patients with impaired renal or hepatic function. The relative risk of glibenclamide accumulation in vivo may lead to the development of severe hypoglycemia, especially when used in supraoptimal dosages. Unfortunately, processes affecting the elimination rate of glibenclamide are incompletely understood. The existence of as yet unknown factors related to the pharmacokinetics of glibenclamide, such as the recent description of its interdependence with the actual degree of metabolic control, seems likely when one considers the inconsistent relationship between prescribed dose and serum levels of glibenclamide in patients with NIDDM.[14,18]

For some of the remaining sulfonylureas, half-lives and other characteristics are given in Table 20–1. Since the mechanism of action of various sulfonylurea compounds is similar, there are no differences in the indications for use of the drugs as related to various subgroups of patients with NIDDM. A possible exception to this statement is that sulfonylurea drugs may differ in their potential for interaction with other pharmaceutical substances. Also, it has been claimed that glisoxepide and gliquidone and also glimepiride and repaglinide may be used, with caution, in patients with certain degrees of renal insufficiency, since these drugs are excreted to a greater extent by the liver than other sulfonylureas (see Table 20–1). Further documentation of these claims is needed before these drugs can be prescribed to patients with kidney disease on a routine basis.

In a recent development, glimepiride has been designated a third-generation sulfonylurea (see Table 20–1). Glimepiride is superior on an effect-to-weight basis; it binds specifically to a 65 kD subunit of the sulfonylurea receptor at the β-cell membrane and stimulates insulin secretion via blockage of the K_{ATP} channels.[21] It has been suggested that glimepiride's specific binding kinetics may result in a particular dependence of its insulinotropic effect on the ambient glucose concentration resulting in a decreased risk of hypoglycemia; hypoglycemic extrapancreatic effects also have been described—whereas its (potentially cardiotoxic) blockage of K_{ATP} channels in extrapancreatic organs may be diminished.[22] No increased risks of hypoglycemia have been seen in patients with renal impairment or in connection with physical exercise. A recent study suggests that glimepiride may be administered once daily only and that its effect is particularly strong on increasing prandial insulinemia/decreasing prandial hyperglycemia.[23]

Although not a sulfonylurea drug, the carbamoyl-methyl-benzoic derivative repaglinide, as recently marketed in several countries, exerts its hypoglycemic action also via a closure of K_{ATP} channels with subsequent depolarization of the β-cell and stimulation of insulin secretion. In line with its specific binding kinetics, repaglinide is characterized by a particularly short half-life and rapid action[24]—these characteristics are suggested to make the drug particularly suitable for several times daily oral administration before main meals. It has been proposed that repaglinide is virtually without risks of severe hypoglycemia and allows a flexibility of mealtime dosing comparable to that of intensified insulin therapy. It is marketed as a fast-acting β-cell mediated prandial glucose regulator.

Clinical Use of Oral Sulfonylurea Therapy

Efficacy in Treating Hyperglycemia. All sulfonylurea drugs listed in Table 20–1 and others previously described can lower blood glucose levels in normals and in many patients with NIDDM. Controversy continues, however, as to what extent and in what subgroups of patients with NIDDM sulfonylurea drugs represent *safe* and *effective* treatment modalities on a long-term basis. Obviously, very few studies of sulfonylureas fulfill the rigid but nevertheless crucial requirements proposed by Jackson and Bressler[14] for valid investigations of the long-term clinical usefulness of such drug therapies. It seems worthy to underscore the requirement for precise definitions of the patient population and the respective goals of treatment in the various (sub-) groups of patients. *Essential is the documentation that diet and exercise therapy have failed (despite adequate weight loss) to reduce glycemia before a double-blind, placebo-controlled, long-term investigation is mounted. Finally, patient adherence to diet and drug therapy has to be documented, and periods of placebo rechallenge (drug versus placebo withdrawal trials) have to be carried out.* With the exception of the UGDP,[3] the UKPDS trial,[4] and the study by Singer and Hurwitz,[25] almost no publications come even close to these essential requirements for a meaningful evaluation of the long-term clinical efficacy of sulfonylurea therapy. The UKPDS[4] has offered new evidence of the efficacy of a treatment policy aiming at (near-) normalizing of glycemic control in newly manifest young (mean age 53 years) type 2 diabetic patients over a mean study period of 11 years. As in the UGDP,[3] there was no effect of optimized blood glucose control on macrovascular endpoints. Unlike in the UGDP,[3] however, the prognosis of microangiopathy was improved, mainly as a result of a significant reduction of the progression of retinopathy (photocoagulation treatments). This success was independent of whether the intensive treatment policy was based on insulin or glibenclamide.[4]

About 20% of all patients with NIDDM show no initial response to sulfonylurea drugs (*primary failures*). Between 5 and 10% of the patients who initially responded satisfactorily develop *secondary failure* during each year of follow-up. It has been shown that after 10 years of sulfonylurea therapy, the drugs continue to be effective in a very small percentage (less than 15%) of those who initially responded. *Since there are no absolute indications for the use of a sulfonylurea, it is crucial*

that rigid selection criteria be enforced before patients with NIDDM are treated with a sulfonylurea. These agents should not be used in patients who have a history of diabetic ketoacidosis, who have been primary or secondary failures on other sulfonylureas, who have kidney or liver disease, or who are pregnant. *Particular caution is warranted in patients with coronary artery disease.* There is universal agreement that some 80% of all overweight patients with NIDDM can—at least early on during the disease—achieve satisfactory metabolic control if they adhere to a hypocaloric diet combined with an exercise program of mild intensity. Thus, there is no indication to treat obese diabetic patients at stable body weight with sulfonylurea drugs. Such treatment is superfluous, and because of possible side effects it may be harmful.

The argument that obese diabetic patients (nonadherent to weight reduction and exercise therapy) should be given the benefit of treatment with a sulfonylurea to prevent the development of hyperglycemic hyperosmolar coma is not based on valid clinical research. Haupt and associates[26] have shown that the discontinuation of sulfonylurea treatment in obese, non-diet-adherent patients in unsatisfactory metabolic control did not increase the level of hyperglycemia.

Unfortunately, *the use of sulfonylurea drugs has become entrenched as the "treatment of laziness" on the part of both the physician and the patient.* How much easier is it to prescribe or swallow a pill than to explain or adhere to a weight-reducing diet in combination with an increase in caloric expenditure? The central problems of the syndrome for which Ethan Sims has coined the term "diabesity" (representing more than 80% of the patients with NIDDM in the industrialized world) are insulin resistance and arterial hypertension associated with obesity/hyperphagia and immobilization.[27] Any rational treatment of this disorder should be based on attempts to *increase* insulin sensitivity. *Thus, hypocaloric dieting and increased physical activity must remain the bases of therapy for overweight patients with NIDDM.*

Recently, we have developed and evaluated a structured treatment and teaching program for NIDDM[28] at the primary health care level (i.e., the office of the practicing physician or an outpatient institution, depending on the characteristics of a given health care system). The principal components of this program are: (1) individual definition of therapeutic objectives for each patient (in contrast to the unspecified global normalization of laboratory values, as attempted by various current policy groups and statements); (2) therapeutic and educational strategies (following earlier recommendations of A. Bouchardat in 1875[29]) based on systematic self-monitoring of glucosuria, simple and flexible nutritional guidelines, and nondrug therapy; (3) emphasis on prevention of acute complications and foot problems; and (4) patient education in structured group sessions. On long-term evaluations based on a prospective controlled trial, this program resulted in a *50% reduction of the use of oral antidiabetic agents, significant weight loss, and substantial improvements of other parameters of diabetes care* in a population of (typically) elderly patients with NIDDM. The efficacy of the program was maintained even after its implementation into Germany's general health care system.[30,31]

Only if patients (without coronary artery disease) are still hyperglycemic despite significant weight loss over several weeks, or if they are already of normal weight and are reasonably physically active, may the use of sulfonylurea drugs be justified—as an alternative to insulin therapy.

Other Effects, Side Effects, Drug Interactions. All currently available sulfonylurea drugs are free of any relevant bacteriostatic activity. However, they may affect a number of other organ systems besides the pancreatic β-cell and the insulin-dependent glucose transport and/or disposition in liver, muscle, and adipose cells, such as through the closure of K_{ATP} channels.

An important question, not yet answered, relates to the *cardiovascular side effects* of sulfonylurea therapy. Earlier animal experiments had suggested a positive inotropic and potentially arrhythmogenic effect of tolbutamide. In 1970, first results from a multicenter trial carried out in the United States (UGPD study) designed to measure the effect of the level of metabolic control on the development of vascular complications in patients with NIDDM were published.[3]

A significant increase in cardiovascular mortality was found in the patients taking tolbutamide, in direct contrast to patients treated with insulin variable dose, insulin standard dose, and placebo. A number of diabetologists discontinued prescribing sulfonylureas, and the use of the drugs fell significantly in the United States as a consequence of the report. Later on, deficiencies in the study design and execution were claimed by a number of critics but were not confirmed by an independent committee appointed by the FDA.

The acrimonious debate that ensued was dominated by drug companies with a vested interest, statisticians, health politicians, lawyers, and the bruised emotions of prescribing physicians and sulfonylurea-consuming patients.[32] Based on present therapeutic strategies and goals for those with NIDDM, the design of the UGDP study left unanswered questions. Neither vigorous attempts to reduce the overweight (a large majority of those studied) nor tolbutamide dose adjustment were included in the design of the trial. Nevertheless, the study and resulting controversy helped reduce, at least in some countries, the excessive use of sulfonylureas. The UGDP study was instrumental in stimulating some national diabetes associations (the American Diabetes Association in 1979 and the German Diabetes Associa-

tion in 1983) to release official policy statements on an optimized treatment of NIDDM. Both highlighted the fundamental importance of hypocaloric diet therapy, weight reduction, and regular physical activity as the bases of a rational approach to the management of NIDDM. Sulfonylurea treatment was described as a potentially beneficial adjunctive treatment in only a limited percentage of patients with NIDDM. However, uncertainty continued to exist about possible cardiotoxic side effects of sulfonylureas.

Despite warnings as to a potential causal relationship between the use of tolbutamide and an increased incidence of cardiovascular mortality in type 2 diabetic patients, sulfonylureas have maintained their worldwide position as the number one oral antidiabetic class of drugs toward the late 1990s. In fact, a whole array of sulfonylurea drugs have been developed and marketed worldwide without having ever been scrutinized to a proof of safety similar to the UGDP study protocol[3] until the UKPDS reported their final results in 1998.[4]

The main reason why the surprising observations of the UGDP study on tolbutamide's cardiotoxicity were looked upon with so much skepticism that they hardly ever transpired into habitual treatment strategies of our health care systems appears to lie in the lack of any pathophysiologic explanation for this phenomenon.[33] Subsequently, the detrimental cardiotoxic side effect of tolbutamide seen in the UGDP[3] has not been reproduced for glibenclamide or chlorpropamide in type 2 diabetic patients (without clinically significant coronary heart disease) in the UKPDS.[4] Unfortunately, the protocol of eligibility for the UKPDS excluded patients with clinically evident heart disease,[4] in contrast to the UGDP,[3] which, with its constituent of a true sample of patients, also newly diagnosed, were admitted without this exclusion. For example, in patients 40–60 years of age, 14–23.1% of the males and 8.6–13.5% of the females in the participating clinical centers had EKG abnormalities and/or a history of angina.[3]

In this context, important experimental findings have been reported in animals and humans. The closure of K_{ATP} channels at various cellular systems of the heart by sulfonylurea drugs could prevent the coronary dilatory response to ischemia, i.e., local vasodilation and mobilization of coronary reserve,[34] to block action potential shortening and to prevent ischaemic preconditioning. Thus, it is through their blockage of K_{ATP} channels that pretreatment with sulfonylureas appears to aggravate the hypoxic damage to the myocardium in the case of coronary occlusion.[11,35] These observations could represent the pathophysiologic plausibility for the UGDP's finding on tolbutamide. In fact, it has been hypothesized that they may explain the different effects of various diabetes treatments on cardiovascular morbidity and mortality seen in the VA CDMS and in the DIGAMI study.[36]

Taken together, these recent findings call for particular caution concerning the use of sulfonylurea drugs in type 2 diabetic patients with coronary artery disease. In fact, it is our opinion that the—albeit incomplete—evidence indicating a cardiotoxic effect of sulfonylurea drugs has become substantial enough to shift the burden of proof to those who are still using sulfonylurea drugs in type 2 diabetic patients with coronary heart disease to document that this is actually safe. Until evidence has been provided to exempt a singular drug from cardiotoxicity, the possibility of an increase of cardiovascular mortality in patients with coronary heart disease applies for all oral antidiabetic agents that exert their β-cytotropic effects via the closure of K_{ATP} channels, i.e., all sulfonylurea and the aforementioned benzoic acid derivatives. Accordingly, the package inserts in the USA include a "Special Warning on Increased Risk of Cardiovascular Mortality" for all of those antidiabetic drugs.[12] In this context, it is worrysome that the ADA's *Consensus Statement: The Pharmacological Treatment of Hyperglycemia in NIDDM* of July 1995[37] does not even mention the danger of a potential cardiovascular toxicity of oral sulfonylurea antidiabetic therapy in patients with type 2 diabetes and coronary heart disease.

To confirm or exclude the persistent suspicion as to cardiotoxicity of oral antidiabetic drugs that work via closure of K_{ATP} channels, a respective randomized prospective study directed to the clinically relevant endpoints comparing insulin and oral antidiabetic drug therapies is urgently required in type 2 diabetic patients with coronary artery disease.[35,36] The results of such a study will be relevant to the treatment of many millions of patients worldwide. The UKPDS is unhelpful in this context, as patients with clinically relevant coronary artery disease were excluded from the trial[4]; furthermore, the power of the study is insufficient to rule out clinically relevant differences concerning cardiovascular morbidity and mortality between the four treatment arms aimed at intensified stepwise metabolic control.

Hypoglycemia is a potentially lethal side effect of sulfonylurea therapy. The high incidence of severe hypoglycemia associated with sulfonylurea treatments actually is a reflection of the excessive and inappropriate use of the agents by physicians and patients.

A number of reviews have summarized the literature and included representative case reports.[14,38,39] Excessive doses of sulfonylureas can precipitate severe hypoglycemia. The highest relative risk is associated with the long-acting drugs chlorpropamide and glibenclamide. The available literature indicates that the incidence of severe hypoglycemia in sulfonylurea-treated patients is disturbingly high, with a majority of the cases occurring in the elderly. It appears that many cases of severe hypoglycemia in these patients are initially diagnosed as cerebrovascular accidents, cerebral arteriosclerosis,

or alcohol and/or drug abuse. Repeated episodes of hypoglycemia may contribute to progressive mental deterioration of elderly patients treated with sulfonylurea drugs. Asplund and coworkers[38] have reported a strong correlation between the use of sulfonylureas in a health care system and the incidences of severe iatrogenic hypoglycemia. It is well known that sulfonylurea-induced hypoglycemia has a high rate of mortality and morbidity (permanent neurologic damage), particularly in the elderly patient. Characteristically, sulfonylurea-induced hypoglycemia is protracted. Patients should be hospitalized. Even though they may respond immediately to IV glucose, they often relapse into profound hypoglycemia and must be treated with parenteral glucose for several days. Risk factors that seem to predispose individuals to the development of severe hypoglycemia include: (1) age above 70 years, (2) history of cerebrovascular accidents or cardiac disorders, (3) impairment of renal or hepatic function, (4) alcohol use, (5) irregular food intake, (6) diarrhea, (7) physical exercise,[40] and, probably of crucial importance, (8) interaction with other drugs, since even small doses of glibenclamide (2.5–5 mg/day) have produced severe hypoglycemia and fatal outcomes.[38] It is claimed that the risk of severe hypoglycemia is substantially reduced or even abolished with the newer drugs glimepiride and repaglinide.

It appears, in general, that neither physicians, patients, nor relatives are adequately educated about the danger of sulfonylurea-induced severe hypoglycemia, its early signs, its therapy, its predisposing factors, and appropriate methods for its prevention. This lack of information on the part of the medical profession and patients appears particularly relevant with regard to the interaction of sulfonylureas with other drugs. In this context it should be noted that the vast majority of those with NIDDM are on at least one additional medication. In a survey of a British diabetes clinic it was discovered that more than 50% of the patients were on one to five other drugs that would interfere with medication.[41] Similar observations were reported from East Germany.[42] Iatrogenically induced side effects of drug interactions now appear to be a major threat to elderly individuals with NIDDM.[43]

Much concern is regularly being voiced with regard to the *weight gain* as a side effect of sulfonylurea treatment. Thus, over a decade of the UKPDS[4] initially normal-weight patients on sulfonylurea treatment gained a mean of 5 kg compared to around 2.5 kg increase in the control (conventional policy) group, whereas overweight patients in the metformin group maintained their body weight. It has been suggested that repaglinide administration is not associated with appreciable weight gain.

Whether—at comparable levels of metabolic and blood pressure control—body weight differences of such a magnitude do play a significant role concerning the prognosis of the patients appears doubtful.[4,44,45]

A number of various, rather nonspecific, side effects have been noted for sulfonylurea drugs. Chlorpropamide and (to a lesser extent) tolbutamide are antidiuretic; sulfonylureas, in particular gliclazide, may reduce platelet aggregation. The clinical significance of those observations is unknown. Some first-generation sulfonylureas were reported to be uricosuric, a finding that was not noted in studies of some of the second-generation drugs. Unconfirmed reports have suggested an increased risk of the development of hypothyroidism associated with sulfonylurea treatment. Disturbing findings indicating low levels of high-density lipoprotein (HDL) cholesterol associated with sulfonylurea treatment, independent of the degree of metabolic control,[46] have remained unconfirmed.

For most of the sulfonylureas, chlorpropamide in particular, isolated cases of toxic side effects such as skin eruptions, aplastic anemia, thrombocytopenia, and cholestatic jaundice have been reported. These severe complications have been rare and are usually reversible on cessation of treatment.

Chlorpropamide has been noted to induce an antabuselike syndrome and/or alcohol-flushing. Similar observations, although less frequent, are reported for most other sulfonylurea drugs. Earlier suggestions that the chlorpropamide alcohol flush was a genetic marker for some subtypes of diabetes mellitus had to be abandoned.[47]

The problem of *drug interactions* as related to sulfonylurea treatment (Table 20–2) was reviewed extensively by Jackson and Bressler[14] and by Hansen and Christensen.[48] The hypoglycemic action of sulfonylureas may be potentiated by pharmacodynamic or pharmacokinetic drug interactions. The list of such interactions with other drugs differs substantially from one sulfonylurea to another. First-generation sulfonylureas are potentiated by anionic-type medications such as aspirin, phenylbutazone, warfarin, and so forth, since these drugs displace first-generation sulfonylureas from albumin-binding sites. No such interactions occur with second-generation sulfonylureas such as glibenclamide, which is bound to albumin by nonionic forces.[49]

Space is not adequate to present a comprehensive list of interactions of sulfonylureas with other pharmaceutical agents. Table 20–2 gives the principles and some examples for such drug interactions. For further details of this complicated field of clinical pharmacology, the reader is referred to two reviews.[14,48] Clearly, the area of drug interactions has been neglected as it relates to the treatment of patients with NIDDM, the majority of whom are being treated by a number of additional medications simultaneously. In addition to numerous potential drug interactions, the problem is further complicated by interindividual differences in the rate of elimination of various drugs (and their combinations) related to the phenomena of polymorphic drug oxidation[50] and pharmacogenetics. All of these unknowns seem to make the assessment of potential risks and benefits of sulfonylurea treatment a labor of Sisyphus. The magnitude of these problems suggests that drug treatment in general and sulfonylurea therapy in particular should be restricted to those NIDDM patients who can really benefit from it.

Combination-Therapy Insulin/Sulfonylurea Drugs

Recently, interest has been revived in an early treatment routine combining sulfonylureas and insulin, which at one time was abandoned as ineffective. It has been suggested that such an approach might facilitate the achievement of adequate metabolic control; that it may reduce insulin requirements, and thus may possibly prevent hyperinsulinemia; that it may render a second (or third) insulin injection unnecessary in NIDDM patients with secondary failure of sulfonylurea drugs; and that it may make the initiation of insulin therapy more easily acceptable, especially for the elderly patient. Of these frequently stipulated expectations, little has been confirmed by adequate clinical trials.

Actually, there are innumerable different strategies of insulin/sulfonylurea combination therapies, depending on which type of insulin is given how many times daily at which times and on which strategy of sulfonylurea treatment is pursued. Recommendations on how to adjust the dosages of the different therapeutic measures are unclear. In general, it appears that the "combination therapies" are justified by some short-term studies[51] directed to the incidence of severe hypoglycemia, metabolic surrogate markers, and practicability- and cost-related scores as well as on the diabetologists' own clinical experience.

Although a reduction of insulin requirements has been unequivocally documented when sulfonylurea drugs are combined with insulin therapy in NIDDM patients with residual β-cell secretory capacity, this has *not* been associated with a reproducible decrease of peripheral serum insulin levels.[52,53] In the majority of trials, combining sulfonylureas with insulin was not associated with an improvement of metabolic control; however, an increased risk of hypoglycemia, a reduction of serum HDL-cholesterol, and (depending on the specifics of the health care system) an increase of the treatment costs were repeatedly reported when sulfonylurea drugs were combined with conventional insulin therapy in NIDDM.

A fundamental problem of the combination therapy of insulin and sulfonylurea drugs is related to the difficulty of an easy adaptation of therapeutic dosage in

TABLE 20–2   Mechanisms of Drug Interactions with Sulfonylureas[a]

Type of Interaction	Hypoglycemic Effects of Sulfonylureas	Examples
Pharmacokinetic Interactions		
1. Change in absorption		
Decrease	Diminished, postponed	Hyperglycemia
Increase	Increased	Cisaprid (?)
2. Change in protein binding		
Decrease	Immediate potentiation, later possible return to normal	Phenylbutazone, salicylate, clofibrate, (some) sulfonamides
Increase	Diminished, possibly prolongation of half-life	Phenobarbitone
3. Change in hepatic metabolism		
Decrease	Potentiated and prolonged	Chloramphenicol
Increase	Diminished	Dicoumarol, phenylbutazone, clofibrate, chronic alcoholism, rifampicine, phenobarbitone
4. Change in renal excretion		
Decrease	Potentiated and prolonged	Probenecid, salicylate, phenylbutazone
Pharmacodynamic Interactions		
1. Change in insulin secretion		
Increase	Potentiated	Monoamino-oxidase inhibitors
Decrease	Diminished	Methysergide, thiazides, phenytoin, non-steroidal anti-inflammatory agents, diazoxide
2. Change in peripheral insulin sensitivity		
Increase	Potentiated	Metformin, thiazolidinedione, ACE inhibitors
Decrease	Diminished	Anabolic steroids, potassium depletion (by diuretics)
3. Change in hepatic glucose production		
Increase	Diminished	Glucocorticoids
Decrease	Potentiated	Methylxanthines, guanethidine, reserpine, ethanol, salicylates, metformin
4. Change in glucose absorption		
Decrease	Potentiated	Acarbose, metformin
5. Inhibition of counterregulation of hypoglycemia	Potentiated	noncardioselective β-blockade (e.g., propranalol)

[a] The examples given in this table are arbitrarily selected from a considerably larger body of information on drug interactions with sulfonylureas; they do not always apply to all sulfonylurea drugs, since these vary considerably with regard to their metabolism, binding to serum albumin, and excretion rates. Source: Ref. 14, with permission.

cases of unsatisfactory metabolic control. At least for the patients, it will be difficult to figure out whether to reduce the dose of their long-acting insulin preparation or their sulfonylurea drug when faced with a tendency of hypoglycemic reactions, e.g., before lunchtime.

Although it *may* be practical to *initiate* insulin treatment in NIDDM patients with secondary failure of sulfonylurea therapy by adding small (stepwise up to maximally 20 U insulin/day) dosages of insulin to the failing sulfonylurea drug, even this frequently advocated therapeutic option needs to be scrutinized in a prospective controlled comparison with the long-term effectivity of a treatment and teaching program based on conventional insulin therapy in patients with NIDDM.[54] Unless such trials have been completed with unequivocally positive results, the combination therapy insulin/sulfonylurea drugs cannot be justified as evidence-based.

Excessive Utilization of Sulfonylurea Drugs

Although there is little doubt of a potential benefit of sulfonylurea treatment in carefully selected patients with NIDDM,[4] the excessive and unjustified use of these drugs has become more and more apparent in recent years. It is of note that substantial differences have always existed from one country to another with regard to physicians' sulfonylurea-prescribing habits,[55] despite comparable prevalence rates for NIDDM. In the United States, doubts concerning the sulfonylureas' effectivity and safety as raised by the UGDP study resulted in a decrease of their use after 1975 with a nadir in 1979. When skepticism was tempered by the revised policy statement of the ADA in 1979,[56] the use of these agents increased quite dramatically: In 1986, 38% of all diagnosed diabetic patients were on oral sulfonylurea therapy. Based on West German sales figures for the mid-1980s, almost every patient with NIDDM not on insulin therapy was on sulfonylurea therapy. Thus, it came as no surprise that glibenclamide was by far the best-selling drug in West Germany with a 1982 turnover of approximately 350 million German marks (based on pharmacy sales figures), almost twice as high as the number two drug on the list (i.e., a cimetidine preparation). It is unlikely that the abuse of oral antidiabetic agents in West Germany was due to the free market health care system, since East German figures also indicated excessive use of sulfonylureas. In 1996, glibenclamide still accounted for 64% of the entire market of antidiabetic agents prescribed to an estimated 2.4 million type 2 diabetic patients in Germany.

One is tempted to hypothesize that physicians, patients, and the public are not well acquainted with the potential risk of excessive sulfonylurea use, which may exert negative effects on the quality of care in various ways. Thus, patients and physicians may fail to even attempt to implement the standard therapies for NIDDM, i.e. hypocaloric nutrition and physical activity. According to the data by Asplund and coworkers,[38] overuse of sulfonylureas will result in increasing incidence rates of side effects of this type of drug treatment, such as severe hypoglycemia, with their potential cardiotoxicity in patients with coronary heart disease representing an additional point of concern. National diabetes associations should educate the medical profession and the public about the dangers and unnecessary financial expenditures associated with the excessive use of sulfonylureas.

Biguanides

Introduced in the mid-1950s, the use of biguanides (see Exhibit 20–2) declined worldwide in the late 1970s; in many countries biguanides were actually banned. Metformin, however, has always remained in use in some countries, and as of the late 1980s it had regained much of its popularity in the context of a marketing campaign coined "metformin renaissance." The drug was approved for U.S. distribution in 1995.

Biguanides do not affect pancreatic β-cell function nor glycemia in normal individuals, but they exert a reproducible antihyperglycemic effect in hyperglycemic patients with NIDDM. The drugs were thought to have an inhibitory action on glucose absorption from the intestinal tract and a stimulatory effect on glucose uptake by peripheral tissues, probably resulting from an inhibition of glucose oxidation.[57] The latter effect is compatible with the observed acceleration of anerobic glycolysis and the tendency of the drugs to increase lactate turnover and plasma lactate levels. Contradictory reports about effects of biguanides on insulin receptor interactions and postreceptor events related to glucose metabolism have appeared. More recently, Stumvoll et al.[58] have shown that metformin's antihyperglycemic effect is almost exclusively due to an inhibition of hepatic glucose production; simultaneously, the drug led to an apparent increase of insulin sensitivity, lowered the rate of conversion of plasma lactate to plasma glucose, and resulted in considerable weight loss. Metformin has gastrointestinal side effects, including loss of appetite and anorexia in up to 40% of patients, and it causes vitamin B_{12} and folate malabsorption. Whether the long-term clinical efficacy of the drug in lowering glycemia is causally related to a decrease in food intake and weight loss, as recently suggested,[59,60] has not been definitively ruled out.

During the 1950s and 1970s, biguanides were used extensively, frequently combined with sulfonylurea or insulin therapy. When the use of sulfonylureas became controversial in the wake of UGDP reports, the use of biguanides boomed. That phenformin was also associated with excess cardiovascular mortality in the UGDP study[3] was hardly noticed; in fact, in this study, phenformin was also found to be associated with an increase in blood pressure, an observation that was confirmed by a significant reduction of blood pressure after withdrawal of biguanides in a study on 118 patients with NIDDM in Finland.[61]

A number of years later, approximately 20 years after the introduction of the biguanides, the association of increased levels of blood lactate during long-term use was rediscovered. This was related to the increased availability of methods to measure blood lactate levels in clinical laboratories. A disturbingly high incidence of lactic acidosis was discovered in patients being treated with biguanides.[62] Lactic acidosis associated with an accumulation of biguanides in the blood and in the liver[62] had a very high fatality rate (from 30% to 90% in different investigations). As a result of these reports, phenformin was banned in most countries in the late 1970s. According to retrospective analyses, the incidence of lactic acidosis in patients on biguanide therapy differed between the various biguanide drugs. Thus, it was claimed that the risk of lactic acidosis was less in patients on metformin than in those on phenformin or buformin. Whether these assessments were actually correct remains questionable. A notable observation was made by Bosisio and colleagues[63] with regard to the apparent heterogeneity of the incidence of biguanide side effects between various surveys. In accordance with the studies by Scott and Poffenbarger,[18] these authors have suggested a genetic polymorphism of the phenformin hydroxylating mechanism that might predispose certain subgroups of patients, i.e., the slow eliminators, to develop high drug levels in the blood and liver and, hence, increase the risk of lactic acidosis.

In any case, the responsible government agencies decided in many European countries to ban phenformin and buformin, whereas metformin remained on the market. As expected, *á la longue* this development reignited interest in metformin.[64,65] Nevertheless, with the exception of Great Britain, France, and some Mediterranean countries, metformin played an insignificant role in the care of NIDDM during the 1980s: only in some diabetes centers was metformin still recommended for overweight patients with diet failure resulting in "refractory" obesity or hypertriglyceridemia. Beginning in the late 1970s, a marketing campaign advocating the use of metformin in NIDDM, particularly in overweight hyperinsulinemic patients, was initiated in Europe, even though new data or arguments in favor of effectivity or safety of the drug were never presented. Nevertheless, the metformin renaissance campaign led to a sharp increase in metformin sales in Germany from 8.9 million prescribed daily doses (DDDs) in 1985 to 119 million DDDs in 1996 (Table 20–3), with metformin accounting for 18% of the entire prescription volume for oral antidiabetic agents. In 1995, metformin was approved for use in the United States and is presently available on a worldwide basis. In parallel, a large number of clinical studies were published describing the well-known antihyperglycemic properties of metformin, as monotherapy, in combination or in comparison with other hypoglycemic therapies, using various clinical protocols[66,67]; with a maximum length of 12 months, mostly carried out for several weeks or months only,

TABLE 20–3 Oral antidiabetic drugs: sales, costs in Germany and in the USA

Oral antidiabetic Drug	Sales in West Germany[a] 1985 (prescribed DDD)	Sales in Germany[b] 1996 (Prescribed DDD) [Percent Change compared to 1995]	Approximate Average cost/ Month of treatment with DDD in 1996[d]	Cost/Month of treatments (USA)
Sulfonylureas				
Glibenclamide	305 million	572 million [−7%]	5 DM	≈17 US$
Glimepride	0	0[c]	35 DM[c]	20.73 US$
Other	97 million	0	0	(chlorpropamide 1.45 US$; tolbutamide 2.75 US$)
Metformin	8.9 million	119 million [+26%]	21 DM	47.20 US$
Acarbose	0	77 million [+8%]	60 DM	41.05 US$
Troglitazone	–	–	–	104.40 US$

[a] Total population 63 million.   DDD = defined daily dosage

[b] Total population 80 million.

[c] Data from 1997.

[d] DM, German marks.

German data adapted from Schwabe U, Paffrath D (Hrsg): Arzeiverordnungsreport '86 and '97. Gustav Fischer Verlag, Stuttgart, 1986, 1997.

U.S. data from Ref. 96 and from Bachman KH, Leviston L: Cost of troglitazone therapy. Arch Intern Med 158:1038, 1998.

these studies were unable to shed any light on efficacy and safety of metformin. Needless to say, no attempts were made to confirm or exclude the potential cardiovascular risk, as indicated during the UGDP study, or to prospectively quantitate the risk of lactic acidosis. No satisfactory documentation of potential patient-oriented outcome benefits and safety of biguanide therapy was ever brought forward until the UKPDS results became available in 1998.[4]

As to the problem of metformin-associated lactic acidosis, meta-analytic calculations based upon data generated under study conditions have estimated an average risk of 0.03 cases per 1,000 patient-years.[66] Suffice it to add that under these conditions, patients are highly selected in order to minimize the risk of lactic acidosis. However, during observational phases of study patients[68] or after introduction of metformin in the routine of the general health care system[69,70] when the surveillance of metformin therapy is bound to be less strict, higher incidence rates of lactic acidosis are to be anticipated. In a recent survey in a German general hospital on consecutively admitted type 2 diabetic patients on metformin therapy, at least one of the contraindications had been neglected in 79% of cases.[71] Furthermore, metformin accumulation may occur for unknown reasons,[72] and some 10% of patients who develop metformin-associated lactic acidosis may not have any of the known risk factors or contraindications to metformin therapy.[73] Consequently, the fear has been voiced that *the renaissance of metformin is being followed by a renaissance of lactic acidosis.*

Furthermore, the risk of a biguanide-associated increase in cardiovascular mortality has still not been excluded for metformin. Albeit metformin monotherapy was not associated with increased blood pressure or an increased cardiovascular mortality risk during the UKPDS,[4] there is still concern over the possibility of untoward cardiovascular side effects of the drug when used in combination with sulfonylurea treatment.[74] In fact, the final results of the UKPDS have confirmed this suspicion as *metformin given in combination with sulfonylureas led to an increase of diabetes-related total mortality.*[4] In the meantime, the issue of metformin's safety has become the subject of an ongoing data-monitoring process in the United States.[75]

In conclusion, first-line pharmacotherapy with metformin as monotherapy in the treatment of overweight seems to be advantageous. However, it needs to be restricted by a formidable list of contraindications, as even authors who advocate limited use of metformin exclude (1) patients with cardiac, hepatic, respiratory, or renal insufficiency/dysfunction; (2) those over age 65 years; (3) those who ingest alcohol regularly; (4) those with chronic or acute infections; (5) pregnant women; (6) those on less than 1,000 calories per day; and (7) those who are "noncooperative" (i.e., who can

not be expected to have blood lactate and creatinine levels and other variables checked on a regular basis). Furthermore, patients who perform physical exercise at anaerobic levels of intensity, patients with intercurrent illness, those on treatment with diuretic drugs, perioperative patients, and patients undergoing hemoconcentration need to be excluded.

In the light of such a *formidable list of contraindications,* there is only a limited number of patients with NIDDM remaining as potential candidates for biguanide therapy, mainly those who are overweight, newly manifest, and do not respond to non-drug-therapy. On the other hand, there may be specific indications for metformin treatment, such as the polycystic ovary syndrome.[76]

On balance, metformin exhibits a substantial antihyperglycemic effect in patients with type 2 diabetes, alone or in combination with other oral antidiabetic agents and/or insulin, and it affects a number of other surrogate markers beneficially. Concerning patient-oriented outcomes substantial benefits and safety have been shown for younger overweight newly manifest type 2 diabetic patients in the UKPDS[4] when metformin is given as monotherapy; the combination of metformin with sulfonylurea treatment appeared to increase mortality in this study.[4] Concerning the risk of potentially fatal lactic acidosis, metformin's safety issue is further complicated by a long list of contraindications. Taking the cost of the drug into account (Table 20–3), metformin seems to be a useful drug for a very limited group of NIDDM patients.

Drugs Delaying or Inhibiting Carbohydrate Absorption

During the past decades, efforts have been made to delay the absorption of complex carbohydrates in order to lower postprandial hyperglycemia in patients with diabetes mellitus. Thus, enrichment of nutrients with indigestible dietary fiber (Lente carbohydrates) has been shown to be useful in delaying intestinal absorption of carbohydrates and thus to diminish hyperglycemia after meals in patients with diabetes.[77]

Antiamylase or amylase-blocking agents, often referred to as "starch-blockers," are not useful in the treatment of patients with NIDDM. An α-glucosid(e hydrol)ase inhibitor (Exhibit 20–2) such as the drug acarbose[78,79] seems more promising. It causes competitive inhibition of disacharidases, delays enzymatic breakdown of polysaccharides and oligosaccharides in the upper gastrointestinal tract, and thus lowers postprandial hyperglycemia by delaying glucose absorption; furthermore, it does not confer any risk of hypoglycemia, lactic acidosis, or weight gain. In fact, a Medline search covering 1978 to June 1998 identified

412 studies on acarbose that—almost invariably—testify for the positive effect of acarbose in lowering glycemia and HbA_{1c} levels, alone or in combination with other hypoglycemic therapies, mostly in type 2, but also in type 1 diabetes—a message that has also been heralded by innumerable (satellite) symposia, congresses, workshops, and other marketing exercises throughout the world. For some groups of patients, e.g., obese hyperinsulinaemic (pre-)diabetic patients, acarbose has even been advocated as first-line drug therapy,[80,81] as it was suggested that the drug would increase insulin sensitivity by a primary decrease of prandial hyperglycemia followed by lower circulating insulin levels—with the potential of primary prevention of type 2 diabetes in high-risk individuals or as a means of delaying sulfonylurea secondary failure in long-term type 2 diabetes.

Nevertheless, the reproducibility of the drug's long-term hypoglycemic effects has not been impressive. In some studies, no consistent effects on HbA_{1c} levels could be demonstrated. In the course of the UKPD study,[82] a randomized, double-blind added-on therapy with acarbose or placebo was performed in some 1900 type 2 diabetic patients. After 3 years HbA_{1c} levels had been lowered by 0.2% in the acarbose group, with only 61% of patients remaining on the treatment because of side effects, with flatulence, crampy abdominal pain, and discomfort representing the main reasons for noncompliance. In fact, throughout several studies the frequency of malabsorption symptoms such as flatulence, abdominal cramps, diarrhea, and so forth was high and disturbingly variable.[83] Accordingly, studies based on carbohydrate turnover measurements in humans have confirmed a significant degree of malabsorption after an oral sucrose load following the administration of acarbose.[84] Other side effects of acarbose include hepatotoxicity[85–87] and a rise in serum acetate levels potentially related to adverse effects on total cholesterol or apolipoprotein B levels.[88]

Subsequently, the following contraindications have been put forward: renal insufficiency (serum creatinine >2.0 mg/dl), liver function abnormalities, inflammatory bowel disease, colonic ulceration or partial intestinal obstruction, pregnancy, and childhood.

Nevertheless, as of 1996 acarbose has been generally approved as an oral antidiabetic drug on a worldwide basis. Acarbose is given with meals in dosages up to 100 mg t.i.d.; should hypoglycemia occur in diabetic patients on acarbose treatment, for effective oral treatment one would have to use glucose (instead of sucrose). As of 1996, acarbose prescriptions made up 15% of the entire volume of oral antidiabetic prescriptions in Germany, and it thus became—due to its high price (costs per DDD are 15 times more expensive than glibenclamide)—the best-selling oral antidiabetic drug in Germany, based upon financial turnover.

More recently, the absorbable α-glucosidase inhibitor miglitol was subjected to short-term evaluations in an attempt to decrease the high rate of malabsorption-related symptoms that are a feature of acarbose therapy.[89]

Based on the considerations of cost-effectiveness and of potential hazards of a drug-induced delay of carbohydrate absorption (especially if associated with malabsorption[90]), physicians and patients should prefer dietary means to decrease postprandial hyperglycemia, if indicated, and more importantly, they should concentrate on attempts to interfere with the *basic* pathophysiologic problems of NIDDM (see Chapters 2 and 16).

Thiazolidinediones (Insulin Sensitizers)

In the course of animal experimentation during the 1980s, the group of thiazolidinediones (Exhibit 20–3) was identified as *insulin sensitizers,* as they were shown to improve peripheral insulin sensitivity; in diabetic animals (with persisting endogenous insulin secretion), these drugs lowered glycemia, serum levels of free fatty acids, triglycerides, and insulin. Such an action profile seemed to render these drugs ideal candidates for a causal treatment of the metabolic syndrome/type 2 diabetes mellitus. Thus, during the early 1990s, troglitazone was intensively studied in type 2 diabetic patients. Alone or in combination with sulfonylureas or insulin treatment, troglitazone increased peripheral glucose disposal via an improved peripheral insulin sensitivity. In a series of studies, it was shown that troglitazone acted beneficially on Hb A_{1c} levels and also lowered elevated triglyceride levels, serum insulin, and proinsulin concentrations, and—in some but not all studies—had a beneficial effect on arterial hypertension. In some studies, there was a tendency of weight gain, however. Even though thiazolidinediones were shown to exert transcriptional effects on fatty acid metabolism by activating a special subclass of PPAR receptor (PPARγ), the mechanism(s) for their overall therapeutic concept to treat (early) type 2 diabetes by improving insulin sensitivity was never fully elucidated. Following a series of positive short- and medium-term studies demonstrating a very benign safety profile and positive efficacy of troglitazone on surrogate markers (HbA_{1c}, risk factors, and markers),[91–93] as well as overall optimistic endorsements by opinion leaders,[94–97] the drug was marketed in Japan, the United States, and Great Britain as of 1997. In fact, within a few months troglitazone became one of the fastest-selling drugs in history.[98] Following reports of (idiosyncratic) *hepatotoxicity associated with the use of troglitazone, the marketing in Great Britain and efforts to get the drug accepted in the European Community were suspended in November 1997; in the United States and Japan a* number of safety restrictions were imposed, but *the drug was not withdrawn* and was still looked upon with great hopes by some.[99]

Even though the thiozolidinediones had looked promising as a innovative drug for potential prevention and treatment of type 2 diabetes to many investigators and opinion leaders, several issues had remained unaddressed before the drug was recommended and accepted for general use: (1) the mechanism(s) of action were incompletely understood and (2) no evidence was provided for long-term efficacy (reductions of excess cardiovascular and/or microangiopathic morbidity and mortality rates) and safety in patients with type 2 diabetes mellitus. Under those circumstances, a somewhat more careful attitude should have been warranted.[100]

Concluding Remarks

Diet therapy, weight reduction, and increased exercise remain the rational therapeutic modalities available for the treatment of NIDDM. In case individual therapeutic goals cannot be achieved, appropriate insulin therapy is the treatment of choice for efficacy and safety reasons. It is estimated that, at a maximum, 20–30% of patients with NIDDM may benefit from the adjunctive use of oral antidiabetic agents. Presently, there are four classes of oral antidiabetic agents: β-cytotropic agents (sulfonylureas, benzoic acid derivatives), biguanides (metformin), disaccharidase inhibitors (acarbose), and thiazolidinediones (troglitazone). The vast majority of type 2 diabetic patients, estimated as 100 million worldwide, is treated with one of these drugs—and increasingly often they are combined in *a stepped-up approach* until all four pharmaceutical principles are being used, in many cases in addition to insulin therapy.

All of the oral antidiabetic drugs have significant antihyperglycemic potencies, and they seem beneficial concerning various additional surrogate markers. For none of these drugs—prescribed alone or in combination—has an improvement of macrovascular morbidity or mortality been documented with the exception of metformin monotherapy in overweight patients newly diagnosed with type 2 diabetes.[4] In younger newly manifest patients beneficial effects with regard to the development of microangiopathy have been documented for glibenclamide (as for insulin), if HbA_{1c} levels can be kept at a medium level of 7.0% over 10 years. Whether this benefit can be reproduced by other oral antidiabetic agents is unknown. For none of these drugs has long-term safety been shown in patients with coronary heart disease. *Metformin in combination with sulfonylurea led to increased mortality* in the UKPDS study.[4]

The expenditure for these drugs in the health care system is formidable. Until the remaining questions regarding endpoint-related effectivity and long-term safety have been resolved, the use of oral antidiabetic agents should be restricted. No doubt, the search for orally effective drugs that are safe will continue. Any trial on oral hypoglyemic drugs developed for long-term clinical use in the future should fulfill the requirements proposed by Jackson and Bressler.[14]

References

1. Loubatières A: The discovery of hypoglycemic sulfonamides and particularly of their action mechanism. Acta Diabetol Lat 6 (Suppl 1):20, 1969.

2. Knowles HC: An historical view of the medical-social aspects of UGDP. Trans Am Clin Climatol Assoc 88:150–157, 1976.

3. UGDP I: Klimt CR, Knatterud GL, Meinert CL, et al.: The University Group Diabetes Program: a study of the effects of hypoglycemic agents on vascular complications in patients with adult-onset diabetes. Diabetes 19 (Suppl 2): 474–830, 1970.

   UGDP V: Evaluation of phenformin therapy. Diabetes 24 (Suppl 1):65–184, 1975.

   UGDP VIII: Evaluation of insulin therapy: Final report. Diabetes 31 (suppl 5):1–81, 1982.

4. UKPDS 1: Effect of diet, sulphonylurea, insulin or biguandine therapy on fasting plasma glucose and body weight after one year. Diabetologia 24:404–411, 1983.

   UKPDS 17: A 9-year update of a randomized, controlled trial on the effect of improved metabolic control on complications in non-insulin-dependent diabetes mellitus. Ann Intern Med 124 (1 pt. 2):136–145, 1996.

   UKPDS 33: Intensive blood-glucose control with sulfonylureas or insulin compared with conventional treatment and risk of complications in patients with type 2 diabetes. Lancet 352:837–853, 1998.

   UKPDS 34: Effect of intensive blood-glucose control with metformin on complications in overweight patients with type 2 diabetes. Lancet 352:854–865, 1998.

5. Berger M: Oral insulin 1922–1992: The history of continuous ambition and failure. In Berger M, Gries FA (eds): Frontiers in Insulin Pharmacology. Stuttgart: Georg Thieme, 1993; pp. 144–147.

6. Bänder A, Creutzfeldt W, Dorfmueller T, et al.: Über die orale Behandlung des Diabetes Mellitus mit N-(4-Methylbenzolsulfonyl) N'-butylharnstoff (D 860). Dtsch Med Wochenschrift 81:823–846, 1956; 887–906, 1956.

7. Levine R: Introduction of the conference chairman. In Butterfield WJH, van Westering W (eds): Tolbutamide . . . after ten years. Excerpta Medica Foundation Internat.

Congr. Series No. 149, Amsterdam, The Netherlands, 1967, p. v.

8. Rollo J: Cases of diabetes mellitus; with the results of the trials of certain acids and other substances in the cure of the lues venera. C. Dilly, in the Poultry, Gillet, Ed. 3. London, 1798.

9. Sturgess NC, Cook DL, Ashford ML, Hales CN: The sulfonylurea receptor may be an ATP-sensitive potassium channel. Lancet 2:474–475, 1985.

10. Boyd E III: Sulfonylurea receptors, ion channels and fruit flies. Diabetes 37:847–850, 1988.

11. Leibowitz G, Cerasi E: Sulfonylurea treatment of NIDDM patients with cardiovascular disease: a mixed blessing? Diabetologia 39:503–514, 1996.

12. Package insert for glibenclamide (Micronase). Washington, DC: Food and Drug Administration, 1984.

13. Kennedy DL, Piper JM, Baum C: Trends in the use of oral hypoglycemic agents. 1964–1986. Diabetes Care 11:558–562, 1988.

14. Jackson JE, Bressler R: Clinical pharmacology of sulfonylurea hypoglycemic agents. Drugs 22:211–245, 1981; 22:295–320, 1981.

15. Gerich JE: Oral hypoglycaemic agents. N Engl J Med 321:1231–1245, 1989.

16. Sartor G, Lundquist I, Melander A, et al.: Improved effect of glibenclamide on administration before breakfast. Eur J Clin Pharmacol 21:403–408, 1998.

17. Groop LA, Luzi L, DeFronzo RA, Melander A: Hyperglycemia and absorption of sulfonylurea drugs. Lancet 2:129–130, 1989.

18. Sartor G, Melander A, Schersten B, et al.: Serum glibenclamide in diabetic patients, and influence of food on the kinetics and effects of glibenclamide. Deabetologia 18:17–22, 1980.

19. Scott J, Poffenbarger PL: Pharmacogenetics of tolbutamide metabolism in humans. Diabetes 28:41–51, 1979.

20. Spraul M, Streek A, Nieradzik M, Berger M: Uniform elimination pattern for glibenclamide in healthy Caucasian males. Drug Res 39:1449–1450, 1989.

21. Draeger E: Clinical profile of glimepiride. Diabetes Res Clin Pract 28(suppl):S139–S146, 1995.

22. Bijlstra PJ, Lutterman JA, Russel FGM, Thien T, Smits P: Interaction of sulfonylurea derivatives with vascular ATP-sensitive potassium channels in humans. Diabetologia 39:1083–1090, 1996.

23. Sonnenberg GE, Garg DC, Weidler DJ, et al.: Short-term comparison of once- versus twice- daily administration of glimepiride in patients with non-insulin-dependent diabetes mellitus. Ann Pharmacother 31:671–676, 1997.

24. Fuhlendorff J, Rorsman P, Kofod H, et al.: Stimulation of insulin release by Repaglinide and Glibenclamide involves both common and distinct processes. Diabetes 47:345–351, 1998.

25. Singer DL, Hurwitz D: Long-term experience with sulphonylureas and placebo. N Engl J Med 277:450–456, 1967.

26. Haupt E, Etti H, Bamberg J, et al.: Blutzuckersenkende Sulfonamide: Eine Placebo Auslaßstudie zur Objek-

tivierung der Wirksamkeit oraler Antidiabetika. Akt Endokrinol Stoffw 5:23–31, 1984.

27. Berger M, Mueller WA, Renold AE: Obesity and diabetes. Some facts, many questions. In Katzen HM, Mahler RJ (eds): Advances in Modern Nutrition, vol. 2. Washington, DC: Hemisphere Publishers, 1978, pp. 211–228.

28. Kronsbein P, Muelhauser I, Venhaus A, et al.: Evaluation of a structured treatment and teaching programme on non-insulin-dependent diabetes. Lancet 2:1407–1411, 1988.

29. Bouchardat A: De la glucosurie ou diabète sucré. Paris: Librairie Germer Baillière, 1875.

30. Grüsser M, Bott U, Ellermann P, et al.: Evaluation of a structured treatment and teaching program for non-insulin treated Type II diabetic outpatients in Germany after the nationwide introduction of reimbursement policy for physicians. Diabetes Care 16:1268–1275, 1993.

31. Berger M, Jörgens V, Flatten G: Health care for persons with non-insulin-dependent diabetes mellitus. The German experience. Ann Intern Med 124(pt 2):153–155, 1996.

32. Kolata GB: Controversy over study on diabetes drugs continues for nearly a decade. Science 203:986–990, 1979.

33. Huupponen R: Adverse cardiovascular effects of sulphonylurea drugs. Clinical significance. Med Toxicol 2: 190–209, 1987.

34. Gasser R, Grisold M, Pokan R, et al.: Blockade of ATP-dependent K^+ channels in myocardium and coronary artery smooth muscle: a possible cause of increased cardiovascular mortality in sulfonylurea-treated patients. Cardiovasc Drug Therapy 11:87–89, 1997.

35. Berger M, Mühlhauser I, Sawicki PT: Possible risk of sulphonylureas in the treatment of non-insulin-dependent diabetes mellitus and coronary artery disease. Diabetologia 41:744, 1998.

36. Berger M, Mühlhauser I, Sawicki PT: Possible risk of sulphonylureas in the treatment of non-insulin-dependent diabetes mellitus and coronary artery disease. Diabetologia 40:1492–1493, 1997.

37. ADA Consensus statement: The pharmacological treatment of hyperglycemia in NIDDM. Diabetes Care 18:1510–1518, 1995.

38. Asplund K, Wilholm BE, Lithner F: Glibenclamide-associated hypoglycemia: a report of 57 cases. Diabetologia 24:412–417, 1983.

39. Jennings AM, Wilson RM, Ward JD: Symptomatic hypoglycemia in NIDDM patients treated with oral hypoglycemic agents. Diabetes Care 12:203–209, 1983.

40. Kemmer FW, Tacken M, Berger M: Mechanism of exercise-induced hypoglycemia during sulfonylurea treatment. Diabetes 36:1178–1182, 1987.

41. Logie AW, Galloway DB, Petrie JC: Drug interactions and long-term antidiabetic therapy. Br J Clin Pharmacol 3:1027–1032, 1976.

42. Schneider H: Untersuchung ueber die Medikation neuentdeckter Typ-II-Diabetiker mit Kardiaka, Antihypertonika, ß-Rezeptorenblockern, Koronartherapeutica und Diuretika. Z Ges Inn Med 38:273–277, 1983.

43. Tattersall RB: Diabetes care in the elderly. Diabetologia 27:167–173, 1984.

44. Klein R, Klein BEK, Moss SE: Is obesity related to microvascular and macrovascular complications in diabetes? Arch Intern Med 157:650–656, 1997.

45. Chaturvedi N, Fuller JH: Mortality risk by body weight and weight change in people with NIDDM. The WHO Multinational Study of Vascular Disease in Diabetes. Diabetes Care 18:766–774, 1995.

46. Lisch HJ, Sailer S: Lipoprotein patterns in diet, sulphonylurea and insulin-treated diabetics. Diabetologia 20:118–122, 1981.

47. Waldhäusl W: To flush or not to flush, comments on the CPAF controversy. Diabetologia 26:12–14, 1984.

48. Hansen JM, Christensen LK: Drug interaction with oral sulphonylurea hypoglycemic drugs. Drugs 13:24–34, 1977.

49. Brown KF, Crooks MJ: Displacement of tolbutamide, glibenclamide and chlorpropamide from serum albumin by anionic drugs. Biochem Pharmacol 25:1175–1178, 1976.

50. Eichelbaum M: Defective oxidation of drugs: kinetic and therapeutic implications. Clin Pharmacokin 7:1–22, 1982.

51. Johnson J, Wolf S, Kubadi U: Efficacy of insulin and sulfonylurea combination therapy in type II diabetes. Archives Intern Med 156:259–264, 1996.

52. Stenmann S, Groop PH, Slorenta C, et al.: Effects of the combination of insulin and glibenclamide in type 2 (non-insulin-dependent) diabetic patients with secondary failure to oral hypoglycaemic agents. Diabetologia 31:206–213, 1988.

53. Ratzmann KP, Berger M: Kombinationstherapie Insulin und Sulfonylharnstoffe: eine kritische Analyse. Zeitschr Aertztl Fortb (Berlin) 84:1105–1107, 1990.

54. Berger M, Joergens V: Praxis der Insulintherapie, 5 Ed., Berlin: Springer, 1995.

55. Bergmann U: International comparison or drug utilization: Use of antidiabetic drugs in seven European countries. In Bergmann U, Grimsson A, Wahba AHW, et al. (eds): Studies in Drug Utilization—Methods and Applications. Copenhagen: World Health Organization, European Series no. 8, 1979.

56. American Diabetes Association: The UGDP controversy (policy statement). Diabetes Care 2:1–3, 1979.

57. Schaefer G: Biguanides: Molecular mode of action. In Cudworth AG (ed): Metformin: Current aspects and future developments. Res Clin Forums 1:4–25, 1979.

58. Stumvoll M, Nurhan N, Periello G, et al.: Metabolic effects of metformin in non-insulin-dependent diabetes mellitus. New Engl J Med 333:550–554, 1995.

59. Paolisso G, Amato L, Eccellente R, et al.: Effect of metformin on food intake in obese subjects. Eur J Clin Invest 28:441–446, 1998.

60. Lee A, Bray GA: Metformin decreases food consumption in obese non-insulin-dependent diabetics. Diabetes 47 (Suppl 2):170 A (abstract), 1996.

61. Sitonen O, Huttunen JK, Jaervinen R, et al.: Effects of discontinuation of biguanide therapy on metabolic control in maturity-onset diabetics. Lancet 1:217–220, 1980.

62. Luft D, Schmuelling RM, Eggstein M: Lactic acidosis in biguanide treated diabetics. Diabetologia 14:75–87, 1978.

63. Bosisio E, Kienle MG, Ciconalli M, et al.: Defective hydroxylation of phenformin as a determinant of drug toxicity. Diabetes 30:644–649, 1983.

64. Cudworth AG (ed): Metformin: Current aspects and future developments. Res Clin Forums 1:1979.

65. Mehnert H, Standl E (eds): Metformin Therapy 1980. Stuttgart: Schattauer, 1980.

66. Bailey CJ, Turner RC: Metformin. New Engl J Med 334:574–579, 1996.

67. Haupt E, Panten U: Die Stellung der Biguanide in der Therapie des Diabetes mellitus. Medizin Klinik 92:472–479, 1997.

68. Innerfield RJ: Metformin-lactic acidosis mortality in US clinical trials. Diabetes 36 (Suppl 2), abst. # 814, 1996.

69. Dalau JD, Lacroix C, Compagnon P, et al.: Role of metformin accumulation in metformin-associated lactic acidosis. Diabetes Care 18:779–784, 1995.

70. Abbasi AA, Kasmikha K: Metformin-induced lactic acidemia. Diabetes 41(Suppl 1):A103, 1998.

71. Nahrwold D, Egberts EH, Holstein A: Contraindications to metformin therapy are generally disregarded. Diabetologia 41 (Suppl 1):A233, 1998.

72. Lalau JD, Race JM, Brinquin L: Lactic acidosis in metformin therapy. Diabetes Care 21:1366–1367, 1998.

73. Al-Jerawi AF, Lassmann MN, Abourizk NN: Lactic acidosis with therapeutic metformin blood level in a low-risk diabetic patient. Diabetes Care 21:1364–1365, 1998.

74. Innerfield RJ: Metformin associated mortality in US studies (letter). New Engl J Med 334:1611–1612, 1996.

75. Stadel BV, Guergiguian J, Fleming GA: Metformin-associated mortality in US studies (letter). New Engl J Med 334:1613, 1996.

76. Nestler JE, Jakubowicz DJ: Decreases in ovarian cytochrome P450c17α activity and serum free testosterone after reduction of insulin secretion in polycystic ovary syndrome. New Engl J Med 335:617–623, 1996.

77. Creutzfeldt W, Foelsch UR (eds): Delaying Absorption as a Therapeutic Principle in Metabolic Disease. Stuttgart: Thieme, 1983.

78. Creutzfeldt W (ed): Proceedings of the First International Symposium on Acarbose. Amsterdam: Excerpta Medica, Excerpta Medica Internat. Congr. Ser. No. 594, 1982.

79. Creutzfeldt W (ed): Proceedings of the 2nd International Symposium on Acarbose. Berlin: Springer, 1988.

80. Hanefeld M, Fischer S, Schulze J, et al: Therapeutic potentials of acarbose as first line drug in non-insulin-dependent diabetes insufficiently treated with diet alone. Diabetes Care 14:732–737, 1991.

81. Mehnert H: Acarbose in der Diabetestherapie. Internist 36:1190–1195, 1995.

82. Holman R, Cull C, Turner R for the UKPDS Study Group: Acarbose improves glycemic control over three years in type 2 diabetes. Diabetes 47 (suppl 1):A93, 1998.

83. Rao RH, Spathis GS: Alpha-glucosidase inhibitor therapy does not improve glycemic control in overweight diabetics poorly controlled on sulfonylureas. Diabetes Nutr Metab 3:17–22, 1990.

84. Radziuk J, Kemmer FW, Morishima T, et al.: The effects of an alpha-glucoside hydrolase inhibitor on glycemia and the absorption of sucrose in man determined using a tracer method. Diabetes 33:207–213, 1984.

85. Carrascosa M, Pascual F, Aresti S: Acarbose-induced acute severe hepatotoxicity. Lancet 349:698–699, 1997.

86. Andrade RJ, Lucena MI, Rodriguez-Mendizábal M: Hepatic injury caused by acarbose. Ann Intern Med 124:931, 1996.

87. Berger M, Köbberling J, Windeler J: Appraisal of effectiveness and therapeutic benefit of Acarbose: a non-consensus conference. Diabetologia 39:873–874, 1996.

88. Wolever TMS, Radmard R, Chiasson JL, et al.: One-year acarbose treatment raises fasting serum acetate in diabetic patients. Diabetic Medicine 12:164–172, 1995.

89. Segal P, Feig PU, Schernthaner G, et al.: The efficacy and safety of miglitol therapy compared with glibenclamide in patients with NIDDM inadequately controlled by diet alone. Diabetes Care 20:687–691, 1997.

90. Cummings JH: Fermentation in the human large intestine: Evidence and implications for health. Lancet 1:1206–1209, 1983.

91. Nolan JJ, Ludvik B, Beerdsen P, et al.: Improvement in glucose tolerance and insulin resistance in obese subjects treated with troglitazone. New Engl J Med 331:1188–1193, 1994.

92. Kumar S, Boulton AJM, Beck-Nielsen H, et al. for the Troglitazone study group: Troglitazone, an insulin enhancer, improves metabolic control in NIDDM patients. Diabetologia 39:701–709, 1996.

93. Ghazzi MN, Perez JE, Antonucci TK, et al., the Troglitazone Study Group, Whitcomb RW: Cardiac and glycemic benefits of troglitazone treatment in NIDDM. Diabetes 46:433–439, 1997.

94. Saltiel AR, Olefsky JM: Thiazolidinediones in the treatment of insulin resistance and type 2 diabetes. Diabetes 45:1661–1669, 1996.

95. Petrie J, Small M, Connell J: "Glitazones," a prospect for non-insulin-dependent diabetes. Lancet 349:70–71, 1997.

96. Dagogo-Jack S, Santiago JV: Pathophysiology of type 2 diabetes and modes of action of therapeutic interventions. Arch Intern Med 157:1802–1817, 1997.

97. Gallwitz B, Schmidt WE, Fölsch UR: Perspectives for future treatment of NIDDM. Endocrinol Metabol 4:293–304, 1997.

98. Mitchell P: Shock as troglitazone withdrawn in UK. Lancet 350:1685, 1997.

99. Imura H: A novel antidiabetic drug, troglitazone—reason for hope and concern. New Engl J Med 338:908–909, 1998.

100. Berger M: To bridge science and patient care in diabetes. Diabetologia 39:749–757, 1996.

21

Pancreas Transplantation for Treatment of Type 1 Diabetes Mellitus

David E.R. Sutherland, Angelika C. Gruessner,
and Rainer W.G. Gruessner

Introduction

Pancreas transplantation is the only treatment of type 1 diabetes that consistently establishes an insulin-independent, normoglycemic state. Currently long-term (>1 year) insulin-independence is achieved in >85% of recipients of pancreas grafts placed simultaneous with the kidney and >80% in recipients of a pancreas after a kidney, and >70% of nonuremic recipients of a pancreas alone. The penalty is immunosuppression, already obligatory for a kidney recipient, but the benefits are improvement in quality of life and the effect that perfect control of glycemia can have on secondary complications.

Pancreas or islet transplant are the only treatments of type 1 diabetes that can establish insulin independence.[1,2] Currently only a pancreas graft does so consistently.[1] The results with this approach to diabetic management are presented in this chapter. The evolving fate of islet transplantation will be presented later.

The Diabetes Control and Complications Trial (DCCT) provided a strong rationale for pancreas and islet transplantation.[3] Tight diabetic control reduces the incidence and severity of secondary complications, but at the expense of an increased frequency of insulin reactions and hypoglycemic episodes. The rigor required is also difficult (finger sticks for blood glucose determinations at least four times per day and multiple insulin injections daily). Even with intense insulin treatment, mean glycosylated hemoglobin levels were a gram percent above normal.[3] Furthermore, some individuals have extreme oscillations of blood glucose no matter what the regimen, and others develop secondary complications even when glycosylated hemoglobin levels were only moderately elevated–good control is not good enough in everyone.

Perfect control is only provided by β-cell replacement. Both islet and pancreas transplantation require a recipient to take immunosuppression. A pancreas transplant also requires major surgery. However, when successful, a pancreas graft makes the recipient euglycemic and glycosylated hemoglobin levels are normal for as long as the graft functions.

Because of the need for immunosuppression, most pancreas transplants are performed either simultaneously or subsequent to a kidney transplant in diabetic patients with advanced nephropathy. Nearly everyone agrees that a kidney transplant is preferable to dialysis in the treatment of uremia (particularly in diabetic patients). Thus in a patient already obligated to immunosuppression there is very little reason not to add a pancreas and only the surgical risks need to be considered. Unfortunately, in uremic diabetic patients, retinopathy and neuropathy are usually far advanced, and the DCCT did not study the effect of instituting strict control on established lesions. Thus, the main value of adding a pancreas to a kidney is the additional improvement in quality of life that accompanies being insulin independent as well as dialysis free.[4] This is not to say that there is not an effect of the pancreas transplant on secondary complications, and improvement in neuropathy and nephropathy has been documented following pancreas transplantation.[5,6,7] Recurrence of diabetic nephropathy in a new kidney is also prevented by a successful pancreas transplant.[8] Nevertheless, advanced retinopathy and vascular disease are unlikely to be affected.

A pancreas transplant should ideally be applied before complications occur, but since there is uncertainty in an individual patient as to whether he or she is complication prone (even with poor control not all get complications), as well as the uncertainty over what the individual side effects of immunosuppression will be, very few pancreas transplants have been done soon after onset of disease. Instead, pancreas transplants alone have largely been employed *in patients with very labile diabetes and hypoglycemic unawareness*, a syndrome that may emerge many years after onset of diabetes, particularly in those with neuropathy. In this situation a pancreas transplant is the most effective treatment, since it completely obviates insulin reactions.[9]

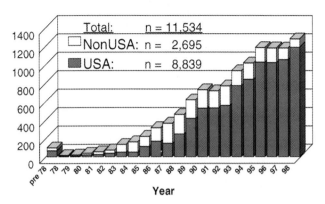

Figure 21–1. Pancreas Transplants Worldwide.

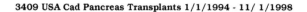

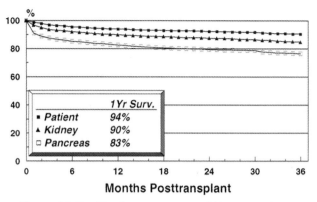

Figure 21–2. Simultaneous pancreas-kidney transplants.

The first pancreas transplant was performed at the University of Minnesota in 1966.[10] By 1998 more than 11,000 had been performed worldwide (Fig. 21–1), including more than 8,000 in the United States.[11] A dramatic increase in the number of cases occurred beginning in the mid-1980s with the introduction of cyclosporine for immunosuppression. The inception of the United Network for Organ Sharing (UNOS) in 1987, facilitating organ procurement and placement, was followed by a steady growth in application. More than 1,000 pancreas transplants are now being done yearly in the United States. Of these approximately 85% are simultaneous with a kidney, 10% are after a kidney, and 5% are pancreas transplants alone. New immunosuppresants were introduced in the 1990s, and results in the latest eras are summarized in the following section.

Pancreas Recipient and Graft Functional (Insulin Independence) Survival Rates

The results of pancreas transplantation have continuously improved over time, as documented in numerous Registry reports.[11] The latest Registry analysis of 1994–98 cases is summarized here. From January 1, 1994 to November 1, 1998, > 4,000 simultaneous pancreas-kidney (SPK), >400 pancreas after kidney (PAK), and >180 pancreas transplants alone (PTA) done in the United States were reported to UNOS. More that 70% of the pancreas transplants were done with bladder drainage (BD) for management of exocrine secretions. Enteric drainage (ED) has increased in frequency, particularly for SPK transplants, from 6% in 1994 to 48% in 1997.

Patient survival rates are similar in all three categories, 94% and 91% at 1 and 3 years, respectively. Pancreas graft survival rates have been 10–20% higher in SPK than the other categories, depending on the duct management technique and immunosuppressive pro-

tocol used. When all cases were included in the analyses and death with a functioning graft was counted as a graft failure, 1 year pancreas graft function (insulin-independence) rates for SPK, PAK and PTA cases were 83%, 71% and 64%, respectively. For SPK cases, kidney graft survival rates at 1 year were 90%. Patient, pancreas and kidney survival rates in the largest category, SPK, are illustrated in Fig. 21–2.

Interestingly, both the patient and the kidney graft survival rates are higher in diabetic recipients for SPK transplants than in type 1 diabetic recipients of cadaver kidney transplants alone (KTA), as documented in the UNOS Registry for 1994–97 cases.[12] The higher patient and kidney survival rates in the SPK cases may reflect selection of healthier patients for the combined procedure, or the positive impact of adding the pancreas on outcome, an hypothesis supported by single center analyses.[13]

When only BD pancreas transplant cases were analyzed, the differences in outcome between the three categories were less than in the overall analysis. With BD, pancreas graft function (insulin-independent) rates at 1 year for SPK (n = 2,369), PAK (n = 261) and PTA (n = 115) cases were 83%, 75% and 68%, respectively. For PAK and PTA cases, these graft survival rates were significantly higher than when the ED technique was used, but for SM cases (n = 912) there was little penalty for using ED, with a 1 year insulin-independent rate of 81%.

The technical failure (TF) rate for 1994–98 pancreas transplants was 9% overall and did not differ significantly by category. The rejection loss rate for technically successful cases, however, did differ significantly by category (all duct management techniques included), at 1 year being 2% for SPIC (n = 2,978), 9% for PAK (n = 307) and 15% for PTA (n = 147) cases. In all categories, however, the rejection rate was much less than in previous eras, and reflects the refinement of immunosuppressive management that has occurred.

With current immunosuppressive regimens the pancreas allograft rejection rate is now lower than the

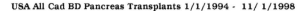

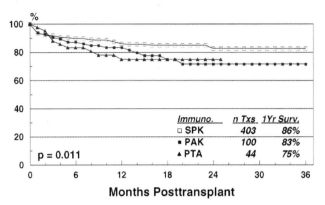

USA All Cad BD Pancreas Transplants 1/1/1994 - 11/ 1/1998

Immuno.	n Txs	1Yr Surv.
□ SPK	403	86%
▪ PAK	100	83%
▲ PTA	44	75%

p = 0.011

Months Posttransplant

Figure 21–3. Pancreas graft function in TAC/MMF treated recipients (see text).

TF rate, and most recipients with a successful graft can expect to remain insulin independent for years or until they die. For 1994–98, US BD pancreas transplant recipients given both of the new immunosuppressant made available during the 1990s, Tacrolimus (TAC) and Mycophenolate Mofetil (MMF) for maintenance therapy, graft survival rates were only slightly different according to category (Fig. 21–3); at 1 year, 86% of SPK ($n = 480$), 83% of PAK ($n = 100$) and 75% of PTA ($n = 44$) recipients were insulin independent.

Surgical Technique

The Achilles' heel of pancreas transplantation is the management of exocrine secretions.[1] ED was used in the very first cases in the late 1960s. Urinary drainage (via the ureter for a segmental graft) was introduced in the early 1970s, and duct injection (DI) with a synthetic polymer in the mid-1970s. All three techniques have been associated with long-term (>10 years) function. But because DI induces gland fibrosis that in some cases may involve the islets and because of a high incidence of infections in association with ED in the early cases, urinary drainage via the bladder became the most popular technique in the 1980s . BD was first used by Sollinger with direct anastamosis, but was modified by Nhgiem, using a whole pancreas duodenal graft with a side-to-side duodenocystostomy, a secure, safe technique. In addition, BD gave the opportunity to directly measure exocrine secretions (amylase in the urine), and a decrease was found to be a sensitive if nonspecific marker of pancreas allograft rejection episodes that could be treated prior to occurrence of hyperglycemia. For solitary pancreas transplants (PAK and PTA), monitoring for rejection episodes is greatly facilitated by BD.

In SPK cases, however, an increase in serum creatinine is a marker for rejection of the kidney, and an increase in creatinine occurs prior to decrease in pan-

creas allograft exocrine function more than 90% of the time. Although the occasional patient will have an isolated rejection of the pancreas that could be missed by using ED, the statistical impact on outcome is that small and bladder-specific complications are avoided (these include dysuria, hemturia, and metabolic acidosis from bicarbonate loss). About 10% of BD pancreas transplants are eventually converted to ED.

Serum pancreatic enzyme levels can also be used to monitor for rejection, an increase being a marker, but probably less sensitive than urinary amylase and no more specific. For solitary pancreas transplants the BD technique is associated with the highest probability of success. For SPK transplants, ED is as successful as BD and is associated with fewer chronic complications (Fig. 21–4).

Immunosuppression

Immunosuppression regimens used for pancreas transplant recipients are no different than those for other solid organ transplants.[1] Since the mid-1980s, cyclosporine in conjunction with either azathioprine, steroids, or both has been the mainstay. However, in the 1990s, two new immunosuppressives have been introduced, FK506 tacrolimus (Prograf®) and mycophenolate mofetil (Cellcept®). Cellcept can replace azathioprine (and prednisone) and can be used in conjunction with either cyclosporine or FK506. The introduction of both has been associated with an improvement in pancreas graft survival rates.[14]

All immunosuppressants have side effects, including increased susceptibility to infection, nephrotoxicity for FK506 and cyclosporine, body habitués, and bone changes with steroids. With the new immunosuppressives, steroid doses can be reduced to very low levels or stopped.[14] There are no protocols yet, however, that will allow discontinuance of immunosuppressants altogether. The side effects must be accepted as a trade-off for insulin independence and must be taken into account in recipient selection.

Effects of Pancreas Transplant on Metabolism and Secondary Complications

A successful pancreas transplant nearly always establishes a completely normoglycemic insulin-independent state in the recipient.[1] Glycosylated hemoglobin levels in pancreas transplant recipients are consistently normal.

Minor metabolic perturbations can exist in some pancreas recipients. Most pancreas transplants are drained via the systemic venous system and thus induce a degree of systemic hyperinsulinemia. Portal drainage

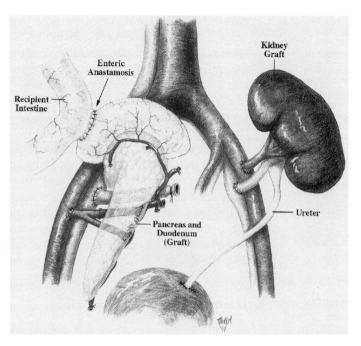

Figure 21–4. Technique for simultaneous cadaver donor primary pancreas and kidney transplants in uremic diabetic patients. A whole pancreaticoduodenal graft is revascularized via the right iliac vessels followed by enteric-drainage via duodeno-enterostomy. The kidney is revascularized via the left iliac vessels followed by ureteroneocystostomy.

of the graft has become more popular in the 1990s, but a clear advantage of one technique over the other has not been shown.

Regarding the effect of secondary complications, given the DCCT results it is clear that a successful pancreas transplant performed early in the course of diabetes would prevent occurrence of secondary complications. The effect on established lesions is less certain, but neuropathy clearly improves in most patients after a successful pancreas transplant,[5,6] and nephropathy can as well.[8]

Numerous quality-of-life studies have been performed in pancreas transplants.[1] All show that patient's satisfaction is higher in SPK and PAK than KTA recipients in regard to many factors, including dietary management as well as impact on family.[4] In PTA recipients, more than 90% of the recipients have stated that management of immunosuppression is easier than management of diabetes. Of course it should be noted that in this patient group nearly all were extremely labile and very dissatisfied with their situation prior to the transplant.

Recipient Selection

Even though it is late in the course of the disease, the most obvious patients to undergo a pancreas transplant are those who also need a kidney transplant and thus are obligated to immunosuppression. For those who do not have a living donor (LD) for the kidney, an SPK transplant from a cadaver donor makes sense. For those that have an LD for the kidney, this option would seem preferable followed later by a cadaver pancreas transplant (PAK). Long-term graft functional survival

probabilities are higher for LD than for cadaver donor kidneys.

The PAK option is probably vastly underutilized, particularly given the high insulin independence rates now achieved with this approach. A LD kidney followed later by a cadaver pancreas avoids long waiting times to get off dialysis or the need for dialysis altogether and gives the highest probability of remaining dialysis-free long-term.

The option of a simultaneous kidney and segmental pancreas transplant from a living donor also exists.[15] Of more than 100 LD pancreas transplants performed at the University of Minnesota since 1978, 26 have been SPK.[16] All of the LD SPK recipients are currently alive with functioning kidneys (100%), and 85% have a functioning pancreas.

Regarding SPK transplants, age has become less of a factor in selection. The patient survival rates are higher in those <45 than those >45 years old.[11] However, the patient and kidney survival rates in KTA are also higher in those <45 years of age than in those >45 years of age, and patient survival rates are still higher for those who receive a transplant than for diabetes patients who remain on dialysis, regardless of age. Furthermore, pancreas graft survival rates are similar in those >45 and <45 years old. It is a matter of informed consent as to what the uremic diabetic patient chooses to do in an attempt to improve quality of life as fully as possible by a pancreas transplant.

Regarding pancreas transplants alone,[17] there is no satisfactory medical treatment for patients with hypoglycemic unawareness. Less strict control is really the only alternative strategy, resulting in high glycosylated hemoglobin levels and an increased risk for secondary complications. A successful pancreas transplant allows such patients to avoid hypoglycemia and gain the freedom of insulin independence. Again, this treatment is probably vastly underutilized.

Should pancreas transplants alone be done early in the course of diabetes before complications occur? No randomized studies have been done to compare long-term complication rates of immunosuppression versus diabetes in comparable populations. However, in patients who have difficulty with diabetic control and are not able to maintain nearly normal glycosylated hemoglobin levels, the risk of secondary complications is at least as great as the risk of complications from immunosuppression. Indeed, a pancreas transplant alone may be a reasonable choice for an individual diabetic who wants to be free of the burden of insulin management and willing to take the risks of immunosuppression.

Summary and Future Considerations

Pancreas transplantation is now performed as a routine for uremic diabetic recipients of kidney transplants either simultaneous with or after the kidney. Such patients are obligated to immunosuppression and with a successful pancreas transplant can achieve insulin independence as well as a dialysis-free state.

Pancreas transplants alone are less commonly applied because of the need for immunosuppression, but the trade-off to achieve an insulin-independent state may be worthwhile for individual patients, particularly those who are labile with hypoglycemic unawareness. This option should certainly be a part of the treatment armamentarium of the modern diabetologist. A positive effect on secondary complications will certainly occur with an early transplant, and even a late transplant can have an impact, as has been shown for neuropathy.

Whether the simpler procedure of islet transplantation will replace pancreas transplants remains to be seen. *Of more than 200 islet allografts performed in the 1990s, <10% of the recipients have achieved insulin independence at 1 year.*[2] Clinical islet trials are ongoing but limited to patients who accept a low individual probability of success to assist in development or those in whom the surgical risks of a pancreas transplant is high. Islet transplantation can be a testing ground for new immunosuppressive protocols, including those with the potential to induce tolerance.

References

1. Sutherland, DER. Pancreas transplantation for treatment of diabetes mellitus In: Turtle JR, editor Diabetes in the New Millennium, In Press.

2. Hering, B.J., Ricordi, C. Islet transplantation for patients with Type 1 diabetes: Results, research priorities and reasons for optimism. Graft 2:12–27, 1999.

3. DCCT Research Group: Diabetes control and complications trial (DCCT): The effect of intensive treatment of diabetes on the development and progression of long term complications in IDDM. New Engl J Med 329: 977–986, 1993.

4. Gross CR, Kangas JR, Lemieux AM, Zehrer CL: One year change in quality of life profiles in patients receiving pancreas and kidney transplants. Trans Proc 27(6):3067–3068, 1995.

5. Kennedy WR, Navarro X, Goetz FC, et al.: Effects of Pancreatic Transplantation on Diabetic Neuropathy. New Engl J Med 322:1031–1037, 1990.

6. Allen DM, Al-Harbi IS, Morris JGL, et al.: Diabetic neuropathy after pancreas transplantation: Determinants of recovery. Transplantation 63:830–838, 1997.

7. Fioretto P, Steffes MW, Sutherland DER, Goetz FC, Mauer SM: Reversal of lesions of diabetic nephropathy after pancreas transplantation. New Engl J Med 339:69, 1998.

8. Bilous RW, Mauer SM, Sutherland DER, et al.: The effects of pancreas transplantation on the glomerular structure of renal allografts in patients with insulin-dependent diabetes. New Engl J Med 321:80–85, 1989.

9. Bolinder J, Wahrenberg H, Linde B, et al.: Improved glucose counterregulation after pancreas transplantation in diabetic patients with unawareness of hypoglycemia. Transplant Proc 23:1667–1669, 1991.

10. Kelly WD, Lillehei RC, Merkel FK, et al.: Allotransplantation of the pancreas and duodenum along with the kidney in diabetic nephropathy. Surgery 61:827–837, 1967.

11. Gruessner A, Sutherland DER: Analysis of United States (US) and non-US pancreas transplants as reported to the International Pancreas Transplant Registry (IPTR) and to the United Network for Organ Sharing (UNOS), in Cecka JM, Terasaki PI (eds): Clinical Transplants 1998, Los Angeles, CA, UCLA Tissue Typing Laboratory, 1999, p 53.

12. Sutherland DER, Cecka M, Gruessner A: Report from the International Pancreas Transplant Registry - 1998. Transplant Proc 31:597, 1999.

13. Tyden G., Bolinder J. Solders, G. et al. Improved survival in patients with insulin-dependent Diabetes Mellitus and end stage nephropathy 10 years after combined pancreas and kidney transplantation. Transplantation 67:645–647, 1999.

14. Gruessner RWG, Sutherland DER, Drangstveit MD, West M, Gruessner A: Mycophenolate mofetil and tacrolimus for induction and maintenance therapy after pancreas transplantation. Transplant Proc 30:518, 1998.

15. Gruessner RWG, Kendall DM, Drangstveit MD, Gruessner A, Sutherland DER: Simultaneous pancreas-kidney transplantation from live donors. Ann Surg 226:471, 1997.

16. Sutherland DER, Najarian JS, Gruessner RWG: Living versus cadaver donor pancreas transplants. Transplant Proc 30:2264, 1998.

17. Gruessner RWG, Sutherland DER, Najarian JS, Dunn DL, Gruessner A: Solitary pancreas transplantation for nonuremic patients with labile insulin-dependent diabetes mellitus. Transplantation 64:1572,1997.

22

Monitoring of Blood and Urine Glucose and Ketone Levels

John K. Davidson and Donald R. Parker

Historical Perspective

More than 100 years ago, chemical (copper reduction), physical (polaroscopic), and fermentative (with yeast) testing methods for sugars were developed. Benedict refined the copper-reduction method (1907)[1] which, because of its relative simplicity and convenience, was used almost exclusively in the home for the next 35 years. Clinitest tablets, introduced in 1941 by Ames, combined copper sulfate, sodium hydroxide, sodium carbonate, and citric acid into a tablet that, when dropped into diluted urine in a test tube, would generate the heat needed to reduce copper sulfate in an alkaline solution and produce a color reaction in the presence of a reducing substance such as glucose. A continuing problem with the copper reduction technique has been its lack of sensitivity and specificity.[2]

Introduction of a method in which the enzyme glucose oxidase was coupled with a chromagen and impregnated onto a "dipstick" (1956) provided another method of self-monitoring. This method was not without problems either, since it was semiquantitative and since it too produced both false-positive and false-negative reactions.[3]

The levels of glucose measured in urine by semiquantitative methods are shown in Figure 22–1. The most sensitive semiquantitative urine testing techniques do not consistently detect levels of less than 0.1% (100 mg glucose/dL). The Beckman analyzer method is specific for glucose in the urine, and it is sensitive and quantitative, i.e., it accurately measures *any* level present in urine (from 1 to 10,000 mg/dL). To satisfy Beer's law and to measure accurately the glucose content of urine samples containing more than

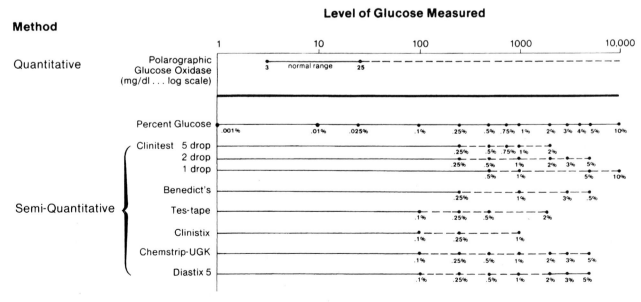

Figure 22–1. Comparison of the level of urine glucose measured by a quantitative method and estimated by several semiquantitative methods. The lowest level of sensitivity of the various semiquanititative methods is 100 mg/dL (0.1%).

500 mg/dL, it is necessary to serially dilute the sample until the measured level is <500 mg/dL.[4] The glucose level measured can then be multiplied by the dilution factor to determine the precise amount of glucose present in the sample being tested. The range of normal for urine is 3 to 25 mg/dL; any level above that is abnormal and is secondary either to *diabetes* or to *renal hyperglucosuria*.

Until a sensitive, specific, quantitative urine glucose measurement method became available (Exhibits 22–1 and 22–2 and Table 22–1) both nondiabetic renal glucosuria and other nondiabetic melliturias (Exhibits 22–3 and 22–4)[5–10] led occasionally to an erroneous diagnosis of diabetes mellitus and to inappropriate insulin treatment.[11] This problem no longer occurs when *specific* urine glucose and follow-up plasma glucose testing methods are used.[4]

Semiquantitative test methods for urine glucose are used to screen newborns, and sometimes others, for glucose and for other nondiabetic melliturias. A positive copper reduction test and a negative glucose oxidase test may be the result of a *nondiabetic mellituria* (see Table 22–1). Follow-up testing to characterize the nature of a nondiabetic mellituria can be carried out as noted in Exhibits 22–5 and 22–6.

Urine testing is aesthetically displeasing to some people, hypoglycemia cannot be evaluated by urine testing, and renal thresholds for glucose vary from one individual to another. These considerations, plus the facts that semiquantitative urine glucose test methods are insensitive and nonspecific, make them unsatisfactory as a sole means of evaluating metabolic control in those who are known to have diabetes.

Immediate and precise answers are needed to evaluate the level of blood glucose control in the home and to permit decision-making by the individual with insulin-dependent diabetes mellitus (IDDM) and non-insulin-dependent diabetes mellitus (NIDDM). The *amplitude of glucose excursions* (AGE) cannot be established without reasonably accurate and fairly frequent home capillary blood or plasma glucose determinations depending on the meter that is used. However desirable, the likelihood of being able to check blood glucose at home seemed remote until Keen and Knight (1962) demonstrated that patients could drop a sample of capillary blood onto filter paper at home and take it to be analyzed later in the hospital laboratory.[12] Introduction of glucose oxidase-chromogen-based reagent strips (Dextrostix) for blood glucose measurement (1964) attracted little attention, since when visually

---

EXHIBIT 22–1   Classification of Glucosurias

Glucosurias (See Figs. 11–1 and 11–2)
Quantitative measurements of urine glucose levels have shown that about 97% of randomly selected individuals not known to have diabetes have random urine glucose (RUG) levels of 3 to 25 mg/dL and that about 3% have levels >25 mg/dL (of these about 72% have diabetes and about 28% do not have diabetes but have renal hyperglucosuria (Fig. 11–2). Since the urine of *all individuals* contains glucose, the term "renal hyperglucosuria" is preferable to the outdated term "renal glucosuria." The term "renal glucosuria" was widely used before sensitive specific urine glucose measurement methodology became available in the 1970s.

A. *Nondiabetic random renal hyperglucosuria*
   The normal tubular transfer maximum for glucose (TM$_G$) is about 300 to 350 mg/min. When the blood glucose level exceeds $\sim$ 180 mg/dL and the plasma glucose level exceeds $\sim$ 200 mg/dL, the amount of glucose presented to the tubules for reabsorption usually exceeds the TM$_G$ of 300 to 350 mg/min, and the amount of glucose in the urine increases. If the TM$_G$ is lower than normal, more glucose will appear in the urine. Rarely, the TM$_G$ is so low that large amounts of glucose (several grams per day) appear in the urine, even after an overnight fast. Renal glucosuria was formerly defined as persistent, including fasting, glucosuria measured by semi-quantitative copper reduction methods that required a level $\geqslant$ 250 mg/dL (0.25%) to produce a positive test. Eighty-five of 50,000 individuals (0.17%) seen at the Joslin Clinic[5] had renal glucosuria according to this definition. This high prevalence probably reflected, at least in part, the prominence of the Joslin Clinic as a referral consultative center.

In the Grady Memorial Hospital (GMH) study of 4,141 randomly selected individuals not known to have diabetes, only 1 had an RUG level >200 mg/DL (317 mg/dL), and this individual's fasting urine glucose was 110 mg/dL. Thus, none of the patients (0/4141, or less than 0.025%) in the GMH series would be classified as having renal glucosuria according to the Joslin Clinic criteria.

On the other hand, since sensitive quantitative random urine glucose measurements have revealed an overlap (26 to 317 mg/dL) between those who are by subsequent testing shown to be diabetic and those who are shown to be nondiabetic, it is useful to classify the nondiabetic group with RUGs >25 mg/dL as nondiabetic random renal hyperglucosurics. In the GMH study, about 0.7% (27 of 4,141 screenees) fell into this category.[4]

B. *Diabetic Random Hyperglucosuria*
   In the GMH study of 4,141 screenees, of the 68 who were on the follow-up testing shown to be diabetic (fasting plasma glucose >140 mg/dL, or sum of fasting and 1-, 2-, and 3-hr venous plasma glucose levels post-100-g glucose load >800 mg/dL), 22 (32.3%) had a screening RUG in the range from 26 to 317 mg/dL, and 46 (67.7%) had a screening RUG in the range of 325 to 10,000 mg/dL (see Fig. 11–2).[4]

C. *Pregnancy*
   Increased urine glucose and lactose in late pregnancy.

EXHIBIT 22–2 Urine Glucose Testing Techniques

I. *Copper reduction tests*

A. As a screening test, the glucose oxidase test will not detect increased levels of galactose or other sugars in urine. It is therefore important that a copper reduction test be used for young pediatric patients.

Of the copper reduction tests used for screening purposes, the qualitative Benedict test (1907)[1] is more sensitive to reducing substances in urine than the single-tablet copper reduction test. Urines containing non-glucose-reducing substances may give positive results. Substances in urine, metabolites, or drug-related metabolites can influence urinary sugar tests. Strong reducing substances such as ascorbic acid, gentisic acid, or homogentisic acid may inhibit the enzyme test while contributing to the positivity of the copper reduction test. The tablet test is not affected as much as the Benedict test. Very large doses of ascorbic acid do not affect the two-drop copper reduction test. In those instances when the copper test is positive and the glucose oxidase test is negative, glucosuria is ruled out; but before investigating for other sugars, the clinical findings and drug history should be evaluated.

B. *Reference values*

Using these tests, the urine of normal children and adults is negative for glucose. Normal neonatal infants during the first 10 to 14 days of life may excrete urine giving a positive reaction due to glucose, galactose, fructose, and lactose. Normal pregnant and postpartum women may give positive reactions to tests for lactose.

C. *Copper reduction tablet test*

Clinitest tablets will react with sufficient quantities of any reducing substances in the urine, including reducing sugars such as lactose, fructose, galactose, maltose, and the pentoses.

Both a five-drop and a two-drop Clinitest method have been described, and corresponding color charts are available for both. The two-drop method was developed in response to the so-called "pass-through" phenomenon, which may occur if more than 2 g/dL of sugar is present in the urine. In the "pass-through" phenomenon, the solution that results after addition of the Clinitest tablet goes through the entire range of colors and back to a dark greenish-brown. The final color does not compare with any section of the color chart; however, it corresponds most closely to a significantly lower result. It is important to observe the entire reaction and for 15 sec after boiling inside the tube has stopped so that the reversion to a different color is not missed and a falsely low result reported. If the "pass-through" phenomenon occurs with the two-drop test, a one-drop test should be done.

D. *Chemistry*

Copper sulfate, sodium hydroxide, sodium carbonate, and citric acid are incorporated into a tablet. Copper sulfate reacts with reducing substances in the urine, converting cupric sulfate to cuprous oxide. Based on Benedict's copper reduction reaction:

$$Cu^{2+} \xrightarrow{\text{hot alkaline solution}} Cu^+$$

$$Cu^+ + OH \rightarrow CuOH \text{ (Yellow)}$$

$$2CuOH \xrightarrow{\text{heat}} Cu_2O \text{ (Red)} + H_2O$$

Heat is caused by the reaction of sodium hydroxide with water and citric acid.

E. *Procedure*

1. *Five-drop method.* Place five drops of urine in a dry test tube and add ten drops of water. Add one Clinitest tablet by easing it into the tube without touching it—it contains strong alkali. Watch while boiling takes place, but do not shake or touch the bottom of the tube; it is hot. Wait for 15 s after boiling stops, then shake the tube gently, and immediately compare the color of the solution with the color scale. Results correspond to the following approximate concentrations: negative; 0.25 g/dL; 0.5 g/dL; 0.75 g/dL; 1.0 g/dL; 2.0 g/dL; pass-through. It is important to watch the solution carefully while it is boiling. If at this time the solution passes through orange to a dark shade of greenish brown, it indicates that more than 2 g/dL sugar is present, and this should be recorded as greater than 2 g/dL without reference to the color scale. Urines showing this "pass-through" phenomenon should be retested with the two-drop method.

2. *Two-drop method.* Place two drops of urine in a test tube and add ten drops of water. Add one Clinitest tablet. Watch while boiling takes place, but do not shake. Wait 15 s after the boiling stops, then shake the tube gently, and compare the color of the solution with the color scale supplied for the two-drop method. The "pass-through" phenomenon may also occur with the two-drop test with a large concentration of sugar, over 5 g/dL. Therefore, it is important to watch the test throughout the entire reaction and waiting period. Report results as negative, trace, 0.5 g/dL, 1 g/dL, 2 g/dL, 3 g/dL, 5 g/dL, and more than 5 g/dL if a "pass-through" reaction occurs.

3. *One-drop method.* If the "pass-through" phenomenon occurs, do a one-drop test (one drop urine, ten drops water).

F. Clinitest reagent tablets will detect >250 mg glucose/dL of urine.

G. *Precautions.* Observe the precautions in the literature supplied with the Clinitest tablets. The bottle must be kept tightly closed at all times to prevent absorption of moisture and kept away from direct heat and sunlight in a cool, dry place. The tablets normally have a spotted bluish-white color. If not stored properly, they will absorb moisture or deteriorate from heat, turning dark blue or brown. In this condition they will not give reliable results. They are also available individually packaged in aluminum foil to help prevent this absorption of moisture. Although more expensive, such packaging is useful when a limited number of tests are performed.

(continued)

EXHIBIT 22–2   *(continued)* Urine Glucose Testing Techniques

II. *Enzymatic Tests* (See Chapter 13.)

Enzymatic methods yield maximum specificity for glucose estimations in urine quantitative glucose oxidase—oxygen electrode method (Beckman), semiquantitative Clinistix, Testape, Diastix, Chemstrip, UG that estimate glucose alone; and Keto-diastix and Chemstrip UGK that esimate glucose and ketones. See Exhibit 22–4. All self-monitored blood glucose methods use glucose oxidase color development, read either visually or with a reflectance meter or electrochemically. (See Exhibit 22–7).

A. In the glucose oxidase method, glucose reacts with the enzyme to produce gluconic acid and hydrogen peroxide. Hydrogen peroxide then reacts with an oxygen acceptor, such as ortho-dianisidine, phenylamine-phenazone, or other chromogenic oxygen acceptors, in a reaction catalyzed by peroxidase to form a color.

(1) β-D-Glucose + O_2 $\xrightarrow{\text{Glucose Oxidase}}$ Gluconolactone $\xrightarrow[O_2]{H_2O}$ Gluconic acid + H_2O_2

(2) H_2O_2 + phenylamine − phenozone (chromogenic O_2 acceptor) $\xrightarrow{\text{peroxidase}}$ Ortho − dianisidine (*or*) color (chromogen) + H_2O

Glucose oxidase is highly specific for beta-D-glucose and any glucose present in the alpha-form must be converted to the beta form before reacting. Some preparations of glucose oxidase contain the enzyme mutarotase, which accelerates this process. The second step involving peroxidase is less specific than the first, and numerous reducing substances inhibit oxidation of the chromogens used in the peroxidase reaction (see Table 22–1). One of the primary advantages of the glucose oxidase method is its low cost.

B. In the glucose oxidase-oxygen electrode method, the reaction of glucose with oxygen is monitored by an oxygen-sensing electrode, with generated H_2O_2 being removed by reaction with ethanol and iodide. By determining the rate of oxygen consumption [see reaction (1) above], the level of glucose in urine and other samples can be measured accurately, since the method is specific, sensitive, precise, linear, and free from important interferences. Results are similar to those obtained by the hexokinase glucose method, the proposed product class standard (see Chapter 13).

C. The main disadvantage of the hexokinase method is its cost, and the fact that when used to measure urine glucose a correction factor for background ultraviolet absorbance by urine must be applied.

[*Sources:* Bradley M, Schumann GB: Examination of urine: glucose and other sugars, pp 401–403; Ketones, p 405. *In* Henry JB (ed): Todd-Sanford-Davidsohn Clinical Diagnosis and Management by Laboratory Methods, Ed. 17. Philadelphia: W.B. Saunders, 1984; Howanitz PG, Howanitz JH: Carbohydrates (glucose measurements), pp 168–169. *In* Henry JB (ed): Todd-Sanford-Davidsohn Clinical Diagnosis and Management by Laboratory Methods, Ed. 17. Philadelphia: W.B. Saunders, 1984. With permission.]

TABLE 22–I   Reactions of Substances Found in Urine to Tests for Glucosuria

Constituent	Glucose Oxidase Reagent Strip	Copper Reduction Tablet Test
Glucose	Positive	Positive
Sugars other than glucose		
Fructose		
Galactose		
Lactose	No effect	Positive
Maltose		
Pentose		
Sucrose	No effect	No effect
Ketones (large amounts)	May depress color	No effect
Creatinine	No effect	May cause false-positive
Uric acid		
Homogentisic acid (alcaptonuria)	No effect	Positive
Drugs[a]		
Ascorbic acid (large amounts)	May delay color	Trace positive
Cephalosporins (Keflin), and so on	No effect	Positive, brown color
L-Dopa (large)	False-negative	No effect
Nalidixic acid glucuronide	No effect	Positive
Probenecid	No effect	Positive
Phenazopyridine hydrochloride	Orange color may affect result	
Salicylate (large)	May lower reading	No effect
X-ray dye (diatrizoates)	No effect	Black color
Contaminants		
Hydrogen peroxide	False-positive	May inhibit positive test
Hypochlorite (bleach)	False-positive	
Sodium fluoride	False-negative	No effect

[a] Other drugs implicated in copper reduction are amino acids, caronamide, chloral hydrate, chloroform chloramphenicol, formaldehyde, hippuric acid, isoniazid, thiazides, oxytetracycline, p-aminosalicylic acid, penicillin, phenols, streptomycin, phenothiazine, and sulibnamides.

[*Source:* Henry JB (ed): Todd, Sanford, Davidsohn, Clinical Diagnosis and Management by Laboratory Methods, Ed. 17. Philadelphia, W.B. Saunders, 1984, p. 401. With permission.]

EXHIBIT 22–3 Urine and Serum Ketone Testing Techniques

Methods of Testing for Ketonuria

The Gerhardt ferric chloride test has been used for many years as a test for acetoacetic acid. However, ferric chloride tests are not very specific and the sensitivity is low—about 25 to 50 mg/dL. The ferric chloride test gives positive results with salicylate and L-dopa.

Acetone and acetoacetic acid react with sodium nitroprusside (nitroferricyanide) in the presence of alkali to produce a purple-colored complex. This reaction was described by Legal (1883) in diabetic urines. In the simplest form of the nitroprusside test, reagent strips (Ketodiastix and Chemstrip UGK) impregnated with sodium nitroprusside and alkali are used, and the color developed in testing urine is compared to a color chart. The reagent strips are not satisfactory in estimating serum, plasma, or blood ketone levels. A tablet form of the test is available and has similar sensitivity. A reagent strip without alkali reacts to acetoacetic acid and not to acetone. The blood level of ketone bodies may be estimated by the nitroprusside test at the bedside. This is especially helpful in determining the severity of ketosis in the treatment of diabetic acidosis, provided that the reagents are fresh.

Stability of Ketones

In urine, bacterial action will cause loss of acetoacetic acid. This may happen in vivo as well as in vitro. Acetone is lost at room temperature but not if kept in a closed container in a refrigerator. If a sample cannot be tested immediately, it should be refrigerated.

Reference Values

Depending on the methods used, total ketone bodies (as acetone) range from 17 to 42 mg/dL. According to Killander (1962), up to 2 mg acetoacetic acid/dL is normal.

Nitroprusside Tablet Test

A tablet test method may be used if the urine has an interfering color. The tablets are very sensitive to humidity and will deteriorate if not stored properly. The Acetest tablet contains sodium nitroprusside (nitroferricyanide), glycine, and a strongly alkaline buffer. It can be used to test whole blood, plasma, serum, or urine.

Procedure

Place the tablet on a clean surface, preferably a piece of white paper. Place one drop of urine, serum, plasma, or whole blood on the tablet. For urine testing, compare the color of the tablet to a color chart at 30 s after application of the specimen. For serum or plasma testing, compare color of tablet to color chart 2 min after application of the specimen. For whole blood testing, 10 min after application of the specimen remove clotted blood from tablet and compare color of tablet to color chart.

If acetone and acetoacetic acid are present, the tablet will show a color varying from lavendar to deep purple. Report the results as negative, small, moderate, or large. If large, a dilution should be made. Report these analyses in a form such as this: undiluted "large," 1:2 dilution "large," 1:4 dilution moderate," and so forth.

Acetest will detect 5 to 10 mg of acetoacetic acid/dL in urine and 20 to 25 mg acetone/dL in urine. As is the case with the reagent strips (Ketodiastix and Chemstrip UGK), it does not react with beta-hydroxybutyrate. It will given positive results with L-dopa and large amounts of phenylketones and with BSP and PSP dyes that react with the alkali in the tablets.

A paper-strip test to measure beta-hydroxybutyrate has been developed.[24]

Rothera's Test

The urine test tube nitroprusside test of Rothera (1908) will detect acetoacetic acid (1 to 5 mg/dL) and acetone (10 to 25 mg/dL).

[*Sources:* Bradley M, Schumann GB: Glucose and other blood sugars. *In* Henry JB (ed): Todd, Sanford, Davidsohn's Clinical Diagnosis and Management by Laboratory Methods, Ed. 17. Philadelphia: W. B. Saunders, 1984, pp. 401–403; Ketones, p. 405. Harano, Y, Suzuki M, Kojima H, et al.: Development of accurate and rapid method for the determination of serum ketone bodies for quantifying ketosis proneness and monitoring metabolic control in diabetic subjects. Diabetes 33(Suppl 1):49A, 1984. With permission.]

read and when prepared by inexperienced individuals they frequently gave grossly inaccurate measurements of the true glucose level.

> *Example:* A comatose female was brought to the emergency room in 1969. A Dextrostix reading indicated that her blood sugar was <50 rng/dL, and she was given 50 mL of 50% glucose (25 g glucose) five times within 30 min (125 g glucose) by IV push since she remained comatose. Thirty minutes after entry, her initial laboratory plasma glucose was reported as 1,700 mg/dL. She was admitted, at which time the laboratory-measured plasma glucose was 2,900 mg/dL and serum osmolality was 450 mOsm. She remained comatose and died 3 hr later in hyperglycemic hyperosmolar coma. It was concluded later that the glucose oxidase in the Dextrostix had been inactivated by alcohol on the stuck finger, and that this in turn accounted for the fact that no color development took place.

> *Another Example (1989):* A 38-year-old woman with IDDM was brought by her family to a hospital treatment room

in stupor with complaints of confusion, weakness, nausea, vomiting, and weight loss of 6 pounds in 2 days. Her capillary blood glucose was measured by an experienced staff nurse who was using an Accu-Chek II. The result reported to the physician was 120 mg/dL. He then ordered an SMA-7 stat. Thirty minutes later, the plasma glucose was reported as 780 mg/dL and the carbon dioxide content as 3 mEq/L. The patient was admitted to the hospital and treated for severe diabetic ketoacidosis (her plasma pH was 6.9) from which she recovered in 24 hr. This case illustrates that when the physician or nurse have *any doubt* about the accuracy of a visually read or meter-read blood glucose strip, a repeat measurement should be done promptly in the hospital laboratory so that critical treatment plans can be implemented as quickly as possible. (See Chapter 24.)

Eyetone meters to measure color development of Dextrostix were introduced in 1970. It then became possible to convert a visually estimated blood glucose level

EXHIBIT 22–4 Urine Testing Products for Ketones and Glucose

Product (Manufacturer)	Packaging	Measures Glucose	Measures Ketones	Readings
TABLETS				
Acetest (Bayer Corporation, Diagnostics Division)	100	no	yes	Small, moderate, large
Clinitest (Bayer Corporation, Diagnostics Division)	36 100 100 (foil wrapped) Kit (36 tablets, test tube, dropper)	yes	no	2-drop method: 0, trace, $\frac{1}{2}$%, 1%, 2%, 3%, 5%+. 5-drop method: 0, $\frac{1}{4}$%, $\frac{1}{2}$%, $\frac{3}{4}$%, 1%, 2%+
STRIPS				
Chemstrip uG (Roche Diagnostics)	100	yes	no	Negative, $\frac{1}{10}$%, $\frac{1}{4}$%, $\frac{1}{2}$%, 1%, 2%, 3%, 5%
Chemstrip uGK (Roche Diagnostics)	100	yes	yes	Glucose: negative, $\frac{1}{10}$%, $\frac{1}{4}$%, $\frac{1}{2}$%, 1%, 2%, 3%, 5% Ketones: negative, small, moderate, and large
Chemstrip K (Roche Diagnostics)	100	no	yes	Negative, small, moderate, large
Clinistix (Bayer Corporation, Diagnostics Division)	50	yes	no	Negative, light, medium, dark
Diastix (Bayer Corporation, Diagnostics Division)	50 100	yes	no	0, $\frac{1}{10}$%, $\frac{1}{4}$%, $\frac{1}{2}$%, 1%, 2%
Ketostix (Bayer Corporation, Diagnostics Division)	20 (foil wrapped) 50 100	no	yes	0, trace, small, moderate, large
Keto-Diastix (Bayer Corporation, Diagnostics Division)	50 100	yes	yes	Glucose: 0, $\frac{1}{10}$%, $\frac{1}{4}$%, $\frac{1}{2}$%, 1%, 2%. Ketones: 0, trace, small, moderate, large

to a meter-read estimate (milligrams of glucose per deciliter or mMol/L).

In 1974 pilot studies among pregnant women using self-monitoring of blood glucose (SMBG) levels correlated well with improved glucose control. (See Chapters 40 and 41.) Such studies stimulated an interest in the development of affordable home blood glucose monitoring methods for individuals with IDDM. As the Stattek (1977),[13] the Glucochek (1978),[14] and the Glucometer (1980)[15] became available, the market became more competitive and cost of meters started to decrease; this trend continues. Visually read Chemstrips (1979) also have been shown to be effective in self-care management.

Jovanovic and Peterson,[16] Howe-Davis,[17] Sonkson,[18] and others reported that SMBG improves glucose control in many patients with IDDM. However, some studies failed to show a positive correlation between home monitoring and glucose control. A study by Mountier and associates[19] suggests that: (1) Many patients do not use devices for glucose monitoring so that appropriate modifications of therapy result, and (2) frequently neither patients nor physicians react satisfactorily to recorded high values.

During the last 20 years, SMBG techniques have improved, and microprocessor based computer devices for blood, plasma, and urine glucose measurements, only for data storage and analysis have become commercially available. See Exhibit 22–7.

Meters that monitor blood glucose levels utilize different methods: (1) reflectance meters (such as the Accu-Chek II) measure reflected light and translate the amount of reflected light into mg/dL (or mM) for blood glucose, (2) two beams of light measure the color change (one touch), (3) a small electric current is produced by the chemical reaction on the strip produced

EXHIBIT 22–5   Melliturias Other than Glucosuria

I. Although it is no longer appropriate to screen the adult population for diabetes with nonspecific copper reduction methods, these tests are useful in screening newborns and others for fructosuria, galactosuria, lactosuria, maltosuria, pentosuria, mannoheptulo-suria, and xylosuria (see Table 22–1). All nonglucose urine sugars can best be identified by thin layer chromatography.

II. *Fructosuria (levulosuria)*[6]

  A. *Hereditary fructose intolerance*

  After ingestion of fructose (in infants fed with milk formulas substituting fructose or sucrose for lactose and in children initially breast-fed, then weaned, then fed with fruits and vegetables), nausea, vomiting, hypoglycemia, and coma may occur and may progress to hepatomegaly, jaundice, cachexia, hepatic failure, and death. Due to fructose-1-phosphate aldolase deficiency in liver, kidney cortex, and small intestine. Incidence estimated at 1 in 20,000. Mode of inheritance autosomal-recessive.

  Between 1956 and 1971, over 100 cases were reported and since then case reports have been numerous. Should detect as early as possible and treat by omitting fructose and sucrose from diet. See Exhibit 22–6 for methods of identifying fructose in the urine and proving the diagnosis.

  B. *Hereditary -1,6-diphosphatase deficiency*

  First reported in 1970, 21 cases reported by 1983. Episodic spells of hyperventilation, apnea, hypoglycemia, ketosis, and lactic acidosis, with a precipitous and often lethal course in the newborn infant. Prove diagnosis by demonstrating deficiency of fructose-1,6-diphosphatase in liver biopsy specimen. Because of the enzyme defect, gluconeogenesis is severely impaired and amino acids, lactate, and ketones accumulate as soon as liver glycogen stores are depleted. Mode of inheritance autosomal-recessive. Treat acute attacks by IV glucose to correct hypo-glycemia; avoid fasting, and eliminate dietary fructose and sucrose.

  C. *Essential fructosuria*

  Asymptomatic, benign, due to absence of fructokinase. Diagnose by observation of fructosuria (on thin layer chromatography) and alimentary hyperfructosuria, with up to 80 to 90% of the administered fructose being retained (normal subjects retain 98 to 99%). First described in 1876, about 80 cases reported by 1969. The term "essential fructosuria," though still used, became obsolete when it was shown in 1962 that the disorder was due to a deficiency of fructokinase. It is an autosomal-recessive trait that occurs in 1 of 130,000 individuals (4 cases seen at Joslin Clinic through 1971) and requires no treatment.

III. *Galactosuria*[7]

  A. *Galactosemia due to galactose-1-phosphate uridyl transferase deficiency*

Characterized clinically by inanition, failure to thrive, vomiting, liver disease, cataracts, and mental retardation secondary to galactose toxicity. Overall prevalence estimated at about 1 in 62,000 newborns. Suspect if urine copper reducing substance present which does not react with glucose oxidase. Prove by absence in the red blood cells of the enzyme galactose-1-phosphate uridyl transferase. Treat by omitting galactose, lactose, and galactose-containing foods from the diet.

  B. *Galactosemia due to galactokinase deficiency*

  Characterized clinically by galactosuria after milk ingestion. Cataracts may be the first and only abnormality. Identify by screening neonate for reducing substance in urine identified as galactose on thin layer chromatography, high blood galactose after milk feedings, absence of galactokinase and normal amount of galactose-I-phosphate uridyl transferase in red blood cells. Prevalence about 1 in 1,000,000 newborns. Treat by omitting galactose from diet.

IV. *Lactosuria*[8]

  A. Late pregnancy and lactation

  B. Intestinal lactase deficiency with lactose intolerance. Abdominal cramping pain, bloating, diarrhea, may appear in childhood or adolescence, very common. Diagnosis made by hydrogen breath test, ^{14}C lactose breath test, oral lactose tolerance test, small intestinal biopsy (lactase deficiency), relief of symptoms when lactose removed from diet.

V. *Essential pentosuria (L-xylulosuria)*

  Prevalence about 1 in 50,000. Joslin Clinic series (1971) 12 patients, all Jews. Benign, requires no treatment. Autosomal-recessive trait. The metabolic block in pentosuria results from reduced activity of L-xylulose reductase, the enzyme that catalyzes the conversion of L-xylulose to xylitol.

VI. *Maltosuria*

  Rare. Of no clinical significance.

VII. *Mannoheptulosuria*

  Appears in urine of some individuals after ingestion of avocado. Of no clinical significance.

VIII. *Xylosuria*

  Appears in urine of some individuals after ingestion of apricots. Of no clinical significance.

IX. *Sucrosuria*

  Rarely reported. May be alimentary, after infusion of sucrose, or may be due to deception by patients who add sucrose to urine thinking that it will give a positive test for glucose in the urine. It will not reduce copper sulfate or give a positive glucose oxidase reaction, but it may increase the urine specific gravity to extremely high levels (i.e., 1.070).

[*Sources:* Gitzelmann R, Steinmann B, Van Den Beighe G: Essential fructosuria, hereditary fructose intolerance, and fructose -1,6-diphosphatase deficiency. *In* Stanbury JB, Wyngaarden JB, Frederickson DS, et al. (eds): The Metabolic Basis of Inherited Disease, Ed. 5. New York: McGraw-Hill, 1983, pp. 1728–1742. Segal S: Disorders of galactose metabolism. *In* Stanbury JB, et al. (eds).: The Metabolic Basis of Inherited Disease, Ed. 5. New York: McGraw-Hill, pp. 1728–1742. Bradley M, Schumann GB: Examination of urine: glucose and other sugars, pp. 401–403; Ketones, p. 405. Howanitz PG, Howanitz JH: Carbohydrate (glucose measurements). *In* Henry JB (ed): Todd, Sanford, Davidsohn's Clinical Diagnosis and Management by Laboratory Methods, Ed. 17. Philadelphia: W. B. Saunders, 1984. With permission.]

EXHIBIT 22–6 Testing Techniques for Nonglucose Melliturias

Some hexoses and pentoses cause positive copper reduction tests in urine when the glucose oxidase test is negative. In some rare cases, it is important to identify the sugars so that the patient with persistent mellituria by copper reduction is not mistakenly labeled as diabetic. Fructose, galactose, lactose, maltose, and L-xylulose (pentose) are found in urine in patients with inherited metabolic disorders. It should be noted that many drug metabolites, e.g., in the form of glucuronides, will also give positive copper reduction tests. If an inherited disorder is suspected, the sugar may be identified by thin layer chromatography. Qualitative confirmatory tests are generally not satisfactory for sugar. The disaccharidase deficiency may be measured on a small intestinal biopsy specimen. Oral tolerance tests and hydrogen breath tests are also used for confirmation. The latter test measures hydrogen gas in expired air 90 min after ingestion of the sugar. Bacterial digestion of the excess unabsorbed sugar causes higher than normal hydrogen levels in enzyme deficiencies.

Small amounts of disaccharides are normally excreted in the urine—about 50 mg in 24 hr. With intestinal diseases such as severe sprue or acute enteritis, the level may rise to 250 mg or more. With high levels of sugars in the gut such as in lactose intolerance, lactose will be absorbed and excreted unchanged in the urine.

Patients with malabsorption of carbohydrate have symptoms relative to the osmotic activity of the sugars in the gut. Cramping pain and fullness occur shortly after ingestion, and watery diarrhea follows. Bacteria metabolize the carbohydrate to form fatty acids, and the stool pH is lowered to less than 6.

Lactose
Lactose may appear in the urine late in normal pregnancy or during lactation.

Intestinal lactase deficiency is present in a large number of people, particularly in Africa and Asia. Intolerance increases with age through childhood to adolescence.

In intestinal disease, lactase activity may be depressed earlier than the activity of other disaccharidases, e.g., maltase and sucrase. Patients with celiac disease, tropical sprue, and kwashiorkor are most affected.

Lactose intolerance in infancy and failure to gain weight may be associated with lactase deficiency and variable lactosuria. In some patients it may occur as a result of a toxic effect of lactose when lactase is not deficient. In these children there is severe vomiting and diarrhea and high levels of lactose in the urine associated with damage to the intestine. Renal tubular dysfunction and aminoaciduria are present. Milk should be removed from the diet immediately in these infants.

Screening for Lactose
Urine is tested with the glucose oxidase reagent strip and a copper reduction test. A qualitative test may also be used. Thin layer chromatography is used to identify lactose in urine. Lactase deficiency may be established by means of oral lactose tolerance tests with analysis of blood glucose levels (lactose splits to form glucose and galactose) at half-hour intervals. Capillary blood may be used. Normal persons may give flat blood glucose levels after lactose loading. A lactase enzyme assay of a biopsy of the small intestine will provide a definitive diagnosis.

Lactose Test (Rubner, 1884)
To 15 mL urine in a test tube, add 3 g lead acetate. Shake and filter. Boil filtrate, add 2 mL concentrated NH_4OH, and boil. Lactose will cause the formation of a brick-red solution and then a red precipitate with clear supernatant. Glucose will cause a yellow solution and yellow precipitate.

Fructose
Fructose appears in urine during parenteral feedings with fructose and in association with inherited enzyme deficiencies that cause benign essential fructosuria and hereditary fructose intolerance associated with severe vomiting and liver and kidney disease (see Exhibit 22–5). Fructose is identified by thin layer chromatography. A qualitative test, the resorcinol test, is found to be useful by some.

Note: Fructose will form from glucose in alkaline urine. When testing for fructose, only freshly collected urine samples should be used.

Quantitative Test
Glucose is removed with glucose oxidase, and a method for inulin (a polyfructose) is used.

Resorcinol Test (Seliwanoff, 1887)
Boil 5 mL urine with 5 mL of 25% HCl. Add about 5 mg resorcinol and boil for 10 s. Fructose will cause the formation of a heavy red precipitate. Separate the precipitate by filtration and dissolve in ethanol. The precipitate should form a red solution in ethanol for the test to be positive. The fructose is converted to hydroxymethyl furfural; this condenses with resorcinol to form a red color. Use a positive control. Lowest level of detection is about 100 mg fructose/dL urine.

Galactose
Galactose appears in urine due to inherited enzyme deficiencies (see Exhibit 22–5). In these diseases, galactose derived from dietary lactose is not converted to glucose. Galactose in urine causes a positive copper reduction test and may be identified by thin layer chromatography.

Pentose
Pentosuria may follow the ingestion of large amounts of fruits (especially apricots), causing the excretion of L-xylose and L-arabinose in amounts up to 0.1 g/day. L-Xylulose is excreted in benign essential pentosuria in amounts of 1 to 4 g/day. At concentrations of 250 to 300 mg/dL, L-xylulose will reduce Benedict's qualitative reagent at 50°C (water bath) within 10 min, or at room temperature in several hours. Fructose will also reduce Benedict's reagent at low temperatures. The pentoses are identified by thin layer chromatography.

Sucrose
Sucrose may appear in the urine after the ingestion of very large amounts of sucrose. Sucrase deficiency is associated with intestinal diseases such as sprue in the same manner as lactase deficiency. Sucrose intolerance is an inherited disorder associated with sucrase and alpha-dextrinase (isomaltase) deficiencies. Symptoms are similar to those seen with lactase deficiency and occur in the first few weeks of life when sweetened food is ingested. Tolerance may develop, but sucrose may have to be avoided permanently.

Factitious sucrosuria may create a high specific gravity urine with negative glucose oxidase and negative copper reduction tests. Sucrose will ferment yeast and can be separated by chromatography but needs to be stained with a substance not dependent on reducing properties. Yeast fermentation and other qualitative tests for sugars (fructose, maltose, and sucrose) give a plus reaction on yeast fermentation, while galactose and lactose give a plus-minus reaction, and pentose gives a negative reaction. Of the other qualitative tests for nonglucose melliturias, fructose is positive on Rubner's lead acetate test, and pentose is positive on Benedict's test at 50°C.

[*Source:* Bradley M, Schumann GM: Glucose and other sugars. *In* Henry JB (ed): Todd, Sanford, Davidsohn's Clinical Diagnosis and Management by Laboratory Methods, Ed. 17. Philadelphia: W. B. Saunders, 1984, pp. 401–403; Ketones, p. 405. With permission.]

by glucose (Precision QID, Glucometer Elite), and (4) the Direct 30/30 has a reusable membrane cartridge that measures glucose in a drop of blood by an electro-chemical sensor.[21]

Different meters vary in: (1) *size* (from less than 1 ounce to 11 ounces), (2) *time for test* (from 30 to 120 s), (3) *ease of use* (some require removal of blood from the strip and timing of the reaction, some do not), (4) *audio readout* (some give test results of values for the visually impaired), and (5) requirement for *periodic calibration* of many meters (confidence strip, control solution).

Many meters have a memory for storing blood glu-cose measurements, and some have full-fledged data management systems. The stored data can be trans-ferred to the physician's computer and translated into graphic or tabular form with statistical analysis to pro-duce calculated means, standard deviations, ranges, and so forth, of blood glucose measurements over time. See Exhibit 22–7.

Test strips may be read visually and by meter, or visually alone (Exhibit 22–7). When a meter is selected, the *cost per test* should be considered. This includes not only the initial cost of the meter, but also ongoing costs of strips, control solutions, finger-sticking supplies (Exhibit 22–8), and other testing supplies.

Exhibit 22–9 lists the names, addresses, and tele-phone numbers of manufacturers of the devices noted in Exhibits 22–7 and 22–8.

Glucose monitoring, and other modes of evaluating metabolic control, should be *assessed individually* based on the needs and motivation of each person. Blood (and plasma) glucose monitoring is a significant advance in diabetes self-care management, which is educational and which can be motivational. It provides the imme-diate feedback needed to permit the patient to make appropriate alterations in a treatment routine, or if indi-cated to contact a professional for immediate advice.

A comparison of differences of glucose measure-ments by the yellow springs instrument (YSI) enzy-matic method on capillary and venous whole blood and plasma during a one year period are shown in Table 22–3. Note the significant differences in sample results.[31]

The American Diabetes Association Concensus Con-ference recommendations on SMBG are listed in Exhibit 22–10. The advantages and disadvantages of SMBG and urine glucose testing are listed in Exhibit 22–11.

On July 28, 1998, the Food and Drug Administration issued a press release[32] which stated "lifescan is recall-ing and replacing its surestep home blood glucose meters manufactured before August, 1997 because the meters may give an error message ("ER-I") instead of "HI" (HIGH) when a person's blood sugar is very high…500 mg/dL or greater. Such a level is very dan-gerous if not recognized and treated and could result in hospitalization or death. FDA has received reports of two deaths in people whose glucose was very high

but who repeatedly got error message readings from the surestep blood glucose meters and who delayed seeking medical care."[11]

Lifescan announced in a letter to professionals (June 15, 1998) that it planned to replace surestep meters made before August, 1997.

The author's recommendation is that if a blood glu-cose meter reading is ≥ 500 mg/dL (plasma glucose equivalent ≥ 575 mg/dL), a doctor or nurse should be contacted *immediately* for treatment recommendations.

It is important to remember that Beer's law and the parabolic color curve limit the accuracy of meter mea-sured blood glucose levels to about 500 mg/dL. It is essential to evaluate such high levels immediately in a central hospital lab or elsewhere with a glucose oxidase polaroscopic or hexokinase enzymatic method. It should be remembered that a conventional blood glucose meter measurement ≥ 500 mg/dL may actually represent a level of >800 mg/dL, >1000 mg/dL, >1200 mg/dL, or even >1500 mg/dL. All patients should learn that the hyperglycemic hyperosmolar state (HHS), defined as a serum osmolality ≥ 350 mOsm/kg due to a markedly elevated plasma glucose level, has an extremely high death rate, almost 1 in 3 in the editor's series of cases (see Chapter 24).

Problem Statement

What methods do individuals and professionals (MD, RN, RD, and others) need to monitor glucose and ketone levels both immediately and over the long term? (See Exhibits 22–4, 22–7 through 22–11.)

Subjective

The selection of tools to be used for SMBG and self-monitoring of urine glucose (SMUG) must be based on a mutually agreeable collaboration between the profes-sionals and the patient concerning what data are to be collected, how the data will be used, and whether or not the patient can afford the costs. (See Exhibits 22–4, 22–7, 22–10, and 22–11.)

Objective

Evaluation of visual acuity, including testing for color blindness, should be done. Individuals who are visu-ally impaired or color blind cannot evaluate tests results on visually-read strips. Eight percent of males and less than 1% of females are affected by red-green color blindness.[22] Devices are available to assist the visually impaired (Exhibit 22–7).[13] It is useful to determine the individual's renal threshold for glucose (Fig. 22–1). Unless renal glucosuria or diabetic nephropathy is pre-sent, the normal renal threshold for plasma glucose is ~ 200 mg/dl and for whole blood is ~ 180 mg/dl. (See Exhibit 22–11.)

EXHIBIT 22–7   Blood Glucose Monitors and Data-Management Systems[20]

Name and Manufacturer	Size (inches)	Wt. (ounces)	Test Strip Used*	Range (mg/dl)	Test Time	Battery
Accu-Chek Advantage (Roche Diagnostics)	3.6 × 2.3 × 0.6	3 with batteries	Accu-Chek Advantage or Accu-Chek Comfort Curve	10–600	40 sec.	(2) 3-volt lithium coin cell
Accu-Chek Complete (Roche Diagnostics)	4.8 × 2.8 × 1.1	4.4	Same as above	10–600	40 sec.	(2) AAA
Accu-Chek Easy (Roche Diagnostics)	4.5 × 2.5 × 0.7	3.4	Accu-Chek Easy Test Strips	20–500	15–60 sec.	Replaceable 6-volt alkaline; good for 1,000 tests
Accu-Chek Instant (Roche Diagnostics)	4.0 × 2.2 × 0.6	1.76	Accu-Chek Instant	20–500	12sec.	(4) 1.5-volt alkaline
Assure (Chronimed)	4.8 × 2.4 × 0.9	5.3	Assure	30–550	35 sec.	1 J-cell (home change)
CheckMate Plus (Cascade Medical)	6.3 × 1.1 × 0.7	1.8 with batteries	CheckMate Plus	25–500	15–70 sec.	(2) 3-volt lithium (6 to 9 months) (replaceable)
Diascan-S (Home Diagnostics)	3.1 × 5.2 × 0.6	4.8	Diascan	10–600	90 sec.	1 J-type (1,500 tests) (home change)
ExacTech (MediSense)	2.2 × 3.6 × 0.4	1.7	ExacTech	40–450	30 sec.	Permanent, no replacement required, 4,000 tests
ExacTech RSG (MediSense)	3.5 × 2.1 × 0.5	1.4	ExacTech RSG	40–450	30 sec.	Permanent, no replacement required, good for a minimum of 4,000 tests
Fast Take (LifeScan)	3.1 × 2.3 × 0.8	1.6	Fast Take	20–600	15 sec.	2 silver oxide #357 (1.5 volt–home change)
Glucometer DEX (Bayer Corporation, Diagnostics Division)	3.2 × 2.6 × 1.0	2.8	Glucometer DEX test sensors; 10-test sensor in one cartridge	10–600	30 sec.	(2) 3-volt lithium (CR-2016)
Glucometer Elite Diabetes Care System (Bayer Corporation, Diagnostics Division)	3.4 × 2.5 × 0.5	1.75	Glucometer Elite	20–600	30 sec.	(2) 3-volt lithium

* These are test strips approved by the manufacturers. In some cases, manufacturers cannot guarantee results or provide assistance if any other test strips are used.

Warranty	How Calibrated	Control Solution	Features
3 yr.	Snap-in code key	yes	No cleaning, wiping, or timing. Two steps to a result. Touchable test strips. Insufficient sample size detection; more blood can be applied if a sufficient sample isn't applied at first. 100-value memory with time and date.
3 yr.	Snap-in code key	yes	No cleaning, wiping, or timing. Large memory that collects, stores, and analyzes up to 1,000 values. Records information such as blood glucose, insulin, carbohydrates, ketones, HbA1c, stress, and exercise.
3 yr.	Snap-in code key	yes	Absorbent test strips with target area for easy dosing outside of the monitor, no timing or wiping of test strips. Large display; 350-value memory with time and date, 14 event codes, 7-day averaging, maximum and minimum values. Comes with carrying case and supplies including test strips, lancet device, and control solutions.
3 yr.	Rocker button coding	yes	Uses fast-acting strip chemistry. Simple two-step procedure. No wiping or timing. Test strips provide visual backup. Nine-value memory. Temperature-warning icon marks test results outside normal operating range. Comes with carrying case and supplies, including test strips, adjustable lancet device, and control solutions.
3 yr.	Calibrator in each box of strips	yes	Data-management system; biosensor technology; 180-test memory; large touch screen display.
Lifetime	Automatic calibration	yes	Display provides words for guidance. Lancing device built in. No wiping, blotting, or timing. Automatic hematocrit and temperature correction. Automatic sample volume check. Stores up to 255 results with time and date and insulin type and dosage. Average glucose reading. Clock with four alarms. Dataport allows downloading to PC. Prompts in 6 languages. Hands-off lancet ejection.
2 yr.	Button calibration (with safety lock) by lot of test strips	yes	Procedure requires no hanging drop of blood; extreme temperature warnings, below 41°F reads *cold* (home change) and above 98°F reads *hot*. Confidence strip supplied. Technique error notification. Automatic memory of last 10 readings. Audio signal emitted during test process can be turned off.
4yr.	Calibrator in each box of strips	yes	Credit card size and shape; simple three-step testing procedure; biosensor technology; no cleaning, wiping, or timing; value-priced test strips; last reading recall and calibration code.
4yr.	Calibrator in each box of strips	yes	Better accuracy; less cost; requires no calibration or coding; simple three-step testing procedure; value-priced test strips; biosensor technology; no cleaning or maintenance required.
3 yr.	Built-in single button	yes	Smallest blood sample; fast test time; compact; 150-test memory with date and time; touchable test strip; near-monitor dosing; 14-day averaging excludes flagged control solution test; warning to check ketones from 240–600 mg/dl.
5 yr.	Automatic calibration	yes 3 levels	Cartridge-based monitor eliminates strip handling. Performs 10 tests without reloading. Cartridge automatically calibrates monitor for 10 tests. Electronic functions automatically validated. Sensor actively draws just the amount of blood it needs. Advanced data management. Download memory for PC tracking. Monitor stores up to 100 results with time, date, and averages.
5 yr.	Strip calibration	yes	No buttons; turned on when test strip is inserted. Blood touched to the tip of the test strip is automatically drawn into the test chamber. Twenty-test memory, and a 3-minute automatic shutoff. Kit includes: blood letting device and lancets, 10 test strips, carrying case, control solution, and log book. Videotape on request.

(continued)

EXHIBIT 22–7 *(continued)* Blood Glucose Monitors and Data-Management Systems[20]

Name and Manufacturer	Size (inches)	Wt. (ounces)	Test Strip Used*	Range (mg/dl)	Test Time	Battery
Glucometer Encore Diabetes Care System (Bayer Corporation, Diagnostics Division)	4.3 × 2.5 × 0.7	3.6	Glucometer Encore	10–600	15 sec.	Permanent; 5-year warranty
MediSense 2 Card (MediSense)	3.6 × 2.2 × 0.4	1.7	MediSense 2 or Precision Q.I.D.	20–600	20 sec.	Permanent, no replacement required, 4,000 tests
MediSense 2 Pen (MediSense)	5.4 × 0.4	1.1	MediSense 2 or Precision Q.I.D.	20–600	20 sec.	Permanent. no replacement required, 4,000 tests
One Touch Basic (LifeScan)	4.8 × 2.6 × 1.1	4.8	Genuine One Touch	0–600	45 sec.	1 J-type (6V) alkaline (home change)
One Touch Profile (LifeScan)	4.3 × 2.6 × 1.2	4.5	Genuine One Touch	0–600	45 sec.	2 AAA alkaline (home change)
PocketLab II (Clinical Diagnostics)	4.9 × 2.1 × 0.7	2.2 with batteries	PocketLab II	40–450	45 sec.	1.55 volt (silver oxide) Eveready No. 357
Precision Q.I.D. (MediSense)	3.6 × 2.2 × 0.4	1.5	Precision Q.I.D	20–600	20 sec.	Permanent, no replacement required, minimum of 4,000 tests
Precision Q.I.D. Pen (MediSense)	5.4 × 0.4	1.1	Precision Q.I.D.	20–600	20 sec.	Permanent, no replacement required
Prestige (Home Diagnostics)	4.5 × 3.1 × 1.3	4.4	Prestige	25–600	10 sec.	6-volt J-cell
Select GT (Chronimed)	4.8 × 2.5 × 1.3	4.7	Select GT	30–600	50 sec.	1 J-cell (home change)
Supreme II (Chronimed)	4.8 × 2.5 × 1.3	4.7	Supreme	30–600	50 sec.	1 J-cell (home change)
SureStep (LifeScan)	3.5 × 2.4 × 0.8	3.8	SureStep	0–500	15–30 sec.	(2) AAA Alkaline (home change)

* These are test strips approved by the manufacturers. In some cases, manufacturers cannot guarantee results or provide assistance if any other test strips are used.

Warranty	How Calibrated	Control Solution	Features
3 yr.	Single button calibration by lot of test strips	yes	Automatic shutoff in 3 minutes. Stores up to 10 results. Includes carrying case, control solution, 10 test strips, and lancets. Spanish instructions available.
4 yr.	Calibrator in each box of strips	yes	Provides all the same features as the MediSense 2 Pen Sensor. Credit card size; extra large display window. Uses same sensor test strips.
4 yr.	Calibrator in each box of strips	yes	Biosensor technology; automatic start with "hands-off" testing; no cleaning, no wiping, no blotting, no timing; pen-size; extended memory; individually wrapped test strips.
3 yr.	Built-in single button	yes	No timing or wiping; large display; English or Spanish; detects most errors in sample application; notifies you when the monitor must be cleaned; recalls your last test result; has 30-day, money-back guarantee.
5 yr.	Built-in single button	yes	Three-step testing with no timing, wiping, or blotting; large display in English, Spanish, or 17 other languages; notifies you when the monitor must be cleaned; automatically stores last 250 results with date and time; provides a 14- and 30-day test average; insulin programming; event labeling.
Lifetime	Automatic calibration	yes	No wiping; one-button operation; large display; store 40 results in memory. Complete starter kit available including 10 strips, a lancing device, lancets, control solution, a quickstart guide in 6 languages, and a log book. Monitor-only package also available.
4yr.	Calibrator in each box of test strips	yes	Eliminates common test errors for clinical accuracy in everyday monitoring. Advanced biosensor technology; simple two-step testing; only requires 2.5 μl of blood; auto-starts when sample is detected; compact size; can apply second blood drop; not affected by many common medications; large display window; data-downloading capability; easy recall of last 10 results.
4 yr. or 4,000 tests	Calibrator in each box of test strips	Precision Q.I.D. high/low and normal control solution	Identical features and benefits as the Precision Q.I.D. hand-held monitor, but in the shape of a pen for portability. Advanced biosensor technology; only requires 3.5 μl of blood. Auto-starts when sample is detected. Ability to add a second drop of blood if necessary. Not affected by common medications; data-downloading capability; recall of last 10 test results.
2yr.	Button	yes	Non-wipe system allows user to apply the blood to test strip outside or inside the monitor; absorbable strip with sample-size verification; extreme temperature warnings; large digital display; universal symbols to guide user through test; videocassettes available in English and Spanish.
3 yr.	Built-in single button	yes	Large display; universal symbols; absorbent test strip; blood can be applied to test strip inside or outside of the monitor; 100-test memory.
3 yr.	Built-in single button	yes	Large display; universal symbols; absorbent test strip; blood can be applied to test strip inside or outside of the monitor; 100-test memory.
3 yr.	Built-in single button	yes	Large display; universal symbols; touchable, absorbent test strip allows maximum flexibility in blood application; blue confirmation dot confirms adequate blood sample; 10-test memory.

EXHIBIT 22–8 Finger-Sticking Supplies[20]

Name (Manufacturer/Distributor)	Features and Supplies
Accu-Chek Softclix Lancet Device (Roche Diagnostics)	Pen-shaped; Comfort Dial provides 11 penetration depth settings to accommodate all skin types; designed to reduce lancet's lateral motion when entering skin; includes 25 lancets and a 30-day refundable guarantee.
Accu-Chek Softclix Lancets (Roche Diagnostics)	Safety lock design for accurate penetration depth: for use with Accu-Chek Softclix lancet device; comes in packages of 100 and 200.
Accu-Chek Soft Touch Lancets (Roche Diagnostics)	28-gauge needle; can be used with Accu-Chek Soft Touch devices, most other lancet devices, or alone; comes in packages of 100 and 200.
Accu-Chek Soft Touch Lancet Device (Roche Diagnostics)	Pen shape; adjustable dial provides five penetration depth settings; 5-year warranty.
Ames Gluco System Lancet 100s (Bayer Corporation, Diagnostics Division)	Can be used in either Autolet or Glucolet.
Ames Glucolet Automatic Lancing Device (Bayer Corporation, Diagnostics Division)	Comes with 10 Gluco System lancets, one opaque regular puncture endcap, multi-lingual instruction insert.
Auto-Lancet (Palco)	Finger-lancing device with tip that adjusts to match different skin types; 1–2 for soft skin, 3 for average skin, 4–5 for skin that is harder to penetrate. Two lancets included. 5-year warranty.
Autolet Mini (Owen Mumford)	Two devices in one package; new extra-depth platforms offer choice of blood flow, new contour grips assist handling, includes 10 Unilet ComforTouch lancets and multi-lingual instructions; compatible with most lancets. Now includes extra-depth platforms and easy-grip contours.
Autolet Platforms (Owen Mumford)	Disposable and ejectable; to be used with Autolet II Clinisafe and Autolet Lite lancing devices to prevent cross-infection and to control penetration depth: choice of three depths: 1.8 mm (white), 2.4 mm (yellow), 3.0 mm (orange).
Autolet Lite (Owen Mumford)	3 platform depths, 1.8 mm, 2.4 mm, 3.0 mm, self-arming; lancet ejection for safety; includes 10 ComforTouch lancets and instructions.
AutoLet Clinisafe (Owen Mumford)	Comes with 20 platforms (10 each of 2 different depths), 10 Unilets, and vinyl wallet.
B-D Lancet Device (Becton Dickinson)	Compatible with most lancets; comes with three B-D Ultra-Fine lancets; 5-year warranty.
B-D Ultra-Fine II Lancets (Becton Dickinson)	30-gauge lancet with cylindrical design for easy handling; fits B-D Lancet Device and most other lancet devices.
Carelet Safety Lancet (Gainor Medical)	Self-contained, single-use safety lancet. After a single use, the needle is encased inside a plastic housing to avoid chance of re-use or re-exposure.
Cleanlet (Gainor Medical)	Now available in 28 gauge. Protective cap snaps securely over lancet tip for safer disposal after a single use. Tri-beveled angle designed for less painful punctures.
Dialet (Home Diagnostics)	Pen-shaped; comes with one regular, one deep tip; for safety, blue dot appears when device is armed.
E-Z Ject Lancets (Can-Am Care)	Fit most lancing devices; available in traditional lite-angle, assorted colors, and thin gauge.
E-Z Lets (Palco)	Tri-beveled sterile lancets for use in most lancing devices.

EXHIBIT 22–8 *(continued)* Finger-Sticking Supplies[20]

Name (Manufacturer/Distributor)	Feutures and Supplies
E-Z Lets II (Palco)	Sterile, single-use, disposable finger-lancing device; automatically retracts; gentle model for regular blood flow; deep puncture for larger blood sample.
E-Z Lets Thin (Palco)	28-gauge lancet.
Gentle-let Lancets, GP Style (Ulster Medical Products)	Fits most automatic lances devices; available in fine-point (23-gauge) or medium-point (21-gauge) needle. Made in U.S.A.
Gentle-let Lancets, Safety Style (Ulster Medical Products)	Can be used in Autolet devices, Glucolet, or for manual use; available in fine-point (23-gauge) or medium-point (21-gauge) needle. Made in U.S.A.
Gentle-let 1 (Ulster Medical Products)	Disposable, single-use lancet device; built-in retractable lancet; normal or extra spring pressure; boxes of 50 or 200. Made in U.S.A.
Haemolance (Chronimed)	Single-use disposable lancet with built-in needle protection system; needle retracts automatically to eliminate risk of cross-contamination and accidental needle punctures.
Lady Lite Lancet (Medicore)	Designed for the feminine fingertip; fine, delicate tip; floral cap; fits most lancet devices.
Lancets (LifeScan)	For use with all Penlet Automatic Blood Samplers from LifeScan and many other blood sampling devices.
Medi-Lance Lancets (Medicore)	Precision tri-bevel comfort tip; fits most lancing devices.
Medi-Lance II Lancets (Medicore)	Tri-bevel comfort tip; extra-long body; fits Glucolet, Autolet, and Medi-Let.
Medi-Let Lancet Device (Medicore)	Kit includes lancing device, 20 platforms, and 10 lancets.
Microlet® Lancets (Bayer Corporation, Diagnostics Division)	For use with Microlet Lancing Device; 25 gauge.
Microlet® Automatic Lancing Device (Bayer Corporation, Diagnostics Division)	Comes with 10 lancets and 2 endcaps; easy cocking mechanism with new ergonomic design.
Microlet® Vaculance (Bayer Corporation, Diagnostics Division)	Vacuum action draws blood to skin surface, allowing patient to choose lancing sites less painful than fingers. No-button simplicity; small blood sample (3 ml); 4 lancing depths; no-touch safety sleeves and protective end caps; extra-small lancet in diamonitor.
Monojector Lancet Device (Can-Am Care)	Works with most lancets, comes with 10 endcaps.
Monolet Original Lancets (Can-Am Care)	Fits most lancing devices; designed for those who have thicker finger pads or have difficulty getting the right amount of blood.
Monolet Thin Lancets (Can-Am Care)	Fits most lancing devices; designed for those who have sensitive fingertips or who easily produce the small sample of blood they need.
One Touch Finepoint Lancets (LifeScan)	25-gauge, single-use lancets fit most lancing devices; available in boxes of 100; protective cap snaps over needle for disposal; polished and coated for less painful blood sampling.
Penlet II Automatic Blood Sampling Device (LifeScan)	Pen-shaped; hands-off lancet removal system to minimize possibility of sticks; comes with LifeScan lancets and two different caps to control the depth of penetration.
Select Lite Lancing Device (Chronimed)	Pen-shaped device is compatible with most lancets; adjustable tip; five settings.

(continued)

EXHIBIT 22–8 *(continued)* Finger-Sticking Supplies[20]

Name (Manufacturer/Distributor)	Features and Supplies
Surelite Lancet (Gainor Medical)	Quality ground lancet tip for smooth penetration; closed-base design prevents needle breakthrough, protecting against accidental needle punctures.
Techlite Lancets (Chronimed)	Fits most devices; available in 21 and 25 gauge; packages of 100 or 200.
Tenderlett (ITC)	Permanently retracting blade, incision controlled to 1.75 mm deep; designed for older children and adults.
Tenderlett Jr. (ITC)	Permanently retracting blade, incision controlled to 1.25 mm deep; designed for children or for smaller blood samples.
Tenderlett Toddler (ITC)	Permanently retracting blade, incision controlled to 0.85 mm deep; designed for older infants and toddlers.
UltraTLC (MediSense)	Available in packages of 50 (with ultraTLC lancing device), 100, and 200; provides a smooth tri-bevel point, 21 gauge.
UltraTLC Adjustable Lancing Device (MediSense)	Adjustable tip provides five penetration depth settings; pen-shaped; includes 50 ultraTLC lancets; 5-year warranty.
Unilet G.P. Lancet (Owen Mumford)	21 gauge; for use with most automatic lancing devices; packages of 100 and 200; blue.
Unilet G.P. Superlite Lancet (Owen Mumford)	23 gauge; for use with most automatic lancing devices; packages of 100 and 200; white.
Unilet Lancet (Long body) (Owen Mumford)	21 gauge; for use with Autolet II Clinisafe, Autolet Lite, and Glucolet lancing devices, or manual use; packages of 200; yellow.
Unilet Superlite Lancet (Long body) (Owen Mumford)	23 gauge; for use with Autolet II Clinisafe, Autolet Lite, and Glucolet lancing devices, or manual use; in packages of 100 or 200; white.
Unilet ComforTouch (Owen Mumford)	26 gauge; for use with most major lancing devices; packages of 100 or 200; purple.
Unistik 1 (Owen Mumford)	Single-use device; lances automatically retracts for safety; needle hidden before and after use; available in two penetration depths: 2.4 mm (yellow) and 3.0 mm (red); 50 per box.
Unistik 2 (Owen Mumford)	Single use for safety and disposability; device and lances are one; punctures and retracts automatically; two puncture depths: 2.4 mm, 3.0 mm; 50 or 100 per box.
Vitalet Lancet (Medical Plastic Devices)	Fits most lancing devices; available with 23- or 26-gauge needle; provides sterile tip for patient's security; tri-bevel stainless steel needle permits smooth skin penetration; made in Canada.
Various store-brand lancets (Can-Am Care)	Retailers (such as Walgreens, Kmart, Wal-Mart, and Rite-Aid) offer their own assortment of store-brand lancets; ask your pharmacist for more information.

EXHIBIT 22–9 Manufacturers & Exclusive Distributors[20]

Activa Brand Products, Inc.
6845 Davand Drive
Missisauga, ONT L5T 1I4
Canada
(905) 565-0223
1-800-991-4464
mark.mpd@pei.sympatico.ca
TUBE-FAB@netcom.ca

Aimsco/Delta Hi-Tech
3762 South 150 East
Salt Lake City, UT 84115
1-800-378-0909

Apothecary Products, Inc.
11531 Rupp Drive
Burnsville, MN 55337-1295
(612) 890-1940
1-800-328-2742

Atwater Carey, Ltd.
339 East Rainbow Blvd.
Salida, CO 81201
(719) 530-0923
1-800-359-1646

Bayer Corporation
Diagnostics Division
511 Benedict Avenue
Tarrytown, NY 10591
1-800-348-8100
www.bayerdiag.com

Becton Dickinson Consumer Products
One Becton Drive
Franklin Lakes, NJ 07417-1883
1-800-237-4554
www.bd.com/diabetes

Bioject, Inc.
7620 SW Bridgeport Road
Portland, OR 97224
(503) 639-7221
1-800-848-2538

Can-Am Care Corp.
Cimetra Industrial Park
Box 98
Chazy, NY 12921
1-800-461-7448

Cascade Medical, Inc.
10180 Viking Drive
Eden Prairie, MN 55344
(612) 941-7345
1-800-525-6718
www.mm.com/cascade

Chronimed
10900 Red Circle Drive

Minnetonka, MN 55343
(612) 979-3600
1-800-444-5951

Clinical Diagnostics, Inc.
2606 Eden Terrace
Rock Hill, SC 29732
(803) 980-1020
1-800-860-9937

Diabetes Support Systems
1868 North University Dr.,
   Suite 106
Plantation, FL 33322
(954) 452-0202
1-800-952-0207

Diabetes Technologies, Inc.
216 W. Jackson Street
Thomasville, GA 31792
(912) 226-7875
1-888-872-2443

Disetronic Medical Systems, Inc.
5201 East River Road, Suite 312
Minneapolis, MN 55421-1014
(612) 571-6878
1-800-280-7801
www.disetronic.com

Eli Lilly and Company
Lilly Corporate Center
Indianapolis, IN 46285
1-800-545-5979

Express-Med, Inc.
3592 Corporate Drive
Columbus, OH 43231-4978
(614) 895-5211
1-800-678-5733

Frio Cooling Products
Freepost SWC0667
Haverfordwest, SA62 522
England
frio@btintemet.com
www.friouk.com

Gainor Medical
2205 Highway 42 North
P.O. Box 353
McDonough, GA 30253
(770) 474-0474
1-800-825-8282

Goldware Medical ID Jewelry
P.O. Box 22335
San Diego, CA 92192
(619) 53-4005
1-800-669-7311

Home Diagnostics, Inc.
2400 NW 55th Court
Ft. Lauderdale, FL 33309
(954) 677-9201
1-800-342-7226

HypOview, Ltd.
146 Belleview Avenue
Adams, MA 01220
(413) 743-8000
1-888-999-1577
sales@hypoview.com
www.hypoview.com

ICN Pharmaceuticals, Inc.
3300 Hyland Ave.
Costa Mesa, CA 92626
(714) 545-0100
1-800-548-5100 Ext. 3232

I.D. Technology, Inc.
117 Nelson Road
Baltimore, MD 21208-1111
(410) 602-1911
www. id-technology.com

Identi-Find
P.O. Box 567
Canton, NC 28716
(7W) 648-6768
labels@primeline.com
www.identifind.com

Insulator
1110 North Olive Avenue
West Palm Beach, FL 33401
(561) 655-9700

ITC
8 Olsen Avenue
Edison, NJ 08820
(732) 548-5700
1-800-631-5945

Jordan Medical Enterprises, Inc.
202 Oaklawn Avenue
South Pasadena, CA 91030
(626) 799-0317
1-800-541-1193

LifeScan, Inc.
1000 Gibraltar Drive
Milpitas, CA 95035-6312
(408) 263-9789
1-800-227-8862
lifescan@lfsus.jnj.com
www.lifescan.com

(continued)

EXHIBIT 22–9   *(continued)* Manufacturers & Exclusive Distributors[20]

The Lighthouse Catalog
111 E. 59th Street
New York, NY 10022
1-800-829-0500

LXN Corporation
5830 Oberlin Drive
San Diego, CA 92121
(619) 546-7500
1-888-596-8378
duet@lxncorp.com
www.lxncorp.com

Mcard Corporation
6320 W. 159th Street, Suite A
Oak Forest, IL 60452
(708) 535-7214
www.mcard.com

Medic Alert
2323 Colorado Avenue
Turlock, CA 95832
1-800-825-3785
postmaster@medicalert.org
www.medicalert.org

Medical Plastic Devices, Inc.
161 Oneida Drive
Pointe Claire, QUE H9R 1A9
Canada
(514) 694-9835
1-888-527-2842

MediCheck International
   Foundation, Inc.
8320 Ballard Rd.
Niles, IL 60714
(847) 299-0620

Medicool, Inc.
23520 Telo Avenue
Suite #6
Torrance, CA 90505
(310) 784-1200
1-800-433-2469
medicool@medicool.com
www.medicool.com

Medicore, Inc.
2337 W. 76th St.
Hialeah, FL 33016
(305) 557-1163
1-800-327-8894

Medi-Ject Corporation
161 Cheshire Lane, Suite 100
Minneapolis, MN 55441
(612) 475-7700

1-800-328-3074
needlefree@mediject.com
www.mediject.com

MediSense, Inc.
4A Crosby Dr.
Bedford, MA 01730
(781) 276-6000
1-800-527-3339

Meditec, Inc.
3322 S. Oneida Way
Denver, CO 80224
(303) 758-6978

MEDport
23 Acorn St.
Providence, RI 02903
(401) 273-0444
medport@medportinc.com
www.medportinc.com

MiniMed, Inc.
12744 San Fernando Road
Sylmar, CA 91342
1-800-933-3322
www.minimed.com

Monroe Specialty
P.O. Box 740
Monroe, WI 53566
1-800-628-0165

Myna Corporation
239 Western Avenue
Essex, MA 01929
(978) 768-9000

Novo Nordisk Pharmaceuticals Inc.
100 Overlook Center
Suite 200
Princeton, NJ 08540
(609) 987-5800
www.novo-nordisk.com

Owen Mumford, Inc.
849 Pickens Industrial Dr. #14
Marietta, GA 30062
(770) 425-5138
1-800-421-6936
owenmumfor@aol.com

Paddock Laboratories
3940 Quebec Avenue N.
Minneapolis, NIN 55427
(612) 546-4676
1-800-546-4676
www.paddocklabs.com

Palco Laboratories
8030 Soquel Avenue
Santa Cruz, CA 95062
(408) 476-3151
1-800-346-4488
www.palcolabs.com

Pharmacy Counter
2655 West Central Avenue
Toledo, OH 43606
(419) 244-9700
1-800-984-1137
diabetesstore@accesstoledo.com

Roche Diagnostics
9115 Hague Road
P.O. Box 50100
Indianapolis, IN 46250-0100
1-800-858-8072

Science Products
Box 888
Southeastern, PA 19399
(610) 296-2111
1-800-888-7400

Scorpio Concepts
HC 54, Box 66
DeTour Village, MI 49725
(906) 297-6506

SOS America, Inc.
P.O. Box 260
Massapequa, NY 11758
(516) 795-3960
1-800-999-1264
info@sosamerica.com
www.sosamerica.com

Transfer-Ease, Inc.
P.O. Box 108
Emerson, NJ 07630-0108
1-888-357-0114

Ulster Medical Products
A Division of Lukens Medical Corp.
3820 Academy Parkway North, NE
Albuquerque, NM 87109-4409
(505) 342-9638
1-800-631-0076
lukens@lukens-med.com
www.lukens-med.com

Whittier Medical, Inc.
865 Turnpike St.
North Andover, MA 01845
(508) 688-5002
1-800-645-1115

TABLE 22–2 Urine Glucose Monitoring Methods

	Glucose Oxidase Methods	Copper Sulfate Reduction Methods

Products	Diastix
	Keto-Diastix
	Testape
	
	Clinistix
	Chemstrip UG
	Chemstrip UGK
		Clinitest
		  Five drops
		  Two drops
		  One drop
		Benedict's solution

Advantages	Convenient	Positive only if high urine glucose (>250 mg/dL), thus useful in IDDM where high urine glucose levels are common and need to be estimated at home
Disadvantages	Ketones may interfere with glucose reading Hard to distinguish between colors Drug interactions False-negative	Materials are cumbersome Mistakes made in urine/water ratio used Drug interactions Toxicity if consumed (mouth and esophageal) burns, particularly in children False-positives False-negatives See Table 11–2 for sensitivity and specificity assessment in relation to quantitative urine glucose measurements

TABLE 22–3 YSI Data Collected on Fresh Bloods from Diabetics.[31]

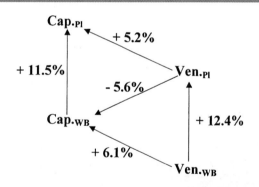

Sample	N =	Mean (mg/dL)	95% CI (mg/dL)	95% Range (mg/dL)
Capillary Plasma	883	206.54	±6.08	199.56 to 211.72
Capillary Whole Blood	883	185.30	±5.43	179.87 to 190.73
Venous Plasma	883	196.38	±5.99	190.39 to 202.37
Venous Whole Blood	883	174.69	±5.25	169.44 to 179.94

Clinical specimen glucose data collected over a period of one year (1997–1998) using the Yellow Springs Instrument (YSI) blood glucose analyzer.[31] Each of 20 studies collected data on 40-50 volunteer diabetics. Capillary and venous samples were collected within 2-3 minutes of each other; plasma was prepared within 90 seconds using a high-speed microcentrifuge; all YSI glucose measurements were made within 10 minutes of sample collection.

Abbreviations: CAP.PI = capillary plasma, CAP.WB = capillary whole blood, VEN.WB = venous whole blood, VEN.PI = venous plasma

EXHIBIT 22–10   American Diabetes Association Consensus Conference Recommendations on Self-Monitoring of Blood Glucose (SMBG)

1. IDDMs should use routinely
2. Continue availability of SMBG systems from multiple sources (Exhibit 22–7)
3. Monitors that are easier to use and that are less dependent on user skill should be developed
4. A reliable system for the visually impaired should be developed
5. Complete *quality-control programs* should be implemented by all users and should be supported by manufacturers and health care providers
6. A glucose monitoring system should be developed that requires the user to complete quality control and calibration functions before accepting a sample

7. Systems should be developed to assure accuracy of SMBG in the hyperglycemic and hypoglycemic ranges and should not be influenced by changes in hematocrit
8. The components of training listed in response to recommendation 6 should be incorporated into professional user and patient user education programs
9. The proper uses of SMBG are: (1) to develop a longitudinal data base related to the patient's blood glucose profile; (2) as an aid in making day-to-day decisions, based on immediately obtained data, regarding various components of the treatment regimen; (3) as an aid in the recognition and response to emergency situations; and (4) as an educational and training tool to enhance understanding of diabetes by patients and their families.

[*Source:* Adapted from: American Diabetes Association Consensus Conference Recommendations on self-monitoring of blood glucose (SMBG). Diabetes Care 10:95–99, 1987. With permission.]

EXHIBIT 22–11   Advantages and Disadvantages of Capillary Blood Glucose Testing and Urine Glucose Testing

ADVANTAGES	DISADVANTAGES
I. Capillary Blood Glucose Testing (SMBG)	
Measure blood glucose levels that are below the renal threshold (≈180 mg/dL for whole blood)	Invasive
Documents hypoglycemia	Uncomfortable
Educational tool for patients to learn variables that influence blood glucose levels	More difficult to learn than urine testing
Allows immediate feedback regarding adjustments in therapy by the patient at home	Expensive
	Results sometimes incorrect and may lead to inappropriate adjustments in therapy
	Some meters do not read above 400 mg/dL unless blood is diluted (see Exhibit 22–7)
II. Urine Glucose Testing	
Noninvasive	Poor correlation between urine glucose levels and plasma or blood glucose levels. Renal threshold in normals ≈200 mg/dL for plasma, ≈180 mg/dL for whole blood, but it may be as low as 100 mg/dL in renal glucosuria and as high as 500 mg/dL in end-stage renal disease
Inexpensive	
Can estimate amount of glucose in urine in specified time period, such as 8 or 24 hours	Unable to detect hypoglycemia

Assessment

The choice of tools to be used for self-monitoring of blood glucose (SMBG), self-monitoring of urine glucose (SMUG), self-monitoring of urine ketones (SMUK) should be determined on an individual basis by the target-zone needs for blood (or plasma) glucose control (see Chapter 18), and available resources (physical, intellectual, professional, and financial).

Both IDDMs and NIDDMs should be educated concerning the importance of testing for urine ketones when ill (such as infection and gastroenteritis) and when capillary glucose levels are ≥250 mg/dL. Also, ketone testing is recommended during pregnancy, not only to detect ketosis due to insulin deficiency, but to

detect *"starvation" ketosis* due to insufficient carbohydrate intake.[23] See Chapters 40 and 41.

Urine ketone levels can be estimated by Acetest (nitroprusside) tablets (Ames), Ketostix (Ames), Ketodiastix (Ames), Chemstrip K (Boehringer), Chemstrip UGK (Boehringer), Kyotest UGK (Kyodex). Ketodiastix, Chemstrip UGK, and Kyotest UGK estimate both urine glucose and urine ketone levels. Serum ketone levels may be estimated using crushed Acetest tablets (Exhibit 22–4). (See Chapter 24.)

None of the tests just noted will detect beta-hydroxybutyrate, but all will detect 5-10 mg/dL acetoacetic acid (upper normal limit = 2 mg/dL) or 20-25 mg/dL acetone (See Exhibit 22–3.) A test strip to measure urine and serum beta-hydroxybutyrate levels has been introduced, but it is seldom used in the United States.[24] Serum beta-hydroxybutyrate levels can be measured by enzymatic methods in a hospital laboratory.

Plan

Methods of testing for urine glucose and ketones are listed in Exhibits 22–2 and 22–4, and methods of testing for ketones are listed in Exhibits 22–3 and 22–4. Substances sometimes found in urine that give *false-positive tests* for glucosuria are listed in Table 22–1. Melliturias other than glucosuria are listed in Exhibit 22–5, and testing techniques for nonglucose melliturias are listed in Exhibit 22–6.

The Committee on Materials and Therapeutic Agents of the American Diabetes Association (1977)[23] made the following recommendations:

1. It is recommended that manufacturers of urine testing devices be encouraged to change scales using "plus" values to "per cent" readings for estimating the urine glucose levels, since the "plus" scales suggest different glucose concentrations when different methods are used (i.e., 1 + by one method may be 3 + by another method, though the urine glucose content may be the same, i.e., 300 mg/dL glucose when measured by a quantitative urine glucose method). Manufacturers complied with this request (see Fig. 22–1), and color-coded charts were provided so that the amount of glucose in the sample can be estimated.

2. It is recommended that the two-drop Clinitest method for urine testing be indicated as the method of choice in labile juvenile diabetes (now designated IDDM).

3. It is recommended that "dipstick" urine testing methods be considered useful in qualitative assessment in stable diabetes (majority of cases now designated NIDDM).

Some have recommended that urines tested for sugar should accumulate in the bladder for only 30 min before collection and be tested (the *"second-void" specimen*) in contrast to the first-voided sample that had accumulated over a longer period of time (the *"first-void" specimen*). This practice has been shown to be of little value.[25] Sometimes is it useful to use a semiquantitative method (Clinitest) to estimate at home the 24-hr glucose spill in grams, or to estimate grams of glucose spilled in each of three 8-hr periods.

Example: Three 8-hr urine samples were collected and the volume of each was measured. The 8 A.M. to 4 P.M. sample contained 650 mL, the 4 P.M. to 12 midnight sample contained 785 mL, the 12 midnight to 8 A.M. sample contained 520 mL (a total 24-hr volume of 1955 mL). By Clinitest estimate, the 8 *a.m.* to 4 P.M. sample contained 1%

glucose (1 g/dL), or a total of 6.50 g (1 g × 6.50 = 6.50 g glucose); the 4 P.M. to 12 midnight sample contained 2% glucose, or a total of 15.70 g (2 g × 7.85 dL = 15.70 g glucose); and the 12 midnight to 8 A.M. sample contained 0.5% glucose, or a total of 2.6 g (0.5 g × 5.20 dL = 2.6 g). Thus, the total glucose spill for the 24-hr period was 24.8 g (6.5 + 15.7 + 2.6 = 24.8 g), or about 10% of the 250 g carbohydrate ingested during the same 24-hr period.

Continuing access to information regarding blood glucose levels is a distinct advantage in assessment of diabetes control, particularly for the intelligent, highly motivated person who desires optimal control and who has an active and variable lifestyle. Exhibit 22–11 compares advantages and disadvantages of urine testing and capillary blood testing.

Symptoms and signs of hypoglycemia may be confirmed by the data provided by the readings. Reactive hyperglycemia, the waning of insulin action, and the dawn phenomenon (see Chapter 18), can also be identified and verified.

The inconvenience and discomfort of blood glucose monitoring may serve to diminish the quality of life for some individuals. Many people are averse to the suggestion that they add another moderately painful procedure, especially if it is done at frequent intervals and is expensive. Blood glucose monitoring may become an additional source of anxiety for individuals with an obsessive-compulsive personality.

Examples: (1) A meticulous elderly women with IDDM arranges her schedule to accommodate eight daily blood glucose readings. Rather than using the tool to enrich her lifestyle, monitoring has become an obsession that elicits a depressive response when results are not "perfect." (2) A college professor with IDDM maintains his capillary blood glucose level (by SMBG) between 50 and 120 mg/dL and his hemoglobin A_{1c} level below 4.5%, despite numerous hypoglycemic episodes, several of which have resulted in generalized convulsions, tongue-biting (with lacerations that required surgical repair), and falling out of bed. His physicians have repeatedly advised him to avoid hypoglycemia, but he has not yet heeded their advice. (3) Of those under "tight glucose control" in the DCCT study, 27% experienced hypoglycemic coma during the first year of the trial, making clear one of the very serious risks of intensive insulin therapy. Several other disadvantages of SMBG are noted in Exhibit 22–11.

Aziz and coworkers,[27] Frindik and associates,[28] Nelson and coworkers,[29] and Reeves et al.[30] measured the statistical correlations between both visually read and meter-read strips and Beckman glucose analyzer measurements. It is important for the physician and the patient to understand that blood glucose monitoring meters provide only an estimate of the true glucose level, with a correlation coefficient of 0.92. Some estimates were more than 30% greater or more than 30% less than the true glucose level.

Long-Term Monitoring and Follow-Up

After the appropriate method or methods of monitoring for the individual with IDDM or NIDDM have been determined, the ongoing monitoring of levels of metabolic control begins.

When the DCCT results were reported in 1993,[33–35] glycohemoglobin testing was in a state of disarray; there were many different assay methods and test results were not easily comparable among the various methods. Even the same assay methods might give widely differing results in different laboratories. After the nine-year DCCT study had shown the relationship between glycemic control and the development and progression of microvascular and neuropathic complications in type I diabetes, it became necessary to standardize glycohemoglobin testing as related to recorded DCCT numbers. By late 1996 the national glycohemoglobin standardization program (NGSP) was in place, and by 1999 some order had emerged from the earlier chaos. Manufacturers of glycohemoglobin testing methods can undergo voluntary testing to document comparability of test results to those obtained by the NGSP laboratory network, which is linked to the DCCT reference method. The College of American Pathologists proficiency testing survey for glycohemoglobin, in which individual laboratories participate, has documented steady improvements in assay quality, in terms of both interlaboratory variability and accuracy in matching the testing target values set by the NGSP laboratory network. The American Diabetes Association recommends that laboratories performing glycohemoglobin testing use only assay methods that are *certified as traceable to the DCCT reference* through the NGSP.[33–35] Standardization of glycohemoglobin testing will make it much easier for major national organizations in the USA that are pushing for better diabetes care (e.g., NIH, CDC, ADA) to monitor results and to promote their *know your number* campaign (goal for glycohemoglobin <7% with *action needed* for levels >8%).

Those with IDDM should be taught that the beta cells of their pancreatic islets are no longer producing enough insulin to keep their blood sugar normal. The endogenous insulin deficit must be replaced by injecting exogenous insulin. SMBG makes it possible to evaluate the response to the insulin replacement program as it develops. (See Chapter 18.) The ideal goal for such a program is to keep the blood glucose in the target range of 80 to 150 mg/dL more than 75% of the time without significant episodes of hypoglycemia. In unstable IDDMs, it may be necessary to raise the upper limit target range to 200 mg/dL.

Since the pharmacokinetics of insulin varies between individuals (rate of absorption from the injected subcutaneous site) and from day-to-day in the same individual, patients need to learn about all factors that influence the blood glucose and how to minimize these variations as much as possible from day to day. See Chapter 18 for a detailed discussion of the pharmacokinetics of insulin and other factors that cause hyperglycemia and hypoglycemia in those with IDDM.

The patient may bring a flow sheet of SMBG to the office to discuss results with the physician and nurse, or may telephone them in order to seek advice concerning changes in the therapeutic routine that may be indicated. It is important that all records be carefully scrutinized by the professionals to assess what has been happening so that suggested changes can be based on adequate data. Eventually, patients can learn from experience how to adjust their insulin doses, exercise patterns, and diets by understanding in more detail how the different variables influence their blood glucose levels. Usually the insulin dose is reduced if blood glucose is below 80 mg/dL (and a missed or delayed meal or excessive exercise is not responsible). Usually, the insulin dose is increased 1 to 2 U if blood glucose is above the upper target level 3 days in a row (if no other reason for the elevation is present).

It is important to the teaching process that professionals allow sufficient time not only for teaching, but for questions to determine that the patient truly understands what is happening and how to adapt.

In a study by Belmont et al.,[36] use of *supplementary regular insulin* based on SMBG did not improve control over a 3-year period; thus, it is inappropriate to make adjustments in the insulin dose based on one measurement.

Results obtained by the glucose monitor used by the patient should be compared with that obtained on the same sample by a Beckman glucose analyzer or similar device to assure appropriate *quality control* of the measurements performed by the patient. If the device being used is giving incorrect measurements, it is dangerous to make adjustments in the insulin dose based on those measurements (See Table 22–3.)[37]

There are many technical errors that should be avoided. These include: (1) not enough blood to cover the strip, (2) diluting blood on the strip with alcohol or moisture from washed hands, (3) perspiration on hands, (4) smearing the blood, (5) timing errors, (6) hand lotion on hands, (7) several small drops of blood on the strip, (8) glucose from food on hands, (9) outdated strips or using wrong type of strip, (10) failing to change the meter calibration code, (11) exposure to excessively hot or cold temperatures, (12) putting the blood on the wrong side of the strip, (13) incorrect visual reading. All of these problems are preventable or correctable with careful initial and follow-up instruction by the diabetes educator and the physician. (See Exhibit 22–10.)

SMBG in those with NIDDM is useful. It quickly reveals the consequences of overeating to overweight

NIDDMs who doubt the value of weight loss from reduced caloric intake. It is also of value when marked hyperglycemia develops because of infection, stress, or overeating in these individuals.

Adherence

Adherence to a prescribed urine and blood glucose testing routine, as to other evaluative and therapeutic modalities, varies greatly between indviduals and their particular circumstances. The care provider may inadvertently encourage nonadherence by requesting unnecessarily frequent monitoring. Allowing the individual's input into the decision-making regarding the choice of tools, frequency of monitoring, and the assumption of appropriate management decisions increases the rate of adherence to a monitoring protocol. Intensive and continuing education is required if monitoring is to be an effective crisis prevention tool and if it is to be an ongoing evaluative tool with the potential to help delay the appearance of, or to prevent, the chronic complications.

Urine and blood glucose monitoring are incentives to achieve and maintain normoglycemia in those with NIDDM or near-normoglycemia in those with IDDM. It provides a measure of self-evaluation that gives the patient a feeling of being an involved team member in the attempt to control his diabetes. Combined with continuing access to optimal follow-up medical care, home monitoring provides a tool that can prevent many avoidable hospitalizations for metabolic decompensation (both hypoglycemia and hyperglycemia).

Standardization of glycohemoglobin testing under the supervision of the National Glycohemoglobin Standardization Program (NGSP) has made chronic monitoring of levels of long-term control much more reliable and should be done every 3-6 months. Normal is <5%, desirable <7%, and action needed if >8%.[21,33–35]

Research Considerations

Much of the research conducted on SMBG in individuals with IDDM shows an improvement in glucose control. The authors have observed many individuals with NIDDM who enthusiastically correlate their weight loss with attainment of normal blood glucose readings. Blood glucose monitoring may serve as an effective reinforcer for individuals whose health beliefs include an understanding of the desirability of glucose control. (See Chapter 14).

The DCCT has shown that aggressive control of blood glucose and hemoglobin A_{1c} levels can prevent or slow the development of microangiopathy and neuropathy in IDDMs, and there is anecdotal and other evidence that good control improves outcomes in NIDDMs. Many studies have been initiated to test this hypothesis. See Chapter 10.

References

1. Pollack H: Stanley Rossiter Benedict: creator of laboratory tests for glycosuria. Diabetes 2:420–421, 1953.

2. Silink M: Home blood glucose monitoring in childhood diabetes mellitus. *In* Peterson CM (ed): The Role of Home Blood Glucose Monitoring and New Insulin Delivery Systems, New York: Physicians Publications, 1982, pp. 176–183.

3. James RC, Chase GR: Evaluation of some commonly used semiquantitative methods for urinary glucose and ketone determinations. Diabetes 23:474–479, 1974.

4. Davidson JK, Reuben MD, Sternberg JC, et al.: Diabetes screening using a quantitative urine glucose method. Diabetes 27:810–816, 1978.

5. Marble A: Non-diabetic mellituria. *In* Marble A, White PA, Bradley RF, et al.: (eds): Joslin's Diabetes Mellitus, Ed. 11. Philadelphia: Lea & Febiger, 1971, pp. 818–829.

6. Gitzelmann R, Steinmann B, Van Den Berghe G: Essential fructosuria, hereditary fructose intolerance, and fructose −1, 6- diphosphatase deficiency. *In* Stanbury JB, Wyngaarden JB, Fredrickson DS, et al. (eds): The Metabolic Basis of Inherited Disease, ed. 5. New York: McGraw-Hill, 1983, pp. 1728–1742.

7. Segal S: Disorders of galactose metabolism. *In* Stanbury JB, et al. (eds): The Metabolic Basis of Inherited Disease, Ed. 5. New York: McGraw-Hill, pp. 167–191.

8. Gray GM: Intestinal disaccaridase deficiencies. *In* Stanbury JB, Wyngaarden JB, Fredrickson DS, et al. (eds): The Metabolic Basis of Inherited Disease, Ed. 5. New York: McGraw-Hill, pp. 1728–1742.

9. Bradley M, Schumann GB: Examination of urine: glucose and other sugars, pp. 401–403; ketones, p. 405. *In* Henry JB (ed): Todd, Sanford, Davidsohn's Clinical Diagnosis and Management by Laboratory Methods, Ed. 17. Philadelphia: W. B. Saunders, 1984.

10. Howanitz PG, Howanitz JH: Carbohydrate (glucose measurements). *In* Henry JB (ed): Todd, Sanford, Davidsohn's Clinical Diagnosis and Management by Laboratory Methods, Ed. 17. Philadelphia: W. B. Saunders, 1984.

11. Asplund J, AhImark G, Gunnarsson R, et al.: Long-term insulin treatment in two nondiabetic patients. JAMA 246:870, 1981.

12. Keen H, Knight RK: Self sampling for blood sugar. Lancet 1:1037–1040, 1962.

13. Bio-Dynamics, Inc., Boehringer-Mannheim Company, Indianapolis, IN, 1983.

14. Larken Industries, Lenexa, KS, 1983.

15. Glucometer Reflectance Photometer Product Profile, Ames Co., Division of Miles Laboratories, Inc., Elkhart, IN, 1980.

16. Jovanovic L, Peterson CM: Management of the pregnant insulin-dependent woman. Diabetes Care 3:63–68, 1980.

17. Howe-Davies S, Holman RR, Phillips M, et al.: Home blood sampling for plasma glucose assay in control of diabetes. Br MedJ 7:596–598, 1978.

18. Sonkson PH, Judd S, Lowy C: Home monitoring of blood glucose: new approach to management of insulin-dependent diabetic patients in Great Britain. Diabetes Care 3:100–107, 1980.

19. Mountier VM, Scott RS, Beaven DW. Use and abuse of glucose reflectance meters. Diabetes 5:542–544, 1982.

20. The American Diabetes Association 1999 resource guide. Supplement to diabetes forecast. Susan H. Law, publisher, Andrew Keegan, managing editor. American Diabetes Association, 1660 Duke St., Alexandria, VA, 22314 phone 703-549-1500.

21. American Diabetes Association: Tests of glycemia. Diabetes care 20 (suppl. 1): 5–18, 1997.

22. Guyton AC: Textbook of Medical Physiology. Philadelphia: W. B. Saunders, 1976.

23. Kohler E: On materials for testing glucose in the urine. Diabetes Care 1:64–66, 1978.

24. Harano Y, Suzuki M, Kojima H, et al.: Development of paper-strip test for 3-hydroxybutyrate and its clinical application. Diabetes Care 7:481–485, 1984.

25. Guthrie DW, Hinnen D, Guthrie RA: Single-voided vs. double-voided urine testing. Diabetes Care 2:269–271, 1979.

26. The DCCT research group: The relationship of glycemic exposure (HbA$_{1c}$) to the risk of development and progression of retinopathy in the diabetes control and complications trial. Diabetes 44:968, 1995.

27. Aziz S, Hsiang Y: Comparative study of home blood glucose monitoring devices: Visidex, Chemstrip, bG, Glu-cometer and Accu-Chek bG. Diabetes Care 6:529–532, 1983.

28. Frindik JP, Kassner DA, Pirkle DA, et al.: Comparison of Visidex and Chemstrip bG with Beckman glucose analyzer determination of blood glucose. Diabetes Care 6:536–539, 1983.

29. Nelson JD, Woelk MA, Shep S: Self glucose monitoring: a comparison of the Glucometer, Glucoscan, and Hypo count B. Diabetes Care 6:262–267,1983.

30. Reeves ML, Forhan SE, Skyler JS et al.: Comparison of methods for blood glucose monitoring. Diabetes Care 4:404–406, 1981.

31. Parker DR and Yip KF: Relationships of glucose concentrations in capillary plasma, capillary whole blood, venous plasma, and venous whole blood. Clinical Chemistry and Laboratory Medicine 37 (Special supplement): S 352, 1999.

32. Food and Drug administration press release (July 28, 1998): Lifescan blood glucose meters recalled.

33. Goldstein DE, Little RR: Bringing order to chaos: Standardizing the hemoglobin A$_{1c}$ assay. Contemporary internal medicine 9:27–32, May 1997.

34. National Glycohemoglobin Standardization Program (NGSP) steering committee: American Diabetes Association, 1997, abstract No. 0584.

35. Goldstein DE, Little RR, Lorenz RA, et al: Tests of glycemia in diabetes. Diabetes care 18:896, 1995.

36. Belmonte MM et al.: Impact of SMBG and control of diabetes as measured by HBA$_1$. Diabetes Care 11:484, 1988.

37. Beckert NM, Belsey R: Reagent strip testing: Blood glucose error in a teaching hospital. Lab Med 19:26–29, 1988.

23

Monitoring Glycosylated Hemoglobin

Judy Ashworth, Charles M. Peterson,
and Lois Jovanovic-Peterson

Two decades have passed since the significance of hemoglobin A_{1c} (HbA_{1c}) for the diabetic patient was elucidated. Now the majority of patients with diabetes mellitus know their most recent HbA_{1c} level equal to the degree that patients with coronary artery disease know their most recent cholesterol level. Not only has this clinical test given clinicians a better means of estimating a patient's average level of glycemia over the prior 2–3 months, but also it has provided diabetic patients with a means of viewing their level of "control" from a wider perspective.

The study of glycosylated proteins, like HbA_{1c}, has also had tremendous impact in other fields of research: from the use of HbA_{1c} levels in the first trimester of pregnancies complicated by diabetes as a predictor of fetal malformations to understanding the role of advanced glycosylation end-products in the normal process of aging as well as the "accelerated aging" process seen in diabetes mellitus.

As the research and application of glycosylated proteins continues to expand and work its way into the realm of routine clinical use, it is essential that clinicians become familiar with the various glycosylation assays available and develop an understanding for their clinical utility as well as their limitations.

Historical Perspective

Glycosylation of circulating proteins, such as hemoglobin, involves the nonenzymatic attachment of glucose or other carbohydrate to the protein. Hemoglobin A_{1c}, specifically, is the nonenzymatic posttranslational modification of hemoglobin A that is formed when the terminal amino group of the β-chain forms an aldimine adduct with glucose (the early Maillard reaction), which then undergoes an Amadori-type rearrangement to form a more stable ketoamine adduct. These chemical reactions are illustrated in Figures 23–1 and 23–2. In 1912, Maillard,[1] for whom the former reaction is named,

suggested that this chemical reaction might be involved in the pathologic mechanisms associated with diabetes mellitus. It was not until 1949, when Linus Pauling and coworkers[2] analyzed hemolysates by moving boundary electrophoresis and discovered that the hemoglobin from a patient with sickle cell anemia had a different mobility from that of a normal individual, that the study of hemoglobin variants emerged, eventually leading to the discovery of HbA_{1c} and its relevance to diabetes mellitus.

In normal human erythrocytes, hemoglobin A (or A_0) comprises about 90% of the total hemoglobin. In 1955, Kunkel and Wallenius[3] separated hemolysates by starch gel electrophoresis and found a minor component that had less negative charge than HbA and comprised about 2.5% of the total. This component, which contained two α- and two β-chains, was named HbA_2 and was found to be elevated in individuals with β-thalassemia.[3,4] In 1958, using column chromatography, Allen et al.[5] separated human hemoglobin into three minor components that, based on the order of their elution from the column, were labeled hemoglobins A_{1a}, A_{1b}, and A_{1c}.

During the 1960s, it was demonstrated that a hexose molecule attaches to the hemoglobin structure in the fast eluting components.[6,7] In 1962, using gel electrophoresis, Huismann and Dozy[8] found an increased level of minor hemoglobin components in a few diabetic patients treated with tolbutamide. However, this finding remained unheeded until 1968 when Rahbar,[9] also using gel electrophoresis, rediscovered this phenomenon in two patients with diabetes mellitus. He later confirmed this observation in 140 diabetic patients.[10] Trivelli et al. (using the column cation exchange chromatographic method that became standard) found that HbA_{1c} concentrations were two to three times higher in diabetic versus nondiabetic individuals.[11] Monozygotic twin studies by Tattersall et al.[12] in 1975 revealed that in twins discordant for diabetes mellitus, only the diabetic twin had an elevated HbA_{1c}.

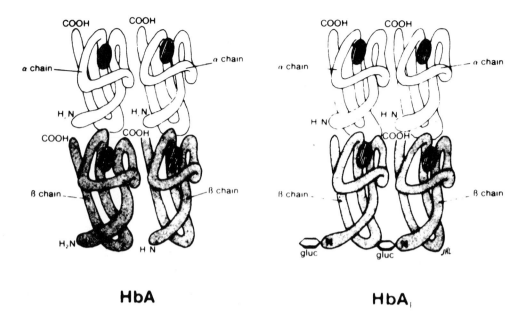

HbA   **HbA$_1$**

Figure 23–1. The schematic adduct formation of glucose with hemoglobin. As can be seen, the hemoglobin molecule consists of a tetramer of two α- and two β-chains of 141 and 146 amino acids, respectively. The amino terminal glycosylation of the β-chains masks a positively charged amino group and accounts for the early elution of hemoglobin A$_{1c}$ on cation exchange chromatography. Certain ε-amino groups of lysines are also glycosylated but are not shown here.

By 1976, it became clear that HbA$_{1c}$ resulted from a posttranslational modification of HbA and that there was a clinical relationship between HbA$_{1c}$ and (1) fasting plasma glucose, (2) peak plasma glucose on the glucose tolerance test, (3) area under the curve of the glucose tolerance test, and (4) mean glucose levels over the preceding weeks.[13–15] It soon became apparent that

an improvement in ambient blood glucose levels resulted in correction of HbA$_{1c}$ levels[16,17] and that these nonenzymatic glycosylation reactions might provide an hypothesis that explains the pathological sequelae of diabetes mellitus via toxicity arising from adduct formation with proteins or nucleic acids.[18] In 1993, the Diabetes Control and Complications Trial (DCCT)[19]

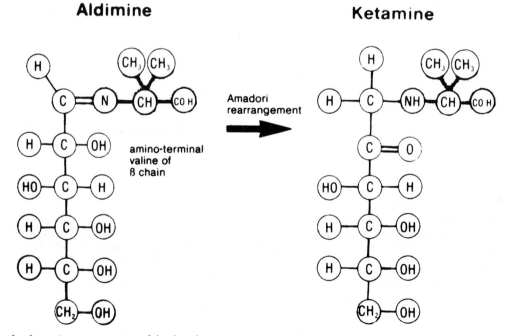

Figure 23–2. A schematic representation of the Amadori rearrangement, whereby the shift of the double bond from carbon 1 of the glucose molecule to carbon 2 results in a stable ketoamine structure rather than the labile aldimine. It is the stability of the rearranged adduct of glucose with proteins that gives the measurement of these adducts clinical utility.

supported this hypothesis by showing that intensive treatment of patients with insulin dependent diabetes mellitus (IDDM) resulted in a mean HbA_{1c} of 7.2% (vs. 9.0% in IDDM patients receiving conventional treatment), and reduced the risk of microvascular complications (retinopathy, nephropathy, and neuropathy) by approximately 60%. The findings brought the utility of the test to the realm of providing confidence limits for outcome variables consistent with the requirements of evidence based medicine.[20]

Since hemoglobin circulates in each erythrocyte for approximately 120 days, there is some opportunity in this cell for late Maillard reactions or nonenzymatic browning to occur (the product of these reactions are referred to as "advanced glycation end-products" or AGEs), and the extent of these changes appear to correlate with glycated hemoglobin values.[21] In formation of AGEs, the Amadori product is degraded into deoxyglucosones that react again with free amino groups to form chromophores, fluorophores, and protein cross-links.[22,23] In tissues that are longer-lived, such as connective tissue, vascular endothelium, and so on, AGEs have been hypothesized to mediate pathology as well as contribute to the normal aging process. The structures of most AGEs are yet to be determined and thus their pathological role remains uncertain, as does their clinical utility.[24,25]

Terminology

Table 23–1 summarizes terminology used for hemoglobin that has been reacted with sugars. HbA_{1c} is one of several minor hemoglobins, but because of its relatively high concentration in normal persons (3–6% of normal hemoglobin), it is the one most extensively studied. Since, after 3 days, circulating erythrocytes are incapable of initiating protein synthesis, HbA_{1c} is produced as a postsynthetic modification of hemoglobin A_0. This modification is nearly irreversible and thus the rate of synthesis of HbA_{1c} reflects the glucose environment of the circulating erythrocyte. Given that the erythrocyte has an average lifespan of 120 days, the HbA_{1c} at any given time reflects the relative level of glycemia over the prior 2–3 months.

Hemoglobin A_1 is a descriptive term that denotes all the fast hemoglobins including acetaldehyde hemoglobin, fetal hemoglobin, as well as HbA_{1c}, HbA_{1a}, and HbA_{1b}. Because many of these hemoglobins have glucose or glucose-breakdown products attached (phosphorylated glycolytic intermediates), they are referred to as glycosylated hemoglobins. They also reflect the average glucose over time; however, the value for glycosylated hemoglobins is about 50% higher than the measurement of HbA_{1c} alone. Thus, the clinician needs to be aware of the specifics of the

TABLE 23–1 Hemoglobin (Hb) Terminology

"Fast" hemoglobin. The total Hb A_1 fractions $(HbA_{1a}, HbA_{1a2}, HbA_{1b}, HbA_{1c})$ that, because of more negative charge, migrates toward the anode on electrophoresis and elutes earlier on cation exchange chromatography than HbA_0.

Fetal hemoglobin (HbF). The major hemoglobin component of newborn blood. HbF may coelute with HbA_{1c} on ion exchange column chromatography.

Glucosylated hemoglobin. Hemoglobin modified by glucose at β-chain valine residues and ε-amino groups of lysine residues.

Glycated hemoglobin. A term favored by biochemists to indicate adducts of sugars and hemoglobin that are formed nonenzymatically.

Glycosylated hemoglobin (glyco-hemoglobin). A generic term for hemoglobin containing glucose and/or other carbohydrate at either valine or lysine residues and thus the sum of glycosyl adducts.

Hemoglobin A. The major adult form of hemoglobin. A tetramer consisting of two α- and two β-chains (α_2, β_2).

Hemoglobin A_0. The major component of HbA identified by its chromatographic and electrophoretic properties. Posttranslational modifications, including glycosylation, do exist, but do not significantly affect the charged properties of the protein.

Hemoglobin A_1. Posttranslationally modified, more negatively charged forms of HbA_0 (primarily glycosylation at the β-chain terminal valine residue) separable from HbA_0 by chromatographic and electrophoretic methods.

Hemoglobin A_{1a1}, HbA_{1a2}, HbA_{1b}, HbA_{1c}. Chromatographically distinct stable components of HbA_1.

Hemoglobin A_{1a1}, HbA_{1a2}, HbA_{1b}: "Fastest," most anionic forms of HbA consisting primarily of adducts of phosphorylated glycoyltic intermediates with HbA_0.

Hemoglobin A_{1c}. Component of HbA_1 that consists of 50–90% hemoglobin (depending on the quality of resolution of the chromatographic system) glucosylated by a ketoamine linkage at the β-chain terminal valine residue.

Pre-hemoglobin A_{1c}. A labile form of glycosylated Hb containing glucose bound in aldimine linkage to the β-chain terminal valine residue.

measurement provided by the laboratory in order to interpret the result meaningfully to patients.

Clinical Applications

Screening

Given that the measurement of HbA_{1c} is indicative of the average blood glucose level for the preceding 2–3 months, there was hope that HbA_{1c} could replace the standard glucose tolerance test as a screening tool for diabetes mellitus. Unfortunately, this was not to be the case. In 1978, Santiago showed that nearly half of patients studied who had diabeteslike glucose tolerance tests had HbA_{1c} levels in the normal range.[25a] Other studies found normal HbA_{1c} levels in 16–65% of patients with abnormal glucose tolerance tests. Therefore, although an elevated HbA_{1c} is highly suggestive of diabetes or impaired glucose tolerance, a normal HbA_{1c} does not exclude either. On the other hand, the test is highly specific. Thus an elevated value (above the laboratory's normal range) combined with an elevated fasting blood glucose is considered by many to be sufficient for the diagnosis of diabetes mellitus.

Monitoring

There is broad consensus that glycated hemoglobin testing be used for routine care of all patients with diabetes mellitus.[26] Beyond its use as a measure of long-term glycemia and risk for chronic complications in diabetes, routine glycated hemoglobin testing has been shown to improve glycemia per se. Larsen et al.[27] assigned 240 patients with IDDM randomly to either a treatment or a control group. GHb testing was performed in both groups quarterly for 12 months; test results were available, however, only to patients and health care providers in the treatment group. There were no other specific differences in management between the two study groups. After 1 year, GHb values were substantially lower in the treatment group than in the control group. The higher the GHb level at baseline, the greater its decrease after 1 year. Thus, knowledge of GHb seems to alter behavior of health care providers and/or patients, with a resultant improvement in glycemia and risk of long-term complications.

The optimum frequency of surveillance for GHb testing is not well established. The current American Diabetes Association (ADA) recommendations[26] are for testing at initial patient assessment and at least quarterly thereafter in patients with IDDM and "as frequently as necessary to assess achievement of glycemic goals in NIDDM." In the DCCT,[19] glycated hemoglobin determinations were performed monthly in the intensive treatment group and quarterly in the standard treatment group. The latter group was not informed of their values. Further studies are needed to determine if current ADA recommendations for testing frequency are appropriate or indeed provide optimum clinical utility. For example, in pregnant women with diabetes, it has been recommended that glycated hemoglobin determinations be performed at least monthly.[28] The most successful programs have described a more frequent performance of the assay.[29]

Although home blood glucose records provide the information needed by the clinician to make changes in the acute management of diabetic patients, the HbA_{1c} value provides a better sense of the average blood glucose concentration over time. Not uncommonly, a dichotomy occurs between self-monitored blood glucose values and HbA_{1c} values, with the latter usually being the more elevated. It is generally found that the HbA_{1c} is more indicative of the true glycemic levels than the self-monitoring diary. As depicted in Figure 23–3, following normalization of blood glucose, HbA_{1c}

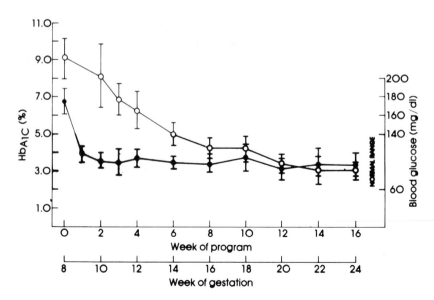

Figure 23–3. The fall in hemoglobin A_{1c} following normalization of plasma glucose levels within 1 week in hospitalized pregnant diabetic patients. As can be seen, the hemoglobin A_{1c} measurement enters the normal range at 8 weeks and reaches a stable plateau at 10–12 weeks following establishment of euglycemia. Reprinted with the permission of the *American Journal of Medicine.*

levels came into the normal range at 8 weeks and reached a stable plateau at 10 weeks. Other authors have found that with stepwise reduction in plasma glucose, 4 months is needed to reach a new steady-state level.[22] Thus, an elevated HbA_{1c} indicates that more intensive effort is required on the part of the health care team and the patient, even in the setting of seemingly acceptable values reported by self-monitoring.

Most often, glycated hemoglobin is used in the routine care of patients as a surrogate mean blood glucose determination during the previous weeks to months. Although several studies, most notably the DCCT, have shown a direct relationship between glycated hemoglobin and average glycemia,[30–32] since glycated hemoglobin assays are not standardized among laboratories, results of these studies are applicable only in the laboratory that performed the test. Thus for most health care providers and patients, it is not possible to relate the glycated hemoglobin test to average blood glucose except in an approximate way. Thus each group should begin to define the relationship between average glycemia and glycated hemoglobin so that the relationship between the two measures can be communicated to patients. If it were only a question of normal versus abnormal test results, standardization of the assays would not be so important; however, glycated hemoglobin values represent a continuum.

Based on the DCCT, some general guidelines in relating glycated hemoglobin to mean blood glucose can be given. In the DCCT, investigators measured glycated hemoglobin and 24-hr, seven-point blood glucose profiles quarterly for 1 year in 278 study subjects.[32] Results were highly correlated ($r = 0180, p < 0.0001$), with a linear relationship between average glycemia and glycated hemoglobin. Roughly, each 1% increase in glycated hemoglobin was related to a 30 mg/dL (1.99 mmol/L) increase in average blood glucose.

Although all of these studies showed a strong statistical relationship between glycemia and glycated hemoglobin, there was considerable scatter, suggesting marked differences among individual patients. Does the regression line closely define the actual relationship between glycated hemoglobin and average blood glucose for all subjects, or are there clinically significant individual variations? Investigators have suggested that there may be "high" and "low" glycators, persons in whom identical glycated hemoglobin levels reflect clinically significant differences in average blood glucose.[33,34] Recent work in rodents documents a different relationship between blood glucose in males versus females,[35] an observation that has not been seen in humans. Thus some investigators argue that if the normal range for glycated hemoglobin can extend over 2% or more, then perhaps, at any average blood glucose level, glycated hemoglobin could vary by as much

among individuals. To date there are no convincing data to support or refute these ideas.

There is a common misconception among both health care providers and patients that since the glycated hemoglobin test reflects mean glycemia during the preceding weeks to months, large changes in glycemia cannot be detected except after many weeks. Mathematical modeling predicts and in vivo studies confirm that although a change in mean blood glucose on day 1 is not fully reflected in the glycated hemoglobin level until 120 days later, a large change in mean blood glucose (up or down) is accompanied by a rapid and large change in glycated hemoglobin. Regardless of the starting level, the time required to reach a midpoint between the starting level and the new steady-state level is accomplished in about 1–2 weeks.[36,37]

When a discrepancy does occur between self-monitoring and the HbA_{1c} level it is helpful to verify the discrepancy by using another method for measuring HbA_{1c}. For example, if the first method used was based on a physical method, such as cation exchange chromatography, then the confirmatory method should utilize a chemical method, such as affinity chromatography or immunoassay. It is possible that HbA_{1c} is falsely elevated. Some hemoglobinopathies, for instance, artifactually raise HbA_{1c}. By the same token, in conditions such as hemolytic anemias or excessive blood-letting on a medical ward, where the average lifespan of erythrocytes is decreased, the HbA_{1c} may be lower than would be predicted for a given level of glycemia. Ingestion of large amounts of vitamins C or E (more than 1 gm/day) also have been reported to lower glycated hemoglobin values.[38,39]

The measurement of glycosylated proteins or hemoglobin is also useful in the detection of potential hypoglycemia. As normal levels of glycemia are approached, the risk of hypoglycemia increases the need for increased surveillance of blood glucose levels throughout the day.[40,41] Individuals with type 1 diabetes or pregnant diabetic women attempting to achieve normoglycemia and normal hemoglobin A_{1c} levels require 8–10 blood glucose self-measurements a day to reach this goal while avoiding hypoglycemia.[42–44]

Predicting Long-term Complications

As earlier discussed, the initial step in the glycosylation of hemoglobin is the early Maillard reaction, whereby an amino moiety undergoes condensation with the aldehyde form of a particular sugar. The product, a labile Schiff base aldimine adduct, is then transformed to a relatively stable ketoamine adduct via the Amadori rearrangement. Since hemoglobin circulates in its erythrocyte for approximately 120 days, there is little opportunity for late Maillard reactions or nonenzymatic "browning" to occur. In these late Maillard

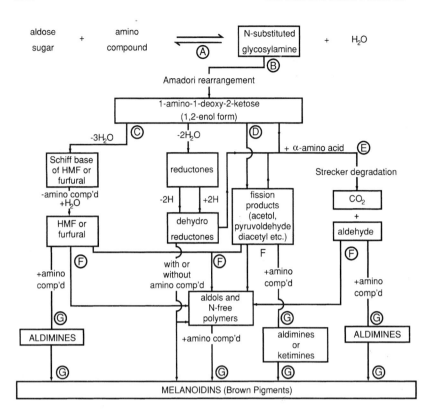

Figure 23–4. A schematic representation of early and late Maillard reactions. The Amadori product may undergo further chemical changes, resulting in browning products, advanced glycosylation end-products, or melanoidins. Modified from Hodge JE: Agric and Food Chem 1:928, 1953. With permission of Helena Laboratories.

reactions, depicted schematically in Fig. 23–4, the Amadori product is degraded into deoxyglucosones, which react again with free amino groups to form chromophores, fluorophores, and protein crosslinks.[24,45] These products are the advanced glycosylation end-products, or AGEs referred to previously. In tissues that are longer lived, AGEs accumulate. Due to their high reactivity in protein cross-linking, their accumulation results in tissue damage that, it is postulated, leads to the pathological conditions seen with diabetes as well as with normal aging.[46]

Table 23–2 summarizes the hypotheses whereby Maillard reactions might contribute to the multiple pathologic conditions associated with hyperglycemia.[47–51] In addition to the numerous studies of early Maillard reactions, the late Maillard reactions have been shown to increase concomitantly with diabetes-related pathologic states.[52–55] Results of the DCCT clearly showed that lowering blood glucose concentration and HbA_{1c} levels slows or prevents the development of retinopathy, nephropathy, and neuropathy in patients with IDDM. It appears reasonable to assume that the same would hold true for NIDDM patients given that the mechanisms by which glucose causes complications is presumed to be the same in both types of diabetes.

Pregnancy

Although HbA_{1c} is an ineffective tool in screening for gestational diabetes,[56–58] it has proved useful in assessing the risk for fetal malformations in pregnancies of type 1 and type 2 diabetic women.[39] Diabetic pregnancies produce infants with congenital anomalies up to five times more frequently than nondiabetic pregnancies. Euglycemia during the first trimester, as evidenced by HbA_{1c} levels within the normal range (<6.1%), reduced the risk of congenital anomalies to near that of the general obstetric population. Diabetic pregnancies with higher HbA_{1c} levels also resulted in spontaneous abortions more frequently than those with lower HbA_{1c} levels.

The use of HbA_{1c} in monitoring pregnancies complicated by diabetes, including those of gestational diabetics, is warranted despite the normal fluctuations in erythropoesis that accompany pregnancy and could consequently affect HbA_{1c} levels (red cell mass increases during the third trimester, which could lead to an artifactual lowering of HbA_{1c}). Although HbA_{1c} reflects relative glycemia over the prior 8–12 weeks, being able to show a downward trend in HbA_{1c} levels measured more frequently, at 2–3 week intervals, provides the clinician and the patient with reassurance that any changes in management are leading to improved control.

Other Glycosylated Proteins

Given the relatively long half-life of hemoglobin, which is dictated by the average lifespan of erythrocytes (120 days), much research has been aimed at identifying other shorter-lived serum or plasma proteins (i.e.,

TABLE 23–2 Hypotheses Regarding the Potential Role of Nonenzymatic Glucosylation and Browning in the Pathology Associated with Diabetes Mellitus

I. **Structural proteins**
   A. *Collagen* : Decreased turnover, flexibility, solubility; decreased ability to bind heparin; increased aggregating potential for platelets, binding of immunoglobulins, crosslinking, and immunogenicity
   B. *Lens crystallins and membrane* : Opacification, increased vulnerability to oxidative stress
   C. *Basement membrane* : Impairment of self-assembly, increased permeability, decreased turnover, increased thickness, decreased ability to bind heparin
   D. *Extracellular matrix* : Changes in binding to other proteins
   E. *Hemoglobin* : Change in oxygen binding
   F. *Fibrin* : Decreased enzymatic degradation
   G. *Red cell membrane* : Increased rigidity
   H. *Tubulin* : Cell structure and transport
   I. *Myelin* : Altered structure and immunologic recognition
   J. *Cellular receptors* : Increased production of growth-promoting cytokines leading to hypertrophy and hyperplasia
II. **Carrier proteins**
   A. *Lipoproteins* : Alternate degradative pathways and metabolism by macrophages and endothelial cells, increased immunogenicity
   B. *Albumin* : Alteration in binding properties for drugs and in handling by the kidney
   C. *IgG* : Altered binding
III. **Enzyme systems**
   A. *Cu-Zn superoxide dismutase* : Vulnerability to oxidative stresses
   B. *Fibrinogen* : Altered coagulation
   C. *Antithrombin III* : Hypercoagulable state
   D. *Purine nucleoside phosphorylase* : Aging of erythrocytes
   E. *Alcohol dehydrogenase* : Substrate metabolism
   F. *Ribonuclease A* : Loss of activity
   G. *Cathepsin B* : Loss of activity
   H. *N-acetyl-D-glucosaminidase* : Loss of activity
   I. *Calmodulin* : Decreased calcium binding
IV. **Coagulation**
   A. *Coagulation cascade* : Increased activity
   B. *Fibrinolysis* : Decreased activity
   C. *Thrombosis* : Increased induction due to increased monokine (TNF,IL-1) secretion from endothelial cells
   D. *Platelets* : Hyperaggregable
V. **Nucleic acids**
   A. *Prokaryotic cells* : Altered gene expression, mutation (insertions and deletions), inhibition of template function
   B. *Eukaryotic cells* : Increased single-strand DNA breaks, DNA excision/repair; age-related changes, congenital malformations
VI. **Potentiation of other diseases of postsynthetic protein modification**
   A. Carbamylation-associated pathology in uremia
   B. Steroid cataract formation
   C. Acetaldehyde-induced changes in alcoholism

albumin, ferritin, globulins, etc.) whose glycosylated fractions could potentially provide an estimate of average glycemia over a much shorter period of time. The fructosamine test, a rapid automated assay for glycosylated serum proteins (GSP), which is largely comprised of albumin and globulins, is less expensive. Its level would reflect average glycemia over the preceding 1–2 weeks. However, the fructosamine value is affected by total serum protein concentration and lipid content and may be influenced by reducing substances in the diet as well. In a study by Parfitt et al.,[59] fructosamine was found to correlate more precisely with mean blood glucose than HbA_1 in well-controlled type 1 diabetic pregnancies. A newer immunoradiometric assay for determining GSP levels, based on an initial study by Gordon and co-workers,[60] appears to be more sensitive than the fructosamine assay, with nearly all diabetic patients showing an elevated GSP level, decreasing the overlap between diabetic and control populations to only 5%. A recent study found that glycosylated plasma protein measurements performed by high-performance liquid chromatography using boronate affinity columns at 24–28 weeks gestation was a better predictor of infant macrosomia than glycated hemoglobin measurements,[61] and glycated albumin is being increasingly investigated.[62] As noted in the ADA Technical Review[63]:

> In summary, the clinical utility of glycated protein determinations to assess short and/or long-term glycemic status in patients with diabetes mellitus remains unclear. Further studies are needed to determine if these assays provide clinical information equivalent to glycated hemoglobin for routine management of patients with diabetes mellitus and if so, do they offer any significant advantages?

A study comparing glycosylated serum albumin (GSA) to HbA_1 and GSP (as determined by the fructosamine test) found that GSA could be a useful alternative to HbA_1 or HbA_{1c} in patients with pathologic conditions affecting their hemoglobin or average erythrocyte lifespan (hemoglobinopathies, hemolytic anemias, etc.). However, some drugs, including sulfonylureas, compete with free glucose at binding sites on albumin, leading to falsely low GSA values, thus lowering the accuracy of this assay, particularly in type 2 diabetic patients, the majority of whom are taking oral agents.[62]

Pros and Cons of Various Assays

Table 23–3 summarizes the available clinical methods of measurement for circulating glycated proteins and the advantages and limitations of each. Measurement of glycosylated hemoglobin, proteins, and HbA_{1c} requires special care on the part of the laboratory to be useful. The measurement of glycosylated hemoglobin and of

TABLE 23–3   Classification of Assays

  I. Physical methods based on changes in pH
    A. Cation exchange chromatography
       Pro: Inexpensive and rapid
       Con: Sensitive to small changes in resin packing,
       ionic strength, pH, temperature, column loading,
       and affected by the labile fraction; variant
       hemoglobins may interfere
    B. High-performance liquid chromatography (HPLC)
       Pro: Dedicated instruments avoid many problems in I.A.
       Con: Relatively expensive
    C. Agarose gel electrophoresis
       Pro: Inexpensive; minimal technician time;
       standardized plates and conditions in kits; less
       sensitive to pH, triglyceride concentrations, and
       temperature
       Con: Precision problems induced by scanner and
       loading variation, sensitive to labile fraction and
       variant hemoglobin
    D. Isoelectric focusing
       Pro: Separates most minor hemoglobin variants
       Con: Precision over time dependent on use of same
       batch of ampholines on standardized plates,
       scanning effects precision
  II. Methods based on chemical principles
    A. Thiobarbituric acid/colorimetric assay

HbA_{1c} is expressed as a percent of the total hemoglobins; therefore, small deviations in measurement can lead to a large percentage change. For example, a 1% change in HbA_{1c} would reflect a change of approximately 35mg/dL in average blood glucose concentration. Thus, precision in the measurement is vital to allow clinicians the comfort of making important clinical decisions based on the results. A National Institutes of Health–sponsored expert committee has recommended that within-laboratory between-run coefficients of variation be maintained at 5% or lower.[64]

Particularly with the publication of the DCCT results,[19] there has been increasing interest in standardization of glycated hemoglobin assays.[65] Each type of assay method measures glycation in a slightly different way and may measure different components. There has been no consensus on a reference method, and there is no single standard available that could be used with all methods. Thus numbers generated in one laboratory cannot be directly compared to numbers generated in another laboratory, even if both use the same basic assay method. A recent College of American

Pathologists survey of glycated hemoglobin assays showed that the interlaboratory coefficient of variation for one HbA_1 method was over 19%.[66] A single quality-control sample gave mean values ranging from 8.6% to 13.8% depending on the glycated hemoglobin component measured and the specific assay method.

A broad-based system of standardization would facilitate the development of uniform goals for blood glucose control in persons with diabetes and has been recommended.[63] Data are available showing that assay precision can be improved by standardization and that standardization among laboratories using a variety of assay methods is feasible.[67–70] *The benefits of standardizing glycated hemoglobin assays to DCCT-reported values would be considerable.*

The clinician needs to be aware of the methods used by the laboratory and be familiar with the pros and cons of the assays used so that she or he can make accurate interpretations of the results and apply them appropriately in the clinical setting.

Conclusions

HbA_{1c} has proved to be an invaluable tool for the management of patients with diabetes mellitus. Though the level at any given time reflects average glycemia over the previous 2–3 months, more frequent measurements are useful when changes in treatment are being made to provide the clinician and the patient with a sense of whether or not they are "winning" with their new regimen. Patients should be aware of their HbA_{1c} level and should be educated by their physician as to the correlation of elevated levels to the development and/or progression of diabetic complications.

Diabetic women contemplating pregnancy should be informed as to the risk of congenital malformations if they have an elevated HbA_{1c} during the first trimester and the higher risk of other complications (i.e., spontaneous abortion, macrosomia) during their pregnancy. Ideally, an effort should be made to normalize the HbA_{1c} level prior to conception.

Current research is promising for the development, refinement, and utilization of other assays for the glycosylated fraction of shorter-lived proteins (GSP, GSA, etc.) that will enable the clinician to better monitor recent changes in blood sugar management, providing us with a larger arsenal with which to wage our ongoing battle against the crippling complications of diabetes mellitus.

References

1. Maillard LC: Reaction generale des acides amines sur les sucres; ses consequences biologiques. CR Acad Sci 154: 66–68, 1912.

2. Pauling L, Itano H, Singer SJ, Wells IC: Sickle cell anemia: A molecular disease. Science 110:543–544, 1949.

3. Kunkel HG, Wallenius G: New hemoglobins in normal adult blood. Science 122:228–229, 1955.

4. Kunkel HG, Ceppellini R, Muller-Eberhard U, Wolf J: Observations on the minor basic hemoglobin components in the blood of normal individuals and patients with thalassemia. J Clin Invest 36:1615–1621, 1961.

5. Allen DW, Schroeder WA, Balog J: Observations on the chromatographic heterogeneity of normal adult and fetal human hemoglobin. J Am Chem Soc 80:1628–1634, 1958.

6. Holmquist WR, Schroeder WA: A new N-terminal blocking group involving a Schiff base in hemoglobin A_{1c}. Biochemistry 5:2489–2503, 1966.

7. Bookchin RM, Gallop PM: Structure of hemoglobin A_{1c}: Nature of the N-terminal beta chain blocking group. Biochim Biophys Res Commun 32:86–93, 1968.

8. Huisman THJ, Dozy AM: Studies on the heterogeneity of hemoglobin. V. Binding of hemoglobin with oxidized glutathione. J Lab Clin Med 60:302–319, 1962.

9. Rahbar S: An abnormal hemoglobin in red cells of diabetics. Clin Chem Acta 22:296–298, 1968.

10. Rahbar S, Blumenfeld O, Ranney HM: Studies of an unusual hemoglobin in patients with diabetes mellitus. Biochem Biophys Res Commun 36:838–843, 1969.

11. Trivelli LA, Ranney HM, Lai H-T: Hemoglobin components in patients with diabetes mellitus. New Eng J Med 248:353–357, 1971.

12. Tattersall RB, Pyke DA, Ranney HM, Bruckheimer SM: Hemoglobin components in diabetes mellitus: Studies in identical twins. New Engl J Med 293:1171–1173, 1975.

13. Bunn HF, Haney DN, Kamin S, et al.: The biosynthesis of human hemoglobin A_{1c}. J Clin Invest 57:1652–1659, 1976.

14. Koenig RJ, Peterson CM, Kilo C, et al.: Hemoglobin A_{1c} as an indicator of the degree of glucose intolerance in diabetes. Diabetes 25:230–232, 1976.

15. Koenig RJ, Peterson CM, Jones RL, et al.: Correlation of glucose regulation and hemoglobin A_{1c} in diabetes mellitus. New Engl J Med 295:417–420, 1976.

16. Peterson CM, Jones RL, Koenig RJ, et al.: Reversible hematologic sequelae of diabetes mellitus. Ann Int Med 86:425–429, 1977.

17. Peterson CM, Koenig RK, Jones RL, et al.: Correlation of serum triglyceride levels and hemoglobin A_{1c} concentrations in diabetes mellitus. Diabetes 26:507–509, 1977.

18. Peterson CM, Jones RL: Minor hemoglobins, diabetic "control" and diseases of postsynthetic protein modification. Ann Int Med 87:489–491, 1977.

19. The Diabetes Control and Complications Trial Research Group: The effects of intensive treatment of diabetes on the development and progression of long-term complications in IDDM. New Eng J Med 329:977–986, 1993.

20. Evidence Based Medicine Working Group: Evidence-based medicine. A new approach to teaching the practice of medicine. JAMA 268:2420–2425, 1992.

21. Makita Z, Vlassara H, Rayfield E, et al.: Hemoglobin-AGE: a circulating marker of advanced glycosylation. Science 258:651–653, 1992.

22. Angyal SJ: The composition of reducing sugars in solution. In Harmon RE (ed), Asymmetry in Carbohydrates. New York: Marcel Dekker, 1979, pp. 15–30.

23. Benkovic SJ: Anomeric specificity of carbohydrate utilizing enzymes. Methods Enzymol 63:370–379, 1979.

24. Hayase F, Nagaraj RH, Miyata S, et al.: Aging of proteins: Immunological detection of a glucose-derived pyrrole formed during Maillard Reaction in vivo. J Biol Chem 263:3758–3764, 1989.

25. Baynes JW, Monnier VM (eds). The Maillard Reaction in Aging Diabetes, and Nutrition. New York: Alan R. Liss, 1989.

25a. Santiago JV, Davis JE, Fisher F: Hemoglobin A_{1c} levels in a diabetes detection program. J Clin Endocrinol Metab 47:578–580, 1978.

26. American Diabetes Association: Standards of medical care for patients with diabetes mellitus position statement. Diabetes Care 17:616–623, 1994.

27. Larsen ML, Horder M, Magensen EF: Effect of long-term monitoring of glycosylated hemoglobin levels in insulin-dependent diabetes mellitus. New Engl J Med 323: 1021–1025, 1990.

28. Santiago JV (ed): American Diabetes Association: Medical Management of Insulin-Dependent (Type I) Diabetes 2ed. Alexandria, VA: American Diabetes Association, 1994.

29. Jovanovic L, Druzin M, Peterson CM: Effect of euglycemia on the outcome of pregnancy in insulin-dependent diabetic women as compared with normal control subjects. Am J Med 71:921–927, 1981.

30. Peterson CM, Jones RL, Dupuis A, et al.: Feasibility of improved blood glucose control in patients with insulin-dependent diabetes mellitus. Diabetes Care 2:329–335, 1980.

31. Nathan DM, Singer DE, Hurxthal K, Goodson JD: The clinical information value of the glycosylated hemoglobin assay. New Engl J Med 310:341–346, 1984.

32. The DCCT Research Group: Diabetes Control and Complications Trial (DCCT): Results of feasibility study. Diabetes Care 10:1–19, 1987.

33. Modan M, Meytes D, Roseman P, et al.: Significance of high Hb A_1 levels in normal glucose tolerance. Diabetes Care 11:422–428, 1988.

34. Yudkin JS, Forrest RD, Jackson CA, et al.: Unexplained variability of glycated hemoglobin in non-diabetic subjects not related to glycaemia. Diabetologia 33:208–215, 1990.

35. Dubuc PU, Scott BK, Peterson CM: Sex differences in glycated hemoglobin in diabetic and non-diabetic C57Bl/6 mice. Diabetes Res Clin Prac 21:95–101, 1993.

36. Beach KW: A theoretical model to predict the behavior of glycosylated hemoglobin levels. J Theor Biol 81: 547–561, 1979.

37. Tahara Y, Shima K: The response of glycated hemoglobin to stepwise plasma glucose change over time in diabetic patients. Diabetes Care 16:1313–1314, 1993.

38. Cerillo A, Giugliano D, Quatraro A, et al.: Vitamin E reduction of protein glycosylation in diabetes. Diabetes Care 14:68–72, 1991.

39. Davie SJ, Gould BJ, Yudkin JS: Effect of vitamin C on glycosylation of proteins. Diabetes 41:167–173, 1992.

40. Mayer TK, Freedman ZR: Protein glycosylation in diabetes mellitus: a review of laboratory measurements and of their clinical utility. Clinica Chimica Acta 127:147–184, 1983.

41. Tahara Y, Shima K: The response of GHb to stepwise plasma glucose change over time in diabetic patients. Diabetes Care 16:1313–1314, 1993.

42. Jovanovic L, Peterson CM, Saxena BB, et al.: Feasibility of maintaining normal glucose profiles in insulin-dependent pregnant diabetic women. Am J Med 68:105–110, 1980.

43. Jovanovic L, Peterson CM, Fuhrmann K (eds): Diabetes and Pregnancy: Teratology, Toxicity and Treatment. New York: Praeger, 1986.

44. Peterson CM, Jovanovic L, Chanoch LH: Randomized trial of computer assisted insulin delivery in patients with type 1 diabetes beginning pump therapy. Am J Med 81:69–72, 1986.

45. Hayase F, Nagaraj RH, Miyata S, et al.: Aging of proteins: Immunological detection of a glucose-derived pyrrole formed during Maillard reaction in vivo. J Biol Chem 263:3758–3764, 1989.

46. Peterson CM (ed): Proceedings of a Conference on Nonenzymatic Glycosylation and Browning Reactions: Their Relevance to Diabetes Mellitus. Diabetes 31(Suppl 3):1–82, 1982.

47. Bunn HF: Non-enzymatic glycosylation of protein: a molecular form of aging. Schweiz Med Wschr 111: 1503–1507, 1981.

48. Peterson CM, Formby B: Glycosylated proteins. In Alberti KGMM, Krall LP (eds): Diabetes Annual 1. New York: Elsevier, 1985, pp. 178–197.

49. Peterson CM, Formby B: Glycosylated proteins. In Alberti KGMM, Krall LP (eds): Diabetes Annual 2 New York: Elsevier, 1986, pp. 137–155.

50. Kowluru RA, Heidorn DB, Edmondson SP, et al.: Glycation of calmodulin: Chemistry and structural and functional consequences. Biochemistry 28:2220–2228, 1989.

51. Arai K, Naguchi S, Fujii S, et al.: Glycation and inactivation of human Cu-Zn-superoxide dismutase. Identification of the in vitro glycated sites. J Biol Chem 262: 16969–16978, 1987.

52. Kaneshige H: Nonenzymatic glycosylation of serum IgG and its effect on antibody activity in patients with diabetes mellitus. Diabetes 36:822–828, 1987.

53. Brownlee M, Cerami A, Vlassara H: Advanced products of nonenzymatic glycosylation and the pathogenesis of diabetic vascular disease. Diabetes Metab Rev 4:437–451, 1988.

54. Monnier VM, Sell DR, Abdul Karim FW, Emancipator SN: Collagen browning and cross-linking are increased in chronic experimental hyperglycemia. Relevance to diabetes and aging. Diabetes 37:867–872, 1988.

55. Cohen MP: Diabetes and Protein Glycosylation: Measurement and Biologic Relevance. New York: Springer-Verlag, 1986.

56. O'Shaughnessey RO, Russ J, Zuspan FP: Glycosylated hemoglobins and diabetes mellitus in pregnancy. Am J Obstet Gynecol 135:783–790, 1979.

57. Fadel HE, Hammond SD, Huff TA, Harp RJ: Glycosylated hemoglobin in normal pregnancy and gestational diabetes mellitus. Obstet Gynecol 54:322–326, 1979.

58. Sheilds LE, Gan EA, Murphy HF, et al.: The prognostic value of hemoglobin A_{1c} in predicting fetal heart disease in diabetic pregnancies. Obstet Gynecol 81:954–957, 1993.

59. Parfitt VJ, Clark JDA, Turner GM, Hartog M: Use of fructosamine and glycated haemoglobin to verify self blood glucose monitoring data in diabetic pregnancy. Diabetic Med 10:162–166, 1993.

60. Gordon A, Glaser B, Wald M, et al.: Glycosylated serum protein levels assayed with highly sensitive immunoradiometric assay accurately reflect glycemic control in diabetic patients. Diabetes Care 15:645–650, 1992.

61. Schrader HM, Jovanovic-Peterson L, Bevier WC, Peterson CM: Fasting plasma glucose and glycosylated plasma protein at 24-28 weeks predict macrosomia in the general obstetric population. Am J Perinatology.

62. Woerner W, Pfleiderer S, Reitbrock N: Selective determination of nonenzymatic glycosylated serum albumin as a medium term index of diabetic control. Int J Clin Pharm, Therapy Toxicol 31:218–222, 1993.

63. Goldstein DE, Little RR, Lorenz RA, et al.: American Diabetes Association technical review on tests of glycemia in diabetes mellitus. Diabetes.

64. Baynes JW, Bunn HF, Goldstein DE, et al.: National Diabetes Data Group: Report of the expert committee on glycosylated hemoglobin. Diabetes Care 7:602–606, 1984.

65. Santiago JV: Lessons from the Diabetes Control and Complications Trial. Diabetes 42:1549–1954, 1993.

66. College of American Pathologists Survey, GHB. Northfield, IL: CAP, 1994.

67. Peterson CM, Jovanovic L, Raskin P, Goldstein DE: A comparative evaluation of glycosylated haemoglobin assays: Feasibility of references and standards. Diabetologia 26:214–217, 1984.

68. Bodor GS, Little RR, Garrett N, et al.: Standardization of glycohemoglobin determinations in the clinical laboratory: Three years of experience. Clin Chem 38:2414–2418, 1992.

69. Little RR, Wiedmeyer HM, England JD, et al.: Interlaboratory standardization of measurements of glycohemoglobins. Clin Chem 38:2363–2364, 1992.

70. Weykamp CW, Penders TJ, Muskeit FAJ, van der Slik W: Effect of calibration on dispersion of glycohemoglobin values as determined by 111 laboratories using 21 methods. Clin Chem 40:138–144, 1994.

Section IV.
Complications

24

Diabetic Ketoacidosis and the Hyperglycemic Hyperosmolar State

John K. Davidson

Historical Perspective

Aretaeus of Cappadocia (81–138 AD) named and described diabetes as "a great flow of wonderfully sweet urine, wasting of the flesh, convulsions, and death not-withstanding all the remedies of a great many famous physicians." Eighteen centuries later, von Mering and Minkowski (1889)[1] discovered pancreatic diabetes in dogs that developed polyuria, glucosuria, hyperglycemia, ketoacidosis, coma, and death following surgical removal of the pancreas. The hypothesis that the pancreas produced a blood sugar-lowering substance (hormone) gradually took hold. Meanwhile, Bouchardat, von Noorden, Allen, Joslin, and others (1870–1923) used short-term fasting to diminish or abolish glucosuria and noted that weight loss on diets low in calories, high in fiber, and high in percentage of complex carbohydrates could suppress ketosis. This approach met with considerable success in those who were hyperglycemic and overweight, and with some success (by prolonging survival time by 1 to 2 years) in those who were not overweight but who were prone to diabetic ketoacidosis (DKA). Mortality rates in the latter group remained 100%, with death occurring either from DKA or from starvation when body weight fell to 60 to 70% of normal.

The discovery and clinical use of insulin by Banting, Best, Collip, Macleod, Campbell, and Fletcher (1921–1922)[2] made DKA "curable" and preventable, and dramatically increased survival rates. Yet DKA mortality rates in different medical centers remained from 12 to 44% until 1941. Since then, the addition of optimal fluid, electrolyte, and antibiotic therapy has reduced mortality rates directly attributable to uncomplicated DKA to less than 2% in most medical centers.

The approach of Mirsky and Soskin (1937–1952),[3,4] who advocated the infusion of up to 500 g glucose IV over the first 24 hr "to ameliorate ketosis by the mass action of the high blood glucose level in restoring tissue glycogen," almost certainly increased the mortality rate due to unappreciated electrolyte (especially potassium) deficits. Root (1944)[5] showed that the death rate decreased if insulin and saline alone (without glucose) were given until the blood glucose level returned to near-normal. Holler, Butler, Sprague, and others (1946–1953)[6–8] recognized the significance of hypokalemia in producing fatal outcomes. Harwood (1951),[9] at the Massachusetts General Hospital, reported the lowest DKA mortality rate (1.5%) attained until that time; he attributed his success to: (1) promptly initiated high-dose insulin therapy, (2) appropriate use of parenteral fluids, and (3) continuous monitoring with prompt recognition and treatment of complications and side effects of therapy by knowledgeable physicians and nurses.

Beigelman (1971–1973)[10] reported 32 deaths in 257 patients during 340 sequential episodes of severe DKA at the Los Angeles County–University of Southern California Medical Center. Only four deaths were attributed to uncomplicated DKA (1.2% per episode, 1.5% per individual), whereas 28 deaths occurred in those with significant complications (8.2% per episode, 10.9% per individual). The overall death rate was 9.4% per episode (32 deaths, 340 episodes). Autopsies were done on 18 of 32 individuals. Diabetes was undiagnosed in seven patients prior to admission, and four of these were chronic alcoholics. Twenty were males, 12 were females. Mean age at death was 52.8 years (range 26 to 84 years). The primary cause of death in 11 patients was vascular (seven myocardial infarction, one congestive heart failure, three stroke), and in 11 it was infection (eight pneumonia, two septicemia, 1 mucormycosis), in two individuals the primary cause of death was renal failure. In two it was acute pancreatitis, in one it was thyroid storm, in one it was carcinoma of the pancreas, and in four it was uncomplicated DKA.

Since the report of Sament and Schwartz[11] of severe stupor, coma, and death in a patient with marked hyperglycemia without ketoacidosis, the hyperglycemic hyperosmolar state (HHS) has become a clearly recognized subset of acutely decompensated diabetes. Also, it is not uncommon for patients to present with coexisting ketoacidosis and hyperosmolality (serum osmolality >350 mOsm). Mortality rates of up to 50% have been reported for HHS, and Young and Bradley (1967)[12] and others found evidence of cerebral edema on autopsy in children who died during treatment of severe DKA. These observations renewed interest in assessing the possible role(s) of rapid shifts of water and electrolytes between extracellular and intracellular spaces during therapy, and of the role that rapid osmolality changes may play in determining otherwise unexplained fatal outcomes.[28a,28b]

Epidemiology

In 1978, of the 226 million individuals in the United States, 5.4 million were known to have diabetes (prevalence = 2.4%). During the same year, there were 56,640 hospitalized cases of DKA (incidence = 1.06% of those with diagnosed diabetes).

In the USA in 1998 15.7 million people (5.9% of the population) have diabetes (10.3 million diagnosed, 5.4 million undiagnosed) and 798,000 new cases are diagnosed each year.[28c] 123,000 children and teen-agers have diabetes, and approximately 40% above the age 20 years are being treated with insulin. In 1995, over 110,000 hospital admissions were for acutely decompensated diabetes (diabetic ketoacidosis or hyperglycemic hypersinolar state or both).

The prevalence of diabetes is higher in the old than in the young, is higher in females than in males, and is higher in African Americans than in Caucasians. The incidence of DKA in those with diagnosed diabetes is higher in the young and in females (see Table 24–2). The *relative risk* of developing DKA in those with diabetes <15 years of age (incidence = 7.31%/year) is 12.4 times the risk of developing DKA in those with diabetes who are 45 to 64 years of age (incidence = 0.59%/year). Yet, because the prevalence of diabetes in those 45 to 64 years of age (5.27%) is 35 times greater than that in those less than 15 years of age (0.15%), there are 2.84 times as many episodes of DKA in the older age group as in the younger age group.

In 1987, DKA accounted for almost 20% of the hospitalizations with diabetes as the primary diagnosis in the United States, and the DKA hospital discharge rate increased with age.

The incidence of DKA in a defined population can be reduced markedly, when quality continuing care is provided (Table 24–1). This table shows that about 4,699 cases of severe DKA and HHS were prevented in a large teaching hospital from 1974–1986 (13 years), and that about 2,401 cases of moderate and mild DKA were prevented from 1975–1986 (12 years) by substituting a

prevention-oriented approach for a crisis-oriented approach (see Chapter 14). This avoidance of 7,100 cases of DKA and HHS that would have necessitated hospitalization resulted in cost-avoidance by the hospital and third-party payers in a 13-year period of 21.3 million dollars (7,100 cases at $3,000 per case = $21,300,000).[13]

In this clinic's population of diabetic patients (data bases were collected on more than 19,000 from 1971 through 1989), a number of audits were done not only to assist the understanding of the incidence and costs of acutely decompensated diabetes, but also to understand the frequency of the different types (DKA, HHS, mixed DKA and HHS), outcomes, and precipitating factors.

An audit from mid-1973 to mid-1975 of 1,000 consecutive cases of acutely decompensated diabetes mellitus revealed that about 67% of the patients had *mild* [total carbon dioxide (CO_2) content of 21 to 28 mEq/L] *or moderate* (total CO_2 content of 11 to 20 mEq/L) *ketoacidosis*; about 25% had severe *ketoacidosis* (CO_2 content ≤10 mEq/L and serum osmolality <350 mOsm/kg); about 5% had *severe* DKA and HHS (CO_2 <10 mEq/L and serum osmolality >350 mOsm/kg); about 2% had a pure HHS (serum osmolality >350 mOsm/kg without ketonemia or ketonuria); and about 1% had almost pure severe DKA (CO_2 ≤10 mEq/L, glucose <150 mg/dL).

An audit (Table 24–1 and Table 24–2) from 1978 through 1985 of 1,074 consecutive cases of severe DKA and HHS (in 455 individuals) revealed that 359 had one episode and that 96 had multiple episodes (totaling 715 episodes with a mean of seven episodes per person and a range from 2 to 34 episodes per person). Thus, 21.1% of the individuals (96) accounted for 66.6% of the episodes of DKA or HHS, or both, and two individuals who had 34 episodes each accounted for 6.3% of the 1,074 episodes.

Fifty-seven deaths occurred during the 8-year period that was audited (5.3% per episode, 12.5% per individual). Patients were divided into those with serum osmolality less than 350 mOsm/kg (1,001) and more than 350 mOsm/kg (73). Twenty-one of the deaths (for a death rate of 28.8% per episode) occurred in those with an osmolality more than 350 mOsm, and 36 of the deaths (for a death rate of 3.6% per episode) occurred in those with an osmolality less than 350 mOsm. The relationship of death rates to chronic complications and to associated diseases was not determined in their series of cases of HHS (>340 mOsm/kg) observed a death rate of 17%, compared to death rates reported by other investigators that ranged from 14% to 42%.[14] They noted three independent predictors of HHS: (1) newly diagnosed diabetes, (2) infection, (3) female gender.

Precipitating causes of DKA and HHS are listed in Exhibit 24–1. The frequency of precipitating causes varies in different populations and is related to: (1) access (or lack of access) to continuing quality education and medical care, (2) early (or delayed) detection of diabetes, (3) adherence (or nonadherence) to

TABLE 24–1 Severe Diabetic Ketoacidosis and Hyperglycemic Hyperosmolar State from 1969, 1974–1986, and Moderate and Mild Diabetic Ketoacidosis from 1974–1986 at Grady Memorial Hospital

Year	No. Severe DKA plus HHS Patients[a]	Episodes per 1,000 Patients[b]	p[c]	Estimated No. Prevented 1974–1986[d]	No. Moderate, Mild DKA[e]	Episodes per 1,000 Patients[b]	p[f]	Estimated No. Prevented 1975–1986[g]	Estimated Total No. Severe, Moderate, and Mild DKAs and HHSs Prevented[h]
1969	502	38.8							
1974	185	14.3	<0.5	317	349	26.9	—	—	317 (No audit for moderate or mild DKA)
1975	174	13.4	<0.01	328	225	17.4	<0.05	124	452
1976	137	10.6	<0.01	365	143	11.0	<0.01	206	571
1977	129	10.0	<0.01	373	142	11.0	<0.01	207	580
1978	112	8.6	<0.01	390	155	12.0	<0.01	194	584
1979	125	9.7	<0.01	377	162	12.5	<0.01	187	564
1980	178	13.7	<0.05	324	150	11.6	<0.01	199	523
1981	136	10.5	<0.01	366	135	10.4	<0.01	214	580
1982	142	11.0	<0.01	360	124	9.6	<0.01	225	585
1983	132	10.2	<0.01	350	174	13.4	<0.01	175	525
1984	107	8.3	<0.01	395	138	10.7	<0.01	211	606
1985	142	11.0	<0.01	360	60	4.6	<0.01	289	649
1986	108	8.3	<0.01	394	179	13.8	<0.01	170	564
Total				4,699	2,136			2,401	7,100
Years	(1974–1986)	(1974–1986)		(1974–1986)	(1975–1986)	(1975–1986)		(1975–1986)	(1975–1986)
Mean (1974–1986)	139	10.7		361.5	148.9	11.5		200.1	565.3
SD (1974–1986)	25.7	2.0		25.9	38.7	3.0		38.7	48.7
SEM (1974–1986)	7.1	0.6		7.2	11.2	0.9		11.2	14.1

[a] Severe DKA = serum CO_2 content $\leq$ 10 mEq/L; HHS = serum osmolality >350 mOsm.

[b] Denominator = 12,950 patients.

[c] Probability (p) that 1969 number of severe DKA plus HHS patients is significantly higher than the number of episodes in subsequent years of comparison.

[d] Estimated number of cases of severe DKA plus HHS prevented in that year (i.e., 502 for 1969 minus 185 in 1974 equals 317 prevented in 1974).

[e] Moderate DKA equals serum CO_2 content 11 to 20 mEq/L, 20 mEq/L mild DKA equals serum CO_2 content >20 mEq/L

[f] Probability (p) that 1974 number of moderate and mild DKAs is significantly higher than the number of episodes in subsequent year of comparison.

[g] Estimated number of cases of moderate and mild DKA prevented in that year (i.e., 349 for 1974 minus 225 for 1975 = 124 prevented in 1975).

[h] Estimated total number of cases of DKA (severe, moderate, mild) and HHS prevented in that year.

TABLE 24–2 Some Demographic and Other Characteristics of 96 Individuals Admitted to Grady Memorial Hospital in 1978 with Severe Ketoacidosis (CO$_2$ Content ≤ 10 mEq/L) and/or with a Hyperosmolar State (Serum Osmolality >350 mOsm)

	Race and Sex[a]						
	Black Female	*Black Male*	*White Female*	*White Male*	**Total**		
Individuals	54	21	12	9	96		
Episodes	61[b]	25	16	10	112		

Age ranges and no. episodes during the year 1978

Age range[c] (years)	≤20	21–30	31–40	41–50	51–60	61–70	71–80
No. individuals	15	12	19	21	15	10	2
No. episodes	19	16	21	22	18	10	4

Treatment routines: All patients were treated with insulin initially and 92 were discharged on insulin; four overweight individuals were discharged on diet therapy alone

Hospital days: Total 727, mean 6.5 (range, 1–84).

Deaths: Total six patients (four severe DKA, two severe HHS)

Undiagnosed prior to admission: 40

Adherence to prescribed therapy:[d] Of the 56 individuals diagnosed prior to admission, 14 were known to be chronic alcoholics, and 36 of the remaining 42 were known to be generally nonadherent in that they frequently discontinued insulin therapy and/or did not adhere to the prescribed diet.

[a] Population of those with known diabetes at GMH: 60.6% BF, 22.6% BM, 11.3% WF, and 5.4% WM.

[b] One episode, 85 individuals; two episodes, 7 individuals; 3 episodes, 3 individuals; 4 episodes, 1 individual.

[c] Age not known in two individuals who each had one episode.

[d] As judged by diabetes clinic attendance, level of plasma glucose control, and weight loss in overweight individuals.

Abbreviations: BF, black female; BM, black male; GMH, Grady Memorial Hospital; WF, white female; WM, white male.

[*Source*: Davidson JK: The United States of America: The Grady Memorial Hospital Experience. *In* Mann JI, Pyorola K, Teuscher A (eds): Diabetes in Epidemiological Perspective, London: Churchill Livingstone, 1983, pp. 243–249. With permission.]

EXHIBIT 24–1 Precipitating Causes of Diabetic Ketoacidosis and the Hyperglycemic Hyperosmolar State

Common
   Delayed diagnosis of diabetes
   Interruption of insulin therapy
   Infection (pulmonary, urinary tract, other)
   Stress (major vascular occlusions, trauma, surgical procedures, burns, and so forth)
   Ethanol abuse

Uncommon
   Down-regulation of insulin receptors (excess adiposity, excessive calorie and sugar intake, inappropriate insulin therapy of non-insulin-dependent diabetes)
   Tube feeding of sucrose (and other sugars) plus water intake inadequate to sustain hyperglycemia-induced osmotic diuresis
   Steroid therapy

Rare
   Immunologic insulin resistance
   Insulin receptors absent
   Insulin receptor antibodies
   Disease states (including tumors) that produce excessive amount of a contrainsulin hormone (glucagon, epinephrine, norepinephrine, cortisol, growth hormone, thyroxin)

prescribed therapy, and (4) infection (presence or absence). Unfortunately, some socially deprived or psychologically disturbed individuals because of disease denial, anxiety, depression, stress, or a desire to manipulate or control parents or professional advisers refuse to accept the responsibility for optimal metabolic control. The prevalence of multiple episodes of DKA or HHS, or both, is common in this group, and the pre-

cipitating cause is usually related to discontinuing insulin therapy (see Chapter 18).

As noted in Table 24–2, it was estimated that the 1978 audited incidence at Grady Hospital could have been reduced by 94% (total DKA from 267 to 17 cases, severe DKA from 12 to 7 cases) *had all undiagnosed cases of diabetes been detected before development of DKA and had all cases been completely adherent to therapy after diagnosis* (no interruption of insulin therapy, no alcohol or addictive drug abuse, no significant failure to adhere to diet, and no failure to self-monitor metabolic state and promptly report significant changes to the primary care physician/nurse team).

Available epidemiologic data are not sufficient to define precisely the incident mortality rates for primary (uncomplicated) and secondary (chronic complications) of acutely decompensated diabetes (DKA, HHS). It was estimated that in the United States in 1982 about 5,000 deaths occurred as a result of primary and (coincident to) secondary episodes of DKA and/or HHS.[15] Mortality rates are higher in those who are older, those who have diabetes of long duration, those who have major vascular or renal complications, and those who have serious infections. Estimated 1989 death rates were: (1) for uncomplicated severe DKA (primary) approximately 1 to 2%, (2) for complicated severe DKA (secondary) approximately 10%, and (3) for HHS approximately 26%.[10,14,15]

The incidence of DKA and HHS and mortality thereunto related can be decreased significantly by early diagnosis coupled with the prompt and optimal use of currently available therapeutic modalities.[16,17] It should be remembered that as the duration of non-insulin-dependent diabetes mellitus (NIDDM) increases, some individuals become insulin dependent and may develop DKA or HHS, or both.

In 1995 in the USA over 110,000 cases of acutely decompensated diabetes (DKA/HHS) were hospitalized.

Pathophysiology

Exhibit 24–2 outlines the pathogenesis of acutely decompensated diabetes mellitus as it may occur in a hypothetical 80 kg adult. In the wake of an insulin deficit, substrate catabolism accelerates, substrate anabolism decelerates, and levels of stress hormones (epinephrine, norepinephrine, glucagon, cortisol, and growth hormone) rise.[18,19,22] Glucose production increases and the plasma glucose level rises; fatty acid release and ketone production increase, and the H^+ level rises. The *rising plasma glucose level increases serum osmolality* (each 100 mg/dL increase above normal in plasma glucose can increase serum osmolality by 5.5 mOsm, see Exhibit 24–3) and this in turn causes water to migrate from the intracellular to the extracellular compartment [the Donnan equilibrium requires that intracellular and extracellular osmolality be balanced (Tables 24–3 and 24–4)]. This initial migration of water from the intracellular to the extracellular compartment may account for *dilutional yponatremia* (i.e., a plasma glucose of 650 mg/dL may increase serum osmolality by 30 mOsm and can account for a lowering of the serum Na^+ from 139.5 to 111.5 mEq/L). A 1998 report[20] suggests that the correction factor for hyperglycemia induced hyponatremia should be *minus* 2.4 mEq/l Na^+ per 100 mq/dl glucose *increase* (above 100 mg/dl), rather than the conventionally used factor of −1.6 mEq/l Na^+. The body tries to compensate for the hyperosmolar state by increased water intake (thirst) and by excretion of excess glucose by osmotic diuresis (kidney). Depending on the relative amount of water lost compared with solute, the result could be *isotonic, hypotonic,* or *hypertonic volume contraction.* When hypovolemia develops, renal plasma flow and glomerular filtration rate decrease, and blood urea nitrogen (BUN) and uric acid rise out of proportion to creatinine. Then oliguria and acute renal failure secondary to acute tubular necrosis may occur.

The body tries to compensate for the increasing H^+ level by hyperventilation to lower PCO_2 (lungs); by buffering the excess H^+ with bicarbonate and other buffering mechanisms (buffers, see Exhibit 24–3); and by excreting more H^+ as free acid, titratable acidity, and NH_3 buffered ketone salts (kidney). Triglycerides and cholesterol may accumulate in the plasma compartment, and can displace plasma water and account for *displacement byponatremia* (lipid content of plasma can rise as high as 10%, and as a result the measured serum sodium could decrease spuriously from 139.5 to 125.5 mEq/L). Electrolytes, especially Na^+ and K^+, are lost in large amounts during the osmotic diuresis. As H^+ production increases, the buffer-kidney-lung compensatory mechanisms are progressively depleted, and the effects of the acidosis become more evident and ominous. The end result of these events, if uninterrupted by appropriate therapy, is severe DKA and death.

Ketone body production and disposal rates in diabetic ketosis and during fasting in nondiabetic individuals have been compared,[21] and the studies have shown that a maximal metabolic disposal rate of about 2.3 mM/min/1.73 m^2 is attained in both groups at concentrations of 10 to 12 mM, which correspond to the highest ketone body levels encountered during prolonged fasting. Thus, fasting ketosis is *self-limited*, but diabetic ketosis is not *self-limited* because the insulin deficit results in higher rates of ketogenesis and higher levels of free fatty acids and glucagon. Since there is no evidence for the existence of a ketone body removal defect specific to diabetes, the *excessive production of ketone bodies* is the main factor leading to uncontrolled hyperketonemia in DKA.[19] Some tissues have a high affinity for ketones at low concentration (muscle extraction 50% at 0.1 mM) with affinity decreasing at high concentration (muscle extraction 1 to 2% at 6 to 7 mM), whereas the affinity for ketones for some tissues remains the same at all concentrations (brain extraction 5 to 10% whatever the concentration).

The biochemical alterations in DKA likely flow from regulation of fructose-2, 6-biphosphate, which in turn determines flux over the glycolytic/gluconeogenic

EXHIBIT 24–2   Pathophysiology of Acutely Decompensated Diabetes Mellitus (Hypothetical 80 kg Adult)

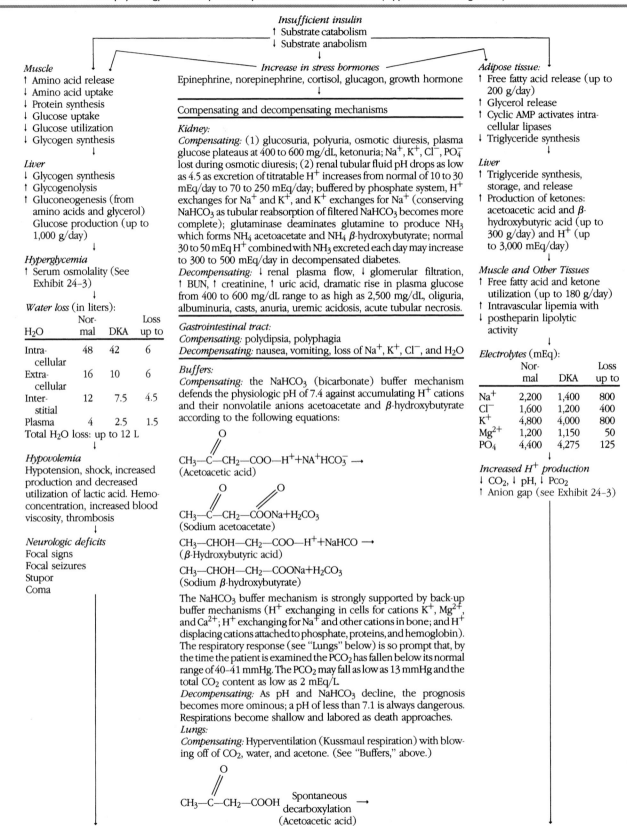

Insufficient insulin
↑ Substrate catabolism
↓ Substrate anabolism

Muscle
↑ Amino acid release
↓ Amino acid uptake
↓ Protein synthesis
↓ Glucose uptake
↓ Glucose utilization
↓ Glycogen synthesis

Liver
↓ Glycogen synthesis
↑ Glycogenolysis
↑ Gluconeogenesis (from amino acids and glycerol) Glucose production (up to 1,000 g/day)

Hyperglycemia
↑ Serum osmolality (See Exhibit 24–3)

Water loss (in liters):

H₂O	Normal	DKA	Loss up to
Intra-cellular	48	42	6
Extra-cellular	16	10	6
Inter-stitial	12	7.5	4.5
Plasma	4	2.5	1.5

Total H₂O loss: up to 12 L

Hypovolemia
Hypotension, shock, increased production and decreased utilization of lactic acid. Hemoconcentration, increased blood viscosity, thrombosis

Neurologic deficits
Focal signs
Focal seizures
Stupor
Coma

Increase in stress hormones
Epinephrine, norepinephrine, cortisol, glucagon, growth hormone

Compensating and decompensating mechanisms

Kidney:
Compensating: (1) glucosuria, polyuria, osmotic diuresis, plasma glucose plateaus at 400 to 600 mg/dL, ketonuria; Na⁺, K⁺, Cl⁻, PO₄⁻ lost during osmotic diuresis; (2) renal tubular fluid pH drops as low as 4.5 as excretion of titratable H⁺ increases from normal of 10 to 30 mEq/day to 70 to 250 mEq/day; buffered by phosphate system, H⁺ exchanges for Na⁺ and K⁺, and K⁺ exchanges for Na⁺ (conserving NaHCO₃ as tubular reabsorption of filtered NaHCO₃ becomes more complete); glutaminase deaminates glutamine to produce NH₃ which forms NH₄ acetoacetate and NH₄ β-hydroxybutyrate; normal 30 to 50 mEq H⁺ combined with NH₃ excreted each day may increase to 300 to 500 mEq/day in decompensated diabetes.
Decompensating: ↓ renal plasma flow, ↓ glomerular filtration, ↑ BUN, ↑ creatinine, ↑ uric acid, dramatic rise in plasma glucose from 400 to 600 mg/dL range to as high as 2,500 mg/dL, oliguria, albuminuria, casts, anuria, uremic acidosis, acute tubular necrosis.

Gastrointestinal tract:
Compensating: polydipsia, polyphagia
Decompensating: nausea, vomiting, loss of Na⁺, K⁺, Cl⁻, and H₂O

Buffers:
Compensating: the NaHCO₃ (bicarbonate) buffer mechanism defends the physiologic pH of 7.4 against accumulating H⁺ cations and their nonvolatile anions acetoacetate and β-hydroxybutyrate according to the following equations:

$$CH_3-\overset{O}{\overset{\|}{C}}-CH_2-COO-H^+ + NA^+HCO_3^- \longrightarrow$$
(Acetoacetic acid)

$$CH_3-\overset{O}{\overset{\|}{C}}-CH_2-\overset{O}{\overset{\|}{C}}OONa + H_2CO_3$$
(Sodium acetoacetate)

$$CH_3-CHOH-CH_2-COO-H^+ + NaHCO \longrightarrow$$
(β-Hydroxybutyric acid)

$$CH_3-CHOH-CH_2-COONa + H_2CO_3$$
(Sodium β-hydroxybutyrate)

The NaHCO₃ buffer mechanism is strongly supported by back-up buffer mechanisms (H⁺ exchanging in cells for cations K⁺, Mg²⁺, and Ca²⁺; H⁺ exchanging for Na⁺ and other cations in bone; and H⁺ displacing cations attached to phosphate, proteins, and hemoglobin). The respiratory response (see "Lungs" below) is so prompt that, by the time the patient is examined the PCO₂ has fallen below its normal range of 40–41 mmHg. The PCO₂ may fall as low as 13 mmHg and the total CO₂ content as low as 2 mEq/L.
Decompensating: As pH and NaHCO₃ decline, the prognosis becomes more ominous; a pH of less than 7.1 is always dangerous. Respirations become shallow and labored as death approaches.
Lungs:
Compensating: Hyperventilation (Kussmaul respiration) with blowing off of CO₂, water, and acetone. (See "Buffers," above.)

$$CH_3-\overset{O}{\overset{\|}{C}}-CH_2-COOH \quad \underset{decarboxylation}{\overset{Spontaneous}{\longrightarrow}}$$
(Acetoacetic acid)

Adipose tissue:
↑ Free fatty acid release (up to 200 g/day)
↑ Glycerol release
↑ Cyclic AMP activates intracellular lipases
↓ Triglyceride synthesis

Liver
↑ Triglyceride synthesis, storage, and release
↑ Production of ketones: acetoacetic acid and β-hydroxybutyric acid (up to 300 g/day) and H⁺ (up to 3,000 mEq/day)

Muscle and Other Tissues
↑ Free fatty acid and ketone utilization (up to 180 g/day)
↑ Intravascular lipemia with
↓ postheparin lipolytic activity

Electrolytes (mEq):

	Normal	DKA	Loss up to
Na⁺	2,200	1,400	800
Cl⁻	1,600	1,200	400
K⁺	4,800	4,000	800
Mg²⁺	1,200	1,150	50
PO₄	4,400	4,275	125

Increased H⁺ production
↓ CO₂, ↓ pH, ↓ Pco₂
↑ Anion gap (see Exhibit 24–3)

(continued)

EXHIBIT 24–2 *(continued)* Pathophysiology of Acutely Decompensated Diabetes Mellitus (Hypothetical 80 kg Adult)

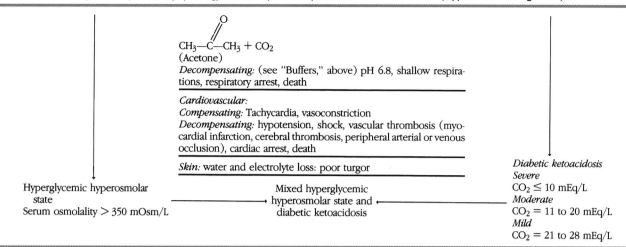

$$CH_3-\overset{\displaystyle O}{\overset{\|}{C}}-CH_3 + CO_2$$
(Acetone)
Decompensating: (see "Buffers," above) pH 6.8, shallow respirations, respiratory arrest, death

Cardiovascular:
Compensating: Tachycardia, vasoconstriction
Decompensating: hypotension, shock, vascular thrombosis (myocardial infarction, cerebral thrombosis, peripheral arterial or venous occlusion), cardiac arrest, death

Skin: water and electrolyte loss: poor turgor

Hyperglycemic hyperosmolar state
Serum osmolality > 350 mOsm/L

Mixed hyperglycemic hyperosmolar state and diabetic ketoacidosis

Diabetic ketoacidosis
Severe
$CO_2 \leq 10$ mEq/L
Moderate
$CO_2 = 11$ to 20 mEq/L
Mild
$CO_2 = 21$ to 28 mEq/L

EXHIBIT 24–3 How to Calculate Serum Osmolality, pH, and Anion Gap

I. *To Calculate Serum Osmolality*
Normal:

$2(Na^+ + K^+) +$ glucose (mg/dL)/18] + [BUN/2.8] $=$ 278 to 302 mOsm/kg

Example:

$2[139.5 + 3.7] + [90/18] + [12/2.8] = 295.7$ mOsm

Abnormal: (hyperglycemic hyperosmolar state):

$2[Na^+ + k^+] +$ [glucose (mg/dL)/18] $+$ [BUN/2.8] > 350 mOsm

Example:

$2[138 + 5.3] + [1080/18] + [60/2.8] = 368.0$ mOsm

Measured serum osmolality (osmometer) may be $\geqq 10$ mOsm/kg higher than calculated serum osmolality, because some of the measured osmotically active particles are not calculated in the above formula.

II. *Henderson-Hasselbalch Equation:*

$$pH = 6.10 + \log \frac{Na^+(HCO_3^-)}{\text{dissolved } CO_2 + H_2CO_3}$$

HCO_3^- is measured as CO_2 content. Dissolved $CO_2 + H_2CO_3$ may be calculated by measuring PCO_2 in mmHg and converting to mEq/L of H_2CO_3 by multiplying PCO_2 (in mmHg) by 0.03.

Normal:

$$pH = 6.10 + \log \frac{CO_2 \text{ content (mEq/L)}}{PCO_2 \text{ (mmHg)} \times 0.03}$$

$$= 6.10 + \log \frac{24 \text{ mEq/L}}{40 \times 0.03} = 6.10 + \log \frac{24}{1.2}$$

$$= 6.10 + \log \frac{20}{1} = 6.10 + 1.30 = 7.40$$

Abnormal: (In severe diabetic ketoacidosis, the following may occur):

$$pH = 6.10 + \log \frac{2 \text{ mEq/L}}{13 \times 0.03} = 6.10 + \log \frac{2}{0.39}$$

$$= 6.10 + \log \frac{5}{1} = 6.10 + 0.70 = 6.80$$

III. *To calculate anion gap:*
Normal: $(Na^+ + K^+) - (Cl^- + HCO_3^-) = 16 \pm 7$ (unmeasured anions)
Example: $(139.5 + 3.7) - (102.1 + 25.1) = 16$
Abnormal: (As may occur in diabetic ketoacidosis because of accumulation of acetoacetate and β-hydroxybutyrate):
Example: $(139.5 + 3.7) - (100 + 5) = 38.2$ mEq. The *anion gap* is 38.2 mEq, or significantly greater than the normal anion gap of 16 ± 7.

---

pathways, and thereby controls hepatic metabolism and ketogenesis[23] (see Chapter 7).

In moderate to severe DKA, β-hydroxybutyrate, acetoacetate, and acetone may be utilized as tissue substrates or excreted in the urine. Also, acetone can be excreted in the breath, and it can contribute approximately 50% as much glucose (acetone → 1-hydroxyacetone (acetol) → 1,2-propanediol (PPD) → pyruvate → oxalacetate → phosphoenolpyruvate → glucose) as does alanine (from gluconeogensis) during DKA. The major fraction of the glucose produced during DKA is derived from recycled lactate and pyruvate and from glycerol.[24,25] During DKA, new glucose synthesized from amino acids (1 g urinary nitrogen equals production of 3 g glucose) is >0.2 mM $\cdot$ min$^{-1}\cdot$1.73 m^{-2} in adults. Glucose derived from acetone $(0.02 \times 0.8 - 1.0 = 0.02$ mM$\cdot$min$^{-1}\cdot$1.73 m$^{-2})$ represents at least 10% of the newly synthesized glucose during DKA $(3$ mg$\cdot$min$\cdot$min$^{-1}\cdot$1.73 m$^{-2})$.

TABLE 24–3   Electrolytes in Intracellular Water Phase

Cations	mEq	mOsm	Anions	mEq	mOsm
K⁺	150[a]	150	Cl⁻	15	15
Na⁺	10	10	HCO₃⁻	10	10
Mg²⁺	40	20	PO₄⁻, PO₄²⁻ and SO₄²⁻	140	94.5
			Protein	35	5
Total	200	180		200	124.5

[a] Dependent on specific tissue analyzed.

[Source: Davidson JK: Diabetic ketoacidosis and hyperglycemic hyperosmolar state. In Schwartz GB, Safar P, Stone JH, et al. (eds): Principles and Practice of Emergency Medicine. Philadelphia: W.B. Saunders, 1985. With permission.]

Although ketones have traditionally been measured by the nitroprusside test, it should be noted that this method measures (or estimates) only the acetoacetate and acetone levels, and it does not measure β-hydroxybutyrate levels, the ketone body that reaches the highest levels during DKA. Accurate measurements of serum acetoacetate and β-hydroxybutyrate may be done using enzymatic methods, but these methods are not available at the bedside. β-Hydroxybutyrate in urine and serum may be measured semiquantitatively by a paper strip that detects levels exceeding 0.1 mmol/L.[26]

It should also be noted that although elevated amylase levels during DKA *may* be secondary to acute pancreatitis, they are usually related to ketone interference with the assay or to amylase activity that originates in another tissue (such as the parotid gland).[27]

A 1990 review of 69 cases (40 from literature 1961–1987, 29 unpublished) of intracerebral crises (herniated brainstem and respiratory arrest precipitated by cerebral edema) revealed that 65% died, 20% had residual brain damage, and 15% recovered.[28a] Sixty-seven of the 69 cases were less than 20 years of age, one was 23 years, and one was 28 years of age.

Subjective or objective warning signs that may lead to a diagnosis of life-threatening cerebral edema are: severe headache, dramatic change in behavior or ability to arouse, increasing obtundation, incontinence, seizures, bradycardia, blood pressure changes, pupillary changes, disturbed temperature regulation, and respiratory arrest. Cerebral edema was usually noted when computed tomography (CT) scanning was done, and postmortem studies on 24 who did not have scans were consistent with cerebral edema and, in most cases, brainstem herniation. Yet CT scanning failed to separate those with DKA who are at risk from those not at risk for an intracerebral crisis. Two risk factors for a subsequent intracerebral crisis were identified: (1) diabetes undiagnosed before DKA developed, and a young age (85% were less than 15 years of age).

Rosenbloom[28b] suggested that, until the precise mechanisms of cerebral edema in DKA are known and can be treated successfully, early diagnosis of diabetes and prevention of DKA (especially in those less than 20 years of age) are the most important means of avoiding intracerebral complications. Also, he expressed the opinion that intervention treatment with hyperventilation, dexamethasone, and mannitol produced better outcomes when started *before respiratory arrest* than when started *after respiratory arrest*. However, early intervention failed to prevent fatal or severe brain damage in nearly half of the patients so treated.

Since the death rate in adults who develop DKA or HHS, or both, is about 25% in those with serum osmolalities more than 350 mOsm and less than 5% in those with serum osmolalities less than 350 mOsm, more studies are needed to define precisely the pathophysiologic mechanisms underlying HHS deaths in adults. Thus, serum osmolality should be *calculated* and *mea-*

TABLE 24–4   Electrolytes in Extracellular Water Phase[a]

Serum (93% Water)						In Water Phase of Serum[b]					
Cations	mEq	mOsm	Anions	mEq	mOsm	Cations	mEq	mOsm	Anions	mEq	mOsm
Na⁺	139.5	139.5	Cl⁻	102.3	102.3	Na⁺	150	150	Cl⁻	110	110
K⁺	3.7	3.7	HCO₃⁻	25.1	25.1	K⁺	4	4	HCO₃⁻	27	27
Ca²⁺	2.8	1.4	PO₄²⁻	1.9	1.0	Ca²⁺	5	2.5	PO₄²⁻	2	1
Mg²⁺	2.8	1.4	SO₄²⁻	1.0	0.5	Mg²⁺	3	1.5	SO₄²⁻	1	0.5
			Protein	14.9	2.0				Protein	16	2
			Organic acid	5.6	5.6				Organic acid	6	6
Total	148.8	146.0		150.8	136.5		162	158		162	146.5

[a] Normal osmolality in intracellular water compartment: cations + anions = 180 + 124.5 = 304.5 mOsm (See Table 24–5).

[b] Normal osmolality in the water phase of serum; cations + anions = 158 + 146.5 = 304.5 mOsm. Normal osmolality of serum (93% water) = 146.0 + 136.5 = 282.5 (range 278–302) mOsm/kg.

Intracellular water osmolality (304.5 mOsm) = extracellular water osmolality (304.5 mOsm).

sured in all individuals with DKA (or HHS) when they are *initially* seen. Serum osmolality may have predictive value in identifying those adults (and possibly children as well) who are at increased risk of death from osmotic dysequilibrium (serum osmolality >350 mOsm) before and during treatment of DKA or HHS, and before symptoms and signs of intracerebral crises (brainstem herniation with respiratory arrest) occur.

A thorough understanding of the pathogenesis in each patient facilitates the planning of therapy so that metabolic homeostasis can be promptly reestablished by replacing insulin, water, electrolyte, and substrate (i.e., glucose) deficits as needed.[17]

Problem Statement: Acutely Decompensated Diabetes Mellitus Subsets: Mild Diabetic Ketoacidosis, Moderate Diabetic Ketoacidosis, Severe Diabetic Ketoacidosis, Hyperglycemic Hyperosmolar State, Mixed Diabetic Ketoacidosis and Hyperglycemic Hyperosmolar State

Initial Data Base and Assessment

An *abbreviated data base* (Exhibit 24–4) should be collected and a preliminary assessment made as quickly as possible (usually within 10 minutes). Blood glucose (visual or meter-read glucose-oxidase-impregnated strip) or plasma or serum glucose (polarographic oxygen-rate glucose oxidase method: Beckman or similar device) and serum acetone (crushed Acetest tablet) and urine acetone and glucose determinations should be done promptly. If these measurements suggest that DKA is mild or moderate, and if the patient is alert (immediate appropriate responses to stimulation), and there are no complications, *treatment on an outpatient basis can be initiated.*

However, if the measurements indicate that the plasma glucose is higher than 500 mg/dL or that DKA is severe ($CO_2 \leq 10$ mEq/L), or that HHS (serum osmolality >350 mOsm/L) is present, or if the patient is *obtunded* (dull indifference requiring increased stimulation to evoke a response), *stuporous* (arousal only by vigorous, including painful, and continuous stimulation), or in *coma* (absent or rudimentary responses to vigorous, including painful, and continuous stimulation), or if significant complications of diabetes or if significant concurrent problems (see Exhibit 24–5, Assessment) are

present, the patient should be hospitalized in an intensive care area with IV 0.9% saline running as soon as possible (within 30 min after the initial evaluation).

Definitive Treatment Plan for Hospitalized DKAs and/or HHSs

The admitting treatment team should promptly collect a *defined data base* (Exhibit 24–5) and should initiate insulin therapy either en route to or immediately on arrival in the intensive care area (Exhibit 24–6). A flow sheet (Exhibits 24–7 and 24–8) should be maintained until the patient has recovered completely.

Hypoglycemia should be excluded during the preadmission initial assessment, and intoxication by beverages, drugs, or poisons, and other causes of metabolic acidosis and coma should be excluded (Exhibit 24–4) as soon as possible.

As early as possible in the course of therapy, the factor (or factors) that precipitated the acutely decompensated diabetes should be identified (see Exhibit 24–1). Complications (Exhibit 24–9) should be noted and appropriately treated. Side effects of therapy (Exhibit 24–10) should be prevented if possible, or treated promptly. A clear airway should be established (using an endotracheal tube if necessary), and oxygen should be given if the patient is hypoxic or cyanotic. The patient should be checked for a distended bladder (catheterized only if absolutely necessary) and a dilated stomach (rarely, a stomach tube must be inserted), and occasionally sideboards and restraints must be applied to prevent the patient from falling out of bed. At least one member of the treatment team should be in *constant attendance* and should *continuously monitor* the patient (see Exhibit 24–6) until alert and the diabetes has compensated. Hypoglycemia (plasma glucose <50 mg/dL) should be prevented by hourly monitoring of the plasma glucose, and hypokalemia (serum $K^+ \leq 3$ mEq/L) should be prevented by hourly monitoring of the serum potassium. Shock should be treated aggressively with prompt and adequate fluid replacement, but fluid overload with congestive heart failure should be avoided. Cardiac or respiratory arrest may occur either secondary to hyperkalemia or hypokalemia (Fig. 24–1), and equipment should be maintained near the patient for either of these emergencies.

Exhibit 24–11 contains a list of the equipment and supplies needed to optimally diagnose and treat acutely decompensated diabetes mellitus. Of even greater importance to optimal diagnosis and treatment is a welltrained team of professionals [MD, RN, registered dietitian (RD), and laboratory technician] who monitor the patient's progress continuously and who

EXHIBIT 24–4   Collection of Abbreviated Data Base with Preliminary Assessment (Differential Diagnosis) of Acutely Decompensated Diabetes Mellitus

Collect *abbreviated data base* as quickly as possible (usually within 10 min) consisting of immediately relevant subjective and objective data (see Exhibit 24–5). In the *comatose* patient, maintain a *patent airway*; in the patient in *shock*, start IV infusion of 0.9% *saline* immediately. Stat plasma glucose (preferably by the Beckman oxygen rate method) and serially diluted plasma ketones (Acetest tables, crushed) will confirm the diagnosis of decompensated diabetes mellitus (or hypoglycemia[a]) in a few minutes. If available *without catheterization*, quantitative urine glucose and ketones should be measured by the same methods.

If the plasma glucose is <50 mg/dL and patient is unable to swallow, give stat up to 50 mL 50% glucose (25 g glucose) IV or 1 mg glucagon IM.[a]

If plasma glucose is <50 mg/dL, and patient is able to swallow, give soft drinks containing sugar, sweetened orange juice, or candy PO.

If plasma glucose is >500 mg/dL and no ketonemia or ketonuria, or if plasma glucose is >150 mg/dL and moderate-to-large ketonuria and/or ketonemia, collect *venous* blood (red top tube) for SMA/6 (Na^+, K^+, CO_2, Cl^-, BUN, glucose), *venous* blood (in plastic syringe wet with heparin, rotate syringe, bend needle, place syringe on cracked ice) for pH,[b] and *venous* blood (red top tube) for measurement of serum osmolality (osmometer).

Patients with severe DKA or HHS, significant complications, or concurrent problems, who are obtunded, stuporous, or in coma, or who have a plasma glucose >500 mg/dL (28 mmol/L), should be hospitalized in an intensive care area with IV 0.9% saline running as soon as possible (see Exhibit 24–5, Assessment).

In patients who are *comatose* or who have *metabolic acidosis*, the following problems should be considered in the differential diagnosis:

I. Intoxication
  A. Beverages
    1. Ethanol
      (a) Hypoglycemia (with or without ketonuria)
      (b) Alcoholic ketoacidosis (uncommon, history of protracted vomiting, prolonged abstention from food, chronic alcoholism, appreciable alcohol intake before admission, blood ethanol may be undetectable, or may be 50 to 500 mg/dL, ketonemia, frequent lactic acidemia, plasma glucose <150 mg/dL)
      (c) Without hypoglycemia or metabolic acidosis
    2. Methanol (formaldehyde, formic acid, metabolic acidosis)
    3. Isopropyl alcohol (transient ketonuria, no acidosis)
    4. Smoke (hypoglycemia)
    5. Antifreeze (ethylene and diethylene glycol metabolized to oxalate, metabolic acidosis)
  B. Drugs
    1. Salicylate (plasma salicylate level > 30 mg/dL, respiratory alkalosis with renal bicarbonate loss hyponatremia, ketoacidosis, dehydration)
    2. Paraldehyde (characteristic odor, metabolic acidosis)
    3. Barbiturates
    4. Opiates
    5. Bromide
    6. Chloral hydrate (metabolic acidosis, respiratory depression, acute hepatic necrosis)
    7. Other sedatives
  C. Poisons
    1. Phenol and other cresols (white burns of mouth)
    2. Fluoride (tetany, hyperglycemia unresponsive to insulin)
    3. Milk sickness (from ingestion of milk or meat of animals poisoned by snakeroot, richweed, or rayless goldenrod; hypoglycemia, acidosis, ketonuria)
    4. Streptozotocin, alloxan, rodenticide (Vacor)
II. Other causes of metabolic acidosis
  A. Lactic acidosis (anion gap otherwise unaccounted for, may be due to phenformin poisoning or shock; draw venous blood without stasis, allow it to clot then separate and freeze serum until assayed for lactate and pyruvate; normal lactate 3.5 to 12.5 mg/dL or 0.4 to 1.4 mEq/L; normal pyruvate 0.6 to 1.2 mg/dL or 0.07 to 0.14 mEq/L; in lactic acidosis serum lactate is > 63 mg/dL or > 7 mEq/L.
  B. Uremic acidosis (anion gap otherwise unaccounted for, elevated BUN and creatinine)
  C. Rhabdomyolysis (renal tubular dysfunction)
III. Other causes of coma
  A. Hypernatremia, hypercalcemia, hypoxia, hepatic coma, myxedema coma, adrenal cortical insufficiency
  B. Severe systemic infection (pneumonia, gram-negative septicemia, typhoid, malaria, meningococcemia)
  C. Shock from any cause, cardiac failure (either may be associated with lactic acidosis)
  D. Hypertensive encephalopathy, eclampsia
  E. Marked hyperthermia or hypothermia
  F. Brain hemorrhage, thrombosis, embolism, or abscess
  G. Epidural or subdural hemorrhage, brain contusion, subarachnoid hemorrhage
  H. Brain tumor, acute bacterial meningitis, viral encephalitis, epileptic seizure
IV. Ketonuria due to starvation ketosis
  This is common in individuals who are ingesting less than 100 g carbohydrate daily. It rarely, if ever, accounts for significant metabolic acidosis. CO_2 content after 7 days of total fasting may decline to 15 mEq/L.

[a] See section on hypoglycemia, in Chapter 18.

[b] Venous pH closely approximates arterial pH in this setting.

EXHIBIT 24–5   Problem Statement: Acutely Decompensated Diabetes Mellitus (Subsets: Severe, Moderate, or Mild Diabetic Ketoacidosis; Hyperglycemia Hyperosmolar State)

Defined Data Base
Subjective (History)
(1) Known diabetes mellitus, previous episodes of acutely decompensated diabetes mellitus, insulin dose and type, missed insulin, diet prescription, gross dietary indiscretion, obesity, weight loss or gain, family history of diabetes mellitus; (2) polyuria, glucosuria, ketonuria; (3) thirst, polydipsia, polyphagia, vomiting, nausea, anorexia, abdominal pain; (4) coma, stupor, obtunded, alert, weakness; (5) rapid breathing, shortness of breath, chest pain; (6) shock, fever, infection, pregnancy, thyrotoxicosis, surgery, trauma, anesthesia; (7) beverage (especially ethanol) or drug abuse, poisoning, medications (steroids, sulfonylurea, phenformin), emotional upset.
Objective
(1) Physical examination: coma, stupor, obtunded, alert, poor skin turgor, weak rapid pulse, hypothermia or hyperthermia, reclining and/or orthostatic hypotension, neck veins, dry, dirty mouth and tongue, fruity odor of breath (acetone) rapid deep respirations (becoming shallow when death approaches), soft eyeballs, dilated pupils, lipemia retinalis diabetic retinopathy, lung rales, pleural friction rub, abdominal tenderness, abdominal distention (dilated stomach), flaccid muscles, weak or absent tendon reflexes, skin or other infection, height, frame, body weight. (2) Laboratory data: glucosuria, ketonuria (acetoacetic

aciduria), possibly albuminuria and/or pyuria, hyperglycemia, ketonemia (acetoacetic acidemia: serially diluted plasma), decreased venous pH (avoid arterial puncture), decreased total CO_2 content, decreased PCO_2, increased serum osmolality (measured, calculated), increased BUN and uric acid, elevated triglycerides, cholesterol, and fatty acids, abnormal lipoprotein typing, leukocytosis, increased hematocrit, serum sodium, potassium, and chloride, phosphorus, plasma lactate and pyruvate, serum magnesium and calcium, amylase, bilirubin, electrocardiogram (ECG), chest x-ray film.
Assessment
(1) Severe diabetic ketoacidosis: $CO_2 \leqq 10$ mEq/L and/or venous plasma pH <7.10; (2) moderate diabetic ketoacidosis: $CO_2 = 11$ to 20 mEq/L and/or pH 7.10 to 7.30; (3) mild diabetic ketoacidosis: $CO_2 = 21$ to 28 mEq/L and/or pH >7.30; (d) hyperglycemic hyperosmolar state: osmolality >350 mOsm/L due primarily to hyperglycemia without ketonemia or ketonuria. Search for *concurrent problems*: infection, gastrointestinal bleeding, acute myocardial infarction, congestive heart failure, arterial or venous thrombosis, uremic acidosis, lactate acidosis. Rule out other causes of coma and/or *metabolic acidosis* (see Exhibit 24–4).
Plan
See Exhibits 24–6 through 24–8.

---

are capable of appropriately modifying standard therapy so as to avoid or treat promptly and adequately side-effects and/or complications.

Insulin

Human regular insulin should be used routinely to treat acutely decompensated diabetes mellitus (see Chapter 18).

Kitabchi, Alberti, and others (1972–1988)[18,30,31] investigated the metabolic effects of low-dose IV regular insulin infusions (3 to 12 U/hr) in the treatment of DKA and showed that such an approach is as *effective* and possibly *safer* (less hypoglycemia, less hypokalemia, maybe less cerebral edema) than was the case with high-dose IV bolus or high-dose subcutaneous insulin therapy routines that had been used since 1951.

Severe Diabetic Ketoacidosis or Hyperglycemia Hyperosmolar State.   With *severe DKA*, and *sometimes in HHS*, in *adults*, an IV bolus of 10 U or more is given by most clinicians initially to avoid under-insulinization during the early phases of therapy (see Exhibit 24–6). This is followed by an IV infusion of 10 U/hr using an IVAC or similar pump piggy-backed to a water and electrolyte infusion line. In poorly responsive (insulin-resistant) patients (usually obese NIDDMs or severe infections), it may be necessary to double the infusion

rate at hourly intervals until the dose is sufficient to lower the plasma glucose at an optimal rate (50 to 100 mg/dL/hr [2.8 to 5.6 mM/hr]).

In *children*, the initial dose is calculated as 0.1 U/kg/hr with the dose being adjusted to a rate of-fall of the plasma glucose of 50 to 100 mg/dL/hr (2.8–5.6 mM/hr).

Obviously, it is not possible in the individual patient to predict in advance how much insulin will be "enough." Some will need more, and some will need less than the amount just noted. The administered dose should be determined by the rate of decline of the plasma glucose level (measured hourly) and by the rate of clearing of ketonuria and ketonemia (which usually occurs more slowly).[15,32] In the early stages of treatment, there may appear to be a paradoxical increase in "ketonuria" and "ketonemia" as measured by the nitroprusside-containing Acetest tablet because of the conversion of large amounts of β-hydroxybutyrate to acetoacetate and acetone. β-Hydroxybutyrate does not produce color with the nitroprusside reaction, but acetoacetate and acetone do. A new paper strip test for measurement of plasma and urine β-hydroxybutyrate has been developed.[26]

In severe DKA or HHS, insulin can also be administered by *IV bolus, intramuscularly,* or *subcutaneously* at a *rate of 10 to 25 U*/hr. The subcutaneous route should be avoided in the markedly dehydrated, hypotensive, or

EXHIBIT 24–6   Outline of Therapy of Acutely Decompensated Diabetes Mellitus[a]

I. *For patients in*
  A. Shock
  B. Coma
  C. Hypotension
  D. Severe ketoacidosis
  E. Hyperglycemic hyperosmolar state (HHS)

Immediately initiate therapy
  1. IV 0.9% saline
  2. Regular insulin
  3. Maintain airway, give oxygen
  4. Urinary catheter if needed
  5. Nasogastric (NG) tube if needed
  6. Monitor continuously; cardiac monitor; hourly glucose; hourly potassium
  7. CVP (central venous pressure) if needed

  Beware of:
    Congestive heart failure
    Pulmonary edema
    Cardiac or respiratory arrest
    Hypokalemia, hyperkalemia
    Cerebral edema with deepening coma

II. *Use of insulin*

Use of U-100 regular human insulin

Dose must be individualized. Mean dose in adults in 1985–1987 in first 24 hr in *severe DKA* at Grady Memorial Hospital by IV infusion was 180 U, in moderate or mild DKA it was 48 U.

  A. *Determine dose by*:
    1. *Rate of decline of plasma glucose* (PG) (hourly levels). Optimal rate is 50 to 100 mg/dL/hr (2.8 to 5.6 mM/hr). When level reaches 200 mg/dL (11.1 mM), begin infusion of 5% or 10% dextrose solution.
    2. *Clearing of ketonemia and ketonuria* (hourly levels)
  B. *Methods of administration*
    1. *In severe DKA or HHS*
      a. *Adults*
        (1) IV bolus 10 U, IV infusion 10 U/hr, adjust to rate of PG decrease
        (2) IV bolus 10 U/hr, adjust to rate of PG decrease
        (3) IM 10 U/hr, adjust to rate of PG decrease
        (4) SC 10 U/hr, adjust to rate of PG decrease
        (5) Avoid SC route in dehydrated and hypotensive patients
      b. *Children*
        (1) Initial dose calculated as 0.1 U/kg/hr, adjust to rate of PG decrease (optimal 50 to 100 mg/dL (2.8 to 5.6 mM/hr); reduce dose to 0.5 U/kg/hr when plasma glucose falls to 200 mg/dL (11.1 mM)
        (2) May administer by IV bolus plus follow-up infusion, IM, or SC (avoid in dehydrated or hypotensive patients)
    2. *In moderate and mild DKA, adults and children*
      a. *Clinic*
        (1) IV bolus (10 U), followed by IV infusion 5 to 10 U/hour, adjust to rate of PG decrease
        (2) IV infusion (10 U/hr), adjust to rate of PG decrease
        (3) SC (10 U/hr), adjust to rate of PG decrease
        (4) IM (10 U/hr), adjust to rate of PG decrease
      b. *Home*
        (1) SC (10 U/hr), adjust to rate of PG decrease
        (2) Self-monitoring blood glucose and urine ketones every hour; telephone report to supervising MD (RN) team
  C. Administer intermediate (NPH human) insulin when plasma glucose level decreases to less than 200 mg/dL (11.1 mM), ketonuria and ketonemia have cleared, and *at least 1 hour before* the IV infusion of insulin is terminated. This will help avoid recurrence of DKA.

III. *Use of Fluids and Electrolytes*
  A. *Severe ketoacidosis or hyperglycemic hyperosmolar coma*

    1. Initially start 0.9% sodium chloride solution. If osmolality >350 mOsm/L, next infusion may be 0.45% NaCl.
    2. If pH < 7.10, may use bicarbonate to raise pH to 7.1. *Note*: Beware of metabolic alkalosis with hypokalemia.
    3. *Potassium*: Begin replacement with second infusion-replace up to 20 to 40 mEq/hr as long as urine flow is >40 mL/hr and there is no evidence of hypokalemia. Replace half the potassium deficit (but usually no more than 400 mEq potassium) in first 24 hr, then use oral route. *Note*: Beware of hyperkalemia, renal failure, fluid overload.

(continued)

EXHIBIT 24–6   *(continued)*   Outline of Therapy of Acutely Decompensated Diabetes Mellitus[a]

B. *Mild or moderate ketoacidosis*	4. Usually it is not necessary to replace magnesium and/or phosphate deficits.
	1. Give oral fluids with sodium chloride and potassium hourly, or more frequently if tolerated, and progress to liquid and soft foods.

IV. *While therapy is proceeding, test and examine for:*
   A. Infection-check urine, sputum, blood, and skin (take suitable cultures). Sometimes dehydrated patients do not become febrile and pulmonary rates do not appear until rehydration has occurred.
   B. May need to repeat chest x-ray examination even if initial x-ray film is clear.
   C. Check for other causes of coma or acidosis (see Exhibit 24–2) and evaluate for other concurrent illness(es) or complication(s) (see Exhibit 24–9).

[a] See text for details.

shocked patient because of delayed absorption and late hypoglycemia.

Moderate and Mild Diabetic Ketoacidosis. Uncomplicated moderate and mild DKA may be treated on an outpatient basis (clinic or home) under careful supervision by the supervising professional. However, if vomiting, fever, obtundation, stupor, or coma are present or develop during treatment, hospitalization is essential.

In the clinic, regular human insulin may be administered *subcutaneously, intramuscularly,* or *intravenously* (usually 10 U/hr in adults) until the plasma (or blood) glucose decreases to 200 mg/dL (11.1 mM). *In the home,* regular human insulin is usually administered *subcutaneously.*

Over a 2-year period (1973–1975) the mean dose of regular insulin administered at Grady Memorial Hospital in the first 24 hours in over 300 cases of severe DKA was 550 U (range, 10 to 5,000 U), and in moderate and mild DKA was 150 U (range, 10 to 1,000 U).

During a subsequent 2-year period (1985–1987), the mean dose of regular insulin administered at Grady Memorial Hospital in the first 24 hours in about 200 cases of severe DKA was 180 U (range, 36 to 360 U), and in about 200 cases of moderate or mild DKA it was 48 U (range, 18 to 240 U). Thus, after intravenous insulin infusion became routine, the total administered dose dropped to less than one third the amount administered in the 1973–1975 period.

Water and Electrolytes

1. *In severe diabetic ketoacidosis and hyperosmolar coma:* The adult may have lost as much as 12 L of water and as much as 800 mEq Na^+ and as much as 800 mEq K^+, somewhat less Cl^-, and smaller amounts of Mg^{++} and phosphate.[34] The first infusion should contain 0.90% NaCl; if the osmolality is >350 mOsm/L and the patient is not in shock, 0.45% NaCl may be given in subsequent infusions until the osmolality has fallen below that level. If the pH is <7.10, $NaHCO_3$ may be given cautiously to raise the pH to 7.1 (more may be needed if

lactic acidosis is present, but the induction of metabolic alkalosis with hypokalemia, which is very dangerous, should be carefully avoided.)[28] Potassium replacement usually is started with the second infusion (with 20 to 40 mEq routinely being mixed with 1 L of infusion fluid); usually 20 to 40 mEq is replaced every hour (if urine flow is as much as 40 mL/hr and there is no evidence of hyperkalemia). K^+ solutions should always be diluted to one liter before infusion, *never injected undiluted,* because *hyperkalemia can produce cardiac arrest.* Serum K^+ should be kept above 3 mEq/L but below 6 mEq/L; about half the K^+ deficit should be replaced (up to 400 mEq K^+) during the first 24 hr, the rest being replaced by the oral route during the next 5 to 10 days. The patient should be carefully monitored for electrocardiographic (see Fig. 24–1) or physical evidence of hypokalemia (muscle flaccidity or paralysis, including respiratory muscle paralysis, cardiac arrhythmias including ventricular fibrillation). Some investigators advocate phosphate replacement, but hypocalcemia and/or hypomagnesemia may be induced.[36] Magnesium replacement may be needed if hypomagnesemia is present or occurs during therapy. The patient also should be carefully monitored for evidence of renal failure (persistent anuria or oliguria) and fluid overload (congestive heart failure). The rate of weight change during therapy is useful in assessing the amount of water retained (Exhibits 24–7 and 24–8).

2. *In mild or moderate ketoacidosis:* Oral fluids containing Na^+ and K^+ given at hourly or more frequent intervals usually are sufficient to replace the water and electrolyte deficits within 24 hr.

Infection

Evidence of urinary tract, pulmonic, and other sites of infection should be sought routinely. If indicated, blood, urine, sputum, and/or other samples should be cultured, and bacterial sensitivity studies should be done. Occasionally, dehydrated patients do not become febrile and pulmonic rates do not appear until rehydration has taken place.

EXHIBIT 24–7   Diabetes Flow Sheet

Patient Identification

Date / /	Physical Examination							Urine			Plasma (1)			Plasma (2)		Serum				Meas. mOsm	Calc. mOsm	Reg. Ins. (units)	Therapy — H_2O (L) and Solutes (mEq)							
	HR	ECG	Wt	T	P	R	BP	Vol	ACE	GLU	ACE	GLU	BUN	pH	PCO_2	Na	K	Cl	CO_2				H_2O	Na	K	Cl	PO_4	Mg	HCO_3	GLU

Abbreviations: HR, hours; ECG, electrocardiogram; Wt, weight; T, temperature; P, pulse; R, respirations; BP, blood pressure; Vol, volume; ACE, acetone; GLU, glucose; BUN, blood urea nitrogen; pH, symbol for hydrogen ion concentration; PCO_2, symbol for CO_2 partial pressure; Na, sodium; K, potassium; Cl, chloride; CO_2, CO_2 content (see Exhibit 24–3, II); Meas., measured; Calc., calculated; mOsm, milliosmols; Reg. Ins., regular insulin; l, liter; mEq, milliequivalent; H_2O, water; PO_4, phosphate; Mg, magnesium; HCO_3, bicarbonate.

EXHIBIT 24–8   Diabetes Flow Sheet, Monitoring Schedule, and Therapeutic Indications[a]

ECG: Record every hour for first 6 hr from fixed monitoring $V_2 - V_3$ electrode, then at indicated intervals thereafter. If available, continuous monitoring may be useful.

Body weight: Record initially, and at indicated intervals thereafter. Weight change is useful in assessing initial water deficit, and its rate of replacement during therapy.

T,P,R,BP: Record every hour.

Urine volume: Measure in polyethylene graduated cylinder, and record at hourly intervals.

Urine acetone: (Acetest or Ketostix) and *urine glucose* (Clinitest): Record at hourly intervals.

Plasma acetone, glucose, and BUN: Determine initially, 1 hr later, then as indicated. Requires 5 ml venous blood in gray top tube. At bedside, determine the highest serial dilution that is positive for acetone (undiluted, 1/2, 1/4, 1/8, 1/16).

Plasma pH and PCO$_2$: Determine initially, 1 hr later, then as indicated. Collect 5 mL venous blood in a plastic syringe that has been wet with heparin, rotate the syringe, bend the needle, place the syringe on cracked ice, and send immediately to the central laboratory.

Serum Na, K, Cl, CO$_2$, and measured serum osmolality: Determine initially, 1 hr later, then as indicated. Requires 5 mL venous blood in red top tube.

Calculate serum osmolality (in mOsm) from the following formula:

$$2(Na + K) + \frac{glucose}{18} + \frac{BUN}{2.8}$$

Therapy: Record the number of units of *regular insulin* and the route of administration (IV, IM, or SC). Record administered *water* in liters (0.5 or 1) and *solutes* (Na, K, Cl, PO2, Mg, HCO$_3^-$, and glucose) in mEq. Therapeutic indications for frequently used solutions are as follows:

Water	%	Solute		mEq/L		mOsm/L	Therapeutic Indication
1 L	0.90	NaCl		Na	154		Use initially. Continue if pH > 7.1, osmolality <350 mOsm.
				Cl	154	308	
1 L	0.45	NaCl		Na	77		Use after 1 L 0.90% NaCl if osmolality >350 mOsm and continue until osmolality <350 mOsm.
				Cl	77	154	
Vials (*Add to full liter of infusion fluid and mix thoroughly*)	—	KCl (10 ml)		K	20		Start when urine flow 40 ml/hr or when ECG (see Fig. 24–1) or clinical evidence of hypokalemia appears.
				Cl	20	40	
	—	KCl (20 ml)		K	40		Infuse at rate of 20 to 40 mEq K/hr to maintain K >3 and <6 mEq/L.
				Cl	40	80	
Vials (50 mL) (Dilute to 0.5 or 1 L)	8.4	NaHCO$_3$		Na	50		When pH < 7.1, may administer *cautiously* to raise pH to 7.1. Avoid hypokalemia and metabolic alkalosis.
				HCO$_3$	50	100	
Vials (15 mL) (Dilute 7.5 ml to 1 L)		KH$_2$PO$_4$		K	66		When hypophosphatemic, may administer *cautiously*. Beware of hypocalcemia and hypomagnesemia.
		K$_2$HPO$_4$	45 mM PO$_4$	PO$_4^-$	24	111	
				PO$_4^=$	42		
Vial (20 mL)		MgSO$_4$	16.5 mM	Mg^{2+}	33		Administer (undiluted) IV over 5-min period for hypomagnesemia.
				SO$_4^=$	33	33	
1 L	5.0	Glucose			278	278	Start glucose infusion when plasma glucose falls to 200 mg/dL, and continue glucose infusion at rate sufficient to maintain plasma glucose level between 100 and 200 mg/dL.
1 L	10.0	Glucose			566	566	

[a] This *diabetes flow sheet* was designed to *suggest* ways to collect data of diagnostic and therapeutic significance to the management of acutely decompensated diabetes mellitus. The recorded *data base* should be modified to conform to the needs of each individual patient. When appropriate, additional physical examination data and laboratory data should be recorded. Additional laboratory data that are sometime needed include hematocrit, white blood cell count and differential, complete urinalysis, plasma lactate and pyruvate, magnesium, calcium, amylase, cholesterol, triglycerides, lipoprotein typing and fatty acids. If lipid is present, measure the lipid layer in a hematocrit tube and correct electrolyte and glucose concentration in plasma water accordingly. Start oral fluid and food and neutral protein Hagedorn (NPH) insulin as soon as the patient can tolerate them. For the majority of patients, this should be within 12 to 24 hr after initiation of therapy.

Abbreviations: See footnote in Exhibit 24–7.

EXHIBIT 24–9   Complications that May Be Encountered During or Immediately After the Treatment of Acutely Decompensated Diabetes Mellitus[a]

I. Malnutrition with substrate deficit(s) (usually occurs in alcoholics and patients poorly nourished because of gastrointestinal surgery and so forth). Give insulin *plus glucose* to abort diabetic acidosis and to replace tissue glycogen; replace protein deficit later.

II. Acute tubular necrosis with renal shutdown

III. Lactic acidosis

IV. Hypernatremia or hyponatremia

V. Hypomagnesemia and hypophosphatemia

VI. Hyperchloremic acidosis (due to administering too much Cl^-)[33]

VII. Cardiac arrhythmias (due to K^+ deficit or excess)

VIII. Acute pancreatitis (due to prior alcohol intake or hypertriglyceridemia)

IX. Immunologic insulin resistance

X. Urinary tract infection (catheter-induced, or other)

XI. Pneumonia (induced by vomiting and aspiration, or other)

XII. Other infections (mucormycosis, tuberculosis, and so on)

XIII. Vascular occlusion(s)
  A. Myocardial infarction
  B. Stroke
  C. Peripheral arterial thrombosis (and gangrene)
  D. Mesenteric thrombosis
  E. Pulmonary embolus
  F. Phlebothrombosis or thrombophlebitis

XIV. Death (designate *primary cause* and *secondary cause[s]*):
  A. Cardiac arrest (myocardial infarction, congestive heart failure, asystole, or ventricular fibrillation [may be induced by hypokalemia or hyperkalemia])
  B. Respiratory arrest (may be induced by hypokalemia)
  C. Brain (stroke, injury, infection, ? cerebral edema, ? cerebral hypoxia)
  D. Infection, overwhelming or uncontrolled [designate organism and site(s)]
  E. Metabolic (uncomplicated DKA or/and HHS; consider hypokalemia, pH < 6.80, rapid osmolality changes during therapy)

[a] See Exhibit 24–10.

EXHIBIT 24–10   Side Effects of Therapy for Acutely Decompensated Diabetes Mellitus[a]

Common

Hypoglycemia (Plasma Glucose <50 mg/dL)

Prevent by monitoring plasma glucose at bedside (Beckman glucose analyzer) at hourly intervals, and starting infusion of 5 to 10% dextrose in distilled water at appropriate rate when plasma glucose has fallen to the 200 mg/dL level.

Hypokalemia (Serum K^+ ≤ 3 mEq/L)

Due to giving too little K^+ or too much $NaHCO_3$ with resultant metabolic alkalosis with hypokalemia. The normal K^+ range is 4.0 to 5.4 mEq/L. Prevent hypokalemia by monitoring serum K^+ and electrocardiogram (ECG) (see Fig. 24–1) at hourly intervals; start K^+ replacement in second liter of fluids (unless contraindicated), or earlier if evidence of hypokalemia is available; and continue K^+ infusion to maintain serum K^+ between 3 and 6 mEq/L.

Uncommon

Metabolic Alkalosis

Due to giving too much $NaHCO_3$. Prevent by using $NaHCO_3$ sparingly, if at all.[34,35]

Fluid Overload with Congestive Heart Failure

Due to giving too much fluid. Avoid by monitoring urine output, dyspnea, pulmonary rates, and, if necessary, central venous pressure.

Recurrent Ketoacidosis

Due to failure to give adequate amounts of insulin at frequent enough intervals during the recovery phase. Avoid by giving appropriate amount of intermediate insulin (NPH) when acidosis has cleared, and by monitoring plasma glucose in postrecovery period so that small amounts of regular insulin can be given every 4 hr if hyperglycemia increases during that period.

Rare

Cerebral Edema[28a,28b]

Prevent by early diagnosis of diabetes and by prevention of DKA, especially in those <20 years old. Intracerebral crises with brainstem herniation, respiratory arrest, and death secondary to cerebral edema *may* be avoided in *some* individuals if recognized and treated by hyperventilation, dexamethasone, and mannitol *before* respiratory arrest (see text for discussion).

Cerebral Hypoxia

In addition to the effect of inadequate ventilation and shock, there is a suggested hypothetic problem that may contribute to cerebral hypoxia. 2,3-Diphosphoglycerate (2,3-DPG) binds specifically to deoxyhemoglobin and lowers its affinity for oxygen. This in turn shifts the oxygen dissociation curve to the right and facilitates the delivery of oxygen to tissues. Loss of phosphates during DKA lowers 2,3-DPG and this shifts the curve to the left, and this may diminish oxygen delivery to the tissues. At the same time, acidosis per se shifts the curve to the right, so that the effects of decreased 2,3-DPG and acidosis on the oxygen dissociation curve cancel each other. During treatment of DKA, acidosis frequently is corrected in a few hours, but when inorganic phosphate is in short supply it may take up to 96 hr for 2,3-DPG to return to normal. This *could* diminish oxygen delivery to tissues and induce hypoxia, and this in turn *may* justify more widespread use of phosphate replacement therapy and more restriction of sodium bicarbonate use in the treatment of DKA. When phosphate therapy is used, it is important to remember that hypocalcemia and/or hypomagnesemia may be induced.[36,37]

[a] See Exhibit 24–9.

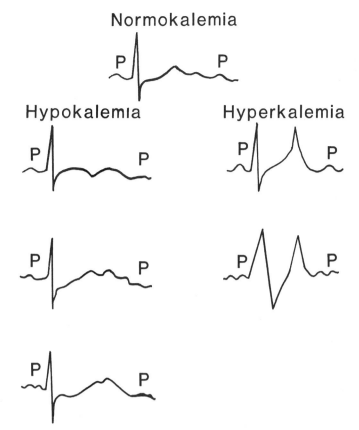

Figure 24–1. Initially, hypokalemia causes flattening and inversion of T waves, ST-segment depression, and the appearance of prominent U waves; later U waves assume the appearance of prolonged, notched T waves and the QU internal is prolonged. This foreshadows the development of dangerous ventricular arrhythmias, especially in those being treated with digitalis or diuretics. Initially, hyperkalemia causes tall peaked T waves. As the K^+ level rises higher yet, the P waves decrease in voltage, the duration of the QRS internal increases markedly, and the S and T waves blend in a sine wave configuration.

The presence of an undiagnosed infection that may become apparent later should be strongly suspected when the neutrophil bands exceed 10%[38] (see Chapter 44).

Other Causes

Other causes of *coma* and *metabolic acidosis* and *concurrent problems* should be sought and appropriately treated if detected (see Exhibits 24–4 and 24–5, Assessment).

Patient Education and Follow-up

Most adequately treated individuals with uncomplicated acutely decompensated diabetes mellitus recover within 24 hr, but those with complications may require several days or weeks to attain maximal benefits from hospitalization. Prior to hospital discharge, appropriate consultation with other professionals (related to chronic complications of diabetes and other problems) should be initiated, and education of the patient and family members concerning the nature of diabetes and its acute and chronic complications should be accomplished. This includes measurement and administration of insulin (if appropriate), continuing optimal diet therapy, and exercise. Thereafter, the patient should be followed-up at frequent intervals in a diabetes clinic or physician's office. Included in follow-up should be optimal changes in life-style, home blood glucose and urine glucose and acetone monitoring, and education in foot care and other relevant matters. The diabetes should be regulated as carefully as possible, and without significant hypoglycemia.

Patient Adherence (or Lack of Adherence) to Prescribed Therapy

Many of the episodes of DKA and HHS that now occur can be prevented by widespread public knowledge of, and prompt response to, the symptoms and signs of diabetes, and by regular systematic screening for and early diagnosis of diabetes in physicians' offices, clinics, hospitals, and nursing homes (see Chapters 11 and 12).

For those who are known to have diabetes, much is yet to be learned about what determines whether or not an individual will adhere to prescribed therapy. Some individuals apparently believe that the *locus of control* of their health is outside themselves and that their actions have little influence on the consequences (morbidity, mortality) of failure to regulate their diabetes. Some use these consequences to control, manipulate, and/or seek the attention of others (professionals, relatives, and friends). Some deny that they have diabetes, or become depressed and harbor a death wish. Professionals should detect early, and deal promptly, effectively, and on a continuing basis with such problems (see Chapters 14, 22, and 47).

EXHIBIT 24–11   Equipment and Supplies Needed to Diagnose and Treat Decompensated Diabetes Mellitus Optimally[a]

In emergency department:
I. To measure plasma glucose stat
   A. Oxygen rate method glucose analyzer (Beckman) (1 min)
   B. SMA/6 (Central Chemistry Laboratory)
   C. Chemstrips (BioDynamics) or Visidex (Ames)—less satisfactory than methods (A) and (B). Deteriorate with aging and exposure to light and moisture. If used, confirm by plasma glucose (SMA/6) in Central Chemistry Laboratory.
II. To measure plasma ketones stat
   A. Acetest tablets, crushed (Ames, Elkhart, IN 46514). Test plasma serially diluted (from undiluted to 1/16 dilution).
   B. Ketostix (Ames). Unsatisfactory for plasma.
III. To measure urine glucose
   A. Oxygen rate method glucose analyzer (Beckman). Measures quantitative urine glucose accurately. Normal level 3 to 25 mg/dL, abnormal level >25 mg/dL.
   B. One-drop, two-drop, and five-drop Clinitest
   C. Testape and Clinistix
IV. To measure urine ketones
   A. Acetest tablets
   B. Ketostix
V. Gray top tube (plasma for glucose and ketones), red top tube (serum for SMA/6 and serum osmolality), blood in plastic syringe with heparin on crushed ice (for pH)
VI. Blood pressure cuff, stethoscope, and thermometer
VII. 0.9% NaCl in 1,000-ml bottles for IV administration
VIII. Oxygen, suction apparatus, oral airway, laryngoscope (two), tubes, local anesthetic, tape, endotracheal tube, cardiorespiratory arrest cart
In intensive care area:
I. Forms to record defined data base (see Exhibit 24–5 and Appendix VII)
II. Flow sheets (see Exhibits 24–7 and 24–8)
III. Gray top tube (plasma for glucose and ketones), red top tube (serum for SMA/6 and serum osmolality), plastic syringe, heparin, and crushed ice (for pH)
IV. Oxygen rate method glucose analyzer (Beckman), Clinitest tablets, Acetest tablets, Ketostix, Testape, and Clinistix

V. Thermometer (rectal), blood pressure cuff, stethoscope, bed scales, tape measure, ECG machine and monitor, polyethylene graduated cylinder (to measure urine volume), infusion pump (IVAC or other), sterile venous pressure tray with inside needle catheter (to measure central venous pressure)
VI. U-100 regular human (rDNA) insulin (U-100 lispro insulin may be used); U-100 NPH human (rDNA) insulin
VII. Fifty milliliter vials of 8.4% NaHCO$_3$ (50 mEq, or 1 mEq/mL)
VIII. One thousand milliliter bottles of 0.45% NaCl, 0.9% NaCl, 5% dextrose in distilled water, 10% dextrose in distilled water, and 50 ml vials of 50% dextrose in distilled water
IX. A. Vials containing 10 ml (20 mEq) and 20 ml (40 mEq) KCl
   B. Vials containing KH$_2$PO$_4^-$ + K$_2$HOP$_4^-$ in 15 ml [66 mEq K + 24 mEq PO$_4^-$ + 42 mEq PO$_4^-$ (45 mM PO$_4$)]
   C. Vials containing 20 ml and 2 g MgSO$_4$ (16.5 mM or 33 mEq Mg^{2+})
X. Oxygen, suction apparatus, oral airway, laryngoscope (two), tubes, local anesthetic, tape, endotracheal tube, cardiorespiratory arrest cart
In central chemistry laboratory:
I. Osmometer to measure serum osmolality
II. Equipment to measure SMA/6 (Na$^+$, K$^+$, Cl$^-$, CO$_2$, BUN, and glucose)
III. Equipment to measure pH
IV. Equipment to measure other indicated chemicals (see Exhibits 24–4 and 24–9), including enzymatic assay for lactate and pyruvate (on freshly drawn, heparinized arterial blood deproteinized promptly with cold perchloric acid and centrifuged in the cold with assays being promptly performed, or on venous blood drawn without stasis clotted on ice with serum being separated and frozen until assayed), enzymatic assay for acetoacetate and β-hydroxybutyrate, β-hydroxybutyrate test strip (for plasma and urine),[26] and suspected intoxicants, drugs, or poisons (collect serum and urine and store in freezer until analyzed by Central Chemistry Laboratory, or by referral laboratory).

[a] See Exhibit 24–8.

Adherence increases with comprehensive patient education in the nature, monitoring, and treatment of insulin-dependent diabetes mellitus, and with continuing access to quality medical care. It decreases with inadequate education, inadequate monitoring of urine and blood glucose levels, and lack of access to, or failure to use continually quality medical care. Inadequate financial resources prevent some from seeking care early. Immaturity, dependence on alcohol or drugs, and serious mental problems without competent continuing supervision by responsible adults at home or in an institution are frequently responsible for precipitating episodes of DKA and HHS.

Process and Outcome Audits

In order to assess comprehensively the consequences of acutely decompensated diabetes, more data on processes (therapy) and outcomes (mortality, morbidity, costs) collected in hospitals, clinics, and physicians' offices are needed. Data should be collected sequentially (monthly and yearly) on all patients, and causes of each episode of DKA and HHS should be determined. Repeaters (more than one episode) should be identified, the reason(s) assessed, and corrective action taken to prevent subsequent episodes.

In 1995 in the USA over 110,000 cases of acutely decompensated diabetes mellitus (DKA/HHS) were hospitalized.

Summary of, and Author's Perspective on Research Underway and Research That Needs to Be Initiated

Research on the therapeutic effectiveness and cost effectiveness of prevention of DKA and HHS by optimal education and follow-up is needed. Theoretically, contemporary knowledge applied universally on a continuing basis can eradicate deaths directly attributable to uncomplicated DKA or HHS.

A continuing national audit to monitor the incidence, causes, morbidity, mortality, and costs related to acutely decompensated diabetes is needed.

Perhaps the greatest need for new research data relates to an evaluation of the safety, therapeutic effectiveness, and cost effectiveness of alternative therapeutic modalities (especially different methods of insulin administration) in current use. Optimal therapy with available therapeutic modalities (insulin, fluid, electrolytes, general support measures, and antibiotics) is safe and effective in approximately 99% of cases of otherwise uncomplicated DKA.

The causes of mortality as a result of (primary) or coincident to (secondary) acutely decompensated diabetes should be determined as accurately as possible by clinical research and by autopsy when possible. The incidence and nature of cerebral edema that terminates fatally and the relationship of such edema to different methods of therapy need particular attention.[28a,28b,39]

Additional data are needed on the biochemical pathophysiology of DKA and HHS. This includes research on substrate, enzyme, hormone, and cell receptor determinants that link and control ketogenesis and gluconeogenesis.

The action of insulin on the liver and how it controls hepatic lipase activity is not yet completely elucidated at cellular and enzymatic levels, nor are the roles that contrainsulin (stress) hormones (glucagon, epinephrine, norepinephrine, cortisol, and growth hormone) play in initiating and sustaining DKA or HHS. The effects of phosphate (red cell 2,3-diphosphoglycerate) and magnesium deficits and repletion on morbidity and mortality are yet to be determined.

References

1. von Mering J, Minkowski O: Diabetes mellitus nach pankreasextirpation. Arch Exp Pathol Pharmakol 26: 371, 1889.

2. Bliss M: The Discovery of Insulin. Toronto: McClellan and Stewart, 1982.

3. Mirsky IA, Heiman JD, Broh-Kahn BH: The antiketogenic action of glucose in the absence of insulin. Am J Physiol 118:290, 1937.

4. Soskin S, Levine R: Carbohydrate Metabolism. Correlation of Physiological, Biochemical, and Clinical Aspects. Chicago: University of Chicago, 1952, p. 314.

5. Root H: Use of insulin and abuse of glucose treatment in diabetic coma. JAMA 127:557–564, 1945.

6. Holler JW: Potassium deficiency occurring during the treatment of diabetic acidosis. JAMA 131:1186–1189, 1946.

7. Butler AM, Talbot NB, Burnett CH, et al.: Metabolic studies in diabetic coma. Trans Assoc Am Physicians 60:102–109, 1947.

8. Sprague RG, Power MH; Electrolyte metabolism in diabetic acidosis. JAMA 151:970–976, 1953.

9. Harwood R: Diabetic acidosis: results of treatment in consecutive cases. N Engl J Med 245:1–9, 1951.

10. Beigelman PM, Warner NE: Thirty-two fatal cases of severe diabetic ketoacidosis, including a case of mucormycosis. Diabetes 22:847–850, 1973.

11. Sament S, Schwartz MB: Severe diabetic stupor without ketosis. S Afr Med J 31:893–894, 1957.

12. Young E, Bradley RF: Cerebral edema with irreversible coma in severe diabetic ketoacidosis. N Engl J Med 276:665–669, 1967.

13. Davidson JK: What does the doctor do when allied health professionals take over? The view of a medical convert. In Larkins R, Zimmet P, Chisholm D (eds): Diabetes 1988. Amsterdam: Elsevier Science Publishers B.V., 1989.

14. Wachtel TJ, Silliman RA, Lamberton P: Predisposing factors for the diabetic hyperosmolar state. Arch Intern Med 147:499–501, 1987.

15. Davidson JK: Diabetic ketoacidosis and hyperglycemic hyperosmolar states. In Schwartz GB, Safar P, Stone JH, et al. (eds): Principles and Practice of Emergency Medicine. Ed. 2. Philadelphia: W.B. Saunders, 1986, pp. 1069–1081.

16. National Diabetes Advisory Board: The Prevention and Treatment of Five Complications of Diabetes: A Guide for Primary Care Practitioners. (5) Detection and Prevention of Acute Hyperglycemia and Acidosis, pp. 33–39, 1983. (Available from the Division of Diabetes Control, Center for Prevention Services, Centers for Disease Control, Atlanta, Ga., 30333.)

17. Drash AL: Acute hyperglycemia and ketoacidosis. A self-study module for use with the prevention and treatment of five complications in diabetes, 1989. Available from:

The Pennsylvania Diabetes Academy, 777 East Park Drive, Harrisburg, PA 17105–8820.

18. Kitabchi AK, Young R, Sacks H, et al.: Diabetic ketoacidosis: reappraisal of therapeutic approach. Annu Rev Med 30:339–357, 1979.

19. Miles JM, Rizza RA, Haymond MW, et al.: Effects of acute insulin deficiency on glucose and ketone body turnover in man: evidence for the primacy of overproduction of glucose and ketone bodies in the genesis of diabetic ketoacidosis. Diabetes 29:926–930, 1980.

20. Hillier TA, Abbott RD, Barrett EJ: Hyponatremia: Evaluating the Correction Factor for Hyperglycemia. Diabetes 47 (suppl. 1):Abs 0267. PA69, May 1998.

21. Fery F, Balasse EO: Ketone body production and disposal in diabetic ketosis: a comparison with fasting ketosis. Diabetes 34:326–332, 1985.

22. Unger RH, Foster DW in Williams: Textbook of Endocrinology, 9th Edition: "Diabetes mellitus," p. 1010–1013, 1998. WB Saunders, Philadelphia.

23. Foster DW: From glycogen to ketones—and back. Diabetes 33:1188–1199, 1984.

24. Owen OE, Trapp VE, Reichard GA, Jr, et al.: Effects of therapy on the nature and quantity of fuels oxidized during diabetic ketoacidosis. Diabetes 29:365–372, 1980.

25. Reichard GA, Skutches CL, Hoeldtke RD, Owen OE: Ketone metabolism in humans during diabetic ketoacidosis. Diabetes 35:668–674, 1986.

26. Harano Y, Suzuki M, Kojuma H, Kashiwagi A, Hidaka H, Shigeta Y: Development of paper-strip test for 3-hydroxybutyrate and its clinical application. Diabetes Care 7:481–485, 1984.

27. Vinicor F, Lehrner LM, Karn RC, et al.: Hyperamylasemia in diabetic ketoacidosis: sources and significance. Ann Intern Med 91:200–204, 1979.

28a. Rosenbloom AL: Intracerebral crises during treatment of diabetic ketoacidosis. Diabetes Care 13:22–33, 1990.

28b. Rosenbloom AL, Hanas R: Diabetic ketoacidosis: treatment guidelines. Clinical Pediatrics (May) 1996, p. 201–206.

28c. "National Diabetes Fact Sheet," released Nov. 1, 1997 by the U.S., Dept. of Health and Human Services, Centers for Disease Control and Prevention, Atlanta, GA.

29. Davidson JK: Transferring patients with insulin-dependent diabetes mellitus from animal source insulins to recombinant DNA human insulin: clinical experience. Clin Ther 11:319–330, 1989.

30. Kitabchi AE, Murphy MB: Diabetic ketoacidosis and hyperosmolar hyperglycemic nonketotic coma. Med Clin North Am 72:1545–1563, 1988.

31. Burghen GA, Etteldorf JN, Fisher JN, et al.: Comparison of high dose and low dose insulin by continuous intravenous infusion in the treatment of diabetic ketoacidosis in children. Diabetes Care 3:15–20, 1980.

32. Carroll P, Matz R: Uncontrolled diabetes mellitus in adults: experience in treating diabetic ketoacidosis and hyperosmolar nonketotic coma with low-dose insulin and a uniform treatment regimen. Diabetes Care 6:579–585, 1983.

33. Oh MS, Banerji MA, Carrol HJ: The mechanism of hyperchloremic acidosis during the recovery phase of diabetic ketoacidosis. Diabetes 30:310–313, 1981.

34. Atchley DW, Loeb RF, Richards DW, Jr., et al.: A detailed study of the electrolyte balances following the withdrawal and reestablishment of insulin therapy. J Clin Invest 12:297–326, 1933.

35. Assal JP, Aoko TT, Manzano FM, et al.: Metabolic effects of sodium bicarbonate in the management of diabetic ketoacidosis. Diabetes 23:405–411, 1974.

36. Winter RJ, Harris CJ, Phillips LS, et al.: Diabetic ketoacidosis. Induction of hypocalcemia and hypomagnesemia by phosphate therapy. Am J Med 67:897–900, 1979.

37. Fisher JN, Katabchi AE: A randomized study of phosphate therapy in the treatment of diabetic ketoacidosis. J Clin Endocrinol Metab 57:177–180, 1983.

38. Slovis CM, Mork VG, Slovis RJ, Bain JR: DKA and infection: leukocyte count and differential as early predictors of serious infection. Am J Emerg Med 5:1–5, 1987.

39. Duck SC, Wyatt DT: Factors associated with brain herniation in the treatment of diabetic ketoacidosis. J Pediatr 113:10–14, 1988.

25

Monitoring the Appearance and Progress of Blood and Vascular Abnormalities

Donald E. McMillan

Circulatory Principles

Circulation, composed of blood and blood vessels, acts to carry oxygen to tissues. It has a role of carrying other sources and products of energy production to their sites of production and excretion—the lungs, liver, and kidneys. The principle under which circulation operates is that the heart does essentially all of the work required to propel the blood through both the lungs, where oxygen is acquired, and the body, where it is delivered. During both passages the pulsatile nature of the heart's action is compensated for by the acquisition of a storage form of energy, called *strain energy*, that is developed by expanding the arterial walls. The walls use their elasticity to store much of the heart's work that actually gave motion to the blood. Much of the kinetic energy generated in the blood during systole becomes elastic strain energy that is returned to the blood during diastole. The circulatory system has controls to maintain the blood pressure at a level appropriate to deliver blood fractionally to different body areas. Blood's distribution in the body depends principally on oxygen demand, a local variable that can change markedly in a number of circumstances. In total body exercise such as running, the muscular system, which normally receives less than one-tenth of the cardiac output, ends up receiving three-quarters of a tripled or quadrupled blood flow. The circulation also depends for its maintenance on the return of blood through the venous system. In the veins, vessel wall tone influences the rate at which blood returns to the heart. The tone in very small veins also exerts an influence over the local presence of white blood cells.

Because so many body processes are affected by diabetes, it is not surprising to find that the circulation is gradually modified. In this chapter we will review the circulatory changes that are produced both acutely and more gradually by the diabetic state. We will focus principally on the major adverse clinical effects and the changes most readily seen to contribute to the acute and chronic pathophysiology of the diabetic state. In doing so, we will also call attention to clinically observable diabetic changes and to physical and laboratory assessment of some of the circulation-influencing substances affected by diabetes.

Circulatory Changes at or Near the Onset of Diabetes (summarized in Exhibit 25–1)

Historical Perspective

Until the discovery of insulin, type 1 diabetes mellitus (IDDM) was a relatively self-limiting disease that had a typical prognosis of 6 months in a young person. Many 19th-century observations of the diabetic state were therefore catalogings of changes that acute and subacute diabetes produced. Naunyn described the anatomic pathology associated with early diabetes

EXHIBIT 25–1 Organ Vascular Changes in Early Diabetes

1. Skin: Vasomotor paralysis in ketoacidosis
2. Adipose tissue: Increased blood flow during poor control
3. Liver: Distention by fatty infiltrates in ketoacidosis
4. Eye: Retinal blood flow may be increased; vasomotor paralysis seen during hyperglycemia
5. Kidney: Early organ and glomerular enlargement, increased GFR and high filtration fraction (type 1), proteinuria with poor control
6. Heart: Slowed ventricular contraction, prolonged preejection phase
7. Large arteries: Greater wall stiffness increases pulse wave propagation velocity, raises the difference between systolic and diastolic pressures
8. Resistance arteries: Tendency to increased arterial blood pressure, diminished control over local blood distribution; tendency to deliver blood to capillaries at higher than normal pressure (similar to hypertension) in long-standing diabetes

in 1898. He found that enlargement of the kidney, in the face of wasting of other tissues and organs, was striking because of its disparity.[1]

Cutaneous Changes

During the period in which insulin treatment was introduced, Weill was able to note that fair-skinned young diabetics had an unusual flushing of their cheeks. He recognized that this appearance was due to a paralysis of tone in the facial blood vessels.[2] The hyperventilation associated with ketoacidosis produces hypocapnia. Lowering of blood carbon dioxide tends to produce vasoconstriction, not vasodilatation, so that the erythema seen in ketoacidosis is likely to be a manifestation of vasomotor paralysis, presumably due to impaired activity of smooth muscle cells in blood vessel walls. Two factors appear to contribute to the acute loss of vascular-wall smooth muscle tension. First, impaired nutritional status associated with the metabolic events leading to ketoacidosis disrupts nitrogen and amino acid metabolism, generating considerable amounts of urea and reducing the availability of amino acids for synthesis of smooth and skeletal muscle actin and myosin. Second, animal experiments suggest that hyperglycemia directly affects local blood vessel tone. The cat's retina fails to respond by vasoconstriction to high oxygen tension during acute hyperglycemia.[3]

Increased Blood Flow to Adipose Tissue

A physiologic concomitant of the disturbed metabolism in diabetic ketoacidosis is mobilization of increased amounts of fatty acids from adipose tissue. The mobilized fatty acids are ultimately converted by the liver to ketoacids in uncontrolled type 1 diabetes. Free fatty acids in body fluids are simple soaps that attack biological membranes. Fatty acids are normally carried by adsorption to albumin and to a lesser extent to plasma lipoproteins. Albumin can become saturated with fatty acids. Low blood flow through adipose tissue would therefore limit the rate of fatty acid delivery into the circulation. Increased blood flow to adipose tissue is one of the major features of uncontrolled diabetes.

While the astute clinician may note increased local heat in adipose areas during uncontrolled diabetes, this blood flow increase is not as recognizable as the enlargement of the liver produced by the conversion of fatty acids delivered to it into neutral fat. Liver distention appears to be responsible for right upper quadrant pain frequently reported in diabetic ketoacidosis. This pain occasionally causes concern that appendicitis is present and can, if not recognized as due to liver enlargement, lead to a dangerous and unnecessary laparotomy.

Retinal Circulation in Early Diabetes

There has been controversy about whether the flow of blood to the retina is increased in early diabetes. It has already been mentioned that vasomotor paralysis impairs retinal vasoconstriction in poorly controlled diabetes.[3] But such a mechanism would not produce an overall flow increase. It is useful to review the physiology of oxygen delivery to the retina in order to appreciate the potential meaning of an increase in retinal blood flow in early diabetes. The retina is the most metabolically active tissue on a weight basis in the body. It exceeds the brain in its oxygen utilization by at least 50%. While the kidneys receive a greater blood supply per gram of tissue, they extract little of the oxygen passing through because they are not as metabolically active.

It is often forgotten that the retina has two circulations. One is visible through the ophthalmoscope, while the other, the choroidal (uveal) circulation, is hidden by the retinal pigment epithelium. The choroid normally carries a total volume of blood flow more than nine times the retinal blood flow. Even though choroidal vein oxygen level is higher than retinal vein oxygen level, the choroid supplies the majority of the retina's oxygen. The retinal circulation that is viewed with the ophthalmoscope is really the backup supply. Because the choroidal circulation is little influenced by changing oxygen demand, the retinal circulation increases strikingly when the oxygen tension of inspired air drops. This occurs both in laboratory experiments and at high altitude. Acute high-altitude exposure in man is often associated with retinal hemorrhage. The majority of individuals who suddenly go to an altitude more than 7000 ft and perform any kind of physical activity will develop flame hemorrhages that can be seen with an ophthalmoscope.[4] These hemorrhages appear to be due to increased retinal blood flow secondary to the sudden decline in arterial oxygen tension.

Because the retinal circulation must meet metabolic needs with wide swings in flow rate compared to the choroidal circulation, either the greater metabolic demand or vasomotor paralysis produced by diabetes can burden the retinal vascular system in a fashion paralleling altitude exposure. This additional burden can become especially important when retinal blood flow is increased by falling arterial oxygen tension, due to a change in posture or a reduction in respiratory efficiency.

Renal Changes in Early Diabetes

Enlargement of the kidney is an essentially universal feature of early and poorly controlled type 1 diabetes that was thoroughly documented in the 19th century.[1] In type 1 diabetes, much more than in type 2, renal enlargement is associated with an increase in glomerular filtration rate (GFR). The two changes, *renal enlarge-ment and GFR increase, are often accompanied by protein-uria*. The proteinuria often disappears promptly with improvement of diabetic control. Potential confusion in a diabetic patient between the proteinuria associated with diabetic nephropathy or other renal disease and this benign proteinuria due to poor control can be resolved by documenting persistence or disappearance of proteinuria as satisfactory control is established. Benign proteinuria is also associated with a slightly low serum creatinine and elevated creatinine clearance, a combination present only very early in diabetic neph-ropathy. Persistent proteinuria requires further evalu-ation, but the clearing of proteinuria associated with poor control by hyperglycemia reduction justifies the label benign. This benign proteinuria is closely associ-ated with the high GFR seen in both early and long-standing uncontrolled diabetes. A similar source of false-positive proteinuria is mediated by vigorous exer-cise during urine collection.

The increased glomerular filtration of poorly con-trolled type 1 diabetes is not associated with a marked increase in blood flow to the kidney. The filtration frac-tion is therefore raised so that the proportion of plasma entering the glomerulus that is actually filtered is ele-vated in poorly controlled diabetes. The mechanism by which this increase in filtration fraction is produced has generated some dispute. It has been proposed that an increase in the local pressure within the glomerulus is required to cause the rise in glomerular filtration rate and filtration fraction. But anatomic studies have noted that the surface area available for filtration is increased even more than the filtration rate.[5] Change in glomeru-lar size by itself may therefore play a large role. The magnitude of the early increase in glomerular filtration may set the stage for the later development of progres-sive renal insufficiency.[6] The earlier 45% overall rate of development of nephropathy is falling, probably due to improved blood pressure management.[7]

The Heart in Early Diabetes

The less favorable outcome when diabetes and coro-nary heart disease are combined has raised concern that diabetes directly affects the vigor of the heart. Asymptomatic coronary disease manifested by an abnormal treadmill test followed by angiography is very frequent in midlife diabetes.[8] Less specific exer-cise studies of the heart in early diabetes have shown modest deficiencies. An increase in the end systolic left ventricular volume suggests impaired cardiac empty-ing in young males with diabetes. The measurement of systolic time intervals, another noninvasive test, has revealed either no abnormality or a tendency to slowed postsystolic relaxation when recognizable microvascu-lar complications are present. Taken together with the

course of active coronary disease in diabetes, these findings may indicate either a direct effect of diabetes on the heart or an effect of damage done by ischemic heart disease.[9] Despite these concerns, the heart appears to function normally in most patients with dia-betes but no serious coronary disease, but the arterial pulse propagation rate and its cardiac load are increased due to arterial stiffening. The altered proper-ties of the large arteries in diabetes may act to burden the heart and generate many of the detected changes.

Blood Pressure Trends in Early Diabetes

It is a clinical maxim that diabetes and hypertension are often seen together, especially in type 2 diabetes.[10] One should keep in mind that the type 1 diabetes patient is also predisposed to hypertension. The efficacy of early and effective management of elevated blood pressure in preventing cardiovascular problems applies at least as much to the diabetic as to the nondiabetic patient. Regular measurements of blood pressure in diabetes, control of salt intake for borderline pressure elevation, prescription of an agent that does not adversely affect carbohydrate and lipid metabolism for mild blood pressure elevation, and more aggressive management of established hypertension are appropriate therapeutic escalations based on frequent blood pressure monitor-ing and evaluation of retinal hypertension findings.

Blood Protein Changes in Early Diabetes

Circulation is composed both of blood vessels and blood. Blood is a complex fluid, composed mainly of plasma and erythrocytes. A small contribution to its bulk is made by white blood cells and an even smaller one by platelets. Plasma's major large molecules are the plasma proteins, including lipoproteins. Lipopro-tein levels are affected by the diabetic state in propor-tion to the impairment of blood glucose control. Very mild prediabetic lipoprotein elevations are markedly aggravated by poor blood glucose control. Diabetics whose prediabetic blood triglyceride level was above 200 mg/dL often have opalescent or milky plasma at diagnosis. The opalescence is due to an increase in very-low-density lipoprotein (VLDL) and the milky appearance to reduced clearance of chylomicra. The elevated lipids can occupy from 1% to 10% of the plasma volume under these circumstances. Because plasma makes up 60% of the volume of blood, the lipid volume increase can have dramatic effects seen in both the laboratory and the retina. Ophthalmoscopic exam-ination will reveal *lipemia retinalis*, a condition in which the retinal veins develop a milky appearance, losing much of their normal reddish-blue color. The obser-vant clinician can therefore decide whether to proceed with laboratory tests that are disturbed by high plasma lipid levels on the basis of the physical examination. Laboratory test abnormalities generated by lipemic plasma are linked both to the opacity produced (light absorbance is increased nonspecifically) and to the volume occupied by the lipid (it will lower the serum sodium if dilution is used in its measurement). In the presence of lipemia, test ordering and interpretation must take into account information about local laboratory methods.

Other plasma protein changes in diabetes are milder, producing their principal effects indirectly. They consist mainly of a decline in serum albumin and increased levels of several members of a group of proteins called the acute-phase reactants. Acute-phase reactants are responsible for a variety of effects including neutralization of the enzymes released by neutrophils during pus formation. As shown in Exhibit 25–2, these protein changes are present early in diabetes and persist in long-standing diabetes. Their relationship to the development of microvascular sequelae has been evaluated and is also shown in Exhibit 25–2. The changes listed have been demonstrated in type 2 diabetes and are a little less striking in type 1 diabetes. Nonetheless, the indicated pattern (Exhibit 25–2) has been shown to be associated with advanced microvascular sequelae. Specific plasma protein changes are discussed further in the section entitled "Routine Laboratory Tests in Early Diabetes." Two blood proteins become elevated in long-standing diabetes; they are discussed in the section "Blood Changes in Long-Standing Diabetes."

Red and White Blood Cells in Early Diabetes

Increased erythrocyte aggregation is seen in the retina and conjunctiva early in diabetes. Retinal arterioles occasionally even display aggregated flow in advanced diabetic retinopathy. When blood flow is sufficiently slowed, erythrocytes regularly aggregate. Anything that slows the retinal circulation can therefore produce visible erythrocyte aggregates. One may test this statement by pressing lightly on the eye while observing retinal blood flow through an ophthalmoscope. This raises intraocular pressure and slows retinal venous flow, causing erythrocyte aggregates to become visible in the retinal microcirculation.

No widely available clinical test of the aggregation propensity of erythrocytes is substantially more sensitive than the *erythrocyte sedimentation rate*. None of the more rapid but more costly tests that have been introduced to supplement the 1-hr erythrocyte sedimentation rate has become established as clearly superior to the sedimentation rate in assessing the tendency of erythrocytes to form rouleaux at low blood flow rates.

EXHIBIT 25–2   Changes in Plasma Protein Levels in Diabetes[a]

Plasma Protein	Early Level	Late Level	Sequelae vs. No Seq
Prealbumin	Decreased	Decreased	No difference
Albumin	Decreased	Decreased	Lower
Alpha-1-acid glycoprotein[b]	Increased	Increased	Slight increase
Alpha-1-antitrypsin[b]	Increased	Increased	No difference
Gc-globulin	Unchanged	Unchanged	No difference
Haptoglobin[b]	Increased	Increased	Higher
Alpha-2-macroglobulin	Unchanged	Increased	No difference
Alpha-2-HS-glycoprotein	Unchanged	Unchanged	No difference
C-reactive protein[b]	Increased	Increased	Slight increase
Hemopexin	Increased	Increased	No difference
Beta-2-glycoprotein I	Increased	Increased	No difference
Transferrin	Unchanged	Unchanged	No difference
Fibrinogen[b]	Increased	Increased	Higher
Complement C3 activator	Increased	Increased	No difference
Compliment C4	Increased	Increased	No difference
Complement C3C	Increased	Increased	No difference
Immunoglobulin A	Unchanged	Increased	No difference
Immunoglobulin M	Unchanged	Unchanged	No difference
Immunoglobulin G	Unchanged	Unchanged	No difference
Immunoglobulin D	Slight decrease	Slight decrease	No difference
Ceruloplasmin[b]	Increased	Increased	No difference

[a] Plasma proteins are listed in order of electrophoretic mobility.

[b] Proteins so marked are acute-phase reactants, commonly elevated in infection and following trauma. The complement components listed usually become elevated at the same time.

In diabetes, glucose attachment by a ketoamine linkage (glycosylation) to the N-terminal valine of the β-chain of hemoglobin increases hemoglobin's affinity for oxygen. In other hemoglobin oxygen-affinity disorders the hematocrit rises. Both such hemoglobin molecule changes and increased blood carbon monoxide due to cigarette smoking produce polycythemia. One might therefore expect that the hematocrit would become elevated in diabetes, but glycosylation affects principally the older erythrocytes. Younger erythrocytes have more normal oxygen-releasing capacities and polycythemia is avoided, although a trend to high-normal hematocrit is seen. While plethora and venous congestion are the clinical correlates of polycythemia, nothing more striking than a marginal increase in polycythemia frequency is seen in early diabetes.

The white blood cell count is commonly elevated in diabetics admitted to the hospital, particularly when they have ketoacidosis or an infection producing poor control. Both my own studies and the absence of contrary reports indicate that the white blood cell count in the ambulatory diabetic is essentially normal.

Immunologic studies have suggested that the functional composition of lymphocytes is altered in early type 1 diabetes. A reduction in the suppressor component of T cells and an increase in islet cell-destroying T cells are apparently linked to the immune process that is destroying the islets. But this change is not reflected in the usual clinical evaluation. The diagnosis of type 1 diabetes normally requires little further support after a high blood glucose has been shown to be associated with substantially elevated levels of serum ketone bodies (acetoacetic acid and acetone) in the presence of an adequate carbohydrate intake.

Polymorphonuclear leukocyte function has been found to be impaired in severely out-of-control diabetes. This deficiency is rapidly corrected by insulin administration. It is not usually detectable in reasonably controlled diabetes.[11] The leukocyte functional defect in severe hyperglycemia combines impaired phagocytosis and diminished generation of oxygen-derived bactericidal compounds—superoxide ions, hydroxyl radicals, and hydrogen peroxide.

Blood Platelet Changes in Early Diabetes

Platelets are present in the bloodstream as small disks about a quarter of the diameter of red blood cells. But they have flat rather than dimpled surfaces. Platelets are able to change their shape abruptly when exposed to certain chemical or physical agents. Their surfaces are converted to irregular projections in a process called *pseudopod formation*. Platelet behavior is altered by the diabetic state. This disturbance is measured in the laboratory as increased in vitro platelet aggregation. In vivo platelet aggregation is the step that forms platelet plugs as more platelets interact with the first-arriving adherent platelets to close a damaged site in the vessel wall that follows venipuncture or mild trauma.

The prominence of platelets in bringing about smooth muscle cell migration in a model of atherogenesis generated intense interest in their behavior in diabetes. Platelet aggregation in diabetes becomes progressively easier to detect as the patient ages and atherosclerosis develops.[12] Developing atheromata create local flow conditions that enhance platelet aggregability. The combination of diabetes and atherosclerosis amplifies the age-associated increase in platelet aggregability seen in nondiabetics.[13] Diabetic platelets act as though they are from a nondiabetic who is 10–15 years older.

The ability of platelets to form aggregation-promoting thromboxanes is decreased by several pharmacologic agents, including aspirin. Antiplatelet treatment has been found useful in several clinical trials, including those in diabetes. At this stage, their use in diabetes for vascular disease prophylaxis is supported but not mandated by the observed data; gastrointestinal upset and bleeding during administration remain problems.

Platelet aggregability is most commonly measured by determining the increased amount of light that passes between platelet clusters in platelet-rich plasma. An agent that favors platelet aggregation, such as adrenalin, collagen, or adenosine diphosphate (ADP), is usually added. This test is important in clinical investigation but has found little use in patient evaluation.

Platelet counts normally have no role in diabetes management, but an exception is the *thrombotic thrombocytopenic purpura* seen occasionally when diabetic vascular disease and overt infection are combined. In this circumstance, bleeding is seen and red cell morphology is strikingly altered (helmet cells, cell fragments, etc.). Blood fibrinogen level, normally mildly elevated in diabetes, can become depressed by fibrinogen's consumption in the coagulation process when this condition is present.

Routine Laboratory Tests in Early Diabetes

Plasma chemical changes are often noted on a diabetic patient's routine laboratory screening panel. High glucose and low normal to low creatinine may be accompanied by a low normal or low serum albumin. The combination of marginally reduced albumin and elevated globulin levels often precedes developing microvascular complications. Two plasma protein components whose levels appear to have prognostic potential are fibrinogen and total globulin. Both are more elevated in patients with diabetes who develop microvascular difficulty.[14] Fibrinogen and total globulin can both be elevated in infection and inflammation, and fibrinogen alone can be elevated following trauma and surgical procedures. This makes their measurement

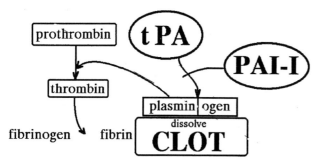

Figure 25–1. The level of all plasma proteins is determined by their rates of production and loss. Fibrinogen is one of the acute phase reactant group, and its production by the liver is influenced by interleukin-6 levels. Its loss is more uniquely influenced by two coagulation-linked paths, mediated by thrombin or plasmin generation. Plasmin attacks fibrinogen as well as fibrin and appears to be more important in shortening the lifespan of fibrinogen in the plasma. Its generation from plasminogen is actively blocked by the endothelial cell product, plasminogen activator inhibitor-1 (PAI-1). Endothelial production of PAI-1 is inhibited by high triglyceride levels, creating a direct linkage between glucose control and high fibrinogen level in diabetic patients with hypertriglyceridemia. Even in diabetes without hypertriglyceridemia, the individual patient fibrinogen level fluctuates with over half the diabetes population value. This degree of fluctuation makes multiple fibrinogen determinations important in attempts to predict future problems.

much more valuable during outpatient ambulatory care. Fibrinogen levels reflect a combination of production rate and intravascular degradation rate (Fig. 25–1). The erythrocyte sedimentation rate is modestly increased in the ambulatory adult diabetic patient; its increase is linked to the aforementioned fibrinogen elevation. Substantial elevation of erythrocyte sedimentation rate in ambulatory adult diabetes without overt infection is prognostically adverse.

Plasma Viscosity Increase in Early Diabetes

The changes in plasma protein composition in diabetes raise *plasma viscosity*. Plasma viscosity measurement has replaced the traditional erythrocyte sedimentation rate in Great Britain but has never achieved popularity in North America. Plasma viscosity is affected by the total plasma protein level. Total plasma protein level is in turn influenced by the patient's hydration state and recent physical activity. A few minutes of vigorous exercise in the upright posture can raise the plasma protein level 10%, leading to a similar degree of increase in plasma viscosity. This increase is as striking as the elevation produced by diabetes and the viscosity disparity between diabetics who do and do not develop early sequelae. Plasma viscosity measurement can be improved by using adjustment for total plasma protein level, but such a test is too difficult to perform for routine clinical use.

Blood Viscosity in Early Diabetes

Even further from current everyday clinical medicine is measurement of the viscosity of diabetic blood. Hematocrit determination measures the major contributor to blood viscosity, the erythrocyte fraction. Blood's viscosity also changes at different rates of flow; it is much more resistant to flow at low shear rate than at high. A viscometer geometry in which shear rate is fairly uniform is therefore highly desirable for blood viscosity measurement. The cone plate viscometer has this feature and therefore has been used fairly widely. It consists of a nearly flat cone rotated just above a flat plate to produce shearing flow in the blood lying between. When the distance between them is properly adjusted, the rotational velocity is twice as great at a point twice as far from the axis, and the distance between the cone and the plate is also doubled. The triangular geometry of the area between the cone and plate creates a constant shear rate from the center outward. Commercial cone plate systems like the Wells Brookfield model (LVT or similar with CP-42 Spindle) can measure blood viscosity satisfactorily from 230 inverse sec down to a shear rate of about 5.6 inverse sec. A modest 5–7% increase in the viscosity of diabetic blood has been reported at 5.6 inverse sec shear rate. In the early reports, this rise seemed to be linked to diabetic vascular complications, but as more diabetic patients were studied, blood viscosity measurement in this shear rate range was found to have little prognostic value.

Subsequent studies showed a 15–30% increase in diabetic blood viscosity in the shear rate range between 0.1 and 1.0 inverse sec. In this shear rate range, blood viscosity measurement requires more sophisticated equipment because the resistive force (stress) that is generated by blood flow becomes extremely small. Blood settles rapidly enough at very low shear rate that the cone plate geometry loses accuracy. A cylinder in cylinder geometry (Couette viscometer) is commonly substituted. Because low friction in the axis of rotation helps in measuring small applied torques, a rotational viscometer equipped with an air bearing gives the best combination of accuracy and a limited displacement during measurement, but cost is higher and operational reproducibility requires automation.

Blood Transient Flow Resistance in Diabetes

The low shear rate viscosity elevation of diabetic blood has been found to be closely associated with a rapidly recovered component of flow resistance, linked to a subtle blood flow property, increased 30% by diabetes, that is called *thixotropy*.[16] The word *thixotropy* is composed of two Greek words that describe the act of changing by touch. Most fluids, like air and water, resist the initiation and maintenance of flow with the same force. When blood and other thixotropic materials are caused to flow after standing, an excess of resistive force, beyond that required to maintain flow, is present only at the start of flow. Thixotropy is therefore a time-based hemorheologic property. While for most thixotropic fluids the resistance returns very slowly, blood is an exception. Complete return of thixotropy requires slow loss of orientation to flow and development of resting structure. Red blood cells lose much of their flow alignment as soon as flow ceases because of their elastic shape and orientation change.

Work must be done to realign the red blood cells as blood flow is reestablished. At low shear rate, an extra force 30% higher at peak than the stable force is required to start blood flowing. We have recently found that over 40% of this added resistance to the onset of flow returns in the period between heartbeats, normally creating a 12% higher brief peak flow resistance between heartbeats.[15] The transient resistance of diabetic blood is a third larger (16%), burdening arterial and venous flow during the initiation or acceleration of blood flow much more than during steady in vitro flow. Blood's higher transient resistance in diabetes is due to a combination of increased erythrocyte aggregability mediated by increased levels of aggregation-promoting blood proteins (reviewed above) and reduced erythrocyte deformability.

Erythrocyte Deformability in Diabetes

Reduced erythrocyte deformability in diabetes is due to a very subtle defect—increased diabetic erythrocyte membrane resistance to changing magnitude of curvature. The diabetic red cell membrane only reacts sluggishly; it is not truly stiff. Like blood's transient resistance and thixotropy, reduced diabetic red cell deformability is therefore a time-based property. Whenever diabetic red cells need to change in shape and when surface curvature change is the principal deformation required, the diabetic red cells resist this kind of shape change about twice as much as normal cells. This property leads directly to a force-mediated model for the development of diabetic microangiopathy.[16] Red cell resistance has been found to be correlated with the blood glucose level at the time the cells are collected. Insulin infusion has been reported to normalize diabetic erythrocyte filterability over a period of 3 hr, even if blood glucose level is kept high by glucose infusion.[17] The ability of insulin infusion to reverse this erythrocyte flow abnormality even when blood glucose remains elevated suggests that insulin directly influences red blood cell membranes.

The complete assessment of low shear rate blood viscosity and transient resistance (thixotropy) is well beyond the scope of all but the most sophisticated research laboratories. Reduced deformability of diabetic erythrocytes is more easily measured using 5 μm (not 3 μm) polycarbonate (Nuclepore) filters. Nickel mesh filters have appeared recently and may be more uniform than Nuclepore. Measurement of the flow rate of red cells accompanied by few or no white cells should be carried out with low pressure and a reduced hematocrit. Any white cells present become permanently embedded in the filter, causing a continuous decline in filtration rate.

Despite its relative simplicity, red cell filtration assessment has achieved little clinical application. We evaluated video-recorded formation of erythrocyte doublets as a simpler possibility.[16] While quite sensitive to diabetic changes, the described technique was at least as difficult to apply as polycarbonate filter studies. If a simple and inexpensive measure of erythrocyte deformability can be developed, clinical evaluation of reduced diabetic erythrocyte deformability might be used more regularly. Low shear rate blood viscosity reflects both the red cell problem and fibrinogen-mediated red cell aggregation, integrating the effects of reduced erythrocyte deformability and increased erythrocyte aggregability. It is likely that such testing will identify diabetic patients with a high susceptibility to vascular problems. Our findings in the Diabetes Control and Complications Trial indicate that vigorous control of hyperglycemia can keep serious complications from developing in patients otherwise shown by increased low shear rate blood viscosity to be at high risk. Viscometry could also help us understand the nature of the burden placed on the circulation by hemorheologic changes in diabetes.

Evaluation of the Circulatory Changes in Long-Standing Diabetes

Historical Perspective

Although lower limb gangrene was already known to be closely associated with diabetes in the 19th century, the concept of diabetic vascular disease was not introduced until 1953. Careful physical evaluations were carried out on residents of Aarhus, Denmark, who had survived diabetes for 15–25 years. The most frequent abnormal findings that were recorded suggested frequent circulatory difficulty, and the term *diabetic angiopathy* was introduced.[18] The term was subsequently divided into microangiopathy and macroangiopathy, based on the size of the vessels affected. Macroangiopathy in diabetes is usually considered to include atherosclerosis both as an increased predilection to ischemic heart disease and to leg artery disease. The concept of diabetic microangiopathy owes a great deal to the introduction of the periodic-acid Schiff (PAS) histochemical technique that is often used to detect increased microvessel glycoprotein content in diabetes.

Histochemical Observations

Blood vessels in long-standing diabetes commonly contain increased amounts of PAS-positive material in their walls. This material is found both in the microvessels and in large arteries. Its deposition appears to be responsible for vascular stiffening (sclerosis). Sclerosis of veins is also seen in long-standing diabetes. It is probably benign; diabetic retinal phlebosclerosis is commonly associated with absence of retinopathy. The PAS-positive material accumulates especially in the intima and media of the walls of the affected vessels.

In capillaries, basement membrane thickening, also PAS-positive, is seen widely, most notably in skeletal muscle and the kidney, but also in the intestine, brain, and heart. Capillary *basement membrane thickening* in diabetes appears to be rather benign, but arteriolar sclerotic changes diminish the ability of resistance arterioles to change in diameter. This loss has been linked to reduced maximal blood flow to skin and skeletal muscle seen in long-standing diabetes.[19] It also affects the ability of organs, including brain and kidney, to maintain a normal rate of blood flow when arterial pressure rises and falls.

Calcification in the walls of arteries that have a prominent elastic and smooth muscle media is an occasionally dramatic radiographic feature of established diabetes; it grows in frequency with its duration. It is very common in diabetic nephropathy and increased in likelihood in diabetic retinopathy. When it is present, arterial calcification can hide associated occlusive changes. Even when present in the leg alone, it diminishes maximal (not resting) blood flow to the lower leg and foot.

Arterial Stiffening

Reduction of the elasticity of arterial walls has been found even in children with diabetes. *Arterial stiffening* is usually demonstrated as an increase in pulse wave velocity, a change that also accompanies the aging process. In aging, vessel-wall thickening is responsible for the stiffening. In diabetes, the change appears to be due to local elastic resistance increase. This could be due to an increase in the proportion of collagen to elastin, to increased stiffness of a normal amount of collagen by chemical cross-linking, or to loss of elastin. The mechanism remains unresolved.

In aging, loss of elasticity of the aorta impairs the storage of elastic (strain) energy following each heartbeat, reducing exercise tolerance.[20] Because aging and the duration of diabetes have additive effects on arterial stiffening, the older individual with long-standing diabetes can have substantial exercise impairment. Adjustment of the exercise prescription for duration of diabetes should be based on concepts established in studies of nondiabetics to help create more effective programs. A 40- to 50-year-old with diabetes of 20 years duration is appropriately exposed to physical conditioning using the exercise load usually prescribed for an individual who is 5–10 years older. It is advisable to recommend exercise conditioning somewhere at or below 80% of the maximal pulse rate assigned on the basis of the age. This level of exercise is capable of establishing and maintaining conditioning without causing the striking rise in blood pressure that accompanies vigorous exercise.

Microcirculatory Deterioration

A major result of diabetic microvessel stiffness is a subtle impairment of the distribution of blood to tissues. Arteriolar stiffness in the retinal and renal microvascular systems appears to contribute to the development of the specific pathology in these two tissues that are seen so frequently in long-standing diabetes. While some studies have suggested future success, we still have no clinical test capable of evaluating the competence of resistance arterioles in various tissues. Arterioles are known to be affected by hypertension as well as diabetes, but in hypertension smooth muscle cell hypertrophy appears to be more important than vessel wall stiffening.

The retinal veins have been observed to dilate progressively over the first decade of diabetes. Their degree of dilatation has a low-grade linkage to the development of diabetic retinopathy. The relationship between retinal vein dilatation and future retinopathy is poor enough that retinal vein size should be noted but not overinterpreted.

Capillary basement membrane thickening (CBMT) is evaluated in skeletal muscle by needle biopsy and tissue examination using the electron microscope. CBMT is known to progress with duration of diabetes. Its assessment has achieved no clinical role. CBMT is not specific to diabetes and has little prognostic value, but CBMT has been reduced by careful glucose control in groups of subjects with diabetes.

Little physiologic impairment is associated with CBMT. Oxygen must diffuse through the thickened membrane to reach nearby mitochondria in skeletal muscle fibers. This passage appears unencumbered, as judged by the essentially normal levels of oxygen in venous blood returning from exercising skeletal muscle in diabetes. Normal oxygen delivery is retained even though the partial pressure of oxygen at which hemoglobin is 50% saturated (P50) of hemoglobin is lowered by increased glycosylation of hemoglobin in diabetes. The last effect is further exaggerated by low levels of 2,3-diphosphoglycerate (DPG). DPG usually falls following meals in diabetes and in diabetic ketoacidosis.

Tests of Blood Vessel Behavior

Inadequate attention has been paid to clinical assessment of the physiologic responses and the reactive behavior of diabetic microvessels. *Limb plethysmography* is a procedure that can be used to measure local blood flow, venous compliance, and the rate of extravasation of fluid from the vascular space. The technique is normally applied to the forearm or the leg below the calf. The circumferential strain gauge has replaced the water-filled chamber in plethysmography, and changes in limb volume are now assessed by recording changes in electrical impedance as the length of the mercury-containing silicone rubber strain gauge increases.

Sudden elevation of venous pressure is produced by inflating a blood pressure cuff to 40–50 mmHg. This causes the blood that is being delivered into the limb, now unable to leave by its veins, to increase the limb size under the strain gauge. The earliest rate of increase in size estimates the rate of entry of blood into the limb. Following the initial blood flow–mediated increase in forearm or leg size, a second rate of increase in size is produced by venous dilatation. The rate of increase in circumference in the second phase is an index of the compliance of the veins as their internal pressure rises. A third phase of forearm circumference increase is seen as fluid is slowly transferred from the vascular to the extravascular compartment in response to the elevated venous pressure. The higher venous pressure with the cuff inflated is transferred back to the capillary bed and small arterioles, causing increased plasma transudation.

The rate of fluid transudation generated by the rise in capillary pressure is quite low. In the forearm, it has actually been found to be reduced in early diabetes, possibly because glucose is an osmotically active agent and the gradient increase produced by hyperglycemia counteracts the pressure rise. One milliosmole of glucose (18 mg/dL) can counteract 19 mmHg pressure. In long-standing diabetes, capillary filtration rate becomes equal to or higher than the nondiabetic transudation rate.

A newer approach to measuring local blood flow is the use of a laser Doppler reflection device on the skin. This technique has allowed the demonstration of impaired maximal local blood flow in different body areas, including the feet, in long-standing diabetes.[21] Maximal local flow is induced by heating the local skin to 44°C, a temperature that overcomes local vasoconstriction.

Persons with both diabetic and nondiabetic neuropathies fail to reduce blood flow to the skin of their feet normally when they stand. Nonneuropathic individuals reduce this flow by about 80%, but diabetics with nerve damage usually fail to reduce leg flow even 50%.[22]

Although tests of limb flow, filtration, and orthostatic responses have not yet achieved clinical utility, one may expect that, as our understanding improves, noninvasive tests will be found that can detect developing diabetic vascular disease in its earliest and most manageable stage.

Microcirculatory Exchange Studies

There is no observation of the microcirculation in diabetes more puzzling than the one made following injection of low molecular weight radioactive substances into the anterior compartment of the leg. Reports from both Scandinavia and the United States have compared nondiabetic and diabetic subjects. The ratio of loss of radioactive xenon, a measure of local blood flow, to that of a number of low-molecular-weight radioactive substances has been studied. Substances such as versenate [ethylenediaminetetraacetic acid (EDTA)], sodium, and iodide are lost by the local tissues at least as rapidly from the diabetic leg as from the nondiabetic leg despite the presumed impairment of local microcirculatory flow. The rate of loss is actually higher when clinically recognizable diabetic sequelae (retinopathy, renal disease) are present,[23] creating a real physiologic riddle.

Leg Artery Disease in Diabetes

One of the most striking problems in chronic established diabetes in the adult over 40 years of age is the development of difficulty with blood flow to the lower extremities. This process can impair lower limb exercise tolerance. More importantly, it sets the stage for leg amputation. In amputation, local arterial disease often acts in conjunction with sensory neuropathic loss. The sensory deficiency favors unrecognized tissue injury. A portal of entry for infection is generated; then reduced arterial pressure allows the infection to compromise the infected tissue's integrity, forcing an amputation.

The distribution of diabetic atherosclerosis in the lower extremity leg contrasts with nondiabetic atherosclerosis. In nondiabetic individuals, occlusive atherosclerosis usually develops mainly in the iliac vessels or in the femoral artery in the adductor (Hunter's) canal. The diabetic patient can have atherosclerotic plaques on these areas, but more obstruction develops in one or more of the three arteries that arise from the popliteal artery in the calf (trifurcation) area: the anterior tibial, posterior tibial, and peroneal arteries. Why these three distal vessels are so susceptible to atherosclerosis in diabetes is unclear, but the failure of blood flow to fall as much on standing in diabetic neuropathy may act to set the stage. Whatever its basis, the development of a low ankle-to-arm ratio (Fig. 25–2) is followed by both regular progression to a lower leg pressure and an increased mortality rate.[24,25]

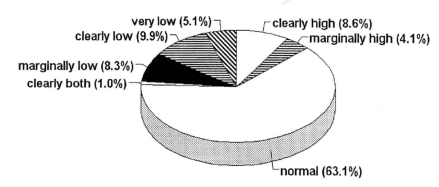

Figure 25–2. The results of screening of unselected diabetic patients using leg blood pressure determination are summarized. The technique applied to the lower leg is detailed in Exhibit 25–4. Using recommendations for screening at age 35 or after 20 years duration of diabetes[24] led to a finding of abnormality (under 0.90 or above 1.30) in 116 of the 314 patients screened. This high result is generated by marginal results at one or two of the four tested sites. It can be reduced by increasing the thresholds to 1.4 and 0.8. This results in 77 distinctly abnormal patterns. One or more values below 0.8 were detected in 46 patients and below 0.6 in 16 patients (15%), while values above 1.4 were seen in 27 patients. The high values were primarily in two groups: middle-aged males and patients with diabetic nephropathy. Leg blood pressure screening is the best means to detect early atherosclerosis in adult diabetes. When findings are less than conclusive, the low risk of serious problems and the slow rate of progression of leg atherosclerosis allow any diagnosis to be deferred until the next examination. When present, a clear diagnosis justifies intensive treatment following NCEP II guidelines.

Leg Blood Pressure Measurement

More than half of the diabetic patients who are found to have leg artery occlusive disease have no claudication. In some, arterial blockage occurs below the blood supply to the major calf muscles and ability to walk is almost unimpaired. Sensory nerve damage robs other people with diabetes of their symptoms. Evaluation of pedal pulses has failed to detect enough cases. Effective detection of leg disease in the midlife adult diabetic requires measurement of leg artery blood pressure (Exhibit 25–3).

The acoustic stethoscope used in arm pressure determination must be replaced by a Doppler ultrasound stethoscope or a similar device.[24] The Doppler ultrasound detector is coupled to the skin over one of the arteries that pass across the ankle using a sound transmission gel. An ordinary arm cuff is most effective when applied just above the ankle (see Exhibit 25–3). The dorsalis pedis and posterior tibial arteries should both be studied for highest detection rates. The peroneal artery needs to be examined only when one cannot detect Doppler pulsation at the other two ankle sites. Once the "whoosh" sound associated with flow is detected, the systolic pressure is determined by inflating the blood pressure cuff to 300 mmHg, letting the cuff pressure out slowly, and reading the cuff pressure at which the sound reappears.

In the supine position, leg systolic pressure is normally equal to or modestly higher than systolic pressure in the arm (Exhibit 25–4). The latter should be recorded just before, during, or just after leg pressure measurement. The same cuff and ultrasound device should be used. An equivocal leg pressure decline is best interpreted by later re-examination. Determination immediately following lower leg exercise may cause leg pressure to drop further when a problem is present, but this maneuver has not proven clinically useful.

A low ankle pressure associated with intermittent claudication usually indicates thigh or lower abdominal arterial disease. This situation is normally further evaluated by determination of local arterial blood pressures and blood flow patterns at multiple sites on each leg and thigh. Proximal obstruction characteristically obliterates the diastolic flow reversal normally present.

Effect of Vascular Calcification

Calcification of the leg arteries in diabetes creates difficulty with leg blood pressure determination. Inflating the blood pressure cuff stops arterial flow by overcoming intraluminal pressure. Rigidity of the vessel wall blocks collapse of the vessel wall against itself so that blood flow fails to stop until enough pressure is applied to collapse the more rigid wall. Local calcification can increase wall rigidity sufficiently to prevent wall collapse entirely, making cuff inflation unable to stop the flow even at 250 or 300 mmHg. Finding either a failure to stop flow or an elevated leg blood pressure ratio (see Exhibit 25–4) is evidence for arterial calcification. Individuals thus identified have a greater than normal risk for future amputation,[25] marking them for intensive foot care education.

Arterial stiffening might cause the examiner to fail to detect occlusive disease using leg blood pressure measurement. While I have found failure to stop flow at 300 mmHg in nearly 10% of persons with diabetes and

EXHIBIT 25–3   Doppler Ultrasound Blood Pressure Technique

Blood Pressure Cuff Application Sites and Cuff Sizes
1. Lower leg—regular arm cuff
2. Calf—oversize arm cuff
3. Thigh—thigh cuff
4. Penis—premature or neonatal infant cuff
5. Arm—arm cuff

Detection Devices
1. Continuous-wave Doppler ultrasound stethoscope
2. Continuous-wave Doppler probe-headphone set
3. Continuous-wave Doppler probe-loudspeaker set

Technique Recommended
1. Detect pulsatile blood flow at an arterial site beyond the cuff using the Doppler device after placing the appropriate cuff at the site selected.
2. Inflate the cuff until the sound at the arterial site being auscultated disappears or until 300 mmHg is reached.
3. Allow the cuff to deflate slowly; the systolic value is the pressure at which sound is first heard regularly.
4. One or two repetitions at each site serve to confirm the values obtained.

Criteria for Interpretation
1. Lower leg (auscultation at dorsalis pedis or posterior tibial artery at the ankle) pressures normally exceed that found in the arm when the subject is supine, due to the velocity of blood in the aorta during systole. Sometimes 0.95 (ankle to arm BP) is used as the cutoff ratio, but less than 0.90 is safer and 0.80 clearer yet. Retesting in 6–18 months should be done in the 0.81–0.94 range.
2. Calf interpretation is essentially the same as lower leg as long as the cuff length is 4/3 or more the diameter of the calf. Failure to use a sufficiently wide cuff will cause falsely high results. The ankle area is preferred for that reason. The calf may be used as an alternate site if the inflated cuff fails to stop ankle flow because of arterial calcification, but this is seldom necessary.
3. Thigh—a few mmHg lower or higher than calf. Lower calf and ankle pressures are seen when the femoral artery is occluded in the adductor canal area or when the popliteal artery is diseased.
4. The systolic pressure in the dorsal penile artery is normally close to that in the arm. A ratio below 0.8 to the brachial systolic pressure is sufficient to support a conclusion of vascular occlusion-based impotence if nocturnal erections are also reduced in firmness.
5. Arm systolic blood pressure values are normally quite close (±5 mmHg) to results obtained using an acoustic stethoscope.

EXHIBIT 25–4   Leg/Arm Blood Pressure Ratio Interpretation

Determine four supine ankle/arm ratios (left and right dorsalis pedis and posterior tibial)

Range of ratios	Interpretation
0.95–1.25	Clearly normal
0.90–0.94	Likely to be normal but not completely
1.26–1.30	Likely to be normal but not completely
0.81–0.89	Not normal atherosclerosis possible, repeat
0.80 or less	Atherosclerosis very likely[a]
0.60 or less (detectable)	Atherosclerosis with high risk for gangrene[a]
1.31–1.39	Marginal evidence for a calcified artery
1.40 or higher	Strong evidence for a calcified artery[a]

[a] At increased risk for an amputation-linked problem

The period between normal and even barely marginal examinations should be 2–3 years because of the slow progression of the early disorder. The initial screening time recommended has been age 35 or 20 years duration of diabetes. High ratios suggest renal disease, particularly in younger patients, and may justify a single youthful screening. A clearly ambiguous pattern justifies a repeat examination in a year or less.

pressure ratios above 1.30 in 5%, I have not experienced true failure to detect occlusion. The pattern of four pressures regularly allows its detection, especially after repeat studies are carried out. This conclusion concurred with by other observers.[24]

Diabetic Impotence

The pressure of blood being delivered to the penis is often reduced in males with diabetes who report impotence and fail to develop an erection when papaverine or prostaglandin is injected into the corpora cavernosa. This problem is commonly combined with reduced nitric oxide production. This reduction is linked in turn to vascular nerve damage. The combination of arterial occlusion and nerve damage/nitric oxide lack is the most frequent cause of impotence in diabetes, accounting for a majority of the cases.[26,27] The systolic pressure in the dorsal penile artery is determined using a Doppler ultrasound detector and a neonatal-sized blood pressure cuff (see Exhibit 25–3). The ratio of the penile artery to arm systolic pressure should exceed 0.80; it is normally about 0.96.

Ultrasound Equipment Sources

Ultrasound Doppler detectors for blood pressure determination may be obtained from a number of manufacturers including Medasonics [stethoscope, model BF4B or Cardiobeat], 38875 Cherry Street, Newark, CA 94560 (phone (800) 227-8076 fax (510) 494-0448), www.medicom.com/medasonics; Parks Medical Electronics [stethoscopes with and without speakers], P.O.Box 5669, Aloha, OR 97006 (phone (800) 547-6427 fax (503) 591-9753), www.parksmed.com; and D.E. Hokanson Inc. [bidirectional pocket stethoscope], Bellevue WA (phone (800) 999-18251 fax (425) 881-1636), www.deh-inc.com.

Wright Medical Corp. [Ultraprobe], 11023 118th Place N.E., Kirkland WA 98033-9919.

Blood Changes in Long-Standing Diabetes

The blood picture changes in chronic diabetes following the development of major diabetic complications. As in other types of renal failure, renal failure due to diabetic nephropathy produces significant to severe anemia.

The level of two serum proteins rises with duration of diabetes even when no serious sequelae develop. For unexplained reasons, serum α-2-macroglobulin, whose level is higher in young females than in young males and declines with age in both sexes, it becomes elevated in long-standing diabetes. Another plasma protein found to be increased in long-standing diabetes is immunoglobulin A (IgA). The IgA elevation exaggerates the rise in IgA with age seen in both nondiabetic and diabetic adults.

No increase in blood viscosity is seen in diabetic children. The diabetic blood viscosity elevation at standard hematocrit is also less striking in long-standing diabetes. The latter viscosity decline with duration may be due to the death of persons with diabetes whose blood viscosity is elevated.

Ischemic Response of Diabetic Nerve

The puzzling resistance to ischemia of diabetic nerve can serve as the basis for a useful early screening test for diabetic neuropathy. When arterial blood flow to an arm is stopped by inflating a blood pressure cuff to 230 mmHg, pain, hypesthesia, and dysesthesia develop in nondiabetics after approximately 18 min. These symptoms are associated with a rapid rise in vibration threshold.[28] People with diabetes undergoing such a test often have no pain or rise in vibration threshold even when the procedure is carried out to a 30 min time limit. Diabetics who fail to develop ischemic sensory loss and spontaneous pain after 30 min are developing sensory neuropathy. Careful control of hyperglycemia appears to prevent the uncoming nerve damage. Detection of resistance to ischemia helps to motivate the diabetic patient who is developing peripheral symptoms to undertake better self-care. Unfortunately for its regular application, many patients complain of discomfort shortly after inflation of the cuff and thus fail to complete the test.

The above clinical testing has been paralleled by laboratory studies showing a well-defined similarity between diabetic neuropathy and nerve damage generated by agents that interfere with oxygen availability. Similar findings are made in hypoxemia due to pulmonary disease, where it can be reversed by oxygen administration. The similarity has led to a formal "hypoxic" model of diabetic neuropathy.[29] This model does not yet allow us to understand the basis for resistance to ischemia.

Diabetic Neuropathy Screening Instruments

Early vibration threshold rise is easily detected using a Biothesiometer, as originally described.[28] This instrument is available for less than $400 from Bio-Medical Instrument Co. 15764 Munn Road, Newbury, Ohio 44065 (phone (440) 564-5461 fax 564-5710). An inexpensive alternative (less than $100), imbedded nylon monofilament threads of varying stiffness was developed by the Long Hansen's Disease Center in Carville, LA. It is now available in different forms from Sensory Testing Systems, 1815 Dallas Dr, Suite 11A, Baton Rouge, LA 70806 (phone (888) 289-9293 fax (225) 923-3670), www.sensorytestingservices.com, Jackson-Hinds Diabetic Foot Clinic Filament Project, Jackson, MS 39216 (phone (601) 982-2650), North Coast Medical, Inc., 187 Stauffer Blvd., San Jose, CA 95125-1042 (phone (800) 821-9319 fax (877) 213-9300), www.ncmedical. com, or Smith and Nephew, PO Box 1005, Germantown, WI 53022-8205 (phone (800) 558-8633), www.smithnephew.com. A more expensive instrument that directly and precisely detects loss of pain sense, the Neurometer, may be obtained for about $8-11,000 from Neurotron, Inc., 1501 Sulgrave Avenues, Suite 203, Baltimore MD 21209 (phone (800) 345-9040 fax (410) 664-0831), www.neurotron.com.

References

1. Naunyn B: Der Diabetes Mellitus. Vienna: A. Holder, 1898.

2. Weil AJ: Das verhalten der kleinsten gefasse beim diabetes mellitus. Klin Wochenschr 3:2093–2094, 1924.

3. Ernest JT, Goldstick TK, Engerman RL: Hyperglycemia impairs retinal oxygen autoregulation in normal and diabetic dogs. Invest Ophthalmol Vis Sci 24:985–989, 1983.

4. McFadden DM, Houston CS, Sutton JR, et al.: High-altitude retinopathy. JAMA 245:581–596, 1981.

5. Osterby R, Parving H, Hommel E, et al.: Glomerular structure and function in diabetic nephropathy. Diabetes 39:1057–1063, 1990.

6. Mogensen CE: Prediction of clinical diabetic nephropathy in IDDM patients. Alternatives to microalbuminuria? Diabetes 39:761–767, 1990.

7. Bojestig M, Arnqvist HJ, Hermannson G, et al.: Declining incidence of nephropathy in insulin-dependent diabetes mellitus. New Engl J Med 330:15–18, 1994.

8. Koistinen MJ: Prevalence of asymptomatic myocardial ischaemia in diabetic subjects. Br Med J 301:92–95, 1990.

9. Crepaldi G, Nosadini R: Diabetic cardiopathy: Is it a real entity? Diabetes/Metabolism Rev 4:273–288, 1988.

10. Felicetta JV, Sowers JR: Systemic hypertension in diabetes mellitus. Am J Cardiol 61:34H–40H, 1988.

11. Valerius NH, Eff C, Hansen NE, et al.: Neutrophil and lymphocyte function in patients with diabetes mellitus. Acta Med Scand 211:463–467, 1982.

12. Dallinger KJC, Jennings PE, Toop MJ, et al.: Platelet aggregation and coagulation factors in insulin dependent diabetics with and without microangiopathy. Diabetic Med 4:44–48, 1987.

13. Scarabin PY, Samama M: Effect of age on ADP-induced platelet aggregation in diabetic and non-diabetic subjects. Thromb Res 22:687–692, 1981.

14. McMillan DE: Blood viscosity and plasma proteins influencing it are increased in type 1 diabetes in the DCCT. Clin Hemorheol 14:473–480, 1995.

15. McMillan DE, Strigberger J, Utterback NG: Rapidly recovered transient flow resistance: a newly discovered property of blood. Amer J Physiol 253:H919–H926, 1987.

16. McMillan DE: The role of the diabetic erythrocyte in the development of microvascular disease. *In* Draznin B, Melmed S, LeRoith D (eds): Complications of Diabetes Mellitus. New York: Alan R. Liss, 1989, pp. 49–58.

17. Vague P, Juhan I: Red cell deformability, platelet aggregation, and insulin action. Diabetes 32(Suppl 2):88–91, 1983.

18. Lundbaek K, Jensen VA: The Aarhus series in long term diabetes. The clinical picture in diabetes mellitus of 15–25 years' duration with a follow-up of a regional series of cases. In Lundbaek K, Jensen VA (eds): Long-Term Diabetes. Copenhagen: Ejnar Munksgaard, 1953, pp. 158–163.

19. Kastrup J: The diabetic arteriole—the impact of diabetic microangiopathy on microcirculatory control. Danish Med Bull 35:334–345, 1988.

20. Yin FCP, Weisfeldt MI, Milnor WR: Role of aortic input impedance in the decreased cardiovascular response to exercise with aging in dogs. J Clin Invest 68:28–38, 1981.

21. Rendell M, Bamisedun O: Diabetic cutaneous microangiopathy. Am J Med 91:611–618, 1992.

22. Rayman G, Hassan A, Tooke JE: Blood flow in the skin of the foot related to posture in diabetes mellitus. Br Med J 292:87–90, 1986.

23. Alpert JS, Coffman JD, Baldimos MC, et al.: Capillary permeability and blood flow in skeletal muscle of patients with diabetes mellitus and genetic pre-diabetes. New Engl J Med 286:454–460, 1972.

24. Orchard TJ, Strandness DE: Assessment of peripheral vascular disease in diabetes. Report and recommendations of an international workshop sponsored by the American Heart Association and the American Diabetes Association. September 18–20, 1992, New Orleans, Louisiana. Diabetes Care 16:1199–1209, 1993.

25. Osmundson PJ, O'Fallon WM, Zimmerman BR, et al.: Course of peripheral occlusive arterial disease in diabetes-vascular laboratory assessment. Diabetes Care 13:143–152, 1990.

26. De Tejada IS, Goldstein I, Azadzoi K, Krane RJ, Cohen RA: Impaired neurogenic and endothelium-mediated relaxation of penile smooth muscle from diabetic men with impotence. New Engl J Med 320:1025–1030, 1989.

27. Zorgniotti AW, Lizza E: Most impotence may be due to vascular abnormalities regardless of etiology—vascular disease as a cause of impotence. Clin Diabetes 6:137–142, 1988.

28. Steiness I: Influence of diabetic status on vibratory perception during ischemia. Acta Med Scand 170:319–338, 1961.

29. Dyck PJ: Hypoxic neuropathy—does hypoxia play a role in diabetic neuropathy? The 1988 Robert Wartenberg lecture. Neurology 39:111–118, 1989.

30. Expert Panel on Detection, Evaluation, and Treatment of High Blood Cholesterol in Adults: Summary of the second report of the National Cholesterol Education Program (NCEP) expert panel on detection, evaluation, and treatment of high cholesterol in adults (adult treatment panel II). JAMA 269:3015–3023, 1993.

Selected Readings

Retinal Circulation and Anatomy

Bill A: Circulation in the eye. In Renkin EM, Michel CC (eds): Handbook of Physiology. Volume 4, part 2. Microcirculation. City, American Physiological Society, New York, 1984, pp. 1001–1034.

Circulatory Mechanics and Dynamics

Fung, Y-C: Biodynamics Circulation. New York: Springer-Verlag, 1984.

Renal Circulatory Physiology

McMillan DE: The microcirculation in diabetes. Microcirculation, Endothelium and Lymphatics 1:3–24, 1984.

Red Blood Cells

Barnes A J: The physical properties of red cells in diabetes mellitus. In Baba S, Kaneko T (eds): Diabetes 1994. Amsterdam: Exerpta Medica, Elsevier, 1995.

Blood Flow Properties

McMillan DE: Hemorheology. In Levin ME, O'Neal LW, Bowker JH (eds): The Diabetic Foot, 5 ed. Mosby Year Book, St. Louis, MO 1993, pp. 115–134.

Leg Artery Disease, Leg Blood Pressure and Flow

Strandness DE: Noninvasive diagnostic techniques. In Bernstein EF (ed): Doppler Ultrasonic Techniques in Vascular Disease. St. Louis, MO: C.V. Mosby Company, 1982, pp. 13–21.

Microcirculatory Pathophysiology in Diabetes

Tooke JE: Microcirculation and diabetes. Br Med Bull 45:1–18, 1989.

26

Diabetic Eye Disease

Nancy M. Holekamp and Travis A. Meredith

Diabetic eye disease is the leading cause of blindness in the United States.[1] However, this need not be the case. Three decades of basic science research, population studies, and carefully controlled national collaborative clinical trials have produced overwhelming data that diabetic eye disease is treatable and visual loss is largely preventable.

Visual loss in diabetes has many causes. Diabetic individuals are at increased risk for developing age-related cataracts, open angle glaucoma, and corneal disease.[2] However, these conditions are not unique to diabetic patients. Retinopathy is the principal, singular cause of visual loss in diabetes mellitus. All physicians involved in the care of diabetic individuals should be thoroughly familiar with diabetic retinopathy and its impact on vision and the patient. Consequently, this chapter will review the pathophysiology of diabetic retinopathy, the clinical presentation and classification of diabetic retinopathy, the epidemiology of diabetic retinopathy, and the medical and ophthalmologic management of patients with diabetic retinopathy.

Pathophysiologic Stages of Diabetic Retinopathy

Although diabetes mellitus is characterized by hyperglycemia and major abnormalities of metabolism, devastating end organ complications arise from its profound affect on blood vessels. Only in the eye can this pathologic process be directly observed. Since the invention of the ophthalmoscope in 1852, the stigmata of diabetic retinal vascular disease—retinal microaneurysms, blot hemorrhages, cotton-wool spots, and hard exudates—have been studied.[3] Through 100 years of observation, it has become clear that diabetic retinopathy is best understood in relation to five fundamental pathologic events: (1) formation of retinal capillary microaneurysms; (2) increased

TABLE 26–1 Five Steps in the Pathophysiology of Diabetic Retinopathy

1. Formation of retinal capillary microaneurysms
2. Increased vascular permeability
3. Microvascular occlusion
4. New blood vessel and fibrous tissue proliferation on the retinal surface
5. Contraction of fibrovascular proliferations

vascular permeability; (3) microvascular occlusion; (4) new blood vessel and fibrous tissue proliferation on the retinal and optic nerve surfaces; and (5) contraction of these fibrovascular proliferations (Table 26–1).[4]

The natural history of diabetic retinopathy is one of progression through each of these five pathophysiologic stages. The visual loss in any one individual, however, depends on the relative contribution of each stage. Retinal capillary microaneurysm formation is the hallmark of diabetic retinopathy and is its earliest detectable sign. It is a benign process without visual consequence. When microaneurysms and/or retinal capillaries become excessively permeable, intraluminal fluid will leak into the retina. Should the resulting intraretinal edema, lipid exudate, and focal hemorrhage involve the retinal center (macula), moderate visual loss ensues. Rather than leaking, retinal capillaries may shut down, becoming nonperfused; visual loss occurs when the macula is involved. Outside the center of vision, progressive and widespread nonperfusion initiates the elaboration of one or more vascular-endothelial growth factors. Abnormal new blood vessel growth follows, first within the retina and then on its anterior surface and on the optic nerve. The abnormal blood vessels bleed easily and are the source of vitreous hemorrhage. The associated fibrous tissue, like all scar tissue, contracts with time and distorts or detaches the retina. This "proliferative" stage of diabetic retinopathy is the most common cause of severe visual loss.

Clinical Stages of Diabetic Retinopathy

Characteristic pathophysiologic findings at each stage of diabetic retinopathy allow for classification of the disease (Table 26–2).[5] Diabetic retinopathy has been divided into nonproliferative and proliferative forms. In nonproliferative diabetic retinopathy the vascular abnormalities and their immediate effects are confined to the retina. In proliferative retinopathy, new blood vessels and scar tissue grow out of the retina to cause more extensive ocular damage. Nonproliferative retinopathy has been further divided into simple background diabetic retinopathy and a more advanced preproliferative retinopathy. Simple background diabetic retinopathy is the clinical manifestation of increased microvascular permeability. It consists of retinal capillary microaneurysms, small intraretinal dot and blot hemorrhages, and lipid exudates. Macular edema is usually seen in the later phases of this stage. Preproliferative diabetic retinopathy is the early clinical manifestation of vascular occlusion. It consists of cotton-wool spots, intraretinal microvascular abnormalities, venous beading, and extensive intraretinal hemorrhages. Macular ischemia may occur in this stage. In proliferative retinopathy, new blood vessels and scar tissue grow out of the retina to cause more extensive secondary ocular damage. This proliferative stage is a response to vascular occlusion and consists of neovascularization, vitreous hemorrhage, fibrovascular proliferation, traction retinal detachment, and rubeosis.

The terminology of each clinical stage of diabetic retinopathy has been standardized to allow for effective communication between physicians treating diabetic patients. What follows is a glossary of terms.

TABLE 26–2   Classification of Diabetic Retinopathy

I. Nonproliferative diabetic retinopathy
   A. Background retinopathy
      1. Microaneurysms
      2. Dot and blot hemorrhages
      3. Hard exudates
      4. Macular edema
   B. Preproliferative retinopathy
      1. Cotton-wool spots
      2. Intraretinal intravascular abnormalities (IRMA)
      3. Venous beading
      4. Extensive hemorrhage
II. Proliferative diabetic retinopathy
   A. Neovascularization of the disc (NVD)
   B. Neovascularization elsewhere in the retina (NVE)
   C. Vitreous hemorrhage
   D. Fibrovascular proliferation
   E. Traction and traction/rhegmatogenous retinal detachment
   F. Iris surface and angle neovascularization

TABLE 26–3   Visual Acuity and Function

20/20	Normal vision
20/40	Common requirement for unrestricted driver's license
20/70	Common requirement for restricted daytime driver's license
20/200	Legal blindness
5/200	Loss of ambulation

Visual acuity.   An arbitrary yet standardized measurement of central retinal function (Table 26–3).

Nonproliferative diabetic retinopathy.   The early clinical stage of diabetic retinopathy in which the vascular abnormalities are confined to the retina.

Background diabetic retinopathy.   The mildest form of nonproliferative diabetic retinopathy characterized by microaneurysms, intraretinal dot and blot hemorrhages, and lipid exudates.

Microaneurysms.   The earliest retinal capillary abnormality seen in background diabetic retinopathy (Fig. 26–1).

Dot-blot hemorrhage.   Small intraretinal accumulations of extravasated blood seen in all stages of diabetic retinopathy (Fig. 26–2).

Lipid exudate.   Intraretinal accumulation of extravasated lipoproteinaceous material, usually in circinate or ring patterns. Also called hard exudate (Fig. 26–3).

Macular edema.   Intraretinal thickening caused by extravasated fluid in the macula or the center of the retina. It is generally seen in patients with nonproliferative diabetic retinopathy. When the thickening occurs in the center of the retina, it is called clinically significant diabetic macular edema and is the most common cause of moderate visual loss. This diagnosis must be

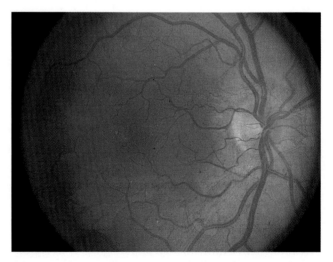

Figure 26–1.   This photograph of the left eye shows numerous pinpoint red microaneurysms in the macula. Visual acuity is 20/20.

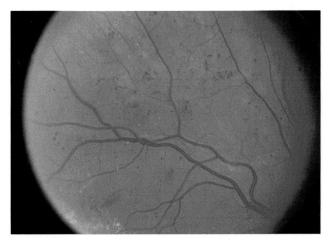

Figure 26–2. This view of the superonasal retina shows numerous dot-blot intraretinal hemorrhages.

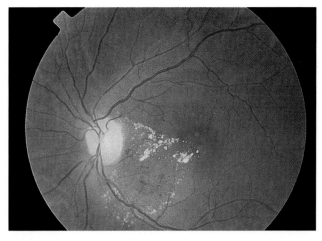

Figure 26–3. This photograph of the right eye shows circinate (ring pattern) lipid surrounding a leaking microaneurysm inferonasal to the optic nerve.

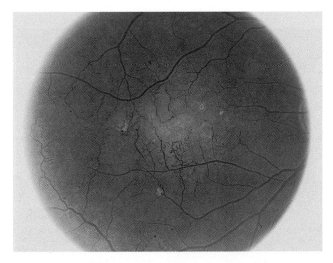

Figure 26–4. This fluorescein angiogram of the right eye shows capillary occlusion and nonperfusion of the blood vessels in the macular zone. Visual acuity is 20/70-1.

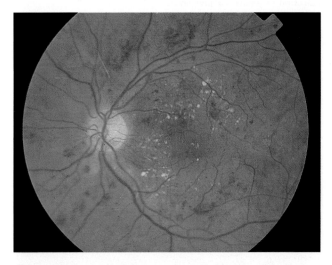

Figure 26–5. In this left eye with preproliferative diabetic retinopathy, extensive intraretinal hemorrhages, intraretinal microvascular abnormalities, lipid deposition and cotton-wool spots are seen.

made with a slit lamp and special ophthalmic lens examinations.

Macular ischemia. Capillary occlusion and nonperfusion in the macular center of the retina. It is generally seen in patients with preproliferative diabetic retinopathy. When it occurs in the central retina, it can cause irreversible visual loss in patients (Fig. 26–4). The diagnosis must be made with a fluorescein angiogram.

Preproliferative diabetic retinopathy. An advanced form of nonproliferative diabetic retinopathy characterized by cotton-wool spots, intraretinal microvascular abnormalities, venous beading, and extensive intraretinal hemorrhages (Fig. 26–5).

Cotton-wool spot. A gray or white abnormality in the inner layer of the retina that is usually the result of an infarction of the nerve fiber layer of the retina. Previously called soft exudate (Fig. 26–6).

IRMA. Intraretinal microvascular abnormalities, seen in preproliferative diabetic retinopathy (Fig. 26–7).

Venous beading. Dilation and tortuosity of retinal veins secondary to retinal ischemia. Seen in preproliferative diabetic retinopathy (Fig. 26–8).

Proliferative diabetic retinopathy. Advanced diabetic retinopathy characterized by neovascularization, vitreous hemorrhage, fibrovascular proliferation, traction retinal detachment, and rubeosis.

Neovascularization of the disc (NVD). New blood vessel growth arising from or close to the optic disc. Seen in proliferative diabetic retinopathy (Fig. 26–9).

Neovascularization elsewhere (NVE). New blood vessel growth arising from the peripheral retina, away from the optic disc. Seen in proliferative diabetic retinopathy (Fig. 26–10).

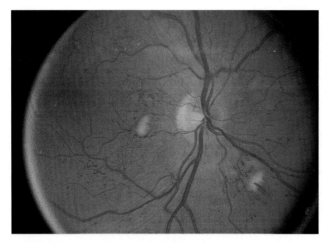

Figure 26–6. This photograph of the left eye shows cotton-wool spots superonasal and directly temporal to the optic nerve. These were previously called soft exudates. They represent infarction of the nerve fiber layer.

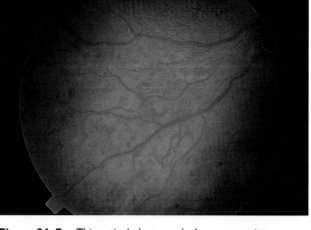

Figure 26–7. This retinal photograph shows extensive intraretinal microvascular abnormalities as seen in preproliferative diabetic retinopathy.

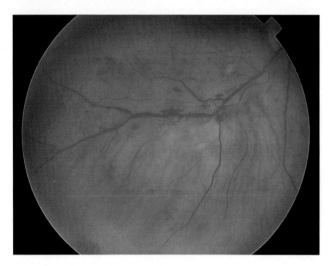

Figure 26–8. The retinal vein along the inferotemporal arcade shows marked venous beading as seen in preproliferative diabetic retinopathy.

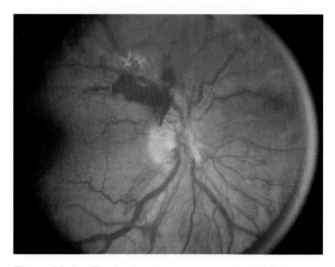

Figure 26–9. The fine lacy but extensive network of blood vessels adjacent to normal retinal blood vessels represents neovascularization of the disc as seen in proliferative diabetic retinopathy. There is associated preretinal hemorrhage superior to the optic nerve.

Vitreous hemorrhage. Blood in the vitreous cavity arising from vitreous traction on neovascular tissue. A common cause of severe visual loss in patients with proliferative diabetic retinopathy (Fig. 26–11).

Fibrovascular proliferation. Translucent, fibrous tissue grows adjacent to neovascularization and becomes increasingly opaque as regression of the new blood vessel occurs (Fig. 26–12).

Traction retinal detachment. Progressive contracture of fibrovascular proliferation on the surface of the retina tractionally elevates and detaches retinal tissue. A common cause of severe visual loss in patients with advanced proliferative diabetic retinopathy.

Rubeosis. Also called iris neovascularization, it is new blood vessel growth on the surface of the iris. It

is the result of severe retinal ischemia and leads to neovascular glaucoma (Fig. 26–13).

Epidemiology of Diabetic Retinopathy

Blindness is 25 times more common in a diabetic person than in a nondiabetic person.[6,7] A large population-based study showed that the principal cause of visual impairment in diabetes was diabetic retinopathy.[8,9] Diabetic retinopathy was the sole or contributing cause of legal blindness in 87% of eyes in younger-onset diabetics and 33% of eyes in older-onset patients. The lower rate of blindness attributable to retinopathy in

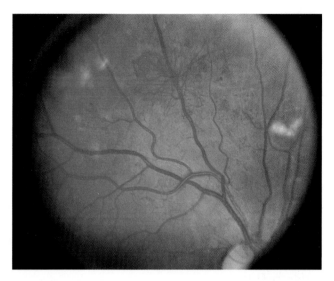

Figure 26–10. The lacy fine network of blood vessels arising from a normal retinal vein represents neovascularization elsewhere.

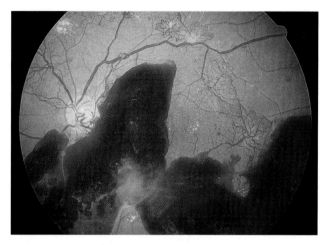

Figure 26–11. Vitreous traction on neovascular tissue in proliferative diabetic retinopathy gives rise to vitreous hemorrhage as seen in this photograph.

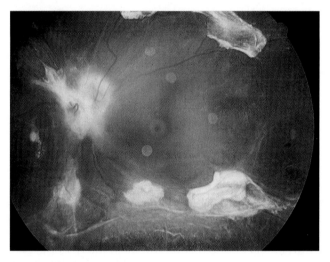

Figure 26–12. Significant fibrovascular proliferation is seen along the major retinal vascular arcades in the left eye of this patient with proliferative diabetic retinopathy.

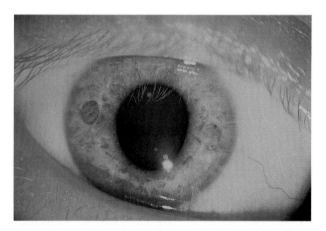

Figure 26–13. Close examination of the iris shows fine new vessel growth along the pupillary rim. Growth of new vessels also occurs in the anterior chamber angle and gives rise to neovascular glaucoma.

older individuals reflects the relatively higher incidence of cataract, glaucoma, and macular degeneration found in that age group.

The epidemiologic statistics for diabetic retinopathy are staggering. Over 35% of any diabetic population will have retinopathy.[11] Diabetic retinopathy is the leading cause of blindness in Americans of working age (20–74 years old).[12] Diabetic retinopathy has been estimated to cause 8,000 cases of legal blindness each year (visual acuity of 20/200 or less in the better eye). Approximately 75,000 new cases of diabetic macular edema and 65,000 new cases of proliferative diabetic retinopathy will occur each year in the United States.[13]

Timely and appropriate intervention for diabetic eye disease depends on knowledge of those patients at high risk for visual loss. Such data comes from a large popula-

tion base cohort study in southern Wisconsin, The Wisconsin Epidemiologic Study of Diabetic Retinopathy (WESDR).[8,9] From 1980 to 1982, 2,366 diabetic subjects were examined. They were classified as younger-onset, i.e., diagnosed at less than 30 years of age and taking insulin (YO-I, $n = 996$), or older-onset, i.e., diagnosed at or after 30 years of age and either taking insulin (OO-I, $n = 674$) or not taking insulin (OO-N, $n = 696$). There is prevalence data from the WESDR baseline examination, and with 10-year follow-up, incidence data (Table 26–4).

Prevalence of Diabetic Retinopathy

In the WESDR, the prevalence of any visual impairment (20/40 or worse in the better eye) was highest in the older insulin-dependent subjects at 18.4%, and

TABLE 26–4   Epidemiology of Diabetic Retinopathy

	Prevalance Data	
	Any Visual Impairment (%)	Legal Blindness (%)
YO-I[a]	7.9	3.2
OO-I[b]	18.4	2.7
OO-N[c]	12.2	2.3

	10-Year Incidence Data	
	Any Visual Impairment (%)	Legal Blindness (%)
YO-I	9.4	1.8
OO-I	37.2	4.0
OO-N	23.9	4.8

	10-Year Incidence Data			
	Any Retinopathy (%)	Progression (%)	Macular Edema (%)	Proliferative Disease (%)
YO-I	89.0	76.0	20.1	30.0
OO-I	79.0	69.0	25.4	24.0
OO-N	67.0	53.0	13.9	10.0

[a] YO-I, younger-onset insulin-dependent.

[b] OO-I, older-onset insulin-dependent.

[c] OO-N, older-onset non-insulin-dependent.

lowest in the younger insulin-dependent subjects at 7.9%. However, the younger insulin-dependent group had the highest incidence of legal blindness (20/200 or worse in the better eye) at 3.2%, and the older non-insulin-dependent group had the lowest at 2.3%.[14] Because a majority of patients with diabetes have older-onset disease, a significant number of diabetic patients encountered by primary care physicians will have experienced some visual impairment. Fewer individuals with diabetes have younger-onset disease, but they are subject to more severe visual loss. It is important to note that blindness is not generally seen in any individual younger than age 25.

Incidence of Diabetic Retinopathy

The 10-year incidence of any visual impairment in the WESDR was 9.4%, 37.2%, and 23.9% in the younger-onset, older-onset taking insulin, and older-onset not taking insulin groups, respectively. Respective 10-year rates of blindness were 1.8%, 4.0%, and 4.8%.[15] Visual loss and blindness are best explained by the incidence of macular edema and proliferative retinopathy. The 10-year incidence of macular edema was 20.1% in the younger-onset group, 25.4% in the older-onset group taking insulin, and 13.9% in the older-onset group not

taking insulin.[16] The 10-year incidence of any retinopathy (89%, 79%, and 67%), progression of retinopathy (75%, 69%, and 53%), and progression to proliferative retinopathy (30%, 24%, and 10%) were all highest in the younger-onset group.[17] One may conclude that older individuals taking insulin are most likely to develop macular edema and associated mild to moderate visual loss, while younger individuals are most likely to develop progressive retinopathy, placing them at higher risk for severe visual loss.

Epidemiologic Risk Factors for Diabetic Retinopathy

Duration of Disease.   Duration of diabetes appears to be the most important determinant of retinopathy for all individuals with the disease. Given a sufficient duration of diabetes, almost 100% of younger-onset diabetic patients and 70% of older-onset diabetic patients will develop some degree of retinopathy.[8,9] Duration of diabetes is predictably linear with development of retinopathy. For example, in younger-onset individuals, none have retinopathy at the time of diagnosis. After 5 years approximately 25% have retinopathy, after 10 years almost 60% have retinopathy, and after 15 years 80% have retinopathy.[8]

Age. The effect of disease duration is not uniform at all ages. Diabetic children are at low risk of retinopathy prior to puberty regardless of the duration of diabetes.[18] Thereafter, the risk becomes appreciable, but age becomes secondary to disease duration as the significant predictor of retinopathy.

Gender. In the WESDR, younger-onset male patients with 10 or more years of diabetes were $1\frac{1}{3}$ times more likely to have proliferative disease than similar female patients.[8] The explanation for this is uncertain. No association was found between gender and diabetic retinopathy in older individuals.[9]

The Internist's Role in Managing Diabetic Retinopathy

Modifying Risk Factors for Diabetic Retinopathy

As stated earlier, the WESDR has identified risk factors for progression of vision-threatening diabetic retinopathy such as age, gender, and duration of diabetes, which cannot be modified. However, the WESDR and other studies have evaluated other possible risk factors that potentially could be modified by conscientious medical care on the part of both doctor and patient. These risk factors include hyperglycemia, blood pressure, aspirin use, smoking, alcohol, physical activity, oral contraceptives, and pregnancy.

Hyperglycemia. One fundamental question in helping people with diabetes manage their disease is the role of hyperglycemia and the development of diabetic retinopathy. Numerous studies in animal models of diabetes[19–21] and epidemiologic studies[8,9,22,23] have implicated hyperglycemia in the long-term complications of the disease, but not until recently has a clinical trial demonstrated a consistent and convincing beneficial effect of intensive glycemic control on them.[24–26]

The Diabetes Control and Complications Trial (DCCT) was a multicenter, randomized, clinical trial designed to compare intensive with conventional diabetes therapy with regard to their effects on the development and progression of the early vascular and neurologic complications of insulin-dependent diabetes mellitus.[27–29] The intensive therapy regimen was designed to achieve blood glucose values as close to the normal range as possible with three or more daily insulin injections or treatment with an insulin pump. Conventional therapy consisted of one or two insulin injections/day. Two different but related questions were asked by the study: Will intensive therapy prevent the development of diabetic retinopathy in patients with no retinopathy (primary prevention), and

will intensive therapy affect the progression of early retinopathy (secondary intervention)?

In the DCCT, 1,441 patients with insulin-dependent diabetes mellitus were followed for a mean of 6.5 years, and the appearance and progression of retinopathy was assessed regularly. In the primary prevention cohort, intensive therapy reduced the adjusted mean risk for the development of retinopathy by 76% compared to conventional therapy. In the secondary intervention cohort, intensive therapy slowed the progression of retinopathy by 54% and reduced the development of proliferative or severe nonproliferative retinopathy by 47%.[30] The study concluded that intensive therapy effectively delays the onset and slows the progression of diabetic retinopathy in patients with insulin-dependent diabetes mellitus.

The DCCT was limited to a small subgroup of people with diabetes—highly motivated patients with insulin-dependent diabetes mellitus between the ages of 13 and 39 years, without hypertension or cardiovascular disease. Do these results hold true for older patients with non-insulin-dependent disease? The answer is probably yes. Treatment that lowers blood glucose concentrations well below those needed to merely relieve symptoms is beneficial, but the best way to achieve this objective may well be different in the two groups of patients. For most patients with insulin-dependent disease, the appropriate treatment is intensive insulin therapy. For most patients with non-insulin-dependent disease, the appropriate treatment may be healthy diet and exercise routines and the use of oral hypoglycemics intended to produce near-euglycemia.[31]

Blood Pressure. Studies of the relationship of high blood pressure to diabetic retinopathy have not produced uniform results.[32–37] In the WESDR, higher blood pressure was associated with an increased prevalence of proliferative retinopathy.[8,9] After controlling for other known risk factors, however, no relationship was found between blood pressure and the incidence of diabetic retinopathy.[38]

One possible reason for failure to find a relationship between blood pressure and the development of proliferative retinopathy may be selective mortality: Individuals with higher blood pressure who developed proliferative diabetic retinopathy may have died before the follow-up examination.[39] Alternatively, high blood pressure may not be related to the development of proliferative retinopathy. Nevertheless, hypertension control is important in people with diabetes. Elevated blood pressure has been shown to be a significant risk factor for cardiovascular disease, stroke, and accelerated renal disease in diabetic patients.

Aspirin Use. Because patients with diabetes mellitus are known to have altered platelet function, it has been postulated that aspirin use might retard the progression of the microvascular angiopathy in diabetic retinopathy. Although not specifically designed to address this question, the WESDR found no relationship between aspirin use and severity of retinopathy. In addition, although the potential for hemorrhagic complications may be more common among aspirin users, no association was found.[40]

The Early Treatment Diabetic Retinopathy Study (ETDRS) was specifically designed to assess the effect of aspirin on ocular events.[41–43] In this multicenter, randomized, clinical trial sponsored by the National Eye Institute, 3,711 patients with retinopathy were assigned randomly to either 650 mg of aspirin/day or placebo. Aspirin did not affect the rate of progression of retinopathy and did not reduce the rate of visual loss, nor did it increase the rate of vitreous hemorrhage from neovascularization.[42] It was concluded that aspirin had no clinically important beneficial effects on the progression of retinopathy. The ETDRS also provided an opportunity to study the effects of aspirin on cardiovascular complications in diabetic patients. Aspirin use and the occurrence of cardiovascular events were not substantially different from the effects observed in other studies that included mainly nondiabetic persons. Furthermore, there was no evidence of harmful effects of aspirin. These findings suggest there are no diabetic ocular contraindications to aspirin when required for cardiovascular disease or other medical indications.[44]

Cigarette Smoking. Little evidence exists for an association between cigarette smoking and the incidence and progression of diabetic retinopathy. In the WESDR, cigarette smoking was not related to prevalence or incidence of proliferative retinopathy.[45,46] However, younger-onset diabetics who smoked were 2.4 times, and older-onset diabetics 1.6 times, as likely to die as those who did not smoke.[39] Diabetic people should be encouraged to abstain from smoking, as it is a significant risk factor for cardiovascular disease, respiratory disease, and cancer.

Alcohol Consumption. Two reports from the WESDR suggest that a moderate degree of alcohol consumption does not affect the prevalence, incidence, or progression of diabetic retinopathy in either younger-onset or older-onset individuals.[47,48] However, it has been shown that diabetic persons with retinopathy who are heavy drinkers do have a greater mortality risk.[39]

Physical Activity. Just as physical activity is associated with lower risks of mortality and cardiovascular disease morbidity in nondiabetic people, the same is true for diabetic individuals. However, diabetic individuals with proliferative diabetic retinopathy may wonder if physical activity places them at greater risk for progressive disease or vitreous hemorrhage. The findings of the WESDR suggest physical activity may be relatively unimportant in the course of proliferative diabetic retinopathy.[49] Furthermore, in another study there was no association between physical activity and subsequent vitreous hemorrhage, with most hemorrhages being noted at rest or upon awakening.[50]

Oral Contraceptives. Data from the WESDR suggest that the use of oral contraceptives by women with insulin-dependent diabetes mellitus is not associated with the presence of proliferative diabetic retinopathy.[51] Oral contraceptives, if not otherwise contraindicated, may be a reasonable approach to preventing pregnancy in diabetic women with retinopathy.

Pregnancy. Pregnancy is known to accelerate progression of both nonproliferative and proliferative diabetic retinopathy in some women.[52] In fact, diabetic retinopathy can become particularly aggressive during pregnancy.[53] With the advent of laser photocoagulation, much has changed in the management of pregnant diabetic women since the 1950s, when women with diabetic retinopathy were encouraged not to become pregnant. Current data suggest that any woman with diabetes who is planning to become pregnant should be examined for retinopathy by an ophthalmologist. All pregnant diabetic women should be examined by an ophthalmologist in the first trimester and thereafter at the discretion of the examiner, but at least every 3 months until parturition.[54] (see Chapters 40 and 41.)

Systemic Co-Morbidity of Diabetic Retinopathy

Diabetic Nephropathy. Diabetic retinopathy and another major microvascular complication of diabetes mellitus, nephropathy, often occur concurrently. Interestingly, the WESDR found a prevalence of proliferative retinopathy in 23% and nephropathy in 22% of a large diabetic population.[55] There is an undeniably high likelihood of retinopathy in patients with nephropathy. In patients with established diabetic nephropathy, over 90% have diabetic retinopathy. In uremic insulin-dependent diabetics, 97% have diabetic retinopathy.[56]

Severity of nephropathy correlates with severity of retinopathy. In a case series of diabetic patients with end-stage renal disease undergoing renal transplantation or dialysis, 75% had proliferative retinopathy and 32% had a visual acuity of 20/160 or worse in the better eye.[57] This association between the presence of diabetic nephropathy and the presence of severe diabetic retinopathy suggests that the diagnosis of one should lead to testing for the other. In fact, finding proteinuria, a known risk indicator for proliferative retinopathy in younger-onset diabetics, identifies patients that will benefit from regular ophthalmologic evaluation.[58]

Diabetic patients on renal dialysis or following renal transplantation usually experience stabilization of visual function.[57] Some nephrologists will be concerned that heparinization during hemodialysis will encourage vitreous hemorrhage in patients with proliferative retinopathy. No increased risk of vitreous hemorrhage has been found comparing patients managed by hemodialysis to those managed by peritoneal dialysis.[57]

Diabetic Neuropathy.   Diabetic retinopathy and its association with diabetic neuropathy is less well studied. Both complications certainly occur with longer duration of disease in both younger and older-onset individuals. In the few studies that have been reported on diabetic neuropathy and retinopathy, most have demonstrated an association of peripheral or autonomic neuropathy with retinopathy. In addition, severity of retinopathy correlates with severity of neuropathy. A 10-year follow-up in the WESDR suggests that men with proliferative retinopathy have a significantly higher incidence of impotence (31%) compared to those without proliferative retinopathy (10%).[59] As with nephropathy, the diagnosis of diabetic neuropathy identifies individuals who will benefit from regular ophthalmologic evaluation.

Morbidity and Mortality.   Retinopathy and other complications of diabetes have been shown to be significant predictors of morbidity and mortality in a diabetic population.[39] This most likely is due to their strong association with systemic conditions that are themselves the underlying cause of illness and death. The diagnosis of significant diabetic retinopathy by an ophthalmologist should alert the primary care physician to initiate vigilant and perhaps more frequent examinations looking for the often associated early renal disease, neuropathy, and cardiovascular disease. Timely intervention may minimize morbidity and mortality.

Indications for Ophthalmologic Consultation

Current Referral Patterns Are Inadequate.   Data from a number of studies suggest that a significant number of Americans with diabetes may not be receiving recommended dilated eye examinations for the detection of retinopathy. Analysis of data collected from the 1989 National Health Interview Survey indicated that only 49% of adults diagnosed with diabetes had had a dilated examination during the previous year.[60] The findings of the WESDR were equally striking. Twenty-six percent of younger-onset diabetics and 36% of older-onset diabetics had never had an eye exam.[61] Fifty-one percent of eyes with proliferative diabetic retinopathy had not been treated with laser photocoagulation. Moreover, based on the WESDR findings, it was estimated that 35,000 Americans with proliferative

retinopathy at risk for severe visual loss and 230,000 Americans with macular edema at risk for moderate visual loss were not under the care of an ophthalmologist in 1980 to 1982.

Problems with Appropriate Referral.   There are numerous medical and nonmedical reasons for inadequate ophthalmologic care for diabetic individuals.[59] Many of the reasons are patient related. First, vision-threatening retinopathy may be asymptomatic. In the WESDR, 18% of younger-onset and 31% of older-onset people with proliferative retinopathy were unaware of their condition.[62] Second, patients may not be properly educated that timely detection of retinopathy and treatment may prevent visual loss. Third, after being told, denial is common. Finally, as with other public health problems, there may be inaccessibility to or inability to pay for ophthalmologic care.[63]

Several important reasons for the lack of dilated eye examinations in diabetic patients are physician related. First, the sensitivity of detecting proliferative retinopathy or macular edema by primary care physicians has been shown to be challenging, even through a dilated pupil under ideal conditions.[64] Specialized equipment such as a slit lamp or contact lens are often not available to the nonophthalmologist. Realistically, most nonophthalmologists routinely choose not to dilate the pupil when doing ophthalmoscopy. Not surprisingly, the sensitivity of detecting retinopathy through an undilated pupil is poor.[65] Diabetic retinopathy in each patient should be not only detected but also classified for purposes of determining appropriate follow-up intervals or deciding to initiate treatment. Secondly, despite national guidelines regarding eye care for people with diabetes, primary care physicians may not be aware of the indications for referral.[66] Third, nonophthalmologists may not be aware of the recently demonstrated efficacy of early detection and laser treatment in preventing visual loss due to macular edema and proliferative diabetic retinopathy.

Recommendations for Ophthalmologic Consultation. The American College of Physicians, American Diabetes Association, and American Academy of Ophthalmology have jointly developed recommendations regarding referral of diabetic patients for ophthalmologic evaluation (Table 26–5).[67] Because it is unusual for

TABLE 26–5 Diabetic Eye Examination Schedule

Age of Onset of Diabetes Mellitus	Recommended Time of First Exam	Routine Minimum Follow-up
0–30	5 years after onset	Yearly
31 and older	At time of diagnosis	Yearly
Prior to pregnancy	Prior to conception or early in first trimester	3 months

younger-onset diabetics to manifest retinopathy at the time of diagnosis, the recommended time of referral to an ophthalmologist for patients between the ages of 0 and 30 is 5 years after onset. In contrast, it is very common for older-onset individuals to manifest retinopathy at the time of diagnosis (in fact, it can be the presenting sign of diabetes). Therefore, recommended time of referral to an ophthalmologist for patients over the age of 30 is at the time of diagnosis. Diabetic women planning on a pregnancy should be referred to an ophthalmologist prior to conception or early in the first trimester.

Ophthalmologist's Role in Managing Diabetic Retinopathy

Once a diabetic patient comes under the care of an ophthalmologist, what can be done to prevent visual loss? Diabetic retinopathy was described in 1967 as "not preventable" and "relatively untreatable."[68] Since then, remarkable advances have been made in the management of diabetic retinopathy. This is largely due to the results of three national collaborative studies sponsored by the National Eye Institute. The first was initiated in 1971, and the last has recently ended. Reports from the Diabetic Retinopathy Study (DRS),[69–82] the Early Treatment Diabetic Retinopathy Study (ETDRS),[83–96] and the Diabetic Retinopathy Vitrectomy Study (DRVS)[97–101] have provided valuable information to the ophthalmologist treating patients with diabetic retinopathy. The following reviews the ophthalmologist's management of diabetic retinopathy according to the results of these clinical trials.

Management According to Stage of Clinical Disease: Results of Clinical Trials

Normal Retina. A diabetic patient with a normal retinal examination, i.e., no evidence of diabetic retinopathy, should be reexamined annually. Within 1 year, 5–10% of patients who are initially normal will develop diabetic retinopathy.[102]

Nonproliferative Diabetic Retinopathy. Patients with retinal microaneurysms and occasional blot hemorrhages or hard exudates should be reexamined within 6-12 months. Disease progression is common. Within 4 years, 16% of insulin-dependent diabetics will progress to proliferative disease.[102]

Nonproliferative Diabetic Retinopathy with Macular Edema. Macular edema is intraretinal thickening due to extravasated fluid. It is commonly seen with nonproliferative diabetic retinopathy. When macular edema affects the center of the retina, it is called clinically significant diabetic macular edema (CSDME) and is a frequent cause of moderate visual loss. Patients with macular edema that is not clinically significant should be reexamined every 4–6 months because they are at risk for developing CSDME.

Because clinically significant diabetic macular edema is a vision-threatening condition, the ETDRS has formulated clear guidelines for its diagnosis and management. CSDME as defined by the ETDRS includes any of the following features:[83] (1) Thickening of the retina at or within 500 microns of the center of the macula; (2) hard exudates at or within 500 microns of the center of the macula, if associated with thickening of the adjacent retina; and (3) a zone or zones of retinal thickening one disc area or larger, any part of which is within one disc diameter of the center of the macula. Those findings must be determined with a slit lamp and special ophthalmic lenses.

This definition attempts to identify pathologic retinal changes that place patients at risk for visual loss. Therefore, anyone with CSDME should be considered for laser surgery even if visual acuity is not yet reduced (substantial recovery of reduced visual acuity is relatively unusual following laser treatment).[85]

Data from the ETDRS show that focal photocoagulation of CSDME substantially reduces the risk of visual loss (Table 26–6). Focal treatment also increases the chance of visual improvement, decreases the frequency of persistent macular edema, and causes only minor visual field losses.[83]

Prior to laser surgery, a fluorescein angiogram is usually performed. Yellow fluorescent dye is injected intravenously through a peripheral vein and

TABLE 26–6 ETDRS Visual Outcome

Severity of Retinopathy	Duration of Follow-up (years)	Control Patients (% with Visual Loss[a])	Treated Patients (% with Visual Loss)
CSDME (center of macula involved)	1	13.3	7.5
	2	26.3	9.4
	3	33.0	13.8

[a] Visual loss is defined as at least doubling of visual angle.

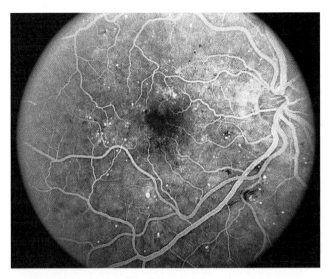

Figure 26–14. In this fluorescein angiogram, pinpoint bright spots denote leaking microaneurysms. There are few, if any, zones of capillary dropout.

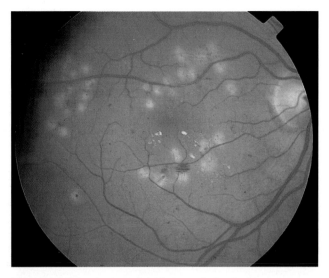

Figure 26–15. In this color photograph, focal white spots denote focal laser treatment to microaneurysms using the argon green laser.

is photographed with a specialized ocular camera as it passes through the retinal vasculature. Leaking microaneurysms and zones of capillary dropout are easily identified (Fig. 26–14). The angiogram is used to guide laser photocoagulation to these areas of leakage. Laser surgery is generally performed in the office under topical anesthesia. It is painless, and there are no postoperative restrictions. Patients should be seen in 2–4 months following surgery. Additional sessions of laser photocoagulation are commonly needed in a single eye to control the leakage from diabetic retinopathy (Fig. 26–15)

Preproliferative Diabetic Retinopathy. Also called severe, nonproliferative diabetic retinopathy, this stage of disease is characterized by the presence of retinal venous beading, large retinal hemorrhages, multiple cotton-wool spots, and extensive intraretinal microvascular abnormalities (IRMA). The risk of progression to proliferative disease is high. Between 10% and 50% of patients with preproliferative changes will develop proliferative diabetic retinopathy within 1 year.[4]

The value of laser surgery for this group of patients was investigated by the ETDRS. The study suggested that panretinal laser photocoagulation not be performed in eyes with mild or moderate preproliferative diabetic retinopathy, provided follow-up every 3–4 months can be maintained. When preproliferative retinopathy is more severe or when reliable follow-up is questionable, laser surgery should be considered.[91]

Proliferative Diabetic Retinopathy. Proliferative diabetic retinopathy is characterized by new blood vessel growth arising from the surface of the retina or optic nerve. The blood vessels are abnormal, causing vitreous hemorrhage, retinal distortion, and retinal detach-

ment. Although the mechanism has never been fully elucidated, it has been suggested since laser photocoagulation was first introduced in 1959[103] and well known since the early 1970s that laser spots applied in a scatter or panretinal distribution throughout the peripheral retina can cause involution of abnormal neovascularization.

The DRS was designed to evaluate the effectiveness of laser photocoagulation in eyes with proliferative diabetic retinopathy. First and foremost, the study identified high-risk characteristics that placed patients at significantly increased risk for severe visual loss: neovascularization of the disc (NVD) greater than $\frac{1}{4}$–$\frac{1}{3}$ disc area, or vitreous or preretinal hemorrhage associated with less extensive NVD, or with NVE $\frac{1}{2}$ disc area or more in size.[71] Second, the study showed that the risk of severe visual loss among patients with high-risk proliferative diabetic retinopathy can be substantially reduced by means of panretinal laser photocoagulation (Table 26–7).[82]

Laser surgery is generally an office procedure (Fig. 26–16). It is common to use retrobulbar anesthesia to keep the patient comfortable during the application of usually 500–1000 laser spots. Laser treatment is applied according to carefully described techniques[82] in a scatter pattern throughout the peripheral retina. Care is taken to avoid the macula, optic nerve, and major retinal vessels (Fig. 26–17). More than one laser session is often required, with each management plan being carefully titrated to each patient. Indications for additional treatment may include inadequate regression of neovascularization, increasing neovascularization, new vitreous hemorrhage, and new areas of neovascularization. Possible side effects of panretinal laser photocoagulation include mild loss of visual

TABLE 26–7 DRS Visual Outcome: Severe Visual Loss[a]

Severity of Retinopathy	Duration of Follow-up (years)	Control Patients (% with Visual Loss)	Treated Patients (% with Visual Loss)
High-risk proliferative	2	14	6
	4	28	12

[a] Severe visual loss is defined as 5/200 acuity or worse.

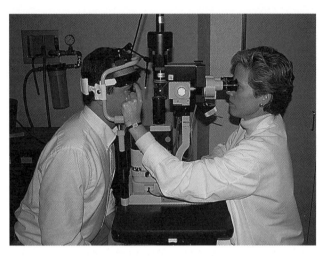

Figure 26–16. Laser surgery is an outpatient office procedure performed under topical or retrobulbar anesthesia.

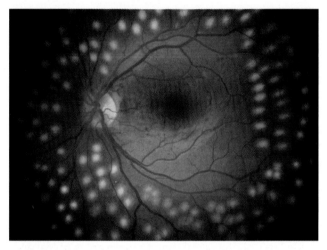

Figure 26–17. This photograph of the left eye shows panretinal laser photocoagulation having been applied to the peripheral retina.

acuity and constriction of peripheral visual field. These harmful effects are generally considered acceptable in eyes at high risk for severe visual loss.[70]

In eyes with proliferative retinopathy without high-risk characteristics, the ETDRS recommended that such eyes be observed at 3- to 4-month intervals for further progression of proliferative disease. Eyes approaching high-risk disease have a 50% chance of reaching it within 12–18 months. Laser treatment should be promptly delivered once high-risk characteristics are present.[94]

Proliferative Retinopathy Not Amenable to Laser Photocoagulation: Vitreous Surgery. It may be impossible to perform laser photocoagulation surgery on some patients with high-risk proliferative diabetic retinopathy due to vitreous hemorrhage or preretinal hemorrhage. In other patients, advanced proliferative diabetic retinopathy may persist despite maximal laser photocoagulation. Vitreous surgery may allow visual rehabilitation in many eyes that are otherwise untreatable (Fig. 26–18).

Vitreous surgery is generally recommended in eyes with traction macular detachment or severe vitreous hemorrhage of 4–6 months duration. The DRVS was designed to identify clinical situations in which patients

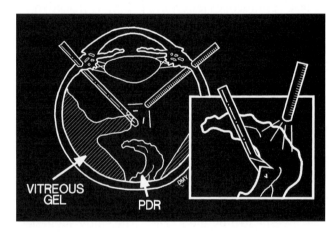

Figure 26–18. Vitreous surgery involves the intraocular manipulation of the vitreous gel, preretinal neovascular and fibrous tissue, and the retina.

might benefit from vitrectomy surgery. Specifically, it investigated the role of vitrectomy in managing eyes with very severe proliferative diabetic retinopathy and found significant benefit of early vitrectomy for eyes with advanced, active proliferative diabetic retinopathy and relatively good visual acuity (Table 26–8).[99] The DRVS also studied the benefits of early vitrectomy (intervention soon after visual loss) for severe vitreous

TABLE 26–8 Vitreous Surgery for Severe Proliferative Retinopathy and Relatively Good Visual Acuity

Visual Acuity	Early Vitrectomy (%)	Conventional Management (%)
20/40 + (2 year)	41.46	30.86
20/40 + (3 year)	47.37	24.66
20/40 + (4 year)	44.14	28.26
NLP (4 year)	Approx. 23	Approx. 19

TABLE 26–9 Vitreous Surgery for Severe Vitreous Hemorrhage

2-Year Visual Acuity (%)	Early Vitrectomy (%)	Deferred Vitrectomy (%)
20/40 +	24.5	15.2
NLP	25.0	29.0

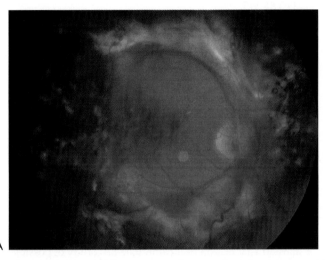

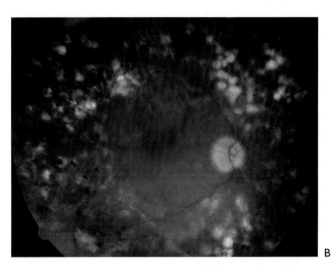

A   B

Figure 26–19. (A) Preoperative photograph of the right eye with severe proliferative diabetic retinopathy and extramacular traction retinal detachment and preretinal hemorrhage. (B) Postoperative photograph of the same eye showing absence of proliferative diabetic retinopathy, no areas of traction retinal detachment, absence of preretinal hemorrhage, and good laser photocoagulation.

hemorrhage and found significant benefit in younger-onset insulin-dependent diabetics, but not in older-onset diabetics, regardless of insulin use (Table 26–9).[98–101]

With advances in vitreoretinal surgical technique, indications for vitrectomy in the management of diabetic eye disease have been expanded. The most common indications for diabetic vitrectomy include (1) severe, nonclearing vitreous hemorrhage; (2) traction retinal detachment recently involving the macula; (3) combined traction and rhegmatogenous retinal detachment; (4) progressive fibrovascular proliferation; (5) dense premacular hemorrhage; and (6) macular edema with premacular traction.[104]

Vitreous surgery is always carried out in the operating room under either general or retrobulbar anesthesia. It has the potential for serious complications, including severe visual loss even to the point of no light perception, phthisis, and pain. The visual success rate will vary according to the indication for surgery and its severity. Overall, the rate of visual improvement in cases of diabetic vitrectomy is about 67% (Figure 26–19).[105,106]

References

1. The National Society to Prevent Blindness, Operational Research Department: Vision Problems in the U.S.: A Statistical Analysis. 1–46 (Abstract), 1980.

2. Klein R, Klein BEK, Moss SE: Visual impairment in diabetes. Ophthalmology 91:1–8, 1984.

3. James WA: Historical aspects of diabetic retinopathy. In Friedman EA, L'Esperance FA (eds.): Diabetic Renal Retinal Syndrome. New York: Grune & Stratton, 1986, pp. 27–42.

4. David MD, Rand LI: Diabetic Retinopathy. In Alberti MM, DeFronzo RA, Keen H, Zimmet P (eds.): International Textbook of Diabetes Mellitus. New York: Wiley, 1992, pp. 1329–1365.

5. Murphy RP: Current status of treatment of non-proliferative and proliferative diabetic retinopathy. In Freidman EA, L'Esperance FA (eds.): Diabetic Renal Retinal Syndrome. New York: Grune & Stratton, 1982, pp. 217–241.

6. Palmberg PF: Diabetic retinopathy. Diabetes 26:703–709, 1977.

7. Kahn HA, Hiller R: Blindness caused by diabetic retinopathy. Am J Ophthalmol 78:58–67, 1974.

8. Klein R, Klein BEK, Moss SE, et al.: The Wisconsin Epidemiologic Study of Diabetic Retinopathy. II. Prevalence in risk of diabetic retinopathy when age at diagnosis is less than 30 years. Arch Ophthalmol 102:520–526, 1984.

9. Klein R, Klein BEK, Moss SE, et al.: The Wisconsin Epidemiologic Study of Diabetic Retinopathy. III. Prevalence in risk of diabetic retinopathy when age at diagnosis is 30 or more years. Arch Ophthalmol 102:527–532, 1984.

10. Klein R, Klein BEK, Moss SE: Visual impairment in diabetes. Ophthalmology 91:1–9, 1984.

11. Klein R, Klein BEK, Moss SE, et al.: The Beaver Dam Eye Study: Retinopathy in adults with newly discovered and previously diagnosed diabetes mellitus. Ophthalmology 99:58–62, 1992.

12. Patz A, Smith RE: The ETDRS in diabetes 2000 (Editorial). Ophthalmology 98:739–740, 1991.

13. Klein R, Klein BEK, Moss SE: The epidemiology of ocular problems in diabetes mellitus. In Feman SS (ed.): Ocular Problems in Diabetes Mellitus. Boston: Blackwell Scientific Publications, pp. 1–51, 1991.

14. Klein R, Moss SE: Visual impairment in diabetes. In Alberti MM, DeFronzo RA, Keen H, Zimmet P (eds.): International Textbook of Diabetes Mellitus. New York: Wiley, 1992, pp. 1373–1384.

15. Moss SE, Klein R, Klein BEK: The ten year incidence of visual loss in the diabetic population. Ophthalmology 101:1061–1070, 1994.

16. Klein R, Klein BEK, Moss SE, et al.: The Wisconsin Epidemiologic Study of Diabetic Retinopathy. XV.: The long term incidence of macular edema. Ophthalmology 102:7–16, 1995.

17. Klein R, Klein BEK, Moss SE, et al.: The Wisconsin Epidemiologic Study of Diabetic retinopathy. XIV.: Ten year incidence and progression of diabetic retinopathy. Arch Ophthalmol 112:1217–1228, 1994.

18. Klein R, Klein BEK, Moss SE, et al.: Retinopathy in young onset diabetic patients. Diabetes Care 8:311–315, 1995.

19. Engerman RL, Bloodworth JM, Nelson S: Relationship of microvascular disease in diabetes to metabolic control. Diabetes 26:760–769, 1977.

20. Engerman RL, Kern TS: Progression of insipient diabetic retinopathy during good glycemic control. Diabetes 36:808–812, 1987.

21. Kohen AJ, McGill PD, Rossetti RG, et al.: A glomerulopathy in spontaneously diabetic rat: Impact of glycemic control. Diabetes 36:944–951, 1987.

22. Klein R, Klein BEK, Moss SE, et al.: Glycosylated hemoglobin predicts the incidence and progression of diabetic retinopathy. JAMA 260:2864–2871, 1988.

23. Chase HP, Jackson WE, Hoop SSL, et al.: Glucose control in the renal and retinal complications of insulin dependent diabetes. JAMA 261:1155–1160, 1989.

24. Crock Collaborative Study Group: Blood glucose control and the evolution of diabetic retinopathy and albuminuria: a preliminary multi-center trial. New Engl J Med 311:365–372, 1984.

25. Lauritzent, Frost-Larsen K, Larsen HW, et al.: Two year experience with continuous subcutaneous insulin infusion in relation to retinopathy and neuropathy. Diabetes 34:74–79, 1985.

26. Brinchmann-Hansen O, Dahl-Jogensen K, Hanssen KF, Sandvik L: The response of diabetic retinopathy to forty-one months of multiple insulin injections, insulin pumps, and conventional insulin therapy. Arch Ophthalmol 106:1242–1246, 1988.

27. The DCCT Research Group: The Diabetes Control and Complications Trial (DCCT): Design and methodologic considerations for the feasibility phase. Diabetes 35:530–545, 1986.

28. The DCCT Research Group: The Diabetes Control and Complications Trial (DCCT): Results of feasibility study. Diabetes Care 10:1–19, 1987.

29. The DCCT Research Group: The Diabetes Control and Complications Trial (DCCT): Update. Diabetes Care 13:427–433, 1990.

30. The DCCT Research Group: The effect of intensive treatment of diabetes on the development and progression of long-term complication in insulin-dependent diabetes mellitus. New Engl J Med 329:977–986, 1993.

31. Lasker RD: The Diabetes Control and Complications Trial: Implications for policy and practice. New Engl J Med 329:1035–1036, 1993.

32. Davis MD: Diabetic retinopathy, diabetic control and blood pressure. Transplant Proc 18:1565–1568, 1986.

33. Barnett AH, Britton JR, Leatherdale BA: Study of possible risk factors for severe retinopathy in non-insulin dependent diabetes. Br Med J 287:529–539, 1983.

34. Ibsen KK, Rotner H, Hougaard P: Blood pressure in children with diabetes mellitus. Acta Paediatr Scand 72:191–196, 1983.

35. Nilsson SE, Nilsson JE, Frostberg N, Emilsson T: The Kristianstad survey. II. Studies in a representative adult diabetic population with special reference to comparison with an adequate control group. Acta Med Scand 469:1–42, 1967.

36. Houston A: Retinopathy in the Poole area: an epidemiological inquiry. In Eschege E (ed.): Advances in Diabetes Epidemiology. Amsterdam: Elsevier, 1982, pp. 199–206.

37. Paisey RB, Arrendondo G, Villalobos A, et al.: Association of differing dietary, metabolic and clinical risk factors with microvascular complications of diabetes: a prevalent study of 503 Mexican type II diabetic subjects. Diabetes Care 7:428–433, 1984.

38. Klein R, Klein BEK, Moss SE, et al.: Is blood pressure a predictor of the incidence of progression of diabetic retinopathy? Arch Intern Med 149:2427–2432, 1989.

39. Klein RE, Moss SE, Klein BEK, et al.: Relation of ocular and systemic factors to survival and diabetes. Arch Intern Med 149:266–272, 1989.

40. Klein BEK, Klein R, Moss SE: Aspirin usage associated with diabetic retinopathy. Diabetes Care 10:600–603, 1987.

41. Early Treatment Diabetic Retinopathy Study (ETDRS) Research Group: ETDRS design in baseline patient characteristics: ETDRS Report 7. Ophthalmology 98:741–756, 1991.

42. Early Treatment Diabetic Retinopathy Study (ETDRS) Research Group: Effects of aspirin treatment on diabetic retinopathy: ETDRS Report 8. Ophthalmology 98:757–765, 1991.

43. Early Treatment Diabetic Retinopathy Study (ETDRS) Research Group: Early photocoagulation for diabetic retinopathy: ETDRS Report 9. Ophthalmology 98:766–785, 1991.

44. ETDRS Investigators: Aspirin effects on mortality and morbidity in patients with diabetes mellitus: Early Treatment Diabetic Retinopathy Study report 14. JAMA 268:1292–1300, 1992.

45. Klein R, Klein BEK, Davis MD: Is cigarette smoking associated with diabetic retinopathy? Am J Epidemiol 118:228–238, 1983.

46. Moss SE, Klein R, Klein BKE: The association of cigarette smoking with diabetic retinopathy. Diabetes Care 14:119–126, 1991.

47. Moss SE, Klein R, Klein BEK: Alcohol consumption and the prevalence of diabetic retinopathy. Ophthalmology 99:926–932, 1992.

48. Moss SE, Klein R, Klein BEK: The association of alcohol consumption with the incidence and regression of diabetic retinopathy. Ophthalmology 101:1962–1968, 1994.

49. Cruickshanks KJ, Moss SE, Klein R, Klein BEK: Physical activity and proliferative retinopathy in people diagnosed with diabetes before age 30 years. Diabetes Care 15:1267–1272, 1992.

50. Anderson B: Activity and diabetic vitreous hemorrhages. Ophthalomology 87:173–175, 1980.

51. Klein BEK, Moss SE, Klein R: Oral contraceptives in women with diabetes. Diabetes Care 13:895–898, 1990.

52. Klein BEK, Moss SE, Klein R: Effect of pregnancy on and progression of diabetic retinopathy. Diabetes Care 13:34–40, 1990.

53. Sunness JS: The pregnant woman's eye. Surv Ophthalmol 32:219–238, 1988.

54. American Academy of Ophthalmology: Policy statement, eyecare of patients with diabetes mellitus. 1991 (Abstract)

55. Klein R, Klein BEK, Demets D, et al.: The Wisconsin Epidemiologic Study of Diabetic Retinopathy. V. Proteinuria and retinopathy in a population of diabetic persons diagnosed prior to 30 years of age. In Freidman EA, L'Esperance FA (eds.): Diabetic Renal Retinal Syndrome. New York: Grune & Stratton, 1982, pp. 245–265.

56. Feldman J, Hirsch S, Friedman EA: Prevalence of diabetic nephropathy at time of treatment for diabetic retinopathy. In Friedman EA, L'Esperance FA (eds.): The Diabetic Renal Retinal Syndrome. New York: Grune & Stratton, 1982, pp. 9–20.

57. Ramsey RC, Knobolch WH, Cantrell HL, et al.: Visual status in transplanted and dialyzed diabetic patients. In Freidman EA, L'Esperance FA (eds.): Prevention and Management: Diabetic Renal Retinal Syndrome. New York: Grune & Stratton, 1982, pp. 427–435.

58. Klein R, Moss SE, Klein BEK: Is gross proteinuria a risk factor for the incidence of proliferative diabetic retinopathy? Ophthalmology 100:1140–1146, 1993.

59. Klein R, Klein BEK, Moss SE: Epidemiology of proliferative diabetic retinopathy. Diabetes Care 15(12):1875–1891, 1992.

60. Brechner RJ, Kowie CC, Howie LJ, et al.: Ophthalmic examination among adults with diagnosed diabetes mellitus. JAMA 270:1714–1718, 1993.

61. Witkin SR, Klein R: Ophthamologic care for persons with diabetes. JAMA 251:2534–2537, 1984.

62. Klein R, Klein BEK, Moss SE, et al.: The validity of a survey question to study diabetic retinopathy. Am J Epidiol 124:104–110, 1986.

63. Klein R: Eye care delivery for people with diabetes: an unmet need. Diabetes Care 17:614–615, 1994.

64. Sussman EJ, Tsiaras WG, Soper KA: Diagnosis of diabetic eye disease. JAMA 247:3231–3234, 1982.

65. Klein R, Klein BEK, Neider MW, et al.: Diabetic retinopathy is detected using ophthalmoscopy, a nonmydriatic camera, and a standard fundus camera. Ophthlmology 92:485–491, 1985.

66. The American College of Physicians and American Academy of Ophthalmology: Screening guidelines for diabetic retinopathy. Ann Int Med 116:683–685, 1992.

67. American College of Physicians AD, American Academy of Ophthalmology: Screening guidelines for diabetic retinopathy, clinical guideline. Ophthalmology 99: 1626–1628, 1992.

68. Duke-Elder S: System of Ophthalmology. St. Louis MO: Mosby, 1967, pp. 410–447.

69. Diabetic Retinopathy Study Group: Preliminary report on effects of photocoagulation therapy. Am J Ophthalmol 81:383–396, 1976.

70. Diabetic Retinopathy Study Research Group: Photocoagulation treatment of proliferative diabetic retinopathy: the second report of Diabetic Retinopathy Study findings. Ophthalmology 97:654–655, 1978.

71. Diabetic Retinopathy Study Research Group: Four risk factors for severe visual loss in diabetic retinopathy: the third report. Arch Ophthalmol 85:82–106, 1979.

72. Diabetic Retinopthy Study Research Group: Photocoagulation treatment of proliferative diabetic retinopathy: a short report of long range results: Report four. Diabetes 28:789–794, 1979.

73. Diabetic Retinopathy Study Research Group: Photocoagulation treatment of proliferative diabetic retinopathy: Relationship of adverse treatment effects to retinopathy severity: Report five. Dev Ophthalmol 2:248–261, 1981.

74. Diabetic Retinopathy Study Research Group: Design, methods and baseline results. Invest Ophthalmol 21: 149–211, 1981.

75. Diabetic Retinopathy Study Reseach Group: Part 7: A modification of the Airlie House classification of diabetic retinopathy. Invest Ophthal 2:210–226, 1981.

76. Diabetic Retinopathy Study Research Group: Photocoagulation treatment of proliferative diabetic retinopathy—clinical application of Diabetic Retinopathy Study (DRS) findings, DRS Report Number 8. Ophthalmology 88: 583–600, 1981.

77. Diabetic Retinopathy Research Study Group: Assessing possible late treatment effects in stopping a clinical trial early: a case study: Report no. 9. Controlled Clin Trials 5:373–381, 1984.

78. Diabetic Retinopathy Study Research Group: Factors influencing the development of visual loss in advanced diabetic retinopathy—report ten. Invest Ophthal 983–991, 1985.

79. Diabetic Retinopathy Study Research Group: Intraocular pressure following panretinal photocoagulation for diabetic retinopathy. Arch Ophthal 105:807–809, 1987.

80. Diabetic Retinopathy Study Research Group: Macular edema in Diabetic Retinopathy Study patients—DRS report twelve. Ophthalmology 94:754–760, 1987.

81. Diabetic Retinopathy Study Research Group: Factors associated with visual outcome after photocoagulation for diabetic retinopathy. Invest Ophthal 23–28, 1989.

82. Diabetic Retinopathy Study Research Group: Indications for photocoagulation treatment of diabetic retinopathy. Int Ophthalmol Clin 27(4):239–253, 1987.

83. Early Treatment Diabetic Retinopathy Study Research Group: Photocoagulation for diabetic macular edema: Study report number one. Arch Ophthal 103:1796–1806, 1985.

84. Early Treatment Diabetic Retinopathy Study Research Group: Report no. 2. Ophthalmology 94:761–774, 1987.

85. Early Treatment Diabetic Retinopathy Study Group: Techniques for scatter and focal photocoagulation treatment of diabetic retinopathy: Report 3. Int Ophthalmol Clin 27:254–264, 1987.

86. Early Treatment Diabetic Retinopathy Study Research Group: Photocoagulation for diabetic macular edema: Report No. 4. Int Ophthalmol Clin 27:265–333, 1987.

87. Early Treatment Diabetic Retinopathy Study Group: Detection of diabetic macular edema ophthalmoscopy versus photography: Early treatment report no. 5. Ophthalmology 96:746–751, 1989.

88. Early Treatment Diabetic Retinopathy Study Group: C-peptide and the classification of diabetes mellitus patients in the early treatment diabetic retinopathy study: Report no. 6. Ann Epidemiol 9–17, 1993.

89. Early Treatment Diabetic Retinopathy Study: Early Treatment Diabetic Retinopathy Study design and baseline patient characteristics: ETDRS report number 7. Ophthalmology 98:741–756, 1991.

90. Early Treatment Diabetic Retinopathy Study Group: Effects of aspirin treatment on diabetic retinopathy: ETDRS report 8. Ophthalmology 98:757–765, 1991.

91. Early Treatment Diabetic Retinopathy Study Research Group: Early photocoagulation for diabetic retinopathy: ETDRS report no. 9. Ophthalmology 98:766–785, 1991.

92. Early Treatment Diabetic Retinopathy Study Research Group: Grading diabetic retinopathy from stereoscopic color fundus photographs—an extension of the modified Airlie House classification: ETDRS report number 10. Ophthalmology 98:786–806, 1991.

93. Early Treatment Diabetic Retinopathy Study Research Group: Classification of diabetic retinopathy from fluorescein angiograms: ETDRS report number 11. Ophthalmology 98:807–822, 1991.

94. Early Treatment Diabetic Retinopathy Study Research Group: Fundus photographic risk factors for progression of diabetic retinopathy: ETDRS report number 12. Ophthalmology 98:823–833, 1991.

95. Early Treatment Diabetic Retinopathy Study Research Group: Fluorescein angiographic risk factors for progression of diabetic retinopathy: ETDRS report number 13. Ophthalmology 98:834–840, 1996.

96. Early Treatment Diabetic Retinopathy Study Research Group: Pars plana vitrectomy in the early treatment diabetic retinopathy study: ETDRS report 17. Ophthalmology 98:1351–1357, 1991.

97. DRVS Research Group: Two-year course of visual acuity in severe proliferative diabetic retinopathy with conventional management. Ophthalmology 92:492–502, 1985.

98. DRVS Research Group: Early vitrectomy for severe vitreous hemorrhage in diabetic retinopathy. Arch Ophthalmol 103:1644–1652, 1985.

99. DRVS Research Group: Early vitrectomy for severe proliferative diabetic retinopathy in eyes with useful vision—results of a randomized trial—DRVS report #3. Ophthalmology 1307–1320, 1988.

100. DRVS Research Group: Clinical application of results of a randomized trial—DRVS study report 4. Ophthalmology 1321–1334, 1988.

101. DRVS Research Group: Early vitrectomy for severe vitreous hemorrhage in diabetic retinopathy—four year results of a randomized trial study report 5. Arch Ophthal 108:958–964, 1990.

102. Klein R: The Wisconsin Epidemiologic Study of Diabetic Retinopathy—four-year incidence and progression of diabetic retinopathy when age at diagnosis is 30 years or more. Arch Ophthalmol 107:244–249, 1989.

103. Diabetic Retinopathy Study Research Group: Preliminary report on effects of photocoagulation therapy. Am J Ophthalmol 81:383–396, 1976.

104. Ho T, Smiddy WE, Flynn HW: Vitrectomy in the management of diabetic eye disease. Surv Ophthalmol 37:190–202, 1992.

105. Michels RG: Vitrectomy for complications of retinopathy. Arch Ophthalmol 96:237–246, 1978.

106. Thompson JT, De Bustros S, Michels RG: Results of vitrectomy for proliferative diabetic retinopathy. Ophthalmology 93:1571–1574, 1986.

27

Diabetes and the Kidney

Barbara S. Daniels and Frederick C. Goetz

Diabetic nephropathy accounts for a large proportion of the increased morbidity and mortality associated with diabetes.[1,2] Even the increased cardiovascular disease associated with diabetes is further accentuated in patients with nephropathy. The enhancement of the understanding of the pathophysiology of diabetic nephropathy that has occurred over the last decade has led to therapies that decrease the incidence of nephropathy, particularly in insulin-dependent diabetes mellitus (IDDM), and slow its progression in both IDDM and non-insulin-dependent diabetes mellitus (NIDDM).

Historical Perspective

Diabetes mellitus was at one time believed to be a disease of the kidneys due to prominent polyuria in the affected individuals. However, proteinuric renal disease in diabetes remained unrecognized until the 20th century, probably because of the short life span of the patient with IDDM in the preinsulin era and the presence of vascular disease and hypertension in the patient with NIDDM. Recognition of the unique structural abnormalities of the diabetic kidney awaited Kimmelstiel and Wilson's landmark paper in 1936, which described unique nodular glomerular abnormalities at autopsy in a group of older diabetic (probably NIDDM) patients with proteinuria, azotemia, and hypertension prior to death. By 1959, renal failure had supplanted ketoacidosis as the major cause of death in youth-onset diabetes due to the better treatment of acute metabolic abnormalities with insulin and the ensuing prolonged life span in these patients. Since then, the understanding of diabetic renal histology and pathophysiology has greatly advanced, and promising therapies aimed at the prevention or amelioration of progressive renal injury are now available. Renal replacement therapy, once considered to be contraindicated in diabetic patients with nephropathy, is now offered routinely to nearly all diabetic patients in the United States.

Epidemiology

Although the initial description of diabetic nephropathy by Kimmelstiel and Wilson utilized information from patients with NIDDM, most epidemiologic studies have focused on IDDM, due at least in part to the ease of better defining the time of onset and the usual absence of coexistent hypertension and vascular disease.

Insulin-Dependent Diabetes Mellitus

Krolewski and his group at the Joslin Clinic and Deckert and colleagues working at Steno Hospital in Denmark have reported extensive epidemiologic studies of patients with IDDM. Both groups have shown that a decrease in the incidence of proteinuria in IDDM has occurred. In the 1930s more than 40% of all newly diagnosed diabetics ultimately developed proteinuria, the hallmark of diabetic nephropathy. With the changing perceptions about glycemic control and availability of longer acting insulin further decrements were seen through the 1960s. There is preliminary evidence to suggest that the last decade has brought with it a further decrease, likely due to increased awareness of the importance of glycemic control. The long "incubation period" for nephropathy, perhaps more than 30 years now, makes it more difficult to interpret the recent decrease in the incidence of new proteinuria in IDDM as a true decrease rather than a delay in onset. Although this apparent decline in incidence of nephropathy in IDDM is very encouraging, the increasing incidence of IDDM among young people may ultimately blunt its impact on the number of patients with diabetic nephropathy.

Glycemic control appears to be the major controllable risk factor for the development of nephropathy in diabetes and recently, improved glycemic control has been demonstrated to decrease the risk of nephropathy. In addition, male diabetics are at increased risk for the development of proteinuria. After 16 years of diabetes, the incidence of proteinuria is 50% greater in males, a pattern that persists even after 40 years of diabetes.

Interestingly, similar gender-related differences are present in experimental diabetic nephropathy as well as some other types of human renal disease. First-degree relatives of patients with diabetic nephropathy have an eightfold increase in their risk of ultimately developing proteinuria and progressive renal insufficiency. Whether this is related to environmental effects, such as parental influence on insulin use and glycemic control, maternal smoking during pregnancy, maternal education,[3] or genetic factors, such as polymorphisms in the genes that control the renin-angiotensin system, is presently unknown. Both a familial history of hypertension and cardiovascular disease are also associated with an increased incidence of nephropathy. In addition, poor glycemic control seems to further accentuate both genetic and environmental risk factors. It has long been known that the patients with the highest levels of blood glucose have the greatest incidence of nephropathy, but it is only recently that improvement in glycemic control has been proven to reduce the incidence.

Non-Insulin-Dependent Diabetes Mellitus

The epidemiology of renal disease in the patient with NIDDM has been more difficult to elucidate because of the inability to date the onset of hyperglycemia and to separate the confounding effects of vascular disease and hypertension. At the time of the initial detection of hyperglycemia, nearly 15% of all NIDDM patients have proteinuria detectable by standard laboratory urinalyses, suggesting the presence of a glomerular disease other than diabetic nephropathy in these patients. Interestingly, this baseline incidence of proteinuria is remarkably constant, regardless of ethnic or socioeconomic background. Since both hypertension and vascular disease are associated with albuminuria in nondiabetics, the specificity of proteinuria for diabetic nephropathy in NIDDM has not been established.

After 15 years, the prevalence of proteinuria in NIDDM has been reported to range from 15% to 50%. It is not yet known whether this time-dependent increase in proteinuria in NIDDM is due to the same process that caused the 15% incidence of proteinuria at the time of diagnosis of diabetes or the occurrence of diabetic nephropathy analogous to that seen in patients with IDDM. However, it is clear that, regardless of the etiology of the proteinuria, it is associated with excess mortality, as is also true in IDDM.

The rate of development of progressive renal insufficiency and end-stage renal disease (ESRD) in NIDDM appears to be less than that for patients with IDDM. Although 85% of all diabetics have NIDDM, only 50% of the diabetics receiving therapy for ESRD have NIDDM, which has been interpreted as evidence that fewer NIDDM patients develop azotemia. Whether this is actually due to a lower incidence of progressive renal insufficiency or increased mortality from other causes before the development of ESRD remains to be defined. In fact, based on the high prevalence of proteinuria and hypertension at the onset of hyperglycemia, it might be expected that renal disease would be more common in NIDDM. Most importantly, the number of patients with NIDDM who are developing nephropathy and requiring treatment for ESRD is increasing rapidly, due in large part to the increasing incidence and prevalence of NIDDM.

Natural History

At the time of presentation, patients with IDDM exhibit an elevated glomerular filtration rate (GFR), nephromegaly, and enhanced renal clearance of albumin detectable by sensitive immunoassay techniques. Following the establishment of glycemic control, GFR declines toward baseline levels and albuminuria acutely abates (Table 27–1).

There are no clinical symptoms or signs or renal dysfunction during the next 10–20 years. During periods of poor glycemic control, an elevation of GFR and microalbuminuria can be detected by sensitive techniques, but routine, standard clinical laboratory studies will be normal. Blood pressure usually remains normal during this "preclinical" period. When patients are randomly studied during this time period without regard for glycemic control, those with elevated GFRs appear to be at the greatest risk for the ultimate devel-

TABLE 27–1 Differences in the Renal Manifestations of IDDM and NIDDM

	IDDM	NIDDM
Glomerular filtration rate at diagnosis	Increased	Normal
Glomerular size	Increased	Normal
Proteinuria during first 5 years	Unusual	10–20%
Proteinuria after 15–20 years	About 20%	About 50%
Hypertension	Accompanies renal disease	Common
Incidence of progressive renal dysfunction	About 20%	<15%

opment of progressive renal insufficiency. Whether this hyperfiltration is solely a marker for poor glycemic control or an independent indicator of hemodynamic glomerular injury is unknown.

Ultimately, in up to 30% of IDDM patients, sensitive immunoassays reveal persistent microalbuminuria, which signals a very high likelihood for the development of diabetic nephropathy. Since maintenance of the glomerular permeability barrier to protein is a sensitive marker of glomerular function, the appearance of even small amounts of albumin in the urine suggests either structural or functional abnormalities within the glomerulus. Using standard human renal clearance techniques, GFR is usually indistinguishable from that in nonmicroalbuminuric patients, but measurements of the intraglomerular pressure, the most important pathogenetic parameter, are impossible in the human. Structural changes such as mesangial expansion and glomerular epithelial cell abnormalities are not discernible on electron microscopic studies of the glomerulus at this early stage, but subtle alterations could escape detection.

Concomitant with the increase in urinary protein excretion, blood pressure may also begin to rise. However, the levels are not yet frankly hypertensive by the standards used to diagnose essential hypertension (140/90 mmHg). During this period, either intensive glycemic control, using an insulin pump, or angiotensin-converting enzyme inhibition may decrease the level of microalbuminuria and ameliorate a progressive rise in protein excretion. It is not known now whether this is due to actual prevention of nephropathy or a delay in its onset.

During the next several years, proteinuria increases and is detectable on routine urinalysis, marking the onset of clinical nephropathy. Concurrently, GFR begins to decrease. Once this process begins, most patients experience an inexorable progression of renal insufficiency. This is reminiscent of the progressive decline in GFR that accompanies many nondiabetic renal diseases and is frequently independent of the disease process that caused the initial damage. Treatment aimed specifically at diabetes, such as improved glycemic control, has less effect on proteinuria at this stage. However, antihypertensive therapy has been very successful in ameliorating the progressive decline in GFR at this stage of diabetic nephropathy, as is true in other types of renal disease.

The natural history of renal disease in NIDDM is not well defined. Glomerular hyperfiltration does not seem to occur, and glomerular hypertrophy, a typical feature in IDDM, is lacking. Proteinuria and hypertension, which are common at the time of diagnosis of NIDDM, are probably not due to diabetic nephropathy per se, but their etiology remains obscure.

Pathophysiology

Renal Hemodynamics

Elevations in GFR in IDDM occur both at the time of diagnosis and during periods of poor glycemic control. The augmentation in GFR is accompanied by an increase in renal plasma flow. In the rat where intraglomerular hemodynamic measurements can be made, an increase in the intraglomerular pressure accompanies these changes. An increase in renal size and glomerular enlargement may be the morphologic equivalent of the hemodynamic findings, and all of these alterations appear to fluctuate, in part, with the level of glycemic control.

The recurrence of an increased GFR during periods of poor control suggests a relationship between either hyperglycemia or insulinopenia and abnormal renal hemodynamics. Insulin appears to have no intrinsic vasoactive or hemodynamic properties, but it could modulate the response to other hormones within the glomerular microcirculation, as has been shown in the glomerulus in vitro for angiotensin II. Recent attention has focused on angiotensin II and prostanoids as mediators of increased intraglomerular flows and pressures, respectively, but additional factors, such as endothelin, nitric oxide, and bradykinin, could also play a role.

In humans, attention has focused on the elevation of GFR, hyperfiltration, as being of primary pathogenic significance, probably due to its ease of measurement. However, elevation of intraglomerular pressure is likely to have a greater damaging effect, as has been demonstrated in experimental models of diabetic nephropathy. In experimental diabetic rats, reversal of glomerular hypertension using either angiotensin-converting enzyme inhibition or dietary protein restriction or protection of the glomerulus from the augmented systemic pressure using a renal artery clamp ameliorates structural renal damage and progressive proteinuria. In all of these models, the beneficial effects occur in the absence of alterations in glycemic control and, in the former two, occur despite maintenance of the elevated GFR. Thus, elevated intraglomerular pressure seems to be the most injurious of the hemodynamic factors in models where it can be measured.

Although diabetic patients are often counseled to moderate their protein intake, their daily protein intake may still be greater than that in normal persons, which may contribute to glomerular hyperfiltration. Elevated ketone levels, comparable to that seen in IDDM, are also associated with an increase in the GFR. As in the rat, a variety of hormonal systems, tubuloglomerular feedback, and the aldose reductase pathway have been implicated in renal hemodynamic changes during the "preproteinuric" stage evidence that those patients with elevated GFRs obtained at random times during the "preclinical" nonproteinuric years are most likely to develop nephropathy. The microalbuminuria that frequently accompanies poor glycemic control in humans may be a marker of glomerular hypertension, as it is in many conditions in the rat. It is at this early preproteinuric stage of diabetic renal alterations that improvement of glycemic control holds the most promise.

Once proteinuria has become established and GFR begins to decrease, the remaining nephrons attempt to compensate for the loss of function in damaged glomeruli. Compensation is accomplished by increased blood flow and augmented intraglomerular pressure in residual "healthy" nephrons, establishing a vicious cycle whereby the remaining functional nephrons are exposed to increasingly damaging hemodynamic forces. In addition, any increment in systemic blood pressure, which occurs concomitantly with the fall in GFR, may be transmitted more directly to the glomerulus due to the dilation of the afferent renal vasculature. This process appears to occur to varying degrees in all types of renal disease and, in diabetic nephropathy, appears to occur independently of the level of glycemic control. Therapy aimed at reducing the intraglomerular hypertension—antihypertensive therapy in general and angiotensin-converting enzyme inhibition in particular—seems to ameliorate the progression of renal failure, further supporting the importance of increased glomerular pressure in the progression of established diabetic nephropathy.

Hyperglycemia

The similarity of renal lesions in patients with IDDM and NIDDM despite differences in insulin production, episodes of ketosis, or mode of therapy suggests the importance of hyperglycemia in the genesis of glomerular damage. Such an effect could be mediated directly through biochemical processes dependent on hyperglycemia or indirectly through the associated alterations in renal hemodynamics that seem to accompany poor glucose control.

Protein glycation, the formation of advanced glycation end-products, the aldose reductase pathway, glucose-induced changes in growth factors mediating a fibroproliferative response, vasoactive hormone receptor function, and others have all been implicated in hyperglycemic renal injury. Our ability to understand and then intercede on the mechanisms responsible may ultimately allow the benefits of "improved glycemic control" without the morbidity associated with hyperglycemia.

Morphology

Glomerular hypertrophy can be documented early in the course of IDDM. During the first several years of dia-betes, thickening of glomerular and tubular basement membranes occurs and the mesangium begins to accumulate periodic acid-Schiff (PAS)–positive material. These changes are related to the diabetic state, since they are not present in the nondiabetic twin of affected individuals. Glomerular morphologic alterations during the years prior to the occurrence of proteinuria have not yet been demonstrated to have pathogenetic or predictive significance, as morphologic changes seem to be present in most patients with IDDM, yet only a minority will ultimately develop ESRD. In patients with microalbuminuria who seem most likely to develop nephropathy, differences in glomerular morphometry are not apparent, so it is not yet clear whether mesangial expansion is the cause or the result of diabetic nephropathy.

Once proteinuria, hypertension, and renal failure ensue, the expansion of the mesangium and its impingement on the glomerular capillary loops, and therefore filtration surface area, correlate well with the loss of glomerular function. It is the diffuse mesangial expansion, rather than nodular glomerular sclerosis usually considered the morphologic sine qua non for diabetic nephropathy, that seems to be of the greatest significance in the pathogenesis of nephropathy. The end-stage diabetic kidney contains many glomeruli that demonstrate marked diffuse sclerosis.

Interstitial fibrosis, usually greatest in the area of sclerotic glomeruli, may be prominent and is highly correlated with progressive renal insufficiency in diabetes. Although it has been tacitly assumed to be due to "death" of a glomerulus with consequent atrophy of the associated tubule, there has been increased attention recently to the causes of interstitial fibrosis in diabetes and the possibility that it may be an important contributor to progressive loss of function. Diabetes may be associated with fibrosis of other tissues, such as tendons of the hand, and may therefore reflect a distinct pathophysiologic process in the kidney (see Chapter 37).

Clinical Evaluation

Diabetes affects the kidney throughout its duration, even in those not destined to develop frank nephropathy. At the onset of hyperglycemia and prior to the development of persistent proteinuria, subtle alterations in either renal structure or function appear to be present in most patients. Since only one-third of patients will ultimately develop nephropathy, it would be ideal to focus therapy on those at risk for this devastating diabetic complication, but that is not yet possible. Current epidemiologic data suggest that poor glycemic control, coexistent hypertension, familial history of diabetic nephropathy, familial history of essential hypertension or cardiovascular disease, maternal smoking during pregnancy, and low level of maternal education or persistent glomerular hyperfiltration are important risk factors and further studies may reveal their usefulness for prospectively identifying patients on whom to focus for intervention.

Most individuals who have IDDM and have persistent macroscopic proteinuria will ultimately develop diabetic ESRD, the major cause of renal failure in the United States. It is in these diabetics with renal disease that the largest increment in morbidity and mortality occurs and the greatest challenge is faced by the clinician.

Subjective Manifestations

Other than the polyuria associated with glycosuria, abnormalities of renal function in diabetes (as for any type of kidney disease) are notoriously silent. Once renal function has deteriorated, symptoms are usually related to salt retention (edema, pulmonary edema, congestive heart failure), hypertension (congestive heart failure, vision loss due to retinal hemorrhage, headache), neuropathy (dysesthesias or loss of sensation), or progressive azotemia (pruritus, nausea, vomiting, insomnia, decline in mental capacity, cramps). The coexistence of uremia and diabetes exacerbates the symptoms of neuropathy and may lead to a marked worsening of symptoms, such as orthostatic hypotension and gastroparesis. Differentiation of the latter from the nausea and vomiting of uremia may be difficult and requires careful attention to the entire clinical picture presented by the patient.

Objective Changes

As with most types of renal disease, blood pressure usually increases as kidney function deteriorates. Occasional IDDM patients may have hypertension early in the course of diabetes, due to coincidental essential hypertension, but an increase in blood pressure in any patient over time should alert the physician to the possible presence of renal disease. While patients with NIDDM have a nearly 50% prevalence of hypertension even in the absence of renal disease, deterioration of hypertensive control may precede the clinical recognition of renal disease. Particularly in young diabetics, blood pressure should be compared to that in either age-matched controls or previously obtained values in the patient, since the conventional "140/90" cutoff for normal blood pressure, based on epidemiologic studies in older patients with normal renal function, may not adequately reflect either the systemic or renal risks of hypertension, as has been shown in nondiabetics with renal disease.

Routine screening for microalbuminuria in preproteinuric patients with IDDM is now widely accepted as a method to identify individuals at high risk to develop nephropathy. However, in patients with NIDDM, interpretation of the values may be further confounded by the presence of essential hypertension, where microalbuminuria may be present even in the absence of identifiable renal disease and may fluctuate with the level of hypertensive control. In addition to the above, the presence of microalbuminuria is associated with increased cardiovascular morbidity and mortality in both IDDM and NIDDM.

Proteinuria that is persistent and detectable by routine screening tests marks the clinical onset of nephropathy. Fractionation of the proteinuria is not needed unless myeloma or light chain nephropathy is suggested by the history or physical examination. Routine or repeated quantitation of the proteinuria from 24-hr urine specimens is not necessary, unless clinical interventions are attempted to decrease proteinuria, in which case, the urine protein to creatinine ratio on a spot urine sample is a convenient mechanism for following proteinuria. Hematuria and red blood cells or red blood cell casts may occur in patients with diabetic nephropathy, but the presence of any of these should alert the clinician to consider alternative diagnoses such as glomerulonephritis or urinary tract malignancy. Particularly in NIDDM, the coexistence of diabetes and other causes of renal failure should be considered.

Renal function is usually monitored by the serum creatinine, but accurate interpretation requires an understanding of creatinine kinetics. Although the relationship between serum creatinine and GFR is an inverse one, it is not linear, because each doubling of the serum creatinine signals a loss of 50% of the renal function. At low levels of serum creatinine, for example, 0.8 mg/dL, an increase in the serum creatinine to 1.6 mg/dL represents a 60 mL/min decrement in GFR or a 50% fall. In some laboratories, a serum creatinine of 1.6 mg/dL is within the "normal" range, so a large reduction in renal function could be disregarded as "insignificant" by the clinician. At higher levels of serum creatinine, such as 4 mg/dL, an increase to 8 mg/dL also represents a 50% fall in GFR, but denotes a 15 mL/min decrement in GFR. Thus, to maximize preservation of renal function and direct therapeutic intervention in patients who have the most renal function to preserve, that is, those with a serum creatinine less than 2 mg/dL, an increased awareness of the implications of even marginal elevations in the serum creatinine is needed. A graphic representation of liter/serum creatinine versus time will follow a linear decline with a slope unique for that patient. Acute accelerations in the slope of the line should alert the clinician to superimposed conditions, such as the use of nonsteroidal anti-inflammatory drugs, urinary tract obstruction, poorly controlled blood pressure, and *papillary necrosis*, or interstitial nephritis from other drugs, and should be interpreted based on the clinical features of the patient. Such a graphic presentation may also be useful in following patients after the introduction of therapy, such as dietary protein restriction or blood pressure control, where the slope should decrease due to a reduction in the rate of progression of renal disease and may serve as positive reinforcement for many patients.

Interpretation of serum creatinine may be further confounded by the fact that the proximal tubule can secrete creatinine, particularly when glomerular filtration is reduced. Thus, symptoms of uremia may occur at serum creatinines much lower than expected due to augmented tubular secretion of creatinine. Cimetidine and trimethoprim inhibit the tubular secretion of creatinine and eventuate in a rise in the serum creatinine despite stable glomerular filtration. Cephalosporin antibiotics and plasma ketoacids (during diabetic ketoacidosis) interfere with the colorimetric assay for creatinine and result in false elevations. Despite these limitations, serum creatinine remains the most useful clinical marker of renal function. If desired, determination of creatinine clearance may be performed once to establish the relationship between serum creatinine and creatinine clearance in any given patient, but repeated measurements are usually not necessary unless the patient's muscle mass changes considerably.

Patients with mild diabetic nephropathy may develop hyperkalemia and metabolic acidosis out of proportion to their level of renal insufficiency due to a type IV *renal tubular acidosis*. This is usually due to hyporenin-hypoaldosteronism, but may be exacerbated by urinary track obstruction, angiotensin-converting enzyme inhibition, and nonsteroidal anti-inflammatory drug use, each of which may independently cause a type IV renal tubular acidosis. Diabetic patients may also develop wide fluctuations in the serum potassium with fluctuations in blood glucose levels, which may further accentuate the hyperkalemia in a type IV renal tubular acidosis.

The *nephrotic syndrome* may amplify the serum lipid abnormalities present in many diabetic patients. In particular, the serum cholesterol level may be elevated and is usually refractory to conservative therapy, such as dietary cholesterol restriction. In most nephrotic patients, hypercholesterolemia is inversely related to the serum albumin and treatment aimed at a reduction in proteinuria, such as dietary protein restriction, angiotensin-converting enzyme inhibition (or other antihypertensive therapy), or nonsteroidal anti-inflammatory drugs, may improve both the lipid profile and the proteinuria. Lipid-lowering agents, including nicotinic acid, cholestyramine, gemfibrozil, or the hydroxymethylglutaryl coenzyme A reductase inhibitors, may also be effective in patients with diabetic nephropathy, but long-term studies establishing efficacy and safety in this patient population are not available.

Assessment

Preclinical Years

Routine monitoring of the patients' blood pressure at each clinic visit is most important. Review of the family history, particularly with respect to hypertension and nephropathy, is also beneficial because a family history of either is a risk factor for the development of nephropathy. Yearly measurement of the serum creatinine and microalbuminuria is adequate, as long as the blood pressure remains normal and proteinuria is absent.

Diagnosis of Nephropathy

For IDDM patients in whom a progressive increase in the serum creatinine and hypertension are first noted within 10 to 30 years of diabetes, the diagnosis of diabetic nephropathy is a clinical one. However, for patients with hematuria, an unusual time course for the development of proteinuria (less than 10 years or more then 30 years), or systemic symptoms, such as myalgias, weight loss, and skin rash, other diagnoses should be considered and a renal biopsy may be necessary. In the past, the presence or absence of retinopathy has been used to determine the presence or absence of nephropathy. However, several studies have shown that greater than 90% of all patients with IDDM have retinopathy within 15 years of diabetes, which greatly diminishes the utility of retinopathy as a marker for renal disease. As many as 10% of patients with a history consistent with diabetic nephropathy may actually have other types of renal disease.

For patients with NIDDM, proteinuria does not appear to be a specific marker for diabetic nephropathy, so decisions about the need for a renal biopsy rest more heavily on the possible presence of a systemic disease with renal manifestations or a treatable primary renal disease. The diagnosis of diabetic nephropathy is further complicated by the increased likelihood of ischemic renal vascular disease, which may be treatable in this patient population. Although the physical examination and noninvasive testing may suggest renal vascular disease, a renal arteriogram must be done to establish the diagnosis (or its absence) if the clinical suspicion is significantly high. As in the nondiabetic population, angioplasty or surgery on the renal artery may have the most benefit in the preservation of renal function rather than the reversal of hypertension.

Progression of Nephropathy

Heightened awareness of serum creatinine and blood pressure are important during this period. As already noted, preservation of renal function is best done early in the course of renal insufficiency when the serum creatinine is less than 2 mg/dL, but a significant impact can still be obtained at higher levels of renal insufficiency. As renal function deteriorates, edema, congestive heart failure, and serum electrolytes (particularly potassium and bicarbonate) should be monitored. Although resistance to insulin is well documented in uremia, hypoglycemia due to decreased renal degradation of insulin is a greater clinical problem and the dose of insulin will usually require reduction.

Plan

Preclinical Phase (Normal Blood Pressure, No Microalbuminuria). Because *only one-third of patients with IDDM ultimately develop nephropathy*, it may be most effective to focus intervention aimed at preventing renal disease on those groups at the greatest risk, as noted earlier in the discussion of epidemiology. The success of any intervention during this prolonged symptom-free period (10–30 years) requires active involvement of all members of the health care team to maintain the patient's interest and enthusiasm.

Intensive Control of Blood Glucose Since several studies have suggested that patients with the greatest likelihood of developing diabetic nephropathy are those with the poorest level of glycemic control, intensive insulin therapy to produce euglycemia has been advanced as a goal for the diabetic patient. However, hypoglycemia and the attendant risk of central nervous system damage, loss of control of an automobile, and so forth must be balanced against the potential benefit. From a population-health viewpoint, a more reasonable goal may be to improve glycemic control in those patients with the greatest hyperglycemia and a number of other risk factors, since those patients appear to have a high risk for nephropathy, and to diminish the focus on euglycemia for those patients with the best control and fewest additional risk factors, recognizing that there may be no glycemic threshold for increased risk.[4]

Prevention of Hypertension The potential efficacy in preventing renal complications through the use of antihypertensive agents in normotensive, nonalbuminuric patients with normal renal function who may have isolated glomerular hypertension has not been reported, and this group represents the largest set of "preclinical" patients. The generalized use of antihypertensive agents in this group of patients should await evidence from clinical trials of a favorable cost, side-effect, and benefit profile.

However, it is reasonable to institute antihypertensive therapy in the small subset of IDDM patients who have essential hypertension, since a family history of hypertension is a risk factor for the development of nephropathy and coexistent hypertension augments the development of nephropathy in experimental models. In this setting, any antihypertensive agent

may be preferable to none, and there is increasing evidence that agents such as angiotensin-converting enzyme inhibitors (ACEIs) that exert effects directly on the renin-angiotensin system should be the agent of first choice.

Long-Term Dietary Protein Restriction. Diabetic patients have higher levels of dietary protein intake than their nondiabetic counterparts, which may exacerbate hemodynamic abnormalities within the diabetic kidney. Tight restriction of dietary protein intake has been advocated, but the potential benefit for the diabetic kidney during the preproteinuric period has not been studied.

Surveillance Yearly evaluation for microalbuminuria and serum creatinine levels and more frequent evaluation of the blood pressure form the cornerstone for the evaluation of renal function during the early years of diabetes.

Microalbuminuria phase. Once microalbuminuria has become persistent, therapy with an ACEI should be initiated to decrease the risk for developing persistent levels of proteinuria and progressive renal disease. The patient is likely to be normotensive at this time, so the therapy is aimed at treating underlying glomerular hypertension, and perhaps interfering with other potentially injurious effects of the renin-angiotensin system.[5] When ACEI cannot be tolerated, usually because of cough, AII receptor antagonists may be alternatives although large trials of their use in this situation are not available.

Proteinuric Patients. Once proteinuria has been established, therapy aimed at ameliorating the progression of renal failure is imperative. Although a very small minority of diabetics may have persistent proteinuria with stable renal function over a several-year period, the majority will ultimately develop ESRD. Antihypertensive therapy is the cornerstone of therapy in this group of patients, and improved glycemic control at this late stage does not appear to have a beneficial effect, probably because progression of the renal failure is dependent on the injurious compensatory processes with the nephron rather than ongoing diabetes-related injury per se.

Parving and collaborators have very convincingly demonstrated the beneficial effects of improved blood pressure control on the progressive decline in renal function in proteinuric patients with IDDM.[5] Using conventional (and, importantly, inexpensive) antihypertensive drugs to maintain the blood pressure at about 140/95 mmHg, these investigators were able to demonstrate a marked decline in the progression of renal failure. With equivalent levels of blood pressure control, ACEIs have an even more beneficial effect on the preservation of renal function than conventional agents such as β-blockers.[6] Thus, ACEIs or angiotensin II receptor antagonists should be included in the antihypertensive regimen in this group of patients. Often, as the renal disease progresses, more than one agent may be required and any of the available agents, if tolerated, are probably equivalent. The use of nifedipine has been controversial in this setting because of its occasional effect of increasing proteinuria and the reports of increased cardiovascular morbidity. Once a day dosing, if possible, improves patient compliance. If the patient has edema or congestive heart failure, loop diuretics such as furosemide will be necessary, as thiazide diuretics are not effective when the serum creatinine is greater than 2 mg/dL.

The level to which the blood pressure should be reduced has not been established. In patients with other types of renal disease, a progressive benefit has been shown with decrease in blood pressures to as low as 120/70 mmHg, but such decrements may be associated with worsened orthostatic hypertension in diabetic patients with autonomic neuropathy. Clearly, the conventional 140/90 mmHg threshold may be appropriate for the prevention of stroke in essential hypertensive patients with normal renal function, but it may not be optimal for a young diabetic with renal disease.[7]

Dietary protein restriction will also reduce proteinuria and slow the progression of diabetic nephropathy. Although a dietary protein intake of about 0.6 g/kg/day is most often prescribed for patients or used in research studies, patient compliance is difficult. Even when patients take as much as 0.9 g/kg/day (determined by urea clearance) beneficial effects of protein restriction can be documented. Formerly, patients with the nephrotic syndrome were encouraged to augment their protein intake to maintain plasma protein levels. Paradoxically, a high-protein diet will often lead to a further decrease in the serum albumin, increased intraglomerular pressure, and the attendant augmentation in proteinuria. A reduction in dietary protein intake will decrease proteinuria and may eventuate in an increment in the serum albumin. A reduction in proteinuria may diminish the hypercholesterolemia associated with the nephrotic syndrome.

For patients with a type IV metabolic acidosis, supplementation with bicarbonate will improve both the acidosis and the hyperkalemia. This is best accomplished by the use of oral sodium bicarbonate or sodium citrate, but diuretics may need to be increased because of the sodium load. Angiotensin-converting enzyme inhibitors or nonsteroidal anti-inflammatory drugs will exacerbate a hyperkalemic metabolic acidosis, which may necessitate their discontinuation if the acidosis and hyperkalemia cannot otherwise be controlled. In patients with wide fluctuations in glycemic control, a type IV renal tubular acidosis will accentuate the hyperkalemia associated with hyperglycemia.

End-Stage Renal Disease. Anticipating the development of ESRD is important so that the patient will have made a selection regarding dialysis modality and/or transplantation months in advance. Once the serum creatinine has risen to about 4 mg/dL (and about 75% of the kidney function has been lost), discussions about ESRD therapy should be initiated. Treatment for ESRD is indicated when the patient has symptoms of uremia, such as pruritus, nausea, vomiting, muscle cramps, refractory edema, hyperkalemia, or acidosis. Although dialysis or transplantation is usually required once the serum creatinine reaches 8–10 mg/dL in nondiabetics, patients with diabetes are less able to tolerate the symptoms of uremia and may require renal replacement therapy before the creatinine rises to that level. *Diabetic patients are now commonly considered as candidates for all types of ESRD therapy: transplantation, hemodialysis, and peritoneal dialysis.*

Of the three modalities for the treatment of ESRD, renal transplantation offers patients the greatest sense of well-being and the best opportunity for a return to a productive lifestyle. However, only recipients of HLA-identical sibling grafts enjoy an increased survival compared with dialysis patients. At the University of Minnesota, long-term (more than 10 years) and patient graft survival statistics are available for diabetic patients transplanted in the late 1960s and 1970s. Forty percent of the 250 diabetic patients receiving renal transplants during that time were alive 10 years later; 75% of those have a functioning graft. As already noted, both patient and graft survival was best in recipients of HLA-identical sibling donor grafts (see Chapter 5).

Following successful transplantation, peripheral and autonomic neuropathy subjectively improves within the first 6–12 months; however, detailed, quantitative neurologic testing fails to show a measurable improvement. Advanced retinopathy remains stable in the majority of the patients. However, nearly 20% of transplanted diabetic patients have lost a limb related to peripheral vascular disease within 5 years after the transplant, which represents a major source of morbidity following transplantation. Cardiovascular disease is a major cause of posttransplantation mortality, and studies are underway at several centers to address strategies to reduce the risk of myocardial infarction after transplantation.

Vascular access for hemodialysis is a major problem for diabetic patients on hemodialysis due to vascular disease and the difficulty in constructing a well-functioning fistula. Therefore, if a patient has selected hemodialysis, a fistula or goretex graft should be placed several months before the likely need for the initiation of dialysis. The use of temporary or even tunneled catheters is not an optimal alternative because of problems with infection, thrombosis, and, often, poor adequacy of dialysis.

In general, diabetic patients tolerate hemodialysis. When good blood pressure control is maintained during the interdialytic period, retinopathy does not accelerate, contrary to beliefs during the 1970s. The neuropathies of uremia and diabetes seem to be synergistic, and subjective improvements in peripheral and autonomic neuropathy following initiation of dialysis are less than those following transplantation.

Peritoneal dialysis is well tolerated in diabetic patients. The high glucose concentrations (ranging from 1,500 to 4,250 mg/dL) in the dialysate may eventuate in worsened hyperglycemia, but insulin can be added to the peritoneal dialysis fluid to minimize this problem. Of note, insulin administered into the peritoneum is absorbed into the portal system, which may have advantageous metabolic effects. Blind patients are able to perform peritoneal dialysis independently because of the availability of equipment that mechanizes the sterile attachment of bags of dialysis fluid to the peritoneal dialysis catheter. Although in the past dialysis has not offered patients the same improvement in quality of life as renal transplantation, the recent introduction of *erythropoietin* may serve to diminish the differences in quality of life between the different treatments.

References

1. Borch-Johnsen K, Andersen PK, Deckert T: The effect of proteinuria on relative mortality in type 1 (insulin-dependent diabetes mellitus). Diabetologia 28:590–596, 1985.

2. Nosadini R, Brocco E: Relationships among microalbuminuria, insulin resistance and renal-cardiac complications in insulin dependent and non insulin dependent diabetes. Exp Clin Endocrinol Diabetes 105(suppl. 2): 1–7, 1997.

3. Rudberg, S, Stattin, EL, Dahlquist, G: Familial and perinatal risk factors for micro-and macroalbuminuria in young IDDM patients. Diabetes 47:1121–1126, 1998.

4. Steffes MW: Glycemic control and the initiation and progression of the complications of diabetes mellitus. Kidney Int 63:S36–39, 1997.

5. Lewis EJ, Hunsicker LG, Bain, RP et al.: The effect of angiotensin-convernting enzyme inhibition on diabetic nephropathy. New Engl J Med 329:1456–1462, 1993.

6. Parving HH, Andersen AR, Smidt UM, Svendsen PA: Early aggressive antihypertensive treatment reduces rate of decline in kidney function in diabetic nephropathy. Lancet 1175–1178, 1989.

7. Breyer JA: Therapeutic interventions for nephropathy in type I diabetes mellitus. Seminars Nephrol 17:114–123, 1997.

28

Cardiovascular Complications of Diabetes Mellitus

Thomas M. Guest, Laurence S. Sperling, David J. Ballard, and William S. Weintraub

Introduction

Diabetes mellitus affects the cardiovascular system in numerous ways, the most apparent of which is a dramatically increased incidence and prevalence of atherosclerotic vascular disease. But diabetes may also directly affect both systolic and diastolic myocardial function in the absence of coronary vasculopathy. Diabetes-associated neuropathies may involve the cardiovascular system, resulting in presyncope/syncope, arrhythmias, and an increased perioperative risk. Each of these topics is presented in Table 28–1.

Atherosclerosis

Epidemiology

Diabetes is clearly a strong and independent risk factor for the development of coronary atherosclerosis. The leading cause of morbidity and mortality in diabetic patients is atherosclerotic cardiovascular disease,[1–3] with the age-adjusted incidence of myocardial infarction being six times greater in diabetic men and four

TABLE 28–1 Cardiovascular Complications of Diabetes Mellitus

Atherosclerosis
  Epidemiology
  Pathophysiology
    Lipid disorders
    Insulin resistance
    Coagulation disorders
    Advanced glycation end-products
  Diagnostic difficulties
  Treatment
Syndrome X
Congestive heart failure
Autonomic neuropathy
Preoperative evaluation and operative risks

times greater in diabetic women than in nondiabetic subjects.[4] Diabetic patients with acute myocardial infarction also suffer significantly higher postinfarction morbidity and mortality.[5–7] More than 75% of hospitalizations for diabetes-related complications are secondary to cardiovascular disease.[8] Intensive glycemic control, while having a favorable effect on the incidence of renal-vascular disease and proliferative retinopathy, has not been conclusively shown to lessen the cardiovascular risk of insulin-dependent diabetes mellitus (IDDM).[9] Hypertension control in those with diabetes is extremely important (see Chapter 38).

Pathophysiology

Lipid Disorders. Both IDDM and non-insulin-dependent diabetes mellitus (NIDDM) are associated with lipid abnormalities that increase the patient's cardiovascular risk (see Chapter 39). Lipid abnormalities in poorly controlled IDDM typically include decreased high-density lipoprotein (HDL) levels, modestly elevated low-density lipoprotein (LDL) levels, and dramatically increased triglycerides. Each of these lipid abnormalities can be significantly improved with adequate glycemic control.[10] Lipid patterns in NIDDM typically include low HDL levels, normal LDL levels, elevated triglycerides, and an increase in very low-density lipoprotein (VLDL)-triglyceride levels. Lipid abnormalities in NIDDM appear to be related to both poor glycemic control and insulin resistance.[11]

Management of lipid disorders in diabetics, as in other patients, needs to include diet and exercise. Bile acid sequestrants and nicotinic acid should be used cautiously in diabetic patients, as these medicines can accentuate hypertriglyceridemia and worsen glucose tolerance, respectively. Therefore, the medication class of choice for the treatment of lipoprotein abnormalities in diabetics is the HMG-CoA reductase inhibitors. These medications will favorably affect LDL and HDL levels. In the Scandinavian Simvastatin Survival Study, treatment of diabetic patients with an HMG-CoA reductase inhibitor was of greater benefit in diabetic subjects than in the complete study population, for the secondary prevention of cardiovascular death and morbidity.[12] When significant hypertriglyceridemia is present, fibric-acid derivatives are often effective.[13] Although increases of LDL levels in both IDDM and NIDDM are modest, there is evidence that glycosylated LDL may be more sensitive to oxidation[14] and uptake by macrophages.[15] These processes are important early events in the development of atherosclerotic plaques.

Insulin Resistance. Resistance to the biological actions of insulin is a common condition, occurring in most patients with NIDDM[16] and in some individuals with normal glucose tolerance. The primary mechanism of insulin resistance appears to involve impairment of tyrosine kinase activity of the insulin receptor.[17] The altered sensitivity to insulin typically involves both a rightward and a downward shift of the insulin dose-response curve.

Recent data suggest that insulin resistance may be a risk factor for atherosclerotic vascular disease, independent of plasma glucose and insulin levels. This large study revealed an inverse relation between insulin sensitivity and atherosclerosis, as measured by ultrasonographic intimal-medial thickness of the carotid artery, in Hispanic and non-Hispanic caucasian Americans but not among African Americans.[18] The relationship between insulin sensitivity and atherosclerosis is only partially accounted for by traditional cardiovascular risk factors. The observed ethnic differences were not explained by the available data.

It is unclear whether insulin resistance and/or hyperinsulinemia accelerate atherosclerosis directly via mitogenic effects on the vascular wall or indirectly through their effects on hypertension, lipid abnormalities, obesity, and possibly coagulation disorders.[19-21] Thiazoliddinediones represent a novel class of drugs that may directly decrease insulin resistance by enhancing insulin sensitivity of skeletal muscle, adipose tissue, and liver. While one of these agents, troglitazone, has proven to have beneficial effects on glycemic control and lipid profiles, no studies evaluating its effect on vascular disease have yet been done.[22-24] This agent should be used cautiously, as it may cause fatal liver disease (see Chapter 20).

Coagulation Disorders. Data from clinical studies have demonstrated a hypercoagulable state in terms of both platelet aggregation and the coagulation cascades in diabetic patients. An imbalance between thrombosis and fibrinolysis exists, favoring not only thrombus formation on a disrupted coronary plaque, but also formation of microthrombi in the arterial wall.

In diabetes, in the presence or absence of vascular disease, there appears to be an ex vivo hyperaggregability of platelets in response to a number of agents.[25-28]

Mechanisms of platelet dysfunction include increased levels of thromboxane A_2 and B_2, decreased platelet cAMP and cGMP, and endothelial release of PGI_2, nitric oxide, and plasminogen-activator inhibitor (PAI). Paired with enhanced platelet aggregation are other factors in the diabetic patient that predispose to thrombosis. These include increased fibrinogen, tissue factor pathway inhibitor and thrombin, and decreased antithrombin III and endogenous heparin. Tissue factor pathway inhibitor levels correlate with serum total cholesterol levels.[29]

Paired with this predisposition to thrombosis is an impairment of endogenous fibrinolytic activity in plasma from diabetic patients. This appears to be secondary to the increased PAI-1 activity, decreased t-PA, activity and $\alpha2$-antiplasmin concentrations present in many diabetic patients.[30,31] Diabetic patients also have elevated plasma concentrations of fibrinogen and von Willebrand's factor and increased factor VIII procoagulant activity, which appear to be sensitive to glycemic control.[32]

In sum, there is enhanced thrombus formation and attenuated fibrinolysis in the diabetic population. This procoagulant state may accelerate acute thrombus formation on a fractured coronary plaque and may also result in the propagation and persistence of microthrombi. Microthrombi prompt the release of platelet-associated vascular mitogens, including platelet-derived growth factor (PDGF), transforming growth factor-beta (TGFβ), and epidermal growth factor (EGF).[33] Thus, the coagulation disorders associated with diabetes likely contribute to the observed accelerated atherosclerosis.

Advanced Glycation End-Products. Advanced glycosylated end-products (AGEs) are the late products of the modification of proteins (and also lipids and nucleic acids) by reducing sugars. Elevated serum levels can be found in diabetic patients, chronic renal failure patients with amyloidosis, and the elderly. AGEs constitute a class of heterologous yellow-brown pigments that have a characteristic fluorescence, tend to form cross-links between themselves, generate reactive oxygen intermediates (ROIs), and have specific cellular receptors.[34,35] There are three general mechanisms by which AGEs may have pathologic effects: (1) intracellular AGEs can directly alter protein and protein function at target tissues; (2) extracellular AGEs can interfere with extracellular matrix function; and (3) extracellular AGEs can induce receptor-mediated soluble ligand production (hormones, cytokines, free radicals).[36,37] AGEs are expressed by endothelial cells and vascular smooth muscle cells (VSMCs) in vitro and have recently been immunolocalized to the medial arterial wall.[38,39]

The role of AGEs in vascular disease is a developing field of study. It has been prompted by the discovery that glycated proteins can generate ROIs,[40,41] a process that is active in the development of atherosclerosis. It also has been shown that AGEs, in both endothelial cell culture and animal models, can produce oxidant stress by a receptor-mediated mechanism, manifest by the appearance of thiobarbituric acid-reactive substances (TBARS) in tissue and malondialdehyde determinants in the vascular wall, and blocked in each case by antioxidants.[42] This oxidant stress has been shown to induce expression of NFκB and VCAM-1,[42,43] thus regulating genes known to be essential to the development of ASCVD.[44,45]

AGEs also play an important role in the regulation of nitric oxide (NO), as AGEs are able to quench NO both in vitro and in rat models. The time course for this closely mirrors that of free radical production by AGEs,[46] supporting the concept of NO quenching by an enhanced free radical load induced by glucose. Also, highly glycosylated hemoglobin, compared to low- or nonglycosylated hemoglobin, inhibits acetylcholine-induced, endothelium-dependent relaxation in rat aorta.[47] A recent study suggests that aging-related vasodilatory impairment and cardiac hypertrophy is prevented by AGE inhibition with aminoguanidine in the rat.[48] AGEs also have been shown to block the antiproliferative effects of NO in rat VSMCs.[49]

AGEs may also contribute to cardiovascular disease by modification of the extracellular matrix (ECM) and/or matrix metalloproteinases (MMPs). AGEs are known to modify ECM molecules, including collagen, laminin, and vitronectin. ECM alteration may result in an expansion of type I collagen packing, an inhibition of type IV collagen association, and decreased EC adhesion. In diabetes, a loss of matrix-bound heparin sulfate proteoglycan is seen in response to AGE-modification of laminin and vitronectin and is thought to stimulate the overproduction of other matrix components. Soluble plasma proteins, such as low-density lipoprotein (LDL) and immunoglobulin G (IgG), can be covalently linked by AGEs on collagen, resulting in the subendothelial accumulation of AGE-linked proteins and contributing to the characteristic diabetic vascular disease. There is abundant evidence that AGEs regulate MMPs in a variety of tissues, but to date no studies looking specifically at the vasculature have been done.

Assessment and Diagnostic Difficulties

The incidence and prevalence of angina, myocardial infarction, sudden death, and congestive heart failure are significantly increased in patients with both type 1 and type 2 diabetes. The premature occurrence of vascular disease, the more extensive disease at initial diagnosis, and the increased morbidity and mortality raise the issue of whether the atherosclerotic process is different in diabetics.[50] Thus, any symptoms suggestive of a cardiac etiology should be thoroughly evaluated.

Symptoms of chest discomfort, dyspnea, and peripheral edema warrant special attention in the diabetic.

Atypical symptoms are frequent. The presence of autonomic neuropathy may alter pain perception related to myocardial ischemia and result in silent ischemia. Unrecognized myocardial infarction is also more common in diabetics.[51] Autonomic neuropathy may affect resting heart rate and parasympathetically regulated heart rate variability. This may be associated with an increased risk of sudden death from cardiac dysrhythmia.[52] Often, the diagnosis of coronary artery disease may be difficult on the basis of the clinical history and examination. The resting 12-lead ECG is commonly normal. Therefore, appropriate noninvasive studies can be beneficial. A standard exercise treadmill test is appropriate for those with a normal baseline ECG and reasonable functional status. In patients with typical symptoms or an abnormal resting ECG a perfusion imaging study[53] or stress echocardiogram should be considered to assess left ventricular function and to provide potential quantitative information. If clinical symptoms of recent onset or of an unstable nature appear, coronary angiography should be considered. Of note, diabetics treated with metformin should withhold this medication for 48 hr following iodinated contrast dye administration, given the known increased risk of potentially fatal lactic acidosis.

Unfortunately, a large proportion of diabetic patients have subclinical coronary artery disease that may rapidly progress to unstable coronary syndromes and/or sudden death. Identification of the patient with subclinical atherosclerosis with diagnostic tools such as electron beam computed tomography or carotid ultrasound may be an important means to reduce future events by aggressive risk reduction. The presence of cerebrovascular and/or peripheral vascular disease often indicates widespead atherosclerotic disease. The presence of microalbuminuria is also a major predictor of underlying atherosclerotic disease. Such patients are at a significantly increased risk for a cardiovascular event, and secondary preventive strategies should be pursued aggressively.

Treatment and Management Considerations

Once the diagnosis of cardiovascular disease has been established, the physician has a wide range of therapeutic options (Table 28–2). Recently, both medical treatment options and revascularization techniques have been greatly improved. Goals of therapy include improvement in symptoms and quality of life as well as reduction in morbidity and mortality. Major efforts should be directed at identifying concomitant cardiovascular risk factors and treating these aggressively. Recent evidence supports optimal treatment of hypertension and reduction in LDL cholesterol in diabetics.

TABLE 28–2 Treatment Options for Diabetics with Coronary Disease

Medical treatment
  β-Blockers
  Nitrates
  ACE inhibitors
  Aspirin
  Lipid-lowering medications (First line: HMG CoA
    reductive inhibitors or fibric acid derivatives)
Angioplasty
  Single vessel disease (Note: increased restenosis rate in
    diabetics)
Bypass surgery
  Proximal, multivessel disease (with/without LV
    dysfunction)
  Left main

Diabetes remains a risk for poor outcome in patients with established coronary disease. In long-term follow-up of diabetics post-myocardial infarction (MI) or revascularization there is a marked increase in death after controlling for other known risk factors. After myocardial infarction there is a higher risk of death, heart failure, and other complications.[54]

Standard medical therapy should include consideration of β-blockers, aspirin, ACEIs, converting enzyme inhibitors, and lipid-lowering therapy.[55] β-Blockers are effective in treating angina and have demonstrated a consistent benefit in the post-MI setting. In the MIAMI trial the reduction in mortality due to metoprolol at 15 days post-MI was four times greater in diabetics than nondiabetics.[56] β-Blockers can be used safely in diabetics; however, their potential for masking hypoglycemic symptoms has unnecessarily limited usage. Unless contraindicated, aspirin should be given to all patients with known vascular disease and potentially all with an increased risk of a cardiovascular event. ACE inhibitors should be considered first line antihypertensive agents in diabetics given the recent data on curbing proteinuria, limiting remodeling after myocardial infarction, and mortality benefit in patients with left ventricular dysfunction.[55] As previously indicated, treatment of lipid abnormalities is critical in patients with known symptomatic disease and early asymptomatic atherosclerosis. A 55% reduction in mortality was noted in diabetics treated with simvastatin followed in the 4S trial,[57] as was a 25% risk reduction confirmed in diabetics treated with pravastatin in the CARE trial.[58]

Thrombolytic therapy, angioplasty, and bypass surgery are other potential treatment options for both stable and unstable coronary disease. Thrombolytic therapy is at least as effective in diabetic patients, possibly more so.[59] It has been found to be most beneficial when administered within the first 6 hr of onset of symptoms. Patients with diabetes account for a signifi-

cant percentage of patients undergoing revascularization procedures. Revascularization options for diabetics pose a challenge because long-term event rates are known to be high. The results of several large angioplasty registries have demonstrated that diabetics undergoing angioplasy have similar initial procedural success rates, but clearly have worse long-term outcomes. Restenosis rates have also been shown to be repeatedly higher in diabetics.[60,61] Diabetes is associated with a higher perioperative morbidity as well as decreased survival following coronary artery bypass surgery. There is an increase in sternal wound infections in diabetics in whom bilateral internal mammary arteries are used for grafts. Although the Emory Angioplasty versus Surgery (EAST) study showed no survival difference between bypass surgery and angioplasty in a small number of treated diabetics.[62,63] Recent data from the BARI[64] and CABRI[66] trials have suggested that diabetics have a higher mortality with angioplasty than surgery. In the BARI study at 5 years survival rate was 65.5% in the angioplasty group versus 80.6% in the bypass group.[64] Presently, evidence-based medicine favors bypass surgery for the diabetic with significant, multivessel coronary disease. Unfortunately, there is often distal vessel disease or small vessel involvement in diabetics, which may be suboptimal for revascularization. Several recent reports have demonstrated important findings that may guide future approaches to the management of diabetics with and without heart disease. The DIGAMI study group[66] reported a 30% 1-year and 11% 3-year reduction in mortality in diabetics with acute MI treated with acute administration of insulin and glucose followed by intensive treatment with multidose subcutaneous insulin. Importantly, diabetic patients without a previous myocardial infarction appear to have as high a risk of MI as nondiabetic patients with a history of a prior MI.[67] Thus, it may be prudent to address all diabetics as intensively in terms of risk reduction goals.

Syndrome X

The original use of the term syndrome X in the cardiac literature was by Kemp in 1967 to describe angina or angina-like chest pain without angiographic evidence of coronary artery disease.[68] *Cardiac syndrome X* probably represents a varied group of vascular pathologies that are characterized by an inability of the coronary vascular bed to adequately respond to increased myocardial oxygen demand. Thus, cardiac syndrome X is frequently referred to as microvascular angina. In 1988, Reaven also used the term syndrome X to describe the metabolic manifestations of insulin resistance and/or chronic hyperinsulinemia in nondiabetic subjects.[20] The *metabolic syndrome X* includes glucose intolerance, hyperinsulinemia, hypertension, and dyslipidemia.

There now exists mounting evidence that the two forms of syndrome X may share a common metabolic etiology. Studies from several groups have suggested that a significant portion of nondiabetic subjects with cardiac syndrome X, or microvascular angina, exhibit insulin resistance and lipid abnormalities.[69–71] These findings raise the possibility that the cardiac syndrome X is merely a manifestation of the metabolic syndrome X.

Cardiomyopathy

Diabetic patients are known to be at an increased risk of *congestive heart failure*.[72,73] This was traditionally thought to be secondary to accelerated coronary artery disease or coronary microangiopathy.[74] However, it has become clear that particular histologic changes also contribute to diabetic cardiomyopathy. The histologic changes include accumulation of PAS-positive material between muscle fibers and collections of collagen and glycoprotein extending into T-tubules.[75] There may also be lipid accumulation within the cardiomyocytes. The myocardial changes can be detected echocardiographically, even before the onset of hemodynamic abnormalities.[76,77] In the absence of vascular disease, these structural changes are felt to account for the clinical observations of reduced diastolic compliance and abnormal systolic function. The onset of diastolic dysfunction typically precedes that of systolic dysfunction.[78] There is also mounting evidence that adrenergic desensitization, metabolic disturbances of free fatty acids and lipids, altered calcium handling, and regulation of myosin light chain phosphorylation also contribute to diabetic cardiomyopathy.[79–82] Given the high incidence of hypertension, coronary artery disease, and multiple cardiovascular risk factors in the diabetic population, it is often difficult to determine the etiology of congestive heart failure in the individual patient. Clinically, congestive heart failure without vascular disease is more common in the diabetic female than in the diabetic male.

Therapeutic modalities for the treatment of diabetic patients with congestive heart failure (Table 28–3) are no different than those for nondiabetics. Patients should follow a low sodium diet and fluid restriction. Systolic dysfunction should include vasodilators (preferably ACE inhibitors), diuretics, and possibly digitalis glycosides as a positive ionotrope. Treatment of diastolic dysfunction in diabetic patients includes the use of calcium-channel blockers (preferably verapamil or diltiazem) to decrease heart rate as a means to increase diastolic filling time and to decrease myocardial contractility, which improves the oxygen supply/demand ratio. Recently, the use of low-dose β-blockers has proven useful in the treatment of both systolic and diastolic heart failure; diabetes is a relative contraindication to the use of this drug, as it can blunt the adrenergic response to hypoglycemia.

Infants born to diabetic mothers have a high incidence of congestive heart failure. This frequently is a transient condition, presumably with a metabolic cause, that resolves spontaneously. However, hypertrophic cardiomyopathy and abnormal ventricular diastolic filling can also occur and seems to be associated with macrosomia and related to poor maternal glycemic control.[83,84]

Autonomic Neuropathy

Diabetic neuropathies of the autonomic nervous system appear to have deleterious effects on the cardiovascular system (see Chapter 36). Under normal conditions the autonomic nervous system regulates heart rate, cardiac contractility, systemic vascular resistance, and venous capacitance. Parasympathetic dysfunction is manifest by an increased resting heart rate and the lack of heart rate variability in response to deep breathing.[85] Sympathetic dysfunction typically follows the parasympathetic changes and results in impaired blood pressure responses to standing or sustained handgrip and a decrease in the resting heart rate from the prior tachycardia.[85]

Diabetic cardiac autonomic neuropathy clinically is associated with an increased incidence of sudden cardiorespiratory death and a greater perioperative risk[86,87] (see Chapter 43). The etiology of these increased risks is postulated to be reentrant ventricular arrhythmias associated with uneven sympathetic denervation and a prolonged QT interval.[88] Other manifestations of diabetic autonomic neuropathy include poor exercise tolerance, loss of diurnal blood pressure regulation, decreased hypoglycemic awareness, abnormal systolic ejection fraction, and diastolic filling at rest and with exercise.[89] Interestingly, autonomic denervation has not been cor-

TABLE 28–3 Heart Failure/Cardiomyopathy in Diabetes

Etiology	Plans	Therapy
Obstructive CAD	Angiography	Revascularization
Diastolic dysfunction	Echo	Calcium blocker, ACE-inhibitor
Systolic dysfunction (without significant CAD)	Echo, functional study, +/− angiography	Vasodiolators (ACE-inhibitor), diuretics, digitalis, β-blocker, limit sodium

related with the phenomenon of silent myocardial ischemia present in many diabetic patients.[90] Evaluation of the cardiac autonomic nervous system in diabetic patients should include measurements of (1) resting pulse rate—greater than 100 bpm is abnormal; (2) pulse rate variation to breathing—acceleration with inspiration of less than 10 bpm is abnormal; (3) pulse rate response to Valsalva maneuver—normally, tachycardia develops with strain and is followed by bradycardia with release; (4) pulse rate response at 15 and 30 sec after standing—normally, tachycardia is followed by reflex bradycardia; (5) systolic blood pressure response 2 min after standing—a decrease of greater than 20 mm Hg is abnormal, a decrease of 10–19 mm Hg is borderline abnormal; (6) diastolic blood pressure response to isometric handgrip—an increase of greater than 16 mm Hg in the relaxed arm is normal; (7) the ECG QT interval—the QT_c should be less than 440 ms. Of these testing modalities, the Valsalva maneuver is likely the best for longitudinally screening for the onset of cardiac autonomic neuropathy.[91] In addition to the above diagnostic tests, a number of investigators have begun to utilize holter monitoring to track patterns of heart rate variability, [123I]metaiodobenzylguanidine (MIBG) to identify patients with early disease,[92] pulse wave velocity to evaluate arterial wall elasticity,[93] and QT dispersion (difference between the longest and shortest intervals) to assess adrenergic denervation and arrhythmic risk.[94]

Diabetic patients should be evaluated on a yearly basis for the development of autonomic neuropathy. Those patients with cardiac autonomic neuropathy need to avoid dehydration or exertion in hot weather conditions and to make certain to avoid the development of foot ulcers (see Chapter 33). Physicians of patients with autonomic neuropathy will need to treat arrhythmias as they develop, manage the increased perioperative risk, and consider relaxing glycemic control to avert hypoglycemic episodes.

Preoperative Evaluation and Operative Risks (see Chapter 43)

Diabetes is a definite predictor of increased perioperative risk in patients undergoing noncardiac surgery. The ACC/AHA task force on perioperative cardiovascular evaluation guidelines[95] classifies diabetes as an intermediate clinical predictor of risk for perioperative myocardial infarction, death, and congestive heart failure. Major predictors of risk include active unstable coronary syndromes, decompensated heart failure, and presence of significant arrhythmias or valvular disease. Other intermediate predictors of increased risk include stable angina, evidence of prior myocardial infarction by history or ECG, or compensated heart failure.[95]

TABLE 28–4 Preoperative Evaluation in Diabetes

Subjective
  Unstable cardiac symptoms (angina, CHF)
  Arrhythmia or syncope
  Valvular disease, previous MI or CHF
  Functional status/exercise tolerance
Objective
  Type and risk of surgical procedure
  Signs of CHF (rales, S3, elevated JVP)
  ECG abnormalities
Plans
  Perioperative risk stratification
  Consider preoperative β-blockers
  Postoperative ECG and cardiac enzymes

Because of the high prevalence of occult obstructive coronary disease in diabetics and the potential for asymptomatic ischemia, a preoperative functional study such as an exercise treadmill, nuclear imaging study, or stress echocardiogram should be considered prior to elective, noncardiac surgery for risk stratification. In particular, an evaluation (Table 28–4) should be strongly considered prior to vascular procedures and prolonged surgical procedures associated with large fluid shifts or significant blood loss. In addition, risk stratification should certainly be considered in diabetics of limited functional capacity.[96] Patients with high risk or equivocal results on noninvasive testing who are reasonable candidates for revascularization should undergo coronary angiographic evaluation prior to intermediate or high-risk surgery. Patients who have recently undergone revascularization or angiography require no additional preoperative evaluation if there has been no interval change in their clinical status.

Perioperative cardiac enzyme and ECG surveillance is recommended in patients with known coronary disease, those who are at high risk, and those undergoing a surgical procedure with a high likelihood of stress. Perioperative β-blockers should be considered in this same population. Diabetics on insulin or oral hypoglycemic agents should have their blood glucose values closely monitored. Perioperative evaluation may identify important cardiovascular problems and risk factors for the first time; appropriate treatment plans and goals therefore should be defined and communicated to the primary care physician.

Summary and Research Considerations

Diabetic patients exhibit multiple abnormalities of the cardiovascular system, resulting in significant increases in morbidity and mortality. A better understanding of the mechanisms by which the cardiac and vascular pathologies develop will guide the evolution of future treatment strategies. Current treatment considerations need to focus on the aggressive control of lipid abnormalities and hypertension, as well as risk factor modification. It is likely that ongoing clinical trials will associate tight glycemic control with a decreased risk of atherosclerotic vascular disease. Trials to evaluate the effects of antioxidants and aminoguanidine on atherosclerosis are planned and may provide a rationale for their use in the near future.

References

1. Cullen K, Stenhouse NS, Wearne KL, et al.: Multiple regression analysis of risk factors for cardiovascular disease and cancer mortality in Busselton, Western Australia: 13 year study. J Chronic Dis 36:371–77, 1983.

2. Eschwege E, Richard JL, Thibult N, et al.: Coronary heart disease mortality in relation with diabetes, blood glucose and plasma insulin levels: the Paris prospective study, ten years later. Horm Metab Res 15(suppl.):41–46, 1985.

3. Fontbonne A, Charles MA, Thibult N, et al.: Hyperinsulinaemia as a predictor of coronary heart disease mortality in a healthy population: the Paris prospective study, 15 year follow-up. Diabetologia 34:356–361, 1991.

4. Pyorala K, Savolainen E, Kaukola S, et al.: Plasma insulin and coronary heart disease risk factor relationship to other risk factors and predictive value during 9.5–year follow-up of the Helsinki policeman study population. Acta Med Scand 701(suppl.):38–52, 1985.

5. Stone PH, Muller JE, Hartwell T, et al.: The effect of diabetes mellitus on prognosis and serial left ventricular function after acute myocardial infarction: Contribution of both coronary disease and diastolic left ventricular dysfunction to the adverse prognosis. J Am Coll Cardiol 14:49, 1989.

6. Herlitz J, Malmberg K, Karlson BW, et al.: Mortality and morbidity during a five-year follow-up of diabetics with myocardial infarction. Acta Med Scand 62:118, 1988.

7. Abbott RD, Donahue RP, Kannel WB, et al.: The impact of diabetes on survival following myocardial infarction in men vs. women. The Framingham Study. JAMA 260:3456, 1988.

8. American Diabetes Association: Consensus statement: Role of cardiovascular risk factors in prevention and treatment of macrovascular disease in diabetes. Diabetes Care 16:72–78, 1993.

9. The Diabetes Control and Complications Trial Research Group: The effect of intensive treatment of diabetes on the development and progression of long-term complications in insulin-dependent diabetes mellitus. New Engl J Med 329:977, 1993.

10. Garg A: Management of dyslipidemia in IDDM patients. Diabetes Care 17:224–234, 1994.

11. Ginsberg NH: Lipoprotein physiology in nondiabetic and diabetic states: Relationship to atherosclerosis. Diabetes Care 14:839–855, 1991.

12. Scandinavian Simvastatin Survival Study Group: Randomized trial of cholesterol lowering in 4444 patients with coronary heart disease: Scandinavian Simvastatin Survival Study (4S). Lancet 344:1383–1389, 1994.

13. Koskinen P, Manttari M, Manninen V, et al.: Coronary heart disease incidence in NIDDM patients in the Helsinki Heart Study. Diabetes Care 15:820–825, 1992.

14. Bowie A, Owens D, Collins P, et al.: Glycosylated low-density lipoprotein is more sensitive to oxidation: Implications for the diabetic patient? Atherosclerosis 102:63–67, 1993.

15. Klein RL, Laiimins M, Lopes-Virella MF: Isolation, characterization, and metabolism of the glycated and nonglycated subfractions of low-density lipoproteins isolated from type I diabetic patients and nondiabetic subjects. Diabetes 44:1093–1098, 1995.

16. Kolterman OG, Gray RS, Griffin J, et al.: Receptor and post-receptor defects contribute to the insulin resistance in non-insulin dependent diabetes mellitus. J Clin Invest 68:957–969, 1981.

17. Kahn CR: Insulin action, diabetogenes, and the cause of type II diabetes. Diabetes 43:1066–84, 1994.

18. Howard G, O'Leary DH, Zaccaro D, et al.: Insulin sensitivity and atherosclerosis. Circulation 93:1809–1817, 1996.

19. Stout RW: Insulin and atheroma: 20–yr perspective. Diabetes Care 13:631–654, 1990.

20. Reaven GM: 1988 Banting lecture: Role of insulin resistance in human disease. Diabetes 1595–1607, 1988.

21. Schneider DJ, Sobel BE: Effect of diabetes on the coagulation and fibrinolytic systems and its implications for atherogenesis. Coron Artery Dis 3:26–32, 1992.

22. Hofmann CA, Colca JR: New oral thiazolidineedione antidiabetic agents act as insulin sensitizers. Diabetes Care 15:1075, 1992.

23. Iwamoto Y, Kuzuya T, Matsudo A, et al.: Effect of new oral antidiabetic agent CS-045 on glucose tolerance and insulin secretion in patients with NIDDM. Diabetes Care 14:1083, 1991.

24. Valiquett TR, Balagtas CC, Whitcomb RW: Troglitazone dose-response study in patients with noninsulin dependent diabetes (abstract). Clin Res 42:400A, 1994.

25. Bern MM: Platelet functions in diabetes mellitus. Diabetes 27:342, 1978.

26. Chirkov YY, et al.: Guanylate cyclase in human platelets with different aggregability. Experientia 46:697–699, 1990.

27. Chen SY, Yu BJ, Liang YQ, et al.: Platelet aggregation, platelet cAMP levels and thromboxane B2 synthesis in patients with diabetes mellitus. Chin Med J 103:312–318, 1990.

28. Trovati M, Anfossi G, Mularoni E, et al.: Desensitization of the platelet aggregation response to adrenaline during insulin-induced hypoglycemia in man. Diabet Med 7:414–419, 1990.

29. Matsuda T, Morishita E, Jokaji H, et al.: Mechanisms on disorders of coagulation and fibrinolysis in diabetes. Diabetes 45(suppl.) 3:S109–110, 1996.

30. Marongiu F, Conti M, Mameli G, et al.: Is the imbalance between thrombin and plasmin activity in diabetes related to the behaviour of antiplasmin activity? Thromb Res 58:91–99, 1990.

31. Morishita E, Asakura H, Jokaji H, et al.: Hypercoagulability and high lipoprotein(a) levels in patients with type II diabetes mellitus. Atherosclerosis 120:7–14, 1996.

32. Kannel WB, D'Agostino RB, Wilson PW, et al.: Diabetes, fibrinogen, and risk of cardiovascular disease: the Framingham experience. Am Heart J 120:672–676, 1990.

33. Schneider DJ, Sobel BE: Effect of diabetes on the coagulation and fibrinolytic systems and its implications for atherogenesis. Coron Artery Dis 3:26–32, 1992.

34. Brownlee M, Cerami A, Vlassara H: Advanced glycosylation endproducts in tissue and the biochemical basis of diabetic complications. New Engl J Med 318:1315–1320, 1988.

35. Schmidt AM, Hori O, Brett J, et al.: Cellular receptors for advanced glycosylation endproducts. Arterioscler Thromb 14:1521–1528, 1994.

36. Brownlee M: Lilly lecture, 1993: Glycation and diabetic complications. Diabetes 43:836, 1994.

37. Hammes HP, Brownlee M: Advanced glycation end products and the pathogenesis of diabetic complications. In LeRoith D, Taylor SI, Olefsky JM (eds.) Diabetes Mellitus. Philadelphia: Lippincott-Raven, 1996, pp. 810–815.

38. Giardino I, Edelstein D, Brownlee M: Nonenzymatic glycosylation in vitro and in bovine endothelial cells alters basic fibroblast growth factor activity. A model for intracellular glycosylation in diabetes. J Clin Invest 94:110–117, 1994.

39. Schleicher ED, Wagner E, Nerlich AG: Increased accumulation of glycoxidation product N-(carboxymethyl)lysine in human tissues in diabetes and aging. J Clin Invest 99:457–468, 1997.

40. Mularkey C, Edelstein D, Brownlee M: Free radical generation by early glycation endproducts: a mechanism for accelerated atherosclerosis in diabetes. Biochem Biophys Res Commun 173:932–939, 1990.

41. Sakurai T, Tsuchiya S: Superoxide production from nonenzymatically glycated protein. FEBS Lett 236:406–410, 1988.

42. Yan SD, Schmidt AM, Anderson GM, et al.: Enhanced cellular oxidant stress by the interaction of advanced glycation end products with their receptors/binding proteins. J Biol Chem 269:9889–9897, 1994.

43. Schmidt AM, Hori O, Chen JX, et al.: Advanced glycation end products interacting with their endothelial receptor induce expression of vascular cell adhesion molecule-1 (VCAM-1) in cultured human endothelial cells and in mice: a potential mechanism for the accelerated vasculopathy of diabetes. J Clin Invest 96:1395–1403, 1995.

44. Cybulsky M, Gimbrone M: Endothelial expression of a mononuclear leukocyte adhesion molecule during atherogenesis. Science 251:788–791, 1991.

45. O'Brien KD, Allen MD, McDonald TO, et al.: Vascular cell adhesion molecule-1 is expressed in human coronary atherosclerotic plaques. Implications for the mode of progression of advanced coronary atherosclerosis. J Clin Invest 92:945–951, 1993.

46. Bucala R, Tracey KJ, Cerami A: Advanced glycosylation products quench nitric oxide and mediate defective endothelium-dependent vasodilation in experimental diabetes. J Clin Invest 87:432, 1991.

47. Rodriguez-Manas L, Arribas S, Girron C, et al.: Interference of glycosylated human hemoglobin with endothelium-dependent responses. Circulation 88:2111, 1993.

48. Li YM, Steffes M, Donnelly T, et al.: Prevention of cardiovascular and renal pathology of aging by the advanced glycation inhibitor aminoguanidine. Proc Natl Acad Sci USA 93:3902–3907, 1996.

49. Hogan M, Cerami A, Bucala R: Advanced glycosylation end products block the antiproliferative effect of nitric oxide: Role in the vascular and renal complications of diabetes mellitus. J Clin Invest 90:1110, 1992.

50. Raman M, Nesto RW: Heart disease in diabetes mellitus. Endocrinol Metabol Clin North Amer 25(2): 1996.

51. Nesto R, et al.: Silent myocardial ischemia and infarction in diabetics with peripheral vascular disease: Assessment by dipyridamole thallium-201 scintingraphy. Am Heart J 120:1073, 1990.

52. Zarich S, et al.: Effect of autonomic nervous dysfunction on the circadian pattern of myocardial ischemia in diabetes mellitus. J Am Coll Cardiol 24:968, 1994.

53. Nesto R, et al.: Angina and exertional myocardial ischemia in diabetic and nondiabetic patients: Assessment by exercise thallium scintigraphy. Ann Intern Med 108:170, 1988.

54. Woodfield S, et al.: Angiographic findings and outcome in diabetic patients treated with thrombolytic therapy after acute myocardial infarction. The GUSTO experience. J Am Coll Cardiol 28(7):1661, 1996.

55. Summary Report from the Consensus Development Conference on Diagnosis of Coronary Heart Disease in People with Diabetes. Diabetes Care 21(9): 1998.

56. Malmberg K, et al.: Effects of metoprolol on mortality and late infarction in diabetics with suspected acute myocardial infarction: Retrospective data from two large studies. Eur Heart J 10:423, 1989.

57. Pyorala K, et al.: Cholesterol lowering with simvastatin improves prognosis of the diabetic patient with coronary heart disease. Diabetes Care 20(4):614, 1997.

58. Goldberg R: Diabetic response to Pravastatin during the care trial. Circulation supp AHA 3159(abstract), 1997.

59. ISIS-2 Collaborative Group: Randomized trial of intravenous streptokinase, oral aspirin, both or neither among 17,187 cases of suspected acute myocardial infarction: ISIS-2. Lancet 2:349, 1998.

60. Rensing B, et al.: On behalf of the CARPORT Study Group: Luminal narrowing after percutaneous transluminal coronary angioplasty. Circulation 88:975, 1993.

61. Stein B, et al.: Influence of diabetes mellitus on early and late outcome after percutaneous transluminal angioplasty. Circulation 91:979, 1995.

62. King SB, et al.: A randomized trial comparing coronary angioplasty with coronary bypass surgery: EAST trial. New Engl J Med 331:1044, 1994.

63. Weintraub WS, et al.: Outcome of coronary bypass surgery versus coronary angioplasty in diabetic patients with multivessel coronary artery disease. J Am Coll Cadiol 31:10, 1998.

64. The Bypass Angioplasty Revascularization Investigators (BARI): Comparison of coronary bypass surgery with angioplasty in patients with multivessel disease. New Engl J Med 375:217, 1996.

65. CABRI Trial: Coronary angioplasty versus bypass revascularization investigation. Lancet 346:1179, 1995.

66. DIGAMI Study Group: Br Med J 314:1512, 1997.

67. Haffner SM, et al.: Mortality from coronary heart disease in subjects with type 2 diabetes and in nondiabetic subjects with and without prior myocardial infarction. New Engl J Med 339:229, 1998.

68. Kemp HG, Elliot WC, Gorlin R: The anginal syndrome with normal coronary arteriography. Trans Assoc Am Physicians 80:59, 1967.

69. Dean JD, Jones CJH, Hutchison SJ, et al.: Hyperinsulinaemia and microvascular angina ("Syndrome X"). Lancet 337:456, 1992.

70. Fuh MM-T, Jeng C-Y, Young MM-S, et al.: Insulin resistance, glucose intolerance, and hyperinsulinemia in patients with microvascular angina. Metabolism 42:1090, 1993.

71. Botker HR, Moller N, Oversen P, et al.: Insulin resistance in microvascular angina (Syndrome X). Lancet 342:136, 1993.

72. Kannel WB, McGee DL: Diabetes and cardiovascular disease: the Framingham study. JAMA 241:2035–38, 1979.

73. Kannel W, Hjortland M, Castelli W: Role of diabetes in congestive heart failure: the Framingham study. Am J Cardiol 34:29, 1974.

74. Sniderman A, Michel C, Racine N: Heart disease in patients with diabetes mellitus. In Draznin R, Eckel RH (eds.): Diabetes and Atherosclerosis: Molecular Basis and Clinical Aspects. New York: Elsevier, 1993, p. 255.

75. Regan FJ, Lyons MM, Ahmed SS, et al.: Evidence of cardiomyopathy in familial diabetes mellitus. J Clin Invest 60:885, 1977.

76. DiBello V, Talarico L, Picano E, et al.: Increased echodensity of myocardial wall in the diabetic heart: an ultrasound tissue characterization study. J Am Coll Cardiol 25:1408–15, 1995.

77. DiBello V, Giampietro O, Matteuccii E, et al.: Ultrasonic videodensitometric analysis in type 1 diabetic myocardium. Coron Artery Dis 7:895–901, 1996.

78. Raev DC: Which left ventricular function is impaired earlier in the evolution of diabetic cardiomyopathy? An echocardiographic study of young type I diabetic patients. Diabetes Care 633–39, 1994.

79. Shimonagata T, Nanto S, Hori M, et al.: A case of hypertensive-diabetic cardiomyopathy demonstrating left ventricular wall motion abnormality. Diabetes Care 19:887–91, 1996.

80. McNeill JH: Role of elevated lipids in diabetic cardiomyopathy. Diabetes Res Clin Pract 31(suppl.):S67–71, 1996.

80. Ranjadayalan K, et al.: Prolonged anginal perceptual threshold in diabetes: Effects on exercise capacity and myocardial ischemia. J Am Coll Cardiol 16:1120, 1990.

81. Liu X, Takeda N, Dhalla NS: Myosin light-chain phosphorylation in diabetic cardiomyopathy in rats. Metabolism 46:71–75, 1997.

82. Lagaadic-Gossmann D, Buckler KJ, Le Prigent K, et al.: Altered Ca2+ handling in ventricular myocytes from diabetic rats. Am J Physiol 270:H1529–37, 1996.

83. Wu PY: Infant of diabetic mother: a continuing challenge for perinatal-neonatal medicine. Acta Paediatr Sinica 37:312–19, 1996.

84. Weber HS, Botti JJ, Baylen BG: Sequential longitudinal evaluation of cardiac growth and ventricular diastolic filling in fetuses of well controlled diabetic mothers. Pediatr Cardiol 15:184–89, 1994.

85. Ewing DJ, Campbell IW, Clarke BF: Heart rate changes in diabetes mellitus. Lancet 1:183–86, 1981.

86. Page M, Watkins PJ: Cardiorespiratory arrest and diabetic autonomic neuropathy. Lancet 1:14–16, 1978.

87. Burgos LG, Ebert TJ, Assiddaoo C, et al.: Increased perioperative cardiovascular morbidity in diabetics with autonomic neuropathy. Anesthesiology 70:591–597, 1989.

88. Ewing DJ, Boland O, Neilson JM, et al.: Autonomic neuropathy, QT interval lengthening, and unexpected deaths in male diabetic patients. Diabetologia 34:182–185, 1991.

89. Zola BE, Vinik AI: Effects of autonomic neuropathy associated with diabetes mellitus on cardiovascular function. Coron Artery Dis 3:33–41, 1992.

90. Koiistinen MJ, Airaksinen KE, Huikuri HV, et al.: No difference in cardiac innervation of diabetic patients with painful and asymptomatic coronary artery disease. Diabetes Care 19:231–233, 1996.

91. Levitt NS, Stansberry KB, Wynchank S, et al.: The natural progression of autonomic neuropathy and autonomic function tests in a cohort of people with IDDM. Diabetes Care 19:751–754, 1996.

92. Matsuo S, Takahashi M, Nakamura Y, et al.: Evaluation of cardiac sympathetic innervation with iodine-123–metaiodobenzylguanidine imaging in silent myocardial ischemia. J Nucl Med 37:712–717, 1996.

93. Okada M, Matsuto T, Satoh S, et al.: Role of pulse wave velocity for assessing autonomic nervous system activities in reference to heart rate variability. Med Inf 21:81–90, 1996.

94. Shiimabukuro M, Chiibana T, Yoshida H, et al.: Increased QT dispersion and cardiac adrenergic dysinnervation in diabetic patients with autonomic neuropathy. Am J Cardiol 78:1057–1059, 1996.

95. Eagle KA, et al.: Guidelines for perioperative cardiovascular evaluation for noncardiac surgery. J Am Coll Cardiol 27:910, 1996.

96. Eagle KA, et al.: Combining clinical and thallium data optimizes perioperative assessment of cardiac risk before major vascular surgery. Ann Intern Med 110:859, 1989.

29

Cerebrovascular Disease

Malachi J. McKenna, Janice M. T. Redmond, and Fred W. Whitehouse

Cerebrovascular disease (CVD) encompasses three distinct syndromes: atherothrombotic brain infarction due to occlusive disease of major intracranial and extracranial arteries; small artery disease resulting in cerebral hemorrhage and lacunar infarction; and aneurysmal disease manifesting as subarachnoid hemorrhage. Stroke—a manifestation of brain infarction due to CVD, cardioembolic disease, or systemic hypoperfusion—challenges the health care professional regarding diagnosis and management, and the neuroscientist regarding etiopathogenesis and prevention. The epidemiology and pathogenesis of each type of CVD in the nondiabetic population differ widely. The purpose of this review is to outline similarities and disparities between diabetic patients and nondiabetic patients and, on the basis of these observations, to offer an approach to CVD in the diabetic patient.

Historical Perspective

It has been recognized for many decades that stroke is a frequent cause of mortality in diabetic patients, albeit less common than coronary heart disease.[1-10] Analysis of death trends at the Joslin Diabetes Center among 34,499 diabetic patients dying between 1897 and 1979 showed that in the years prior to the discovery of insulin in 1922 death was caused by stroke in about 4% and by heart disease in about 8%. Since the 1940s, the trend has been remarkably consistent: stroke accounted for death in nearly 12% of patients, about fourfold less than coronary heart disease.[4] This analysis included patients with insulin-dependent DM (IDDM) and non-insulin-dependent DM (NIDDM). Recent studies are in broad agreement. In three populations of patients with IDDM the frequency of stroke as a cause of death varied from 1 to 7%, whereas cardiac disease accounted for 23 to 26%.[1-3] The Framingham Study, predominantly including patients with NIDDM (type II DM) and impaired glucose tolerance, noted stroke as a cause of death in 17% and coronary heart disease in 62% of

diabetics.[6] The Honolulu Heart Study found stroke as a cause of death in 8% of diabetic men (NIDDM only) compared with coronary heart disease in 38%.[11] Numerous epidemiologic surveys have identified DM as a risk factor for stroke.[10-12] In addition, hyperglycemia has an adverse effect on ischemic damage and long-term outcome.[6-9,15-18]

Epidemiology

In stroke populations from every region of the world, patients with DM or impaired glucose tolerance are represented in greater numbers than expected by chance alone.[10-12,19-21]

Information regarding the epidemiology of stroke is summarized in the following categories: the prevalence of DM in stroke populations and effect of DM on subsequent outcome, the incidence and mortality of stroke in DM compared with the general population, risk factors for stroke in DM, acute ischemic stroke management, and preventative measures.

Prevalence of Diabetes in Stroke Populations and Outcome

It is estimated that the prevalence of DM, both known and unrecognized, in patients admitted with stroke varies from 11 to 44%.[9,20,22-26] DM is known to be present in about 2.5% of the general population, and an equal number of persons are thought to have unrecognized disease. The documented prevalence of recognized diabetes at the time of stroke is similar for most studies at about 8%, but there is divergence of findings regarding the frequency of unrecognized DM, varying from 6 to 42%. Most studies assign the term "unrecognized DM" if there is an elevated glycosylated hemoglobin at the time of stroke in the absence of a history of DM. So variations in findings may be explained, in part, by different methodologies. Also, none of these studies established the correct diagnosis by oral glucose tolerance testing following recovery from stroke. Stress hyperglycemia, defined in the acute setting as elevated random glucose without a rise in glycosylated hemoglobin, is reported to occur in nearly 10% of stroke cases.[26] Stress hyperglycemia may be more apt to occur following brainstem infarction due to damage of glucose regulatory centers, similar in etiology to diabetes pique.[22]

Whatever discordancies there may be in determining the frequency of DM (both recognized and unrecognized) and of stress hyperglycemia, there is uniformity of opinion that both mortality, immediate and remote, and morbidity are adversely altered by any degree of glucose intolerance.[7–9,20,22–26] The presence of heart disease rather than hypertension seemed responsible for excess mortality. Moreover, long-term recovery is also limited. One study reported that 43% of patients with a random blood glucose of greater than 120 mg/dL returned to work compared with 76% of patients with a value below 120 mg/dL.[8]

Mortality and Incidence

Three prospective epidemiologic studies of population-based cohorts in the United States have shown similar findings of increased stroke risk in diabetic patients.[10–12] The Framingham study, a community-based prospective survey of 5,209 persons followed over 20 years, reported that the incidence of stroke was significantly higher in diabetic versus nondiabetic patients.[10] The relative risk of stroke (after adjusting for age, systolic blood pressure, cigarette smoking, cholesterol, and left ventricular hypertrophy) for both men and women with DM was 2.2. In the Honolulu Heart Study conducted over 12 years on nearly 7,000 men, the relative risk of mortality from a thromboembolic stroke in subjects with DM was 2.0.[11] Furthermore, in nondiabetic men with blood glucose response to 50 g load at the 80th percentile compared with men with a value at the 20th percentile, the relative risk of stroke was 1.4. In the Rancho Bernardo Study of 3,778 adults followed for 10 years, the relative risk of stroke for diabetic men was 1.8 and for diabetic women it was 2.2 after adjusting for age, systolic blood pressure, cholesterol level, obesity, smoking habits, and excluding persons with a previous history of heart attack, heart failure, or stroke.[12]

It has now been established by a number of investigators that the risk of thromboembolic infarction but not cerebral hemorrhage is greater in the diabetic population than in comparable nondiabetic subjects,[11,20,27,28] an observation that is all the more remarkable since hypertension is common in diabetic subjects. Indeed, the likelihood of subarachnoid hemorrhage seems to be diminished in DM.[29,30]

EXHIBIT 29–1   Risk Markers for Stroke in the Diabetic Patient[a]

Hypertension	Cigarette smoking
Age	Poor glycemic control
Male gender	Hyperinsulinemia
Hypercholesterolemia	Macroangiopathy (at other sites)
Hypertriglyceridemia	Microangiopathy
Obesity	

[a] See text for discussion.

Risk Factors

A variety of different risk factors are invoked in the genesis of stroke (Exhibit 29–1). Seven risk factors for stroke in the general population have been identified by the Framingham study, namely, age, impaired cardiac function, current smoking history, serum cholesterol, systolic blood pressure, gender, and historical or laboratory findings indicating glucose intolerance. Raised blood pressure is the strongest risk factor for stroke in the general population. Regarding risk factors for stroke in DM, information has been acquired from two categories of studies: comparison of diabetic with nondiabetic patients in stroke populations, and comparison of diabetic patients with and without stroke. There are inconsistencies in the findings of these studies, quite diverse in design and sample. It is apparent that the likelihood of thromboembolic stroke is associated with an atherogenic profile. DM, per se, is associated with such a profile.[10–12] It is debated whether these attendant risk factors entirely account for stroke or if the diabetic state has an independent role. At least, an interaction of risk factors is suggested to be more important than a single factor.

Blood Pressure.   Three large prospective studies about the incidence of stroke in DM have confirmed hypertension to be more common in diabetics compared with nondiabetics, two referring to systolic blood pressure, and the other to a combined abnormality in systolic and diastolic blood pressure.[11,12,19] In studies comparing diabetic patients with and without stroke, similar findings have been documented. The WHO Study of Vascular Disease in Diabetes (3,583 subjects, including IDDM and NIDDM, from nine different countries) measured a significantly higher mean systolic blood pressure of 147 mmHg in stroke patients versus 137 mmHg in those without stroke.[31] In a cross-sectional study of 448 Japanese patients with NIDDM systolic blood pressure but not diastolic blood pressure was found to be associated with stroke.[32] The Rochester Epidemiologic Study reported a TIA or stroke in 16% versus 12% of diabetic patients if blood pressure exceeded 160/95 mmHg.[33] One study of stroke death in younger diabetic patients reported hypertension in 64%.[2]

Age and Race. Stroke is primarily a disease of the aged population. The Framingham Study reported a fivefold increase of stroke incidence in diabetic men from age ranges 45 to 54 years compared to 65 to 74 years in men and a ninefold increase in diabetic women.[10] In comparing diabetics with nondiabetics, the Rochester Epidemiologic Study discovered no age difference; the average age of TIA being 70 years and of stroke being 75 years.[27] By comparison, the WHO Study[31] and the Nagasaki RERF[19] observed that diabetics with stroke were older. Substantial racial differences have been recorded: stroke is common in Japanese and in African Americans, but no data on this matter are available in diabetic populations in the United States.

Gender. As for all types of macrovascular disease in the nondiabetic population, including stroke, there is a preponderance of men over women. However, this is not the case in the diabetic population[12] and may even be reversed.[10]

Hyperlipidemia. Although hypercholesterolemia is recognized to be an important risk factor for myocardial infarction in the general population, its association with stroke is weaker. The Honolulu Heart Study did find an association between both hypercholesterolemia and hypertriglyceridemia and stroke in diabetic patients,[13] but neither the Rancho Bernardo Study[12] nor the Nagasaki RERF[19] could detect any association between hypercholesterolemia and stroke risk in diabetic patients. The WHO Study recorded similar serum cholesterol and triglyceride levels in diabetics with and without stroke.[31] However, on comparing diabetics with a high serum cholesterol (exceeding 280 mg/dL) to those with a normal value (less than 200 md/dL), the rate of stroke was significantly higher, 5.7% versus 2.4%.

Weight. Obesity is defined in many different ways in the various studies, namely, by absolute body weight, relative body weight, percent of ideal body weight, and the body mass index. The Honolulu Heart Study, comprising men only, did find a significant association between stroke and obesity as defined by the body mass index.[11] This is not in accordance with all other studies, either comparing diabetics to nondiabetics or comparing diabetics with stroke versus those without, regardless of the method of defining obesity.[12,19,31–33]

Cigarette Smoking. The Honolulu Heart Study found that diabetics were less likely to smoke than nondiabetics, 38.8% versus 44.4%.[11] The Rancho Bernardo had a similar finding in men (24.6% versus 31.0%) but not so in women with DM, 19.9% of whom smoked versus 16% of nondiabetic patients.[12] The Framingham Study could not determine an association between smoking and stroke in women, but did consider it to be a factor for men, the attributable risk being 14-fold less than that of hypertension.[10] In the only study comparing diabetics with stroke to those without, the prevalence of smokers was exactly equal at 37%.[31] A British study of younger diabetic patients noted a history of smoking in 79% of patients who died of a stroke.[2]

Diabetic Complications. Associations between stroke risk and other diabetic complications have been sought. In the Rancho Bernardo Study there was a significant association with prior stroke in both sexes, and with coronary heart disease in men.[12] The Rochester Epidemiologic Project found a higher frequency of stroke and TIA if the electrocardiogram (ECG) was abnormal.[33] In the Honolulu Heart Study the presence of proteinuria in diabetics was twice as likely to be associated with stroke.[11] No link between stroke and proteinuria or ECG abnormalities was evident in the Nagasaki RERF.[19] One clinical survey noted microvascular lesions and peripheral vascular disease in less than 10% of stroke patients but heart disease in 81%, findings more commonly noted than in either a diabetic group without stroke or in a nondiabetic stroke group.[7] In that study atrial fibrillation was present in one fourth of patients in all groups. Regarding a family history of macrovascular disease, diabetic women with a family history of coronary heart disease (but not stroke) appear to have a greater risk of developing stroke.[12]

Hyperglycemia. Data regarding indices of glycemic control and stroke risk are sparse. The WHO Study noted an insignificant rise in fasting plasma glucose (based on only one estimation per patient) in diabetics with stroke versus those without (196 mg/dL versus 189 mg/dL).[31] However, on comparing subjects with highest values (greater than 250 mg/dL) to those with the lowest values (150 mg/dL), the rate of stroke was significantly higher at 4.0% versus 2.2%. In a smaller study in Japan, there was no difference between both fasting blood glucose and postprandial blood glucose in diabetics with stroke versus those without, whereas these indices were significantly related to retinopathy, proteinuria, and absence of patellar tendon reflex.[32] A lower frequency of stroke was noted in the Rochester Epidemiologic Project in subjects with good glycemic control (if more than 50% of fasting blood glucose values were below 150 mg/dL) compared with those with poor control (if more than 50% of values exceeded 150 mg/dL).[33] In the DCCT, none of the patients during the active treatment period in either arm manifested with stroke, although two patients in the intensive arm reported one transient ischemic attack each (34). Further information is awaited from the ten-year observational extension project.

Summary. Thus, diabetic patients have an increased incidence of stroke and of several risk factors. Recent epidemiologic studies, with few exceptions, are in agreement that DM is an independent risk factor for stroke. Two exceptions are the Rochester Epidemiologic Project, which showed hypertension accounting for all excess mortality from stroke,[33] and the Nagasaki RERF, which reported after multivariate analysis that age, systolic hypertension, and male gender, but not DM were significant risk factors for stroke.[19] Three major prospective studies in the United States reached a contrary conclusion.[10-12] The Framingham Study quantified the attributable risk of DM for stroke to be significant but sevenfold less than hypertension in both men and women.[10] This may in part be explained by the lower prevalence of DM compared with hypertension; conversely, it may reflect an underestimation of DM in the population studied and the potentially adverse effect of even minor abnormalities of glucose tolerance. The Honolulu Heart Study concluded that DM was an independent risk factor for stroke.[11] The Rancho Bernardo Study demonstrated that the relative risk of stroke in diabetes was still apparent after stratification for blood pressure, using both univariate and multivariate analyses.[12]

Pathology

Two major differences have been noted between diabetic and nondiabetic patients: one, the unlikely occurrence of cerebral hemorrhage; second, the substantial increase in frequency and number of lacunes, small foci of infarction that usually cavitate.

In contrast to epidemiologic studies, autopsy series reveal only a modest increase in classic stroke in diabetics but a marked increase in lacunes.[35-37] Two detailed pathologic studies have noted lacunes to occur at least twice as frequently in diabetic patients.[36,37] Multiple small lacunar lesions were found predominantly in the pons, basal ganglia, and the thalamus, territories perfused by branches of the small paramedian perforating arteries. The term *"lacune"* refers to a small deep infarct attributable to a primary arterial disease that involves a penetrating branch of a large cerebral artery. This does not include lesions of nonvascular origin, or infarction that is due to embolism or that is a component of a larger stroke. Typically, areas supplied by small perforating arteries in the infratentorium are involved. Unlike cerebral surface vessels, these penetrators share two features that are considered to predispose to lacune formation. First, these arteries are exposed to pronounced hemodynamic influences; they have a luminal diameter of less than 500 μm, whereas the parent vessels have a luminal diameter greater than 6 mm. Second, they do not communicate with a collateral system, and the territory supplied is usually small. The lacunar state is conventionally associated with hypertension, although lacunes have been discovered in the absence of a history of hypertension. A synergistic effect between hypertension and DM in the occurrence of lacunes has been suggested.[37]

Pathophysiology

The pathophysiology of stroke in DM is complex and involves many different disease processes (Exhibit 29–2).

EXHIBIT 29–2 Pathophysiology of Stroke in Diabetes Mellitus (A Simplified Schema)

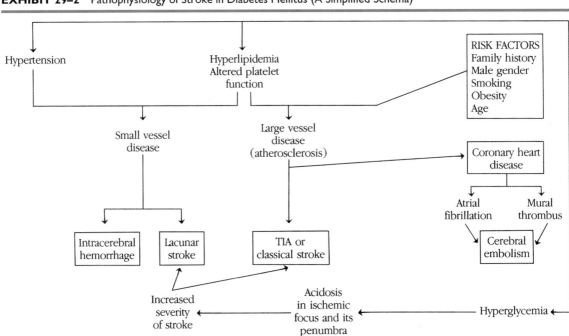

Clearly, there is a state of accelerated atherosclerosis in the cerebral circulation in DM, as there is in other major arteries.[38] This is related to a variety of disturbances, most notably alterations in endothelial and platelet function as well as lipoprotein metabolism.[38] These aspects are discussed in great detail in Chapters 25, 30, 38, and 39. Only factors germane to the genesis of stroke in DM will be addressed here, in particular the development of lacunes and the adverse influence of hyperglycemia on cerebral metabolism following ischemia.

Lacunes

The pathogenesis of these minute areas of infarction (*encephalomalacia*) in the diabetic is uncertain. Small arteries in DM are more likely to exhibit proliferative changes, microatheromas, and lipohyalinization that may compromise vessel wall function as well as luminal diameter. It has generally been explained that infarction in regions supplied by nonoccluded vessels results from hemodynamic factors, either local or systemic. A sudden cardiac arrhythmia or episode of hypotension may compromise flow to the region. Alternatively, local vascular spasm could seriously curtail perfusion. Impaired cerebral autoregulation has been documented in DM; vessels fail to respond when stressed by changes in oxygen and carbon dioxide tensions. One study noted abnormal cerebrovascular reactivity in 59 diabetic patients when compared with 28 control subjects; 36 of 59 diabetic patients failed to show an increase in cerebral blood flow after inhalation of 5% carbon dioxide.[39] The authors concluded that a *"diminished cerebrovascular reserve"* makes the diabetic vulnerable to stroke because of an inability to increase cerebral blood flow following usual stimuli. Indeed, patients with DM have a reduced prevalence of migraine, consonant with the observation of vessels having an impaired vasodilatory capacity.[40]

Hyperglycemia and Ischemia

The increased mortality and morbidity following infarction in diabetic patients compared with nondiabetic patients is unexplained. As mentioned before, there is substantive data from clinical surveys implying that even minor elevations in serum glucose, less than levels necessary to make a diagnosis of DM, herald a poor outcome.[8,9,22–26] The mechanism of this association is poorly understood. One study postulated that hyperglycemia predisposed to cerebral edema, as measured by computed tomography (CT), and thereby promoted greater brain damage.[17] Analysis of cases collected in the Pilot Data Bank of the National Institute of Neurological and Communicative Disorders showed an apparent threshold level of blood glucose (equal to 100 mg/dL), which predicted poor outcome, but no linear relationship with mortality or with variables having therapeutic implications for infarcts.[41]

Similarly, a recent study of serum glucose testing in stroke patients on admission to the hospital could find no relationship between glucose and either volume of infarct on CT and immediate neurologic deficit, the main determinants of long-term outcome in this study.[18] Nonetheless, there is widespread belief that events in the zone of ischemia and its penumbra are adversely influenced by even a minimal rise in blood glucose.[13–16] Treatment is an attempt to salvage the ischemic penumbra.

The Problem in Summary

One can summarize from published reports on stroke in diabetic patients the following:

1. Coronary heart disease clearly outstrips stroke as a cause of mortality and morbidity in all diabetic patients.

2. The incidence of stroke in the diabetic population is about twice that of the nondiabetic population.

3. Although the relative risk of both stroke and TIA are increased in DM, the risk of both cerebral hemorrhage and subarachnoid hemorrhage are not, and risk for the latter may even be reduced.

4. With regard to risk factors, diabetic patients with stroke tend to have an atherogenic profile of hypertension, hyperlipidemia, advanced age, and cigarette smoking. Nonetheless, it has been shown that DM per se is an independent risk factor for stroke, but of lesser magnitude than hypertension.

5. There is limited information regarding the relationship between the degree of glycemic control and the risk of stroke. Indices of glycemic control, based on blood glucose measurement, demonstrate a connection between higher concentrations and stroke risk. However, the relationship of glycosylated hemoglobin or of other glycated proteins to stroke risk has not yet been reported.

6. Hyperglycemia at the time of stroke, whether due to DM or stress hyperglycemia, has an adverse influence on immediate and remote outcome.

Clinical Aspects

The clinical presentation of stroke in diabetics differs in no way from that of nondiabetic patients. Typical manifestations are outlined in Exhibit 29–3. *In the diabetic patient receiving insulin or a sulfonylurea, hypoglycemia must always be considered* because its features are protean and may serve as a concomitant of a stroke syndrome in patients with a preexisting ischemic focus. Other conditions can be confused with

EXHIBIT 29–3　Some Clinical Manifestations of Stroke

Symptoms and signs may be transient (hr), progressive (days), or fixed	Cortical bindness, homonymous hemianopia
Carotid artery territory	Vertigo
Contralateral paresis or sensory loss	Horner's syndrome
Ipsilateral blindness (amaurosis fugax)	Lacunes
Aphasia	Pure motor or sensory stroke
Vertebrobasilar artery territory	Ataxic hemiparesis
Hemiplegia, quadriplegia	Dysarthria-clumsy hand syndrome
"Drop" attacks without loss of consciousness	Parkinson's disease, hemiballismus
Crossed cranial nerve palsies in the brainstem giving rise to diplopia, dysarthria, dysphagia, and perioral paresthesia	Systemic hypoperfusion (border zone ischemia)
	Lightheadedness, blurring of vision, dizziness, confusion, focal signs uncommon

EXHIBIT 29–4　Differential Diagnosis of Stroke in the Diabetic Patient

Hypoglycemia[a]	Dural sinus thrombosis
Embolism	Cortical vein thrombosis
Subdural hematoma	Multiple sclerosis
Neoplastic disease (primary or secondary)	

[a] Hypoglycemia may precipitate ischemic cerebral symptoms, and its presence must be considered at the onset of stroke symptoms.

stroke (Exhibit 29–4). Rarer causes of stroke must also be considered (Exhibit 29–5).

Diagnosis and Assessment

General

CVD should be suspected whenever a diabetic patient presents with an acute neurologic event, especially in patients over age 50 years and in those who have long-duration disease. Clinical evaluation should include a careful inquiry into symptoms suspicious of TIAs, documentation of the presence of hypertension, and careful examination of the neck for carotid artery bruits and of the retina for vascular abnormalities (arteriolar spasm or Hollenhorst plaques). The presence of clinical syndromes such as amaurosis fugax, monoparesis, transient aphasia, or hypoglycemia associated with ischemic symptoms should alert the clinician to symptomatic CVD. Since true vertigo rarely is a symptom of hypoglycemia, its occurrence in association with brain-

stem ischemia will suggest symptomatic vertebrobasilar insufficiency.

Our approach to a patient is depicted in Exhibit 29–6. Apart from the initial clinical examination, it is essential to exclude hypoglycemia promptly, since this will require immediate management. We request neurologic consultation for urgent evaluation of acute stroke patients. Subsequent investigation is determined by the clinical findings. It is not sufficient to categorize a stroke according to the time course, namely, completed stroke, stroke-in-evolution, or TIA. One must attempt to define the cause and mechanism of the stroke, the exact sites of damage, and the type of neurologic deficit. Initial clinical evaluation guides the use of procedures to confirm and elaborate on the diagnosis. Neuroimaging depicts the lesion and its pathologic anatomy, whereas studies of vessels aid in determining the cause of stroke.

Brain Imaging

An intracerebral hematoma is recognized within a few hours as a discrete area of high density, it is essential that a CT be performed as soon as possible after symptomatic onset. Cerebral infarction may not be seen in the first 48 hours. After a week, the infarct may appear isodense, and demonstration of contrast enhancement may be necessary to exclude malignancy. In the acute stages of ischemic infarction, CT will identify the presence and degree of edema extending into both gray and white matter. CT should exclude subdural hematoma, subarachnoid hemorrhage, and dural sinus thrombosis.

EXHIBIT 29–5　Rare Causes of Stroke

Amyloid angiopathy	Genetic and hereditary diseases
Narcotic drugs (cocaine, amphetamine, heroin)	Marfan's syndrome
Arterial dissection	Homocysteinuria
Fibromuscular dysplasia	Fabry's disease
Sickle cell disease	Menkes's kinky hair disease
Giant cell arteritis	Mitochondrial encephalomyelopathy
Migraine and vasospasm	Hypercoagulable states

EXHIBIT 29–6   How We Handle a Diabetic Patient Suspected of Having a Stroke

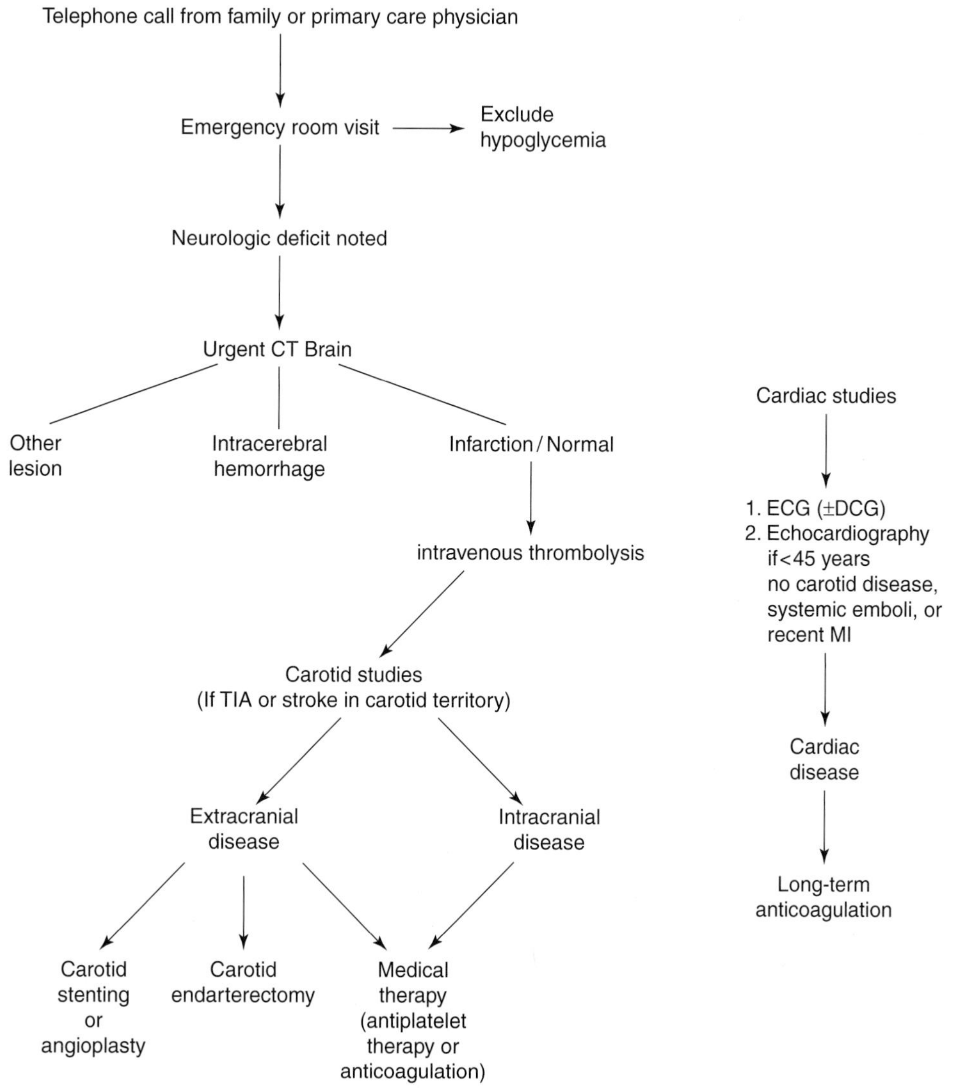

Telephone call from family or primary care physician

↓

Emergency room visit → Exclude hypoglycemia

↓

Neurologic deficit noted

↓

Urgent CT Brain

Other lesion   Intracerebral hemorrhage   Infarction / Normal

↓

intravenous thrombolysis

↓

Carotid studies
(If TIA or stroke in carotid territory)

Extracranial disease   Intracranial disease

Carotid stenting or angioplasty   Carotid endarterectomy   Medical therapy (antiplatelet therapy or anticoagulation)

Cardiac studies

↓

1. ECG (±DCG)
2. Echocardiography if < 45 years no carotid disease, systemic emboli, or recent MI

↓

Cardiac disease

↓

Long-term anticoagulation

Abbreviations: CT: computed tomography; EC-IC: extracranial-intracranial; ECG: electrocardiogram; MI: myocardial infarction; MRI: magnetic resonance imaging; TIA: transient ischemic attack.

CT can also identify lacunar infarcts, appearing as hypointense lesions.[58] The resolution of CT limits the visualization of lacunes only a few millimeters in size, but larger foci measuring 0.5 to 1.0 mm can be detected. Their recognition aids in resolving issues regarding correlation between the lacunar syndromes and anatomic defects. To date, there is no neuroradiologic study in diabetic patients that has systematically sought to define the prevalence of lacunes, symptomatic or not. Another limitation of CT, apart from detecting small lesions, is the site of the lesion. Bone-related artifacts impair imaging of infarcts in the middle and posterior fossa. Brainstem infarcts, typically small and devastating, are apt to elude CT detection.

Fortunately, magnetic resonance imaging (MRI) is particularly well-suited to study these regions.[59] In addition, MRI provides better anatomic definition of a stroke, is superior in identifying stroke during the subacute stage, and has greater spatial resolution facilitating the detection of lacunes. However, MRI does not distinguish readily between hemorrhage, tumor, and infarction and is not practical as an emergency investigation. Neither CT nor MRI shed light on the mechanism of stroke or on the nature of the intravascular process.

Cardiac Studies

A 12-lead resting ECG with rhythm strip will identify the majority of cases with arrhythmia and infarction. The value of continuous monitoring of cardiac rhythm is uncertain. The value of routine cardiac echocardiography for patients with focal cerebral ischemia is limited by the finding of false-positive results.[60] Patients should be chosen using selective criteria such as age under 45 years, absence of carotid artery disease on angiographic study, evidence of hemorrhagic infarction, CT evidence of infarction in more than one territory, other sites of systemic embolization, or cardiac disorders associated with thrombus formation. Two-dimensional echocardiography is preferable to an M-mode study in the detection of mural thrombi in the ventricle and segmental dyskinesia, but neither are sensitive enough to detect all atrial thrombi.

Carotid Artery Studies

Appropriate diagnostic studies include noninvasive flow analysis of the carotid system followed by cerebral angiography in selected patients. The clinical state of the patient, the progressive nature of the symptoms, the presence of complicating systemic vascular disease, and the patient's point of view will naturally guide the diagnostic workup. Noninvasive studies carry no risk, but one must be prepared to address the issue of invasive studies when positive or inconclusive data emerge from these no-risk studies.

Disease of the carotid arteries is best studied by contrast angiography. This is a procedure not without risk of stroke, renal failure, and even death. A variety of noninvasive methods are also available (Exhibit 29–7), including duplex ultrasonography, carotid Doppler ultrasound, transcranial Doppler ultrasound, and digital substraction angiography (DSA).[42] Currently for diabetic patients there are no specific guidelines for when and how to perform studies.

Duplex ultrasonography can be useful. This combines two different ultrasound techniques: a pulsed echo or B-mode ultrasonogram to obtain an image of the vessel; and a pulsed Doppler mode to examine flow at sites of interest.[42] Carotid Doppler ultrasound, using either a pulsed-wave or continuous-wave machine, detects changes in blood flow velocity but not alterations in anatomy. Transcranial Doppler ultrasound is done with a probe positioned over either the temporal squama or over the foramen magnum orbit. Arterial pressure and flow are measured so that narrowing can be estimated, the presence of collateral channels can be identified, and changes can be monitored over the

course of a patient's illness. Intravenous DSA is a computerized technique in which precontrast images are subtracted from postcontrast images of arteries. Contrast media must be injected into a central vein, thus eliminating risks of intra-arterial catheterization but not of contrast side effects.

Conventional arteriography permits selective examination of both carotid and vertebral arteries and of the intracerebral circulation, providing extensive data on arterial disease. The risk of contrast complications must be carefully weighed against benefit of the procedure. *Radiocontrast nephrotoxicity* is apt to occur in diabetics with coexisting renal disease in about 10% of cases.[43]

Treatment

Thrombolytic Therapy

The major thrust in acute stroke management is to restore perfusion to hypoperfused brain tissue in the ischemic penumbra. Reperfusion must be initiated while tissue is still viable. Substantial progress has been made in defining the role of thrombolytic therapy, namely recombinant tissue plasminogen activator (rt-PA) and alteplase. In 1995, the European Cooperative Acute Stroke Study[44] and the National Institute of Neurologic Disorders and Stroke rt-PA Study Group[45] showed benefit in treatment of patients with acute ischemic stroke with intravenous rt-PA which was given within 3-6 hours of symptom onset. There was a positive outcome difference in both studies in favor of treatment at 90 days; but, the studies showed a 3- to 10-fold increase in intracerebral hemorrhage, respectively.

It is clearly important that the correct diagnosis is reached in the emergency room and that treatment guidelines are followed. Conditions such as migraine, tumor and subdural hematoma may mimick stroke that will be excluded by CT scanning. As mentioned above, early in the course of an ischemic stroke the CT scan may be normal even though there may be a large stroke-in-evolution; such patients have a high risk of hemorrhagic stroke following rt-PA. Patients should not receive therapy if blood pressure is over 185/100 or if on aspirin or on anticoagulant therapy. Up to one-third of patients who present with a stroke might be eligible for thrombolysis. In patients receiving thrombolytic therapy, innovative tests are being employed to identify early reversible areas of ischemia: diffusion weighted MRI, perfusion MRI, SPECT scan, and PET.[46] The role of electroencephalography and transcranial doppler studies is also being evaluated. Screening patients for treatment means that the appropriate personnel and tests are available on a 24-hour basis. A definitive algorithm to ensure safety and efficacy is not yet agreed on.

EXHIBIT 29–7 Carotid Artery Studies

Duplex ultrasonography	Transcranial Doppler ultrasound
Carotid Doppler ultrasound	Digital substraction angiography
	Carotid angiography

Glycemic Control

Poor metabolic control may contribute to the progression of stroke.[47] Patients are at increased risk of developing hyperosmolar nonketotic coma, particularly if care is not given to achieving good glycemic control.[48] This is likely to emerge in elderly patients or in those with a severe neurologic deficit who readily become dehydrated, especially if diuretic therapy or intravenous dextrose are administered inadvertently. The development of a hyperosmolar state, whether iatrogenic or serendipitous, can only be deleterious to a patient with stroke.

The issue of tight glycemic control during the early phase of stroke is certainly intimated by studies showing a direct relationship of glucose level at the time of stroke to subsequent outcome. At the very least, *during the acute phase all patients with hyperglycemia should be managed with insulin therapy.* The dose of short-acting insulin, administered subcutaneously every 4 to 6 hours, should be dependent on fingerstick blood glucose measured at the bedside. The exact dose should be regulated according to individual needs. When the blood glucose falls below 180 mg/dL in the unconscious patient, who is not able to be fed, intravenous glucose should be infused at about 5 g/hr. A glucose/insulin infusion is best to achieve stable glycemic control: an insulin infusion should be started at 1 U/hr and altered according to the blood glucose response, and glucose infusion (5 g/hr) is started when blood glucose declines below 180 mg/dL. Regardless of approach, blood glucose levels should be maintained between 80 and 150 mg/dL. Not until there is further information concerning the benefit of euglycemic control on outcome should one aim for more stringent control. (See Chapters 17 and 18.)

Antiplatelet Therapy

Antiplatelet therapy given to subjects with DM has been tested in one double-blind placebo-controlled trial. The VA Cooperative Study, was a randomized multicenter trial on the effects of placebo versus aspirin (325 mg) and dipyridamole (75 mg) given thrice daily to 231 men with NIDDM and either a recent amputation for gangrene or active gangrene, a very late secondary intervention trial.[49] No beneficial effect was noted in the major endpoints: opposite side amputations or death due to cardiovascular disease. In fact, the total death rate was higher in the treated group because there was a significant increase in unexplained, sudden, or unobserved deaths. However, on subgroup analysis, a significant beneficial effect on CVD was noted. The prevalence of strokes and TIAs over the 6-year observation period was 8% in the treated group and 19% in the placebo group. This observation was considered all the more striking, since the percentage of prior ischemic events was 19% for treated versus 7% for untreated patients.[50] This observation is in agreement with secondary prevention trials in the general population where prolonged antiplatelet therapy can avoid about one third of future strokes.[51]

A role for aspirin in the acute management of stroke has been claimed following the results of the International Stroke Trial, which used 300 mg daily, and the Chinese Stroke Trial, which used 160 mg daily.[52,53] It is projected that the early use of aspirin would reduce the number of strokes and deaths in the first month by 10 per 1000 treated patients. It is suggested that aspirin be started as soon as an ischemic stroke has been verified by CT scanning.

A new antiplatelet agent called ticlopidine may be even more potent than aspirin. A randomized double-blind trial compared patients who had either a TIA or a more prolonged, but reversible, deficit with 90 days of treatment.[55] The Ticlopidine Aspirin Stroke Study showed that ticlopidine significantly reduced the risk of fatal and non-fatal stroke by 24% from 18.1 to 13.8 per 100 patients followed for 5 years compared to aspirin.

Anticoagulant Therapy

There is no role for unfractionated heparin in acute stroke based on the recent findings of the International Stroke Trial.[52] Preliminary results of low molecular weight heparin are not encouraging. Prolonged anticoagulation is required to prevent cardioembolic ischemia due to atrial fibrillation, valvular disease, and dilated cardiomyopathy. The duration of therapy is indefinite for these conditions, although there is some suggestion that a clustering of strokes occurs in the first few months after the initial diagnosis of atrial fibrillation.[55] The risk of bleeding must be balanced against the benefits for each patient. Clearly, a patient with a cerebral embolus and a predisposing cardiac condition needs intervention. Anticoagulation should be deferred until cerebral hemorrhage is excluded by CT after 48 hours and should be avoided if hypertension is extant in order to prevent conversion of an ischemic region to a hemorrhagic one.

Surgical Intervention

In high-grade stenosis of the carotid artery, carotid endarterectomy (CEA) has been shown to be better than medical management, including patients with symptoms in the ipsilateral carotid circulation or without symptoms. Three recent trials - North American Symptomatic Carotid Endarterectomy Trial[56], the European Carotid Surgery Trial[57], the VA Cooperative

Symptomatic Carotid Stenosis Trial[58] - each showed that CEA improved outcome in selected patients with high-grade extracranial carotid artery stenosis when performed in centers with low morbidity and mortality. In these studies, there were some differences in design, methods of measuring stenosis and endpoints. In a recent metaanalysis using the primary data, CEA was associated with lower rate of non-fatal stroke at 30 days, an higher rate of non-fatal myocardial infarction, but no significant effect on mortality; the benefit of surgery increased with the degree of stenosis.[59] Men and women had equal benefit.

Three recent trials have looked at asymptomatic stenosis: Mayo Clinic,[60] VA Cooperative Study.[61] Asymptomatic Carotid Atherosclerosis Study.[62] The major risk appears to be perioperative stroke and myocardial infarction but followed by a decreased risk of stroke, transient monocular blindness and death. There was no significant difference with increasing degrees of stenosis.

While clinical studies of CEA report a perioperative complication rate of about 3%, community-based surveys describe a higher rate of 6 to 20%. Surgical complications are increased in cases of re-stenosis. The role of non-surgical alternatives such as angioplasty and stenting is being explored. One study suggests that angioplasty with stenting is safe and well tolerated; patients were maintained on aspirin and ticlopidine after the procedure.[62] Further evaluation is underway to define the role of interventional neuroradiology in stroke management and the clinical scenarios where it would be most useful.

Education and Rehabilitation

Education of the diabetic patient and family members in mitigating risk factors for stroke and in methods of assuring adherence to a medical program should be a component of clinical care. The need for urgent assessment on the occurrence of a stroke should be emphasized. Many diabetic patients after a stroke have diminished cerebral function that adversely affects recall and attention span. Proper self-management of diabetes may not be possible, particularly if insulin-requiring. Family support helps the patient adhere to a treatment regimen better than artificial devices, such as pill dispensers, check-off lists, or memory joggers. The humanism of this support adds to the quality of the patient's ambience. Regular visits by the patient to the physician permit appropriate adjustment of the medical program. In a large metropolitan area, visits by nursing personnel when a patient is home-bound have been an invaluable aid in maintaining a successful treatment program. Nurses are often responsible for early identification of inchoate medical problems, which are then corrected with greater ease. The management of stroke and its complications should not stop with surgery or drug therapy. Indeed, patients recovering from stroke should be offered the full array of specialty support and advice. These specialists include psychiatrists and physical therapists as well as occupational and speech therapists. It may be necessary to spend some time at a rehabilitation center. It is important to help the patient understand that recovery may be slow, erratic, and not always complete.

1. Krolewski AS, Kosiniski EJ, Warram JH, et al.: Magnitude and determinants of coronary artery disease in juvenile-onset, insulin-dependent diabetes mellitus. Am J Cardiol 59:750–755, 1987.

2. Tunbridge WMG: Factors contributing to deaths of diabetics under fifty years of age. Lancet 1:569–572, 1981.

3. Deckert T, Poulsen JE, Larsen M: Prognosis of diabetics with diabetes onset before age thirty-one. Diabetologia 14:363–370, 1978.

4. Entamacher PS, Krall LP, Krancer SN: Diabetes mortality from vital statistics. *In* Marble A, Krall LP, Bradley RF, Christlieb AR, Soeldner JS (eds): Joslin's Diabetes Mellitus. Philadelphia: Lea & Febiger, 1985, pp. 278–297.

5. Kessler I: Mortality experience of diabetic patients. Am J Med 51:715–724, 1971.

6. Garcia M, McNamara P, Gordon T, et al.: Morbidity and mortality in diabetics in the Framingham population. Diabetes 23:105–111, 1974.

7. Asplund K, Hagg E, Helmers C, et al.: The natural history of stroke in diabetic patients. Acta Med Scand 207:417–424, 1980.

8. Pulsinelli WA, Levy DE, Sigsbee B, et al.: Increased damage after ischemic stroke in patients with hyperglycemia with or without established diabetes mellitus. AmJ Med 74:540–544, 1983.

9. Oppenheimer SM, Hoffbrand BI, Oswald GA, et al.: Diabetes mellitus and early mortality from stroke. Br Med J 291:1014–1015, 1985.

10. Kannel WB, McGee DL: Diabetes and cardiovascular disease. The Framingham study. JAMA 241:2035–2038, 1979.

11. Abbot RD, Donahue RP, MacMahon SW, et al.: Diabetes and the risk of stroke. The Honolulu Heart Program. JAMA 257:949–952, 1987.

12. Barret-Connor E, Khaw K-T: Diabetes mellitus: an independent risk factor for stroke? Am J Epidemiol 128: 116–123, 1988.

13. Nedergaard M, Astrup J: Infarct rim: effect of hyperglycemia on direct current potential and [^{14}C]2-deoxyglucose phosphorylation. J Cereb Blood Flow Metabol 6: 607–615, 1986.

14. Chopp M, Frinak S, Walton DR, et al.: Intracellular acidosis during and after cerebral ischemia: in vivo nuclear

magnetic resonance study of hyperglycemia in cats. Stroke 18:919–923, 1987.

15. Levine SR, Welch KMA, Helpern JA, et al.: Prolonged deterioration of ischemic brain energy metabolism and acidosis associated with hyperglycemia: studied by serial ^{31}P NMR spectroscopy. Ann Neurol 23:416–418, 1988.

16. Prado R, Ginsberg MD, Dietrich WD, et al.: Hyperglycemia increases infarct size in collaterally perfused but not end-arterial vascular territories. J Cereb Blood Flow Metab 8:186–192, 1988.

17. Berger L, Hakim AM: The association of hyperglycemia with cerebral edema in stroke. Stroke 17:865–871, 1986.

18. Adams HP, Olinger CP, Marler JR, et al.: Comparison of admission serum glucose concentration with neurologic outcome in acute cerebral infarction. Stroke 19:455–458, 1988.

19. Toyama K, Neriishi S, Kawamoto S, et al.: Risk factors of cerebro-vascular disorders in mild diabetes. Tohoku J Exp Med 141 (Suppl):535–540, 1983.

20. Lindegard B, Hillbom M: Associations between brain infarction, diabetes and alcoholism: observations from the Gothenburg population cohort study. Acta Neurol Scand 75:195–200, 1987.

21. Salonen JT, Puska P, Tuomilehto J, et al.: Relation of blood pressure, serum lipids, and smoking to the risk of cerebral stroke. A longitudinal study in Eastern Finland. Stroke 13:327–333, 1982.

22. Melamed E: Reactive hyperglycaemia in patients with acute stroke. J Neurol Sci 29:267–275, 1976.

23. Riddle MC, Hart J: Hyperglycemia, recognized and unrecognized, as a risk factor for stroke and transient ischaemic attacks. Stroke 13:356–359, 1982.

24. Samanta A, Burden AC: Diabetes mellitus and early mortality from stroke. Br Med J 291:1349, 1985.

25. Cox NH, Lorains JW: The prognostic value of blood glucose and glycosylated haemoglobin estimation in persons with stroke. Postgrad Med J 62:7–10, 1986.

26. Gray CS, Taylor R, French JM, et al.: The prognostic value of stress hyperglycaemia and previously unrecognized diabetes in acute stroke. Diabetic Med 4:237–240, 1987.

27. Roehmholdt ME, Palumbo PJ, Whisnant JP, et al.: Transient ischemic attack and stroke in a community-based diabetic cohort. Mayo Clin Proc 58:56–58, 1983.

28. Kagan A, Popper JS, Rhoads GG: Factors related to stroke incidence in Hawaiian Japanese men. Stroke 11:14–21, 1987.

29. Mohr JP, Caplan LR, Melski JW, et al.: The Harvard Cooperative Stroke Registry: a prospective study. Neurology (New York) 28:754–762, 1978.

30. Adams HP, Putman SF, Kassell NF, et al.: Prevalence of diabetes mellitus among patients with subarachnoid hemorrhage. Arch Neurol 41:1033–1035, 1984.

31. West KM, Ahuja MMS, Bennett PH, et al.: The role of circulating glucose and triglyceride concentrations and their interactions with other "risk factors" as determinants of arterial disease in nine diabetic population samples from the WHO multinational study. Diabetes Care 6:361–369, 1983.

32. Ishihara M, Yukimura Y, Yamada T, et al.: Diabetic complications and their relationship to risk factors in a Japanese population. Diabetes Care 7:533–538, 1984.

33. Palumbo PJ, Elveback LR, Whisnant JP: Neurologic complications of diabetes mellitus: transient ischemic attack stroke and peripheral neuropathy. Adv Neurol 19:593–601, 1978.

34. The DCCT Research Group. Effect of intensive diabetes management on macrovascular events in the Diabetes Control and Complications Trial. Amer J Cardiol 75:894–903, 1995.

35. Bell ET: A postmortem study of vascular disease in diabetes. Arch Pathol 53:444–455, 1952.

36. Alex M, Baron EK, Goldenberg S, et al.: An autopsy of cerebrovascular accident in diabetes mellitus. Circulation 25:663–673, 1962.

37. Aronson SM: Intracranial vascular lesions in patients with diabetes mellitus. J Neuropathol Exp Neurol 23:183–196, 1973.

38. Colwell JA, Lopes-Virella MF: A review of the development of large-vessel disease in diabetes mellitus. Am J Med 85(Suppl 5A):113–118, 1988.

39. Dandona P, James IM, Newbury PA, et al.: Cerebral blood flow in diabetes mellitus: evidence of abnormal cerebrovascular reactivity. Br Med J 2:325–326, 1978.

40. Burn WK, Machin D, Waters WE: Prevalence of migraine in patients with diabetes. Br Med J 289:1579–1580, 1984.

41. Mohr JP, Rubenstein LV, Tatemichi TK, et al.: Blood sugar and acute stroke: the NINCDS Pilot Stroke Data Bank. Stroke 16:143, 1985.

42. Feussner JR, Matchar DB: When and how to study the carotid arteries. Ann Intern Med 109:805–818, 1988.

43. Parfrey PS, Griffiths SM, Barrett BJ, et al.: Contrast material-induced renal failure in patients with diabetes mellitus renal insufficiency, or both. N Engl J Med 320:143–149, 1989.

44. Hacke W, Kaste M, Dieschi C, et al.: Intravenous thrombolysis with recombinant tissue plasminogen activator for accurate hemispheric stroke: The European Cooperative Acute Stroke Study (ECASS). JAMA 274:1017–59, 1995.

45. The National Institute of Neurological Disorders and Stroke r-TPA Stroke Study Group. N Engl J Med 333:1581–1593, 1995.

46. Heiss W-D, Grond M, Thiel A, et al.: Ischaemic brain tissue salvaged from infarction with alteplase. Lancet 349:1599–1560, 1997.

47. Asplund K, Erikson S, Hagg E, et al.: Hyperosmolar nonketotic coma in diabetic stroke patients. Acta Med Scand 212:407–411, 1982.

48. Weir CJ, Murray GD, Dyker AG, et al.: Is hyperglycaemia an independent predictor of poor outcome after acute stroke? Results of a long term follow up study. BMJ 314:1303–1306.

49. Colwell JA, Bingham SF, Abraira C, et al.: The Cooperative Study Group: Veterans Administration Cooperative Study on antiplatelet agents in diabetic patients after amputation for gangrene. II. Effects of aspirin and dipyridamole on athersclerotic vascular disease rates. Diabetes Care 9:140–148, 1986.

50. Colwell JA, Bingham SF: VA Cooperative Study on antiplatelet agents in diabetic patients after amputation for gangrene. Haemostasis 16:433–438, 1986.

51. Antiplatelet Trialists' Collaboration: Secondary prevention of vascular disease by prolonged antiplatelet treatment. Br Med J 296:320–331, 1988.

52. International Stroke Trial Collaborative Group. The International Stroke Trial (IST): a randomised trial of aspirin, subcutaneous heparin, both, or neither among 19435 patients with acute ischaemic stroke. Lancet 349:1569–1581, 1997.

53. CAST (Chinese Acute Stroke Trial) Collaborative Group. CAST: randomised placebo-controlled trial of early aspirin use in 20000 patients with acute ischaemic stroke. Lancet 349:1641–1649, 1997.

54. Ticlopidine Aspirin Stroke Study Group. Ticlopidine versus aspirin for stroke prevention: on-treatment results from the Ticlopidine Aspirin Stroke Study. J Stroke Cerebrovasc Dis 3:168–176, 1993.

55. Petersen P, Boysen G, Gotfredsen J, et al.: Placebo-controlled, randomized trial of warfarin and aspirin for prevention of thromboembolic complications in chronic atrial fibrillation. Lancet 1:175–179, 1989.

56. North American Symptomatic Carotid Endartertectomy Trial Collaborators. Benefits of carotid endartertectomy in symptomatic patients with high-grade carotid stenosis. NEJM 325:445–453, 1991.

57. European Carotid Surgery Trialists Collaborative Group. MRC European carotid surgery trial: interim results for symptomatic patients with severe (70 to 99%) or with mild (0 to 29%) carotid stenosis. Lancet 337:1235–1243, 1991.

58. Mayberg MR, Wilson E, Yatsu F, et al.: Carotid endarterectomy and prevention of cerebral ischemia in symptomatic carotid stenosis. JAMA 226:3289–3294, 1991.

59. Goldstein LB, Hasselblad V, Matchar DB, et al.: Comparison and meta-analysis of randomized trials of endarterectomy for symptomatic carotid stenosis. Neurology 45:1965–1970, 1995.

60. Mayo Asymptomatic Carotid Endarterectomy Study Group. Results of a randomized controlled trial of carotid endarterectomy for asymptomatic carotid stenosis. Mayo Clinic Proceedings 67:513–518, 1992.

61. Hobson II RW, Weiss DG, Fields WS, et al.: Efficacy of carotid endarterectomy for asymptomatic carotid stenosis. N Engl J Med 328:221–227, 1993.

62. Executive Committee for the Asymptomatic Carotid Atherosclerosis Study. Endarterectomy for asymptomatic carotid artery stenosis. JAMA 273:1421–1428, 1995.

63. Yadav JS, Roubin GS, King P, et al.: Angioplasty and stenting for restenosis after endarterectomy. Stroke 27:2075–2079, 1996.

30

Peripheral Vascular Disease in Diabetes Mellitus

John A. Colwell

Historical Perspective

Past Eras (400 BC–AD 1922)

According to the Gospel of St. Matthew: "If thy right hand offend thee, cut it off and cast it from thee." In 400 bc, Hippocrates reportedly "cut away the mortified parts," largely in patients with gangrene following vascular occlusion. In the 1st century ad, Celsus advised that amputation should be done at or immediately above the separation of the dead from the living flesh. Cautery was used in the 11th century to control the serious problems of hemorrhage, and in the 16th century, ligatures and the tourniquet were first successfully used.

The first published picture of an amputation appeared in 1517 in the *Field Book of Wound Surgery* by Hans von Gersdorff. He used a tourniquet; stopped bleeding with a styptic composed of vitriol, lime, alum, aloes, and nutgalls; and enclosed the stump in the bladder of a bull, ox, or hog. By the 17th century, it is known that amputations were performed not only because of traumatic wounds or fractures, but also for foot ulcers and abscesses. In 1842, Symes first performed his celebrated amputation at the level of the ankle joint, and the first major amputation under general anesthesia (ether) was performed in 1846 by Robert Liston. In 1852, Marchal was the first to point out the association of diabetes with gangrene. In 1867, Lister described his antiseptic methods, but it was almost 20 years later, at about the time that von Mering and Minkowski described pancreatic diabetes in dogs, that antisepsis was completely accepted by the medical and surgical community. By 1891, Heidenhain had published a thorough review of diabetes and arteriosclerosis of the legs and had defined appropriate levels for amputation to be performed if gangrene occurred.

Gradually, over the next 30 years, amputations were performed in diabetic patients with gangrene, but it was not until the discovery of insulin in 1921–1922 that extensive data began to appear regarding this procedure for the diabetic patient.

Modern Era (1922–Present)

Prior to the discovery of insulin, vascular disease was reported to cause less than 20% of deaths in diabetic patients. Nevertheless, it was recognized that people with diabetes had more arteriosclerotic vascular disease when compared with those without diabetes. Autopsy studies prior to 1930 in diabetic patients showed that 29% of them had gangrene at the time of death, and while these figures improved somewhat over the next two decades, about 20% of the deaths in one large series were still due to gangrene between 1931 and 1955. At the Joslin Clinic, over 40% of 16,382 operations in diabetic patients were major or minor amputations from 1923 to 1945; this fell to a rate from 31% to 36% between 1945 and 1964 and to 22% by 1969, as vascular reconstructive procedures became more popular.[1] Nevertheless, even in recent years, amputation for diabetic gangrene is frequently performed in all large hospitals with an adult diabetic population.

A modern historical perspective on the medical and surgical evaluation and management of peripheral vascular disease in diabetes mellitus is given in Table 30–1. Since the discovery of insulin, there has been a steady trend to lower the percentage of fat prescribed for a diabetic diet and to decrease the amount of saturated fat in the diet. This has been accompanied by a trend to increase the percentage of carbohydrate, with a recent emphasis on the use of increased amounts of fiber in the dietary prescription. For about 20 years after the discovery of insulin, much of the clinical research concentrated on modifying insulins in such a way as to prolong the timing of regular insulin. This led to the development of protamine zinc insulin (PZI), PZI-regular insulin mixtures, and the intermediate insulin: neutral protamine Hagedorn (NPH), globin, and the Lente insulins in the 1950s (see Chapter 18).

During this period, advances in anesthetic and fluid management of surgical patients were made, and the antibiotic era began. Late in the 1950s, the oral

TABLE 30–1   Medical and Surgical Evaluation and Management of Patients with Peripheral Vascular Disease and Diabetes Mellitus

| Year | Diet (%)[a] | | | Major Medical Advances | Diagnostic Procedure | Surgical Procedures |
	C	P	F			
1920–1930	30	20	50	Insulin discovered	History; physical examination	Above-knee amputation Sympathectomy
1931–1940				Insulins modified (timing)	X ray film	
1941–1950	35	20	45	Anesthetics improved; IV fluid therapy		Below-knee amputation; transmetatarsal amputation; venous bypass procedure
1957–1960	40	20	40	Antibiotics; oral hypoglycemic agents	Arteriography	Endarterectomy
1961–1970	45	20	35	Rehabilitation procedures		
1971–1980	50	20	30	Purified insulins; exercise	Noninvasive testing	Transluminal angioplasty
1980–1989	55	20	25	Insulin pumps; self-monitoring of blood glucose; human insulin	Vascular laboratories	
1990–	55	15	30	Prevention and treatment of risk factors	MRI	Laser

[a] C, carbohydrate; F, fat; P, protein.

hypoglycemic agents were introduced and were widely used for non-insulin-dependent diabetic (NIDDM) patients thereafter. Improved rehabilitation procedures helped the amputee patient. In the 1970s, it was found that the older insulins contained many impurities, and highly purified insulins were developed. This era culminated in the development of synthetic and semisynthetic human insulin preparations, which were first marketed in the 1980s.

In recent years, there has been an intense national interest in the value of exercise as a regular part of the lifestyle of many individuals. This has been adopted by most physicians as a new point of emphasis in diabetic management. In addition, new techniques of medical management have emerged, including self-monitoring of blood glucose and insulin pump therapy, particularly for insulin-dependent diabetic patients.

Diagnostic procedures for peripheral vascular disease were relatively crude until recent years. Thus, in the first half of the century, evaluation was limited to history, physical examination, and X-ray examination for vascular calcification. Recent advances with noninvasive and invasive procedures done in modern vascular laboratories have improved diagnostic sensitivity and specificity in peripheral vascular disorders.

Early surgical management of the diabetic patient with gangrene of a lower extremity usually consisted of above-knee amputation. Sympathectomy was discovered in the 1920s and was widely practiced for a few decades, but was found to be generally unsuccessful in diabetics with peripheral vascular disease who required surgery. As time progressed and medical and prosthetic management improved, it became apparent

that rehabilitation was more successful when distal amputations were performed, and the procedures of transmetatarsal and below-knee amputations were developed. The latter procedure has replaced above-knee amputations in most diabetic patients. Arterial bypass procedures, with or without endarterectomy, have been performed since the 1950s in diabetic as well as in nondiabetic patients and have been serially modified so that they remain procedures of choice if limb survival is predicted. In very recent years, the technique of transluminal angioplasty has attained some popularity in the management of some forms of peripheral vascular disease (see Chapter 34).

The 21st century will see additional advances. It is likely that the emphasis will gradually shift to preventive strategies that are directed at major risk factors. Examination of the feet, foot care education, and guidelines for care will be accepted as cost-effective strategies. Control of systolic and diastolic hypertension without adverse side effects is now possible with new antihypertensive agents, and control of hyperlipidemia is also materially aided by new dietary and pharmacologic approaches. Collaborative trials are planned or are underway to assess these preventive approaches, and the issue of the need for intensive glycemic control may also be resolved in the next decade. Thus, while surgical procedures such as amputation, bypass, endarterectomy, angioplasty, and laser therapy may still be used, there should be a diminished need for these procedures in the future. The net effect will be a marked saving in health care costs and improved quality of life for people with diabetes.

Epidemiology

Scope, Impact, and Costs

West has described the information available about peripheral vascular disease in diabetes mellitus as an "epidemiologist's nightmare." In general, standardization of methods was minimal in the past, and modern epidemiologic techniques and interpretation were lacking. Recent studies are providing excellent epidemiologic information in some populations.

The toll of peripheral vascular disease in diabetes mellitus is enormous. It has been estimated to be 30 times more common in diabetic than in nondiabetic individuals, and the risk of gangrene is increased markedly in diabetic patients. In a classic 1950 autopsy series,[2] Bell studied autopsy records on 2,130 diabetic persons who had died from 1911 through 1955. Deaths occurred most frequently between ages 61 and 80. Gangrene was found in 21% of the deaths in diabetic patients and was 53 to 71 times more common in diabetics than in nondiabetics. Equal numbers of diabetic males and females were found to have atherosclerotic gangrene at autopsy. No significant difference in the frequency of hypertension in diabetic and control groups was found, and there was no relationship between duration of diabetes and the development of gangrene. About 37% of the patients had required insulin at any time. Causes of death were primarily vascular, with 46% due to gangrene, 20% to coronary artery disease, and 13% to cerebrovascular accident or renal atherosclerosis.

In hospital studies of diabetic patients, peripheral vascular disease may account for 25% of their admissions, and hospital stays are typically very long. Whether conservative medical management, bypass surgery or angioplasty, or amputation is chosen, prolonged hospitalization is usually necessary. In an effort to save a leg, often a stepwise approach to management is used, which is time consuming and costly. About 50% of amputations of the lower extremity in the United States are done in diabetic patients. When diabetes is mentioned as a cause of death on death certificates, gangrene is also mentioned frequently—at a frequency 20 times greater than in persons dying of other causes.

Diabetes is a major contributor to peripheral vascular disease in most populations, but the magnitude of this contribution is quite variable. In various reports, it has ranged from 15% among females with arteriosclerosis obliterans in Oslo, to 23% among Australian amputees, to 45–65% among amputees in series reported from the United States.[2]

The total cost of caring for foot problems in people with diabetes in not known. However, estimates of the hospitalization costs for foot ulcers and for amputations can be made.[3] In 1990, it was estimated that 54,000 amputations were done in diabetic individuals in the United States. In 1992, 39,287 bills were submitted to Medicare for lower limb amputations. Average length of stay was 18.4 days, and average reimbursement to the hospital was $10,969. Reimbursement from private insurance was $26,940 for this procedure. While these data illustrate the difficulty in estimating exact costs for caring for foot problems in diabetes, it is clear that these chronic problems are a major drain on health care resources (see Chapter 50).

Prevalence

Investigators in early series were obliged to use such insensitive estimates of peripheral vascular disease as amputations, diminished or absent peripheral pulses, or leg-vessel calcification to provide evidence of the disease in diabetic versus nondiabetic populations. Gangrene is about 100 times more common among diabetic patients in the United States than in Japan. Peripheral vascular disease is present in only 9% of diabetics in India, but still exceeds the prevalence in nondiabetic patients. In two well-controlled series in Sweden, absent pulses were found in about 10% of diabetics but in only about 2.6% of age and sex-matched control patients. In the Tecumseh Study, foot pulses were absent about twice as often among subjects with blood glucose ranges in the upper quintile of the population than in other groups.[4] Vascular calcification of the lower extremities occurred in about 4% of control subjects, but in 9–11% of diabetics of short duration and in 18–53% of those of long duration. In insulin-dependent diabetics with disease of 35 years duration, vascular calcification may be seen in 90% of patients. In a study from Minnesota,[5] the age-adjusted prevalence of clinical peripheral vascular disease in a population-based cohort of diabetic patients was 3.3/1,000 population in 1970. In patients ages 60–79, it was 7.2 (females) to 9.2 (males)/1,000 population.

Large series of diabetics have been studied with noninvasive techniques. In 506 diabetics, peripheral vascular disease was found in 24% of insulin-dependent and in 38% of non-insulin-dependent patients.[6] In the latter group, the male-to-female ratio was about 1.5:1, whereas it was almost equal among insulin-dependent patients.

In West Germany, the prevalence was somewhat less in a study of 623 diabetic outpatients.[7] A prevalence of 15.9% of peripheral vascular disease was found—14.4% in females and 18% in males. As in most series, there was a greater yield of peripheral vascular disease in older patients (over 30% above the age of 70) when compared with younger patients (under 5% in those under 50).

Incidence

Data regarding incidence of peripheral vascular disease in the general population and among patients with diabetes mellitus are somewhat limited. Some of the earliest population-based data were the reports from the Scandinavian countries, in which 12% of insulin-dependent patients in Denmark were found to require amputation.[8] The annual rate of diabetes-related amputations in Sweden was estimated at 10/100,000 population[9] and in Denmark at 7/100,000 population.[8] It is estimated that from 30,000 to 54,000 amputations are performed each year in the United States in people with diabetes.[3,10–12]

Davidson et al.[13] provided data that illustrated the value of a coordinated program of diabetic education, prevention, and management. In their program, the amputation rate decreased from 13.3/1,000 patients in 1973 to 6.7/1,000 patients in 1980. Improved foot care programs have led to a 49–85% reduction in amputation rates after their implementation.[12]

In a Rochester, Minnesota, study,[5] the incidence of peripheral vascular disease, as defined by absent or markedly diminished pulses or gangrene, was 21.3/1,000 patient-years in males and 17.6/1,000 patient-years in females. It was estimated that in diabetic patients free from arteriosclerosis obliterans the cumulative incidence of subsequent peripheral vascular disease was about 15% at 10 years and 45% at 20 years after the diagnosis of diabetes.

Beach et al. have provided excellent data on the progression of lower extremity arterial occlusive disease (LEAOD) in diabetic subjects.[14] At baseline, 22% of NIDDM had LEAOD, whereas only 3% of controls had it. The incidence of new LEAOD was 14% in 2 years, and progression occurred in 87% of patients over the same period.

In another longitudinal study,[15] 24.8% of diabetic women and 18.9% of diabetic men had acquired early peripheral vascular disease, as detected by Doppler examination, in 5 years of follow-up.

In Sweden the annual incidence of hospitalization for peripheral vascular disease in diabetes mellitus was 1%/year in the sixth decade, and rose 1%/year through the ninth decade. In a prospective study using noninvasive techniques in a large series of NIDDM patients in the United States, a 9.8% incidence of peripheral vascular disease was found in a little over 2 years of the study.[16] In diabetic patients, the Framingham Study showed that the incidence of intermittent claudication among diabetic subjects was about 4.5 times that of control subjects.[17]

Risk Factors (Table 30–2)

Age.   Age is one of the most important risk factors for peripheral vascular disease in diabetes mellitus. In most reports, gangrene and amputation are rarely found in patients under the age of 40 years. In Bell's autopsy series, only 3 of 1,878 diabetic patients who were found to have atherosclerotic gangrene were under the age of 40.[2] In most cross-sectional studies, the mean age of patients with gangrene or amputation is close to 60 years.

In recent studies, in which noninvasive techniques have been used to diagnose peripheral vascular disease, age has also been found to be an important risk factor. Highly significant correlations between age and the presence of vascular disease have been found in the United States and West Germany.[5–7,10] Vascular calcification is also influenced by age as well as by duration of diabetes.

Duration of Diabetes.   Radiographic evidence of calcification was found about twice as often among dia-

TABLE 30–2   Risk Factors and Peripheral Vascular Disease in Diabetes Mellitus (DM)

Risk Factor	Method Used			
	Noninvasive Testing	Claudication	Vessel Calcification	Gangrene or Amputation
Age	Yes	[a]	Yes	Yes
Duration of DM	Yes	[a]	Yes	Yes
Lipids/lipoproteins	Yes	Yes	[a]	[a]
Hypertension	Yes/no	Yes	[a]	[a]
Smoking	Yes	Yes	[a]	[a]
Race				
Caucasian	Yes	[a]	[a]	[a]
African American	[a]	[a]	[a]	Yes
Sex	[b]	[b]	[b]	[b]
Obesity	[b]	[b]	[b]	[b]
Hyperglycemia	[b]	[b]	[b]	Yes

[a] Not determined or negative.

[b] No correlation.

betics of short duration and about 3.7 times as often in diabetics of long duration when compared with age- and sex-matched control subjects in one series.[18] The findings of diminished or absent pulses in the lower extremities also correlated highly with duration of diabetes. Using noninvasive techniques, a correlation with duration was found in two series when diabetics treated with insulin were studied,[6,7] but this correlation was less significant in one other population.[16] Several recent studies have indicated that duration of diabetes is a predictor of lower extremity amputation.[19,20]

Plasma Lipids/Lipoproteins. Hyperlipoproteinemia is frequently seen in diabetic populations with peripheral vascular disease. Prevalence ranges from 39% to 60%, depending on the series under study. Hypertriglyceridemia appears to be seen more frequently than hypercholesterolemia, but this may relate only to the general use of a relatively high cutoff point for "normal" serum cholesterol levels. A positive relationship between hypertriglyceridemia and peripheral vascular disease has been reported.[21]

In a very thorough study, it was reported that the risk factors for peripheral vascular disease (as defined by noninvasive testing) in insulin-treated NIDDM and insulin-dependent (IDDM) patients were very-low-density lipoprotein (VLDL), triglyceride, and low-density lipoprotein (LDL) cholesterol levels.[6] Age and duration of diabetes were also highly correlated. In the insulin-treated NIDDM group, high-density lipoprotein (HDL) cholesterol levels had an inverse relationship to peripheral vascular disease. These investigators have reexamined these questions and have found that elevated plasma triglyceride and decreased plasma HDL cholesterol levels are significant risk factors.[14] Support for lipids/lipoproteins as risk factors for peripheral vascular disease was provided from a study in Finland, where increased total and LDL cholesterol, increased total and VLDL triglycerides, and low HDL cholesterol correlated with claudication in IDDM and NIDDM.[22]

Increased serum cholesterol concentration was associated with the appearance of peripheral vascular disease (as assessed by noninvasive studies) in one report of a 2-year longitudinal study.[16] This was also true in the Framingham Study,[17] as assessed by intermittent claudication.

Hypertension. In the Framingham Study, hypertension was also found to be a risk factor for the appearance of intermittent claudication in diabetic patients.[17] In studies in India and Australia, blood pressure had little effect on peripheral vascular disease in diabetic patients. Blood pressure was not found to be one of the most important factors in one recent prospective study in the United States,[16] but systolic hypertension was defined as an important risk factor for peripheral vascular disease in a West German study.[7] It is apparent that conflicting data exist on this point, but the collective impression is that elevated blood pressure levels may have only a modest effect on the risk of peripheral vascular disease in diabetes mellitus when compared with other risk factors such as age, duration of diabetes, and lipid or lipoprotein abnormalities.

Smoking. Smoking was the strongest risk factor for intermittent claudication among diabetic patients in the Framingham Study.[17] In two recent reports, smoking was found to be an important risk factor in one group of diabetics with peripheral vascular disease,[7] but not in another.[16] Smoking was found to favor above-knee amputation, whereas diabetes appeared to favor below-knee amputation.[23]

Race. In two studies, opposite results have been obtained regarding the influence of race on peripheral vascular disease in diabetes mellitus. In one of six states in the United States survey,[10] African Americans diabetic subjects were found to have an amputation rate 2.3 times greater than Caucasian diabetic persons. It was not possible to determine whether this related to health care patterns or to inherent differences in the natural history of the disease. In a brief report,[16] however, multivariate analysis in a cohort of 163 NIDDM patients showed that Caucasian race was among the most significant risk factors for the development of arteriosclerosis obliterans, as determined by noninvasive techniques. However, recent data from California indicate that African-American diabetic individuals have the highest amputation rate (95.2/10,000 people) when compared to Hispanics (44.4/10,000) or non-Hispanic Caucasians (56/10,000).[24]

Risk factors for lower extremity amputations have now been reported from a 12-year follow-up in the Pima Indian population.[25] Altered lipid/lipoprotein profiles were not predictive of amputation, whereas duration of diabetes, medial arterial calcification, retinopathy, nephropathy, peripheral neuropathy, and hyperglycemia all emerged as risk factors. The rate of amputation among Pima Indians with diabetes was 3.7 times greater than control diabetic populations elsewhere in the United States. Whether this reflects an increased risk or more complete ascertainment is not clear. If the latter is true, rate and costs of amputations in diabetic individuals may be much higher than previously reported.

Gender. In nondiabetic subjects, there is a male predominance in peripheral vascular disease of about 4:1. This ratio is reduced to about 2:1 or less in diabetic subjects with peripheral vascular disease.[5,7,10] It has been unclear in epidemiologic studies whether sex is an independent risk factor for peripheral vascular disease among diabetic patients. High rates of smoking or other unrecognized factors in males may contribute to the apparent male predominance in various populations studies for peripheral vascular disease.

Obesity. In many studies, a large proportion of diabetic patients with amputation have had a history of long-standing obesity. Obesity may coexist with hyperinsulinemia, insulin resistance, decreased exercise, and other factors that may contribute to atherosclerosis. In studies published to date, there has been little or no evidence that obesity is a major independent risk factor for peripheral vascular disease in diabetes mellitus.

Hyperglycemia. Recent epidemiologic studies have established that fasting glucose or hemoglobin A_{1c} are important predictors for amputation in NIDDM, even after adjustment for other cardiovascular risk factors.[19,20] In support of the view that glycemia is an important risk factor for amputation was the finding that the small vessel and neuropathic complications of diabetes (retinopathy, neuropathy, nephropathy) were also predictors of amputation.[19] A dose–response relationship was seen between glycated hemoglobin and amputation risk.[20]

Thus, a strong case can be made from epidemiologic studies that prolonged hyperglycemia is an important contributor to amputation in diabetes. However, prospective intervention trial data are lacking, and a separation of the relative influences of neuropathy and of arteriosclerosis is difficult.

Morbidity and Mortality

Amputations and Deaths

There is abundant evidence that significant morbidity and mortality occur in diabetic patients who have had amputation for gangrene. Between 1952 and 1970, from 51 to 60% of patients had a second amputation within 5 years of the first in five different series (Table 30–3). Improved figures have been reported in one more recent large series of amputations: 32% in 5 years.

These patients usually have advanced vascular disease of a generalized nature. This leads to high mortality, with in-hospital deaths as high as 33–50% before 1950. These figures fell to between 7% and 25% from

TABLE 30–3 Amputation of Opposite Leg in Diabetic Patients—% After One Amputation

Observer	Year	By 1 Year	By 3 Years	By 5 Years
Silbert[37]	1952		30	51
Goldner[38]	1960	23	40	66
Hoar[39]	1962		36	50
Cameron[40]	1964	44		57
Ecker[41]	1970		61	
Roon[42]	1976			32

TABLE 30–4 Amputation in Diabetic Patients: Death Rates

Observer	Year	Patients Dying(%) In-hospital	1–3 Years	3–5 Years
Levin[43]	1935	50		
Pearse[44]	1940	32		
Mendelberg[45]	1944	33		
Smith[46]	1956	12		52
Hoar[39]	1962	7	45	
Cameron[40]	1964	25	40	50
Baddeley[47]	1965	15	44	52
Warren[48]	1968	25		
Whitehouse[49]	1968	10	49	70
Haimovici[50]	1970	9	35	59
Ecker[41]	1970	23	39	
Kahn[51]	1974	9		
Roon[42]	1976	3	57	61
Huston[52]	1980	15	41	
Colwell[53]	1986		33	
Pohjalainen[54]	1988	27[a]		
Waugh[55]	1988		50	

[a] Within 3 months of surgery.

1950 to 1970. Later studies have yielded figures in a slightly lower range (Table 30–4). Like the data for amputations, there is remarkable consistency regarding deaths in the years after amputation: 33–57% within 3 years and 50–70% within 5 years. Despite marked advances in medical and surgical management and in diagnostic techniques (see Table 30–1), there is no evidence of a substantial improvement in the 3- or 5-year mortality figures in the recent literature.

Pathways to amputation in people with diabetes have been studied,[26] and seven major factors have been identified. Amputations were usually from multiple causes, with minor trauma being the pivotal event in 86% of cases. Other causes, usually in combination, were ulceration, faulty wound healing, gangrene, infection, neuropathy, and ischemia.

In another study,[27] significant risk factors for amputation in diabetes were decreased cutaneous circulation, ankle-brachial index less than .45, absent vibration sensation, and decreased plasma HDL cholesterol level.

Three variables were found to be predictive of foot ulcer in a separate study: absent Achilles reflex, absent sensation to a monofilament test, and decreased oxygenation $(TcPO_2)$. These studies indicated that both neuropathic and vascular abnormalities were independently associated with increased risk for ulceration.[28]

Finally, it became apparent that peripheral vascular disease in people with diabetes is a significant predictor of future vascular events. In the Framingham Study, intermittent claudication in diabetes was a predictor of cardiovascular events in diabetes.[29] Medial calcification was an independent predictor of cardiovascular mortality in type 2 diabetic subjects in Finland.[30]

Reduction for Risk Factors for Amputation

A well-controlled prospective study indicated that risk factors for lower extremity amputation could be reduced by a multifaceted intervention.[31] Patients received foot-care education, entered into a contract for desired self-care, and received reinforcement by telephone and other reminders. Health care providers were given practice guidelines and flow sheets and were reminded to ask patients to remove footwear, perform foot examination, and provide health care education. Patients receiving the intervention were less likely than control patients to have serious foot lesions in this 1-year study. They were also more likely to report good foot-care behaviors and to have foot examinations and education at office visits.

Pathophysiology of Atherosclerosis in Diabetes Mellitus

There have been recent reviews of this subject that should be consulted for detailed information.[32,33] Current ideas about the pathogenesis of atherosclerosis [32,33] suggest that the process may begin with endothelial injury. Monocyte-derived macrophages adhere to the site of injury and may accumulate lipids, resulting in foam cell and fatty streak development. This is then followed by platelet adhesion to the site of injury and platelet aggregation and release of intracellular materials that may cause further aggregation, vasoconstriction, and smooth muscle proliferation. Platelet survival may be shortened, platelet turnover may be accelerated, and platelet-plasma interactions may occur. In the area of injury, there may be accumulation of cholesterol esters, and HDL cholesterol may exert a protective influence, while atherogenic lipoproteins (LDL cholesterol and VLDL remnants) may promote the process. Arterial wall accumulation of advanced glycation products may occur, and vascular wall stiffness may eventually compromise the ability of the vasculature to adapt to these new stresses. Finally, hypercoagulability and decreased fibrinolysis may be present and contribute to thrombosis and vascular occlusion.[33]

Although it is by no means clear what the sequence of events is in atherosclerosis in diabetes mellitus, it is likely that some or all of these processes may be involved. Accordingly, each will be briefly considered.

Endothelial Injury

This may occur via a number of mechanisms, including hypertension, hypercholesterolemia, immunologic injury, viral infection, and local trauma. In the diabetic state it is not clear which, if any, of these mechanisms occur. However, it is clear that endothelial injury is probably present in many diabetic patients, as indicated by elevated levels of von Willebrand factor, an endothelial glycoprotein. Furthermore, there is decreased endothelial release of prostacyclin, a vasodilator and antiplatelet aggregating agent, as well as of inhibitors of plasminogen activator, an activator of fibrinolysis, and decreased release of lipoprotein lipase by vascular endothelium. It can be predicted that the net effects of these endothelial alterations would be to favor atherosclerosis and thrombosis, and it is likely that they are contributory in diabetes mellitus.

Platelet Function

Increased adhesiveness and aggregability of platelets in patients with diabetes have now been demonstrated on many occasions.[32,33] Increased aggregability, like endothelial damage, may occur very early in the diabetic state in animals and humans, suggesting that it could contribute to, as well as result from, vascular disease. Platelets from diabetic subjects release increased amounts of proaggregatory prostanoids, such as thromboxane. Platelet–plasma interactions with plasma proteins, including glycated LDL, immune complexes, and fibrinogen, have been shown to occur. In patients with advanced vascular disease, platelet survival is shortened and turnover is rapid. In vivo evidence of altered platelet function is provided by elevated levels of the platelet specific proteins, platelet factor 4, and β-thromboglobulin. Studies have indicated that platelets from diabetics release increased amounts of growth-promoting factors similar to the smooth muscle cell mitogenic factor described by Ross.[34] It has been postulated that this platelet-derived growth factor activity plays an important role in atherosclerosis by promoting smooth muscle cell production.

Lipids and Lipoproteins

It has long been recognized that elevated plasma cholesterol and triglyceride levels may be found in diabetes mellitus, particularly when metabolic control is poor. More recently, it has become clear that elevated plasma VLDL and LDL levels and suppressed HDL concentrations are also frequently seen in the diabetic state.[32,33] In IDDM patients, this appears only in the presence of significant hyperglycemia, whereas in NIDDM patients it may be seen even when glycemia is minimal. This combination is clearly an atherogenic mix and could contribute in a significant way to the accelerated atherosclerosis of diabetes mellitus. In peripheral vascular disease, this is supported by epidemiologic data (see Table 30–2).

Work has focused on precisely what lipid or lipoprotein defects might exist. The atherogenic particles that accumulate are not simply LDL; rather, they may emerge from accelerated VLDL production and diminished peripheral clearance of VLDL remnants. Furthermore, it appears that LDL particles may be glycosylated and carry excess triglyceride. It is possible that these alterations may impair cellular handling and metabolism of atherogenic lipoproteins, lead to lipid accumulation, and promote atherosclerosis.[35]

It is now recognized that glycosylated LDL, whether produced in vitro or separated from plasma of patients with diabetes, can interact with macrophages to increase their cholesterol update and deposition of cholesterol esters.[35] The net result is foam cell production. In addition, it has now been demonstrated that glycosylated LDL will interact with platelets to promote hypersensitivity to agonists and increased release of thromboxane.[33] These are two mechanisms by which protein glycosylation may accelerate atherosclerosis in diabetes.

Arterial Media

To complicate the process, it is clear that increased arterial wall stiffness often accompanies the diabetic state. Advanced glycation products have been found to accumulate in excess and may trap lipoproteins locally. In any case, it is likely that the arterial wall stiffening seen in diabetes also contributes to the complicated process of atherosclerosis.

Coagulation

Although elevated plasma levels of a variety of coagulation factors—V, VII, VIII, IX, X, XII—have been reported in the diabetic state, the significance is not clear. Of probable importance, however, are the consistently reported elevated plasma fibrinogen levels, an accelerated fibrinogen turnover, a decreased plasminogen activator activity due to an increased activity of plasminogen activator inhibitor (PAI-1).[33] Generally, these findings are seen in diabetic patients with consistent hyperglycemia or with advanced vascular disease, but elevated PAI-1 levels are seen in some individuals with impaired glucose tolerance. Disseminated intravascular coagulation may occur, and fibrin thrombi are seen histopathologically in advanced cases of peripheral vascular disease and neuropathy in diabetes mellitus.

Thus, it is likely that altered endothelial and platelet function, lipid and lipoprotein metabolism, and coagulation contribute to the problem of accelerated peripheral vascular disease in diabetes mellitus. The process is accentuated by the classic risk factors of hypertension and smoking, and the hyperglycemia of diabetes may contribute through protein glycosylation and other mechanisms.

Research Considerations

The following areas are suggested for additional research in the problems of peripheral vascular disease in diabetes mellitus.

Epidemiology

Recommended are standardization of methods of diagnosing and assessing peripheral vascular disease in epidemiologic studies, population-based studies on incidence and prevalence of peripheral vascular disease, multivariate analyses of baseline cardiovascular risk factors and peripheral vascular disease endpoints in a variety of populations, and coordination of ongoing epidemiologic studies to yield maximal information in a short time frame.

Clinical Research

Suggested courses of research include prospective studies on the effect of altering one or more risk factors on the rate of progression of peripheral vascular disease in diabetic patients, controlled clinical trials to properly assess various surgical techniques in the prevention and/or progression of peripheral vascular disease, short-term trials of promising agents (prostanoids, fibrinolytic agents, and so forth) and acute thrombosis in peripheral arterial circulation in the legs, and investigation of improved techniques for the early recognition and monitoring of progression of peripheral vascular disease in diabetes mellitus.

Disease Mechanisms

Areas of study are factors that promote endothelial injury and control endothelial function in the diabetic state, the relationship of altered platelet and macrophage function to atherosclerosis, mechanisms by which lipids and lipoproteins contribute to accelerated atherosclerosis in the diabetic state, and assessment of the contributions of the vascular wall and the hemodynamic and prothrombotic changes of the diabetic state to peripheral vascular disease.

An important consensus development conference on the prevention and treatment of macrovascular disease in diabetes was sponsored by the American Diabetes Association.[36] Support for these and other research initiatives was provided from the consensus document that emerged from this conference.

References

1. Wheelock FC, Marble A: Surgery and diabetes. In Marble A, White P, Bradley RF, et al. (eds): Joslin's Diabetes Mellitus, Ed. 11. Philadelphia: Lea & Febiger, 1971, pp. 599–620.

2. Bell ET: Incidence of gangrene of the extremities in nondiabetic and diabetic persons. Arch Pathol 49:469–473, 1950.

3. Reiber GE, Boyko EJ, Smith DG: Lower extremity foot ulcers and amputations in diabetes. In National Diabetes Data Group: Diabetes in America, Ed. 2. Washington, DC: National Institutes of Health, National Institute of Diabetes and Digestive and Kidney Disease (NIH Publications No. 95-1468), 1995, pp. 409–427.

4. Epstein FH, Ostrander LD, Johnson BC, et al.: Epidemiological studies of cardiovascular diseases in a total community—Tecumseh, Michigan. Ann Intern Med 62:1170–1187, 1965.

5. Melton IJ, Machen KM, Palumbo PJ, et al.: Incidence and prevalence of clinical peripheral vascular disease in population-based cohort of 56 diabetic patients. Diabetes Care 3:650–654, 1980.

6. Beach KW, Brunzell JD, Conquest LL, et al.: The correlation of arteriosclerosis obliterans with lipoproteins in insulin-dependent and noninsulin-dependent diabetes. Diabetes 28:836–840, 1979.

7. Janka HU, Standle E, Mehnert H: Peripheral vascular disease in diabetes mellitus and its relation to cardiovascular risk factors: Screening with the Doppler ultrasonic technique. Diabetes Care 3:207–213, 1980.

8. Hierton T, James H: Lower extremity amputation in Uppsala County 1947–1969: Incidence and prosthetic rehabilitation. Acta Orthop Scand 44:573–582, 1973.

9. Christensen S: Lower extremity amputation in the county of Aalborg, 1961–1971: Population study and follow-up. Acta Orthop Scand 47:329–334, 1976.

10. Most R, Sinnock P: The epidemiology of lower extremity amputations in diabetic individuals. Diabetes Care 6:87–91, 1983.

11. Center for Economic Studies in Medicine: Direct and Indirect Costs of Diabetes in the United States in 1987. Alexandria, VA: American Diabetes Association, 1988, pp. 1–20.

12. Bild DE, Selby JV, Sinnock P, et al.: Lower-extremity amputation in people with diabetes. Epidemiology and prevention. Diabetes Care 12:24–31, 1989.

13. Davidson JK, Alogna M, Goldsmith M, et al.: Assessment of program effectiveness at Grady Memorial Hospital. In Steiner G, Lawrence PA (eds): Educating Diabetic Patients. New York: Springer, 1981, pp. 329–348.

14. Beach KW, Bedford GR, Bergelin RO, et al.: Progression of lower-extremity arterial occlusive disease in type II diabetes mellitus. Diabetes Care 11:464–472, 1988.

15. Janka HU, Walter H, Standl E, et al.: Relation between daily insulin dose and development of arterial occlusion in insulin-treated diabetics. Aktuel Endokrinol Stoffwechsel 8:10–14, 1987.

16. Kuebler TW, Bendick PJ, Norton JA, Jr: Risk factors for atheriosclerosis obliterans found in longitudinal study of type II diabetes. Diabetes 32(Suppl 1):11A, 1983.

17. Garcia ML, McNamara PM, Gordon T, et al.: Morbidity and mortality in diabetes in Framingham population: Sixteen year follow-up study. Diabetes 23:105–111, 1974.

18. Nilsson SE, Lindholm H, Bulow S, et al.: The Kristianstad Study Survey 1963–1964. Studies in a normal adult population for variation and correlation in some clinical, anthropometric, and laboratory values, especially the peroral glucose tolerance test. Acta Med Scand 177(Suppl 428)1:54, 1964.

19. Selby JV, Zhang D. Risk factors for lower extremity amputation in persons with diabetes. Diabetes Care 18:509–516, 1995.

20. Lehto S, Ronnemaa T, Pyorala K, et al.: Risk factors predicting lower extremity amputations in patients with NIDDM. Diabetes Care 19:607, 612, 1996.

21. Sorge F, Schwardtzkopff W, Nanhaus GA: Insulin response to oral glucose in patients with a previous myocardial infarction and patients with peripheral vascular disease: Hyperinsulinism and its relationships to hypertriglyceridemia and overweight. Diabetes 25:586–594, 1976.

22. Laakso M, Pyorala K: Lipid and lipoprotein abnormalities in diabetic patients with peripheral vascular disease. Atherosclerosis 74:55–63, 1988.

23. Stewart CPU: The influence of smoking on the level of lower limb amputation. Prosthet Orthot Int 11:113–116, 1987.

24. Lowery LA, Ashry HR, van Houtum W, et al.: Variation in the incidence and proportion of diabetes related amputations in minorities. Diabetes Care 19:48–52, 1996.

25. Nelson, RG, Gohdes DM, Everhart JE, et al: Lower-extremity amputations in NIDDM. 12 year follow-up study in Pima Indians. Diabetes Care 11:8–16, 1988.

26. Pecoraro RE, Reiber GE, Burgess EM. Pathways to diabetic limb amputation. Basis for prevention. Diabetes Care 13:513–521, 1990.

27. Reiber, GE, Pecoraro RE, Koepsell TD. Risk factors for amputation in patients with diabetes mellitus. Ann Int Med 117:97–105, 1992.

28. Mc Neely MJ, Boyko EJ, Abroni JH, et al.: The independent contributors of diabetic neuropathy and vasculopathy in foot ulceration. Diabetes Care 18:216–219, 1995.

29. Brand FN, Abbott RD, Kannel WB. Diabetes, intermittant claudication, and risk of cardiovascular events. Diabetes 38:504–509, 1989.

30. Niskanen L, Siitonen, O, Suhonen M, et al.: Medial artery calcification predicts cardiovascular mortality in patients with NIDDM. Diabetes Care 17:1252–1256, 1994.

31. Litzelman DK, Slemanda CW, Langefeld CD, et al.: Reduction of lower extremity clinical abnormalities in

patients with non-insulin dependent diabetes mellitus. Ann Int Med 119:36–41, 1993.

32. Colwell JA, Lyons TJ, Klein RL, Lopes-Virella MF. New concepts about the pathogenesis of atherosclerosis and thrombosis in diabetes mellitus. In Levin MJ (ed): The Diabetic Foot. St. Louis, MO: Mosby, 1992, pp. 79–114.

33. Colwell JA, Jokl, R: Vascular thrombosis in diabetes. In Porte D, Sherwin R, Rifkin H. (eds.): Diabetes Mellitus; Theory and Practice, Ed. 5. Norwalk, CT: Appleton and Lange, 1996, pp. 207–216.

34. Ross R: The pathogenesis of atherosclerosis—an update. New Engl J Med 314:488–500, 1986.

35. Lopes-Virella M, Klein RL, Lyons TJ, et al.: Glycosylation of low-density lipoprotein enchances cholesteryl ester synthesis in human monocyte-derived macrophages. Diabetes 37:550–557, 1988.

36. Colwell JA: Consensus statement on role of cardiovascular risk factors in the prevention and treatment of macrovascular risk factors in the prevention and treatment of macrovascular disease in diabetes. Diabetes Care 12:573–579, 1989.

37. Silbert S: Amputation of the lower extremity in diabetes mellitus. Diabetes 1:297–299, 1952.

38. Goldner MD: The fate of the second leg in the diabetic amputee. Diabetes 9:100–103, 1960.

39. Hoar CS, Torres J: Evaluation of below-the-knee amputation in the treatment of diabetic gangrene. New Engl J Med 266:440–443, 1962.

40. Cameron HC, Lennard-Jones JE, Robinson MD: Amputations in the diabetic: Outcome and survival. Lancet 2:605–607, 1964.

41. Ecker ML, Jacobs BS: Lower extremity amputation in diabetic patients. Diabetes 19:189–195, 1970.

42. Roon AJ, Moore WS, Goldstone J: Below-knee amputation: A modern approach. Am J Surg 134:153–158, 1977.

43. Levin CM, Dealey FN: The surgical diabetic, a five-year survey. Ann Surg 102:1029–1039, 1935.

44. Pearse HE, Zeigler HR: Is the conservative treatment of infection of gangrene in diabetic patients worthwhile? Surgery 8:72–78, 1940.

45. Mendelberg A, Sheinfield W: Diabetic amputions: Amputation of lower extremity in diabetes: Analysis of 128 cases. Am J Surg 71:70–75, 1944.

46. Smith BD: A twenty-year follow-up in fifty below-knee amputations for gangrene in diabetes. Surg Gynecol Obstet 103:625–630, 1956.

47. Baddeley RM, Fulford JC: A trial of conservative amputations for lesions of the feet in diabetes mellitus. Br J Surg 52:38–43, 1965.

48. Warren R, Kihn RB: A survey of lower extremity amputations for ischemia. Surgery 63:107–120, 1968.

49. Whitehouse FW, Jergensen C, Black MA: The later life of the diabetic amputee. Another look at fate of the second leg. Diabetes 17:520–521, 1968.

50. Haimovici H: Peripheral arterial disease in diabetes mellitus. In Ellenberg M, Rifkin H (eds): Diabetes Mellitus, Theory and Practice. New York: McGraw-Hill, 1970.

51. Kahn O, Wagner W, Bessman AN: Mortality of diabetics treated surgically for lower limb infection and/or gangrene. Diabetes 23:287–292, 1974.

52. Huston CC, Bivins BA, Ernst CB, et al.: Morbid implications of above-knee amputations. Report of a series and review of the literature. Arch Surg 115:165–167, 1980.

53. Colwell JA, Bingham SF, Abraira C, et al. VA Cooperative Study on antiplatelet agents in diabetic patients after amputation for gangrene. II. Effects of aspirin and dipyridamole on atherosclerotic vascular disease rates. Diabetes Care 9:140–148, 1986.

54. Pohjalainen T, Alaranta H: Lower limb amputations in southern Finland 1984–1985. Prosthet Orthot Int 12:9–18, 1988.

55. Waugh NR: Amputations in diabetic patients—a review of rates, relative risks and resource use. Community Med 10:279–288, 1988.

Selected Readings

History

Lawson RA: Amputations through the ages. Aust NZ J Med 42:221–230, 1973.

Davis NS Jr: Diabetic gangrene. JAMA 31:103–105, 1989.

Epidemiology and Reviews

Levin MJ (ed): The Diabetic Foot. St. Louis, MO: Mosby, 1992.

West KM: Epidemiology of Diabetes and Its Vascular Lesions. New York: Elsevier, 1978.

Most RS, Sinnock P: The epidemiology of lower-extremity amputations in diabetic individuals. Diabetes Care 6:87–91, 1983.

Pathophysiology of Atherosclerosis in Diabetes Mellitus

Reaven GM, Steiner G (eds): Proceeding of a conference on diabetes and atherosclerosis. Diabetes 30(Suppl 2):1–110, 1981.

Moskowitz J (ed): Diabetes and Atherosclerosis Connection. New York: Juvenile Diabetes Foundation, 1981.

Lopes-Virella MG, Jokl R, Colwell JA: Rheology and clotting factors in diabetes mellitus. In Howe PD, Marshall SM, Alberti KGMM, Krall LP (eds): The Diabetes Annual 7. Amsterdam: Elsevier, 1993, pp. 83–106.

Klein RL, Colwell JA. Altered endothelial function in diabetes. An overview. In Conn PM, Sowers JR (eds): Contemporary Endocrinology: Endocrinology of the Vasculature. Totowa, NJ: Humana, 1996, pp. 125–134.

Jokl R, Colwell JA: Clotting disorders in diabetes. In Alberti KGMM, DeFronzo RA, Zimmet P, Keen, H (eds): International Textbook of Diabetes Mellitus, Ed. 2. Chichester, Sussex: Wiley, 1997, pp. 1543–1557.

31

The Diabetic Foot

William C. Coleman

In 1991 the United States Department of Health set a goal of reducing the number of lower extremity amputations performed annually on people with diabetes by 40% by the year 2000.[1] We have an increasing amount of evidence in the professional literature to prove that lower extremity amputation rates can be dramatically reduced by programs that stress patient education, techniques of prevention, and early identification and treatment of injuries.[2–4] The Centers for Disease Control and Prevention in Atlanta records that during the years 1990–1994 there were 56,000 lower extremity amputations performed on diabetic patients.[5] Studies reported by the National Center for Health Statistics cite that for the years 1994 and 1995 the rate of amputation was 67,000 annually.[6] These figures would indicate that current national efforts to lower the rate of amputation are not having an effect on this epidemic.

Diabetic patients can experience sensory loss and diminished circulation in their lower extremities. Of these two, it is often the insensitivity that misleads both patient and physician into a state of lower motivation to find immediate solutions to foot injuries.

Three factors that complicate attempts to manage injuries on the feet of persons with diabetes are:

(1) Without pain, the patient does not take small wounds seriously.

(2) Physicians often wait for the patient to complain and fail to remove shoes routinely to have a look.

(3) Surgeons are sometimes fatalistic about infected diabetic feet and advise amputation too readily.

All three attitudes are demonstrated by the case of a 45-year-old diabetic woman who came to our clinic in a panic because a surgeon had just told her she would have to have her leg amputated. The foot she showed us was swollen, hot, and red; there was a profuse discharge of pus from an ulcer under the first metatarsal head. The patient had cut her shoe open to accommodate the swollen foot and the dressings were soaked in pus, yet she walked into the room without limping. She had stepped on a thumbtack while clearing up Christmas decorations and had not discovered the tack until she went to bed that evening. The wound had enlarged to the size of an ulcer, and she had walked with a large bandage over the ulcer for the previous 3 months. During this time she had visited her physician twice for advice about her diet and medication but had not bothered to tell him about her foot problem. The physician had not asked her about her feet even though she was having increasing problems controlling her insulin requirements. When the infection in her foot suddenly became severe, accompanied by osteomyelitis, septic arthritis, and a spreading cellulitis, she went to a surgeon who asked her if she was a diabetic. He then told her that this was a common problem in diabetes, that it indicated impending gangrene, and that she would be better to have the leg amputated. When we saw her she had good pulses at ankle level and had no problem with her vascular supply. A week in bed on antibiotics after her wound was debrided resulted in rapid reduction of swelling and the discharge. Her foot finally healed in a plaster cast, and she is walking well in a shoe with a molded insole (see also Chapter 33).

Pain is such a fundamental part of the normal interaction between a patient and a physician that the whole system of asking for and receiving help from a physician breaks down when wounds and infections of the foot are unaccompanied by pain. When a patient walks briskly into a physician's office without a limp and asks questions about diet, it doesn't even occur to the physician that the patient may be walking on an open, infected wound or may have a fracture developing into a neuropathic joint disintegration. Physicians who deal with diabetics must make it *an absolute routine to insist that patients take off their shoes.* The feet may be inspected by a nurse or a therapist, but it is only by regular inspection that the earliest problems will be picked up and later amputations will be prevented.

Fundamental to the management of diabetic foot problems is the patient's attitude toward his insensate feet. From birth a person defines the outer limits of their body by the sensations at the surface of the skin. Body image is built on the sensations of touch and pain. When sensation is lost identity with the insensate part is diminished significantly. It is not enough that a person can see his foot and know that it is attached to his own leg. It is not enough even that the patient can wiggle his toes and know that his foot will move when he tells it to. The patient does not really accept a foot as part of his body if, when it is touched, the brain does not recognize that a touch has occurred.

Clinicians who frequently treat patients with insensate feet often are frustrated by the frequent incidents of poor patient compliance with clinical instructions. Recommendations of proper footwear or wound care are often ignored by persons who feel no pain in injured feet.[7] The clinician needs to understand that these people do not deserve less respect or attention for this behavior. Some of the most intelligent people have done the same kind of things, and many physicians would act just as "stupidly" if their foot felt like a block of wood tacked on to the end of their leg. Anybody who undertakes to be responsible for a diabetic must come to terms with the profound differences in attitude these patients have toward their feet when compared with all those who have normal sensations of touch and pain. To come to terms with this attitude means to accept it and then help the patients develop a sensible, objective attitude toward their feet in place of the subjective attitude that accompanied the sensory feelings that have been irretrievably lost. It also means with coming to terms with oneself and trying to identify compassionately with the patient who seems to have disowned his or her feet.

Levels of Sensation

It is rare that the foot of a person with diabetic neuropathy becomes totally insensitive. In fact, the loss of sensation is gradual and partial, and there is no clearly recognizable point or level at which the foot becomes vulnerable because of insensitivity. It is possible to lose 50% of all the nerve endings in a segment of skin before they become aware of any sensory loss at all. At that stage the patient may still have all the modalities of sensation. A stronger stimulus is simply required for the patient to recognize that sensation exists. A good question is not why the foot so often breaks down in diabetes, but why it does *not* break down more often in normal individuals. It is a stimulating mental exercise to consider the skeleton of a normal human foot while thinking about the stress it bears. A metatarsal bone is about the diameter of a pencil. An individual

metatarsal shaft can be snapped in half by the bare hands. Yet at every step a jogger is lifting his heel and putting his entire weight on five metatarsals that stand up on end and sustain his weight and thrust him forward while enduring torsional and angulating stress across each metatarsal shaft. Each metatarsal head is rounded, and when the skeletal foot rests on a board the head only touches the surface of the board by less than a square cm of bone contact. The pressure under each metatarsal head, loaded with its share of the whole weight of a person, is enormous, enough to crush the delicate tissues of the sole. Yet fine septa of fibrous tissue, anchored to the skeleton and to the skin, lock hundreds of small globes of fat into position so that when the bone comes down and bears weight, each globe of fat is compressed and thrusts the stress in all directions. Thus by the time the skin takes weight, the area of stress has spread out so that the pressure is not so high.

These anatomical and functional provisions for keeping the foot undamaged would still be inadequate but for one more factor—sensory feedback. The design of the foot has kept the bones slender and the bulk of viscoelastic tissue to a reasonable minimum so that it is not necessary to have a great heavy foot on the end of each leg. The sensory feedback system keeps the foot alert to any excess of stress that would endanger the bones or break the skin. Just before the stress is fully accepted the body feels it and adjusts the way the foot is placed, so that a greater area of the foot can share the stress or so that the stress itself is minimized. This protective sensory feedback is rarely enough to be called pain; it is a whisper of discomfort, mostly at a reflex level, that is a constant monitor of the buildup of stress. That is what makes it safe to walk on the fragile, beautiful feet with which humans are born.

Before discussing the ways in which diabetic feet can be preserved, one final comment on "normal" feet is in order. Although normal feet are beautiful, it is the exception to find normal feet in the United States or in other "developed" countries. The common image of feet is that they are ugly and that they smell. Both the ugliness and the smell are the products of occlusive or compressive fashion footwear. Hands would smell and become ugly if the fingers were compressed into streamlined compressive gloves from morning till night. The clenched fingers of stroke victims become offensive if regular opening and cleansing is not performed. In doing so the interdigital skin is found to be macerated and easily torn. The feet of diabetic patients suffer not only because of their specific problems of denervation and vascular change, but also from the grossly insulting constraints that "civilized" fashion imposes on the feet of all who submit to it. All health professionals who learn about feet and take care of diabetic feet should feel it their duty to extend their influence and advise nondiabetic patients and friends to recognize the beauty of normal feet and to renounce the tyranny of foot fashions that harm them.

Clinical Evaluation

The first bastion of defense for the diabetic foot is an awareness by both the patient and physician that a problem exists.

Not every diabetic has a foot problem. It is not the diabetes itself that destroys a foot, but either the lack of blood supply or the failure of sensation. All diabetics should have the pulses checked at ankle level and should have a sensory check of the feet at least every year, so that they may know when they have become vulnerable and when special precautions have become necessary. If the clinician cannot feel a pulse, a noninvasive test of the circulation should be performed.

Eighty percent of persons with diabetes who have a foot injury have peripheral neuropathy as the major complicating factor in wound management.[8,9] Sensory testing has been a problem in the past for two reasons. The first is that traditional sensory testing (such as pinprick, light touch, tuning forks, proprioception, and temperature) has not been a useful clinical tool. Diabetic patients who don't feel large open wounds on the bottom of their foot can respond normally to these tests. This would indicate that these tests are not revealing the absence of protective levels of sensation (protective sensation being the retention of enough nerve function to prevent injury by feeling a threat and adequate feeling to prevent the use of an injured part). The second reason is that the resultant findings from sensory tests would not change the treatment recommended for the patient.

A simple, inexpensive test to quantify the presence or absence of protective sensation is now being accepted as the clinical standard. Semmes-Weinstein nylon monofilaments that bend at a pressure of 10 g may identify the protective threshold for most diabetic patients.[10] It is as effective as and is less time consuming than other clinical methods of sensory evaluation to identify foot vulnerability.[11] Other new techniques using bioesthesiometers[12] or isolating specific types of nerve fibers may be moving clinical evaluation of sensation closer to useful quantification of nerve function.[13]

Since loss of protective sensation has been identified as a factor that greatly increases the diabetic patient's likelihood of foot injury, a test capable of revealing this loss will set this higher-risk group of diabetics apart from those who have normal protective mechanisms. This higher-risk group can then receive special attention and education about footwear and footcare.[14] In a recent survey of factors that place a person with diabetes at greater risk of foot ulceration, risk increased when neuropathy was present in conjunction with the presence of diabetes for more than 10 years, poor blood sugar control, foot deformity, male gender, a history of previous amputation, and higher pressures under the foot.[15] The risk of developing a foot ulcer was not found to correlate to ethanol use, peripheral vascular disease, less formal education, retinopathy, obesity, or tobacco use.

Vascular problems are dealt with elsewhere in this book (see Chapter 34), but it should be noted here that diabetic feet with diminished blood supply will often last for many years and even for a lifetime if wounds and infections can be prevented. It is commonly the onset of infection that places so much demand on the blood supply of a diabetic, dysvascular foot that the balance is disturbed and gangrene may set in. Thus the special care that we describe here is equally important for the diabetic whether the foot has primarily a defect in blood supply, primarily in the sensory nerves, or both.

Common Causes of Foot Damage

We will describe four special dangers, each of which needs to be explained to each patient who has diminished sensation as well as to their wives or husbands and to every member of the staff of a diabetic clinic.

Direct Damage

This may occur most commonly from sharp objects that are stepped on or from heat. The skin of the sole is tough. It can tolerate pressures of more than 500 lb/sq in. (psi) without breaking or tearing. The danger comes from projecting points or edges that have an area of less than a .25 sq in. When the patient takes a step, his whole weight may rest on a point or edge so small that the pressure or shear stress rises high enough to allow penetration of the skin. In the absence of pain sensation a person will go on walking all day with a splinter imbedded in the skin.

Pressures high enough to break the skin never occur while the patient is wearing shoes that have a hard or thick sole. The direct mechanical forces of running, jumping, or kicking will never break the skin while the patient is wearing a shoe. They may break a bone but not the skin. However, skin can be broken if a sharp object has fallen into the shoe before it is put on or if nails used in the making of a shoe later penetrate the insole and then the foot. Direct damage to the sole occurs only when walking barefoot, in socks, or in thin slippers.

Therefore, although barefoot walking is good for most feet, it must never be allowed for an insensitive foot. Once pain sensation is lost, the rule is to never walk barefoot and to always shake out and inspect the inside of shoes before putting them on. Some form of open sandal that has a hard undersole and allows air to circulate is good for the foot. It may be worn at home by those who have to wear full shoes outdoors.

When most forms of low-heeled footwear are worn, the pressures under the foot are lower than under the barefoot or while socks are worn.[16] Older or heavier persons do not generally have significantly higher pressures under their feet. Persons with diabetes usually have greater pressures than nondiabetics under their feet while walking.[17]

Heat is a hidden danger. Diabetics should be careful of the floor of automobiles and trucks. It is worth checking the floor, especially during a long drive that may heat up the engine and exhaust pipe. I have known diabetics to suffer very severe loss of the sole of the foot from this cause, especially the heel of the driver of the car. While visiting Indian Health Service clinics in the southwestern United States I visited patients who had burned the bottom of their feet while walking on hot black-top roadways.

Diabetics should never sit facing a fire or heater with the feet extended and should never step into a hot bath without first testing it with a sensitive part of the body or a thermometer.

Ischemia, or Local Bloodlessness

Pressure sores are caused by external pressure that is sustained for a long time. True low pressure sores almost never occur on the soles of the feet. This is because the pressures of walking are intermittent, and the sole gets its blood supply every time the foot is lifted. Pressure sores result from "continuous" pressure maintained for many hours. The pressure is commonly quite low, about 2 or 3 psi, enough to blanch the skin and keep out the blood supply. This pressure is exceeded at every step on the sole of the foot, but it is very rare for anybody to stand still for long enough to get a pressure sore. The only common causes of low pressure sores in diabetes are from tight shoes or bed sores. One of the earliest signs of loss of sensation is that the patient begins to buy smaller size shoes. The patients may not yet know that they lack sensation, but they notice that they do not feel the normal sense of support of the shoe, so they assume the shoe is too loose and they ask for a tighter one. Female patients often like to wear as small a shoe as they can tolerate, and they are the first to get into this kind of trouble when they have diabetes. Eighty-eight percent of women in a recent study were found to be wearing shoes 1.2 cm narrower than the size of their foot.[18]

Ischemic pressure sores occur on the edges or margins of the feet, where the fabric of the shoe takes a bend, rather than on the sole. This is especially likely where there is a double curvature, as at a bunion. Dia-

betics need to take special care when they buy new shoes. They need to know that shoes must have plenty of room around the forefoot and toes but should have a snug fit around the heel (to prevent rubbing the heel and the formation of blisters). They also should be advised to buy leather shoes rather than plastic because leather will gradually conform to the foot, even when the original fit was not too good. It is difficult for the patient to be sure about pressure in the shoe, so we suggest that no new shoe be worn for more than 2 or 3 hours at a time for the first day or two. The feet must be inspected when the new shoes are removed, and any red flush must be taken seriously. A red spot, or hot spot, probably means that the pressure there was too high to allow blood supply to the skin, and a sore would have occurred if the shoe had been worn all day. Even when shoes are not new it is a good idea to change shoes twice a day. A pair of shoes should be kept at the workplace and used as a change at midday. On return home in the evening a second change is made, and houseshoes worn all evening. Thus no shoe is worn continuously for more than 5 or 6 hours at a time. Even if one shoe is somewhat tight, it will not cause low-pressure ulceration in that period of time.

Inflammation from Repetitive Stress

Ulceration from this cause is far more common than from either of the first two causes. The amount of pressure involved is much higher than that needed to cause low pressure sores, but not nearly high enough to cause direct damage. We have performed many experiments on the footpads of rats to determine the patterns of damage that result from different levels of stress at different patterns of time and repetition. For example, pressures of 20 psi, which are common in ordinary walking, were applied 10,000 times a day, day after day, to rat footpads. This is about equivalent, in an average human, to jogging 7 miles every day on hard surfaces. As the result of ulceration the footpads of the rats showed only a rise of temperature and some swelling by the second and third days and began to show blisters and signs of necrosis later in the week. By the end of the week most rat footpads had broken down and ulcerated. The histology of the footpads showed that this kind of repetitive stress causes a gradual buildup of inflammation with edema and incursion of inflammatory cells until the whole tissue is stiff and turgid. It is quite different, in a mechanical sense, from what it was before. It lacks compliancy, so that localization of stress becomes more severe than in the normal sole. The final necrosis begins deep in the tissues and gives the appearance of an enzymatic autolysis.

In the normally sensate foot inflammation results in discomfort. As inflammation increases pain increases to warn of damage. Without pain as a warning that the inflammation is intensifying, the person with insensate feet continues the damaging activity. The inflammation continues to levels far greater than a person with normal protective sensation would ever allow.

The whole process of inflammation and then of necrosis occurs more rapidly if the pressure is higher or if there are more repetitions/day. The process may be slowed down or reversed by lowering the pressure or simply by having fewer repetitions/day. In one batch of rats we used the same pressure (20 psi), but used 8,000 repetitions/day instead of 10,000, and also gave them the weekend off. These rats went through a period of swelling and mild inflammatory reaction, but that subsided and after several weeks the footpads actually improved over their original state. At the end of 6 weeks the pads were well keratinized, hypertrophied, and strong.

The important lesson from all of this is that we now know that the stress of one day causes histologic change in the sole that remains on into the next days, and it renders the affected part of the foot more vulnerable to further stress. If, however, the stress is moderated and spaced out, the foot can be conditioned to become stronger and better able to survive.

The most consistent sign of developing inflammation is local heat. We tell our patients to feel their feet every night when they go to bed. If one part feels hot compared to the rest, that may be a sign that it is in danger of breakdown within a few days if the stress is allowed to continue at the same level. If the patient also has loss of sensation in his hands, it is best to get a friend or family member to do the daily test. A device capable of quantifying surface skin temperature is essential in a clinic designed for the management of problems commonly encountered on diabetic feet.[19,20] The surface skin temperature will elevate in correlation with underlying inflammation over a small area of skin. If the temperature of this area is 2°C (3.5°F) greater than the rest of that foot or the same location on the other foot, the underlying soft tissue or bone has been damaged. This measurement should be taken after the foot has been rested and uncovered for 20 min. Infrared thermometers are the most rapid and accurate means of quantifying surface skin temperature.[19]

The best way to reduce the level of pressure on the sole of the foot is to spread the thrust of weight-bearing over a larger area of sole. This can be done by using a soft, compliant insole or a molded insole. Because it is not possible for the foot to feel for errors in placement of shoe corrections, we do not ever prescribe modular inserts, such as arch supports or scaphoid pads. It is so easy to make total-contact, custom-molded inserts of expanded polyethelene materials such as Plastazote that off-the-shelf molded inserts should never be used.

To have room for a molded insole, it is usually necessary to purchase an extra-depth shoe. There are a number of companies who market good leather shoes with added vertical space within the shoe to make room for special insoles.

The greatest stress on the sole of the foot occurs at the level of the metatarsal heads, across the ball of the foot. The moment of highest stress occurs as the heel is lifted and the foot flexes at the base of the toes. Since the other foot is off the ground at that moment, all the weight of the body comes on the one forefoot while the foot is bending. The result is shear stress, which can be very harmful. For this reason, in patients who tend to get into trouble at this part of the forefoot, we recommend a rigid-soled shoe, with the toes turned up a little, and a thickening under the sole, called a rocker. This allows the foot to pivot on the rocker and avoid taking weight on the end of the foot. It also prevents the foot from bending at the metatarsal heads level, and thus avoids much shear stress (Fig. 31–1).

Shoes with higher heels cause higher pressures under the metatarsal heads:[21]

(1) A shoe with a 1.9 cm heel height results in a 22% higher pressure.

(2) A shoe with a 5 cm heel height results in a 57% higher pressure.

(3) A shoe with a 8.3 cm heel height results in a 76% higher pressure.

In the case of feet that have already had some damage and have healed with some irregularity of bone structure, it is important to make the foot as even and plantigrade as possible so that it will not be necessary to use custom-made shoes. Bony projections may have to be surgically removed and other deformities corrected, such as tight calf muscles or inversion of the

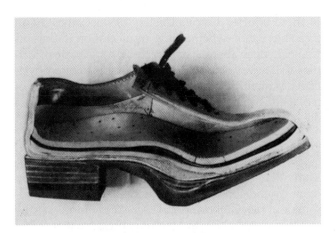

Figure 31–1. Construction detail of custom-made rigid-sole rocker shoe that minimizes pressure in vulnerable forefoot area.

foot. It is dangerous to attempt to correct foot deformities by means of footwear, as this involves pressure on surface tissues that may result in pressure sores.

Infection

The result of damage from one of the three causes already outlined are wounds or ulcers through the skin. The really severe damage to the diabetic foot does not occur until later. The wound or ulcer gets infected, then the patient goes on walking on it, spreading the infection or fluids into deeper tissues, bones, joints, and tendon sheaths. The gross infections that occur by walking on infected tissues may destroy the foot by uncontrolled infection and gangrene, which demand more blood supply than the reduced blood vessels can supply. Walking on infected tissues may also result in the loss of bone to an extent that it makes the foot inadequate to walk on and bear weight.

It is important to prevent wounds and ulcers whenever possible, but it is still more important to help the patient understand that if ever a wound occurs, it is an emergency that must be healed before any more walking takes place. This is a hard lesson to learn, but it becomes easier if the patient also understands that his foot will heal very well if only it is rested. Diabetics often have the idea that their feet are just bad feet. They use terms such as "nonhealing flesh" and get these ideas from other diabetics—even from doctors who have a tendency to amputate diabetic limbs rather freely because they think the prospect for healing is poor and the prospect for recurrence is very high. In fact, most neuropathic ulcers heal very promptly in a plaster cast if they are given the chance to do so.

Treatment

With the knowledge that inflammation is a major factor in further destruction in insensate feet, cessation of the causes of inflammation is essential in the management of these injuries. Once an injury has occurred on an insensitive foot, whether it is an ulceration in the soft tissues, a deep abscess, or a fracture, some basic principles will always apply. From the first instant a physician has identified that damage is present in the foot of a diabetic he needs to begin to ensure that four factors are addressed by his treatment.

Relief of Direct Mechanical Stress

Many diabetics with foot injury continue to walk on open wounds on the bottom of their feet. Fluids accumulate at the wound site and each step compresses the soft tissues, resulting in hydraulic pressure that forces the fluids into previously uninvolved tissues. Compression of the injury site also further damages tissues

directly. In addition, the back-and-forth motion of the foot in gait tears the tissues by shear stress.

Immobilize Joints and Tendons

Sometimes contamination can enter damaged joint capsules and tendon sheaths. Also, there are potential spaces between tissue layers in the foot that can facilitate the movement of contaminated fluids. Many diabetic foot infections that have been difficult to manage may be attributable to the inability of the body's defenses to localize the problem. Motion of tendons and muscles can continually expand the area of involvement in the infection.

Control Pedal Edema

Excessive interstitial fluids interfere with many of the mechanisms needed for healing. One of the primary problems created by edema is a decrease in density of the capillary network at the wound site. The additional interstitial fluid spreads the capillaries apart. This results in less oxygen, nutrients, and removal of metabolites/g of tissue around the injury.

Examine for Systemic Response to Infection

The presence of infection alters any management decisions regarding foot care. This will not change the need to address the previous three factors, but the form of treatment will probably be altered.

Acute Ulcers

When an ulcer or wound is new or when it is acutely inflamed, has profuse discharge, or is accompanied by fever and tender glands in the groin, it is designated as "acute." Patients with such ulcers should be treated by bed rest and antibiotics for a few days until the acute phase has passed. While the ulcer is acute, bed rest must be strictly enforced. It is not safe for the patient to walk even to the bathroom, because one single step may squeeze the infected tissues of the sole and force infected material into previously uninfected areas. Patients often say that they can use crutches or hop on one leg to the bathroom. Indeed they can, but most will forget and will put their weight on the infected foot.

During this time the foot and leg should be placed in a rigid posterior splint. Although direct stress and edema will be minimized by bed rest, the insensate patient may actually move the foot more than usual to ensure that it still works as before.

Chronic Ulcers

Once the fever is down, the foot less swollen, the discharge is reduced, the ulcer may be designated "chronic." The patient may be allowed moderate ambulation, and the ulcer will heal. At no time should the foot be subjected to unequal pressure until it is fully epithelialized. By far the best way to ensure rest and healing to the foot is to put it in a plaster cast.

Many physicians are reluctant to enclose a wound in a cast. They want to be able to see it every day, and they think the dressings need to be changed. Even before the age of antibiotics, Orr[22] and Trueta[23] proved that infected wounds and tissues affected by osteomyelitis did very well when enclosed in a plaster cast. It is still true today that infections and wounds heal best if they are not looked at and if dressings are not changed, as long as they are not made worse by mechanical stress.

In 1989, a controlled clinical trial of total contact casting performed at Barnes Hospital in St. Louis[24] compared casting with traditional wound management of diabetic plantar ulcers. It found casting to be significantly more effective and reliable in healing these ulcers. Also, fewer infections developed during the course of treatment. Myerson reported that 90% of 71 ulcers averaging 3.5 cm in diameter healed within a mean of $5\frac{1}{2}$ weeks.[25]

The plaster cast provides protection from external stress and frees the patient to ambulate without harm to the wound.[26] One or two exceptions and precautions are necessary. A wound should not be enclosed in a cast if:

(1) It is deep, with only a small opening at the surface. It may heal overquickly and leave a deep abscess inside. This kind of wound should be widened until it is as wide as it is deep. The edges may be kept apart by loose vaseline gauze and then enclosed in a cast.

(2) There is profuse discharge. This often indicates the presence of dead bone or slough in the wound. This should be debrided and treated with the patient in bed (acute ulcer) until the acute phase subsides.

(3) The foot is very swollen. The danger here is not that the swelling will increase but that it will decrease and result in a loose cast. Loose casts allow the leg to move and rub, causing blisters and ulcers. This can be avoided by leaving the cast on for only a few days.

(4) There are signs of gangrene. If the foot is cold and blue, it is wise to keep the patient in bed for observation until it is determined whether amputation may be indicated. A posterior splint would be advisable at this time too.

Total Contact Plaster Cast

The features that differentiate this type of cast are:

(1) The patient lies face down with the knee bent.

(2) A small dressing is placed over the ulcer (Fig. 31–2).

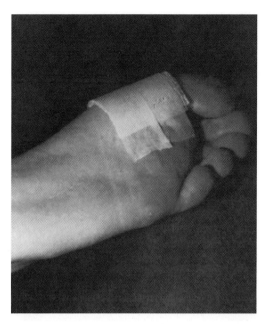

Figure 31–2. Gauze dressing over ulcer is secured by paper surgical tape.

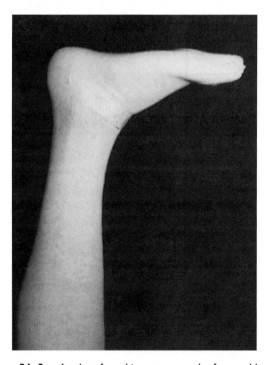

Figure 31–3. A tube of stockinette covers the foot and leg. Wrinkles occurring in the stockinette anterior to the ankle can be eliminated by making a transverse cut in the stockinette and overlapping and securely taping the edges.

(3) A sleeve of stockinette is worn up the leg to the knee (Fig. 31–3).

(4) Felt padding with bevelled edges is placed over each malleolus, over abnormal bony prominences, and down the front of the tibia (to make it easy to remove the cast later) (Fig. 31–4).

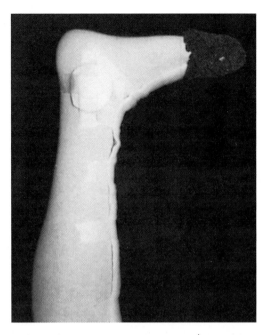

Figure 31–4. Orthopedic felt about 6 mm ($\frac{1}{4}$ in.) thick covers both malleoli. Edges are beveled. Similar felt about 4 cm (1$\frac{1}{2}$ in.) wide with beveled edges protects the tibial crest and facilitates cast removal. Plastic foam protects the toes.

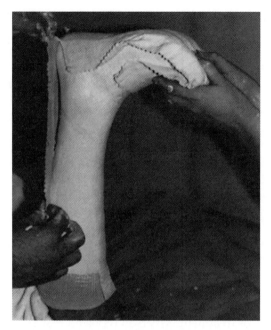

Figure 31–5. Assistance is required to hold ankle at 90° and toes in extension. Toes are held in extension to prevent toe-ground contact later during walking. After the eggshell-thin, total-contact first layer has set, slabs (five layers of plaster splint) are applied to provide support. These are followed by circular plaster bandages.

(5) A foam pad is placed around the toes.

(6) A single fast-setting plaster bandage of fine quality (Gypsona is preferred) is loosely applied around foot, ankle, and lower leg. It is immediately rubbed into every hollow and around every contour of the foot until it has set (Fig. 31–5).

(7) Once the inner eggshell-thin layer has set in total contact, slabs of plaster and circular bandages are rapidly applied, followed by a supporting plywood sole and rocker support (Figs. 31–6 and 31–7). No weight bearing is allowed for 24 hr.

If there has been any swelling in the foot, the plaster cast must be changed after a few days, or it will be loose and cause friction. Most times we change the first cast in about 1 week. The second cast is likely to be kept on for 2 weeks. Casting continues until the ulcer has healed.

A corrected shoe must be ready to wear when the plaster cast is removed. When ulcers recur, it is usually in the first week or two after healing, when the tissues are fragile. It is inexcusable to allow a patient to walk in his old shoes at this stage. If new definitive shoes are not ready, a quick-molded sandal may be formed on the foot, using Plastazote heated to 280°F (it will not burn the foot because it is mostly air bubbles, but it is safest to form it over a sock). Straps are attached, and the patient may walk in this until proper shoes are ready.

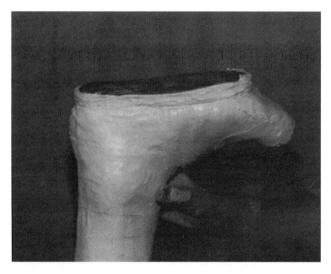

Figure 31–6. A $\frac{1}{4}$ in. (about 6 mm) plywood sole plate is placed from the heel to the metatarsal heads to prevent localized pressure under the walking heel that could collapse the cast. Gaps between plywood and cast should be filled with plaster.

Neuropathic Bone and Joint Damage

The physician should always be aware of the possibility of a broken bone or collapsed joint in a patient who does not complain of pain. Any swollen foot or hot foot should be investigated by X-ray examination at once.

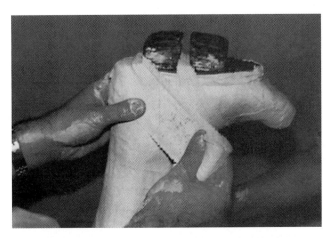

Figure 31–7. A rubber heel (rocker support) is placed just behind the center of the sole. No weight-bearing is allowed for 24 hr. Cast removal is accomplished by splitting the cast along the tibial crest.

If neuropathic breakdown is diagnosed promptly it can usually be healed. If the patient goes on walking on it, the damage becomes more and more gross until amputation is inevitable.

There have been many cases in which physicians have given antibiotics to a patient who complained of a hot swollen foot or who treated it as an insect bite, because it did not occur to them that a person could fracture a bone with no history of trauma or pain.

After a hospital stay of 1 month the foot service was consulted for assistance in the management of a 56-year-old black male with a 15-year history of diagnosis of type 2 diabetes. He had originally been admitted for IV antibiotic treatment of a suspected foot infection. The foot had been red, hot, and swollen for 3 weeks, while being treated with oral antibiotics prior to admission. There was no history of recent open foot wound. After admission, radiologic studies showed bone changes on the top of the tarsal bones, and an opinion of possible osteomyelitis was given by the radiologist. The patient had been taken to surgery during this hospital stay for incision and drainage (no abscess was found) and bone biopsy (negative for bacteria). After the general surgery and orthopedic services insisted that below-knee amputation was the only reasonable course of future care the patient insisted on another opinion.

The initial evaluation by the foot service resulted in findings of a red, hot, swollen foot with a 1×4 cm superficial postsurgical wound dorsally. Radiologic films revealed a neuropathic fracture consistent with the medial pillar pattern of tarsal disintegration described by Brand.[27]

The foot was placed in a posterior splint until the dorsal wound healed 3 weeks later. Erythemia and edema reduced significantly. After wound closure he was placed in a below-knee cast for 4 weeks; afterward, a CAM walker boot with Velcro straps and custom molded footbed was used. Thermometry indicated that inflammation was reducing, and changes were made in his supportive devices. After 13 weeks he was provided with a pair of depth, oxford shoes with custom-made orthoses. He has remained injury free for 8 years and returns to the clinic every 2 months to monitor his condition.

Surface skin temperature is the most important sign the clinician has in the early detection of injury of insensitive feet. If no other cause of inflammation is identified, the foot should be casted as a fracture. Temperature will reveal injuries prior to ulceration and can be used to determine the progression of rehabilitation after injury and postoperatively.

Immobilization of all neuropathic fractures by casting is recommended. Too often physicians fail to cast these "Charcot" problems and the bone structure of the foot progressively disintegrates.

Conclusion

The history of insensate foot care is filled with the medical community embracing the newest topical agent, oral medication, and surgical intervention. However, successful management of the foot problems of people with diabetes has repeatedly been proven to come as the result of addressing the psychologic, mechanical, and biological factors through multidisciplinary cooperation. Epidemiologic data on the cost of managing diabetic foot injury justifies expense of programs focused on prevention. The failure to develop these programs during the 1990s will result in the failure of the achievement of a 40% reduction in lower extremity amputations by the year 2000 (see Chapter 33).

References

1. Department of Health and Human Services: Healthy People 2000, National Health Promotion and Disease Prevention Objectives. Washington, DC: Government Printing Office, 1991.

2. Davidson, JK, Alogna M, Goldsmith M, Borden J: Assessment of program effectiveness at Grady Memorial Hospital—Atlanta. In Steiner G, Lawrence PA (eds): Educating Diabetic Patients. New York: Springer-Verlag, 1981, pp. 329–348.

3. Runyan JW: The Memphis Chronic Disease Program. JAMA 231:264–267, 1975.

4. Assal JP, Muhlhauser I, Pernat A, et al.: Patient education as the basis for diabetes care in clinical practice. Diabetologia 28:602–613, 1985.

5. Reiber GE, Boyko EJ, Smith DG: Lower extremity foot ulcers and amputations in diabetes. In Harris ML, Cowie CC, et al. (eds): Diabetes in America, Ed. 2. Washington, DC: Department of Health and Human Services (NIH publication no. 95–1468), 1995, pp. 409–428.

6. National Center for Health Statistics: Healthy People 2000 Review, 1995–96. Hyattsville, MD: Public Health Service, 1996.

7. Edmonds ME, Blundell MP, Morris HE, et al.: The diabetic foot: Impact of a foot clinic. Q J Med 232:763–771, 1986.

8. Pecoraro RE, Reiber GE, Burgess EM: Pathways to diabetic limb amputation: Basis for prevention. Diabetes Care 13:513–521, 1990.

9. Boulton AJM: The diabetic foot: Neuropathic in aetiology? Diabetic Med 7:852–858, 1990.

10. Birke JA, Sims DS: Plantar sensory threshold in the Hansen's disease ulceratic foot. Proc Int Conf Biomech Clin Kines Hand and Foot Madras, India, Dec 1985, pp 332–336.

11. Sosenko JM, Kato M, Soto R, Bild DE: Comparison of quantitative sensory threshold measures for their association with foot ulceration in diabetic patients. Diabetes Care 13:1057–1061, 1990.

12. Boulton AJM, Kubrusly DB, Bowker JH, et al.: Impaired vibratory perception and diabetic foot ulceration. Diabetic Med 3:335–337, 1986.

13. Masson EA, Fernando D, Veves A, Boulton AJM: A critical independent evaluation of the "Neurometer(R)" in the assessment of diabetic peripheral neuropathy. Neurometer(R) CPT Abstracts. Diabetes 38(Suppl. 2): Detroit, 1989, p. 130A.

14. Coleman WC: Footwear in a management program of injury prevention. In Levin WM, O'Neal LW (eds): The Diabetic Foot, Ed. 4. St. Louis, MO: Mosby, 1987, pp. 293–309.

15. Lavery LA, Armstrong DG, Vela SA, et al.: Practical criteria for screening patients at high risk for diabetic foot ulceration. Arch Intern Med 158:157–162, 1998.

16. Sarnow MR, Veves A, Guirini JM, et al.: In-shoe foot pressure measurements in diabetic patients with at-risk feet and in healthy subjects. Diabetes Care 17(9):1002–1006, 1994.

17. Veves A, Masson EA, Fernando DJS, Boulton AJM: Use of experimental padded hosiery to reduce foot pressures in diabetic neuropathy. Diabetic Med 7:324–326, 1990.

18. Frey C, Thompson F, Smith J, et al.: American Orthopedic Foot and Ankle Society women's shoe survey. Foot Ankle 14:78–81, 1993.

19. Bergtholdt HT, Brand PW: Temperature assessment and plantar inflammation. Lepr Rev. 47:211–215,1976.

20. Chan AW, Macfarlane IA, Bowsher DR: Contact strenonography of painful diabetic neuropathic foot, Diabetes Care. 14:918–924, 1991.

21. Snow RE, Williams KR, Holmes GB Jr: The effects of wearing high heeled shoes on pedal pressure in women. Foot Ankle. 13:85–92, 1992.

22. Orr HW: The principles involved in the treatment of osteomyelitis and compound fractures. Lancet 54: 622–624, 1934.

23. Trueta J: Treatment of war wounds and fractures. Br Med J 1:616–617, 1942.

24. Mueller MJ, Diamond JE, Sinacore DR, Delitto A, Blair III VP, Drury DA, Rose SJ: Total contact casting in treatment of diabetic plantar ulcers: Diab Care 12:384–388, 1989.

25. Myerson M, Papa J, Eaton K, Wilson K: The total contact cast for management of neuropathic plantar ulceration of the foot. *J Bone Joint Surg.* 74–A(2):261–269, 1992.

26. Coleman WC, Brand PW, Birke JA: The total contact cast: a therapy for plantar ulceration on insensitive feet. *J Am Podiatr Med Assoc* 74:548–552, 1984.

27. Harris JR, Brand PW: patterns of disintegragion of the tarsus in the anaesthetic foot. *J Bone Joint Surg.* 48–B(1): 4–16, 1966.

32

Pathophysiology of Diabetic Foot Lesions

Marvin E. Levin

In the 39th year of his reign, King Asa became affected with gangrene of his feet; he did not seek guidance from the Lord but resorted to physicians. He rested with his forefathers in the 41st year of his reign.
—*II Chronicles XVI*, 12–14

Historical Perspective

Whether or not King Asa did indeed suffer from diabetic gangrene of the feet remains a moot point. In King Asa's time the Lord certainly had more to offer than King Asa's physicians. Furthermore, in those times and until the discovery of insulin, most diabetic patients did not live long enough to develop the problems that now affect the diabetic foot. Today, with added years of life, the diabetic complications of vascular disease and neuropathy have had time to develop. Nowhere else in the body do we so clearly see the ravages and magnitude of these diabetic complications as in the diabetic foot. Today physicians have a great deal to offer the diabetic patient with a foot lesion. Saving the foot is a realistic goal. To achieve this goal the treating physician must understand the pathogenesis of diabetic foot lesions. Intervention in the cascade of events (Fig. 32–1) leading to amputation can prevent this catastrophe.

Epidemiology

A primary cause for hospital admission of the patient with diabetes is a foot ulcer. Six percent (162,500) of the diabetic patients admitted to the hospital annually in the United States are admitted because of a foot ulcer.[1] At the India Institute of Diabetes in Bombay, India, more than 10% of all admissions for diabetes are primarily for foot management.[2] Seventy percent required surgical intervention, and >40% of those interventions were either a toe or limb amputation.[2] In the United Kingdom, >50% of the bed occupancy of diabetic patients is due to foot problems.[3] A large survey in the United Kingdom showed that of 6,000 patients attend-

ing diabetes clinics, >2% had an active foot ulcer and 2.5% were amputees.[4] Data from the National Hospital Discharge Summary in the United States showed that the average number of amputations per year from 1989 to 1992 was 51,605. This data included amputations of the toes, 12,427 (24%); midfoot, 2,967 (5.8%); below-the-knee (BK), 20,028 (38.8%); and above-the-knee, 11,048 (21.4%). The remaining 10% included hip, pelvis, knee, and sites not listed.[1] These figures are similar to those compiled by the division of Diabetes Translation of the Centers for Disease Control and Prevention.[5] The average length of stay for amputation reported by Reiber et al.[1] was 20.3 days for patients with private insurance and only 12.4 days for patients on Medicare. Similar differences occurred in diabetic patients hospitalized for foot ulcers. Those with private insurance averaged 17.8 days and those on Medicare, 12 days.

The exact cost of an amputation is difficult to ascertain because of the differences in payment by Medicare and other third-party carriers. Reimbursement for patients with private insurance averaged $26,000, while reimbursement for Medicare patients averaged $10,969, less than half.[1] Eckman et al.[6] reported the average cost for initial hospitalization for amputation of a toe to be $22,026; for a transmetatarsal, $22,373; and for a BK amputation, $22,419. The cost for a toe amputation was essentially the same as that for a BK amputation. For patients that had amputation but died during the initial hospitalization, the costs were astronomical—$59,017 for a toe, $59,365 for a metatarsal, and $59,410 for a BK amputation.[6] Assuming 51,000 amputations, the annual costs would be more than $1 billion. This does not include physicians' charges, rehabilitation costs, disability payments, and, frequently, loss of job.

Today it is estimated that there are more than 16 million diabetics in our country. That is a total of 160 million diabetic toes, less those lost to amputation: enough to keep every podiatrist, family practitioner, surgeon, internist, and diabetologist busy for a lifetime. Furthermore, we can expect to see the problems increasing

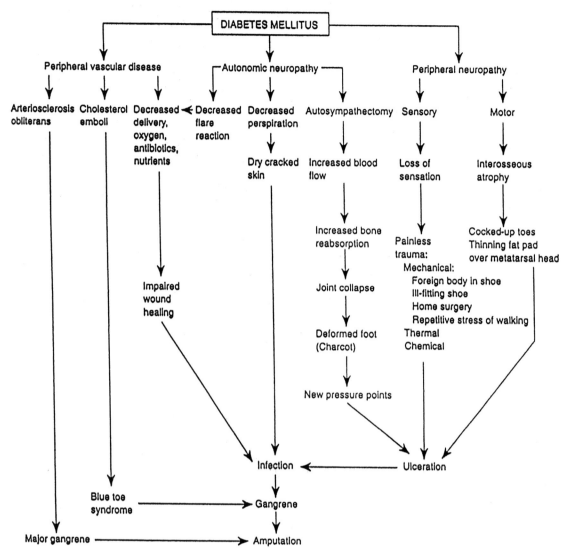

Figure 32–1.   Pathogenesis of diabetic foot lesions. [*Source:* Levin ME: Medical evaluation and treatment. In Levin ME, O'Neal LW, Bowker JH (eds.): The Diabetic Foot, Ed 5. St. Louis MO: Mosby, 1993. With permission.]

since the diabetic population is growing by 6%/year, doubling every 15 years. By the turn of the century, we can expect to have 20 million diabetics. In addition, the diabetic population is aging. Approximately 90% of the diabetic population is over 40 years, and most foot problems occur after age 40 and increase with age. Amputation is more common in African Americans.[7] There is a greater incidence of amputations in men.[8] Reiber et al. found the risk factors for amputation to be insufficient cutaneous circulation below the knee and in the foot, ankle/brachial blood pressure index below 0.45, absent vibratory perception, low levels of high-density lipoprotein (HDL), and lack of previous outpatient diabetes education.[9] Selby and Zhang found additional risk factors to be the level of glucose control, duration of diabetes, and systolic blood pressure.[10]

Interestingly they did not find African Americans to be at increased risk for diabetes related amputation when their access to medical care was good.[10] McNeely et al. found impaired cutaneous oxygenation was a strong risk factor for ulceration. However, in a clinical setting, sensory examination with the 5.07 Semmes-Weinstein monofilament remained the single most practical measure of risk assessment.[11]

In 3 years, following amputation of a limb, approximately 40% of these patients will have amputation of the contralateral limb. This figure rises to approximately 55% after 5 years. This is not surprising since the remaining lower limb has peripheral neuropathy (PN) and peripheral arterial disease (PAD). In addition, the foot of the contralateral limb now bears increased pressure. In fact, even a great toe amputation leads to significantly higher pressures under the first metatarsal head, lesser metatarsal heads, and toes and increased pressure under the heel of the contralateral foot.[12]

Increased pressure plays a significant role in plantar ulceration.[13] Limited joint mobility also can lead to increased pressure and ulceration.[14]

Pathophysiology of Diabetic Foot Lesions

The human foot is truly a mechanical marvel. It consists of 29 joints, eight of which are major, 26 bones, and 42 muscles. In a lifetime these feet walk over 100,000 miles, the equivalent of four times around the world. The sole of the foot contains the largest area of keratinized epidermis in the body. Additional stresses and repeated walking increase this keratinization, resulting in callus formation. These highly thickened callus areas are prone to ulceration. Most neuropathic ulcerations occur over the planter surface of the great toe and over the heads of the metatarsals, particularly the first, second, or fifth metatarsal heads. These ulcerations are usually painless. Ulcerations over the lateral aspect of the foot are most often due to ill-fitting shoes. Ulcerations on the dorsum of the foot are usually secondary to trauma. Small painful ulcers at the tip of the toes or around the ankle are usually ischemic in origin.

Figure 32–1 is a schematic outline of the pathophysiology of diabetic foot lesions that can lead to amputation. Anyone who sees even a small number of diabetic patients will eventually be faced with the many problems of the diabetic foot, peripheral neuropathy (PN), peripheral arterial disease (PAD), foot ulcers, infection, gangrene, amputation, and rehabilitation. In the diabetic foot the signs and symptoms of either ischemia or neuropathy may predominate.

Gavin reported pure PN to be present in 60% of all diabetic patients with ulceration, pure ischemia in 20% and a combination of PN and PAD in 20%.[15]

Vascular disease may ultimately lead to gangrene and amputation, but most diabetic foot lesions are initiated by painless neuropathic lesions. While pain and paresthesias are the patient's chief complaint, it is the loss of sensation and subsequent development of the insensitive foot that allows prolonged painless trauma and results in major foot lesions. The PAD prevents healing.

Infection in the ulcerated areas initiates the final cataclysmic events, that of gangrene and amputation. Infection is more significant in the diabetic because elevated blood sugar levels interfere with the leukocyte function: to move toward the bacteria, engulf it, digest it, and kill it. Blood sugars should be maintained under 200 mg/dL in diabetic patients with infection. Sugars over 200 mg/dL appear to interfere with leukocyte function. Infection is also more difficult to treat in the

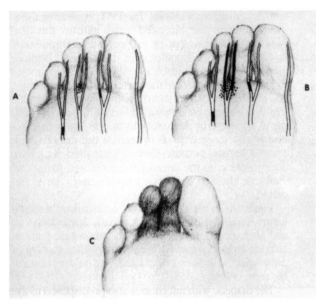

Figure 32–2. Schematic drawings of the mechanism whereby advancing infection causes obliteration of small arteries that have been converted into endarteries by the arteriosclerotic disease process, with resultant gangrene. A. Early web space infection in foot with patchy segmental arteriosclerotic occlusion of digital and metatarsal vessels. B. Thrombosis of arteries adjacent to web space infection. C. Gangrene of second and third toes. [*Source:* O'Neal LW: Surgical pathology of the foot and clinicopathologic correlations. In Levin ME, O'Neal LW, Bowker JH (eds.): The Diabetic Foot, Ed. 5. St. Louis: Mosby, 1993. With permission.]

diabetic with atherosclerosis because there is impaired leukocyte transportation to the areas of infection, oxygen and antibiotic therapy delivery to the infected site is also impaired.

Infections in the diabetic foot are usually of a mixed nature, featuring both aerobes, usually Staphylococcus and Streptococcus, and frequently anaerobes, particularly *Bacteriodes fragilis*. It is therefore critical that any of these infected lesions be cultured, not only aerobically but also anaerobically.

The diabetic with infection is also predisposed to the formation of microthrombi. In the nondiabetic, infection usually produces increased blood flow and a large amount of erythema and warmth. However, in the diabetic there is a tendency toward microthrombi formation. These microthrombi create further ischemic changes, resulting in gangrene or increasing necrosis (Fig. 32–2).

Vascular Disease

PAD in diabetes mellitus involves both large and small vessels. The pathology of PAD in the large vessels, macroangiopathy, differs slightly, if at all, in the diabetic when compared with the nondiabetic. The changes in the vessel wall, both in the media and intima, consisting

EXHIBIT 32–1   Differences in Diabetic and Nondiabetic Periperal Vascular Disease

	Diabetic	Nondiabetic
Clinical	More common	Less common
	Younger patient	Older patient
	More rapid	Less rapid
Male/female	M = F	M ≫ F
Occlusion	Multisegmental	Single segment
Vessels adjacent to occlusion	Involved	Not involved
Collateral vessels	Involved	Usually normal
Lower extremities	Both	Unilateral
Vessels involved	Tibial	Aortic
	Peroneal	Iliac
		Femoral

of deposits of lipid, cholesterol, calcium, platelets, and smooth muscle cells, are qualitatively the same in both groups although quantitatively greater in the diabetic. Exhibit 32–1 lists the important differences between diabetic and nondiabetic PAD. It should be stressed that in the diabetic the vessels involved are primarily those below the knee. In the series of Janka and coworkers[16] the overall prevalence of isolated proximal vascular disease involving femoral and iliac vessels was 5.8% in the diabetic, the same percentage as in the general population. They concluded that proximal vascular disease in the diabetic may represent the atherosclerotic process with coexisting diabetes but did not necessarily represent diabetogenic macroangiopathy. While this may be true, it is my own personal clinical feeling that there is some acceleration of this atherosclerotic process even in these larger vessels in the diabetic. Atherosclerotic involvement of the larger proximal vessels, the iliacs and femorals, is definitely accelerated by smoking. For example, we recently saw a 27-year-old patient with insulin-dependent diabetes mellitus (IDDM), diabetic since age 5 years, who had been a heavy smoker since age 13. At age 27 years, he developed intermittent claudication in his right leg and was found on angiography to have occlusion of the femoral artery.

As noted, one of the major differences between the nondiabetic and the diabetic is the vessels involved. This is demonstrated by the type of vascular surgery that is performed in these patients. Although vascular surgery of all types is more common in the diabetic than the nondiabetic, the procedure most frequently performed in the diabetic is tibioperoneal bypass surgery, involving the vessels below the knee. Vascular procedures performed on the diabetic lower extremity are approximately 10% aortofemoral bypass, 40% femoropopliteal bypass, and 70% tibioperoneal bypass.[17] Percutaneous angioplasty is less applicable in the diabetic because the atherosclerotic process occurs most often in the smaller vessels.

It should also be noted that large- and small-vessel disease do not necessarily progress at the same rate. For example, small vessels in the toes often have far-advanced atherosclerosis compared with the more proximal vessels. Thus, the dorsalis pedis or posterior tibial pulses may be present and of adequate quality, yet the toes may show evidence of significant vascular insufficiency. This accounts for the fact that approximately one-third of diabetics may have small areas of gangrene with palpable dorsalis pedis and/or posterior tibial pulses.

Figure 32–3 is an example of a patchy area of gangrene in the medial aspect of the left great toe incurred in a patient with diabetes of 16 years duration. The posterior tibial pulse in this patient was palpable.

Microangiopathy is not a signifcant factor in the pathogenesis of diabetic foot lesions. Although there may be some capillary basement membrane thicken-

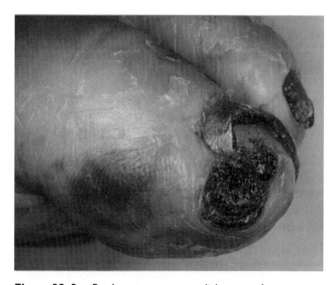

Figure 32–3.   Patchy gangrene on medial aspect of great toe caused by small-vessel disease. [*Source:* Levin ME: Medical evaluation and treatment. In Levin ME, O'Neal LW (eds.): The Diabetic Foot, Ed. 3. St. Louis MO: C.V. Mosby, 1983. With permission.]

ing, there is no evidence that this contributes to the foot lesions. This has been particularly stressed by LoGerfo and Coffman.[18] They further suggested that in many instances there are enough patent vessels in the foot to allow vascular surgery.

Gangrene of the toes can result from atherosclerosis and thrombosis or from microthrombi caused by infection (see Fig. 32–2) or from microemboli that break off from atheromatous plaques in the larger vessels of the lower extremity, resulting in cyanotic toes or the blue toe syndrome.[19,20] The foot may also show petechiae from these cholesterol emboli (Fig. 32–4). These frequently are painful. The toe takes on a deep purplish discoloration, and this can result in gangrene and amputation. These toes can, on occasion, be revascularized. The atheromatous plaques may be present in the aorta, iliac, or more distant vessels. The syndrome is characterized by the sudden onset of pain in the toe and occasionally by leg and thigh myalgias if muscular arteries are involved. When digital artery blood flow becomes impaired, the toe may become bluish-purple. A sharp demarcation occurs between normally per-

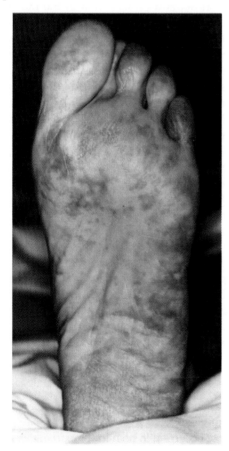

Figure 32–4. Note purplish discolorization of fifth toe and reticular pattern in skin of the foot. These areas do not blanche and are painful. This is indicative of ischemia and is due to cholesterol emboli from atherosclerotic plaques in the more proximal larger arteries. (Courtesy Dr. Gregorio A. Sicard, Washington University School of Medicine, St. Louis, Missouri.)

fused skin and ischemic areas. Many of these patients have received anticoagulation therapy with warfarin. This has been the case in most of the patients that I have seen with this syndrome. Thrombolytic therapy, streptokinase,[21] and tissue plasminogen activator[22] can also be associated with the blue toe syndrome. It is therefore extremely important to check periodically the toes and feet of patients receiving anticoagulants. However, all patients with this syndrome are not on anticoagulant therapy.

Repeated attacks of acute ischemic changes, particularly those occurring in both lower extremities and the development of painful cyanotic toes, suggest microemboli. Older reports suggested that atheromatous embolization stems from the aortic iliac segments. Currently, the treatment of choice is vascular surgery to remove these plaques, thereby preventing further embolization. In the study of Fisher et al.[23] patients with multilevel atherosclerotic occlusive disease had their peripheral lesions treated first. In their small series the authors had no morbidity or mortality. Recurrent embolization did not occur during the follow-up period of 8–24 months.

Some of the impaired blood flow in the diabetic results from an increase in blood viscosity due to elevated levels of fibrinogen, von Willebrand's factor, increased platelet adhesion, and aggregation.[24] Diabetics are also predisposed to thrombosis formation. McGill et al. have shown a threefold increase in tissue plasminogen activator inhibitor type I.[25] Increase in red blood cell rigidity has also been demonstrated.[26] All of these factors lead to an increase in blood viscosity and a decrease in blood flow.

Risk Factors

Listed in Exhibit 32–2 are the risk factors in the development of diabetic macrovascular disease. Age, duration, and genetic factors, of course, cannot be corrected. However, certain risk factors can be altered. Smoking is a definite risk factor that can be corrected, and it is critically important that the diabetic patient does not smoke. Smoking a single cigarette can narrow the arteries and reduce blood flow for as long as an hour.[27] Although the nicotine and carbon monoxide content of cigarette smoke has been believed to be the major risk, a recent article by Kaufman and colleagues[28] has shown that patients who smoked cigarettes with a reduced

EXHIBIT 32–2 Vascular Disease: Risk Factors

Genetics	Cholesterol
Age	Triglyceride
Duration of diabetes	Hyperglycemia
Smoking	Hyperinsulinemia
Systolic blood pressure	Truncal obesity
Diastolic blood pressure	

amount of nicotine and carbon monoxide did not have any lower risk factor for myocardial infarction than did those who smoked the cigarettes containing a larger amount of those substances.

Hypertension is also a risk factor than can be controlled. Control of both systolic and diastolic pressure is important. There is no question that a strong correlation exists between hypercholesterolemia and cardiovascular disease. However, not all authorities have found a correlation between PAD and hypercholesterolemia.[29] Nevertheless, any patient with elevated cholesterol values should be treated. The role of hyperglycemia in the pathogenesis of PAD is also debatable. Nelson et al.[29] have found a correlation between hyperglycemia and PAD. Others, however, have not found a strong correlation.[30] Hyperinsulinemia can also be a factor in the pathogenesis of atherosclerosis. Hyperinsulinemia is common in patients with non-insulin-dependent diabetes mellitus (NIDDM) who have insulin resistance. It is also common in patients with IDDM because the insulin is administered subcutaneously and does not initially pass through the liver for removal. Fifty percent of insulin secreted by the pancreas is removed by one pass through the liver.

Insulin is a growth-promoting factor and has been found by several investigators to stimulate the duplication of smooth muscles and their migration into the lumen.[31,32] Duplication of smooth muscle cells and their migration into the vessel lumen is a critical event in the formation of the atherosclerotic plaque. In addition, there are, as noted, increased clotting factors in diabetes. Even though platelet factors of increased adherence and adhesion have been demonstrated in diabetics, clinical trials to date with antiplatelet drugs in diabetic PAD have not yet been reported to be totally effective.[33]

Subjective and Objective Data of Peripheral Vascular Disease

The subjective (symptoms) and objective (signs) findings of PAD are listed in Exhibit 32–3. Intermittent claudication is a common symptom of PAD. The word "claudication" comes from the Latin, meaning to limp. The patient with claudication may begin to limp when ischemic symptoms develop. However, more characteristically, he stops to rest. Therefore the pain resulting from intermittent claudication is characterized by pain associated with walking, relieved by cessation of walking without the need to sit down. In the assessment (differential diagnosis), intermittent claudication must be distinguished from the pain resulting from degenerative arthritic changes, disk disease, tumors of the spinal cord, particularly the cauda equine, thrombophlebitis, anemia, and even myxedema. Pain with walking due to these causes is referred to as pseudoclaudication. The differential from ischemic claudication can be made by history alone. The patient with claudication due to ischemia simply needs to stop walking and rest for a moment or two and then proceed. Patients with pseudoclaudication usually require 15–20 minutes of rest and frequently give a history of having to sit down and change position, flex, or extend their back to get relief. The symptoms of intermittent claudication depend on ischemia in the muscle; thus, despite extensive involvement of the small vessels of the diabetic foot, symptoms of claudication are infrequent because of small muscle mass. Some investigators believe the claudication does not occur in the foot. The most common area for claudication to occur is in the calf. Diabetics with severe PAD may not have symptoms of claudication because of PN and the loss of sensory pain perception.

Improvement in intermittent claudication can be achieved with supervised training and exercise programs.[34]

Cold feet are a common complaint in patients with PAD. It is cold feet that prompt the diabetic to resort to the use of hot water bottles and heating pads. This can result in severe burns to a foot that has become insensitive to heat due to PN.

Rest pain usually indicates at least two hemodynamically significant arterial blocks in a series. Rest pain is caused by nerve ischemia and is persistent with peaks of intensity. It is worse at night and may require the use of narcotics for relief. Rest pain is decreased by

EXHIBIT 32–3   Signs and Symptoms of Vascular Disease in the Diabetic Lower Extremity

Intermittent claudication	Delayed venous filling after elevation of extremity
Cold feet	Dependent rubor
Nocturnal pain	Atrophy of subcutaneous fatty tissues
Rest pain	Shiny appearance of skin
Noctural and rest pain relieved with dependency of extremity	Loss of hair on foot and toes
Absent pulses	Thickened nails, frequently with fungus infection
Blanching on elevation	Gangrene

dependency of the lower extremity but is aggravated by heat, elevation, and exercise. Because of the relief produced by dependency, the patient often sleeps in a chair, and edema of the leg secondary to constant dependency is common. In the diabetic, rest pain may be absent despite the ischemia because diabetic PN has destroyed the sensory perception.

Nocturnal ischemic pain is a form of neuritis that usually precedes rest pain. It occurs at night or during sleep because the circulation is essentially of the core variety, with very little perfusion of the lower extremity. Ischemic neuritis thus produced becomes intense and disrupts sleep. The patient invariably gains relief by standing up or dangling his feet over the edge of the bed and on occasion by walking a short distance. This activity increases his cardiac output, leading to improved perfusion of the lower extremities and relief of the ischemic neuritis. If lesions that produce nocturnal rest pain are not corrected, tissue necrosis and gangrene almost always develop, necessitating amputation. Rest pain and nocturnal pain are therefore indications for angiography and possible vascular surgery to relieve the arterial occlusions. Absent pulses are of course significant evidence of PAD. Examination of the patient with intermittent claudication involving the calf muscle may reveal both a femoral and pedal but no popliteal pulse. The pedal pulses are present because of the collaterals in these patients. After a brisk walk, the foot will pale and become pulseless.

Pallor of the foot on elevation is an important sign of ischemia. With the patient in the supine position, the feet are elevated to a 45° angle and held in this position until one or both feet blanch. The patient is then instructed to sit upright with the feet in a dependent position. Venous and capillary filling time is usually less than 15 sec but prolonged to minutes in the ischemic extremity. The extremity with severe PAD will develop rubor after dependency. It should be remembered that patients with varicose veins may also have dependent rubor on the basis of venous stasis. Pallor on elevation, prolonged filling time, and dependent rubor are hallmarks of significant lower extremity vascular insufficiency.

Further ischemic changes are characterized by shiny, atrophic cool skin. As vascular insufficiency progresses, there is loss of hair on the dorsum of the foot. Thickening of the nails is also influenced by the vascular insufficiency, and the nails have frequent secondary fungal infection. In addition, the nails tend to grow more slowly when the blood supply is decreased. Further ischemia leads to atrophy of the subcutaneous tissue. The skin appears to be tightly drawn over the foot, and ulceration can occur from minor trauma to this atrophic skin. Figure 32–5 illustrates the typical diabetic foot afflicted with PAD and neuropathy.

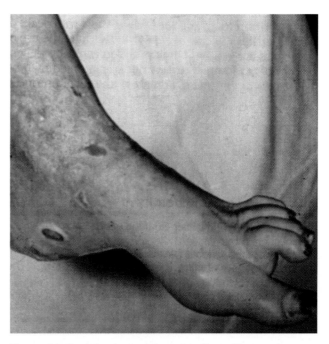

Figure 32–5. The classic diabetic foot: loss of hair on the dorsum of foot and toes, shiny atrophic skin, loss of subcutaneous fat, and atrophy of the interosseous muscles with resulting turned-up toes (hammer toes). (Courtesy John F. Fiarbairn II, M.D., Mayo Clinic, Rochester, MN., and The Upjohn Company, Kalamazoo, MI.)

In the diabetic, most of the changes of ischemia occur slowly, although the possibility of sudden occlusion from emboli or complete thrombosis must always be considered. The signs and symptoms of acute occlusion are usually called the "five Ps." These are listed in Exhibit 32–4.

The extent of ischemia and the final outcome depend on collateral circulation and the time elapsing from the onset of acute occlusion and treatment. Most sudden occlusions are the result of emboli, but they can also result from thrombosis at the site of an atherosclerotic plaque. These occlusions must be treated as soon as possible since peripheral nerves and skeletal muscle have less resistance to ischemia than skin and bone. Malan and Tattoni[35] have indicated that irreversible changes of skeletal muscle and peripheral nerves occur after 4–6 hr of severe ischemia. Pain from embolism is usually more severe and more sudden in onset than pain from thrombosis. Pallor is also more severe with embolism than with thrombosis. With embolism the

EXHIBIT 32–4 The Five Ps of Acute Arterial Occlusion

Pain	Sudden onset
Pallor	Waxy
Paresthesia	Numbness
Paralysis	Sudden weakness
Pulseless	Absent pulses

affected extremity is waxlike and lemon yellow in color. With thrombosis, the extremity is less cadaverous in appearance and tends to be somewhat cyanotic. The paresthesias are due to peripheral nerve ischemia.

Neuropathy

As noted in Fig. 32–1, the neuropathy can ultimately result in amputation through various pathways. These include the loss of autonomic, sensory, or motor nerve function. Autonomic involvement results in decrease in perspiration. This leads to dryness, cracking, and fissuring of the skin, which can become infected.

The most important neuropathic abnormality is the loss of sensation and the development of an insensitive foot. Such a foot is vulnerable to painless trauma, which can be mechanical, thermal, or chemical. The most common mechanical problems that I see result from home surgery. Despite frequent warnings against this by the physician, many patients find it impossible to resist and try to cut out their ingrown toenails, frequently cutting nails and calluses too deeply. These wounds then become infected. Walking barefoot can also result in foot lesions. Figure 32–6 illustrates such

an example. In this case a nail is embedded in the foot of a diabetic patient. The patient had noted a painless, reddened area on his foot for approximately 2 months. Because the area was enlarging, he went to see his physician. A radiograph of this area demonstrated the nail and marked osteomyelitis. The foot ultimately required amputation. Figures 32–7 and 32–8 are examples of massive foreign objects found in the shoes of patients who were totally unaware of their presence and walked on them for an entire day. Other mechanical problems result from improperly fitted shoes.

Thermal injuries are common. Patients with vascular insufficiency have cold feet and commonly the uneducated patient will use a heating pad or hot water bottle on them with disastrous results (Fig. 32–9).

Changes in the shape of the foot lead to new pressure points and callus buildup at these new areas,

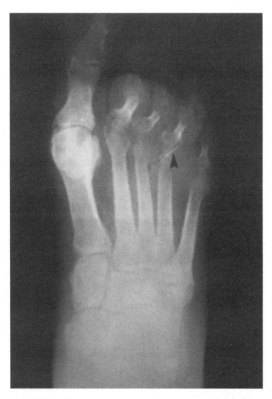

Figure 32–6. Carpenter's nail present for approximately 2 months in tissues of foot of an insulin-requiring diabetic patient. He had no knowledge of having stepped on this nail nor did he have any pain or discomfort (Photograph courtesy of Dr. Joseph Marr, Division of Infectious Disease, Department of Medicine, University of Colorado at Denver.) [*Source:* Levin ME: Medical evaluation and treatment. In Levin ME, O'Neil LW, Bowker JH (eds.): The Diabetic Foot, Ed. 5. St. Louis, MO: Mosby, 1993. With permission.]

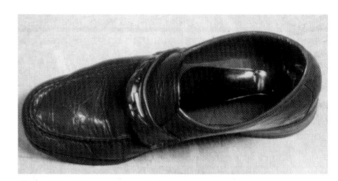

Figure 32–7. Shoehorn in shoe worn by patient who, because of an insensitive foot resulting from diabetic neuropathy, was unaware of its presence until removing shoe at end of day. [*Source:* Levin ME: Medical evaluation and treatment. In Levin ME, O'Neal LW, Bowker JH (eds.): The Diabetic Foot, Eds 5. St. Louis, MO: Mosby, 1993. With permission.]

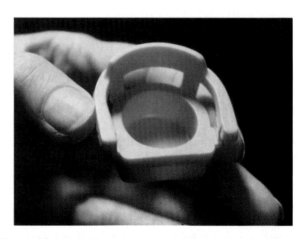

Figure 32–8. Doll's chair measuring 2.5 × 3.8 cm found in patient's shoe. He had worn the shoe all day without being aware of chair's presence because of an almost total absence of sensory perception produced by severe diabetic neuropathy. [*Source:* Levin ME: Medical evaluation and treatment. In Levin ME, O'Neal LW, Bowker JH (eds.): The Diabetic Foot, Ed. 5. St. Louis, MO: Mosby, 1993. With permission.]

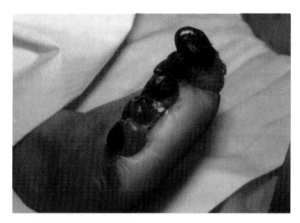

Figure 32–9. Gangrene in toes of patient who had soaked his cold foot in hot water. [*Source:* Levin ME: Medical evaluation and treatment. In Levin ME, O'Neal LW, Bowker JH (eds.): The Diabetic Foot, Ed. 5. St. Louis, MO: Mosby, 1993. With permission.]

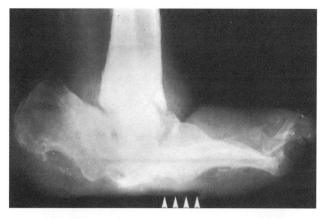

Figure 32–10. Radiograph of Charcot's foot. Severe osteolytic and destructive changes are seen with gross disorganization of the ankle joints and loss of volume of the tarsal bones. There is subluxation at the metatarsal phalangeal joints. The arrows points to the ulcerated areas seen in Figure 32–11.

which then break down and ulcerate. Muscle atrophy due to involvement of the motor nerves leads to an imbalance of the muscles in the foot. This frequently leads to cocked up toes and ulceration may occur on the tips and tops of the toes and frequently, because of thinning of the fat pad, underneath the first metatarsophalangeal head. Prevention of ulceration in these areas requires straightening out of these cocked up or claw toes at a time when circulation is good. However, if this cannot be done, then it is critically important to make sure the toe box of the shoe is large enough to accommodate these deformed toes. An in-depth shoe that can accommodate a plastic insole is frequently required to decrease pressure over the metatarsal heads, especially the first, and the plantar tips of the toes.

The development of Charcot's foot is not unusual. Classically, Charcot's foot presents as acutely hot and swollen with bounding pulses and prominent veins. Despite what is written in some textbooks, these patients frequently have some pain and discomfort. It may be difficult to differentiate the warm, reddened Charcot's foot from that of cellulitis. However, the patient with Charcot's foot is afebrile, and the white blood cell count is normal. The sedimentation rate may be slightly elevated. The neuropathic component related to the development of Charcot's foot probably stems from involvement of the autonomic nervous system. The result is the equivalent of sympathectomy of the nerves in the feet. The arteries dilate and arteriovenous shunts have been demonstrated in these feet.[36] Young et al. felt that minor trauma in patients with PN might result in fractures in those with reduced bone density.[37] Edmonds et al. felt that the increased blood flow in the feet of these patients led to increased osteoclastic activity and reduced bone density.[38] These patients with PN had a greater frequency of tripping and falling.[39] Patients with PN may have a tendency to sway and an inability to maintain pos-

ture.[40] Patients who develop Charcot's foot frequently give a history of mild trauma, such as tripping. Radiographic examination in the acute stage reveals no bony abnormality. If the patient is allowed to continue to walk, there can be gradual dissolution and fragmentation of the distal ends of the metatarsals and frequently involvement of the tarsometatarsal joint. The radiographs also show the absence of calcification in the interosseous arteries, further evidence that there is no significant vascular insufficiency. Because there is relative insensitivity in these feet, patients continue to walk, subsequently developing so-called *stress fractures* and further bone destruction. The treatment for these patients in the acute stage is nonweight-bearing, frequently with the use of a contact cast. If the process is allowed to progress, the arch collapses (Fig. 32–10), the foot becomes everted and shortened, the arch is lost and takes on a rockerbottom configuration. It is the planter area of the arch that frequently breaks down and becomes ulcerated (Fig. 32–11). Ulceration on the planter surface in the area of the arch is a classic sign of Charcot's foot.

Changes in gait with new pressure points may occur from muscle atrophy or from a sprain. I recently examined a patient with long-standing diabetic neuropathy and PAD who had stepped into a hole and sprained his ankle. This caused him to limp and to place additional pressure on his foot. He developed a painless ulcer that did not heal. It became infected, and he ultimately required a BK amputation.

Listed in Exhibit 32–5 are the signs and symptoms of neuropathy of the diabetic foot. Neuropathy in the lower extremity is frequently bilateral and tends to be symmetrical. Sensory involvement is characterized by two major symptom complexes: one consists of pain and paresthesia, the other, paradoxically, of a decreased sensation of pain and temperature. The paresthesias may be manifested as pain, tingling, or burning and

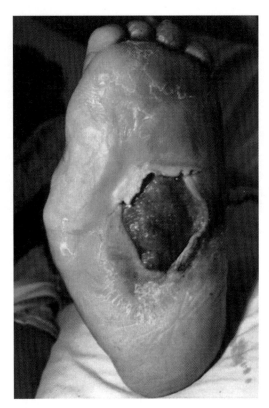

Figure 32–11. A massive planter ulcer on the left foot of a 69-year-old man with diabetes of 17 years duration. He had severe peripheral neuropathy and bilateral Charcot's joints. He ultimately had to have a left BK amputation.

EXHIBIT 32–5 Signs and Symptoms of Neuropathy in the Diabetic Foot and Leg

Paresthesia
Hyperesthesia
Hypoesthesia
Radicular pain
Loss of deep tendon reflexes
Loss of vibratory and position sense
Anhydrosis
Heavy callus formation over pressure points
Trophic ulcers
Infection complicating trophic ulcers
Foot drop
Changes in shape of foot produced by:
   Muscle atrophy
   Changes in bone and joints
Radiographic signs
   Demineralization
   Osteolysis
   Charcot's joint

may be severe and knifelike or shooting in nature. At times it is almost constant, and frequently it is most severe at night. In some instances it is severe enough to require narcotics for relief. A wide variety of medications have been used to relieve these painful symptoms. The tricyclics are the most commonly used.[41] A recent treatment is Capsacian (Axain).[42] This topi-

EXHIBIT 32–6 Causes of Peripheral Neuropathy

Diabetes mellitus	Malignancy
Alcoholism	Pressure neuropathy
Herniated nucleus pulposus	Uremia
Heavy metals	Porphyria
Vitamin deficiencies	Hansen's disease (leprosy)
Collagen disease	Drugs
Pernicious anemia	

cally applied cream depletes substance P in the nerves, thus decreasing pain.

The importance of blood sugar control in preventing or decreasing the progression of neuropathy has been well established by the Diabetes Control and Complications Trial (DCCT).[43]

It must be kept in mind that peripheral neuropathy may have many causes, and these must also be considered in the diabetic (Exhibit 32–6).

The heel of the diabetic is particularly vulnerable to trauma. The heel is exposed to a great deal of pressure, resulting in callus buildup. As the callus becomes thicker, it tends to crack and becomes a source of infection. When the heel is infected, the infection tends to penetrate deeply. The skin of the heel is tightly bound by numerous vertical septa extending through the subcutaneous tissue to the surface of the calcaneous. These septa result in formation of small cylinders that are packed with fatty tissue. These small honeycombed fat-containing tubes become cushions and in effect act like shock absorbers on heel impact. With ischemic changes there is atrophy of the subcutaneous fatty tissue, thus decreasing the effectiveness of the shock-absorber-like effect.

When the patient requires bed rest for any length of time, such as when hospitalized, particular attention must be paid to the heel. Because of the loss of sensation, the patient tends to keep the heels in the same position. In addition, the heel suffers friction trauma when the patient uses it to change his or her position. This results in pressure necrosis, causing the skin to break down (Fig. 32–12). Infection and gangrene can follow. These patients should have their heels inspected at least once and preferably twice a day. The presence of even slight erythema is a warning of impending pressure necrosis. Prevention is critical. This is best accomplished by heel protectors or pressure-reducing mattresses.

Infection

Infection is the third major factor in the pathogenesis of diabetic foot lesions leading to amputation. Breaks in the skin, which may be almost imperceptible, cracks or fissures in calluses, or major wounds, such as diabetic foot ulcers, act as portals of entry for bacteria. It is not unusual to culture four or five different organisms from these wounds. These may be gram-negative and grampositive organisms, aerobes and anaerobes.

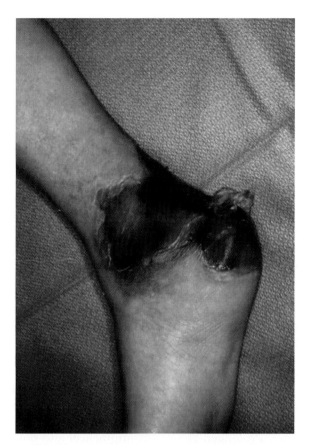

Figure 32–12. Gangrene of the heel in bedridden diabetic patient caused by the weight of the immobile neuropathic foot on the mattress. [*Source:* O'Neal LW: Surgical pathology of the foot and clinicopathologic correlations. In Levin ME, O'Neal LW, Bowker JH (eds): The Diabetic Foot, Ed 5. St. Louis, MO: Mosby 1993. With permission.]

EXHIBIT 32–7   Management of Diabetic Foot Ulcers

1. Evaluation
   a. Clinical appearance
   b. Depth of penetration
   c. X-rays to detect
      (1) Foreign body
      (2) Osteomyelitis
      (3) Subcutaneous gas
   d. Location
   e. Biopsy
   f. Blood supply (noninvasive vascular studies)
2. Debridement, radical
3. Bacterial cultures (aerobic and anaerobic)
4. Metabolic control
5. Antibiotics
   a. Oral
   b. Parenteral
6. Do not soak the feet
7. Decrease of edema
8. Non-weight-bearing
   a. Bedrest
   b. Crutches
   c. Wheelchair
   d. Special sandals
   e. Contact casting
9. Improve circulation (vascular surgery)

Adapted from Levin ME: The diabetic foot: Pathophysiology, evaluation, and treatment. In Levin ME, O'Neal LW, Bowker J (eds.): The Diabetic Foot, Ed. 5. St. Louis, MO: Mosby Year Book, pp. 17-60, 1993.

The success in obtaining the proper culture depends on technique. Simply swabbing the wound to obtain material for culture can give a false result. After debriding the wound a culture should be taken by curettage from the base of the wound. Special techniques are required when obtaining material for anaerobic culture. Infection in the diabetic foot is difficult to treat for many reasons. Hyperglycemia impairs leukocyte function. The infection can be polymicrobial. Aerobes and anaerobes are frequently present requiring special culturing techniques and appropriate antibiotics. Inadequate debridement leaves necrotic material, which impairs eradication of the infection. Osteomyelitis is common. Finally, peripheral arterial disease impairs the delivery of oxygen and antibiotics.

Management of Diabetic Foot Ulcers

Exhibit 32–7 lists steps in the management of diabetic foot ulcers.[44] Management of a foot ulcer requires establishment of the size and depth of the ulcer. What appears to be a superficial ulceration may be only the tip of the iceberg. Penetration may extend deep into the tissues.

X-rays are necessary to rule out osteomyelitis, gas formation, the presence of foreign objects, and asymptomatic fractures. Therefore, any foot with ulceration or infection should be X-rayed.

Vigorous sharp debridement of the ulcer to establish the degree of penetration and to remove all necrotic tissue should be done. Debridement should be carried down to healthy bleeding tissue. The ulcer after debridement will in all probability be larger than it was at presentation. Eschars should be completely removed if there is adequate circulation. Whirlpool is not the method of choice for debridement. In some instances the patient has to be taken to the operating room for adequate debridement.

Biopsy should be considered when the ulcer is in an atypical location, not over the metatarsal heads or the plantar surface of the hallux, when it cannot be explained by trauma, and when it is unresponsive to aggressive therapy. On occasion, biopsy of an atypical ulcer has revealed malignancy, both primary and metastatic.

Antibiotic therapy should begin immediately after obtaining the cultures with a broad-spectrum antibiotic, then changed accordingly depending on the organisms and sensitivities. The selection of an oral antibiotic or parenteral antibiotic for the treatment of a diabetic foot infection depends on medical judgment. Many diabetic foot infections contain gram-negative organisms. Therefore, the oral antibiotic chosen should be effective for gram-positive and gram-negative organisms.

If an oral antibiotic is selected, it is my opinion that the diabetic patient should not be told to take the medication and return in 1 week. Infection in the diabetic patient can deteriorate rapidly within 24–48 hr. Therefore, the diabetic patient on oral therapy should be seen within a few days after institution of therapy. The patient must be instructed to notify the physician at once should there be an increase in redness, drainage, or evidence of lymphangitis. While many of these patients have insensate feet, the development of pain is indicative of deep infection and requires immediate attention. The development of a bad odor also indicates worsening infection and frequently the presence of anaerobes.

It is very important that patients with infection monitor their blood glucose levels closely. A rising blood glucose level strongly suggests worsening infection, even though other signs and symptoms are absent.

The patient with what appears to be a minor infection on the plantar surface of the foot who develops erythema and edema on the dorsum of the foot should be hospitalized. Even though the patient is not septic, there is high probability that the infection on the plantar surface has penetrated deep into the tissues and has spread to the dorsum of the foot. Patients with infection and severe PAD should be hospitalized and evaluated for vascular surgery. The worst scenario leading to amputation is infection and ischemia. TcPo2 <20 mmHg measured below the knee and in the foot is a significant risk for amputation.[9] Patients with PAD should be given parenteral antibiotics to achieve a higher concentration of antibiotics in the peripheral tissues than can be achieved by oral therapy alone. Furthermore, the antibiotic of choice frequently can only be given parenterally. Patients who are toxic and have significantly elevated blood sugars should be admitted to the hospital. The wound must be surgically debrided, parenteral antibiotics must be started, and blood sugars must be brought under control. Consultation with a diabetologist and infectious disease specialist is recommended. If the circulation is impaired, a vascular surgeon should be consulted.

When infection is not responding to aggressive treatment, the wound should be debrided again and recultured, as the flora may have changed. Chronic recurrent or resistant infection suggests the presence of osteomyelitis.

Osteomyelitis is a frequent complication of diabetic foot ulcers and infection.[45,46] Osteomyelitis may be difficult to detect on a clinical basis. Newman et al.[45] showed that in biopsy-proven osteomyelitis, only one-third of the patients had clinically suspected osteomyelitis. If bone is visible or the ulcer can be probed to the bone, the probability of osteomyelitis is very strong.[46] Scanning techniques for osteomyelitis are not always successful. The triple-phase scan with technetium lacks specificity. Scans with Indium III can be helpful. Magnetic resonance imaging (MRI) is proving to be a helpful technique.[47]

Because diabetic foot infection can be very complex, consultation with an expert in infectious disease may be extremely helpful.

Soaking the feet has no benefit, although it has been a traditional approach. Soaking can lead to maceration and infection. Because the foot is insensitive, soaking may take place in water that is too hot, resulting in severe burns. Chemical soaks can result in chemical burns.[48]

Edema is frequently present and can contribute to vascular insufficiency by compression of the capillaries. Elevation of the feet to the thickness of one pillow can be beneficial. Higher elevation may impede circulation.

Avoidance of weight-bearing is essential. These patients have insensitive feet, and, because the ulcer is not painful, they continue to walk. The result is an increase in pressure necrosis that can delay healing. Weight-bearing can also force bacteria deeper into the tissues. Prolonged bed rest is impractical and potentially dangerous because of possible venous thrombosis and pulmonary emboli. The use of crutches and/or a wheelchair is seldom successful in achieving total and consistent non-weight-bearing. Many patients with PN have ataxia, making the use of crutches potentially dangerous. The best method for achieving non-weight-bearing in the appropriately selected patient is the contact cast.[49] The contact cast allows the patient to be ambulatory but essentially non-weight-bearing by decreasing the pressure on the ulcerated area. The contact cast is contraindicated for patients who are ataxic, blind, pathologically obese, and/or have severe PAD.[49]

The healing of a foot ulcer in the immunosupressed patient with diabetes is markedly impaired, and these patients also have a higher amputation rate.[50] Immunosuppression is common because of the increasing frequency of kidney and pancreas transplants.

When an ulcer does not heal despite good metabolic control, adequate debridement, parenteral antibiotic therapy, and avoidance of weight-bearing, the impaired healing may be the result of vascular insufficiency. Ankle or brachial indexes of <0.50 or transcutaneous oxygen pressure <30 mmHg and certainly those <20 mmHg are highly predictive that the infection will not resolve and that the ulcer will not heal. The importance of peripheral arterial reconstruction was demonstrated by LoGerfo et al.[51] In 2,883 extreme distal arterial reconstructions, they found a statistically significant decrease in every category of amputation, a decrease that correlated precisely with increasing the rate of dorsalis pedis artery bypass.

Other indications for vascular surgery is night pain or rest pain and impending gangrene due to ischemia. Most PAD in the patient with diabetes occurs below the knee or below the trifurcation and affects the smaller tibial and peroneal arteries. For this reason, end-arterectomy and angioplasty can rarely be accomplished in these smaller vessels. The most successful surgery in these patients is tibial-peroneal bypass. This is accomplished by using the patient's own saphenous vein and microvascular surgical techniques to hook up vessels above the knee to the pedal vessels, which are frequently patent.[52,53] (See Chapter 34.)

Topical Therapy of Foot Ulcers

The proper dressing of a wound depends on the type of wound, its location, size, depth, and the amount of drainage.[54]

The use of topical therapy for wounds goes back to ancient times, when an unbelievable number of substances, ranging from wine to human excreta, were used to treat wounds. Today the available topically applied agents to prevent and treat wounds number greater than 2,300.[55] The use of resins and enzyme therapy to help debride is advocated by some. Although these can be beneficial, they represent adjunct therapy and should not be substituted for aggressive surgical debridement. In the past, it has been common practice to use a number of bactericidal topical agents such as povidone-iodine (Betadine), acetic acid, hydrogen peroxide, and sodium hypochlorite (Dakin's solution). Although these substances will destroy surface bacteria, they can be cytotoxic to granulation tissue. Rodeheaver et al.[56] have recently reviewed the controversies in topical wound management. Other topical antibiotics such as silver sulfadiazine (Silvadene) can be very effective but only for removing surface bacteria. The use of topical preparations alone and allowing these patients to bear weight puts them at great jeopardy for amputation.

The latest addition to topical therapy is wound-healing growth factors. Platelet-derived growth factor (PDGF) can be an important adjunct to healing wounds that have shown resistance to comprehensive approaches. A recent report by Steed and the Diabetic Ulcer Study Group[57] has shown that recombinant PDGF can also be effective in wound healing.

Post-Treatment of Healed Diabetic Foot Ulcers

Once a diabetic foot ulcer is healed, the job is not complete. The underlying etiology that caused the ulceration in many instances still exists. Therefore special means are necessary to prevent recurrence. This frequently requires reeducation of the patient in walking, in taking shorter steps, and frequently in a change of jobs. Special shoes are very important.

Special Shoes

Special shoes are indicated in patients who have cocked-up toes and need an enlarged toe box to prevent irritation of the tips on the tops of the toes. Patients with markedly deformed feet such as Charcot's foot need specially molded shoes. Special shoes are critically important to prevent ulcerations or recurrence of ulcers. This frequently requires extra depth shoes with a plastic-like material, frequently Plastazote inserts to redistribute the weight. A study at King's College in London demonstrated an 83% recurrence of ulcers when patients returned to wearing their regular shoes. However, with the use of special shoes, there was only a 17% recurrence.[58]

Foot Inspection

Foot inspection is one of the most essential parts of the physical examination of the diabetic. However, this is frequently neglected. In a study by Cohen,[59] in a clinic setting, only 16% of the patients' feet were examined. Bailey et al.[60] found that only 12% of the patients had their feet examined. It is mandatory that shoes, socks, trousers, and pantyhose be removed at every visit and that feet and legs be thoroughly examined. Instruction to the patient on foot care should be carried out at this time.

Teamwork

Problems of the diabetic foot are extremely complicated. Prevention and treatment of these problems can only be achieved by the teamwork of multiple disciplines. Teamwork as depicted in Fig. 32–13 is not the type of teamwork I am referring to.

Members of the team include the generalist, diabetologist, radiologist, vascular surgeon, a specialist in infectious disease, a neurologist, podiatrist, and orthotist. In some cases, the services of a social worker are required. If amputation cannot be avoided, the expertise of the specialist in rehabilitation becomes necessary.

Failure to seek consultation from one or more of these experts can deprive the patient of a skill that could save his foot and leg. Today, the podiatrist plays an increasingly important role in the diabetic patient's care. It is common for the podiatrist to make the initial diagnosis of diabetes. Many podiatrists have blood sugar–measuring devices in their offices and frequently stress to patients the need for taking better care of themselves. Initiation and reinforcement of good foot care is

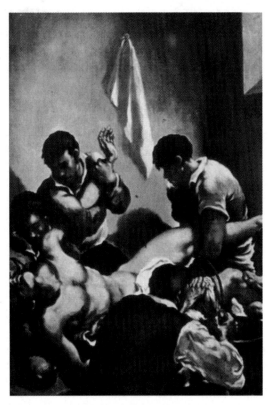

Figure 32–13. This painting depicts the agonies of a patient undergoing amputation in ancient times. Formerly, amputations were performed only for gangrene, with alcohol as an anesthetic. Many people died during this guillotine operation; some even died of shock and terror before the operation began. [*Source:* International Museum of Surgical Sciences and Hall of Fame. International College of Surgeons, Chicago, Illinois (Hall of Fame). The painting was done by the Italian Count Gregorio Calvi de Bergolo in 1953. With permission.]

done frequently by the podiatrist. In addition, surgical procedures such as removal of pressure exostosis can prevent recurrent tissue breakdown at these areas.

Patient Education

Of all the techniques discussed in this chapter, none is more important than patient education on proper foot care. Until a cure for diabetes has been found, we will be faced with angiopathy and neuropathy. The major therapeutic approach to saving the foot continues to be patient education in the care of the foot. To accomplish this, a major effort is required from both physician, whether a generalist, internist, diabetologist, or podiatrist, and the patient. The physician must inspect the patient's feet at every visit. No examination of the diabetic patient is complete until the shoes and stockings have been removed and the feet carefully examined by either the physician or the nurse. It is important to inspect between the toes daily since interdigital ulceration is common in the diabetic. At the time of foot inspection, the physician must thoroughly and repeatedly educate the patient in the care of his feet. Included in Exhibit 32–8 are the major teaching points that I use.

Because poor vision, blindness, and obesity are so common in the diabetic, the patient may not be able to see the feet, and it may be necessary for another member of the family to make daily inspections of the feet and to cut the nails when necessary. Daily bathing of the feet is important. The patient must be instructed to dry the feet carefully, especially between the toes, avoiding residual wetness and subsequent maceration of the tissues. It must also be stressed repeatedly to the patient to test the temperature of the water before bathing. Because of poor circulation, the diabetic patient's feet often feel cold, and the patient resorts to the use of a hot water bottle or heating pad to warm them. However, this can result in disaster. Because the diabetics frequently have neuropathy, they may not be aware of extreme heat. Thermal burns from hot water bottles and heating pads are extremely common in the diabetic. The patient with cold feet should be instructed to wear warm socks at night.

Chemical agents such as keratolytic preparations are widely advertised for the treatment of corns and calluses, but the use of these agents can result in chemical burns. The patient must be warned against their indiscriminate use and should use only those medications prescribed by the physician or podiatrist.

It is imperative that the patient inspect inside the shoes for foreign objects before putting them on. It is common for the patient with the loss of sensory perception to be unaware of small pebbles, nails, or other foreign objects in the shoe and to walk on them for long periods of time, even days. The result is ulceration and frequently infection, gangrene, and amputation.

To avoid pressure Spots, the patient should avoid mended stockings or those with seams. Garters should not be worn because they prevent venous return and lead to the development of peripheral edema. Shoes must be properly fitted, and new shoes must be broken in gradually. Shoes made of leather are preferable to those made of plastic materials. Because of the extreme vulnerability of the diabetic foot, the patient should never walk barefoot. Nails should be cut straight across after soaking the feet in tepid water for approximately 5–10 min to soften the nails. Corns and calluses should be cared for only after explicit instructions from the physician or podiatrist. Because the skin of the diabetic foot, deprived of autonomic innervation, does not perspire and frequently is dry, the use of moistening creams such as aqueous lanolin, hand lotions, or even vegetable shortening decreases the tendency for cracks and fissures to occur. These creams should be applied in a very thin coating after bathing to seal in the moisture. It should be stressed that the skin

EXHIBIT 32–8   Patient Instructions for the Care of the Diabetic Foot

1. Inspect the feet daily for blisters, cuts and scratches, or reddened areas. The use of a mirror can aid in seeing the bottom of the feet. Always check between the toes. A family member can help with the inspection.
2. Wash feet daily. Dry carefully, especially between the toes.
3. Avoid extremes of temperatures. Test water with hand or elbow before bathing.
4. If feet feel cold at night, wear socks. Do not apply a hot water bottle, electric blanket, or heating pad.
5. Do not walk on hot surfaces such as sandy beaches or on the cement around swimming pools.
6. Do not walk barefoot.
7. Do not cut corns. Do not use chemical agents for the removal of corns and calluses. Do not use corn plasters. Do not use strong antiseptic solutions on your feet.
8. Do not use adhesive tape on the feet.
9. Inspect the inside of shoes daily for foreign objects, nail points, torn lining, and rough areas.
10. If your vision is impaired, have a family member inspect feet daily, trim nails, and buff down calluses.
11. Do not soak feet unless specifically instructed.
12. For dry skin, use a very thin coat of a lubricating oil or cream. Apply after bathing. Do not put the oil or cream between the toes. Consult your physician for type of lubricant and detailed instructions.
13. Wear properly fitting stockings. Do not wear mended stockings. Avoid stockings with seams. Change stockings daily. Do not wear garters.
14. Shoes should be comfortable at the time of purchase. Purchase shoes in the afternoon when feet tend to be the largest. Do not depend on them to stretch. Shoes should be made of leather. Running or walking shoes may be worn after checking with your physician.
15. Inform your shoe salesman that you are diabetic.
16. Do not wear shoes without stockings.
17. Do not wear sandals with thongs between the toes.
18. Ask about therapeutic shoes if you have a foot deformity, such as bunions or claw toes, or if you have had a previous foot ulcer.
19. In wintertime take special precautions. Wear wool socks and protective foot gear, such as fleece-lined boots.
20. Cut nails straight across or follow the curve of the nail.
21. Do not cut corns and calluses. Follow special instructions from your physicians or podiatrist. If the nails are thick or difficult to cut, have a family member, physician, or podiatrist do this.
22. See your physician regularly and be sure that your feet and between the toes are examined at each visit.
23. Do not smoke.
24. Notify your physician or podiatrist at once should you develop a blister or sore on your foot.
25. Be sure to inform your podiatrist that you are diabetic.

Adapted from Levin ME: The diabetic foot: Pathophysiology, evaluation, and treatment. In Levin ME, O'Neal LW, Bowker JH (eds.): The Diabetic Foot, Ed. 5. St. Louis, MO: Mosby Year Book, 1993.

should merely be moistened with a small amount of cream, and it should be rubbed well into the skin; a heavy or greasy coating of the skin should be avoided. These creams must not be placed between toes, since this can lead to maceration of the tissues, tissue breakdown, and infection. Calluses can be planed down daily with an emery board, pumice stone, or special file after patient instruction.

Figure 32–14 demonstrates a technique for trying shoes to avoid pressure on the dorsalis pedis artery.

At the time of the office visit, while the shoes and socks are off, the nurse and/or the physician should inspect the feet and review the "do's and don'ts" of foot care with the patient. A successful educational program on foot care cannot be accomplished by simply handing the patient a list of instructions. The instructions should be explained and questions encouraged so that the patient can attain a better understanding of the importance of foot care. These instructions should be carried out at least once a year, preferably more often. The effectiveness of an educational program in reducing amputation has been well documented.[61–63]

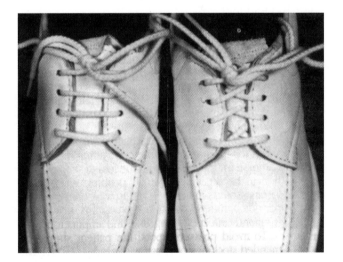

Figure 32–14.   Left: shoelaces tied in manner that avoids compression over dorsalis pedis artery; right: crisscross method of tying shoes that results in potential compression of dorsalis pedis artery. [*Source:* Levin ME: Medical evaluation and treatment. *In* Levin ME, O'Neal LW (eds): The Diabetic Foot, Ed 4. St. Louis: C.V. Mosby, 1988. Whit permission.]

Exercise for Diabetic Patients with Foot Problems

Exercise is an important modality in the management of diabetes. However, in patients with PAD, PN, previous ulceration, or deformed feet, weight-bearing exercises such as jogging, prolonged walking, and treadmill and step exercises may need to be curtailed or avoided. The presence of an active foot ulcer is an absolute contraindication for weight-bearing exercise. Even patients who have a healed ulcer must take special precautions when exercising. Patients with PN and an insensate foot can do a variety of non-weight-bearing exercises such as swimming, bicycling, rowing, and upper body exercises.[64]

Patients, particularly those with PAD, PN, and previously healed ulcerations, should have specific and detailed instructions in foot care and in techniques for decreasing foot pressure before undertaking an exercise program.

Patient Adherence

Patient adherence to foot care depends primarily on the patient's education regarding its importance. The responsibility for the patient's education in foot care falls primarily on the physician and his assistants. To achieve patient adherence, the feet must be examined at each visit to the physician's office, and foot-care instruction must be given at every visit, constantly reinforcing the importance of foot care, with explicit explanation of why these techniques should be carried out, along with emphatic instructions on what constitutes good and bad foot care.

Despite the most detailed and repeated instructions, many patients will not adhere to good foot care. For instance, it is very difficult to convince some women to forego wearing high-heeled shoes despite their lament that "these shoes are killing me," which in fact may be more truth than fiction. As noted earlier, many patients have an irresistible urge to do "home surgery." For many patients, "going barefoot feels too good to give up," or they are just simply not motivated enough to put on their shoes for their own protection.

Cessation of smoking is almost impossible for many patients, even after having had a leg amputated for vascular insufficiency resulting in gangrene. It is not a rare experience for a physician to visit his patient postamputation and find him lying in bed smoking. When the danger and risk to the remaining limb is explained for the hundredth time, the response is usually, "You're right, Doc. I know smoking can cause the loss of the other leg. I am going to quit smoking—some day."

For all the above reasons, and despite the constant efforts of health care professionals, patient adherence is difficult to accomplish. The problem is compounded even further by the fact that many patients do not keep their appointments. Without patient cooperation, adherence cannot be achieved, but with continued effort on the part of the physician and assistants, patient adherence to good foot care can be improved.

Audits

The institution of diabetes foot centers and intensified programs on foot care and patient education has resulted in a significant decrease in amputation rate by a variety of authors. Davidson and colleagues from Grady Memorial Hospital have demonstrated that an intensified program in foot care reduced amputation rate by 50% (see Chapter 33).[61] Edmonds[58] also decreased the amputation rate by 50%, and Assal et al.[62] have reported a decrease of 83% in their amputation rate. Although figures may vary, I think it is now well established that the institution of aggressive diabetes foot care programs can reduce the amputation rate by 50%.

Conclusions

As was noted at the beginning of this chapter, the problems of the diabetic foot are increasing. The diabetic population is increasing and aging; over 50,000 major amputations are performed on diabetic patients every year in the United States.

The ultimate goal is, of course, the cure of diabetes, but until that has been accomplished, we will have to deal with angiopathy, neuropathy, foot ulcers, infection, gangrene, and amputation. To date, there is no single factor or combination of factors that will prevent vascular disease or neuropathy. More precise control of the blood sugar, while helpful, is not the complete answer. Understanding the pathophysiology of how these lesions occur makes it possible through a variety of prophylactic and therapeutic means to interrupt the various pathways leading to diabetic foot problems. Teamwork by the specialists involved in the care of the diabetic is critically important in saving the diabetic foot. However, the foremost modality in saving the foot is through repeated patient education. The importance of this cannot be emphasized too strongly.

References

1. Reiber GE, Boyko EJ, Smith DG: Lower extremity foot ulcers and amputation in individuals with diabetes. In Harris MI, Cowie CC, Stern MP, et al. (eds.): Diabetes in America, Ed. 2 (DHHS Pub. no. 95-1468). Washington, DC: U.S. Government Printing Office, 1995, pp. 408–428.

2. Sathe SR: Managing the diabetic foot in developing countries. IDF Bull 38:16–18, 1993.

3. Waugh NR: Amputations in diabetic patients: a review of rates, relative risks, and resource use. Comm Med 10:279–288, 1988.

4. Mac Leod AF, Williams DRR, Sonken PH, Boulton AJM: Risk factors for foot ulceration in hospital clinic attenders (Abstract). Diabetologia 34(Suppl. 2):A39, 1991.

5. Centers for Disease Control and Prevention: Diabetes Surveillance. Atlanta, GA: U.S. Department of Health and Human Services, Public Health Service, 1993.

6. Eckman MH, Greenfield S, Mackey WC, et al.: Foot infections in diabetic patients: Decision and cost-effective analyses. JAMA 273:712–720, 1995.

7. Centers for Disease Control and Prevention: Diabetes Surveillance. Atlanta, GA: U.S. Department of Health and Human Services, Public Health Service, 1991.

8. Reiber GE: Epidemiology of the diabetic foot. In Levin ME, O'Neal LW, Bowker JH (eds.): The Diabetic Foot, Ed. 5. St. Louis, MO: Mosby, 1993, pp. 1–15.

9. Reiber RE, Pecoraro RE, Koepsell TD: Risk factors for amputation in patients with diabetes mellitus: a case-control study. Ann Int Med 117(2):97–105, 1992.

10. Selby JV, Zhang D: Risk factors for lower extremity amputation in persons with diabetes Diab Care 18(4):509–516, 1995.

11. McNeely MJ, Boyko EJ, Ahroni JH, et al.: The independent contributions of diabetic neuropathy and vasculopathy in foot ulceration: How great are the risks? Diabetes Care 18(2):216–219, 1995.

12. Lavery LA, Lavery DC, Quebedeax-Farnham TL: Increased foot pressures after great toe amputation in diabetes Diabetes Care 18:1460–1462, 1995.

13. Caputo GM, Cavanagh PR, Ulbrecht JS, et al.: Current concepts: Assessment and management of foot disease in patients with diabetes New Engl J Med 331:854–860, 1994.

14. Fernando DJS, Masson EA, Vevas A, Boulton AJM: Relationship of limited joint mobility to abnormal foot pressures and foot ulceration Diabetes Care 14:8–11, 1991.

15. Gavin L: A comprehensive approach to sidestep diabetic foot problems Endocrinologist 3:191–203, 1993.

16. Janka HU, Standl E, Mehnert H: Peripheral vascular disease in diabetes mellitus and its relation to cardiovascular risk factors: Screening with the Doppler ultrasonic technique. Diabetes Care 3:207–213, 1980.

17. Levin ME, Sicard GA: Evaluating and treating diabetic peripheral vascular disease, part I. Clin Diabetes 5:62–70, 1987.

18. LoGerfo F, Coffman JD: Vascular and microvascular disease of the foot in diabetes New Engl J Med 211:1615–1619, 1984.

19. O'Keefe ST, Woods BB, Reslin DJ: Blue toe syndrome: Causes and management. Arch Intern Med 152:2197–2202, 1992.

20. Peace WH, Wiet SP: Noninvasive evaluation of atherosclerotic emboli. In Yao JST, Pearce WH (eds.): The Ischemic Extremity: Advances in Treatment. East Norwalk, CT: Appleton & Lange, 1995, pp. 303–311.

21. Queen M, Biem HJ, Moe GW, Sugar L: Development of cholesterol embolization syndrome after intravenous streptokinase for acute myocardial infarction. Am J Cardiol 6:1042–1043, 1990.

22. Shapiro LS: Cholesterol embolization after treatment with tissue plasminogen activators (Letter). New Engl J Med 321:1270, 1989.

23. Fisher DF Jr, Clagett GP, Brigham RA: Dilemmas in dealing with the blue toe syndrome: Aortic versus peripheral source. Am J Surg 148:836–839, 1984.

24. Colwell JA, Lopes-Virella MF, Winocour PD, Halushka PV: New concepts about the pathogenesis of atherosclerosis in diabetes mellitus. In Levin ME, O'Neal LW (eds.): The Diabetic Foot, Ed 4. St. Louis, MO: Mosby, 1988, pp. 51–70.

25. McGill JB, Schneider DJ, Arfken CL, Lucore CL, Sobel BE: Factors responsible for impaired fibrinolysis in obese subjects and NIDDM patients. Diabetes 43:104–109, 1994.

26. Sargent WQ: Hemorheology. In Levin ME, O'Neal LW (eds.): The Diabetic Foot, Ed 4. St. Louis, MO: Mosby, 1988, pp. 71–75.

27. Fairbairn JF II, Juergens JL: The principles of medical treatment. In Juergens JL, et al. (eds.): Peripheral Vascular Disease. Philadelphia: W.B. Saunders, 1980, pp. 855–878.

28. Kaufman DW, Helmrich SP, Rosenberg L: Nicotine and carbon monoxide content of cigarette smoke and the risk of myocardial infarction in young men. New Engl J Med 308:409–413, 1983.

29. Nelson RG, Gohdes DM, Everhart JE, et al.: Lower extremity amputations in NIDDM: 12-yr follow-up study in Pima Indians. Diabetes Care 11:8–16, 1988.

30. Beach KW, Strandness DE Jr: Arteriosclerosis obliterans and associated risk factors in insulin dependent diabetics. Diabetes 28:882–888, 1980.

31. Capron L, Jarnet J, Kazandjian S, Housset E: Growth promoting effects of diabetes and insulin on arteries: an in vivo study of rat aorta. Diabetes 35:973–978, 1986.

32. Sato Y, Shiraishi S, Oshida Y, et al.: Experimental atherosclerosis-like lesions induced by hyperinsulinism in Wistar rats. Diabetes 38:91–96, 1989.

33. Colwell JA, Bingham SF, Abraira C, et al., and the Cooperative Study Group: Veterans Administration Cooperative Study on antiplatelet agents in diabetic patients after amputation for gangrene: II. Effects of aspirin and dipyridamole on atherosclerotic vascular disease rates. Diabetes Care 9:140, 1986.

34. Gardner AW, Poehlman ET: Exercise rehabilitation programs for the treatment of claudication pain: a meta-analysis. JAMA 274:975–980, 1995.

35. Malan E, Tattoni G: Physioanatomopathology of acute ischemia of the extremities. J Cardiovas Surg 4:212–225, 1963.

36. Boulton AJM, Hardisty CA, Betts RP, et al.: Dynamic foot pressure and other studies as diagnostic and management aids in diabetic neuropathy. Diabetes Care 6:26–33, 1983.

37. Young MJ, Marshall A, Adams JE, et al.: Osteopenia, neurological dysfunction, and the development of Charcot neuroarthropathy. Diabetes Care 18:34–38, 1995.

38. Edmonds ME, Clarke MB, Newton S, et al.: Increased uptake of bone radiopharmaceutical in diabetic neuropathy. Quart J Med 57:843–855, 1985.

39. Cavanagh PR, Derr JA, Ulbrecht JS, et al.: Problems with gait and posture in neuropathic patients with insulin dependent diabetes mellitus. Diabetic Med 9:469–474, 1992.

40. Uccioli L, Giacomini PG, Monticone G, et al.: Body sway in diabetic neuropathy. Diabetes Care 18:339–344, 1995.

41. Sindrup SH, Gram LF, Brosen K, et al.: The selective serotonin reuptake inhibitor paroxetine is effective in the treatment of diabetic neuropathy symptoms. Pain 42:135–144, 1990.

42. Capsaicin Study Group: Treatment of painful diabetic neuropathy with topical capsaicin: a multicenter, double-blind, vehicle-controlled study. Arch Intern Med 151:2225–2229, 1991.

43. The Diabetes Control and Complications Trial Research Group. The effect of intensive treatment of diabetes on the development and progression of long-term complications in insulin-dependent diabetes mellitus. New Engl J Med 329:977–986, 1993.

44. Levin ME: Preventing amputation in the patient with diabetes. Diabetes Care 18:1383–1394, 1995.

45. Newman LG, Waller J, Palestro CJ: Unsuspected osteomyelitis in diabetic foot ulcers. JAMA 266:1246–1251, 1991.

46. Grayson ML, Gibbons GW, Balogh K, et al.: Probing to bone in infected pedal ulcers: a clinical sign of underlying osteomyelitis in diabetic patients. JAMA 273:721–728, 1995.

47. Durham JR: The role of magnetic resonance imaging in the management of foot abscess in the diabetic patient. In Yao JST, Pearce WH (eds.): The Ischemic Extremity: Advances in Treatment. Norwalk, CT: Appleton & Lange, 1995, pp. 257–268.

48. Levin ME, Spratt IL: To soak or not to soak. Clin Diabetes 4:44–45, 1986.

49. Sinacore DR, Mueller MJ: Total-contact casting in the treatment of neuropathic ulcers. In Levin ME, O'Neal LW, Bowker JH (eds.): The Diabetic Foot, Ed. 5. St. Louis, MO: Mosby, 1993, pp. 283–304.

50. Fletcher F, Ain M, Jacobs, R: Healing of foot ulcers in immunosuppressed renal transplant patients. Clin Orthop Relat Res 296:37–42, 1993.

51. LoGerfo FW, Gibbons GW, Pomposelli FB Jr: Trends in the care of the diabetic foot: Expanded role of arterial reconstruction. Arch Surg 127:617–621, 1992.

52. Leather RP, Chang BB, Darling RC III, Shah DM: Not all in situ bypasses are created equal. In Yao JST, Pearce WH (eds.): The Ischemic Extremity: Advances in Treatment. Norwalk, CT: Appleton & Lange, 1995, pp. 391–403.

53. Cronenwett JL, Colen LB: Ischemic limb salvage by revascularization and free tissue transfer. In Yao JST, Pearce WH (eds.): The Ischemic Extremity: Advances in Treatment. Norwalk, CT: Appleton & Lange, 1995, pp. 405–418.

54. Alvarez OM, Gilson G, Auletta MJ: Local aspects of diabetic foot ulcer care: Assessment, dressings, and topical agents. In Levin ME, O'Neal LW, Bowker JH (eds.): The Diabetic Foot, Ed. 5. St. Louis, MO: Mosby, 1993, pp. 259–281.

55. Rodeheaver G, Baharestani MM, Brabec ME, et al.: Wound healing and wound management: Focus on debridement: an interdisciplinary round table, September 18, 1992, Jackson Hole, WY. Adv Wound Care 7:22–36, 1994.

56. Rodeheaver G: Controversies in topical wound management. Ostomy/Wound Manage 20:58–65, 1988.

57. Steed DL, The Diabetic Ulcer Study Group: Clinical evaluation of recombinant human platelet-derived growth factor for the treatment of lower extremity diabetic ulcers. J Vasc Surg 21:71–81, 1995.

58. Edmonds ME, Blundell MP, Morris ME, et al.: Improved survival of the diabetic foot the role of a specialized foot clinic. Quart J Med 60:763–771, 1986.

59. Cohen SJ: Potential barriers to diabetes care. Diabetes Care 6:499–500, 1983.

60. Bailey TS, Yu HM, Rayfield EJ: Pattern of foot examination in a diabetic clinic. Am J Med 78:371–374, 1985.

61. Davidson JK, Alogna M, Goldsmith M, et al.: Assessment of program effectiveness at Grady Memorial Hospital, Atlanta, Georgia. In Steiner G, Lawrence PA (eds.): Educating Diabetic Patients. New York: Springer-Verlag, 1981, p. 329.

62. Assal JP, Muhlhauser I, Pernat A, et al.: Patient education as the basis for diabetes care in clinical practice. Diabetologia 28:602–613, 1985.

63. Litzelman DK, Slemenda CW, Langefeld CD, et al.: Reduction of lower extremity clinical abnormalities in patients with non-insulin-dependent diabetes mellitus. Ann Intern Med 119:36–41, 1993.

64. Levin ME: Exercise in diabetic patients with foot complications. In Handbook of Diabetes and Exercise. Alexandria, VA: American Diabetes Association, 1995, pp. 135–142.

33

Conservative Therapy of Foot Abnormalities, Infections, and Vascular Insufficiency

Edwin Hobgood

Historical Perspective

In the 14th century a guild of barber-surgeons existed in northern Europe. Their work consisted of blood-letting, pulling teeth, cutting corns, trimming nails and hair, applying leeches and cups, and compounding ointments and other preparations for the sake of beauty or relief of pain. These individuals were the forerunners of present-day chiropodists and podiatrists.

In 1774 a Dr. Low of London wrote a treatise dealing with the "cause of corns, warts, bunions, and other painful and offensive cutaneous excrescences," in which the term "chiropodologia" (from the Greek meaning study of the hand and foot) first appeared.[1] Chiropody developed into a general term for foot care of the above-mentioned sort. Later the name was changed to podiatry (from the Greek words for foot and healing), particularly in the United States. The name was changed for a number of reasons including the fact that the care involved was generally confined to the foot or lower extremities, and there was a desire to avoid confusion with chiropractic. Podiatry evolved in part in the United States due to the need for performance of certain limited types of medical care of the feet and lower extremities, services that physicians were unable or unwilling to perform. Podiatrists today, however, emphasize that they are trained and capable of doing all forms of foot care and not just the treatment of corns, calluses, and the like.[2,3]

Chronic diseases, one of which is diabetes, are now responsible for many serious health problems. The podiatrist has long been recognized as an important member of the medical team in the management of complications of diabetes affecting the feet. Among the first podiatrists to serve on a clinical, hospital, or group practice staff was Dr. Paul L. Tarara, a 1917 graduate of the New York College of Podiatric Medicine, who moved to Rochester, Minnesota, to establish his practice. Among his patients were the Mayo brothers—Charles and William—who invited Dr. Tarara to join their staff at the Mayo Clinic in 1926.[4] In 1928 Dr. Elliott P. Joslin appointed Dr. John F. Kelly to supervise a foot-care clinic for diabetics, and Dr. Kelly became a pioneer of hospital podiatry when he was named to the staff of the New England Deaconess Hospital and the Massachusetts General Hospital. He provided care for patients in both institutions until his retirement in 1964.[5]

Epidemiology

With the increasing incidence of diabetes in an aging population, there is a parallel increase in the incidence of complications of diabetes. Of these, foot problems are among the most common and disabling, and they often lead to gangrene and amputation.

In a retrospective cohort study from 1 Jan. 1993 through 31 Dec. 1994 in Tayside, Scotland, patients with diabetes had a 12.3 risk of an amputation compared with non-diabetic residents.[6]

It is important to recognize that there is no standardized routine for the care of the diabetic foot. It must be treated conscientiously, tenderly, and continuously on the basis of *individual need*.

At Atlanta's Grady Memorial Hospital, for example, beginning in 1973, a program of comprehensive foot care involving a podiatrist and other health care professionals resulted in a reduction from 13.3 lower extremity amputations per 1000 patients with diabetes in 1973 to 5.8 amputations per 1000 patients in 1986, a decrease of more than 50%. Over a 13-year period (1974-1986) an estimated 996 amputations were avoided, resulting in an estimated avoidance of 15.936 million dollars). Average mean cost of hospitalization, rehabilitation, etc. was $16,000 per amputation).

In the last decade, many observers have confirmed that fact that risk factors for lower extremity amputation in diabetic persons can be identified,[7] and that amputations can be avoided in many individuals.[8]

When amputation is performed for gangrene, the other leg will begin to have problems within 18 to 36 months in 50% of patients[9] (see Chapter 30). Prevention and prophylactic measures are thus doubly important for the second foot. If amputation can be avoided, many patients can remain at least partially self-sufficient until the consequences of coronary artery or other vascular disease develop, thereby avoiding the great cost of hospitalization, surgery, prosthesis fitting, rehabilitation, and dependence on the family or society for the duration of the amputee's life (see Exhibit 33–1).

A minor problem in the nondiabetic patient can be a major problem in a patient with diabetes who has lower-extremity neuropathy and/or arteriopathy. Tberefore, early detection, preventive foot care, proper education, and appropriate continuous therapy are required to prevent the development and progression of foot lesions.[10,11]

Pathophysiology

See Chapters 30, 31, and 32.

Problem Statement

Lower-extremity problems may present in one or more ways, as noted in Exhibit 33–2.

Subjective

In the individual patient, the initial subjective findings presented in Exhibit 33–2 may consist of single or multiple components from items I, II, III, or IV. Pain is frequently minimal or absent in patients with advanced neuropathic ulcers, even in patients with extensive cellulitis and tissue necrosis.[13] When neuropathic pain is present, it can be extraordinarily severe. It should be distinguished from ischemic pain as to location, nature, duration, severity, and relation to exercise. Neuropathic pain is often more severe at night. Getting out of bed and walking sometimes provides relief. In peripheral vascular disease with ischemia, pain is increased by walking. The importance of ischemic rest pain, since it is a symptom of impending gangrene, should be noted.

Objective

Dermatologic, musculoskeletal, neurologic, and circulatory examinations should be done as outlined in Exhibit 33–3.

EXHIBIT 33–1   Lower-Extremity Amputations in Patients with Diabetes Mellitus at Grady Memorial Hospital 1973–1986[a]

Year	No. Amputations	No. Patients	NO. Amputations Per 1000 Patients	No. Patients With Amputations Per 1000 Patients[b]	P[b]	Estimated No. Amputations Prevented[c]
Pre-1973	Est. 150–200/yr					
1973	172		13.3			
1974	108		8.3		<0.01	64
1975	88		6.8		<0.01	84
1976	88		6.8		<0.01	84
1977	100		7.7		<0.01	72
1978	86	68	6.6	5.3	<0.01	86
1979	92		7.1		<0.01	80
1980	87		6.7		<0.01	85
1981	100		7.7		<0.01	72
1982	117	98	6.6	5.5	<0.01	75
1983	120	98	6.8	5.5	<0.01	71
1984	110	84	6.2	4.7	<0.01	85
1985	141	104	7.9	5.9	<0.01	42
1986	103	83	5.8	4.7	<0.01	96
						996

[a] Estimated number of patients with diabetes served by Grady Memorial Hospital increased from 12,950 (1973–1980) to 17,750 (1982–1986). Calculations were based on a denominator of 12,950 for the years 1973–1981, and a denominator of 17,750 for the years 1982–1986.

[b] Probability that 1973 amputation number was significantly higher than number in subsequent year of comparison. The mean decrease in incidence of amputations over the 13-year period was 40%.

[c] Estimated number of amputations avoided from 1974–1986 (13 years) is 996. At an estimated cost of $16,000 each, this represents a cost avoidance from prevented amputations of 15.936 million dollars. See Davidson[10,11] and Bild et al.[12]

EXHIBIT 33–2   Lower-Extremity Problems in Diabetes Mellitus

I. Neuropathy[10]
  A. Diminished sensation (makes lower extremities much more susceptible to trauma)
  B. Neuropathic ulcers
  C. Mechanical abnormalities (hallux valgus, hammer toe, arthropathy) may result in neuropathic joints
II. Diminished blood supply[10]
  A. Large blood vessels (macroangiopathy or arteriopathy)
  B. Small blood vessels (microangiopathy)
  C. Both
III. Infection[10]
  A. Fungal

  1. Hypertrophic mycotic toenails
  2. Tinea pedis (athlete's foot)
  B. Bacterial
  1. In skin disruptions
    (a) Secondary to fungus infection
    (b) Under corns or callosities
    (c) Around bone or joint deformities
    (d) Trauma
IV. Decreased host resistance
  A. Uncontrolled diabetes
  B. Local ischemia
  C. Other, including renal failure and hematologic disorders (See Chapters 25 and 27.)

EXHIBIT 33–3   Objective Findings That May Be Noted in Lower Extremities of Patients with Diabetes Mellitus

I. Dermatologic[14,15,16]
The skin and nails should be examined by noticing hair changes, nail changes, scars, sweating, color change, dermatoses, temperature, nevi, infections, tumors, dermatitis factitia (due to pruritus), diabetic dermopathy, necrobiosis lipoidica diabeticorum, corns, calluses, and ulcers. The patient with advanced vascular disease will frequently have skin that is dry, tight, and shiny in appearance.

II. Musculoskeletal
The bones, joints, and muscles should be examined for presence of pain, edema, heat, rubor, stiffness, or deformity. Bunions, hammer toes, prominent metatarsals, and other mechanical abnormalities causing excessive pressure on, or excessive weight-bearing by, any part of the foot can produce calluses and/or neuropathic ulcers. Abnormal pressure on the weight-bearing surface of the foot may be assessed by using a Harris footprint mat or thermister readings (see Chapters 30, 31, and 32).

III. Neurologic
All components of the nervous system should be evaluated including sensory, including use of 10-g (5.07) SEMMES-WEINSTEIN MONOFILIMENT for sensory examination of a professional and at home by the patient,[15,16] motor, tendon reflexes, and pilomotor (or sweating). Special attention should be given to the sensory system and the patient's ability to perceive vibration, position, touch, temperature, and pain sensation.

IV. Circulatory system
The arterial pulses (dorsalis pedis, posterior tibial, popliteal, and femoral) should be palpated and correlated with the presence of claudication, rest pain, ulceration, and/or gangrene. The skin temperature, color, texture, hair, and nail status are also checked. The venous filling time is also noted (ordinarily veins fill within 15 s when a foot is placed in a dependent position after elevation). Venous filling may occur in those with ischemia plus venous insufficiency in less than 15 s. In patients with diabetes the concurrent presence of pedal pulses and tissue necrosis is common, indicating microvascular angiopathy.
A. Signs of circulatory impairment may be:
  1. Mild: decreased or absent pulse(s)
  2. Moderate: nutritional changes, e.g., loss of subcutaneous tissue, shiny skin, tapering of toes, decreased hair, and changes in the nails
  3. Severe: marked decrease in temperature, increased capillary and venous filling time (>15 s). Rubor, in the dependent position, blanching on slight elevation, tissue breakdown (i.e., ulcers and/or gangrene)
  4. Laboratory evaluation of lower-extremity circulation includes noninvasive (Doppler ultrasonography, plethysmography) and invasive (angiography) tests. See Chapters 30, 31, and 32.
B. The venous and lymphatic systems should be evaluated for competency.

Assessment

All abnormalities listed in Exhibits 33–2 and 33–3 should be noted and assessed to determine the nature and extent of the patient's foot problems.

Initial Plans

Since most adult patients with diabetes develop minor foot lesions requiring occasional attention, the initial plan should encompass preventive education and prophylactic treatment for all. Also, on each visit to the health care provider, the patient's plasma glucose and body weight should be measured and diet and/or insulin therapy revised as needed to maintain the best attainable metabolic control. In some patients, initial plans may need modification to deal promptly with the consequences of trauma, infection, inadequate circulation, and peripheral neuropathy, as shown in Exhibit 33–4.

EXHIBIT 33–4 Initial Plans for Patients with Trauma, Infection, Inadequate Circulation, and Peripheral Neuropathy

I. Decrease local trauma
  A. Bed rest
  B. Redistribute weight bearing (i.e., corrective shoes and/or removable appliances consisting of compressible materials of rubber, cork, urethane foam, Spenco, or Plastazote)[11,12]
  C. Correction of biomechanical and/or orthopedic deformities if indicated
II. Control of infection
  A. After bacterial culture and antibiotic sensitivity studies, appropriate systemic antibiotic therapy (see Chapter 45)
  B. Roentgenographic evaluation to distinguish between bone destruction from infection and bone destruction and/or dissolution from neuropathic changes
  C. Local debridement
III. Improve circulation
  A. Indications for referral of patients to vascular surgeon for evaluation.
    1. History of claudication
    2. Sudden change in temperature, motor, or sensory function associated with sudden onset of pain (acute occlusion of major artery)
    3. Absent pedal pulses
    4. Decreased femoral pulse
    5. Signs and symptoms of severe ischemia
    6. Unilateral edema or swelling
    7. Extensive osteomyelitis with ulcer or gangrene and systemic infection
  B. Position of the limb: avoid elevation if there are signs and symptoms of severe ischemia.
  C. In presence of edema and infection, the foot should be kept on level with the heart, since the dependent position aggravates the edema and infection.
  D. Angiography if indicated
  E. Endarterectomy if indicated
  F. Bypass grafting if indicated
IV. Role of surgery (see Chapter 34)
  A. Drainage of localized abscesses
  B. Local debridement of necrotic tissue which may result in amputation of one or more toes
  C. Vascular reconstruction is indicated in patients with ischemia and a localized obstruction in a major artery demonstrated by angiography. Depending on the site of the occlusion, a femoropopliteal or an aortofemoral bypass operation is performed. Only a small proportion of diabetic patients require vascular reconstruction. The outcome of these procedures is much more favorable if they are done prior to the onset of gangrene.
  D. Major amputation—below knee (BK) or above knee (AK)—for extensive gangrene involving the dorsum of the foot or severe ischemia in absence of a correctable vascular lesion.

Patient Education[34]

Foot Hygiene When initially evaluated, patients should be instructed in proper foot hygiene. This includes careful cleaning between the toes and proper trimming of nails by patients (who are able to do so) or by a relative or friend. The patient should be instructed to wash the feet daily with a mild soap and warm–*never hot*–water, washing gently between the toes and being careful not to break the skin. Feet should be thoroughly dried by patting with a soft towel, paying special attention to the area between the toes. Nails should be cleaned with absorbent cotton wrapped around an orangewood stick. Nails should be cut straight across, never shorter than the tops of the toes, and smoothed by filing away from the toes. Razor blades or knives are prohibited for nail trimming. Only sharp, properly shaped scissors and safe abrasive wheels should be used.

Patients are advised to avoid extremes of temperature—especially hot bath water. The temperature of water may vary between 80° and 100°F. The patient should *never* apply hot water bottles, heating pads, electric heaters, or any other form of mechanical heating device that might burn the skin. To warm the feet, the patient should wrap them with a blanket or towel already slightly warmed (not over 100°F) before going to bed.

Patients should be taught proper skin care, including proper bathing and foot lubrication. If the feet are dry or scaly, they should be rubbed lightly with a skin emollient or moisture-restoring cream or lotion once a day until they are soft, taking care not to put cream between the toes which might result in maceration. If the feet perspire and are moist, or if toes are cramped, a small amount of foot powder should be used and small pieces of lamb's wool should be placed between the toes.

Patients should be encouraged to examine their feet daily. They should check for bruises, swelling, discoloration, corns, calluses, cuts, puncture wounds, local tenderness, and excessive dryness that may lead to fissures. Fissure and callus formation on the heel is one of the most common problems. Fissured calluses may be infected with fungus. Callus formation on the weight-bearing plantar surface of the foot is a sign of excessive pressure over bony prominences due to excessive weight-bearing by the affected part (or parts) of the foot. Proper shoes (which distribute evenly the weight borne by the plantar aspect of the feet) should be used. The use of improperly fitting shoes such as bedroom slippers or open-heeled shoes causes excessive dryness of the skin and fissures may develop. Calluses with fissures should be treated by gently filing with a pumice stone or emery cloth followed by use of a moisture-restoring agent.

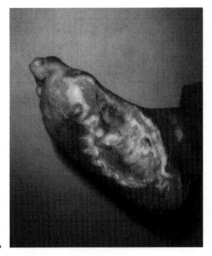
A

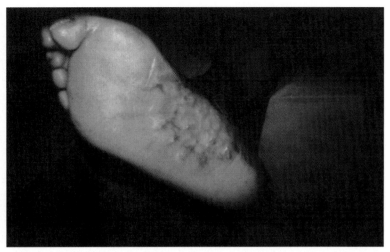
B

Figure 33–1 A. Fifty-eight-year-old woman with infected neuropathic ulceration of right foot after walking a long distance in improper shoes. Due to diminished pedal pulses (arteriopathy), patient had been advised to have below-the-knee amputation. B. Six months later, lesions shown in A completely healed by conservative therapy using antibiotics, control of diabetes, and suitable extradepth protective shoes with soft-density Plastazote appliance.

Creams and ointments are principally mixtures (emulsions) of greases and water or inert oils. The relative amounts of grease and water determine the type of emulsion. Oil in water (O/W) is one in which oil droplets (discontinuous phase) are suspended in water (continuous phase), and a water in oil (W/O) emulsion is one in which the water droplets are suspended in oil. The addition of emulsifiers (Tween 80, tyloxapol) and the use of high-speed blenders create highly satisfactory "tailored" products. The inert oils are principally Carbowax (polyethylene glycol bases), lanolin, and mineral oil. Long ago materials such as goose grease, lard, mutton fat, and so forth were used. Modern technology has made available a number of variations of emulsifiers and W/O or O/W mixtures. It is important to remember that heavy creams and ointments should never be used on oozing or infected areas where drainage is needed, and that oils and greases may produce folliculitis if used in heavily hirsute areas.

Lukewarm soapy water will usually soften the skin of the feet so that corns and callosities can be removed or reduced in thickness with an emery cloth or pumice stone. Application of the emollient after bathing holds the moisture in the dry skin. If the skin of the feet is extremely dry and thickened with callosities, application of a skin emollient to the feet and covering the feet with a plastic covering successively each night when retiring will retain the moisture in the skin and cause the callosities to peel off, eventually leaving the skin soft and smooth. The procedure is contraindicated if there is a problem with excessive perspiration (hyperhidrosis), or with tinea pedis or other fungus infections of the skin of the feet.

Patients should be warned not to use chemical agents that destroy tissue such as salicylic acid, carbolic acid (phenol), add iodine. Certain antiperspirants should not be used because they irritate the skin and cause tissue damage or chafing. All corn and callus remedies are taboo for patients who have neuropathy and/or arteriopathy. Once there is a loss of tissue or a skin break, infection easily results. The patient should check with his physician before using any over-the-counter material on his feet.

Patients should be warned not to apply adhesive tape to the skin of the toes, feet or legs, since the hazards to the patient with neuropathy and/or impaired circulation of tearing the skin while removing the tape are considerable. Tape should be used only over gauze. Even micropore paper tape can tear the skin when removed improperly. If it is necessary to remove any adhesive material from the skin, the area should be soaked in lukewarm water and the adhesive material gently removed without tearing the skin.

Patients should be warned not to cut corns, calluses, ingrown toenails, or other foot lesions ("bathroom surgery"), never to walk barefoot (because those with diabetes often have loss of sensation in the feet and may not feel a cut or blister), and to avoid temperature extremes (both cold and hot).

Proper Shoes Patients should be advised to wear foot gear that is comfortable, well-fitted, and that has firm counters to protect the heels. Shoes that have been worn by others should not be used. When standing or working long hours, shoes that distribute weight equally over the plantar aspect of the feet should be worn rather than bedroom slippers or loafers. Arch supports should be fitted by professionals (pedorthists or others), making sure that rough areas do not press against the soles of the feet. New shoes should be fitted

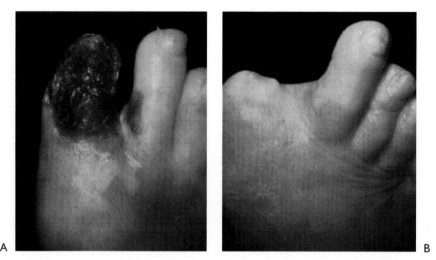

Figure 33–2 A. Seventy-one-year-old woman with absent pedal pulses and ischemic changes of foot developed dry gangrene following removal of loosened great toe nail. Patient had been advised to have below-the-knee amputation. B. Four months later, complete healing after spontaneous amputation of toe. Patient required to keep foot dry and to exercise foot intermittently by rolling soft drink bottle gently under bottom of foot.

in the afternoon to compensate for swelling of feet that may occur after standing. New shoes should be broken in slowly by wearing them initially for 1 hr/day. For men a plain oxford, blucher style, with steel shank and rubber heel is recommended. Men's shoes constructed of stiff cordovan, of very stiff calf leather, and of vinyl are nonporous, cause moisture and heat to accumulate, and should not be used. Shoes made of polyurethane have some "breathability," but are not ideal.

Leather has natural pores that enable moisture and heat to escape and air to enter, and it conforms to the shape of the foot. Leather soles are highly resistant to punctures. Leathers differ in quality, depending on the age and condition of the hide. Top grain leather from cowhide or calfskin is sturdy and scuff-resistant.

Kidskin is lighter, softer and more pliable than calf and is more easily scuffed. The flesh side of calf or kidskin is suede, which has a fine nap. Patent leather has a varnishlike coat; if it is of good quality, the grain of the leather is visible.

Leather conforms to the curves and protuberances of the feet, but synthetic materials tend to snap back to their original shape when the shoe is removed.

Soft calf, vice kid, or kangaroo leather are preferred for the upper surface of men's shoes in order to prevent pressure on the dorsum of the foot and toes. A bluchertype oxford of soft leather, fabric, garbardine, or suede should be recommended for women. Wearing of tight-fitting straps, high heels, open-toe or open-heel shoes, and oxfords without tongues should be discouraged. When shoes are fitted, the patient should stand on a

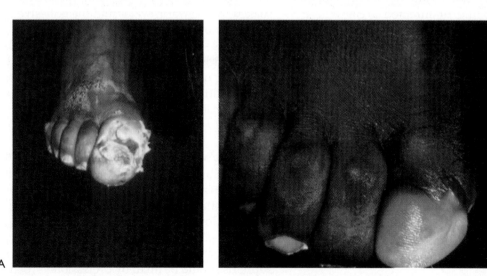

Figure 33–3 A. Seventy-two-year-old man with osteomyelitis of right great toe following infected ingrowing great toe nail. B. Three months later, complete healing resulted from appropriate debridement, antibiotics, control of diabetes, and wearing of extradepth shoes with soft-density Plastazote appliance.

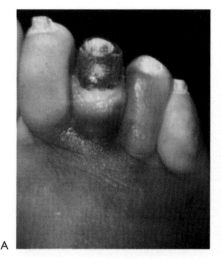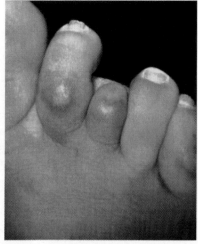

A   B

Figure 33–4   A. Sixty-two-year-old woman developed gangrene of middle toe of right foot after stubbing her toe. Due to diminished pedal pulses, patient had been advised to have transmetatarsal amputation. B. Five months later, complete healing followed spontaneous amputation and local therapy using daily applications of diluted povidoneiodine solution plus optimal control of diabetes.

piece of paper and draw an outline of the bare foot. The foot outline should not be visible when the shoe is placed on top of the outline.

Protective sensation of the foot has been lost if the patient cannot consistently feel the touch of a 10-g (5.07) SEMMES-WEINSTEIN MONOFILIMENT. All patients with loss of protective sensation should at least wear and athletic shoe or a shoe of similar design. Medicare and Medicaid have been mandated to provide one pair of extra-depth shoes and three pairs of inserts or one pair of custom-molded shoes plus two additional pairs of inserts each year for patients with high-risk feet.[15] By preventing a significant number of avoidable amputations, these protective shoes will almost certainly save lives, limbs, suffering, and money.

Patients should be taught to avoid constriction of the lower extremities by not sitting with legs crossed or hanging over the sharp edge of a table or chair, and by not wearing circular garters or tight socks. Panty hose may suffice. Where indicated, support stockings may be prescribed by the physician or podiatrist.

Patients should be admonished not to use tobacco in any form because it aggravates vascular insufficiency.

Patients with inadequate lower-extremity blood flow (i.e., intermittent claudication) should be instructed in a program of regular foot and leg exercises to promote development of collateral circulation. Three daily walks of about 30 min (covering about 1.5 miles each) are recommended with the patient stopping to rest should intermittent claudication occur.

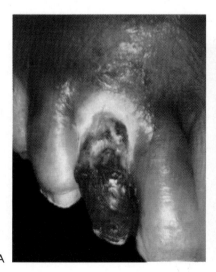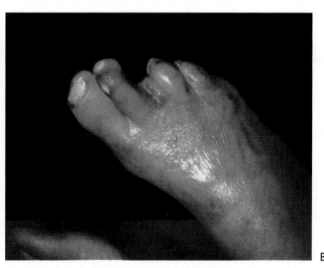

A   B

Figure 33–5   A. Fifty-seven-year-old man with severe neuropathy and arteriopathy developed gangrene of right middle toe after stepping on a nail. Due to diminished pedal pulses, patient had been advised to have below-the-knee amputation. B. Three months later, complete healing followed spontaneous amputation, optimal control of diabetes, and appropriate antibiotic therapy.

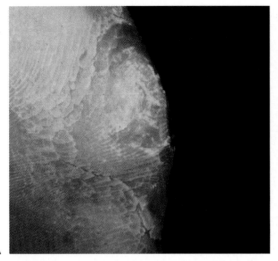
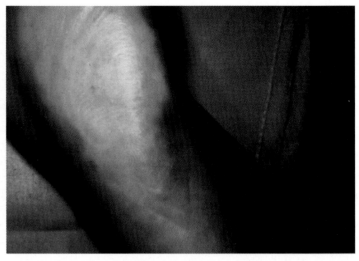

Figure 33–6 A. Fifty-year-old man with hematoma under thickened callus due to improper weight distribution (note crack in skin due to dryness). This patient was seen in diabetes clinic after having below-the-knee amputation of the other foot resulting from same type of callus and subsequent bacterial infection following breakdown of callus and osteomyelitis. Diabetes mellitus was diagnosed at time of admission for amputation. B. Same foot 2 weeks after reduction of thickened callus.

Follow-up

Metabolic control should be assessed on each visit to the podiatrist, since hyperglycemia decreases healing ability and increases the risk of infection. Patients should be taught the difference between pain caused by neuropathy and pain caused by ischemia. Neuropathic pain is often accentuated by uncontrolled diabetes and can be extraordinarily severe.

Patients should be taught to recognize and report promptly all subjective or objective changes in the lower extremities. Since almost all adult patients with diabetes develop minor foot lesions requiring occasional attention, and since many develop lesions that can lead to loss of a foot or leg, preventive and/or prophylactic continuing foot care is the ideal form of therapy.

Assessment and management of foot disease of those with diabetes has been reviewed[15,16] and new approaches to treatment of ulcers[24,25,29] and osteomyelitis[21] are being evaluated.

Audits

An ongoing audit of amputations since 1973 in those with diabetes at Grady Memorial Hospital has shown that the amputation rate can be decreased significantly by an effective foot-care program (see Exhibit 33–1). Runyan et al.,[22] Assal et al.,[23] and others[24–29] have reported similar observations. Delaying and/or preventing amputations can lead to significant cost-avoidance while improving the quality of the patient's life.

The St. Vincent Declaration for Care and Research in Diabetes was drafted in 1989 by patients with diabetes, health-care professionals, and representatives of government, diabetes associations, and industry. In the St. Vincent Declaration program of 1992,[30] a number of

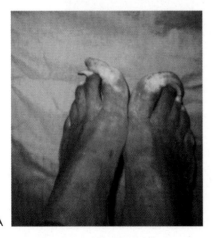
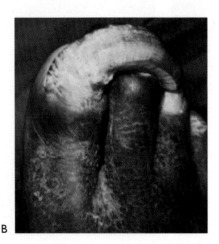
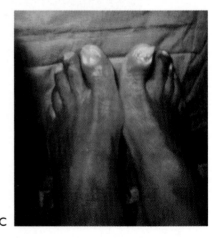

Figure 33–7 A. Fifty-five-year-old man with hypertrophic mycotic toenails (onychomycosis) and subsequent onychogryphosis of great toe nails. B. Closer view of right great toe demonstrating onychogryphosis and dermatophytosis. C. Same patient following palliative reduction of hypertrophic mycotic: toenails.

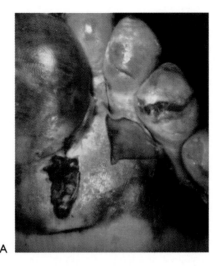
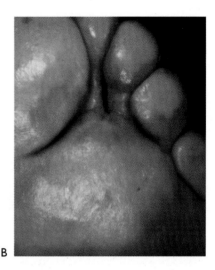

Figure 33–8 Fifty-six-year-old man with severe neuropathy and necrosis from second-and third-degree burns sustained after putting foot on heater. B. The same foot 6 weeks later.   A   B

five-year targets were outlined, one being to reduce by one-half the rate of lower extremity amputations (LEAs). Nearly all European countries have developed task forces to research and create long-term initiatives to prevent or delay the development of the chronic complications. Several regions have reported significant decreases in the amputation rate. For instance, a regional study in Denmark of 2848 major LEAs from 1982 to 1993 revealed an overall incidence decrease of 40%.[31] As excellent foot care programs become available to those with diabetes throughout the world, it seems reasonable to expect that the rate of lower extremity amputations will decrease.

The St. Vincent group is planning a 10th anniversary meeting for October 1999.

Adherence

In some patients, gangrene develops before diabetes is diagnosed. Some amputations occur in those who are nonadherent to prescribed podiatric or medical therapy (Exhibit 33–5). If diabetes is diagnosed as early as possible, and if all who have diabetes are well educated and appropriately treated, the present world-wide amputation rate would almost certainly decrease significantly.[27,31,32,33]

Research Considerations

See Chapters 25, 30, 31, 32, and 34.

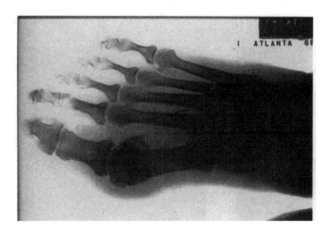

Figure 33-9 X-ray film of foot taken to rule out osteomyelitis of first metatarsal head secondary to neuropathic (malperforans) ulcer under first metatarsal head. Presence of needle in foot unknown to patient

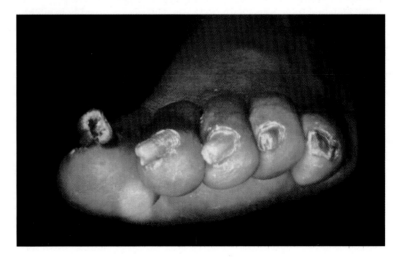

Figure 33-10 Seventy-one-year-old man with arteriopathy and hypertrophic mycotic incurvated toenails. This type of nail easily hooks bedding or socks causing avulsion of nail and subsequent infection.

EXHIBIT 33–5 Some Demographic and Other Characteristics of 68 Individuals with Diabetes Mellitus Who Had Lower-Extremity Amputations at Grady Memorial Hospital in 1978

	Black Female	Black Male	White Female	White Male	Total
Individuals	41	23	2	2	68
No. amputations	47	33	3	3	86
Age (years) at diagnosis: Mean (range)	60.5 (15–89)	42.6 (15–75)	56 (44–78)	52.5 (44–61)	
Age (years) at amputation: Mean (range)	71.6 (42–96)	57.8 (16–84)	73 (68–78)	58.5 (49–68)	
Not known to have diabetes on admission	8	6	1	0	15
Known to have diabetes on admission	33	17	1	2	53
Mean duration (years) and range (years)	11.4 (1–36)	11.9 (1–25)	24 (one patient only)	6 (5–7)	

	Toe(s)	Transmetatarsal	Syme's	Below Knee	Above Knee	Above-Knee Stump Revision
Level of initial amputation	12	1	2	42 (1 bilateral)	12	—
Level of follow-up amputation				6	9 (1 bilateral)	2

Treatment routines: diet alone in 63, diet plus insulin in 23 (mean dose, 23 U/day; range, 3–60).
Podiatric care less than 1-year preamputation: Yes, 18; no, 50
Adherence to prescribed therapy: Good, 8; fair, 4; poor, 33; not known, 23 (including 15 undiagnosed on admission)
Deaths: 0 during surgery, 5 in hospital, 6 less than 10 months after hospital discharge.
Causes: cardiac arrest in 9, renal failure in 1, septic shock in 1.
Days in hospital: mean (range): 5 who died in hospital, 15.2 (6–30); 63 who left hospital alive: 18.9 (4–55). Total days: 1,266

References

1. Krauz CE: History of chiropody (mineographed). Philadelphia: 1947, p. 135. Cited in J Am Podiatry Assoc 64:279, 1974.

2. Lerner HJ: Steps in the development of the profession of podiatry. J Am Podiatry Assoc 64:279–297, 1974.

3. Fowler RE: President's message. J Natl Assoc Chirop 46:172, 1956.

4. Zych D (ed): Retirement? How Sweet It Is! APH Report, April 1983, p. 14.

5. Chernyak EL: A tribute to three men. In Papazian HZ (ed): An Overview of the Podiatry Service and Podiatry Residence Program at the New England Deaconess Hospital. The Hospital Podiatrist 12(10), 1977, pp. 4–9.

6. Morris AD, McAlpine R, Steinke D, et al.: Diabetes & Lower Limb Amputation in the Community. *Diabetes Care* 21:738–743, 1998.

7. Selby JV, Zhang D: Risk Factors for Lower Extremity Amputation in Persons with Diabetes. *Diabetes Care* 18:509–516, 1995.

8. Levin ME: Preventing Amputation in the Patient with Diabetes. *Diabetes Care* 18:1383–1394, 1995.

9. Goldner MG: The fate of the second leg in the diabetic amputee. Diabetes 9:100, 1960.

10. Davidson JK: The Grady Memorial Hospital diabetes programme. In Diabetes in Epidemiological Perspective. London: Churchill Livingstone, 1983, pp. 243–249.

11. Davidson JK: What does the doctor do when allied health professionals take over? The view of a medical convert. In Larkins R, Zimmet P, Chisholm D (eds): Diabetes 1988. Amsterdam: Elsevier Science Publishers B.V. 1989, pp. 955–958.

12. Bild D, Selby J, Sinnock P, Browner W, Braveman P, Showstack J: Lower-extremity amputation in people with diabetes: epidemiology and prevention. Diabetes Care 12:24–31, 1989.

13. Brand P, Yancey P: The Gift Nobody Wants. *The Southern Sugar Club.* Harper Collins Perennial. Zondervan. New York, NY, 1995, pp. 180–197.

14. Whitehouse FW, Block MA: The problem of the 'diabetic foot.' J Am Geriat Soc 12:1045–1050, 1964.

15. American Diabetes Association Position Statement: "Foot Care in Patient with Diabetes Mellitus, 1997." *Diabetes Care* 21(Suppl. 1) Jan. 1998, pp. 554–555.

16. Birke JA, Rolfsen RJ: "Evaluation of a Self-Administered Sensory Testing Tool to Identify Patients at Risk of Diabetes-related Foot Problems." *Diabetes Care* 21:23–25, 1998.

17. Anderson MH: A Manual of Lower Extremities Orthotics. Springfield, IL: Charles C Thomas, 1972.

18. Hertzman CA: Use of Plastazote in foot disabilities. Am J Phys Med 52:289–303, 1973.

19. Capurto GM, Cavanaugh PR, Ulbrecht JS, Gibbons GW, Karchmer AW: "Assessment and Management of

Foot Disease in Patients with Diabetes." N Engl J Med 331:854–860, 1994.

20. Steed DL for the Diabetic Ulcer Study Group: "Clinical Evaluation of Recombiant Human Platelet-Derived Growth Factor for the Treatment for Lower Extremity Diabetic Ulcers." J. Vasc. Surgery 21:71–81, 1995.

21. Grayson ML, Gibbons GW, Balogh K, Levin E, Karchmer AW: "Probing to Bone in Infected Pedal Ulcers: A Clinical Sign of Underlying Osteomyelitis in Diabetic Patients." JAMA 273:721–728, 1995.

22. Runyan JW, Vander Zwaag R, Joyner MB, et al.: The Memphis diabetes continuing care program. Diabetes Care 3:382–386, 1980.

23. Assal JP, Gfeller R, Ekoe JM: Patient Education in Diabetes. *In* Recent Trends in Diabetes Research, Symposium September 22–24, 1981. Stockholm: Almqvist and Wiksell, 1982.

24. Peter-Reisch B, Assal JP, Reiber G: "Pivotal Events: A Neglected Field of Factors Leading to Diabetic Foot Complications." Diabetologia 39(Suppl. 1), A 1008, 1996.

25. Tanudjaja T, Chautelau E: "Recurrent Foot Ulcer Disease in Diabetes Mellitus." Diabetologia 39(Suppl. 1), A 1002, 1996.

26. Sproul M, Schönbach AM, Mülhauser I, Berger M: "Evaluation of Foot Care and Amputation in Elderly Patients Treated with Insulin." *Diabetologia* 39(Suppl. 1), A 996, 1996.

27. New JP, McDowell D, Young RJ: "Amputations in Newly Diagnosed Diabetics – a Substantial Problem." *Diabelotogia* 39(Suppl. 1), A 994, 1996.

28. Abbott CA, Vitelkyte L, Carrington A, Boulton AJM: "Morbidity and Mortality in Peripheral Vascular Disease Patients with Unilateral Lower Limb Amputation." *Diabetologia* 38(Suppl. 1), A 1046, 1995.

29. Dargis V, Pantalejeve O, Jonushaitea A, Vileikyte L, Boulton AJM: "Benefits of a Multidisciplinary Approach in the Management of Recurrent Diabetic Foot Ulceration." *Diabetologia* 41(Suppl. 1), A 1077, 1998.

30. Krause HMJ, Porta M, Keen H: "Diabetes Care and Research in Europe: The St. Vincent Declaration Action Programme." *International Diabetes Federation Europe*, 1992.

31. Ebskov B, Ebskov L: Major Lower Limb Amputation in Diabetic Patients: Developments During 1982–1993. *Diabetologia* 39 1607–1610, 1996.

32. Helfand AE: Practice guide for podiatric programs in extended care facilities. J Am Podiatry Assoc 56:220–230, 1966.

33. Levin MD, O'Neal LW: The Diabetic Foot. St. Louis: C.V. Mosby, 1993.

34. Hobgood E: Care of the feet and lower extremities. *In* Steiner G, Lawrence PH (eds): Educating Diabetic Patients. New York: Springer-Verlag, 1981, pp. 40–46.

34

The Role of Vascular Surgery in the Management of Arterial Insufficiency in Diabetes

Atef A. Salam

A wide range of manifestations of arterial insufficiency is seen in diabetic patients. At one end of the spectrum are those who have mild symptoms that do not interfere with the quality of life and represent no immediate danger to the extremity involved. At the other end are those who are disabled by the symptoms of arterial insufficiency and in whom the ischemic changes may rapidly progress to actual gangrene unless the blood supply of the leg is restored. One of the important goals of the total care of the diabetic patient is to identify these circulatory changes and treat them before they cause irreversible complications.

Clinical Assessment of Arterial Insufficiency

The clinical manifestations of arterial insufficiency are well known. Intermittent claudication, usually in the calf and less frequently in the buttocks, is the most common presenting complaint in patients with major arterial disease. The characteristic sequence, exercise-pain-rest-relief, helps to distinguish claudication from other types of musculoskeletal pain. The length of the claudication distance is a reliable measure of the degree of arterial blood flow impairment and is a crucial factor in determining whether or not the patient is severely disabled by his disease. Another important factor that enters into this determination is the general condition of the patient with particular emphasis on any medical or physical illness that might continue to curtail the patient's ability to walk even after symptoms of arterial insufficiency are relieved.

As the ischemia advances, the patient's ability to walk progressively lessens until he reaches the point where resting does not relieve his foot or leg pain. Ischemic rest pain is an ominous symptom that indicates that tissue perfusion has fallen below the critical level necessary to meet the oxygen requirements of the nonexercising muscle cell. Patients with this degree of ischemia often hang their feet over the side of the bed, particularly at night, to alleviate this pain. This often causes foot swelling, particularly in patients with coexisting hypoproteinemia or congestive heart failure. The increased extracellular pressure, secondary to edema in such patients, further impedes tissue perfusion. This vicious circle rapidly leads to whole-thickness necrosis of the skin of the foot's dorsal surface, where most of the fluid accumulation takes place. This is a tragic complication, because even with successful bypass the foot cannot be salvaged once these ischemic changes have occurred. Thus, rest pain associated with edema of the foot is an indication for aggressive management of any systemic factor contributing to the swelling and is an indication for urgent evaluation for vascular reconstruction.

Ischemic rest pain should not be mistaken for such conditions as diabetic neuropathy, root compression, night cramps, plantar abscess, or atherosclerotic microembolization. Foot pain at rest, unassociated with any evidence of nutritional changes in the skin or subcutaneous tissue or appropriate reduction of ankle Doppler blood flow, is usually due to nonischemic causes.

Since atherosclerosis is a generalized disease, all patients presenting with symptoms of arterial insufficiency should be screened for coexisting carotid or coronary artery disease. A history of transient ischemic attacks or stroke is often obtained in these patients and is frequently associated with correctable extracranial carotid artery disease. Neck examination for bruit and appropriate vascular laboratory tests are indicated in these patients. Similarly, any patient with a history of angina or other evidence of heart disease should undergo a complete cardiac workup and, if warranted, heart catheterization.

The local findings in patients presenting with chronic arterial insufficiency vary according to the extent of ischemia. In mild cases absence of pulse at the ankle level may be the only evidence of circulatory deficiency. In advanced cases nutritional changes become noticeable. These include tapering of toes, retardation of toenail growth, and loss of hair on the distal third of the leg. Color and temperature changes are seen in patients with severe arterial insufficiency and are usually associated with rest pain. In advanced cases the precapillary arterial sphincter loses its function; hence, the foot changes color from pink in the dependent position to waxy-white with elevation. Other clinical tests that are useful in assessing the degree of severity of ischemia include measurement of refilling time in the capillary bed of a digit or one of the foot veins.

Noninvasive Vascular Laboratory Studies

Several techniques have been introduced to evaluate limb blood flow noninvasively in recent years.[1-12] The two methods most commonly used are Doppler ultrasound pressure measurements and pneumoplethysmography.

The Doppler method is used to measure segmental blood pressure by listening with the probe over one of the pedal vessels, dorsalis pedis, or posterior tibial, with pressure cuffs applied at the high thigh level, above the knee, and at ankle level. As the cuff is deflated, arterial flow resumes and is immediately heard with the Doppler instrument. This point represents systolic pressure at the level of cuff application. An index is obtained by dividing the segmental pressure by the brachial systolic pressure. This index correlates directly with the level of arterial blood flow. The ankle pressure reading may be erroneously elevated in patients with calcified vessels because of the high cuff pressure level that is needed to obliterate blood flow in such cases. Calcified vessels are often seen in diabetic patients who present with manifestations of peripheral vascular disease.

The other method that is commonly used for noninvasive testing is segmental plethysmography. In this technique, a cuff with a pressure sensor is used to measure and record variation in arterial volume in a specific limb segment during each cardiac cycle. This measurement should not be confused with absolute blood flow. The wave obtained is similar to the arterial pulse contour and contains information regarding the degree and level of occlusive disease.

Noninvasive tests serve as an objective means for documenting circulatory changes. They help to differentiate true from false claudication and ischemic from nonischemic rest pain. They are also useful in the postoperative evaluation and follow-up of patients after vascular reconstructive procedures. Noninvasive tests, however, can be misleading at times unless the information provided by them is carefully correlated with the results of a complete clinical evaluation (See Chapter 25.)

Angiography

The role of angiography is to provide the surgeon with a vascular map that outlines the distribution of the disease and determines its suitability for operative treatment. Angiographic studies are not needed in patients for whom operative intervention is unnecessary because the symptoms are nondisabling or for patients at high risk due to the presence of severe heart disease. Evaluation of operative risk is further discussed under individual operations.

Advocates of balloon angioplasty recommend angiography for any patient who is disabled by his ischemic symptoms regardless of his general condition, since, according to them, balloon angioplasty can be done safely even in poor risk patients. Balloon angioplasty, however, is not without danger, and, as discussed later, most of the complications of this technique require surgical intervention. One should, therefore, anticipate the potential need for operative treatment in assessing the patient's suitability for this method of treatment.

Treatment of Arterial Insufficiency in Diabetics

Preventive Measures

The tragic loss of an extremity in a diabetic patient is often triggered by a seemingly minor injury, such as irritation secondary to an improperly trimmed nail or transient compression caused by wearing ill-fitting shoes.[13] Diabetic patients have a tendency to underestimate the danger of such injuries because they often have neuropathic changes, hence they usually experience very little pain. Other risk factors in regard to the complications of arterial insufficiency in diabetes include cigarette smoking, high blood pressure, and high blood glucose levels due to inadequate diabetes control.

Patient education is one of the most important aspects of the overall management of diabetics, particularly if one is dealing with elderly or rural patient populations. The teaching sessions should focus on foot protection against trauma, proper control of diabetes and hypertension, frequent medical checkups, and early detection of limb ischemia manifestations. Close cooperation between the physician, nurse specialist, social worker, and podiatrist is essential to achieve this goal.

Criteria for Selection of Patients for Vascular Reconstruction

While this discussion is focused on arterial reconstruction in diabetics, it should be emphasized that this type of surgery is needed in only a small segment of this patient population. In most instances arterial insufficiency is either asymptomatic or too mild to justify operative treatment. Restoration of blood flow does not protect the patient against further progression of atherosclerosis distally. Hence, it is not expected to alter the natural course of the disease, nor is there any basis for recommending arterial reconstruction in patients with nondisabling claudication as a means of protecting them against a future amputation. Only 7.2% of such patients are at risk for losing an extremity in 5 years, and the percentage only reaches 12.2% in 10 years.

Conversely, vascular reconstruction is very valuable in relieving patients with disabling claudication. In patients with pregangrenous changes, operative restoration of blood flow is of crucial value in averting an amputation.

Using these general principles, patients with diabetes and manifestations of circulatory insufficiency may be classified into clinically identifiable groups that share certain criteria that may serve as general guidelines for selection of a method of treatment.

Group 1-Clinical Features: Asymptomatic arterial insufficiency as revealed by nonpalpable ankle pulses. The fact that these patients are able to exercise without developing claudication negates the possibility of them having any significant femoral or popliteal artery disease. Such patients usually have either a palpable popliteal pulse or only a minimal reduction of their ankle Doppler pressure (ischemic index of 0.8 or more). This type of asymptomatic arterial insufficiency is commonly seen in patients who have had diabetes for more than 5 years. Obviously, neither surgery nor angiography has a place in the management of these patients.

Group 2-Clinical Features: Neuropathic ulcer of the foot; no claudication; palpable ankle pulse or ankle ischemic index greater than 0.8. Peripheral arterial disease is not a major problem in patients with such findings. Consequently, they do not need angiographic evaluation. Reconstructive vascular surgery is unlikely to be of any benefit in healing the ulcer in this type of patient. Management of neuropathic ulcers is discussed in Chapters 31, 32, and 33.

Group 3-Clinical Features: Mild claudication; no skin loss. This picture is seen in patients with atherosclerosis of the major arteries which is either mild or partially compensated for by collateral circulation. Noninvasive tests in this clinical setting usually show an ankle ischemic index of not less than 0.8. Although these patients may have reconstructible arterial disease, their symptoms are considered too mild to justify operative intervention. Consequently, angiographic studies are not needed in such patients.

Group 4-Clinical Features: Mild claudication associated with a nonhealing toe or foot ulceration in a nonpressure-bearing location. Again, claudication indicates that circulatory insufficiency is due at least in part to major artery disease. Unlike group 3 patients, these patients have a nonhealing ulcer, which is an added risk factor because of the danger of bacterial invasion and worsening of ischemia secondary to inflammation. Decreased tissue perfusion is an important factor in the development of these ulcers, but from the therapeutic point of view it is essential to determine whether reduction of foot blood flow in such patients is due primarily to small artery or major artery disease. Noninvasive vascular laboratory studies are useful in this regard. A near-normal ankle Doppler pressure is an indication that foot ischemia is mainly due to small-vessel disease. Patients with such findings do not usually benefit from operative correction of an angiographically demonstrable lesion. Conversely, patients with decreased ankle blood flow should be considered for surgical treatment.

Group 5-Clinical Features: Either disabling claudication or rest pain associated with signs and symptoms of impending gangrene. These symptoms are clear indications for angiographic evaluation and operative treatment unless the patient has a medical contraindication to operative management or the angiographic studies reveal noncorrectable arterial disease.

Group 6-Clinical Features: Rest pain with or without ischemic foot or toe ulcer; palpable popliteal pulse and absent Doppler signals or markedly reduced ankle ischemic index (0.2 to 0.4). These findings signify severe tibial artery disease. There is some controversy regarding the place of bypass operations in this group of patients. This controversy will be further discussed in the section on femorotibial bypass operations.

Vascular Reconstructive Procedures

The past three decades have witnessed successful development of the surgical treatment of arterial occlusive disease. Several operative techniques are now available for the management of diabetic patients with symptomatic limb ischemia secondary to associated atherosclerotic disease. The following is a brief description of the basic features, indications, and results of these operative procedures.

Aortobifemoral Bypass Operation

In this operation an inverted Y-shaped Dacron graft is used by bypass aortoiliac occlusive disease (Fig. 34–1).

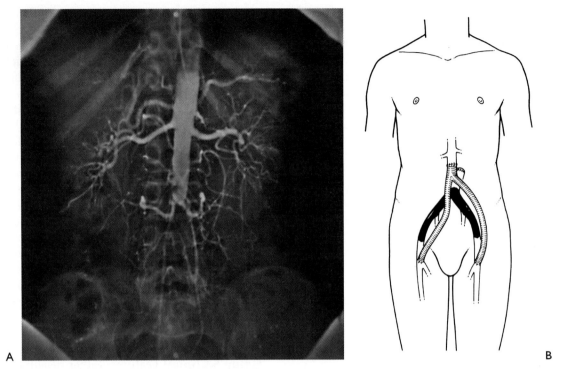

Figure 34–1.   A. Aortoiliac occlusive disease. B. Aortobifemoral bypass graft.

The abdominal aorta is transected below the renal arteries, its distal end oversewn, and its proximal end anastomosed to the stem of the dacron graft. One limb of the graft is then anastomosed end-to-side to each of the common femoral arteries. The aorta is not transected when the proximal end of the graft is anastomosed using the end-to-side rather than the end-to-end technique.[14-21]

Aortobifemoral bypass operation is indicated in patients with disabling claudication or impending gangrene secondary to aortoiliac occlusive disease. All such patients should be screened for evidence of heart disease. In some instances it might be advisable to do a coronary bypass operation first and defer the aortobifemoral bypass until the patient has recovered from his heart operation. In properly selected patients, an aortobifemoral bypass procedure can be performed with an operative mortality of less than 2%. This mortality is largely due to cardiac complications; hence, a thorough preoperative evaluation of myocardial function in these patients is important.

Excellent results can usually be achieved by the aortobifemoral bypass operation. Immediate postoperative graft failure occurs in less than 1% of the patients and is usually due to poor performance of a distal anastomosis to a diseased arterial segment with a compromised outflow. Late patency rate, as determined by life expectancy table analysis, is 88% at 5 years and 75% at 10 years. Late failure is usually due to progressive atherosclerotic changes of the profunda femoris artery and is usually preceded by gradual shortening of the claudication distance and progressive reduction in Doppler pressure measurement in the extremity involved. Patients who are not relieved by the aortobifemoral procedures and those with recurrent symptoms should be studied angiographically to assess their suitability for a femoropopliteal or femorotibial bypass operation.

Axillary-Femoral Bypass

This is an alternative technique for the treatment of patients with bilateral aortoiliac disease in whom an aorta bypass operation is considered too risky because of advanced heart disease (Fig. 34–2).

In this operation the axillary artery is used as a source for arterial inflow. The graft is interposed between it and the common femoral artery with a side limb extended to the common femoral artery of the opposite side. The graft is placed in a subcutaneous tunnel; hence, there is no need to open the abdomen or clamp the aorta in this operation. Since axillary-femoral bypass grafts have a lower patency rate than the aortobifemoral bypass, the latter operation is still considered the procedure of choice in good-risk patients.

Femorofemoral Bypass

Like the axillary-femoral operation, this procedure is indicated in patients with iliac occlusive disease in

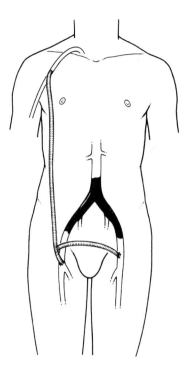

Figure 34–2. Axillary-femoral bypass with crossover graft to the other groin.

whom a major operation is unsafe because of coexisting heart disease (Fig. 34–3). Since the common femoral artery is used for inflow, this procedure is only suitable for patients with unilateral iliac disease. The crossover bypass is placed in a subcutaneous tunnel, which is made suprapubically in the abdominal wall. The long-term patency rate of this operation is superior to axillary-femoral bypass because of the short length of the graft, and in some reports it approaches that of the aorto-bifemoral operation.

Fentoropopliteal and Femorotibial Bypasses (22–29)

This operation is indicated in patients with disabling claudication or rest pain and angiographic demonstration of femoropopliteal occlusive disease (Fig. 34–4). Other prerequisites for recommending this operation are the absence of any significant aortoiliac disease and the demonstration of an adequate outflow. The reversed saphenous vein is the most frequently used graft for femoropopliteal or femorotibial bypass operation. It has a superior patency rate compared with other graft material, particularly when, due to the extent of the disease, the distal anastomosis is made distal to the level of the knee joint. In some instances, however, the surgeon may be forced to use other graft material because the saphenous vein is anatomically unsuitable or has already been used surgically for previous bypass operation. The umbilical vein, dacron, or polytetrafluoroethylene (PTFE) grafts may be used in these situations.

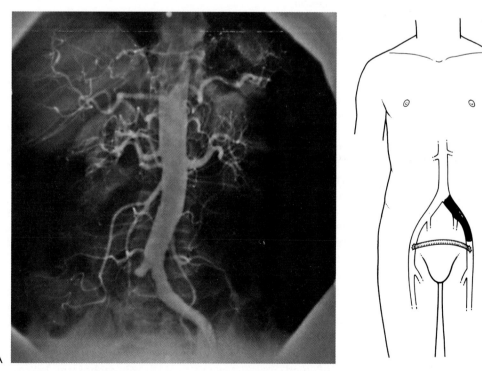

A   B

Figure 34–3.   A. Unilateral iliac artery occlusion suitable for femorofemoral bypass. B. Femorofemoral bypass graft.

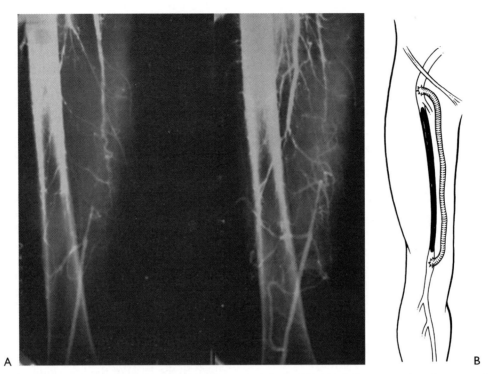

Figure 34–4.   A. Atherosclerotic occlusion of superficial femoral artery. B. Femoropopliteal bypass graft.

Early failure (within 4 weeks) of femoropopliteal bypass operations in patients with adequate runoff is usually due to technical reasons and is an indication for urgent reexploration. On the other hand, reexploration is rarely useful in patients in whom graft occlusion is secondary to severe tibioperineal atherosclerotic disease. As for long-term results, reversed saphenous vein femoropopliteal bypass grafts have a 5-year patency rate in the range of 50 to 60% with an annual attrition rate of approximately 5%. Late occlusion after this operation is usually due to distal progression of the disease.

More recently the in-situ saphenous vein by-pass technique has become increasingly popular in the surgical treatment of infrapopliteal occlusive arterial disease. In this procedure the saphenous vein is left in place but the valves are destroyed using a special valvulotome. Veins which are too small to be used for reversed by-pass operations are suitable for the in-situ techniques. The available data suggest that the in-situ technique is superior to reversed vein grafts and results in high initial patency rates even in limited outflow tracts.

There is some controversy in regard to the advisability of femorotibial bypasses in diabetic patients. Some surgeons question the value of these procedures in diabetics on the basis of the high incidence of small vessel disease in this patient population. Others report

no differences in the long-term patency rate of femorotibial bypasses in comparable series of diabetic and nondiabetic patients (Fig. 34–5).

Percutaneous Transluminal Angiography (30–33)

As an alternative to bypass procedures, Gruentzig[30] has proposed the use of a special balloon catheter to dilate atherosclerotic stenotic lesions in patients with symptomatic peripheral arterial disease. The catheter used in this technique is a double-lumen balloon catheter with unique physical characteristics. The outer layer of the balloon catheter and the balloon itself are constructed of polyvinyl chloride, material that when inflated up to 6 atmospheric pressure will remain within the optimal dilation range for the specific balloon. This allows substantial inflation under high pressure while maintaining the cylindrical balloon shape and avoiding overdilation.

Balloon dilation of atherosclerotic lesions in peripheral arteries is being evaluated in many centers at the present time. Its attractive features include reduced cost and relative simplicity compared with surgical bypass procedures. Several investigators have reported good success rates with this technique, but most of these series consist of a relatively small number of patients

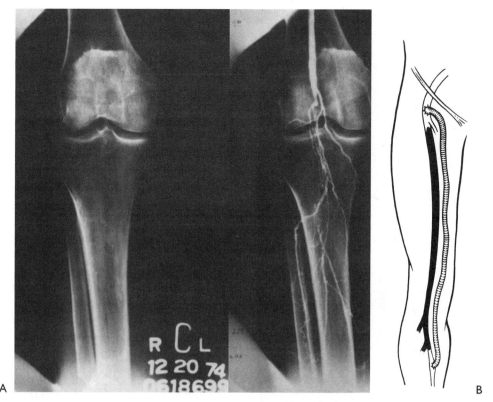

Figure 34–5.   A. Atherosclerotic occlusion of the popliteal and proximal tibial artery. B. Femorotibial bypass graft.

with follow-up of no more than 15 years.[30–32] Until its long-term efficacy is well documented, transluminal angioplasty should be attempted only in patients with disabling claudication or ischemic rest pain.

High-grade isolated iliac stenosis (Fig. 34–6) with a pressure gradient of more than 10 mmHg is generally considered as the most favorable lesion to dilate transluminally. At times, dilation of such lesions is done to improve inflow in preparation for a femoropopliteal bypass operation in patients with combined proximal and distal disease.

Balloon dilation has also been advocated for the treatment of short stenosis, single or multiple, in the femoropopliteal system, provided the occluded segment does not exceed 10 cm in length (Fig. 34–7). Generally, the longer the length of the lesion, the higher the failure rate and the higher the incidence of complications. Also, calcification of the vessel wall as demonstrated fluoroscopically or radiologically is considered an ominous finding regarding the success of this technique.

The complications of balloon dilation include subintimal dissection, thrombosis, embolization, disruption of the artery, and puncture site hematoma. Because of these potentially serious complications, balloon dilation should be reserved for patients with limb-threatening ischemia or disabling claudication. It should be empha-

sized that most of the complications of this technique require surgical intervention; hence, the importance of judicious assessment of the value versus the potential risk of this therapeutic approach, particularly in high-risk patients (Exhibit 34–1).

The concept of dilating atherosclerotic vessels raises several questions. First, what happens to the plaque or the diseased area? Since no direct way of imaging the dilation site other than angiography is available, this question may never be resolved. Second, is the effect, or are the results of this form of therapy durable long enough to justify their use in lieu of bypass surgery in properly selected patients? The answer to this question will have to await long-term studies of a sufficient number of patients, since most of the published reports represent short-term preliminary impressions largely influenced by the postdilation appearance of the arterial lesion and the early response to this form of treatment.

Arterial Stents

This technique has been introduced in recent years to enhance the long term patentcy rate after balloon angioplasty. The preliminary results seem to support the use of stents in the management of iliac artery stenotic lesions. Less clear however, is the role of stents in the management of more distal lesions. At present, by-pass

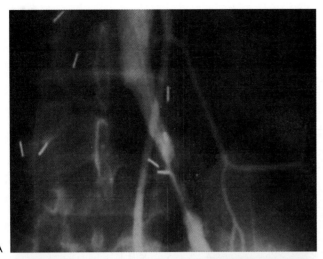

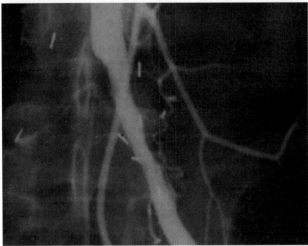

Figure 34–6.   A. High-grade stenosis of the left common iliac artery before balloon angioplasty. B. Same lesion in (A) after balloon dilation.

surgery remains the treatment of choice for obstructive lesions involving the superficial femoral, popliteal or tibial arteries. Stenting of such lesions should be reserved for patients who present with rest pain and are not considered candidates for surgical revascularization.

Laser in the Treatment of P.V.D. (34–39)

Applications of laser energy for treatment of vascular disease have recently received much attention in the media and in medical publications. Initial data show that recanalization of iliac, femoral and popliteal lesions can be accomplished in a majority of cases with the chance of success being inversely proportional to the length of occlusion. Results in the tibial vessels are disappointing. Techniques which are still in the developmental stage are aimed at improving the results and reducing the complications of laser canalization techniques.

Other Endoarterial Recanalization Techniques

Several mechanical devices have been recently introduced for the treatment of arterial occlusive disease. One such device is the atherectomy catheter which is introduced percutaneously and advanced to the occluded segment under fluoroscopic control. Another device consists of a catheter with a high speed rotating tip which is used to drill a canal in the occluded artery. These devices are still in the investigative stage and their wide scale use should await further evaluation.

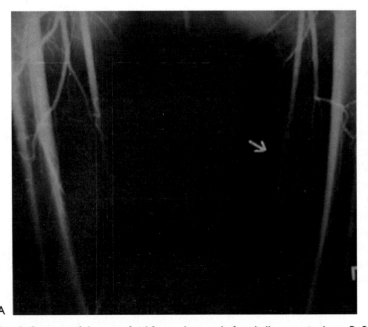

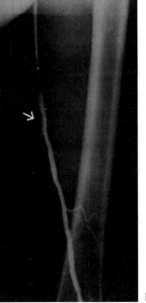

Figure 34–7.   A. Stenosis of the superficial femoral artery before balloon angioplasty. B. Same lesion shown in (A) after balloon dilation.

EXHIBIT 34–1   Complications of Transluminal Angioplasty

I. Arterial puncture and other side effects from catheter manipulation
  A. Hematoma at puncture site
    1. Neurologic deficit
    2. Mural thrombi
  B. Spasm with local ischemia
  C. Atherosclerotic plaque emboli
II. Local reactions at the dilation site
  A. Dissection of arterial wall due to subintimal passage of contrast media
    1. Arterial blockage
  B. False passage of the guidewire
  C. Rupture of intima, and media
    1. False aneurysms (pulsating hematomas)
    2. Fatal bleeding
  D. Arterial rupture
  E. Thrombosis of dilated segment
  F. Periarterial fibrosis
  G. Circumferential tearing of balloon
III. Hemodynamic effects
  A. Hypotension
  B. Anemia
  C. Myocardial infarction
IV. Effects of contrast media
  A. Acute tubular necrosis
V. Effects of heparinization
  A. Fatal bleeding if artery is perforated or ruptured

References

1. Bernstein EF, Rhodes GA, Stuart SH, et al.: Toe pulse reappearance time in prediction of aortofemoral bypass success. Ann Surg 193:201–205, 1981.

2. Fronek A, Coel M, Bernstein EF: The importance of combined multisegmental pressure and Doppler flow velocity studies in the diagnosis of peripheral arterial occlusive disease. Surgery 84:840–847, 1978.

3. Heintz SE, Bone GE, Slaymaker EE, et al.: Value of arterial pressure measurements in the proximal and distal part of the thigh in arterial occlusive disease. Surg Gynecol Obstet 146:337–343, 1978.

4. Hummel BW, Hummel BA, Mowbry A, et al.: Reactive hyperemia vs. treadmill exercise testing in arterial disease. Arch Surg 113:95–98, 1978.

5. Kozloff L, Collins GJ, Jr, Rich NM, et al.: Fallibility of postoperative Doppler ankle pressures in determining the adequacy of proximal arterial revascularization. Am J Surg 139:326–329, 1980.

6. Nicholas GG, Myers JL, DeMuth WE, Jr: The role of vascular laboratory criteria in the selection of patients for lower extremity amputation. Ann Surg 195:469–473, 1982.

7. O'Donnell TF, Lahey SJ, Kelly JJ, et al.: A prospective study of Doppler pressures and segmental plethysmography before and following aortofemoral bypass. Surgery 86: 120–129, 1979.

8. Raines JK, Jaffrin MY, Rao S: A noninvasive pressure pulse recorder: development and rationale. Med Instrum 7:245–250, 1973.

9. Strandness DE, Jr: The use and abuse of the vascular laboratory. Surg Clin North Am 59:707–717, 1979.

10. Strandness DE, Jr: Doppler ultrasonic techniques in vascular disease. In Bernstein EF (ed): Noninvasive Diagnostic Techniques in Vascular Disease. St. Louis: C.V. Mosby, pp. 13–21, 1982.

11. Bergan JJ, Yao JST: Invited overview: role of the vascular laboratory. Surgery 88:9–16, 1980.

12. Yao JST, O'Mara CS, Flinn WR, et al.: Postoperative evaluation of graft failure. In Bernhard VM, Towne JB (eds): Complications in Vascular Surgery. New York: Grune & Stratton, 1980, pp. 1–19.

13. Boyd MA: The natural course of arteriosclerosis of the lower extremities. Angiology 11:10–14, 1960.

14. Malone JM, Moore WS, Goldstone J: The natural history of bilateral aortofemoral bypass grafts for ischemia of the lower extremities. Arch Surg 110: 1300–1306, 1975.

15. Mozersky DJ, Sumner DS, Strandness DE: Long-term results of reconstructive aortoiliac surgery. Am J Surg 123:503–509, 1972.

16. Blaisdell FW, Hall AD, Lim RC, Jr, et al.: Aortoiliac artery substitution utilizing subcutaneous grafts. Ann Surg 172: 775–780, 1970.

17. Butcher HR, Jaffe BM: Treatment of aorto-iliac arterial occlusive disease by endarterectomy. Ann Surg 173: 925–937, 1971.

18. Kouchoukos NT, Levy JF, Balfour JF, et al.: Operative therapy for aortoiliac arterial occlusive disease; a comparison of therapeutic methods. Arch Surg 96:628–635, 1968.

19. Mannick JA, Williams LE, Nabseth DC: The late results of axillofemoral grafts. Surgery 68:1038–1043, 1970.

20. Dick LS, Brief DK, Alpert J, et al.: A 12 year experience with femorofemoral crossover grafts. Arch Surg 115: 1359–1365, 1980.

21. Bergan JJ, Veith O, Bernhard VM, et al.: Randomization of autogenous vein and polytetrafluoroethylene (PTFE) grafts in femoro-distal reconstruction. Surgery 92:921–930, 1982.

22. Burnham Sli, Flanigan DP, Goodreau JJ, et al.: Non vein bypass in below-knee reoperation for lower limb ischemia. Surgery 84:417–424, 1978.

23. Corson JD, Johnson WC, LoGerfo FW, et al.: Doppler ankle systolic blood pressure. Prognostic value in vein bypass grafts of the lower extremity. Arch Surg 113:932–935, 1978.

24. Dardik H, Ibrahim IM, Dardik I: Evaluation of glutaraldehyde-tanned human umbilical cord vein as a vascular prosthesis for bypass to the popliteal, tibial and peroneal arteries. Surgery 83:577–588, 1978.

25. De Weese JA, Robb CG: Autogenous venous grafts ten years later. Surgery 82:775–784, 1977.

26. Mannick JA, Jackson BT, Coffman JD, et al.: Success of bypass vein grafts in patients with isolated popliteal artery segments. Surgery 61:17–25, 1967.

27. Reichle FA, Rankin KP, Tyson RR, et al.: Long-term results of femoroinfrapopliteal bypass in diabetic patients with severe ischemia of the lower extremity. Am J Surg 137:653–656, 1979.

28. Veith FJ, Moss CM, Fell SC, et al.: Comparison of expanded polytetrafluoroethylene and autologous saphenous vein grafts in high risk arterial reconstruction for limb salvage. Surg Gynecol Obstet 147:749–752, 1978.

29. Leather RP, Shah DM, et al: Resurrection of the in-situ vein bypass, 1000 cases later. Ann Surg 208:435-442, 1988.

30. Gruentzig A, Hopff H: Perkutane Rekanalisation chronischer arterieller Verschlusse mit einem neuen Dilatations-Katheter. Dtsch Med Wochenschr 99:2502–2505, 1974.

31. Kumpe DA, Jones DN: Percutaneous transluminal angioplasty: radiological viewpoint. Vasc Diagn Ther 3:19, 1982.

32. Spence RK, Freiman DB, Gatenby R, et al.: Long term results of transluminal angioplasty of the iliac and femoral arteries. Arch Surg 116:1377–1386, 1981.

33. Loerum F, Castaneda-Zunigo WR, Amplatz KA: Complications of transluminal angioplasty. *In* Casteneda-Zunigo WR (ed): Transluminal Angioplasty. New York: Thieme-Stratton, 1983, pp. 41–44.

34. White RA, White GH: Laser thermal probe recanalization of occluded arteries. Vas Surg 9:598–608, 1989.

35. Perler BA, Osterman FA, et al: Percutaneous laser probe femoropopliteal angioplasty. Vas Surg 10:3551–7, 1989.

36. Newman GE, Miner DB, et al: Peripheral artery atherectomy-Description of technique and report of initial results. Radiology 169:677–680, 1988.

37. Thomas E. Brothers, M.D., Jacob G. Robinson, MD., and Bruce M. Elliot, M.D.: Diabetes Mellitus in the major risk factor for African Americans who undergo peripheral bypass graft operation. Journal of Vascular Surgery 29(2):352–357, 1999.

38. J.P. Becquemin, M.D., E. Allaire, M.D., P. Qvarfordt, M.D., P. Desgranges, M.D. PhD., H. Kobeiter, M.D., and D. Melliere, M.D.: Surgical transluminal iliac angioplasty with selective stenting: Long term results assessed by means of duplex scanning. Journal of Vascular Surgery 29(3):422–429, 1999.

39. R.D. Murphy, C.E. Encarnacion, A. LeVan, J.C. Palmaz: Iliac artery stent placement with the Palmaz Stent: Follow-up study. Journal of Vascular Intervention Radiology, 6:321–329, 1995.

35

Peripheral and Cranial Neuropathy in Diabetes

David S. H. Bell and John Ward

Historical Perspective

For almost two centuries, pains and paresthesias in the lower limbs have been associated with diabetes, and at one time this association led to the theory that diabetes mellitus was a disorder of the nervous system. However, the reverse was recognized by deCalvi in 1864.

At the turn of the century clinical descriptions of mononeuropathies (Althus 1890), neuropathic pain and nocturnal hyperesthesia (Auch's 1890), loss of deep tendon reflexes (Bouchard 1884), and the steppage gait of foot drop (Charcot 1890) appeared in the literature.[1,2]

It has only been in the last 20 years, however, that the extent of the morbidity and mortality that result from diabetic neuropathy has been appreciated. This renewed awareness is largely due to the development of significant diagnostic methods to quantify the severity of the disease. On the other hand, these techniques are extremely sensitive and have led to the diagnosis of diabetic neuropathy in patients without signs or symptoms of the disease. We prefer to restrict the term diabetic neuropathy to the latter group of patients.

Epidemiology

Problems with definition and with the variety of clinical syndromes that occur, coupled with the clear fact that many syndromes develop relatively suddenly, lead to difficulties in producing reliable prevalence statistics. One fact is clear—*diabetic peripheral neuropathy is common*. Whether we need large numbers of prevalence studies is arguable, although there is always the hope that such studies may not only measure prevalence but would also identify those who are at risk of developing neuropathy, which would then lead to an insight into the pathogenesis of diabetic neuropathy.

Applying the clinical definition, 18.5% of patients have a clinical problem.[3] More epidemiologically based studies produce higher numbers. In the Diabetes Control and Complications Trial (DCCT), between 35% and 54% of those with IDDM were deemed to have neuropathy on the basis of a very meticulous examination by a neurologist.[4] Interestingly, the occurrence of neuropathy was more likely in those developing diabetes after puberty. In the DCCT cohort, the features of those developing neuropathy were as follows—male smokers who were taller than usual with retinopathy and low insulin secretion. There was no correlation with glycosylated hemoglobin in this study.

In a recently analyzed study in Europe aiming to assess the rate of complications of insulin-dependent diabetes mellitus (IDDM) in Europe, *EURODIAB*, a 40% prevalence was seen.[5] Here age, duration of diabetes, and poor quality of blood glucose control were the important factors, with an interesting previously described association with microalbuminuria.[6] In an extensive epidemiologic study in Pittsburgh, the prevalence of diabetic peripheral neuropathy by clinical examination was shown to be 31%, relating to abnormal Vibration Perception Threshold (VPT) of 69% and an abnormal Temperature Discrimination Threshold (TDT) of 41%. Measurement of conduction velocity produced an instance of neuropathy of 43% appertaining to sural sensory measurements and 53% in motor measurements.[7]

It is equally important to realize the prevalence of diabetic neuropathy in populations with non-insulin-dependent diabetes mellitus (NIDDM). It is not at all clear as to whether there is any significant difference in the syndromes of diabetic neuropathy between the two groups of diabetic patients, but studies certainly have indicated very significant prevalence of neuropathy in such subjects.[8] In a British study the prevalence was 41.6% in subjects screened in the community, but not in special diabetic clinics.

Pathogenetic Mechanisms

Basically we do not have a clear understanding of the mechanisms that lead to nerve damage in human diabetes. Animal work has formed the basis of the theories concerning abnormalities of metabolic pathways that are also present in humans. Human studies consist of observations in nerves exhibiting advanced and often destructive tissue damage.

The Metabolic Hypothesis

Abnormalities of the polyol pathway have been seen in studies in relation to diabetic neuropathy for well over 20 years now, and no satisfactory agreement or evidence of beneficial treatment resulting from such theories is yet available.[9,10] In the animal models relating directly to hyperglycemia, the following pathway is produced:

Sorbitol elevated

Myoinositol depressed

NaK++ATPase depressed

All of this is controlled by the enzyme aldose reductase. It is thought that abnormalities of these pathways lead to the well-known slowing of nerve conduction velocity (CV) and to some pathologic change. Hence, an exciting possibility exists in that inhibition of the enzyme aldose reductase regardless of the blood glucose would prevent these biochemical abnormalities, normalize nerve conduction velocity, and prevent changes. In diabetic rats this is undoubtedly true.

However, in human studies the picture is far less clear following the use of a variety of aldose reductase inhibitors (ARIs). In a large diabetic population, treatment for 1 year resulted in an improvement in CV of around 1m/sec.[11] In clinical trials specifically aimed at studying symptoms and physiologic measures, some CV improvement is apparent between 1–2 m/sec, but very little benefit in terms of symptoms has been reported with marginal improvements in autonomic function tests.[12] A more recent study looked at the effect of withdrawal of an ARI after 3 years of treatment. The expected deterioration in CV did not occur in those subjects who remained on active treatment compared to placebo, but there was some return of symptoms in the treated group.[13]

There has been one biopsy study in a small number of patients in which an increase in nerve fiber count was demonstrated in those treated with an ARI, although whether these fibers were functional and effective is not clear.[14]

In many ways after so many years of research this story is very disappointing, and *it leaves physicians with no certainty that these agents are worthwhile*. In defense of ARIs, it must be said that when they have been administered to advanced neuropathy, the nerve is already very severely damaged and ischemic and it seems unlikely that a metabolic agent designed to block a fundamental and possibly initiating factor would be effective, particularly since most of the trials have been

very short in comparison to the natural history of diabetes and diabetic neuropathy. Unfortunately, truly long-term preventive studies in patients with no disease or minimal disease have not been carried out for the understandable reasons of cost and time.

The situation of the moment is that available ARI agents produce a small improvement in CV and prevent demonstrable deterioration in CV. Whether this justifies their long-term use in patients with no more than a marginal depression of conduction velocity has not been decided.

The Microvascular Hypothesis

Fagerberg (1959) was the first to suggest that disease of nerve microvessels was important.[15] Over the years descriptions of endothelial capillary abnormalities have appeared. More recently, a large body of evidence has been produced indicating that profound microvascular changes are present in human diabetic neuropathy—grossly so in well established neuropathy but also in minor ways much earlier in the course of diabetes. Considerable evidence from animal work also exists. The case in human diabetic peripheral neuropathy is as follows:

1. Abnormalities of endoneurial capillaries are present in neuropathic sural nerve compared to controls, the degree of abnormality correlating with the clinical state. These changes consist of endothelial swelling, occlusion of the lumen, and significant thickening of the basal lamina. Changes of this nature, although present in skin and muscle, are not so severe as in the nerve itself, suggesting a neurovascular interaction.[16]

2. Ischemia of the sural nerve has been demonstrated by insertion of electrodes in vivo.[17]

3. Magnified photography of sural nerve vessels demonstrates attenuated epineurial arteries, venous distension and tortuosity, and direct arteriovenous shunting[18] (Figs. 35–1 to 35–3).

4. Injection of intravenous fluorescein appears very slowly in neuropathy nerve.

5. CV does not increase with exercise in neuropathy compared to the 5 m/sec improvement seen in controls.[19]

6. Insulin neuritis. This is a fascinating clinical state in which, following a period of poor blood glucose control, improvement in control, usually with insulin, is followed within 6 weeks by the development of a very painful neuropathy. In vivo photographic examination of five such nerves has revealed loss of all normal vessel anatomy with multiple arterio venous shunts and whirls of proliferating new vessels—"neural new vessels"[20] (Fig. 35–4).

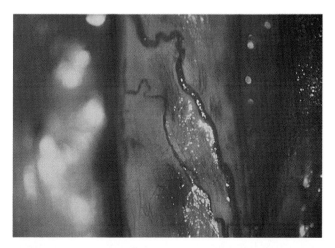

Figure 35–1. Human sural nerve in diabetic peripheral neuropathy showing attenuated arterial and distended distorted vein with arteriovenous shunt, bottom right.

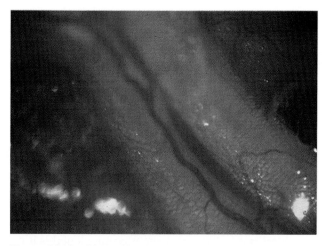

Figure 35–2. Normal human sural nerve, artery and vein, direct in vivo photography.

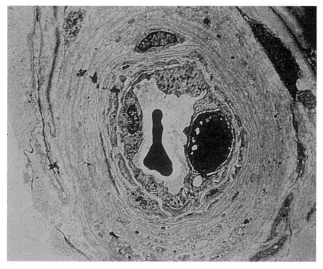

Figure 35–3. Gross basal laminar thickness in capillary of sural nerve—electron microscope.

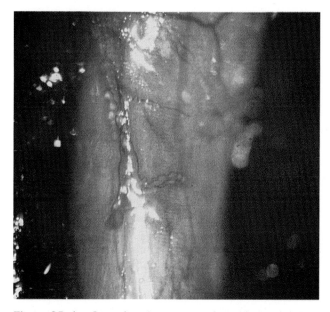

Figure 35–4. Case of insulin neuritis with proliferating new vessels—neural new vessels in response to ischemia.

7. Animal work. Animal work provides equally powerful evidence that:
   a. Animals placed in hypoxic chambers develop vessel and nerve changes similar to those seen in diabetic neuropathy. Oxygen supplementation prevents this change.[21]
   b. Nerve blood flow is distinctly abnormal in diabetic animals.
   c. Nerve blood flow can be returned to normal by the use of a number of agents[22]—α-blockers, calcium-channel blockers, and ACE inhibitors (ACE inhibitors improve CV in humans).

Clearly, there is a very great need to carry out clinical studies with a number of these agents, many of which are established in medical practice for other indications.

Other Areas

1. Nerve proteins are undoubtedly glycated, and reversal of such glycation in animals has been demonstrated by the administration of aminoguanidine. Human clinical trials are underway.[23]

2. Growth factors are obviously fundamentally important in repair and development of nerve and may play an important part in diabetic neuropathy, but research is at a very fundamental and early stage.[24]

3. γ-Linolenic acid has profound effects on fatty acid cycles within vessels and is known in animals and humans to result in significant improvement in conduction velocity. Again, trials are underway.[25]

Neuropathology

Slowly in the life of a nerve in a diabetic environment, pathologic changes occur that eventually lead to an end-stage disease with very severely damaged nerves. The exact time sequence for this is not clearly understood, but it does seem that subtle changes are present in many diabetic subjects at an early stage of their disease. The most striking feature on cross-sectional examination of a diabetic peripheral nerve is the very significant loss of fibers. Other changes consist of demyelination and subsequent remyelination, new fiber development, axonal atrophy, and a variety of changes in the paranodal area.[26] As time goes on, both structural and functional changes occur; all of this is on a background of glycation of nerve proteins. This is clearly an extremely complex picture, possibly denying the fact of one unifying pathogenetic mechanism.

Definition

In clinical practice, damage to peripheral nerve in diabetes causes much morbidity and unhappiness. Many unpleasant clinical syndromes occur—e.g., the production of the anesthetic foot and its potential for frequent foot ulceration, the development of impotence—all underlying the devastating effects of this tissue damage. Sadly, our knowledge of the mechanisms that lead to nerve damage and the lack of fundamental effective treatment leave physicians frustrated as to how to help their patients, other than offering them considerable sympathetic support and advice as to how to prevent clinical problems.

Despite years of study and clinical observation, no generally agreed-upon definition of diabetic peripheral neuropathy is available. There are many clinical syndromes, and these are described in detail later in this chapter. At this point, it is reasonable to raise the question as to whether the same pathogenetic mechanism is responsible for all of these different clinical pictures. Why does the peripheral nervous system respond in different ways?

There is indeed a need for a generally agreed-upon definition of neuropathy so that clinical studies and trials from different centers may be compared and contrasted. There are moves now to agree to a consensus, and a personal view of this will be given later. The definition of diabetic neuropathy will be somewhat different depending on the situation—routine clinical practice, epidemiologic studies, or scientific studies and trials.[27]

Routine clinical practice

The following definition is offered: a state of nerve damage in diabetes resulting in symptoms or problems that bring a patient to seek medical help or physical signs indicating a vulnerable state of the peripheral nerves that is likely to lead to tissue breakdown—i.e., anesthesia leading to ulceration.

This is a practical working clinical approach that should allow physicians to help those with problems and prevent future disease.

Epidemiology

Where large populations are to be studied, measures and assessments must be limited, accurate, and reproducible. Thus, a simple symptom score with a limited examination (e.g., knee and ankle jerks, a measure of muscle strength) will identify many people with a problem. Added to this should be a measure of VPT and one or two measures of autonomic function (heart rate response to standing and different phases of respiration). Measurement of nerve conduction velocities are usually too complex and costly for large epidemiologic studies.

Scientific trials and studies

It has been customary in such studies to obtain measures of great complexity that take hours to carry out in each individual. Requirements for such studies, therefore, are:

- Very detailed neurologic symptom score
- Very detailed neurologic disability score
- multiple electrophysiologic measures of motor and sensory conduction velocities with peripheral latencies and action potentials
- VPT (Vibration Perception Threshold)
- TDT (Temperature Discrimination Threshold)
- A package of autonomic function tests

If such a detailed approach is taken, there is a possibility of grading neuropathy as suggested by Dyck:[28]

0   No neuropathy, no symptoms or signs, and less than two abnormal tests

1   No symptoms or signs, more than two abnormal tests

2   Minor symptoms and signs with more than two abnormal tests

3   Severe symptoms and signs with more than two abnormal tests

It seems likely that even in important clinical trials and studies a much simplified protocol could and will be devised to allow realistic standardization among centers that lean heavily on clinical assessment. Such a modification is therefore suggested:

- A limited series of important symptoms
- Basic physical signs such as reflexes
- Sensory change and power
- Two or three autonomic function tests
- A limited electrophysiological measure (VPT and TDT are possibilities)

The aim should be to provide an assessment that can be carried out accurately, effectively, and uniformly within 1 hour.

Measurement

Reproducible measurements are essential in clinical trials. However, in clinical practice it is usually not necessary to resort to electrophysiologic investigation and to allow diagnosis to be based on symptoms and signs. However, in difficult cases, to obtain a diagnosis, detailed neurologic, electrophysiologic, and other physiologic measurements must be available. *A constant concern in clinical practice is the possibility of overlooking another cause of nerve damage or a spinal cord lesion.*

Conduction velocity

This is the one measure that is known to correlate very significantly with the degree of nerve damage.[29] It is also the most reproducible of all investigations, giving a reasonable degree of specificity, and is the one measure that could be regarded as a gold standard.[30] If in the course of electrophysiologic investigation good peripheral latencies and action potentials are available then they correlate very satisfactorily with nerve fiber numbers. Thus, a conduction velocity is a distinct indication of the state of the nerve.

However, there are problems with this measure. Standardization of temperature is vital (2 m/sec increase for every 1°C), and the procedure requires highly trained skill for accuracy. The metabolic state affects the measure (a 3 m/sec change may be achieved in healthy and diseased nerves following lowering of the blood glucose). It must also be remembered that CV is a measure of the function of myelinated fibers, which constitute only 25% of the fiber population. CV's major disadvantage in clinical practice is that good electrophysiologic testing takes considerable time and expertise.

A major question in diabetic neuropathy circles is whether an impairment of CV constitutes "diabetic neuropathy." Since impairment relates to nerve damage, the answer should be yes, and if we had effective interventional therapy it would seem reasonable to treat an impaired CV. Moreover, the DCCT has shown an enormous benefit of blood glucose control in relation to nerve function, suggesting that impairment

should be looked upon as a risk factor for the future development of neuropathic syndromes necessitating better metabolic control.[31] There is a known and predictable deterioration in CV with duration of diabetes, and physiologic blood glucose control certainly will prevent this.

Vibration perception threshold

VPT is a measure of large fiber function. It is reasonably reproducible and accurate and very useful for large epidemiologic studies.[32] Since impairment is associated with points of high pressure in the feet known to be a risk factor for foot ulceration, this measure is a good way of identifying those at risk of foot ulceration.

Temperature discrimination threshold

TDT is a sensitive measure of small fiber function.[33] It does not correlate as clearly with clinical syndromes, is time consuming, and is difficult to carry out.

Sural nerve biopsy

Biopsy might be regarded as the ultimate measurement in the assessment of a peripheral nerve, and of course it has an important part to play in differential diagnosis. Generally only one biopsy possibility exists in an individual, although clinical trials involving two time-separated biopsies have now been carried out. The ethics of two biopsies must be considered even though some drug regulatory authorities require repeat biopsy evidence to assess the efficacy of treatment. However, a wide body of neurologic opinion would not agree with this requirement because measures of CV supported by clinical and other physiologic measures are sufficient to decide on clinical benefit.

Diabetic Mononeuropathies

Problem Statement

The diabetic mononeuropathies involve either a single or multiple discreet cranial or peripheral nerve and constitute approximately 15% of diabetic neuropathies. Mononeuropathies occur primarily in the older age group in whom the other manifestations of diabetic neuropathy may not be present. The mononeuropathies (with the exception of entrapment mononeuropathies) are usually abrupt in onset and tend to heal spontaneously. Since mononeuropathy can occur as a consequence of many diseases other than diabetes mellitus, other causative factors should be excluded. Diabetic mononeuropathies, in direct contrast to distal symmetrical polyneuropathy, are the direct result of ischemic events. In the cranial nerves, ischemic damage to the central portion of the nerve with preservation of the peripheral fibers has been described.[34] Multiple discrete microinfarctions of the obturator, femoral sciatic, and posterior tibial nerves have also been described.[35] These infarcts are thought to be due to occlusion of the vasa nervorum. With the availability of magnetic resonance imaging (MRI), it has been suggested that the infarct is in the brain stem rather than in the cranial nerve[36]

Cranial Mononeuropathies

Problem Statement. The most common form of diabetic mononeuropathy is involvement of the cranial nerves, with the nerves to the extraocular muscles being preferentially afflicted. The third cranial nerve is the most commonly affected, followed by the fourth, sixth, and seventh cranial nerves. Cranial nerve involvement is usually unilateral and isolated but can be bilateral and involve more than one nerve (mononeuropathy multiplex). When mononeuropathy multiplex occurs, other etiologies such as a collagen vascular disease should be suspected.

Subjective. The onset is usually abrupt, and, in about 50% of cases, diplopia is preceded by pain in the distribution of the ophthalmic and maxillary branches of the ipsilateral trigeminal nerve. The patient, however, does not usually present to a physician until diplopia develops (Fig. 35–5).

Objective. With a third nerve palsy there is ptosis and paralysis of the extraocular muscles innervated by the third nerve. With sparing of the lateral rectus and superior oblique muscles, the patient can move the eye only outward and downward and in looking in any other direction will experience diplopia. However, in the majority of patients whose third nerve palsy is due to diabetes mellitus, the pupillary response to light is maintained due to the peripheral placement and different vascular supply of the somatomotor fibers of the

third nerve.[34] In the sixth nerve palsy the eyeball is deviated inwardly and diplopia is evoked by lateral gaze. With a facial nerve involvement there is the typical Bell's palsy with ipsilateral facial weakness including the muscles of the forehead. In diabetic patients with Bell's palsy, ipsilateral loss of taste does not usually occur, suggesting that the lesion is more distal in the diabetic population and occurs after the chorda tympani leaves the seventh nerve.[37] Bilateral facial nerve involvement, which is usually only associated with sarcoidosis or Guillain-Barré Syndrome, has been reported to occur more frequently in diabetic patients.

Assessment. With all of the diabetic cranial mononeuropathies, other physical signs that may suggest a more central lesion should be sought with a thorough central nervous system examination. The diagnosis of diabetic cranial mononeuropathy can only be made when other etiologies are excluded. Apart from diabetes mellitus, the most common cause of cranial nerve palsies are trauma, tumor, and vascular abnormalities. Myasthenia gravis, thyroid disease, and multiple sclerosis need to be ruled out by history, physical examination, and appropriate tests. The sixth nerve palsy is of particular concern since the long intracranial course of this nerve renders it vulnerable to many intracranial disease processes. Trauma and tumor can be ruled out with computed tomography (CT) scans or MRI. If the history is suggestive of an intracranial aneurysm with a sudden onset of severe headache, then angiography may be necessary.

The single exception is with an isolated third nerve palsy with preserved pupillary response. In this case the odds are 3:1 that the lesion is due to diabetes, and a prudent physician may prefer to simply follow the course of the disease.

Plan. Once the diagnosis of diabetic cranial mononeuropathy has been made, the patient should be reassured that there will be spontaneous, complete, or partial resolution within 3–6 months. Whether this course will be shortened with the use of antiplatelet agents or rheolitics is not known and has never been subjected to clinical trial. However, since the etiology is vascular, aspirin 625 mg daily and/or Pentoxifylline 400 mg t.i.d. may be helpful. Until the diplopia disappears use of a patch to cover the affected eye may help the patient subjectively, and for the first 1 or 2 weeks adequate analgesia should be prescribed.

Diabetic Radiculopathy

Problem Statement

Diabetic radiculopathy is a form of diabetic mononeuropathy that involves a single nerve root but may afflict multiple nerve roots and may be recurrent. Diabetic

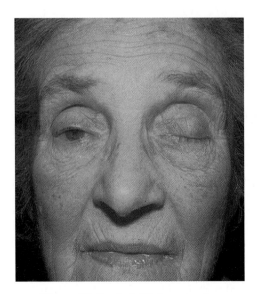

Figure 35–5. Left third nerve palsy.

radiculopathy most often occurs in older individuals who are known to have diabetes.[38]

Subjective

The patient presents with unilateral and often severe pain in the thorax or abdomen, which is often worse at night, causes insomnia, and is of rapid onset, and the distribution is that of a single dermatome that does not cross the midline.

Objective

Areas of tenderness in the abdomen or thoracic wall can often be detected. In the abdomen the tenderness is not changed or worsened by contracting the abdominal wall musculature, in contrast to intraabdominal lesions, where the tenderness is often relieved by this maneuver. Often hyperesthesia or in some cases hypoesthesia in the affected dermatome can be elicited with a careful objective sensory examination. In severe cases there is obvious motor involvement with hypotonia and atrophy in the affected dermatome so that on attaining the upright posture there is bulging of the abdominal wall.[39] In almost all cases objective evidence of distal symmetrical polyneuropathy is also present.

Assessment

The importance of a diabetic radiculopathy is that the condition is not misdiagnosed as an intraabdominal or intrathoracic lesion such as pneumonia, pulmonary embolus, myocardial infarct, cholecystitis, appendicitis, or diverticulitis.[40] An electrophysiologic determination of the neural origin of the pain is required with nerve conduction velocities and (EMGs) to avoid inappropriate therapeutic or surgical procedures. However, other causes of radiculopathy, such as herpes zoster, collagen vascular disease, or lesions of the spine or spinal canal, may need to be ruled out with radiographs or MRI. In this way, compression of the nerve root by a tumor, cyst, or granuloma can be ruled out. Polycythemia vera is a rare and easily excluded cause of radiculopathy.

Plan

The patient can be reassured that even though the pain is severe, it will resolve within 6 weeks to 3 months. Usually the more severe the pain the more rapid the resolution. Therapy for neuropathic pain, as described later in the discussion of the treatment of the painful symptoms of distal symmetrical polyneuropathy, is indicated. A regional local anesthetic block may give prolonged relief and negate or lessen the need for oral analgesia. As with the cranial mononeuropathies, antiplatelet therapy or rheolytic therapy with aspirin or pentoxifylline may shorten the course or improve the symptoms associated with diabetic radiculopathy.

Entrapment and Pressure Neuropathies

Problem Statement

In the diabetic patient, peripheral nerves are more prone to damage from external pressure. In addition with the glycosylation of protein and cross-linking of collagen, a less elastic, stiffer, and more voluminous connective tissue is formed and results in a higher incidence of entrapment neuropathies.[41]

Subjective

Entrapment of the median nerve in the carpal tunnel is the most common entrapment neuropathy seen in the diabetic patient. Often the patient will have objective findings without symptoms and the entrapment will be found on a routine physical examination. More commonly, the patient presents with tingling and, later, pain in the hand that is worse at night and somewhat relieved by hanging the affected hand over the side of the bed. In various situations patients may note wasting in the hands or that they are dropping objects frequently.

In a similar fashion, the ulnar nerve is susceptible to pressure at the elbow and in the Pisohamate tunnel with paresthesias and numbness of the lateral aspect of the hand. The patient may also notice wasting of the interosseous muscles of the hand and weakness of the hand with loss of grip strength and a tendency to drop objects.

Occasionally the radial nerve can be compressed in the axilla or as it crosses the humerus in the upper arm or at the wrist. This results in pain and paresthesias of the medial dorsal portion of the hand.

In the lower extremity compression of the lateral femoral cutaneous nerve at the inguinal ligament gives rise to pain, numbness, and paresthesia on the lateral part of the thigh (*meralgia paresthetica*). Similarly, entrapment of the femoral nerve leads to pain, numbness, and paresthesia involving the anterior surface of the thigh. Peroneal compression at the level of the head of the fibula (*crossed-leg palsy*) not only causes pain, paresthesias, and numbness on the dorsum of the foot but can also in severe cases give rise to unilateral foot drop. Rarely, compression of the posterior tibial nerve in the tarsal tunnel leads to pain, paresthesia, and numbness on the plantar surface of the foot.

Mononeuropathies involving the phrenic, long thoracic, and obturator nerves have been described in patients with diabetes mellitus. Whether these lesions are caused by external pressure from the local anatomy, by infarction, or purely by glucose intolerance is unknown.

Objective

With carpal tunnel syndrome there may be wasting of the thenar imminence, decrease in sensation over the distribution of the median nerve in the hand, a weakness of abduction of the thumb, and a positive Tinel's sign (symptoms reproduced by percussion over the carpal tunnel).

With ulnar entrapment there may be loss of pinprick sensation over the lateral aspect of the hand including the little and ulnar aspect of the ring finger. The major clinical finding in severe ulnar entrapment is wasting of the interossei and loss of grip and interdigital strength.

With lateral cutaneous and femoral entrapment there is characteristic loss and decrease in sensation over the lateral and anterior part of the thigh, respectively. With peroneal compression there may be loss of sensation in the dorsum of the foot as well as weakness of dorsiflexion of the foot. In the compression of the posterior tibial nerve in the tarsal tunnel, there is often loss of sensation on the plantar surface of the foot.

Assessment

Isolated peripheral mononeuropathies are likely to give rise to diagnostic insecurity, and clinical findings are usually confirmed with suitable nerve conduction studies.[42] However, with a background of distal symmetrical polyneuropathy, a decrease in nerve conduction velocity may be difficult to detect. Therefore, when electrical studies conflict with solid clinical findings, a negative electrical study should not delay appropriate therapy. One exception is an isolated femoral nerve mononeuropathy where lesions such as an inguinal hernia, retroperitoneal hematoma, or tumor should be excluded by pelvic ultrasound or computerized axial tomography.[43]

Plan

If only mild sensory symptoms are present, treatment with mild analgesia, night splinting in the case of carpal tunnel syndrome, removal of weight-bearing from the elbows with ulnar neuropathy, and the avoidance of leg-crossing with a common peroneal neuropathy are all that is required.

When atrophy of muscle either due to the neuropathy itself or to lack of utilization of the affected part is present, active physical therapy is essential whether or not surgery is performed. If symptoms are severe and/or muscle wasting is present, then surgical decompression of the affected nerve is indicated. This is particularly true of carpal tunnel syndrome and ulnar entrapment. A local nerve block may temporarily relieve the situation, but injection of steroids is discouraged because of the adverse effect on diabetic control. While many entrapment neuropathies are self-limiting, recovery takes much longer than with cranial mononeuropathies or with diabetic radiculopathies.

Diabetic Amyotrophy and Neuropathic Cachexia

Problem Statement

The syndromes of amyotrophy and neuropathic cachexia are uncommon and poorly understood forms of diabetic polyneuropathy. It has been postulated that there are two forms of this syndrome. A more common acute form is thought to be due to multiple infarcts in the proximal nerve trunks and lumbosacral plexus, whereas a rarer and more slowly evolving variety is thought to be due to metabolic factors.[44,45]

Subjective

The disease usually occurs in an older male with a recent onset of diabetes and often with a history of heavy alcohol intake. As a rule, weight loss of as much as 40% of the initial body weight is followed by depression, emotional lability, and severe pain and weakness in the muscles of the thigh. Patients complain of being unable to climb stairs, having difficulty arising from a sitting position, and falling due to their "knees giving way."[46]

Objective

There is invariably marked wasting of the quadriceps muscles that predominantly involves the iliopsoas, quadriceps, and adductor muscles. This is accompanied by absent knee jerks in a depressed and cachectic patient. Almost invariably, the objective signs of distal symmetrical polyneuropathy are present in the lower limb.

Assessment

Weight loss accompanied by neuropathic pain in an older diabetic male causes the patient and physician to think of an occult malignancy. Thus in most cases, a full cancer work-up is undertaken. In addition, other neuromuscular diseases, collagen vascular diseases, and pathology of the spinal cord or cauda equina need to be ruled out as well as the endocrine myopathies of thyrotoxicosis and Cushing's disease and Guillain-Barré syndrome. The diagnosis of diabetic amyotrophy is thus confirmed by a process of elimination. The only positive diagnostic information comes from the typical history, physical findings, abnormal nerve conduction velocities, and elevation of protein and myoinositol concentrations in the cerebrospinal fluid.[46]

Plan

The patient should be counseled to abstain from alcohol intake. Euglycemia, which is usually easily achieved with insulin in these patients should be sought. A high calorie diet with, if necessary, liquid caloric supplements should also be prescribed. Intensive physical therapy to prevent or ameliorate muscle atrophy should be undertaken as soon as possible. Treatment of pain is as outlined later in the discussion of the treatment of the pain of distal symmetrical polyneuropathy. Many of these patients have severe depression, and a high dose of tricyclic antidepressants may help both the depression and neuropathic pain.

While this condition resolves spontaneously in 1–3 years, recovery is not always complete. Generally severe symptoms persist for more than 6 months, weight loss is resolved in 1 year, and muscle strength is maximized in 2–3 years. Patients need to be reassured that they will recover from the disease but that recovery will take time.

Distal Symmetrical Polyneuropathy

Problem Statement

Distal symmetrical polyneuropathy is the most common and widely recognized form of diabetic neuropathy. Usually decreased nerve conduction velocities of the peripheral nerves and signs of peripheral nerve disease precede the development of symptomatic distal symmetrical polyneuropathy. Less commonly, the symptoms of distal symmetrical polyneuropathy may precede the development of objective signs and may even precede the clinical recognition of carbohydrate intolerance. This is thought to be due to the late diagnosis of diabetes in an older person with an insidious and asymptomatic onset of NIDDM.[47]

Subjective

Around two-thirds of patients who have objective findings of distal symmetrical polyneuropathy have no symptoms. Occasionally, following stress, trauma, or change in the diabetic regimen, the onset can be acute, but as a rule symptoms of distal symmetrical polyneuropathy present in an insidious and monotonously predictable pattern.[48] The symptoms start distally and gradually proceed proximally with the patient noting numbness and paresthesias in the feet. These symptoms may occur over the entire foot or may involve a discreet area such as a toe. Paresthesias may be described as feelings of coldness, itching, burning, or tingling. The complaints are invariably worse at night and often become less severe when the patient arises and walks around. When the patients arise from bed, especially at night, they describe a feeling that they are walking on cottonwool, or even of the floor feeling strange. At this early stage patients may also describe a deep aching sensation in the legs and experience cramps in the calves at night.

As the disease progresses, pain in the lower extremities becomes the outstanding feature. Patients describe a deep pain in the foot that is likened to a toothache and that again is worse at night and is helped by arising and walking around. At this stage there is often hyperesthesia of the feet and legs that precludes contact with bedclothes or the weight of one leg on top of the other. At a later stage, shooting pains described as an "electric shock traveling down the leg" are often experienced.

Objective

Signs of distal symmetrical polyneuropathy are usually first found during an annual physical examination in a patient with established diabetes. However, in 15% of patients with type 2 diabetes, signs of distal symmetrical polyneuropathy are present at the onset of diabetes, presumably due to a delay in diagnosis.[47] Usually long fibers are affected first so that loss of vibration sense is the earliest finding, followed by the loss of ankle jerks. Later with the involvement of shorter fibers there is loss of pinprick sensation in a stocking distribution. The level to which short fiber pain and temperature sensation is lost is usually lower than the level to which large fiber vibration and joint position sense are lost.

Assessment

Nerve conduction velocities are not necessary to confirm the diagnosis of distal symmetrical polyneuropathy. However, nerve conduction velocities may be useful when a superimposed entrapment neuropathy is clinically suspected.

Plan

Treatment of the symptoms of distal symmetrical polyneuropathy can be difficult and frustrating for both the patient and the physician. Usually through a process of trial and error a medication is found that will at least partially relieve the symptoms. The patient should be reassured that usually the more acute and severe the symptoms are, the more quickly they are likely to disappear.

In mild cases, use of a TENS machine, warm baths, or ice in conjunction with simple analgesia such as acetaminophen may be all that is required. In addition, rigid control of the diabetes has been shown to elevate the threshold for neuropathic symptoms and is indicated in all patients.[49] When hyperesthesia is present, the application of capsaicin cream in 0.025 or 0.075% concentrations can be helpful.[50] Capsaicin is a derivative of red peppers that is antagonistic to the action of Substance P, the neurotransmitter involved in pain sensation. Care should be taken to apply the cream in a thin layer so that erythema can be avoided. Tachyphylaxis is common so that capsaicin's use may be self-limited.

In those patients with less localized symptoms, tricyclic antidepressants are the cornerstone of therapy.[51] If symptoms are not relieved by the tricyclic antidepressant, addition of a phenothiazine such as fluphenazine 3–6 mg daily may result in symptomatic control.[52] Antiepileptic drugs have been used to treat symptoms of distal symmetrical polyneuropathy. Dilantin, long advocated in this situation, has been shown in a randomized and blinded study to be ineffective.[53] In a similarly designed study, carbamazepine has been shown to be effective[54] but limited by its potential toxicities, especially suppression of the bone marrow. Clonazepam is widely used despite a lack of objective evidence for its efficacy.

In severe cases, the use of a lidocaine infusion (5 mgs/kg over 30 min) has been shown to provide symptomatic relief for 3–21 days.[55] Mexilitine, an oral antiarrhythmic agent with an action on the nerve membrane similar to lidocaine, has in a double-blind trial been shown to be effective in relieving neuropathic symptoms.[56] In this situation, mexilitene can be used in a dose of up to 10 mg/kg/day, but side effects may limit its use.

Other unproven but widely utilized treatments of symptomatic distal symmetrical polyneuropathy include metoclopramide, 10 mg t.i.d., clonidine 0.1–0.5 mg daily, and pentoxifylline 400 mg t.i.d.

Although presently in use in some countries for the treatment of distal symmetrical polyneuropathy, the aldose reductase inhibitors have so far not shown efficacy in the treatment of the symptoms of distal symmetrical polyneuropathy.[57] Other therapies that are based on the proposed etiologies of distal symmetrical polyneuropathy and partially proven or unproven including 800 mg or 1600 mg[58] daily of brewer's yeast to correct neuronal myoinositol level and the replacement of neuronal γ-linolenic acid deficiency with a daily intake of 480 mg evening primrose oil or other supplements high in γ-linolenic acid.[33] In the future, aminoguanidine, which reverses glycation of protein and stimulates nitric oxide production, may be helpful in treating distal symmetrical polyneuropathy.[31]

In general, the use of stronger analgesics such as those containing oxycodone and propoxyphene have little effect on neuropathic symptoms, have a great potential for addiction, and are best avoided.

Motor Involvement of Distal Symmetrical Polyneuropathy

Subjective

In patients with severe sensory symptoms, muscle weakness of the lower extremities is an almost universal concomitant, but as a rule this weakness is not appreciated by the patients since it is essentially limited to the interosseous musculature of the foot. Occasionally the extensors of the foot will also be involved so that foot drop results. Involvement of the thigh musculature is more common in the older diabetic man who complains of difficulty in climbing stairs or rising from a chair.

Objective

Wasting of the interossei results in a disequilibrium between the flexors and the extensors of the toes leading to cocking up and retraction of the toes. Shoes that were previously comfortable become uncomfortable, and corns and ulceration of the dorsal surfaces of the toes may be present. Because of clawing of the foot, the metatarsal head moves posteriorly relative to their protective plantar metatarsal fat pad so that the heads of the metatarsals can be easily palpated under the skin. In combination with a loss of pain sensation, pressure ulcers develop under the metatarsal heads, particularly the first metatarsal head, which takes nearly twice as much weight as the other metatarsal heads and is the most common site of neuropathic ulceration. While a similar foot deformity occurs in rheumatoid arthritis, foot ulcers are unusual because pain sensation is not lost.

Assessment

In an occasional situation, differentiation of motor involvement due to distal symmetrical polyneuropathy may have to be differentiated from femoral entrapment, diabetic amyotrophy, and common peroneal entrapment. In such cases, nerve conduction velocities

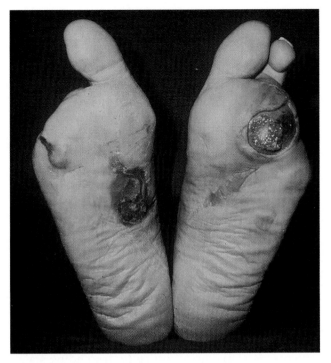

Figure 35–6. Tragedy of diabetic neuropathy with digital ischemia and neuropathic ulcers.

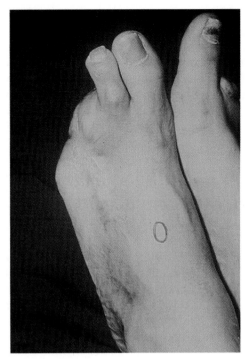

Figure 35–7. Typical neuropathic foot. Bounding visible pulse next to venous distension—sign of arteriovenous shunting near ischemic and amputated toes.

and EMGs are necessary, as well as an accurate clinical assessment. In assessing the patient who has a diabetic foot ulcer, it is important to assess the arterial supply to the foot since healing is unlikely in the absence of a reasonable blood supply (Figs. 35–6 and 35–7).

Plan

In 80% of diabetic amputees, minor trauma to the feet is the initiating event, leading to ulceration, infection, ischemia, gangrene, and amputation; a lack of education in diabetic foot care was a positive factor for amputation.[59] In addition, it has been shown that the amputation rate can be halved in 1 year when an education program in foot care is provided to a group of diabetic patients.[60] It is therefore essential that patients with diabetic neuropathy be repeatedly educated in the care of their feet and in the necessity of seeking medical help when even mild infections or skin breakdown occurs.

With other than a superficial foot ulcer, antibiotics will be necessary to control infection; if cellulitis develops, an intravenous antibiotic becomes necessary. Selection of antibiotics is empirical since cultures of the base of an ulcer reveal a wide spectrum of gram-negative, gram-positive, aerobic, and anaerobic bacteria.[61] An initial broad-spectrum antibiotic regimen is therefore mandatory. Later, more specific therapy can

be chosen from culture and sensitivities obtained from blood culture or from a culture taken at the time of debridement (see Chapter 44).

The most important facet of foot ulcer therapy is surgical debridement, which may include debridement of osteomyelitic bone. The frequency of osteomyelitis is underestimated[63]—higher with deeper ulcers–and its presence impairs healing.

With adequate debridement and elimination of infection, only a lack of weight-bearing is necessary to achieve healing. This can best be achieved with bed rest but other methods such as the use of total contact casting may be necessary (see Chapter 31).[63]

Slow or inadequate healing of foot ulcers may be due to an inadequate blood or oxygen supply to the foot. Hyperbaric oxygen is of unproven value, but an arterial bypass of the tibial vessels from the femoral or iliac artery to a patent dorsalis pedis artery has recently been shown to be effective in improving oxygenation and healing of the foot. The use of growth factors, including the use of the patient's own platelet derived growth factors, may accelerate healing. When foot ulcers are recurrent, surgical flattening of the heads of the metatarsals can avoid further ulceration.

Long-term antibiotic therapy may be necessary when osteomyelitis is diagnosed. However, noninvasive diagnosis of osteomyelitis is difficult since osteopenia due to distal symmetrical polyneuropathy is easily confused with osteomyelitis on a foot X-ray. In the presence of an ulcer or neuropathic osteoarthropathy, a thallium bone scan will show increased activity.[64] MRI with galladium enhancement (a white cell–labelled scan in conjunction with the bone scan), at one time were thought to be helpful, have been shown to be less accurate in diagnosing osteomyelitis than serial foot X-rays in conjunction with clinical assessment by an experienced clinician and (see Chapters 30, 31, 32, 33, 34).

Upper Limb Involvement of Distal Symmetrical Polyneuropathy

In those patients with severe distal symmetrical polyneuropathy disease, and predominantly in men, motor involvement will extend to the upper extremities and will involve the interosseous musculature of the hands. In addition, sensory involvement is also present and is almost invariably asymptomatic.

Subjective

Because of denervation involvement of the small muscles of the hand, everyday tasks that involve fine movements of the hands, such as tying shoelaces, writing, brushing teeth, shaving, and holding a cup by the handle, become difficult. If fine hand movements are an essential part of a patient's occupation, the patient may become disabled and seek help. However, usually patients do not seek help for problems of fine movement but will readily admit to these problems when asked directly.

Because of sensory loss, patients may present with burns on the hands from cigarettes or from handling hot objects such as irons and cooking utensils. For this reason, diabetic patients who lose their vision can seldom be taught to read Braille.

Objective

In the upper limbs, temperature, pain, vibration, or joint position sense is lost in a glove distribution and not in the distribution of the median ulnar and radial nerves. Wasting of the interossei is invariably present with weakness of interdigital strength and obvious difficulty with fine movements of the hands.

Assessment

Care must be taken to distinguish between distal symmetrical polyneuropathy and entrapment neuropathy involving the hand. This can best be achieved with careful clinical examination and confirmed if necessary by nerve conduction velocities. Since decompression of the median and ulnar nerve can lead to restoration of

hand strength, it becomes very important to differentiate between the entrapment neuropathies and the manifestations of distal symmetrical polyneuropathy in the upper limb.

Plan

Patients need to be educated to avoid contact with potentially hot objects.

Proprioceptive Difficulties with Distal Symmetrical Polyneuropathy

Subjective

With more severe forms of sensory loss, proprioception may be lost. In this situation the patient is dependent upon visual stimuli to establish the spatial position of the body. As a result, walking in a dimly lit room or closing the eyelids while showering may result in falls. Patients also have great difficulty descending stairs. Patients compensate for their disability by adopting a broad-based gait, avoiding stairs or supporting themselves with both hands when descending stairs, and using a night light.

Objective

These patients have a positive Romberg's sign with passive and active unsteadiness when standing with their feet together and eyes closed. In addition, there is invariably severe distal symmetrical polyneuropathy with absolute loss of vibration sense and joint position sense in the lower limb.

Assessment

Other causes of severe proprioceptive difficulty such as pernicious anemia and syphilis need to be ruled out.

Plan

The major goal of therapy is to avoid falls. Use of a walker and alterations in the home, especially with regard to adequate lighting, are very important.

Diabetic Neuropathic Osteoarthropathy (Charcot's Joints)

In the patient with distal symmetrical polyneuropathy, autonomic denervation is almost always present. For example, medial calcific arteriosclerosis, which characterizes the peripheral arteries in the diabetic patient,

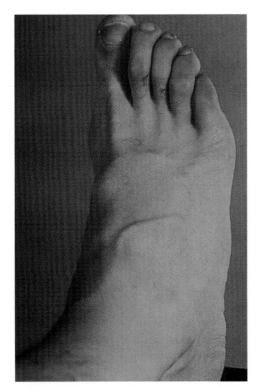

Figure 35–8. Gross venous distension in the diabetic neuropathic foot. Warm foot with palpable pulses.

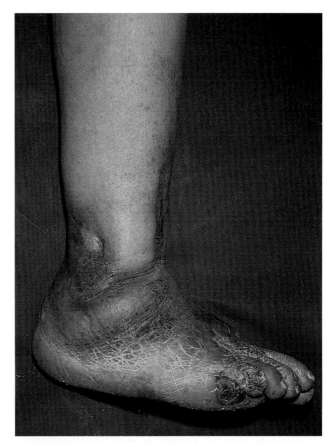

Figure 35–9. Gross example of Charcot's foot. Collapsed mid tarsal arch and subluxation of ankle joint.

can also be caused by lumbar sympathectomy and is therefore due to autonomic neuropathy.

Another manifestation of autonomic denervation is arteriovenous shunting causing hyperdynamic circulation and increased temperature of pedal skin, which may cause the physician to believe that infection, in particular osteomyelitis, is present.[65,66] Arteriovenous shunting also causes osteopenia and stress fractures, which, because of the lack of pain sensation, are unappreciated by the patient. Continued ambulation of the patient despite pedal trauma and stress fractures leads to destruction of the phalangeal, tarsal, metatarsal, and ankle bones with obliteration of the joint space. As a result there is a loss of the longitudinal arch and broadening of the foot. Eventually a characteristic rockerbottom sole develops due to dislocation at the tarsal metatarsal joints and the foot literally becomes a bag of bones[42] (Figs. 35–8 and 35–9).

Subjective

Patients present with deformity of the foot and difficulty getting suitably fitted shoes. Because of repeated stress fractures the patients may also present with swelling of the foot that is usually unilateral.

Objective

Examination of the foot may be normal. However, there may be swelling without evidence of deep vein

thrombosis or infection and an increased temperature of the skin of the foot. The characteristic clawing of the foot with the characteristic rockerbottom sole may also be present.

Assessment

Treatment is most successful when started at an early stage. Even before any X-ray changes occur, patients may present with unilateral foot swelling. At that time other causes of swelling, such as deep venous thrombosis, should be ruled out and the patient referred to an orthopedist for conservative treatment.

Plan

Treatment of Charcot's joint is a combination of conservative and surgical treatment and involves all members of the diabetic team. With early diagnosis, conservative treatment with casting is successful. However, at a later stage surgical intervention may be necessary to achieve an acceptable anatomic result so that the patient may be mobile without the risk of further foot damage. The use of extra-depth shoes with a molded insole and a rockerbottom sole is helpful (see Chapter 31).[67]

References

1. Rundles RW: Diabetic neuropathy. Medicine (Baltimore) 24:111–116, 1945.

2. Thomas PK, Eliasson SG: Diabetic neuropathy. Dyck PJ, Thomas PK, Lambert et al. (eds.): In Peripheral Neuropathy. Philadelphia: W.B. Saunders, 1984, pp. 1773–1810.

3. Boulton AJM, Knight G, Drury J, Ward JD: The prevalence of symptomatic diabetic neuropathy in an insulin treated population. Diabetes Care 8:125–128, 1985.

4. DCCT Research Group: Factors in development of diabetic neuropathy; baseline analysis of neuropathy and feasibility phase of Diabetes Control and Complications Trial (DCCT). Diabetes 70:476–481, 1988.

5. Tesfaye S, Malik R, Harris N, Jakubowski JJ, Mody C, Rinnie IG, Ward JD: Arterio-venous shunting and proliferating new vessels in acute painful neuropathy of rapid glycaemic control (insulin neuritis). Diabetologia 39(3):324–335, 1996.

6. Bell DSH, Ketchum CH, Robinson CA, et al.: Microalbuminuria associated with diabetic neuropathy. Diabetes Care 15:528–531, 1992.

7. Maser RE, Becker DJ, Drash AL, et al.: Pittsburgh epidemiology of diabetes complications study. Measuring diabetic neuropathy follow-up results. Diabetes Care 15:525–527, 1992.

8. Kumar S, Ashe HA, Parnell LN, et al.: The prevalence of foot ulceration and its correlates in type 2 diabetic patients: Population based study. Diabetic Med 11:480–484, 1994.

9. Greene DA, Lattimer SA, Sima AAF: Sorbitol phosphoinositides and the NaK+ATPase in the pathogenesis of diabetic complications. New Engl J Med 316:599–606, 1987.

10. Tomlinson DR: The pharmacology of diabetic neuropathy. Diabetes Metab Rev 7:67–84, 1992.

11. Judzewitsch RG, Jaspan JB, Polonsky KS, et al.: Aldose reductase inhibition improves nerve conduction velocity in diabetic patients. New Engl J Med 308:119–123, 1983.

12. McLeod AF, Boulton AJM, Owens DR, et al.: A multicentre trial of the aldose reductase inhibitor Tolrestat in patients with symptomatic peripheral neuropathy. Diabetes Metabol 18:14–20, 1992.

13. Santiago JV, Sonksen PH, Boulton AJM, et al.: Withdrawal of the aldose reductase inhibitor Tolrestat in patients with diabetic neuropathy: Effect on nerve function. J Diabetes Complications 7:170–178, 1993.

14. Sima AAF, Bril V, Nathaniel V, et al.: Regeneration and repair of myelinated fibers in sural nerve biopsies from patients with diabetic neuropathy treated with Sorbinil, an investigational aldose reductase inhibitor. New Engl J Med 319:548–555, 1988.

15. Fargerberg SE: Diabetic neuropathy: a clinical and histological study on the significance of vascular affection. Acta Med Scan 345: (Suppl) 1–97, 1959.

16. Malik RA, Newrick PG, Sharma AK, et al.: Microangiopathy in human diabetic neuropathy: Relationship between capillary abnormalities and the severity of neuropathy. Diabetologia 32:92–102, 1989.

17. Newrick PG, Wilson AJ, Jakubowski JJ, et al.: Sural nerve oxygen tension in diabetes. Br Med J 293:1053–1054, 1986.

18. Tesfaye S, Harris N, Jakubowski JJ, et al.: Impaired blood flow and arteriovenous shunting in diabetic neuropathy: a novel technique of nerve photography and fluorescein angiography.

19. Tesfaye S, Harris N, Wilson RM, Ward JD: Exercise induced conduction velocity increment. A marker of impaired peripheral nerve blood flow in diabetic neuropathy. Diabetologia 35:155–159, 1992.

20. Tesfaye S, Harris N, Jakubowski JJ, et al.: Microvascular shunting and neural new vessel formation in insulin neuritis. (submitted for publication).

21. Low PA, Schmelzer JD, Ward KK, Yao JK: Experimental chronic hypoxic neuropathy: Relevance to diabetic neuropathy. American Journal of Physiology 250:94–99, 1986.

22. Cameron NE, Cotter MA: Potential therapeutic approaches to the treatment or prevention of diabetic neuropathy: Evidence from experimental studies. Diabetic Med 10:593–605, 1993.

23. Brownlee M, Cerami A, Vlasara H: Advanced glycosylation end products in tissues and the biochemical basis of diabetic complications. New Engl J Med 318:1315–1321, 1988.

24. Schmit RE: The role of nerve growth factor in the pathogenesis and therapy of diabetic neuropathy. Diabetic Med 10 (Supp 2): 10S–13S, 1993.

25. The Gamma Linolenic Acid Multi-Centre Trial Group, Keen H, Payan J, Allawi J, et al.: Treatment of diabetic neuropathy with gamma linolenic acid. Diabetes Care 16:8–15, 1993.

26. Llewelyn JG, Thomas PK, Gilbey SG, et al.: Pattern of myelinated fibre loss in the sural nerve in neuropathy related to type 1 (insulin-dependent) diabetes. Diabetologia 31:162–167, 1988.

27. Feldman EL, Stevens MJ, Thomas PK, et al.: A practical two-step quantitative clinical electrophysiological assessment for the diagnosis and staging of diabetic neuropathy. Diabetes Care 17:281–289, 1994.

28. Dyck PJ: Detection, characterization and staging of polyneuropathy assessed in diabetics. Muscle Nerve 11:21–31, 1988.

29. Veves A, Malik RA, Lye RH, et al.: The relationship between sural nerve morphometric findings and measures of peripheral nerve function in mild diabetic neuropathy. Diabetic Med 8:917–921, 1991.

30. Daube JR: Electrophysiologic testing in diabetic neuropathy. In Diabetic Neuropathy. Dyck PJ, Thomas PK, Asbury, Winegrad, Porte. Philadelphia: W.B. Saunders, 1987.

31. The Diabetes Control and Complications Trial Research Group: The effect of intensive treatment of diabetes on the development and progression of long-term compli-

cations in insulin-dependent diabetes mellitus. New Engl J Med 321:683–689, 1993.

32. Bloom S, Till S, Sonksen P, Smith S: Use of a biothesiometer to measure individual vibration thresholds and their variations in 519 diabetic subjects. Br Med J 288:793–797, 1984.

33. Sosenko JM, Kato M, Soto RA, et al.: Specific assessment of warm and cool sensitivities in adult diabetic patients. Diabetes Care 11:481–483, 1988.

34. Asbury AK, Aldredge H, Hershberg R, Fisher CM: Occulomotor palsy in diabetes mellitus: a clinico-pathological study. Brain 93:555–566, 1970.

35. Ruff MC, Ashburg AK: Ischemic mononeuropathy and mononeuropathy multiplex in diabetes mellitus. New Engl J M 279:17–22, 1968

36. Hopf HC, Guttman L: Diabetic 3rd nerve palsy: Evidence of a mesencephalic lesion. Neurology 40:1041–1045, 1990.

37. Pecket P, Schuttner A: Concurrent Bell's palsy and diabetes mellitus: a diabetic mononeuropathy? J Neurol Neurosurg Psy 45:652–655, 1982.

38. Ellenberg M. Diabetic truncal mononeuropathy—a new clinical syndrome. Diabetes Care 1:10–13, 1978.

39. Boulton AJ, Angus E, Aggar DR, Weiss DR: Diabetic thoracic polyradiculopathy presenting as abdominal swelling. Br Med J 298:789–799, 1984.

40. Harati Y, Niakan E: Diabetic thoracoabdominal neuropathy. A cause of chest and abdominal pain. Arch Int Med 146:1493–1494, 1986.

41. Fraser DM, Campbell IW, Ewing DT, Clarke BF: Mononeuropathy in diabetes mellitus. Diabetes 28:96–106, 1979.

42. Clements RS Jr, Bell DSH: Diagnostic, pathogenic and therapeutic aspects of diabetic neuropathy. In Cohen MP, Foa PP (eds.): Special Topics in Endocrinology and Metabolism Volume 3. New York: Alan R. Liss, 1981, pp. 1–43.

43. Calvarley JR, Mulder PW: Autogenous mono-neuropathy: Diagnosis, treatment and clinical significance. Med Clin N Amer 44:989–999, 1960.

44. Garland HT: Amyotrophy due to hypoglycemia. Br Med J 1:707–708, 1955.

45. Asbury AK: Proximal diabetic neuropathy. Ann Neurol 2:179–180, 1977.

46. Chokroverty S, Reyes MG, Rubinof A, Tonaki H: The syndrome of diabetic amyotrophy. Ann Neurol 2:181–194, 1977.

47. Fruser DM, Campbell IW, Ewing DJ, et al.: Peripheral and autonomic nerve function in newly diagnosed diabetes mellitus. Diabetes 26:546–550, 1977.

48. Archer AG, Watkins PJ, Thomas PK, et al.: The natural history of acute painful neuropathy in diabetes. J Neurol Neurosurg Psy 46:491–499, 1983.

49. Morley GK, Mooradian AD, Levine AS, Morley JE: Mechanism of pain in diabetic peripheral neuropathy. Effect of glucose or pain perception in humans. Amer J Med 77:79–82, 1984.

50. Tundun R, Lewis G, Krusiniski P, et al.: Topical Capsaicin in painful diabetic neuropathy: Controlled study with long-term follow-up. Diabetes Care 15:8–14, 1992.

51. Young RJ, Clarke BF: Pain relief in diabetic neuropathy: the effectiveness of Imipramine and related drugs. Diabetic Med 2:363–366, 1985.

52. Mendel CM, Klein RF, Chappel DA, et al.: A trial of Amitriptyline and Fluphenizine in the treatment of diabetic neuropathy. JAMA 255:637–639, 1986.

53. Saudek CD, Werns S, Reidenberg MM: Phenytoin in the treatment of diabetic symmetrical polyneuropathy. Clin Pharmacol Therapeutics 22:196–199, 1977.

54. Rull JA, Quibrera R, Gomzalez-Millan H, Loranzo-Castaneda O: Symptomatic treatment of peripheral diabetic neuropathy with carbamazepine (Tegretol): Double-blind crossover trial. Diabetologia 5:215–218, 1969.

55. Kustrup J, Peterson P, Deggard A, et al.: Intravenous Lidocaine infusion—a new treatment of chronic painful diabetic neuropathy. Pain 28:69–75, 1987.

56. Deggard A, Petersen P, Kustrup J: Mexiletine for treatment of chronic painful diabetic neuropathy. Lancet 1:8575–8576, 1988.

57. Jaspan JB, Towle VL, Maselli R, Herold K: Clinical studies with an aldose reductase inhibitor in the autonomic and somatic neuropathies of diabetes. Metabolism 35:83–92, 1986.

58. Clements RS, Vourganti B, Kaba T, et al.: Dietary myoinositol intake and peripheral nerve function in diabetic neuropathy. Metabolism 28:477–483, 1979.

59. Brand P, Yancey P (eds.): The Gift Nobody Wants. New York: Harper-Perennial; 1995.

60. Davidson JK: The Grady Memorial Hospital Diabetes Program in Mann JI, Pyorala K, Teuscher A (eds.): Diabetes in Epidemiological Perspective. New York: Longmon (Churchill Livingstone), 1983, pp. 332–341.

61. Louie TJ, Bartlett JG, Tally FP et al.: Aerobic and anaerobic bacteria in diabetic foot ulcers. Ann Intern Med 85(4):461–463, 1976.

62. Newman LG, Waller J, Palestro CJ, et al.: Unsuspected osteomyelitis in diabetic foot ulcers. Diagnosis and monitoring by leukocyte scanning with indium in 111 oxyquinoline. JAMA 266(9):1246–51, 1991.

63. Boulton AJ, Bowker JH, Gadia M, et al.: Use of plaster casts in the management of diabetic neuropathic foot ulcers. Diabetes Care 9(2):149–152, 1986.

64. Edmonds ME, Clarke MB, Newton S, et al.: Increased uptake of bone radiopharmaceutical in diabetic neuropathy. Quart J Medicine 57:843–855, 1985.

65. Boulton AJM, Scarpello JHB, Ward JD: Venous oxygenation in the diabetic neuropathic foot: Evidence of arteriovenous shunting. Diabetologia 22:6–8, 1982.

66. Ward JD, Simms JM, Knight G, et al.: Venous distension in the diabetic neuropathic foot (physical sign of arteriovenous shunting). J Roy Soc Med 76:1011–1014, 1983.

67. Clements RS, Jr., Bell DSH: Diagnostic, pathogenic and therapeutic aspects of diabetic neuropathy. In Cohen MP, Foa PP (eds.): Special Topics in Endocrinology and Metabolism Volume 3. New York Alan R. Liss, 1981, pp. 1–43.

36

Diabetic Autonomic Neuropathy
Aaron I. Vinik and Leonard C. Glass

Peripheral sensory and motor neuropathy is now recognized as the most frequent life-spoiling complication of insulin-dependent (type 1) and non-insulin-dependent (type 2) diabetes, and its prevalence increases with the duration of diabetes and the level of hyperglycemia.[1] In recent years there has been an increasing amount of interest in the effects of diabetes on the autonomic nervous system. Autonomic neuropathy (AN) affects every system in the body. It may be central, e.g., cardiac, or peripheral, with impaired sweating, poor hydration, and reduced cutaneous blood flow. Once symptomatic, life expectancy may be reduced 50% within $2\frac{1}{2}$–5 years.[2] Effects on the sympathetic and parasympathetic nervous systems may be diverse; there may be impotence, delayed gastric emptying, impaired glucose counterregulatory function, and nocturnal diarrhea. There may be an early functional phase, e.g., hypoglycemia unresponsiveness, wherein there is no structural abnormality in the sympathetic nervous system. Usually, however, clinical manifestations arise at a late stage in the pathologic process. This late appearance with severe neuronal loss reduces the likelihood of reversibility.

In the past, a vast amount of research has gone into the study of diabetic neuropathy and into trying to find simple, noninvasive tests to detect autonomic and peripheral neuropathy before obvious symptoms occur. Before suitable tests were designed for assessing the nervous system, neuropathy was thought of as a late complication of diabetes,[3] but in recent years new tools and techniques have been developed that offer the opportunity to recognize problems before subjective symptoms appear.

In this chapter we will review the epidemiology and clinical presentations of the various forms of autonomic nerve dysfunction. For a detailed report on therapy of this condition, the reader is referred to the review by Vinik and Suwanwalaikorn.[4]

Epidemiology

Although the incidence of AN is greater in type 1 than in type 2 diabetes, its prevalence seems to be greater among type 2 patients, and certainly the absolute number with AN is considerably higher among type 2 patients. Prevalence figures range from 10% to 95% after 10 years of diabetes.[1] The range of prevalence estimates are wide and underestimation is likely to be due to patients usually not being tested for autonomic dysfunction until symptomatic, and not being treated in a setting with the equipment necessary to perform the necessary tests. Thus they may not be identified until later in the disease process.

Independent risk factors for AN include hypertension, raised low-density lipoprotein cholesterol (LDL-C), reduced high-density lipoprotein cholesterol (HDL-C), and female sex. Age is a more important determinant than duration of diabetes. Although it is commonly stated that AN is a disease of lean people, AN occurs more frequently in people with a higher body mass index.[5]

The 5-year survival of patients with clinically overt AN is 40–60%, compared to 99% in patients without neuropathy. Nearly 100% of all diabetic patients show minor abnormalities in autonomic function tests (e.g., pancreatic polypeptide response to hypoglycemia or loss of the heart beat-to-beat [R-R] variation with deep breathing), but it may be that only those patients with symptoms of AN are at increased risk of sudden death, myocardial infarction (MI), or renal failure.[6,7]

Pathophysiology

The autonomic nervous system (ANS) consists of an afferent and an efferent system, with long efferents in the vagus and short postganglionic unmyelinated fibers in the sympathetic nervous system (SNS). AN may be classified as organic or functional. In organic AN, there is a diffuse lesion affecting small fibers of the cholinergic, noradrenergic, and peptidergic nervous systems. The impairment in sympathetic and parasympathetic function is accompanied by impaired warm thermal perception or sudomotor dysfunction (C-fibers), impaired cold perception (A.-δ fibers), and decreased neurogenic thermal flare (mediated by neuropeptides, substance P, calcitonin gene-related peptide [CGRP], neuropeptide K, and possibly others). Organic AN may be subdivided into subclinical (before the appearance of clinical symptoms) and clinical (in which symptoms appear).

In functional AN there is no apparent organic lesion. Functional AN may be subdivided as occurring (1) after hypoglycemia, (2) after intensive diabetes control, or (3) after hyperglycemia.

Diabetes can cause dysfunction of every part of the ANS. The areas of dysfunction that are most important to the clinician include cardiovascular reflexes, gastrointestinal function, genitourinary function, and certain metabolic functions such as glucose counterregulation and awareness of hypoglycemia.

Specific System Involvement

Because almost all body organs are innervated by the ANS, any organ can be affected by diabetic autonomic neuropathy. Once clinical autonomic neuropathy is established the patient often has other complications of diabetes,[8] including coexistence with somatic neuropathy. Therefore, subclinical abnormalities of the ANS may be present, yet the disorder may never be suspected, and when clinical symptoms become present, they may be severe and confined to a single organ, which may become the focus of intense diagnostic and therapeutic attention (Table 36–1).[9] Also, studies have shown that it is very unusual for spontaneous improvement to occur once clinical disease is apparent.[8]

Tests of the ANS generally stimulate reflex arcs. The reflex arc involves a stimulus, one or more sensors, afferent fibers, ganglionic or central processing, efferent fibers, nerve endings, and effector organs. Tests of the ANS measure end-organ response. Because they stimulate the entire reflex arc, these tests cannot locate specific defects within the reflex arc. Opposing sympathetic and parasympathetic fibers dually innervate many organs; thus, any given result may reflect a decrease of function in one pathway or an increase in another. Furthermore, the nerves of the autonomic system are not easily accessible for nerve conduction studies because they are widely dispersed in a "weblike"[9] fashion. Therefore, the testing of the ANS is complicated by dual innervation, composite reflex arcs, and anatomical dispersion. There are, however, certain areas in the body, e.g., the skin or pupil, where direct access to functional testing is more feasible.

TABLE 36–1   Clinical Manifestations of Autonomic Neuropathy

Cardiovascular
  Tachycardia, exercise intolerance
  Cardiac denervation
  Orthostatic hypotension
  Heat intolerance
  Skin temperature reversal, dry skin, and dependent
    edema

Gastrointestinal
  Esophageal enteropathy
  Gastroparesis diabeticorum
  Constipation
  Diarrhea
  Fecal incontinence

Genitourinary
  Neurogenic bladder
  Impotence
  Cystopathy
  Retrograde ejaculation

Sweating Disturbances
  Areas of symmetrical anhydrosis
  Gustatory sweating

Metabolic
  Hypoglycemia unawareness
  Hypoglycemia unresponsiveness
  Hypoglycemia-associated autonomic failure (HAAF)

Pupillary
  Decreased diameter of dark-adapted pupil
  Argyll-Robertson type pupil

Cardiovascular Abnormalities (Table 36–2)

Cardiac AN is characterized by resting tachycardia, impaired exercise-induced cardiovascular responses, cardiac denervation, orthostatic hypotension, heat intolerance, impaired vasodilation, and impaired venoarteriolar reflex (dependent edema).

Resting Tachycardia. Preganglionic parasympathetic fibers reach the ganglionic neurons through cervical and thoracic branches of the vagus nerve. Postganglionic fibers are distributed to the sinus and atrioventricular (AV) nodes. No parasympathetic fibers reach the ventricles. Preganglionic fibers of the sympathetic division arise from the intermediolateral nucleus of T1–T4. Postganglionic axons originate from the three cervical and the upper four to six thoracic paravertebral ganglia. These postganglionic sympathetic axons are widely distributed throughout the heart: They supply all structures that receive parasympathetic innervation plus coronary arteries and ventricular myocardial fibers. The cerebral cortex, particularly the limbic cortex, sends efferents to the vasomotor center, thereby accounting for the tachycardia associated with emotions.[10] The lat-

TABLE 36–2 Cardiovascular Autonomic Neuropathy

Clinical Evaluation
  Symptoms
  Decreased effort tolerance
  Heat intolerance
  Arrhythmias
  Orthostasis
  Signs
  Tachycardia
  Loss of sinus arrhythmia
  Orthostasis and perioperative hypotension
  Dry, scaly feet
Diagnostic Test
  Resting heart rate >100 bpm
  R-R variation >15 bpm, expiration to inspiration ratio
    <1.0
  Valsalva ratio <1.2
  30:15 ratio <1.02
  SBP fall with standing >20 mmHg
  DBP response to hand grip <16 mmHg with 30% max for
    5 min
  QTc interval >440 msec
Treatment
  Supervised exercise programs
  Care with heat exposure (i.e., hydration)
  Perioperative—informed anesthesiologist
  Scrupulous foot care
  Relaxation of diabetes control
  Manage arrhythmias
  Regulate nocturnal BP

eral adrenergic and the ventromedial nuclei of the hypothalamus may be important sensors of hypoglycemia and activation of the sympatho-adrenal response. With repeated episodes of hypoglycemia there appears to be down-regulation of autonomic responses for reasons that remain to be elucidated.

The basal heart rate is set by the chronotropic properties of the heart through its intrinsic pacemaker, the sinus node. Autonomic influences on heart rate under basal conditions, beat-to-beat variations, and changes associated with breathing are mediated by the parasympathetic system. Consequently, these variations can be abolished by atropine, but not by β-blockade. These tonic vagal impulses originate in the cardioinhibitory center in the medulla, which is formed partially by the nucleus ambiguus. Cardioinhibitory impulses also originate in the dorsal motor nucleus of the vagus and the nucleus of the tractus solitarius.

Sympathetically mediated tachycardia originates in the vasomotor center, a large diffuse area in the reticular formation of the medulla. Stimulation of its rostrolateral portions causes tachycardia and vasoconstriction. Under basal conditions there is little if any tonic discharge in the cardiac sympathetic fibers.

The earliest manifestations of impaired autonomic denervation of the heart are due to vagal denervation. Frequently, a resting tachycardia of >90–100 beats/min is observed, and more rapid rates of up to 130 may occur.[3,7,11] As the condition evolves, there is sympathetic loss resulting in a fixed, slightly elevated rate, unresponsive to maneuvers that influence it reflexively. This is similar to that following blockade with atropine and propranolol or the denervated transplanted heart.[11] Because diabetics as a group have faster heart rates than controls, resting tachycardia is not a reliable indication of autonomic neuropathy.

Cardiac Denervation Syndrome. The increased prevalence of painless myocardial infarction, coronary artery spasm, and sudden death in diabetic patients has been attributed to AN.[7,9,11] The state of nearly total cardiac denervation is indicated by a pulse rate of 80–90 beats/min that does not change with exercise, sleep, or stress.[9] Cardiac denervation has been suggested as an explanation for the increase in incidence of painless myocardial ischemia and infarction in diabetic patients, with early studies showing an incidence of 42% of painless myocardial infarction in diabetics, as compared with 6% in nondiabetics.[12] In this series, patients with silent myocardial infarction presented with symptoms of congestive heart failure (CHF), uncontrolled diabetes, hiccups, or weakness and tiredness. Moreover, painless myocardial infarction has been considered the cause of sudden death in diabetics,[3,7,11] but recent evidence suggests that adrenergic supersensitivity may be secondary to cardiac denervation as a cause for sudden death.[3] Therefore, chest pain in any location in a patient with diabetes should be considered of myocardial origin until proven otherwise.[13] Moreover, unexplained fatigue, confusion, tiredness, edema, hemoptysis, nausea and vomiting, diaphoresis, arrhythmias, cough, or dyspnea should alert one to a possible silent myocardial infarct.

Exercise-Induced Cardiovascular Responses. Usually, with exercise, cardiac sympathetic tone increases and cardiac output is augmented, while cardiac parasympathetic tone is decreased. Both the heart rate and peripheral resistance are increased so as to divert blood flow from the viscera to skeletal muscle.[9] Near the stage of exhaustion, release of epinephrine is intensified, further increasing cardiac stimulation. In diabetic AN, tolerance to exercise is limited by impairment of the sympathetic and parasympathetic functions that normally augment cardiac output and redirect peripheral blood flow to skeletal muscles.

Postural Hypotension (Fig. 36–1). When one stands, a pooling of approximately 500–700 ml of blood volume is sequestered in the lower extremities and

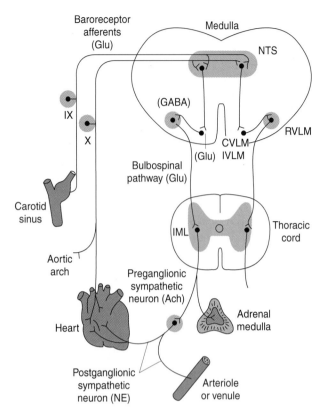

Figure 36–1. Basic autonomic pathways involved in the regulation of blood pressure. The baroreceptors are stretch receptors in the walls of the heart and blood vessels. The carotid sinus and the aortic arch receptors monitor the arterial circulation, and the receptors in the atria and the pulmonary circulation monitor the cardiopulmonary circulation. The baroreceptors are stimulated by distention structures in which they are located and discharge at an increased or decreased rate as appropriate. The afferents travel via the glossopharyngeal (IX) and vagus (X) nerves to the medulla to the nucleus of the tractus solitarius (NTS) and thence to the caudate, intermediate, and rostral ventromedulla (CVLM, IVLM, RVLM). Efferents then travel to the intermediolateral nucleus of the spinal cord and preganglionic sympathetic neurons synapse at the ganglia. Postganglionic sympathetic neurons terminate in the heart, arteriole, or adrenal medulla and are responsible for changes in heart rate, vasoconstriction, and epinephrine release, all of which are important to maintain blood pressure in the change from the horizontal to the vertical position. Not shown is the afferent vagus to the heart responsible for slowing of the heart, for example with deep breathing. Testing of the baroreceptor arc is central to evaluation of the cardiopulmonary autonomic integrity.

abdominal viscera through gravitational pull. When there is a normal baroreflex arc, this fall in blood pressure is rapidly corrected by peripheral vasoconstriction and tachycardia.[7,9,11] The consequent drop in cardiac output plus the gravitational influence on blood flow to the structures above the heart create diminished pressure levels in the blood vessels. The system that responds most rapidly to these changes in blood pressure is the arterial "baroreceptor" system, which is

induced by nerve receptors located mainly in the walls of the aorta in the chest and in the walls of the internal carotid arteries in the neck.[14]

When the baroreceptors detect a drop in arterial pressure, their firing rate decreases. The cardioinhibitory center then decreases its output of vagal impulses, permitting the unopposed influence of the previously masked sympathetic tone. At the same time, the baroreceptors influence the vasomotor center by increasing its rate of firing of sympathetic impulses. Therefore, blood pressure shifts caused by postural changes are maintained by two opposing mechanisms; first, vasomotor tone is augmented, thus increasing peripheral resistance or afterload, and second, cardiac output is increased by a faster heart rate and increases in stroke volume.[7,9,11] Furthermore, venoconstriction occurs, increasing venous return, further contributing to enhanced cardiac output.

In diabetic AN, there is interruption of the compensatory mechanisms responsible for maintaining blood pressure homeostasis. This interference causes postural hypotension. Weakness, dizziness, visual impairment, and syncope are all symptoms of postural hypotension, which is perhaps the most noticeable feature of cardiovascular AN. A decrease of 10 mmHg diastolic blood pressure or 30 mmHg systolic blood pressure when one changes from a lying to a standing position accompanied by symptoms is considered the accepted criteria for the diagnosis of postural hypotension.[3,7,9,11]

Assessment of Postural Hypotension. Two pathophysiologic states cause orthostatic hypotension: autonomic insufficiency and intravascular volume depletion. Physical examination and history should easily rule out volume depletion states.

An important point is the exclusion of contributing factors that may be aggravating or unmasking the orthostatic hypotension of diabetic AN origin. Prominent among these are volume depletion secondary to diuretics, excessive sweating, diarrhea, or polyuria. Other problems occur with antihypertensive medications, β-blockers, tricyclic antidepressants, and phenothiazines. β-blockers impair heart rate responses, and the last two act through their α-adrenergic-blocking properties impairing vasoconstriction.

Insulin therapy has been shown to aggravate the orthostatic changes. This may be mediated by mild intravascular depletion secondary to increased capillary permeability caused by insulin or by a direct effect on the neuromuscular junction. It now appears that insulin may directly stimulate endothelial release of nitric oxide (NO), a potent vasodilator, and sensitize smooth muscle to the relaxant effects of prostacyclin and NO, thereby causing vasodilatation unopposed by the action of norepinephrine. This effect, which usually occurs within 10 min following insulin administration, is progressive and may last for several hours. The similarity of the symptoms (confusion, lightheadedness, and/or syncopy) and the close relationship to insulin administration may lead to an erroneous diagnosis of hypoglycemia, but the proximity of symptoms to the injection should dispel the notion. This distinction however, may be troublesome with Humalog® insulin, which acts within 15 min (see Chapter 18).

Marked decreases in both systolic and diastolic supine blood pressure have recently been described in patients with idiopathic autonomic dysfunction following food ingestion. This effect may be mediated by release of gastrointestinal hormones, triggered by food, which may lead to sequestration of blood in the splanchnic circulation. Obviously, such changes can exaggerate orthostatic hypotension in the postprandial state. More frequent small feedings and indomethacin may ameliorate these postprandial blood pressure changes. If resistant meal-induced orthostasis occurs, this can often be relieved by octreotide treatment. This long-acting somatostatin analog redistributes blood volume between the splanchnic and systemic circulations.

Multiple tests are available for the evaluation of cardiovascular reflexes. A simple and reliable test is the variation of heart rate with respiration, termed "beat-to-beat variation." The afferent input is not clear but may be related in part to the baroreceptors. The efferent limb is parasympathetic through the vagal nerve. The absence of beat-to-beat variation in a resting diabetic patient during slow, deep respiration is highly suggestive of autonomic dysfunction.

The sustained handgrip test is an easily performed and useful test that has a high sensitivity for detection of sympathetic dysfunction in diabetic AN. An abnormal test is indicative of extensive damage to the autonomic pathways subserving the cardiovascular responses. A point of caution is that it is an effort-dependent test, and subjects must be cajoled and encouraged to exert their maximum effort. A standardized test has been described: The maximum voluntary contraction (MVC) is determined with a handgrip dynamometer. Handgrip is then maintained at 30% of maximum voluntary capacity for as long as possible to a maximum of 5 min. During this period of isometric exercise, blood pressure is recorded on the opposite nonexercising arm. The best discriminator between normal individuals and diabetics with AN is the increase in diastolic pressure. The difference between the mean of three preexercise diastolic readings and the last reading prior to release of handgrip (blood pressure readings being obtained every minute during the isometric exercise) in normal males (age 25–45) was 33 ±9 mmHg: in females, 24 ± 9 mmHg. A rise in diastolic pressure of 10 mmHg or less is considered abnormal. Presently this rest is the only simple way to evaluate for damage of the efferent sympathetic component of the baroreceptor reflex.

The Valsalva maneuver may be useful as a test of both sympathetic and parasympathetic function. This maneuver, originally described by Antonio Valsalva, a surgeon from Bologna,[15] consists of a forced expiration against a resistance that must be maintained for at least 7 sec for the normal circulatory responses to occur. During the maneuver, the heart rate is characterized by four phases. As the patient attempts to maintain a pressure of 40 mmHg while blowing into a mouthpiece connected to an aneroid manometer, the following four phases occur:

Phase 1. Increased intrathoracic pressure is transmitted to the aorta, causing a rise in arterial blood pressure by mechanical aortic compression.

Phase 2. There is a gradual decrease in systolic and diastolic pressure, secondary to a reduction in venous return. Shortly thereafter, the blood pressure reaches a nadir and then begins to return to baseline. These latter changes are due to splanchnic vasoconstriction and tachycardia generated by stimulation of the baroreceptors.

Phase 3. This is characterized by a transient fall in mean blood pressure, occurring 1–2 sec after release of the strain. It is due to the reverse of the phenomenon seen in phase 1, i.e., the release of the pressure compressing the aorta.

Phase 4. Systolic and mean blood pressure rise above the resting baseline level within 10 sec after strain release. The increasing venous return upon release of strain acting synergistically with the lingering splanchnic vasoconstriction and tachycardia of phase 2 accounts for this overshoot of the blood pressure. In response to this pressure overshoot, a reflex bradycardia is mediated by the baroreceptor mechanism (through heightened vagal efferent impulses).

Patients with autonomic neuropathy affecting the baroreceptor mechanism will show a continual downward drift of the blood pressure in phase 2 (absence of splanchnic vasoconstriction). There will be no overshoot in phase 4 (same mechanism) and no reflex bradycardia in response to the blood pressure overshoot. The problems with this test are twofold: It is effort dependent and, more importantly, in order to measure adequately the above-described phasic blood pressure changes, the test is invasive, i.e., arterial catheterization is required.

A simple evaluation of the overshoot in phase 4 of the Valsalva maneuver may be used: The patient is asked to perform the maneuver under close observation for approximately 8–10 sec. Inflation of the blood pressure cuff is started within 2–3 sec of the onset of the strain. Inflation should be completed just about the time of the release of the maneuver. The recording thereby obtained coincides with the time of occurrence of the blood pressure systolic overshoot. An intact baroreceptor is present when such overshoot compared with a baseline blood pressure systolic reading is ≥ 20 mmHg.

The Valsalva ratio test obviates the invasive component of the formal Valsalva maneuver. The heart rate is continuously monitored with an electrocardiograph while the patient performs the maneuver. The Valsalva ratio is that of the longest pulse interval after the maneuver (determined from the R-R interval) to the shortest pulse interval during the maneuver. A ratio of <1:10 is abnormal, 1:10–1:20 is borderline, and ≥1:21 is defined as normal. Although it is a simple, noninvasive test for the integrity of the baroreceptor mechanism, it may be less sensitive than the formal invasive testing and probably measures only the vagal part of the reflex. It has been shown to be very reproducible and has been used successfully to predict premature demise.[6]

This test is effort dependent and therefore subjects can cheat, but aside from this limitation, it is a useful test, being simple, easy to perform, noninvasive, and reproducible.[16] Also, the test should be avoided in patients with diabetes with proliferative retinopathy, as intraocular pressure increases during the maneuver.[15]

Another simple noninvasive test for reflex vasoconstriction is the cold pressor test: The patient is asked to immerse his or her arm in a 4°C icebath for 1 min. The response is an increase in systolic pressure of ≥15 mmHg. Recently, another simple cardiovascular test for diagnosis of diabetic AN (standing-to-lying heart rate variation) has been described. The test is usually done in combination with tests for orthostasis when supine and erect catecholamines are measured. This is particularly useful to distinguish degrees of sympathetic nerve dysfunction for example, the modest reduction in catecholamines in Shy Drager syndrome (MSA), and diabetic DAN and the severe reduction with idiopathic orthostatic hypotension (IOH) accompanying pure autonomic failure. More recently, Goldstein et al.[17] have proposed a classification based upon 6-[18F] fluorodopamine positron emission tomography and neurochemical analysis that allows clearer distinction between central and peripheral sympathetic and parasympathetic dysfunction.[18]

Gastrointestinal Disorders

Gastrointestinal complaints are prevalent among diabetic patients. These complaints often reflect diabetic gastrointestinal AN, and even though the entire gastrointestinal tract may be involved with generally hypotonic and poorly contractile smooth muscle, the patient is often asymptomatic.[9,11] Parasympathetic, sympathetic, and afferent sensory fibers innervate the gastrointestinal tract, but the relative role of damage to these innervations is not clearly understood.

The gastrointestinal manifestations of diabetic AN are diverse (Table 36–3). Therefore, symptoms and pathogenic mechanisms can be categorized according to which section of the gastrointestinal tract is affected.

TABLE 36–3   Summary of Manifestations of Autonomic Gastrointestinal Dysfunction in Diabetes

Esophageal enteropathy
   Disordered peristalsis
   Abnormal lower esophageal sphincter function
Gastroparesis diabeticorum
   Nonobstructive impairment of gastric propulsive activity, brady/tachygastria, pylorospasm
Diarrhea
   Impaired motility—bacterial overgrowth syndrome
   Increased motility and secretory activity (choleretic diarrhea)
Constipation
   Decreased or absent gastrocolic reflex
Fecal incontinence
   Abnormal internal anal sphincter tone
   Impaired rectal sensation
   Abnormal external sphincter
   Gallbladder atony and enlargement

Esophageal Atony.   Esophageal immotility is well recognized, but symptoms such as inability to swallow (dysphagia), retrosternal discomfort, and heartburn are uncommon.[11] Manometry shows the absence of normal interdigestive motor cycles in the stomach with antral hypermotility after indigestion of a solid meal.[19] These motility changes are similar to that following vagal section in animals and consistent with vagal neuropathy. Often this is discovered accidentally with barium esophageal swallows. Recently developed radionucleotide diagnostic techniques that are more sensitive and less invasive than manometry may reveal a greater prevalence of esophageal motor dysfunction.[9] Damage to preganglionic fibers rather than the myenteric plexus has been implicated because of lack of denervation hypersensitivity.[11] If disordered motility or lower esophageal sphincter flaccidity can be demonstrated, the symptoms may subside when treated with a dopamine antagonist.[9] Recognition of esophageal dysfunction is becoming increasingly important, especially with drugs that have the potential to cause esophageal erosion and performation with dire consequences, e.g, the oral bisphosphonates.

Gastroparesis Diabeticorum.   Diabetic AN can impair gastric acid secretion and gastrointestinal motility. Impairment of gastric acid secretion may be due to vagal damage since normal secretory response is produced by direct parietal-cell stimulation.[9] This reduction in acid secretion leads to elevation of gastrin that in time can stimulate proliferation of enterochromaffin (EC) cells to form the "gastric carcinoid." This presents with gastric polyps and bleeding from the gastrointestinal tract and causes dyspepsia. The condition has been referred to as *"diabetic pseudogastrinoma syndrome"* (gut hormones in diabetic autonomic neuropathy).[20]

When gastric dysmotility is present, the patient may be anorexic and may experience vague upper abdominal fullness soon after eating, vomiting, and early satiety. Furthermore, a gastric splash may be present upon physical examination. The patient may have frequent hypoglycemic episodes that make diabetes control more difficult and lead to weight loss.

Disorders that can mimic diabetic gastroparesis include peptic ulcer disease, gastritis, gastric carcinoma, and ingestion of anticholinergic agents. Therefore, a careful history, including medications (ganglionic blockers and psychotropic drugs), is imperative.

Gastric emptying can be assessed either by the standard method of barium-meal radiography or by the more sensitive radionuclide techniques,[9] which distinguish between solid-phase and liquid-phase emptying disorders. Furthermore, gastroduodenoscopy should be performed to exclude pyloric obstruction or other mechanical causes of obstruction.

It is of interest to note that about 60% of patients attending a diabetes clinic have symptoms of gastroparesis, but only rarely is gastroparesis found (less than 10%). Paradoxically, as many as 25% of asymptomatic patients with diabetes have been found to have some degree of gastroparesis with sophisticated testing.[4]

Treatment should stress improvement of glycemic control and correction of other metabolic abnormalities. It also includes dietary modification (small, low–fat, and/or liquid meals), gastric suction, metoclopramide (5–20 mg every 6-8 hr by IV or oral suspension), domperidone (10–20 mg every 1/2 hr before meals and at bedtime), cisapride (10–20 mg 1/2 hr before meals), bethanechol (10–20 mg every 6–8 hr), or the antibiotic erythromycin (250 mg 1/2 hr before meals). In some severe cases, jejunostomy may be needed to provide for feeding and resting the stomach until such time that it recovers its function.

Colonic Atony and Diabetic Constipation/Diarrhea Syndromes.
Constipation is the most frequent gastrointestinal symptom in diabetic AN, occurring in >60% of patients.[9] It may be associated with atony of the large bowel and rectum and sometimes with megacolon.[11] Other patients suffer from diabetic diarrhea and some have alternating bouts of constipation and diarrhea.[9]

The symptoms of diabetic diarrhea are characteristic, with intermittent episodes lasting from hours to days. The patient may have nocturnal diarrhea and fecal incontinence, expelling more than 300 g of stool,[9] and may have as many as 20–30 bowel movements in 24 hr.[9,11] Diarrhea may result from intestinal hypermotility due to diminished sympathetic inhibition, hypomotility with bacterial overgrowth, pancreatic insufficiency, steatorrhea with a mucosal histologic pattern ("*diabetic sprue*"), or bile-salt malabsorption.[9,19]

After exclusion of other possible causes of diarrhea (drugs, celiac disease, colitis, tumor), therapy may require polypharmacy to achieve relief. Codeine phosphate and loperamide should be avoided.[19] If acute and severe, fluids and electrolytes should be prescribed. It is important to recognize that stasis is the major problem and that diarrhea is generally a consequence of the stasis, bacterial overgrowth, malabsorption, and bile-induced electrolyte secretion and loss. Even though the resulting bile-salt malabsorption can contribute to diabetic diarrhea, there is no evidence that gallbladder atony predisposes to gallstones.[9,11] The first line should be to drive the bowel, e.g., with propulsid 10 mg q 4-6h. This is better than metaclopramide since it targets the large intestine. The patient should be warned that diarrhea will initially worsen.

Bacterial overgrowth can be treated with a 3-week course of metronidazole (250 mg t.i.d.). The intestinal disorder together with its treatment can raise blood glucose levels; therefore, close monitoring should be enforced.

Urogenital System Disorders

Bladder Atony. Sympathetic, parasympathetic, and somatic fibers enervate the normal bladder. Parasympathetic nerve fibers are responsible for maintaining contraction of the bladder fundus during urination, while the involuntary relaxation of the internal urethral sphincter and the trigone is controlled by sympathetic fibers. Voluntary control of the bladder is provided by somatic pudendal innervation of the external sphincter through sacral segments S2-4.

In diabetic AN, the motor function of the bladder is unimpaired, but afferent fiber damage results in diminished bladder sensation. Damage to parasympathetic innervation results in decreased tone and weakness of the detrusor urinae, and loss of sympathetic innervation of the internal urethral sphincter and the trigone causes sphincter dysfunction.[9,11] The urinary bladder can be enlarged to more than three times its normal size.[11] Patients are seen with bladders filled to their umbilicus, yet they feel no discomfort.

Loss of bladder sensation occurs early with diminished voiding frequency, and the patient is no longer able to void completely. Consequently, dribbling and overflow incontinence are common complaints.[9] Because of residual urine (greater than 150 mL), there is a predisposition to recurrent urinary tract infections.

Sexual Dysfunction. The prevalence of sexual dysfunction is about 50% in diabetic males and about 30% in women,[9,11] but limitations in assessing female sexual dysfunction may be the cause for the sex-related difference.

Neuropathy can produce loss of penile erection or retrograde ejaculation, or both, in diabetic men, while libido, potency, and orgasmic function are normal.

Retrograde ejaculation is caused by damage to efferent sympathetic innervation, which coordinates the simultaneous closure of the internal vesicle sphincter and relaxation of the external vesicle sphincter during ejaculation. Lack of spermatozoa in the semen and presence of motile sperm in a postcoital specimen of urine confirm the diagnosis.[9]

Neurogenic erectile impotence is the most common form of organic sexual dysfunction in diabetic men, but impotence may have causes other than AN, and so it should be attributable to diabetes only if the possibility of other causes has been excluded. Impotence due to AN has a gradual onset with progression to complete impotence over a period of 6 months to 2 years.[11] Organic impotence can be confirmed by the documentation, in a sleep laboratory, of penile tumescence and erection during rapid eye movement (REMs) sleep. The absence of erections during REMs sleep would confirm organic impotence.

There is no evidence that endocrine dysfunction contributes to organic impotence,[9,11] but vascular insufficiency has been reported as a cause of impotence in diabetic patients.[9] Penile vascular insufficiency can be assessed by direct measurement of penile blood pressure with a Doppler monitor, and, if confirmed, vascular insufficiency might be surgically correctable[9] (see Chapter 25).

Viagra is a GMP type 5 phosphodiesterase inhibitor that enhances blood flow to the corpora cavernousae with sexual stimulation. It is effective in diabetic men about 40–50% of the time. *Before it is prescribed, it is important to exclude ischemic heart disease. It is absolutely contraindicated in patients being treated with nitroglycerine or other nitrate-containig drugs.* Direct injection of prostacyclin[21] into the corpus cavernosum will induce satisfactory erections in a significant number of men.[19] Also, surgical implantation of a penile prosthesis may be appropriate. The less expensive type of prosthesis is a semirigid, permanently erect type that may be embarrassing and uncomfortable for some patients. The inflatable type is three times more expensive and subject to mechanical failure,[9] but it avoids the embarrassment caused by other devices. Therefore, it is important to begin treatment with a detailed assessment of the patient's sexual attitudes and lifestyle.

Metabolic Dysfunction

Hypoglycemia Unawareness (Table 36–4). Blood glucose concentration is normally maintained during starvation or increased insulin action by an asymptomatic parasympathetic response with bradycardia and mild hypotension, followed by a sympathetic response with glucagon and epinephrine secretion for short-term glucose counterregulation and growth hormone and cortisol in long-term regulation.[22] The release of catecholamines alerts the patient to take the required mea-

TABLE 36–4 Hypoglycemia Unawareness and Unresponsiveness

Clinical Evaluation
  Symptoms
  Hyperadrenergic
  Palpitation, tremor, anxiety, diaphoresis, irritability
  Neuroglycopenic
  Headache, dizziness, tingling, hunger, blurred vision, difficulty thinking, faintness
  Signs
  Convulsions, loss of consciousness
Diagnostic Test
  Insulin infusion test (overnight normalization of plasma glucose, insulin 0.67 mU/kg/min, plasma glucose 2.0 mmol/L ± neuroglycopenia)
  Stepped hypoglycemic clamp (insulin 1.0 mU/kg/min, glucose level of 5.0, 4.4, 3.9, 2.8, and 2.2 mmol/L)
Treatment
  "Attentive" avoidance of hypoglycemia
  Less stringent glucose control

sures to prevent coma due to low blood glucose. The absence of warning signs of impending neuroglycopenia[15] is known as "*hypoglycemic unawareness.*" The failure of glucose counterregulation can be confirmed by the absence of glucagon and epinephrine responses to hypoglycemia induced by a standard, controlled dose of insulin.[9,22] See Chapter 21.

In patients with type 1 diabetes, the glucagon response is impaired with diabetes duration of 1–5 years, and after 14–31 years of diabetes, the glucagon response is almost undetectable.[9,11] It is not present in those with AN. However, a syndrome of hypoglycemic autonomic failure occurs with intensification of diabetes control and repeated episodes of hypoglycemia.[23] The exact mechanism is not understood, but it does represent a real barrier to physiologic glycemic control.

Pupillary Abnormalities

Normally, sympathetic stimulation dilates the ocular pupil, and parasympathetic stimulation constricts it. Patients with diabetic AN show delayed or absent reflex response to light and diminished hippus,[11] accounted for by decreased sympathetic activity[9] and a reduced resting pupillary diameter.[11]

Distal Autonomic Function Disturbance

Sudomotor Dysfunction. Sudomotor activity is influenced reflexively by changes in skin temperature and directly by central hypothalamic receptors that monitor body core temperature.[11] Diabetic autonomic sudomotor dysfunction can be manifested by distal anhidrosis (diminished or absent sweating) following damage to sympathetic innervation of eccrine glands. The anhidrosis usually has a patchy distribution over the lower extremity that diminishes thermoregulatory reserve and, in severe cases, may involve the lower trunk and arms. Loss of lower body sweating can lead to dry, brittle skin that cracks easily and predisposes to ulcer formation. Although clinical evaluation is usually sufficient, impaired sweating may be evaluated using simple starch, iodine, or more sophisticated measurements of iontophoresis and by electromyographic evaluation of small nerve fiber function.

The characteristic distal and symmetrical pattern of diabetic autonomic sudomotor dysfunction suggests a pathogenic relation to distal symmetrical somatic polyneuropathy, which is also present at time of diagnosis. It has been suggested that the reason for this relationship is that the damage to sympathetic innervation of the sweat glands is localized to postganglionic fibers,[11] that accompany peripheral nerves. Hyperhidrosis (compensatory sweating) of the trunk and face is also present following decreased ability of the lower extremities to dissipate heat.

QSART, sweat beads, and thermoregulatory control are tests that have proved, useful in evaluating sweat gland function. During the test a slain thermistor probe is attached to the dorsum of the left foot at midfoot level, and the foot is warmed to 31°C using an infrared lamp. Four sites on the foot are studied with the patient supine.

Sweat beads count the number of sweat glands that are innervated. This test is qualitative rather than quantitative, although the number of glands can be used as a quantitative index. Thermoregulatory control evaluates the amount of surface area that does not sweat after standard heating. It is less precise than the previous two tests.

An uncommon symptom of sudomotor dysfunction is *gustatory sweating* within seconds of eating a particular food.[9,11] There is no current medication available to treat this problem, but symptomatic relief can be obtained by avoiding the specific inciting food, and some people have received benefit from a scopolamine patch placed behind the ear.

Alterations in Cutaneous Blood Flow. Microvascular insufficiency has been proposed as a cause of diabetic neuropathy by several research teams.[24–27] Studies have suggested that absolute or relative ischemia may exist in the nerves of patients with diabetes secondary to altered function of the endoneural and/or epineural blood vessels. Furthermore, histopathologic studies have shown the presence of different degrees of endoneurial and epineurial microvasculopathy, mainly thickening of the blood vessel wall or occlusion.[25,28,29] Several functional disturbances are found in the microvasculature of the nerves of diabetic subjects.[24] These disturbances include decreased neural blood flow,[30] increased vascular resistance,[31] decreased pO_2,[31,32] and altered vascular permeability. The decrease in neural blood flow and increased vascular resistance could result from changes in microvascular reactivity, such as impaired dilator responses for substance P, calcitonin gene-related peptide, and reactive hyperemia.

Microvascular skin flow is under the control of the ANS and is regulated by both the central and peripheral components of the ANS. In a recent study, it was shown that vasomotion, the rhythmic contraction of arterioles and small arteries, is disordered in diabetes.[24,33] Microvascular blood flow can be accurately measured noninvasively using laser Doppler flowmetry (Fig. 36–2). Smooth muscle microvasculature in the periphery reacts sympathetically to a number of stressor tasks. These may be divided into those dependent upon the integrity of the central nervous system (orienting response and mental arithmetic) and those dependent upon the distal sympathetic axonal response (handgrip and cold presser tests).

At present there are no therapeutic interventions that specifically reverse autonomically mediated abnormalities in microvascular blood flow.

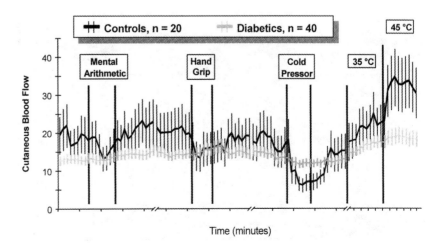

Figure 36–2. Skin blood flow measured from the index finger in diabetic (shaded line) and age-matched healthy subjects (solid line). (From Stansberry et al: Diabetes Care 20:1711–1716, 1997.) What is important to note is that the abnormalities in blood flow to the pulpar surface of the fingers are under the control of the adrenergic nervous system and that this may be the first detectable abnormality in peripheral autonomic function. Impairment of cutaneous blood flow reduces the delivery of important nutrients to the skin and is the precursor of the ulcer and infection with subsequent gangrene.

Differential Diagnosis

The differential diagnosis of AN includes idiopathic orthostatic hypotension, Shy-Drager syndrome (orthostatic hypotension, pyramidal and cerebellar signs including tremor, rigidity, hyperreflexia, ataxia, and urinary and bowel dysfunction), panhypopituitarism, pheochromocytoma, hypovolemia (due to poor glycemic control or diuretics), and medications such as insulin, vasodilators (nitrates, calcium channel blockers, hydralazine), and sympathetic blockers (methyldopa, clonidine, prazosin, guanethidine, phenothiazine, tricyclic antidepressants). Alcoholic neuropathy may also cause orthostatic hypotension.

A careful history for diabetes, cancer, drugs, alcohol, HIV, family history for familial amyloidosis and travel history to South America and exposure to Trypanosoma cruzi (Chagas disease), medication review, and clinical evaluation and physical examination will usually rule out other conditions. Norepinephrine responses to hypoglycemia may be of value in idiopathic orthostatic hypotension as well as Shy–Drager syndrome, and screens for heavy metals, as well as serologic tests for Chagas disease, may be helpful. The diagnosis of diabetic AN is thus one of exclusion.[4]

References

1. Vinik AI, Mitchell BD, Leichter SB, et al.: Epidemiology of the complications of diabetes. In Diabetes: Clinical Science in Practice. Leslie RDG, Robbins DC, (eds): Cambridge: Cambridge University Press, 1995, pp. 221–287.

2. Vinik AI, Zola BE: The effects of diabetic autonomic neuropathy on the cardiovascular system: New horizons in diabetes mellitus and cardiovascular disease. In Marteke VJ (ed): Current Science. Delran, NJ: Weekly Reader Corporation, 1995, pp. 159–171.

3. Vinik AI, Holland MT, Le Beau JM, et al.: Diabetic neuropathies. Diabetes Care 15(12):1926–1975, 1992.

4. Vinik AI, Suwanwalaikorn S: Autonomic neuropathy. In deFronzo R (ed): Current Therapy of Diabetes Mellitus. St. Louis, MO: Mosby-Year Book, 1997, pp. 165–176.

5. Maser R, Pfeifer M, Dorman J: Diabetic autonomic neuropathy and cardiovascular risk. Arch Intern Med 150:1218–1222, 1990.

6. Levitt NS, Stansberry KB, Wynchanck S, et al.: Natural progression of autonomic neuropathy and autonomic function tests in a cohort of people with IDDM. Diabetes Care 19(7):751–754, 1996.

7. Ewing DJ, Campbell IW, Clarke BF: Assessment of cardiovascular effects in diabetic autonomic neuropathy and prognostic implications. Ann Intern Med 92:308–311, 1980.

8. Abraham RR, Levy DM: Diabetic neuropathy: Measurement and quantitation. In Goto Y, War J (eds): Diabetic Neuropathy. Wiley, 1990, pp. 259–268.

9. Greene DA, Pfeifer MA: Diabetic neuropathy. In Olefsky JM, Sherwin RS, (eds): Diabetes Mellitus: Management and Complications. New York: Churchill Livingston, 1985, pp. 223–254.

10. Guyton AC: Rhythmic excitation of the heart. In Guyton AC (ed): Textbook of Medical Physiology, 6 ed. Philadelphia: W.B. Saunders, 1981, pp. 165–175.

11. Clarke BF, Ewing DJ, Campbell IW: Diabetic autonomic neuropathy. Diabetologia 17:195–212, 1979.

12. Bradley R, Schonfeld A: Diminished pain in diabetic patients with acute myocardial infarction. Geriatrics 17:322–326, 1962.

13. Cohen S, Snape W: Movement of the small intestine and large bowel. In Sleisinger M, Fordtram J (eds): Gastrointestinal Disease, 3 ed. Philadelphia: W.B. Saunders, 1983, pp. 859–871.

14. Guyton AC: Blood pressure control: Special role of the kidneys and body fluids. Science 1813–1816, 1991.

15. Glass LC: A study of nerve function in diabetes mellitus and normal individuals. Biology. 1992; University of Miami. BS.

16. Clarke B, Ewing D, Campbell I: Diabetic autonomic neuropathy. Diabetologia 17:195–212, 1979.

17. Goldstein DS, Holmes C, Cannon RO, et al.: Sympathetic cardioneuropathy in dysautonomias. New Engl J Med 336(10):696–702,

18. Mathias CJ: Autonomic disorders and their recognition. Editorial. New Engl J Med 336(10):721–724,

19. Ward JD: Clinical features of diabetic peripheral neuropathies. In War J, Goto Y (eds): Diabetic Neuropathy. Wiley, 1990, pp. 281–296.

20. Vinik AI, Glowniak J: Hormonal secretion in diabetic autonomic neuropathy. NY State J Med 82:871–886, 1982.

21. Vinik AI, Richardson DW: Erectile dysfunction in diabetes. Clinical Diabetes 14(5):111–120, Sept/Oct 1996.

22. Havel PJ, Taborsky GJ Jr: The contribution of the autonomic nervous system to changes of glucagon and insulin secretion during hypoglycemic stress. Endocrine Rev 10:332–350, 1989.

23. Cryer PE, Binder C, Bolli GB, et al.: Hypoglycemia in insulin dependent diabetes mellitus. Diabetes 38: 1193–1199, 1989.

24. Vinik AI, Milicevic Z: Recent advances in the diagnosis and treatment of diabetic neuropathy. Endocrinologist 6(6):443–461, 1996.

25. Malik RA, Newrick PG, Sharma AK, et al.: Microangiopathy in human diabetic neuropathy: Relationship between capillary abnormalities and the severity of neuropathy. Diabetologia 32:92–102, 1989.

26. Dyck PJ, Hansen S, Karnes J, et al.: Capillary number and percentage closed in human diabetic sural nerve. Proc Natl Acad Sci USA 82:2513–2517, 1985.

27. Low P, Lagerlund T, McManis P: Nerve blood flow and oxygen delivery in normal, diabetic, and ischemic neuropathy. Int Rev Neurobiol 31:355–438, 1989.

28. Powell H, Rosoff J, Myers R: Microangiopathy in human diabetic neuropathy. Acta Neuropathol (Berl) 68:295–303, 1985.

29. Yasuda H, Dyck PJ: Abnormalities of endoneurial microvessels and sural nerve pathology in diabetic neuropathy. Neurology 37:20–28, 1987.

30. Tuck RR, Schmelzer JD, Low PA: Endoneurial blood flow and oxygen tension in the sciatic nerves of rats with experimental diabetic neuropathy. Brain 107:935–950, 1984.

31. Newrick PG, Wilson AJ, Jakubowski J, et al.: Sural nerve oxygen tension in diabetes. Br Med J 293:1053–1054, 1986.

32. Zochodne DW, Ho LT: Normal blood flow but lower oxygen tension in diabetes of young rats: Microenvironment and the influence of sympathectomy. Can J Physiol Pharmacol 70:651–659, 1992.

33. Stansberry KB, Shapiro SA, Hill M, et al.: Impaired peripheral vasomotion in diabetes. Diabetes Care 19(7):715–721, 1996.

37

Bone, Joint, Tendon, and Muscle Problems in Diabetes

W. Hayes Wilson and C.H. Wilson, Jr.*

Historical Perspective

An association between diabetes mellitus and gouty arthritis has been suggested since the 18th century, although a direct link has not been confirmed. Other diabetic conditions, described in the 1800s, merit clear distinction from systemic collagen vascular diseases. Scleredema was first described in 1861 by Arning,[1] and by Piffard in 1871[2]; however, it was not until 1902 that Buschke clearly described scleredema,[3] which was later distinguished from scleroderma in 1967 by Holubar and Mach.[4] In 1932, Davis et al. reported an association between Dupuytren's contractures and diabetes mellitus.[5] In 1936, Jordon first described the association of diabetes mellitus with the neuropathic joint.[6] More than a decade later, in 1950, Forestier and Rotes Querol[7] described a distinct type of ankylosing hyperostosis of the anterior longitudinal ligaments of the spine. By 1954 an association between diabetes mellitus and hyperostotic spondylosis was recognized and was later confirmed by Harris et al.[8] in 1974. Lundbeck[9] described hand stiffness in young patients with diabetes in 1957; since that time Rosenbloom et al.[10] have described limited joint mobility in large cohorts of young patients. Although associations have been noted between diabetes mellitus and collagen vascular/musculoskeletal disease for more than a century, it was not until the last two or three decades that we have come to understand and appreciate the significance of these associations.

Pathophysiology

A combination of pathophysiologic changes are responsible for the articular and periarticular abnormalities found in patients with diabetes mellitus. As discussed in Chapters 25, 30, 35, and 36, significant vascular changes and microvascular changes are key components of not only visceral pathology but also neurologic and musculoskeletal pathology (see Chapters 31, 32, 33, and 34). Clearly, neuropathic changes are responsible

for Charcot joints and diabetic feet. In addition, there are increased amounts of type III collagen identified in the palmar fascia of patients with Dupuytren's disease (DD) and particularly in the nodular tissue. This active deposition of connective tissue is due to myofibroblasts, which are also noted with proliferation of fibroblasts in adhesive capsulitis (frozen shoulder) and hip capsulitis. A defect in microcirculation is likely to be the common denominator between patients with limited joint mobility from diabetes mellitus as well as limited joint mobility associated with hypertension and patients with scleroderma. There may be localized deposition of excess connective tissue in the flexor tendon sheath of fingers of patients with diabetes mellitus causing painful "triggering." This is often associated with a palpable nodule over the flexor tendon. The term *"tenosynoviosclerosis"* has been used to describe this as inflammatory changes in the tendon sheath.

Problem Statement

One of the challenges in attempting to understand the musculoskeletal manifestations of diabetes is that the nomenclature is often unclear and overlapping. Particularly confusing is the terminology describing abnormalities of the upper extremity, *diabetic hand, diabetic shoulder-hand syndrome, stiff hand syndrome, and limited joint mobility.* One reason for this lack of clarity is that there are common pathophysiologic changes that are manifested in varying degrees and in various components of the connective tissues. Also, because of common pathophysiology a simultaneous occurrence of more than one condition is frequently present in any one patient (e.g., carpal tunnel syndrome and DD).

The following discussion attempts to sort out and explain some key differences and similarities of the various syndromes, as well as compare and contrast similar problems in the nondiabetic population. The discussion will begin with a general overview of the approach to evaluation of musculoskeletal complaints, followed by disease or syndrome specific discussions.

*Deceased

Subjective

Subjective complaints involving the bones, joints, tendons, and muscles most often include complaints of pain. It is important in patients with diabetes mellitus to frame these complaints in an overall picture that focuses on the whole patient and not just one confined area. The reason for this approach is that, as mentioned earlier, the pathophysiologic process is similar all over the body. It is equally as important to investigate neuropathic symptoms such as anesthesia as well as pain. We are concerned about the time the pain has been present (hours, days, weeks, months, years) and whether the pain is constant or intermittent. What is the quality of the pain (sharp, dull, burning, tingling), and does it radiate or are there radicular type symptoms? The intensity of the pain can be graded on a scale of 0–10, with 0 being no pain at all and 10 being the worst possible pain. Ameliorating and exacerbating factors are helpful. For instance, in the case of crystalline arthritis there is often an indiscretion with alcohol that precedes an episode of gout. We can further categorize musculoskeletal complications of diabetes regionally, meaning that oftentimes the complications are predominantly in the hands, such as in DD, or confined to the hand and shoulder, as in shoulder-hand syndrome. Certainly there are more diffuse musculoskeletal syndromes such as osteoarthritis and rheumatoid arthritis that may, debatably, have some unique attributes in the diabetic patient.

For purposes of illustration and discussion, emphasis will be directed not only on structure (bones, joints, tendons, and muscles), but also location. Location helps frame the investigation in the diabetic patient.

EXHIBIT 37–1   Bone, Joint, Tendon, and Muscle Problems Associated with Diabetes

Bone
  Osteoporosis
  Diabetic osteoarthropathy
  Diffuse idiopathic skeletal hyperostosis (DISH)
Joint
  Neuroarthropathy (Charcot's joint)
  Stiff hand syndrome
  Limited joint mobility (LJM)
  Adhesive capsulitis (frozen shoulder)
  Shoulder-hand syndrome/reflex sympathetic
    dystrophy (RSD)
  Osteoarthritis
  Gout/pseudogout
  Carpal tunnel syndrome (diabetic hand)
Tendon
  Flexor tenosynovitis
  Dupuytren's disease
Muscle
  Fibromyalgia
Skin
  Scleredema diabeticorum

Exhibit 37–1 illustrates the different musculoskeletal problems in diabetes by structure; Exhibit 37–2 categorizes them by region. The regions can be thought of as upper extremity, lower extremity, and diffuse or axial complaints. In assessing the patient the clinician may find that the patient is most concerned about one specific area when in fact the problem is more diffuse (e.g., Charcot's joint with more widespread neuropathy). For this reason there will inevitably be some overlap.

EXHIBIT 37–2   Regional Approach to Connective Tissue Manifestations of Diabetes Mellitus

	Unique to Diabetes	Common in Diabetes
Upper Extremity		
Shoulder		
Adhesive capsulitis		X
Shoulder-hand syndrome		X
Hand and Wrist		
Stiff hand syndrome	X (type 1)	
Limited joint mobility	X	
Dupuytren's disease		X
Flexor tenosynovitis		X (type 1)
Carpal tunnel syndrome		X
Lower Extremity		
Neuroarthopathy/Charcot's joint		X
Forefoot osteolysis	X	
Diffuse/Axial		
Diffuse idiopathic skeletal hyperostosis (DISH)		X (type 2)
Osteoporosis		X (type 1)
Scleredema diabeticorum	X	

Adapted from Kaye T: Watching for and managing musculoskeletal problems in diabetes. J Musculoskel Med 11(9):24–37, 1994.

Objective

Initial inspection can reveal a great deal about a patient. It begins with watching the patient walk and observing any gait abnormalities. With the patient properly draped, the examiner can look for asymmetry, muscle wasting, redness, warmth, or swelling. Loss of hair over the extremity may be a clue to vascular disease that coexists with musculoskeletal and neuropathic problems. Muscle wasting may be readily apparent or subtle. A thorough neurologic examination is important (details on this are found in Chapters 35 and 36). Range of motion is important to assess, particularly in the shoulders and hands, as they have a predilection for contracture. Asking a patient to place both palms together as tightly as possible may reveal a "prayer sign" (Figure 37–1), which indicates that there are flexion contractures at the metacarpophalangeal and proximal interphalangeal (PIP) joints characteristic of limited joint mobility (LJM).

The Upper Extremity

Pain in the Shoulder

Adhesive Capsulitis/Frozen Shoulder. One cause of painful shoulder in patients with diabetes mellitus is rotator cuff dysfunction with a "frozen shoulder," also known as adhesive capsulitis or calcific periarthritis. This is characterized by an extreme limitation of motion,

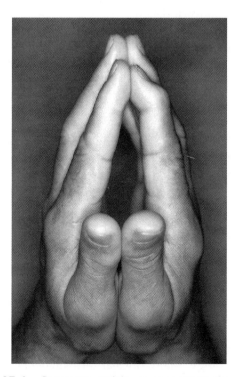

Figure 37–1. Prayer sign, inability to approximate the palmar surfaces, indicative of limited joint mobility.

which is frequently self-limited. In a review of the medical records of 800 diabetics, Bridgeman[11] found evidence of adhesive capsulitis in 11% of patients. This number is nearly five times the incidence in the nondiabetic control group. Connally et al.[12] have noted that diabetics have an eight times greater incidence of bilateral adhesive capsulitis than controls. With this statistic, patients with adhesive capsulitis, and no other obvious cause, should be checked for diabetes, particularly if the adhesive capsulitis is bilateral.

Adhesive capsulitis is found more commonly in the nondominant extremity, in women, and in individuals over 40 years of age.[12] Patients complain of gradual onset of pain, with progressive loss of range of motion. The pathologic process is not well understood; however, capsular fibrosis and thickening have been found.[13] This is usually treated with physical therapy, heat, range of motion, ultrasound, and sometimes local corticosteroid injection. In one study intraarticular injection and exercise were the most efficacious treatment.[14] Left untreated adhesive capsulitis may progress to near total immobility.

Diabetic Shoulder-Hand Syndrome. In the case of the painful shoulder it is important to explore events leading up to and preceding the onset of pain. As noted earlier, the classic presentation of adhesive capsulitis is thickening of the joint capsule with adhesion and loss of volume. In diabetes, adhesive capsulitis has a rarer but finite association with swelling, erythema, tenderness, decreased temperature, and hyperhidrosis of the hand, consistent with reflex sympathetic dystrophy (RSD). Adhesive capsulitis may precede, accompany, or follow diabetic shoulder-hand syndrome, referred to as RSD or as Sudek's dystrophy. The symptoms of RSD have three phases. Initially there is a hyperemic and swollen phase. The second phase includes loss of range of motion and often a waxy appearance to the skin. The third phase has atrophy and loss of function of the limb. In a period of weeks to months the symptoms usually resolve; however, they may persist and be accompanied by frozen shoulder, atrophy of the shoulder muscles, and osteoporotic changes of the hand and shoulder.[15] In fact, studies indicate that frozen shoulder is common in diabetes but that RSD is rare.[16]

Physical therapy is helpful in treating RSD, specifically for mobilization of the limb to preserve function and range of motion. Other measures include stellate ganglion block or intravenous guanethidine blockade.

The Hand

Limited Joint Mobility. Dr. Arlan Rosenbloom was the first to describe the syndrome of LJM, and he has described the key differences between the abnormalities associated with the diabetic hand (see Exhibit 37–3). The initial observation was limitation of flexion and

EXHIBIT 37–3   Differential Diagnosis in the Diabetic Hand

Condition	Association with Diabetes	Involvement	Comments
Shoulder-hand syndrome (reflex dystrophy)	10–20% of older patients with IDDM/NIDDM have frozen shoulder, few have SHS	All fingers	Severe pain and muscle atrophy
Limited joint mobility	Exclusively; 25–50% IDDM (greatest over 5 yr duration, postpubertal); 25–75% NIDDM	Starts in fifth digits, extends radially; wrist and elbow, rarely knee	Painless, muscles and nerves normal
Stiff hand syndrome	Exclusively with diabetes; rare; IDDM >20 years	All fingers	Painful, paresthesia but normal vibratory and tactile sense
Dupuytren's disease	40% over age 40; 16% present at time of diagnosis	Third and fourth digits	Painless, muscles normal
Flexor tenosynovitis	One-third associated with diabetes, predominantly female	First, third, and fourth digits	Painful, muscles and nerves normal
Carpal tunnel syndrome (diabetic hand)	5–16% due to diabetes	All fingers	Ulnar as well as median nerve conduction delay, intrinsic and thenar muscle atrophy

Adapted from Ref. 34 and from Rosenbloom AL: Skeletal and joint manifestations of childhood diabetes. Ped Clin N Amer 31:572, 1984.

extension of the interphalangeal, metacarpophalangeal, and wrist joints, in association with short stature, thick waxy skin, delayed sexual maturations and early microvascular complications.[17] Reported prevalence in various studies is 8–55% among insulin-dependent diabetic patients. In one large study of 309 patients, ages 1–28 years, 30% had contractures and one-third had dermal sclerosis.[10] LJM is more closely linked to attained age than to duration of diabetes or to age of onset of diabetes.[18] After the detection of mild LJM there is a range of 3 months to 4 years before the onset of moderate to severe changes, and mild changes often persist. After 5 years duration, half of young patients with diabetes will have moderate to severe limitation. LJM is not limited to children and young adults with insulin-dependent diabetes mellitus (IDDM), but is found also in adult-onset IDDM and non-insulin-dependent diabetes mellitus (NIDDM).[19] The fact that as much as 20% of the nondiabetic population may have finger contractures due to age related conditions, such as osteoarthritis, confounds somewhat the estimate of LJM in the adult population. In children, however, it is uncommon to see finger contractures without diabetes.

In fact, LJM is not confined to the hand but may also involve larger joints, including the wrists, elbows, ankles, and cervical and thoracolumbar spine. The changes are painless and therefore the impairment is loss of function resulting from lost range of motion. The significance of LJM is less related to the effect on function and more related to its association with microvascular complications.[10] In a study of 169 patients LJM was associated with an 83% risk of retinopathy and nephropathy after 16 years of diabetes, whereas the risk was 25% in the absence of LJM.[10] LJM has been associated with a 4.3-fold relative risk of clinical neuropathy in IDDM.[19]

In the differential diagnosis of the diabetic hand are DD, carpal tunnel syndrome, flexor tenosynovitis, stiff hand syndrome, LJM, and diabetic shoulder-hand syndrome (reflex sympathetic dystrophy). There are distinct differences that separate these conditions, although more than one may coexist in the same patient. One distinguishing characteristic is pain/paresthesia that occurs in all of the conditions associated with the diabetic hand except for LJM and DD, which are painless. LJM involves the fifth digit and extends radially, while DD involves the third and forth digits and is associated with palmar fascia thickening and nodules. As described earlier, LJM characteristically occurs in children, while DD does not.

Stiff Hand Syndrome.   Stiff hand syndrome was first described by Lundbaek in 1957 in five patients with long-standing IDDM.[9] The initial description was of a severe form of vascular disease of the hand. This condition is found exclusively in patients with diabetes and is felt to have a vascular, and possibly a neurovascular, etiology. Many unclear terms have been used, such as *diabetic cheiroarthropathy*, from the Greek meaning "hand", and *diabetic hand syndrome*. The five initial patients were described as having burning paresthesia of the hands with progressively limited mobility. The hands appear thick and tight with a waxy appearance, much like the changes found in scleroderma. The subcutaneous tissues of the hands are thickened and stiff, with microangiopathic changes such as thickening of the basement membrane. The thickened skin extends to the wrist, unlike in LJM, where it may extend up the forearm. Calcification of the arteries of the hand were noted on radiographs in all initial five patients. In contrast to RSD, there is no evidence of atrophy of the muscles. Despite paresthesia, these patients had normal tactile and vibratory sense.

Management of stiff hand syndrome centers around good diabetic control. Beyond this, physical therapy and symptomatic treatment is available to patients.

Dupuytren's Disease

DD is diagnosed by palpating thickened palmar fascia with skin tethering, which eventually leads to contracture. In patients without diabetes, DD is primarily a disease of white males of European decent. The incidence of DD in the adult diabetic population approaches 40%, with an equal incidence men to women, and may be present when diabetes is first diagnosed. Women may present with knuckle pads, nodules, and skin tethering without contractures. Ten to fifteen percent of patients with DD have diabetes. In patients with diabetes there is a predilection for involvement of the third and fourth digits, as opposed to those patients without diabetes, who generally have involvement of the fourth and fifth digits. It is important to contrast this involvement of the third and fourth digits with the onset of LJM, which always begins in the fifth finger and moves radially, with the palmar fascia and knuckle pads being normal.

DDs treated with surgery reveal increased type III collagen, as well as increased hydroxylation and glycosylation of reducible cross-links, typical of granulation and scar tissue.[20] Baird et al.[21] have found a T-cell-mediated autoimmune mechanism in individuals with diabetes and DD.

Flexor Tenosynovitis

Flexor tenosynovitis, known as "trigger finger," is characterized by proliferation of fibrous tissue in the tendon sheath, particularly where it goes through a fibrous band of tissue, the flexor retinaculum. Tissue distally swells and may form a nodule that is painful with flexion of the digit, due to constriction moving through the fibrous band. The analogy can be made that it is like a knot on a line that is pulled back and forth through a pulley, occasionally sticking. This so-called "triggering" refers to the extra effort needed to pull the nodule through the flexor retinaculum. Like a six-shooter in the Old West, there is a threshold with the squeezing

motion, similar to a finger on a trigger, which releases when the hammer falls and the gun fires. Conservative therapy includes splinting, occupational therapy, and local corticosteroid injection. If this fails to resolve the problem surgical release may be necessary.

Carpal Tunnel Syndrome

Diabetes is found in 5–16% of patients with carpal tunnel syndrome.[15] Typically carpal tunnel syndrome is the result of compression of the median nerve as it courses through the carpal tunnel at the wrist. It is the most common entrapment neuropathy, characterized by paresthesia of the thumb, index finger, and middle finger. Patients often complain of pain in their hands that awakens them at night and is relieved by shaking their hands. Carpal tunnel syndrome in patients with diabetes has evidence of an intrinsic lesion of the median nerve that is attributable, at least in part, to intrinsic median nerve neuropathy or myoneural dysfunction.[22] In addition to delays in median nerve conduction velocity, about 50% of patients with diabetes and carpal tunnel syndrome have similar conduction delays in ulnar nerve conduction on the same hand. There is an association as well with flexion contractures at the interphalangeal and metacarpophalangeal joints. Jung et al.[22] noted in their patients that flexion contractures of the fingers, whether or not associated with DD, were associated with an increased degree of neuropathy. In fact, if digital contractures are present muscle atrophy is noted to be more severe. It is uncertain as to whether the digital contractures contribute to or are the result of neuropathy. Nevertheless, one important consideration, particularly when ulnar as well as median nerve conduction delays are present, is a need for caution in considering surgical release of the carpal tunnel because intrinsic diabetic or other neuropathy may mimic entrapment. There is some evidence to suggest that vitamin B$_6$ (pyridoxine) deficiency may play a part in the neuropathy; however, reports have failed to demonstrate an improvement with vitamin B$_6$ supplementation in diabetic carpal tunnel syndrome.

Lower Extremity

There are multiple problems that may affect the lower extremities. The diabetic foot is discussed in Chapters 31, 32, and 33. In general, two main contributing causes for lower extremity problems are diabetic osteoarthropathy and neuroarthropathy.

Diabetic Osteoarthropathy (Osteolysis)

Diabetic osteoarthropathy applies to osteolysis, which may be localized or generalized, involving primarily the distal metatarsus. Diabetic osteoarthropathy occurs as a late complication of diabetes and may be manifested as pain and erythema at the proximal metatarsalphalangeal (MTP) joint. Diabetic osteoarthropathy is reported in 0.1–0.4% of diabetic patients.[23] In general it occurs in the sixth and seventh decade of life and is evenly distributed among men and women.

Forgacs[24] has described the clinical signs and symptoms and has classified them into four groups: neurologic symptoms, skin involvement, loose joints/articular swelling, and deformities. Universally peripheral neuropathy is present and manifested as symptoms of paresthesia and reflex disorders. Various skin changes from erythema to frank ulceration may be present. Painless articular swelling with subluxation of the MTP is characteristic of diabetic osteoarthropathy. In advanced stages contracture and foreshortening of the foot is found due to destruction of the MTP joint and collapse of the arch resulting in the so called *rockerbottom sole.*[24]

The differential diagnosis must include other causes of lytic bone lesions, such as infection and tumor. The lesion is commonly misdiagnosed as osteomyelitis. CT and MRI scans may be helpful in defining infection or differentiating it from diabetic osteoarthropathy. In diabetic osteoarthropathy spontaneous recovery often occurs, and therefore prognosis is generally good. Because no specific treatment is yet available, local measures and tight control of diabetes are the mainstays of therapy. Osteolysis is due to neuropathy more frequently than inflammation or infection. Therefore, surgical intervention and amputation should be considered with caution and should be reserved only for cases with gangrene or other serious complications.

Neuroarthropathy (Charcot's joint)

Neuropathic arthropathy (Charcot's joint) is generally a chronic, destructive arthropathy associated with peripheral neuropathy/sensory loss. It most often involves the tarso-metatarsal joints, MTP joints, tibiotalar joints (60%, 30% and 10%, respectively), and the knee.[25] Attempts to experimentally re-create neuropathic arthropathy have demonstrated a "neurogenic acceleration" of joint degeneration in patients with diabetic neuropathy.[26] It has been shown that anterior cruciate ligament transection in dogs only causes nonprogressive osteoarthritic changes, unless they have undergone dorsal root ganglionectomy, the functional equivalent to diabetic neuropathy. Slowman-Kovacs et al.,[25] describe three patients with longstanding IDDM in whom neuropathic arthropathy developed within weeks following minor trauma to the foot and ankle. The differential diagnosis of diabetic neuropathic arthropathy includes infection, osteoarthritis, and reflex sympathetic dystrophy. Plain X-rays and cultures are helpful initially. Over time the characteristic appearance of hypertrophic destructive changes with periar-

ticular debris and periosteal reaction are typical of neuropathic arthropathy.

Although the pathophysiology is not completely understood, what is clear is that even minor trauma in a patient with long-standing diabetic neuropathy may have the serious consequence of a rapidly developing neuroarthropathy (Charcot's joint) and that early treatment with immobilization may minimize the damage.[27]

Diffuse/Axial

Scleredema

Scleredema is a rare disorder characterized by diffuse symmetric thickening of the skin, most often over the neck and upper back. There are two forms of scleredema. One is postinfectious, and the other is associated with diabetes. The salient distinction between *scleredema* and *scleroderma* is in their histology and histochemistry. In scleredema the epidermis is normal with dermal thickening, sometimes as much as three to four times normal. This is caused by the size of the collagen bundles and separation of these bundles by clear spaces. Appendageal structures usually remain intact. Scleroderma later in the disease has atrophy of the adnexa, prominent dermal sclerosis, and a few elastic fibers. Additional clinical features are also present such as Raynauds, skin atrophy, and, notably, hand and foot involvement.

Scleredema Adultorum of Buscke

The postinfectious type of scleredema is *scleredema adultorum of Buscke.*[28] This is a disease that, contrary to its name, occurs primarily in children and young adults. There is likewise neither sclerosis nor edema. There is a 2:1 predilection for females over males.[29] More than 50% of the cases are reported in patients under 20 years of age.[30] The cause for scleredema adultorum of Buscke is unknown; however, in two-thirds of cases the disease is preceded by a prodromal infection.[29] Streptococcus is the most often associated pathogen,[29] although viruses and other bacteria have been associated as well. Skin involvement is most commonly on the posterior and lateral aspects of the neck, upper back, and shoulders; however, it may also involve the face and, infrequently, the lower back, abdomen, upper arms and thighs. It is a very important distinction that the hands are rarely affected and the feet are never involved.[31] This is in contradistinction to scleroderma, which typically begins in the fingers and almost universally involves the distal extremities, particularly when there is central involvement.

There is no pain, and symptoms involve limitation of motion. Scleredema adultorum of Buscke usually resolves spontaneously in 6 months to 2 years in the reverse order that it developed.[32] In some patients the scleredema persists indefinitely. There may be an association with diabetes in this population of patients.

Scleredema Diabeticorum

Jelinek[33] reviewed 54 reported cases of *scleredema diabeticorum* and noted that there are important distinctions compared to the adultorum type of scleredema, as shown in Exhibit 37–4. The physical characteristics are similar in both diseases; however, the patient population and clinical features are significantly different. Scleredema diabeticorum has a 4:1 predilection for males.[34] It has been reported in childhood; however, it is primarily a disease of middle-aged adults, with the average age being 51.[33] The onset is usually insidious. It always appears on the neck and upper back and, unlike the adultorum type, it often extends to the face as well as the anterior trunk and may involve most of the body.[33] Unlike the adultorum type, when associated with diabetes, scleredema does not have spontaneous remission and is most often progressive.[33] Scleredema diabeticorum is found primarily in obese middle-aged men.

Usually the diabetes, both type 1 and type 2, is long standing and precedes the scleredema by several years. Typically, all patients with scleredema diabeticorum are obese. Unfortunately, it is also associated with internal organ involvement, including ischemic heart disease and retinopathy.[35] Thus the two types of scleredema have unique features. One important difference is that scleredema associated with diabetes is, as yet, untreatable and permanent (see Exhibit 37–4).

Osteopenia/Osteoporosis

Osteopenia has been described in IDDM and NIDDM, although there is controversy regarding its significance.[34] The technique for testing the bone mineral density varied in different studies and primarily detected decreased bone density in the appendicular skeleton. Auwerx et al.[36] found that with longstanding IDDM there is loss of bone density in the peripheral skeleton of both men and women; however, women also had decreased bone density in the spine. In clinical studies, a significantly increased relative risk for fracture has not yet been shown. This is perhaps the most significant point, in that the burden of care is not increased due to diabetes. Nevertheless, osteoporosis is a silent disease, and every postmenopausal woman should have a bone density test for detection of osteoporosis. Statistically the relative risk of osteoporotic fracture is significant for all women in their fifth and sixth decades of life. The comorbidity of diabetes would surely not improve their outcome.

Hyperostosis (Forestier's disease)

Forestier et al.[7] first described ankylosing hyperostosis, also known as diffuse idiopathic skeletal hyperostosis (DISH), and its distinctive X-ray findings. This first description noted osteophytes in the right and lateral aspect of the thoracolumbar spine that over time become exuberant with a "flowing" pattern connecting multiple vertebral bodies. In contrast to ankylosing spondylitis and osteoarthritis, disc spaces and apophyseal joints are normal in DISH.

There are extra spinal sites of hyperostosis, including the pelvis, heel, foot, and elbow, as well as the poles of the patella and the distal tibia and fibula. Rarely the shoulder, metacarpals, and skull may be involved. It is not unusual for DISH to be an asymptomatic finding. Symptoms when present in DISH are not a result of inflammation, but rather relate to discomfort from direct effect of the hyperostosis, such as limitation of motion in the spine. Dysphagia had been described in 16% of patients with osteophytosis in the cervical spine, due to direct esophageal impingement. In one study ankylosing hyperostosis was found in 21% of 122 elderly patients with diabetes, compared with 4% of 148 control patients.[37] Half of patients with hyperostosis have evidence of diabetes.[34]

EXHIBIT 37–4 Scleredema Adultorum vs Scleredema Diabeticorum

Feature	Scleredema Adultorum of Bushke	Scleredema Diabeticorum
Demographic	Predominantly girls and young women	Predominantly middle-aged men
Prodromal infection	Common; streptococci, or other bacteria or viruses	Uncommon
Association with diabetes	None	Always associated with diabetes, generally long-standing and poorly controlled; insulin resistance is common, may occur in NIDDM
Treatment	None effective	None effective; generally does not respond to antidiabetic therapy
Resolution	75% resolve spontaneously within 2 years	Almost always unremitting

Adapted from Ref. 33.

Common Systemic Diseases in Diabetic Patients

Osteoarthritis.   Osteoarthritis is more prevalent in young and middle-aged patients with diabetes.[38] Furthermore, joint damage occurs earlier and is more severe in patients with diabetes. The increased propensity for joint damage may be due to loss of glycosaminoglycans in cartilaginous tissue.[38]

Gout/Pseudogout.   Correlation between gout or pseudogout and diabetes has not been proven. Hyperuricemia, hyperlipidemia, and hyperglycemia are a well-recognized combination, although it is felt that obesity is the linking factor. In nonobese patients with diabetes and normal renal function, there is no increased propensity for gout or pseudogout[39] compared to normal subjects.

Rheumatoid Arthritis.   Thomas et al.[40] have noted an association with HLA-DR3 and/or DR4 in both rheumatoid arthritis and IDDM. In rheumatoid arthritis and IDDM antibodies are found to islet cells as well as other organ-specific antibodies. There is clustering of these two diseases in families. The combination of rheumatoid arthritis and IDDM has an unfavorable effect with more aggressive erosive articular disease. It can be postulated that, just as noted earlier with neuropathic arthropathy, diabetic neuropathy plays a role in this accelerated destructive process.[41]

Fibromyalgia.   There is no direct correlation with fibromyalgia and diabetes other than the fact that both are common disorders and, if only by chance, occur together. More importantly, many of the symptoms attributable to fibromyalgia are common in diabetes. Because fibromyalgia is a diagnosis of exclusion, other possible diagnoses must be ruled out before arriving at the diagnosis of fibromyalgia. Having made a proper diagnosis the diabetic patient may still have symptoms of and fulfill the criteria for fibromyalgia: (1) diffuse pain above and below the waist and on either side of the body that has been present for at least 3 months and (2) at least 11 of 18 characteristic tender points. The tender points are bilateral at the lateral epicondyles, second intercostal space, anterior sternocleidomastoid, occiput, upper trapezius, upper medial scapula, posterior superior iliac spines, and trochanteric and medial knee areas. Pragmatically speaking, many of the therapies for treating fibromyalgia would have a beneficial effect on the diabetic patient, e.g., stretching, aerobic exercise, improving stage four restorative sleep, and relaxation techniques. Additionally, medications such as antidepressants may also help treat underlying diabetic neuropathy. Caution should be exercised in using nonsteroidal anti-inflammatory drugs (NSAIDs), as they may diminish renal blood flow and exacerbate renal insufficiency.

Assessment

There are many components that factor into the equation when coming to a conclusion regarding a patient with diabetes and musculoskeletal symptoms. The "big picture" is essential in arriving at a correct diagnosis, so that an appropriate plan of treatment can be formulated. With all we know about the pathophysiology of diabetes as well as collagen vascular disease, we still do not have the most rudimentary etiopathogenic information, and therefore our diagnoses are often descriptive. As our knowledge of the molecular and genetic intricacies improves, we will become better not only at characterizing these diseases, but also at treating them.

Plan

Initial.   Diagnostic procedures are limited regarding diagnosis of rheumatologic manifestations of diabetes. Clinical awareness and experience are essential to solving the problems. Clearly, radiographs are important in confirming the diagnosis of Charcot's joint, forefoot osteolysis, diffuse idiopathic skeletal hyperostosis, and calcific periarthritis. Dual energy X-ray absorptiometry (DEXA) is the gold standard for measuring osteoporosis at the present time. In the case of reflex sympathetic dystrophy, a three-phase bone scan may be helpful. Limited joint mobility, stiff hand syndrome, DD, flexor tenosynovitis, and adhesive capsulitis are clinical diagnoses. Carpal tunnel syndrome is investigated with electromyogram and nerve conduction testing.

Therapy begins with strict control of blood sugar. Physical therapy and occupational therapy are instrumental in maintaining and improving mobility in the majority of musculoskeletal syndromes, as they tend to limit mobility. Judicious use of local corticosteroid injections is helpful in adhesive capsulitis of the shoulder as well as carpal tunnel syndrome. Splinting is often helpful in carpal tunnel syndrome and may be helpful in neuroarthropathy. Surgical intervention may become necessary in both of these conditions.

Follow-up.   As previously mentioned, close monitoring and treatment with the goal of maintaining near-normal blood glucose are the cornerstones of therapy. From a musculoskeletal standpoint, coordination of care with a therapist, an orthopedist, a neurologist, and a rheumatologist is sometimes necessary to best address the complex complaints related to the bones, muscles, joints, and tendons. The primary goal is to minimize pain and discomfort while maximizing range of motion and function. These goals are synergistic.

Education. Education regarding the importance of good diabetic control includes exercise. Exercises with stretching are essential for decreasing pain and increasing mobility. This has a dual benefit of not only strengthening and maintaining flexibility but also helping control of blood glucose.

Adherence. As with any chronic illness, patients need encouragement and coaching to maintain their therapy program. A positive outlook on minimizing complications and maximizing independence is paramount to having a patient comply with the therapeutic plan.

Audit. Clear communication between consultants, therapists, and the diabetologist is the key to maintaining control of care to achieve a successful outcome.

Side Effects of Therapy. In general, because of the vasculopathy associated with diabetes, which is often associated with renal insufficiency, NSAIDs are relatively contraindicated. If used, it is important to monitor renal function and discontinue NSAIDs if there is worsening. The majority of therapeutic modalities are non-pharmacologic and only run the risk of overstretching or straining a joint or muscle group. Of course, if corticosteroids are used, blood sugars are often elevated and additional hypoglycemic therapy may be required. Local corticosteroid injection also has an approximate 1 in 1,000 chance of infection; this may be slightly elevated in the diabetic.

Research Considerations

Clearly the goal in treating the connective tissue disorders in diabetes mellitus is founded in treating the underlying disease process involved in diabetes. As outlined earlier, the rheumatologic manifestations are outward signs and symptoms of a myriad of macromolecular and microvascular complications that alter the very fabric that makes up the bone, joint, tendon, and muscles of diabetic patients—the connective tissue. As with all rheumatologic diseases we are searching for the precipitating trigger that begins the cascade of molecular changes that cause the complications noted. One area of research that is on the near horizon is the development of more specific immune regulators that specifically target inflammation and cause fewer side effects. Until a cure is found for diabetes, research is directed toward treatments that will have as few side effects as possible.

References

1. Arning E: Beitrag zur Lehre vom Sclerema Adultorum. Wurzburg Medicin Zeitschr 2:186, 1861.

2. Piffard HG: Acute scleriasis; spontaneous recovery, NY Med Gazette 7:51, 1871..

3. Buschke A: Ueber Scleroedem. Berl Klin Wochenschr 39:955–957, 1902.

4. Holubar K, Mach KW: Scleredema (Buschke) Acta Derm Venereol 47:102–110,1967.

5. Davis JS, Finesilver EM: Dupuytren's contraction—with a note on the incidence of the contraction in diabetes. Arch Surg 24:933–989, 1932.

6. Jordan WR: Neuritic manifestations in diabetes mellitus. Arch Intern Med 57:307–366, 1936.

7. Forestier J, Rotes-Querol J: Senile ankylosing hyperostosis of the spine. Ann Rheum Dis 9:321–330, 1950.

8. Harris J, Carter AR, Glick EN, et al.: Ankylosing hyperostosis I. Clinical and radiologic features. Ann Rheum Dis 33:210–215, 1974.

9. Lundbaek K: Stiff hands in long-term diabetes. Acta Med Scand 158:447, 1957.

10. Rosenbloom AL, Silverstein JH, Lesotte DC, et al.: Limited joint mobility of childhood diabetes mellitus indicates increased risk for microvascular disease. New Engl J Med 305:191–194, 1981.

11. Bridgeman JF: Periarthritis of the shoulder and diabetes mellitus. Ann Rheum Dis 31:69–71, 1972.

12. Connally J, Regen E, Evans OB: The management of the painful stiff shoulder. Clin Orthop 84:97–103, 1972.

13. Neviasser JS: Adhesive capsulitis of the shoulder: A study of the pathological findings in periarthritis of the shoulder. J Bone Joint Surg 27:211–222, 1945.

14. Lee PN, Lee M, Haq AMM, et al.: Periarthritis of the shoulder. Ann Rheum Dis 33:116–119, 1974.

15. Bland JH, Frymoyer JW, Newberg AH: Rheumatic syndromes in endocrine disease. Semin Arthritis Rheum 9:23, 1979.

16. Pal B, Andersen J, Dick WR, et al.: Limitation of joint mobility and shoulder capsulitis in insulin- and non-insulin dependent diabetes mellitus. Br J Rheumatol 25:147, 1986.

17. Rosenbloom AL, Frias JL: Diabetes, short stature and joint stiffness—a new syndrome. Clin Res 22:92A, 1974.

18. Rosenbloom AL, Silverstein JH, Lezotte DC, et al.: Limited joint mobility in diabetes mellitus in childhood: Natural history and relationship to growth impairment. J Pediatr 101:874, 1982.

19. Starkman HS, Gleason RE, Rand LJ, et al.: Limited joint mobility of the hand in patients with diabetes mellitus: Relation to chronic complications. Ann Rheum Dis 43:251–257, 1984.

20. Bazin JH, LeLouis M, Duance VC, et al.: Biochemistry and histology of the connective tissue in Dupuytren's disease lesions. Eur J Clin Invest 10:9, 1980.

21. Baird KS, Crossan JF, Alwan WH, et al.: T-cell mediated response in Dupuytren's disease. Lancet 341:1622, 1993.

22. Jung Y, Hohmann TC, Gernerth JA, et al.: Diabetic hand syndrome. Metabolism 20(11), 1008–1015, 1971.

23. Sinha S, Munichodappa C, Kozak G: Neuroarthropathy in diabetes mellitus. Medicine 51:191–210, 1972.

24. Forgacs S: Clinical picture of diabetic osteoarthropathy. Acta Diabetol Lat 13:111–129, 1976.

25. Slowman-Kovacs SD, Braunstein EM, Brandt KD: Rapidly progressive Charcot arthropathy following minor joint trauma in patients with diabetic neuropathy. Arth Rheum 33:412–417, 1990.

26. O'Conner BL, Palmoski MJ, Brandt KD: Neurogenic acceleration of degenerative joint lesions. J Bone Joint Surg 67A:562–572, 1985.

27. Bruckner FE, Howell A: Neuropathic joints. Semin Arthritis Rheum 31:171–1573, 1988.

28. Buschke A: Verhandlungen der Berliner dermatologischen Gesellschaft. Arch Dermatol Syph 53:383–386, 1900.

29. Greenberg LM, Geppert C, Worthen HG, Good RA: Scleredema in children. Three cases with histochemical study and review of the world's literature. Pediatrics 32: 1044–1054, 1963.

30. Margolis J, Broadrick B: Scleredema and diabetes mellitus. J Am Geriatr Soc 22:541–546, 1974.

31. Curtis AC, Shulak BM: Scleredema adultorum. Arch Dermatol 92:526–541, 1965.

32. Monk BE, Pembroke AC, Vollum DI: Scleredema of Buschke and diabetes mellitus. A report of 2 cases. Clin Exp Dermatol 8:389–391, 1983.

33. Jelinek JE: Collagen disorders in which diabetes and cutaneous features coexist. In Jelinek JE (ed): The Skin in Diabetes. Philadelphia: Lea& Febiger, 1986 .

34. Rosenbloom AL, Silverstein JH: Connective tissue and joint diseases in diabetes mellitus. Endocrin Metab Clin North Amer 25:473–475, 1996.

35. Cole GW, Headley J, Skowsky R: Scleredema diabeticorum: A common and distinct cutaneous manifestation of diabetes mellitus. Diabetes Care, 6:189–192, 1983.

36. Auwerx J, Dequeker J, Bouillon R, et al.: Mineral metabolism and bone mass at peripheral and axial skeleton in diabetes mellitus. Diabetes 37:8, 1988.

37. Julkumen H, Karava R, Viljamen V: Hyperostosis of the spine in diabetes mellitus and acromegaly. Diabetologia 2:123–126, 1966.

38. Crisp AJ, Heathcoate JG: Connective tissue abnormalities in diabetes mellitus. J R Coll Physicians Lond 18:132–141, 1984.

39. McCarty DJ, Silcox DC, Coe F: Diseases associated with calcium pyrophosphate dihydrate crystal deposition. Am J Med 56:704, 1974.

40. Thomas J, Young A, Gossuch A: Evidence for an association between rheumatoid arthritis and autoimmune endocrine disease. Ann Rheum Dis 42:297–300, 1983.

41. Forgacs S. Diabetes mellitus and rheumatic disease. Clin Rheum Dis. 12:729–53, 1986.

Selected Readings

Gray RG, Gottlieb NL: Rheumatic disorders associated with diabetes mellitus. Sem Arthr Rheum 6:9–34, 1976.

Crisp AL: Diabetes mellitus and the rheumatologist. Br J Rheum 25:135–137, 1986.

Rosenbloom AIL: Skeletal and joint manifestations of childhood diabetes. Pediatr Clin North Amer 31: 569–589, 1984.

Larkin JG, Frier BM: Limited joint mobility and Dupuytren's contracture in diabetic, hypertensive and normal populations. Br Med J 292:1494, 1986.

Trapp RG, Soler NG, Spencer-Green G: Nailford capillaroscopy in type I diabetes with vasculopathy and limited joint mobility. J Rheum 13:917–920, 1986.

Nepom BS, Palmer J, Kim SJ, et al.: Specific genomic markers for the HAL-DQ subregion discriminate between DR 4 insulin-dependent diabetes mellitus and DR4 seropositive juvenile rheumatoid arthritis. J Exp Med 164:345–50, 1986.

Boyle JA, McDiddie M, Buchanan KD, et al.: Diabetes mellitus and gout. Ann Rheum Dis 28: 374–378, 1969.

Sherry DD, Rothestein RRL, Petty RE: Joint contractures preceding insulin-dependent diabetes mellitus. Arthr Rheum 11:1362–1364, 1982.

Rosenbloom AL: Joint manifestations of diabetes in the young. In Serrano-Rios M, Lefebvre PJ (eds): Diabetes 1985. Amsterdam: Elsevier, 1986, pp. 762–766.

Heath M, Melton LJ, Chic GP: Diabetes mellitus and risk of skeletal fracture. New Engl J Med 303:567–570, 1980.

Lawson PM, Maneschi F, Kohner EM: The relationship of hand abnormalities to diabetes and diabetic retinopathy. Diabetes Care 6:140–143, 1983.

Garza-Elizondo MA, Diaz-Jouanen E, Franco-Casique JJ, Alacron-Segovia D: Joint contractures and scleroderma-like skin changes in the hands of insulin-dependent juvenile diabetics. J Rheumatol 10:797–800, 1983.

Seibold J: Digital sclerosis in children with insulin dependent diabetes mellitus. Arthritis Rheumatol 265:1357–1361, 1982.

Rosenbloom AL, Silverstein JH, Riley WH, Maclaren NK: Limited joint mobility in childhood diabetes: Family studies. Diabetes Care 6:370–373, 1983.

Buithieu M, Rosenbloom AL, Conlon M, Thomas JL: Joint mobility and control in IDDM patients. Diabetes 37:129A, 1988.

Grgic A, Rosenbloom AL, Weber FT, et al.: Joint contracture—common manifestation of childhood diabetes mellitus. J Pediatr 8:584, 1976.

Hanna W, Freisen D, Bombardier C, et al.: Pathologic features of diabetic thick skin. J Am Acad Dermatol 16:546, 1987.

Pastran RS, Cohen AS: The rheumatologic manifestations of diabetes mellitus. Med Clin North Am 62:829, 1978.

Schulte L, Roberts MS, Zimmerman C, et al.: A quantitative assessment of limited joint mobility in patients with diabetes: Goniometric analysis of upper extremity passive range of motion. Arthritis Rheumatol 36:1429, 1993.

Van De Staak WJBM, Bergers AMG: Ultrastructrual abnormalities in the skin nerves of a patient with scleroderma adultorum (Buschke) and diabetes mellitus. Dermatologia 151:223, 1975.

Resnick D, Shaul S, Robins J: Diffuse idiopathic skeletal hypertosis (DISH). Forestier's disease with extraspinal manifestations. Radiology 115:513–524, 1975.

Yosipovitch G, Yosipovitch Z, Karp M, Mukamel M: Trigger finger in young patients with insulin-dependent diabetes. J Rheumatol 17:951–952, 1990.

Section V.
Concomitant Problems

38

Hypertension in the Patient with Diabetes

W. Dallas Hall

Historical Perspective

The association of hypertension, hyperglycemia, obesity, and arteriosclerosis was recognized by Prebble[1] and Herrick[2] in 1923. By 1927, Fineberg[3] reported that diabetes was especially prevalent (33%) in patients with isolated systolic hypertension (ISH). The high prevalence of diabetes (26%) in patients with ISH was subsequently confirmed by Colandrea and associates.[4]

A strong association between diabetes, hypertension, obesity, and atherosclerosis thus has been known for more than 75 years. Today, it is established that both the incidence and prevalence of systolic and diastolic hypertension occur with an increased frequency in diabetic patients.[5]

Epidemiology

In a study of 662 diabetics and 662 sex- and age-matched control subjects, Pell and D'Alonzo[6] reported that hypertension (repeated systolic pressure 150 mmHg or higher or diastolic pressure 95 mmHg or higher) was 54% more likely in diabetics. A strong relationship between hypertension and obesity is well known,[7] but in these 662 diabetics, hypertension occurred disproportionately even when patients were categorized into five groups of percent ideal body weight from −10% to ≥40%.

The Framingham study included 239 adults with diabetes.[8] Both blood pressure and relative body weight were significantly higher than in the population as a whole. The average blood pressure was 6/3 mmHg higher in diabetic men and even more (12/5 mmHg) in diabetic women. The prevalence of hypertension (160/95 mmHg or higher) was also greater in both diabetic men and women. Study of two large populations in London has shown a higher systolic blood pressure in newly diagnosed and borderline diabetics.[9]

Elevation of blood pressure is an early feature of diabetic nephropathy, and the majority of these patients have hypertension.[10–12]

Pathophysiology

Observations by Weidmann and coworkers[13] suggest that, unlike nondiabetic patients with hypertension,[14] total body exchangeable sodium is increased in adult hypertensive diabetics with normal renal function. The hypertension associated with diabetes is thus a "volume-dependent" type of hypertension.[15] Plasma levels of renin and aldosterone are typically normal or low rather than elevated.[13,16–19]

Increases in plasma insulin concentration within the physiologic range stimulate sodium reabsorption by the thick ascending limb of Henle.[20,21] This is a specific effect of insulin, independent of hyperglycemia. Ingestion of as little as 75 g carbohydrate can stimulate insulin levels (moreso in hypertensives)[22] and abruptly reduce urinary sodium excretion.[23] Metabolic balance studies on high-carbohydrate diets also demonstrate hyperinsulinemia and transient sodium retention in normal subjects.[24] Tedde and coworkers[25] demonstrated that a 30–50% reduction in insulin dosage was associated with natriuresis and improvement in blood pressure in six women with non-insulin-dependent diabetes mellitus (NIDDM).

Insulin also acts on the sympathetic nervous system to increase vascular tone and blood pressure. During experiments with insulin infusion using the euglycemic clamp, plasma norepinephrine increases in animals[26] and humans.[27,28] Insulin may also increase sympathetic discharge from the central nervous system.[29]

Recent studies have further examined the relation between hyperinsulinemia and hypertension in patients with obesity and NIDDM. Hypertension often precedes the diagnosis of NIDDM, indicating that elevated blood glucose per se is not the cause of the hypertension. Nondiabetic, obese, and nonobese patients with essential hypertension often have hyperinsulinemia or insulin resistance.[30–32] Insulin resistance (i.e., abnormal nonoxidative glucose disposal) may be the primary abnormality, with reflex hyperinsulinemia as a surrogate marker.[33] DeFronzo[20] postulated that primary insulin resistance would result in hyper-insulinemia, sodium retention, sympathetic stimulation, and elevated blood pressure. Chronic infusion of insulin, however, does not raise blood pressure,[34] suggesting that factors other than hyperinsulinemia may be responsible for blood pressure elevation in obese nondiabetic patients with essential hypertension.[35]

Insulin resistance per se is an established risk factor for cardiovascular disease.[36–38] Hyperinsulinemia has been associated directly with the level of blood pressure,[39] the risk of ischemic heart disease,[38] and the level of triglycerides[39] and small dense low-density lipoprotein (LDL) particles.[36,40] Hyperinsulinemia is associated inversely with the level of high-density lipoprotein (HDL).[39,41] Also reported are associations between insulin resistance and carotid wall thickness,[42] left ventricular hypertrophy,[43,44] and microalbuminuria.[44,45] Most of these associations have been shown to be independent of confounding variables such as age, obesity, or the presence of diabetes. One common mechanistic theme for these associations is that insulin stimulates endothelium-derived, nitric oxide–dependent vasodilation that is impaired in insulin-resistant states.[46,47]

These observations do not explain the hypertension observed in insulin-dependent diabetics who are insulin deficient. However, insulin-deficient diabetics who have developed mild renal insufficiency have a volume-dependent hypertension with an inability of the kidney to excrete salt and water adequately because of impaired renal function rather than hyperinsulinemia.

Diabetic patients often demonstrate defects of both the sympathetic and parasympathetic autonomic nervous systems. Clinical recognition of these defects is important for the proper selection and monitoring of antihypertensive drug therapy. Bennett and associates[48] found asymptomatic orthostatic hypotension with 20–40 mmHg reductions in the standing blood pressure in 8 of 21 diabetics (mean age 45 years). Those without orthostasis had the expected rise in standing heart rate (i.e., 11–13 beats/min), whereas those with orthostasis had either exaggerated (up to 30–40 beats/min), normal, or subnormal heart rate responses to standing, associated with a variety of defects in clinical tests of autonomic function. Symptomatic orthostatic hypotension with more than a 50/20 mmHg reduction in standing blood pressure is common in patients with diabetic nephropathy and is typically associated with defective release of renin in the upright posture.[49]

Many patients with diabetes, especially those with autonomic neuropathy, microalbuminuria, or established nephropathy, have a reversed circadian blood pressure rhythm with blunting or absence of the usual nocturnal dip.[50–53] This may relate to the association between microalbuminuria and the risks of both cardiovascular disease and progressive nephropathy.

The levels of plasma catecholamines are generally similar in diabetic and normal subjects, but diabetics demonstrate an exaggerated blood pressure response to infusion of either norepinephrine or angiotensin II.[54]

Problem Statement: Hypertension

Subjective Symptoms

Essential hypertension is generally considered to be an asymptomatic disorder, although Bulpitt and coworkers[55] noted an excess of nocturia, unsteady gait, waking headaches, and depression in untreated hypertensive individuals compared with normotensive subjects. Also, the classic triad of symptoms of pheochromocytoma (headaches, palpitations, excessive sweating) can masquerade as worsening hyperglycemia in a diabetic with resistant hypertension. Prevalent symptoms of target organ complications in hypertensive diabetics include visual disturbances, transient ischemic attacks, angina, dyspnea from heart failure, claudication from peripheral vascular disease, and dysuria due to urinary tract disorders. Sexual dysfunction is very common in both diabetic men and women.[56,57] It often worsens following antihypertensive therapy with diuretics, β-blockers, or centrally acting α-agonists.

Objective Findings

Blood pressure should be measured with an adult obese cuff when the midarm circumference exceeds 33 cm; thigh cuffs are usually necessary when the midarm circumference exceeds 38 cm. If the regular adult cuff is used on obese arms, falsely elevated readings can be obtained with the patient misdiagnosed as hypertensive. Because of the common occurrence of orthostatic hypotension in diabetics, both blood pressure and heart rate should be measured in the standing as well as the supine or sitting position. Adequate funduscopic examination usually requires dilation to differentiate hypertensive from diabetic retinopathy. Microaneurysms, blot hemorrhages, neovascularity, multiple small exudates, and large hemorrhages point to diabetes, whereas arterial narrowing, a few large exudates, and slit hemorrhages relate more specifically to hypertension. Evidence of either left ventricular hypertrophy or congestive heart failure indicates a poor prognosis. Bruits over the carotid, renal, iliac, or femoral arteries provide evidence of peripheral atherosclerosis.

The diagnosis of hypertension generally requires confirmation of seated or supine diastolic blood pressure of 90 mmHg or higher (phase V) or systolic blood pressure of 140 mmHg or higher on three consecutive occasions. ISH is defined as a repeated systolic pres-

TABLE 38–1   Clinical Clues to Secondary Causes of Hypertension—Often Attributed to Diabetes or Its Complications

Clinical Clue	Attributed To	HBP Etiology	Diagnostic Screening Test
Worsening HBP	Poor dietary compliance or medication adherence	Renoparenchymal disease (diabetic nephropathy)	Test for microalbuminuria (>20–30 ug/min or 20–30 mg/L) and recheck serum Cr; switch from thiazide type to loop diuretic if serum Cr $\geq$ 2 mg/dL
Rising serum Cr	Diabetic nephropathy	Bilateral renal artery stenosis	Positive captopril scintiscan
Worsening hyperglycemia	Poor dietary compliance	Cushing's syndrome, hyperthyroidism, pheochromocytoma	Elevated 24 hr urinary free cortisol Low TSH Elevated 24 hr urinary metanephrine
Hypokalemia	Diuretics, vomiting	Primary aldosteronism	Saline suppression test (see text)
Palpitations, PVCs, SVT[a]	Ischemic heart disease	Pheochromocytoma	Elevated 24 hr urinary metanephrine

[a] Supraventricular tachycardias.

sure 140 mmHg or higher and a diastolic pressure less than 90 mmHg.

The initial laboratory examination recommended by the Joint National Commission on the Detection, Evaluation and Treatment of High Blood Pressure includes a complete urinalysis, complete blood count, fasting blood chemistry profile (potassium, creatinine, fasting glucose) cholesterol, HDL cholesterol, and electrocardiogram.[58]

Assessment for Secondary Causes of Hypertension

The vast majority of hypertensive diabetics do not have specific correctable underlying cause for their hypertension. Those few who have a correctable cause, however, often remain undiagnosed because of symptoms that overlap with their diabetes or its complications. These "sneaky" symptoms or events are outlined in Table 38–1, along with suggested diagnostic screening tests.

Renoparenchymal Hypertension (Diabetic Nephropathy)   Renoparenchymal hypertension due to diabetic nephropathy is the most common secondary cause of hypertension in diabetics (Table 38–2). It should be suspected if the level of serum creatinine exceeds 1.4 mg/dL, if there is macroproteinuria in excess of

TABLE 38–2   Secondary Causes of Hypertension in Patients with Diabetes Mellitus

Renoparenchymal hypertension
  Diabetic nephropathy
  Other intrinsic renal diseases
Renovascular hypertension
Cushing's syndrome
Primary aldosteronism
Pheochromocytoma
Sleep apnea

200–300 mg/day, or if there is reproducible (three occasions) microalbuminuria exceeding 16–30 ug/min in a timed collection or 16–30 mg/L in a spot collection.[59]

Renovascular Hypertension   Atherosclerotic renovascular hypertension is the second most common secondary cause of hypertension in a diabetic and should be suspected by worsening hypertension and the finding of a bruit in the upper abdomen (approximately 40–60% of patients).[60] One autopsy study reported that 10% of patients with diabetes and hypertension had anatomic renal artery stenosis (bilateral in 43%), a prevalence more than twice that (i.e., 4.3%) of the general population.[61] Evaluation for possible renal artery stenosis generally proceeds with captopril renography.[62,63] Aortography has more than the usual risk of complications (including contrast-induced acute renal failure) in diabetic patients, particularly those with proteinuria or serum creatinine levels above 2 mg/dL.[64–66]

Cushing's Syndrome   Cushing's syndrome should be considered when an obese, hypertensive, and somewhat hirsute diabetic develops sudden weight gain with worsening hypertension and hyperglycemia. An excellent screening test is the 24 hr urinary excretion of free cortisol and creatinine. An alternate screening method is the overnight dexamethasone suppression test where the level of plasma cortisol should normally be below 5 ug/dL at 8:00 AM after taking 1 mg dexamethasone at 11:00 PM the prior evening.

Primary Aldosteronism   Primary aldosteronism should be excluded in hypertensive diabetics with spontaneous hypokalemia. Hedeland and associates[67] reported a twofold increase in the frequency of adrenocortical adenomas found at autopsy of diabetics, compared with nondiabetics. A diagnosis of primary aldosteronism is supported strongly by lack of suppression of the plasma aldosterone level to below 10 ng/dL after the infusion of 2 L of normal saline over 4 hr.[68]

Pheochromocytoma Pheochromocytoma typically presents with the triad of headache, palpitation, and sweating in a patient with tachycardia and hypertension that is difficult to manage. A timed urine collection for metanephrine and creatinine is one of the most useful screening tests. The metanephrine (expressed in micrograms) to creatinine (expressed in milligrams) ratio is usually below 1.0 in essential hypertension and above 2.2 with pheochromocytoma. Another useful screening procedure is the clonidine suppression test.[69] With pheochromocytoma, elevated levels of plasma norepinephrine do not suppress by 50% or more 3 hr after an oral dose of 0.3 mg clonidine. An abdominal computed tomography (CT) scan will demonstrate an adrenal mass in 90% of proven cases.[70]

Sleep Apnea Sleep apnea is a recently acknowledged secondary cause of hypertension. It occurs most often in obese men and is suspected by marked fatigue and daytime sleepiness in a patient whose partner provides a history of nocturnal snoring and gaspy breathing. Nocturnal home oximetry monitoring is very sensitive for the detection of transient desaturation, but the specificity is poor.[71]

Initial Plan of Therapy

Control of stage 1, 2, or 3 hypertension reduces the risk of stroke, congestive heart failure, and renal failure. Elevations of systolic pressure contribute as much or more to cardiovascular risks as do elevations of diastolic blood pressure.[72] The randomized, placebo-controlled Systolic Hypertension in the Elderly (SHEP) study demonstrated a 36% reduction in the risk of stroke following diuretic-based therapy for ISH.[73] The trial included 583 NIDDM patients (mean age 71 years) in whom the absolute risk reduction for cardiovascular events was twice as great as nondiabetic patients.[74]

Early control of intrarenal hemodynamics can be a critical factor in retarding the initiation and progression of diabetic nephropathy.[75] For example, control of blood pressure to levels of 140/95 mmHg or less was shown by Mogensen[76] to reduce proteinuria and slow the progression of diabetic nephropathy by 50% following reduction of blood pressure with a combination of a vasodilator, β-blocker, and furosemide as needed. More recent studies suggest that angiotensin-converting enzyme (ACE) inhibitors have a specific action in decreasing proteinuria and slowing the progression of renal failure in the early diabetic nephropathy of IDDM[77] and NIDDM.[78,79] In the often-quoted study of captopril versus placebo, however, progression was

improved markedly but not halted or reversed.[77] The actively treated patients did much better than the placebo-treated group, but progression of renal failure remained rapid with an average decrease in creatinine clearance of about 8 mL/min/year (i.e., from 84 to 59 mL/min over the 3 years).

JNC-VI,[58] the National High Blood Pressure Working Group on Hypertension in Diabetes,[80] and the American Diabetes Association[81] have recently recommended a blood pressure treatment goal of 130/85 mmHg or less in hypertensive diabetics. Excellent review articles expand on these recommendations.[82–88]

Diuretics Despite the risk of exacerbating diabetes, diuretics are not contraindicated in patients with reasonably well-controlled diabetes. In fact, the previously mentioned volume-dependent nature of diabetic hypertension often requires that diuretics be an integral part of the antihypertensive regimen. Although some reports indicate that long-term diuretic therapy can lead to worsening of glucose tolerance and clinical events,[89–92] others show no increased incidence of clinical diabetes relative to the use of other antihypertensive drugs.[93] The thiazide and thiazidelike diuretics have been most incriminated as having a diabetogenic effect, although furosemide can exert similar effects.[94] Little recognized is that a large component of any diuretic-mediated worsening of glucose intolerance is mediated through hypokalemia with impaired release of insulin.[95] Cautious but aggressive supplemental oral potassium therapy to maintain normokalemia can improve both the hyperglycemia[96] and the blood pressure. Kaplan et al.[97] reported significant decreases in blood pressure when serum potassium levels were raised by about 0.5 mEq/L with the use of oral potassium supplements in nondiabetic hypertensive patients with serum potassium levels below 3.5 mEq/L.

Relatively high doses of diuretics should not be used routinely because of the risk of hypokalemia, hypomagnesemia, ventricular arrhythmias, and sudden death in susceptible patients.[98–100] In addition, short-term trials have shown that most diuretics cause a rise in both serum cholesterol and triglycerides, which could impose additional risks to the hypertensive diabetic.[101] However, in longer-term trials these elevated lipid levels usually return to normal, although not all agree.[102] Table 38–3 provides recommended initial and maximal doses of various diuretics in hypertensive diabetics. Loop diuretics such as furosemide, bumetamide, or torsemide are usually required to accomplish an effective diuresis in patients with renal insufficiency and a serum creatinine level above 2–3 mg/dL. Furosemide should generally be given at least twice daily. Indapamide is a thiazidelike diuretic that is effective in low doses that do not usually adversely effect glucose control or lipid metabolism.[103–105]

TABLE 38–3 Recommended Initial and Maximal Diuretic Doses in Diabetic Patients with Hypertension

Diuretic Type	Initial Daily Dose (mg)	Maximal Daily Dose (mg)
Thiazide or thiazide-like diuretics		
Chlorthalidone	12.5	50
Hydrochlorodiazide	12.5	50
Indapamide	1.25	5
Metolazone (Mykrox)	0.5	1
Metolazone (Zaroxolyn)	2.5	10
Loop diuretics		
Bumetanide	0.5	4
Furosemide	40	240
Torsemide	5	100
Potassium-sparing diuretics[a]		
Amiloride	5	10
Spironolactone	25	100
Triamterene	25	100

[a] Potassium-sparing diuretics should be used only with caution in diabetic patients because of an increased risk of hyperkalemia.

β-Blockers

Patients with diabetes mellitus have a higher incidence than nondiabetics of acute myocardial infarction,[106] double and triple vessel coronary artery disease,[107] silent ischemia,[108] silent myocardial infarction,[109] and mortality following myocardial infarction.[110] Long-term β-blocker therapy is generally indicated after myocardial infarction.[111] In a non-randomized trial, Kjekshus et al.[112] reported a 1-year post–myocardial infarction mortality of 10% in diabetics discharged on β-blockers versus 23% for diabetics not receiving β-blockers, suggesting that patients with diabetes mellitus also benefit from chronic β-blocker therapy following myocardial infarction.

However, β-blockers, by a direct inhibition of pancreatic insulin release and a decrease in serum insulin levels, can worsen glucose tolerance in the diabetic patient. This effect is more apparent with nonselective (e.g., propranolol, nadolol) than with more cardioselective agents (e.g., acebutolol, atenolol, bisoprolol, metoprolol).[113,114] Moreover, nonselective β-blockers also can delay the recovery of blood glucose toward normal following hypoglycemia. Recovery of blood glucose from hypoglycemic levels is partly a function of B_2-mediated glycogenolysis.

β-blockers can also mask the tachycardia and palpitations that are part of the usual response to hypoglycemia. Presumably by allowing unopposed α-stimulation, hypoglycemia (in the presence of β-blockade) can be associated with a *rise* in diastolic blood pressure and a reflex bradycardia.[115] Nonselective β-blockade with propranolol is associated with an increase rather than a decrease in sweating during hypoglycemia.[116] The amplitude of physiologic tremor is primarily a B_2-mediated response that is blocked by nonselective β-blockers.[117] Hence, nonselective β-blockers can mask the palpitations, tachycardia, and tremor (but not the sweating) associated with hypoglycemia. They also prolong the time for recovery of blood glucose toward normal following hypoglycemia. All of these deleterious effects are less with the selective compared to the nonselective β-blockers.[118] Table 38–4 summarizes these effects of nonselective and selective β-blockers on hypoglycemia.

Serum lipids can also be adversely affected by β-blockers. Nonselective β-blockers can elevate triglyceride levels and reduce HDL levels in some patients. This effect may be less if cardioselective agents are used. The increasing clinical use of potent lipid-altering agents may make this issue relatively moot.

When therapy with a β-blocker is necessary, it is rational to choose only the cardioselective β-blockers in diabetic patients, particularly those who are insulin dependent. Remember, however, that β-blockers are relatively contraindicated in patients with bronchospasm.

Sympatholytic Agents A sympatholytic agent can be added if diastolic blood pressure remains 90 mmHg or more or systolic blood pressure remains 140 mmHg or more following 2–4 weeks of therapy with a thiazide, ACE inhibitor, β-blocker, or calcium-channel antagonist. Clonidine and guanabenz are centrally acting sympatholytic agents. The starting dose for clonidine is 0.1 mg twice daily; for guanabenz, 4 mg twice daily.

TABLE 38–4   Effect of Nonselective versus Cardioselective β-Blockers on the Response to Insulin-Induced Hypoglycemia

Event	Normal Response	Nonselective β-Blockers	Selective β-Blockers
Palpitations	↑	↓	↓
Sweating	↑	↑	?
Tremor	↑	↓	±
Heart rate	↑	↓	±
Diastolic pressure	↓	↑	±
Recovery time	–	↑↑	↑

Noncompliant patients may be at risk of "rebound hypertension" following abrupt discontinuation of either of these drugs. Guanfacine is a long-acting central sympatholytic agent that may be given once daily (1–2 mg), with a low risk of "rebound hypertension."[119]

Vasodilators   Hydralazine is a direct vasodilator that is effective when used in combination with a diuretic and a β-blocker. Initial doses are usually 10–25 mg twice daily. Use in combination with a sympatholytic agent helps prevent the hydralazine-induced reflex stimulation of the sympathetic nervous system with elevated catecholamines, tachycardia, and increased myocardial oxygen demand.

α-Blockers   Prazosin, terazosin, and doxazosin are selective blockers of postsynaptic α-receptors, indirectly producing vasodilation. Initial doses can be associated with dizziness or orthostatic hypotension. Terazosin and doxazosin are once-daily selective α_1-blockers; their starting dose is 1 mg daily. α-blockers tend to improve insulin sensitivity,[120–122] decrease total cholesterol, and increase HDL cholesterol.[101,123]

Calcium-Channel Antagonists   Amlodipine, diltiazem, felodipine, isradipine, nicardipine, nifedipine, nisoldipine, and verapamil are currently marketed calcium-channel antagonists that are useful in selected patients with hypertension, angina, or arrhythmias. They decrease the elevated peripheral vascular resistance that is characteristic of diabetic patients with hypertension. They also induce a transient natriuresis that may be apparent to the patient during initial therapy. They generally have no adverse effect on serum lipids[101] or insulin sensitivity.[121,122]

Recent controversy has surrounded reports suggesting that the use of short-acting calcium-channel antagonists might be associated with an increase in the risk of cardiovascular events.[124–126] There are no current data, however, on which to convey concern about the long-acting, once-daily forms of calcium-channel antagonists used most often in clinical practice. A recent case-control study reported no excess in the risks of cardiovascular events when therapy with long-acting calcium-

channel antagonists was compared to β-blockers.[127] Results of the Systolic Hypertension in Europe (SYST-EUR) trial became available in the fall of 1997.[128] Elderly patients (n = 4,695) with ISH were randomized to placebo versus the long-acting calcium-channel antagonist nitrendipine (plus enalapril and hydrochlorothiazide as needed). After a median follow-up period of 2 years, the group receiving nitrendipine had a 42% reduction in fatal or nonfatal stroke and a 31% reduction in all cardiovascular events. Other long-term, randomized, controlled clinical trials are ongoing.[129]

A number of reports suggest that the nondihydropyridine calcium-channel antagonists may have a role for the reduction of proteinuria or stabilization of renal function in patients with diabetic nephropathy.[130–133]

Converting Enzyme Inhibitors   Benazepril, captopril, enalapril, fosinopril, lisinopril, moexipril, quinapril, ramipril, and trandolopril are currently marketed ACE inhibitors that have several distinct advantages for the hypertensive patient with diabetes. They do not cause sodium retention and do not adversely affect lipids. There is also evidence that many of the ACE inhibitors may increase insulin sensitivity with a beneficial effect on metabolic control in NIDDM.[134,135] Another advantage of ACE inhibitors is their benefit on progression of renal function and proteinuria in diabetics with early or incipient nephropathy. Several studies have shown a decrease in proteinuria in diabetics treated with ACE inhibitors,[136–140] as well as a stabilization of glomerular filtration rate that may be independent of the systemic blood pressure–lowering effect.[77,141,142] The mechanism by which this occurs is believed to be a reduction of glomerular capillary hydrostatic pressure by inhibition of the vasoconstrictive effect of angiotensin II on efferent glomerular arterioles. Of note is that a high dietary salt intake can abolish the beneficial effect of ACE inhibitors on proteinuria.[143,144]

Adverse effects of ACE inhibitors are few, primarily a nonproductive cough that occurs in about 15% of patients, especially women.[145,146] A rare but more serious adverse effect is angioedema, which may be more common in African Americans.[147] Acute deterioration of renal function can occur in the setting of bilateral renal artery stenosis or stenosis of a renal artery in a solitary kidney.

Hyperkalemia is uncommon in clinical trials using ACE inhibitors in patients with serum creatinine levels of 2.5 mg/dL or less. The risk of hyperkalemia, however, merits special caution in elderly diabetics because of the age-related decline in glomerular filtration rate (often not obvious from just the serum creatinine level),[148] the increased prevalence of hypoaldosteronism in elderly diabetics,[17] the frequent use of nonsteroidal anti-inflammatory agents,[149] and the concomitant use of potassium supplements.

Angiotensin II Receptor Blockers (ARB) The angiotensin II receptor antagonists (e.g., losartan, valsartan) interfere with binding of angiotensin II to angiotensin type 1 receptors. They are often useful in patients with ACE inhibitor–induced cough. A recent 1-year trial of losartan (50 mg/day) versus captopril (50 mg three times/day) reported a significant decrease in mortality (9% vs. 13% respectively) in elderly patients with congestive heart failure.[150] There also are preliminary data suggesting reduction in proteinuria.[151] Data also suggest that ARBs promote regression of left ventricular hypertrophy (LVH).[152,154] Like the ACE inhibitors, these drugs should not be used in pregnancy.

Patient Education and Follow-up Educational plans should be established at the onset of antihypertensive therapy in the diabetic. These include not only the usual content for education of hypertensive patients (e.g., the asymptomatic nature of the disease and the importance of adherence to medications and compliance with dietary instructions and appointments), but also attention to unique situations in the hypertensive diabetic. Examples include meticulous attention to home glucose monitoring during the initial week of diuretic therapy, when patients with previously borderline control can sometimes become uncontrolled or rarely develop hyperosmolar coma, or the observation for any change in symptoms of hypoglycemia when the patient begins β-blocker therapy after myocardial infarction.

Patients should also be advised concerning common adverse effects of antihypertensive therapy that might otherwise be attributed to their diabetes. Examples include fatigue, dyspnea, cold extremities, or claudication, sometimes associated with β-blocker therapy, or impotence, which can occur with the diuretics or sympatholytic drugs.

Consultations are particularly relevant to the hypertensive diabetic. The dietitian is important for maintenance of weight reduction and a low-sodium diet (generally a diet below 2,300 mg sodium is adequately low); the ophthalmologist to help assess ocular compli-cations; the cardiologist to help evaluate and manage chest pain; the nephrologist for renal failure; and the vascular surgeon and podiatrist to evaluate and treat symptoms of peripheral vascular disease.

Process and Outcome Audits

The most difficult part of any audit is defining the population on which the audit is to be conducted. Begin by making an alphabetized or numerical list of all the hypertensive diabetic individuals in the practice or group setting. Then set certain standards of optimal care that you would like to see in all patients. Examples might include:

1. Office visit within the last 6 months.

2. Repeat chemistries performed within the last 12 months.

3. Last measured cholesterol less than 200.

4. Last measured systolic blood pressure less than 140 mmHg.

5. Last measured diastolic blood pressure less than 90 mmHg.

6. Last measured blood glucose less than 150 mg/dL.

7. Hb A_{1c} value less than 8%.

Next, consider what percent exceptions to the standards that you would reasonably allow. For example, you might desire less than a 10% exception to the question concerning an office visit within the preceding 6 months, whereas you might be content to maintain control of systolic blood pressure below 140 mmHg and diastolic blood pressure below 90 mmHg in 80% of patients. Once standards and exceptions are established, review of office charts can be done by office personnel.

Audits will help identify deficiencies in care of the hypertensive patient with diabetes. Additional efforts in tracking patients for follow-up will allow calculation of an annual mortality and morbidity rate that can be compared to previous outcome data before and after a revision of your therapeutic strategy.

Research Considerations

Biochemical and Physiologic Studies

As previously mentioned, Weidmann and coworkers[13] found an expansion of total body sodium in hypertensive diabetics, and DeFronzo[20] and others[21] have provided an explanation of how high-carbohydrate intake and hyperinsulinemia can cause retention of sodium by the kidney. Meanwhile, Baron[46] and Sowers[47] have described that insulin resistance is primarily associated with endothelial dysfunction whereby nitric oxide-dependent vasodilation is impaired. Further investigation into the nature of this defect could provide insight into the mechanism and therapeutic implications for accelerated atherosclerosis in the diabetic patient with hypertension. The finding of a renal protective effect of ACE inhibition has also led researchers to pursue the relationship between angiotensin II, prostaglandins, and glomerular capillary pressure.

References

1. Prebble WE: Obesity: Observations on one thousand cases. Boston Med Surg J 88:617–621, 1923.

2. Herrick WW: Hypertension and hyperglycemia. JAMA 81:1942–1944, 1923.

3. Fineberg MH: Systolic hypertension. Its relationship to atherosclerosis of the aorta and larger arteries. Am J Med Sci 173:835–843, 1927.

4. Colandrea MA, Friedman GD, Nichaman NZ, et al.: Systolic hypertension in the elderly. An epidemiologic assessment. Circulation 41:239–245, 1970.

5. Klein R, Klein BEK, Lee KE, et al.: The incidence of hypertension in insulin-dependent diabetes. Arch Intern Med 156:622–627, 1996.

6. Pell S, D'Alonzo CA: Some aspects of hypertension in diabetes mellitus. JAMA 202:104–110, 1967.

7. Havlik RL, Hubert HB, Fabitz RR, et al.: Weight and hypertension. Ann Intern Med 98:855–859, 1983.

8. Garcia MJ, McNamara PM, Gordon T, et al.: Morbidity and mortality in diabetics in the Framingham population. Sixteen year followup study. Diabetes 23:105–111, 1974.

9. Jarrett RJ, Keen H, McCartney M, et al.: Glucose tolerance and blood pressure in two population samples: Their relation to diabetes mellitus and hypertension. Int J Epidemiol 7:15–24, 1978.

10. Morgensen CE: Progression of nephropathy in long term diabetes with proteinuria and effect of initial antihypertensive treatment. Scand J Clin Lab Invest 36:383–388, 1976.

11. Parving HH, Smidt UM, Friisberg B, et al.: A prospective study of glomerular filtration rate and arterial blood pressure in insulin-dependent diabetics with diabetic nephropathy. Diabetologia 20:457–461, 1981.

12. Mehler PS, Jeffers BW, Estacio R, et al.: Associations of hypertension and complications in non-insulin-dependent diabetes mellitus. Am J Hypertens 10:152–161, 1997.

13. Weidmann P, Beretta-Piccoli C, Keusch G, et al.: Sodium-volume factor, cardiovascular reactivity and hypotensive mechanism of diuretic therapy in mild hypertension associated with diabetes mellitus. Am J Med 67:779–784, 1979.

14. Tarazi RD, Frohlich ED, Dustan HP: Plasma volume in men with essential hypertension. N Engl J Med 278:762–765, 1968.

15. O'Hare JA, Ferriss JB, Brady D, et al.: Exchangeable sodium and renin in hypertensive diabetic patients with and without nephropathy. Hypertension 7(Suppl II): II-43–II-48, 1985.

16. Christlieb AR, Kaldany A, D'Elia JA: Plasma renin activity and hypertension in diabetes mellitus. Diabetes 25:969–974, 1976.

17. Perez GO, Lespier L, Knowles R, et al.: Potassium homeostasis in chronic diabetes mellitus. Arch Intern Med 137:1018–1022, 1977.

18. Fernandez-Cruz A Jr, Noth RH, Lassman MN, et al.: Low plasma renin activity in normotensive patients with diabetes mellitus: Relationship to neuropathy. Hypertension 3:87–92, 1981.

19. Trujillo A, Eggena P, Barrett J, et al.: Renin regulation in type II diabetes mellitus: Influence of dietary sodium. Hypertension 13:200–205, 1989.

20. DeFronzo RA: The effect of insulin on renal sodium metabolism. A review with clinical implications. Diabetologia 21:164–171, 1981.

21. Kageyama S, Yamamoto J, Isogai Y, et al.: Effect of insulin on sodium reabsorption in hypertensive patients. Am J Hypertens 7:409–415, 1994.

22. Zavaroni I, Mazza S, Dall'Aglio E, et al.: Prevalence of hyperinsulinemia in patients with high blood pressure. J Intern Med 231:235–240, 1992.

23. Hodges RE, Rebello T: Carbohydrates and blood pressure. Ann Intern Med 98:838–841, 1983.

24. Affarah HB, Hall WD, Heymsfield SB, et al.: High-carbohydrate diet: Antinatriuretic and blood pressure response in normal men. Am J Clin Nutr 44:341–348, 1986.

25. Tedde R, Sechi LA, Marigliano A, et al.: Antihypertensive effects of insulin reduction in diabetic-hypertensive patients. Am J Hypertens 2:163–170, 1989.

26. Liang C-S, Doherty JU, Faillace R, et al.: Insulin infusion in conscious dogs. Effects on systemic and coronary hemodynamic regional blood flows and plasma catecholamines. J Clin Invest 69:1311–1326, 1982.

27. Rowe JW, Young JB, Minaker KL, et al.: Effects of insulin and glucose infusions on sympathetic nervous activity in normal men. Diabetes 30:219–225, 1981.

28. Anderson EA, Hoffman RP, Balon TW, et al.: Hyperinsulinemia produces both sympathetic and neural activation and vasodilation in normal humans. J Clin Invest 87:2246–2252, 1991.

29. Kwok RPS, Juorio AW: The effect of insulin on rat brain noradrenaline. Neurochem Res 13:887–892, 1988.

30. Ferrannini E, Buzzigoli G, Bonnadonna R, et al.: Insulin resistance in essential hypertension. N Engl J Med 317:350–357, 1987.

31. Slater EE: Insulin resistance and hypertension. Hypertension 18(Suppl I):I108–I114, 1991.

32. Reaven GM, Lithell H, Landsberg L: Hypertension and associated metabolic abnormalities. The role of insulin resistance and the sympathoadrenal system. N Engl J Med 334:374–381, 1996.

33. Flack JM, Sowers JR: Epidemiologic and clinical aspects of insulin resistance and hyperinsulinemia. Am J Med 91 (Suppl 1A):11S–21S, 1991.

34. Hall JE, Coleman TG, Mizelle HL: Does chronic hyperinsulinemia cause hypertension? Am J Hypertens 2:171–173, 1989.

35. Hall JE, Brands MW, Dixon WN, et al.: Obesity-induced hypertension: Renal function and systemic hemodynamics. Hypertension 22:292–299, 1993.

36. Sowers JR, Standley PR, Ram JL, et al.: Hyperinsulinemia, insulin resistance, and hyperglycemia: Contributing factors in the pathogenesis of hypertension and atherosclerosis. Am J Hypertens 6:260S–270S, 1993.

37. Davidson MB: Clinical implications of insulin resistance syndromes. Am J Med 99:420–426, 1995.

38. Despres J-P, Lamarche B, Mauriege P, et al.: Hyperinsulinemia as an independent risk-factor for ischemic heart disease. N Engl J Med 334:952–957, 1996.

39. Manolio TA, Savage PJ, Burke GL, et al.: Association of fasting insulin with blood pressure and lipids in young adults. The CARDIA study. Arteriosclerosis 10:430–436, 1990.

40. Austin MA, Mykkanen L, Kuusisto J, et al.: Prospective study of small LDLs as a risk factor for non-insulin-dependent diabetes mellitus in elderly men and women. Circulation 92:1770–1778, 1995.

41. Laws R, Reaven GM: Evidence for an independent relationship between insulin resistance and fasting plasma HDL-cholesterol, triglyceride and insulin concentrations. J Intern Med 231:25–30, 1992.

42. Suzuki M, Shinozaki K, Kanazawa A, et al.: Insulin resistance as an independent risk factor for carotid wall thickening. Hypertension 28:593–598, 1996.

43. Diez J, Laviades C, Mayor G: Effects of antihypertensive therapy on left ventricular hypertrophy of essential hypertension: A role for insulin-like growth factor? J Human Hypertens 7:479–484, 1993.

44. Tomiyama H, Doba N, Kushiro T, et al.: The relationship of hyperinsulinemic state to left ventricular hypertrophy, microalbuminuria, and physical fitness in borderline and mild hypertensives. Am J Hypertens 10:587–591, 1997.

45. Bianchi S, Bigazzi R, Galvan AQ, et al.: Insulin resistance in microalbuminuric hypertension: Sites and mechanisms. Hypertension 26:789–795, 1995.

46. Baron AD: Insulin and the vasculative—old actors, new roles. J Invest Med 44:406–412, 1996.

47. Sowers JR: Insulin and insulin-like growth factor in normal and pathological cardiovascular pathology. Hypertension 29:691–699, 1997.

48. Bennett T, Hosking DJ, Hampton JR: Cardiovascular control in diabetes mellitus. Br Med J 2:585–587,1975.

49. Christlieb AR, Munichoodappa C, Braaten JT: Decreased response of plasma renin activity to orthostasis in diabetic patients with orthostatic hypotension. Diabetes 23:835–840, 1974.

50. Nakano S, Ishii T, Kitazawa M, et al.: Altered circadian blood pressure rhythm and progression of diabetic nephropathy in non-insulin dependent diabetes mellitus subjects: An average three year follow-up study. J Investig Med 44:247–253, 1996.

51. Berrut G, Hallab M, Bouhanick B, et al.: Value of ambulatory blood pressure monitoring in type I (insulin-dependent) diabetic patients with incipient diabetic nephropathy. Am J Hypertens 7:222–227, 1994.

52. Equiluz-Bruck S, Schnack C, Kopp HP, et al.: Nondipping of nocturnal blood pressure is related to urinary albumin excretion rate in patients with type 2 diabetes mellitus. Am J Hypertens 9:1139–1143, 1996.

53. Mitchell TH, Nolan B, Henry M, et al.: Microalbuminuria in patients with non-insulin-dependent diabetes mellitus relates to nocturnal systolic blood pressure. Am J Med 102:531–535, 1997.

54. Beretta-Piccoli C, Weidmann P: Exaggerated pressor responsiveness to norepinephrine in nonazotemic diabetes mellitus. Am J Med 71:829–835, 1981.

55. Bulpitt CJ, Dollery CT, Carne S: Change in symptoms of hypertensive patients after referral to hospital clinic. Br Heart J 38:121–128, 1976.

56. Lipson LG: Treatment of hypertension in diabetic men: Problems with sexual dysfunction. Am J Cardiol 53:46A–50A, 1984.

57. Leedom L, Feldman M, Procci W, et al.: Symptoms of sexual dysfunction and depression in diabetic women. J Diabetes Complications 5:38–41, 1991.

58. Joint National Committee on Prevention, Detection, Evaluation, and Treatment of High Blood Pressure (JNC VI): The Sixth Report of the Joint National Committee on Prevention, Detection, Evaluation, and Treatment of High Blood Pressure. Arch Intern Med 157:2414-2446, 1997.

59. Mueller PW, Hall WD, Caudill SP, et al.: An in-depth examination of the excretion of albumin and other sensitive markers of renal damage in mild hypertension. Am J Hypertens 8:1072–1082, 1995.

60. Shapiro AP, Perez-Stable E, Moutsos SE: Coexistence of renal arterial hypertension and diabetes mellitus. JAMA 192:813–816, 1965.

61. Sawicki PT, Kaiser S, Heinemann L, et al.: Prevalence of renal artery stenosis in diabetes mellitus: an autopsy study. J Intern Med 229:489–492, 1991.

62. Sfanianakis GN, Bourgoignie JJ, Jaffe D, et al.: Single-dose captopril scintigraphy in the diagnosis of renovascular hypertension. J Nucl Med 28:1383–1392, 1987.

63. Taylor A, Nally J, Aurell M, et al.: Consensus report on ACE inhibitor renography for detecting renovascular hypertension. J Nucl Med 37:1876–1882, 1996.

64. Harkonen S, Kjellstrand CM: Exacerbation of diabetic renal failure following intravenous pyelography. Am J Med 63:939–946, 1977.

65. Schwab SJ, Hlatky MA, Pieper KS, et al.: Contrast nephrotoxicity: A randomized controlled trial of a non-ionic and an ionic radiographic contrast agent. N Engl J Med 320:149–153, 1989.

66. Moore RD, Steinberg EP, Powe NR, et al.: Nephrotoxicity of high-osmolality versus low-osmolality contrast media: Randomized clinical trial. Radiology 182:649–655, 1992.

67. Hedeland H, Östberg G, Hövfelt B: On the prevalence of adrenocortical adenomas in an autopsy material in relation to hypertension and diabetes. Acta Med Scand 184:211–214, 1968.

68. Holland OB: Primary aldosteronism. Semin Nephrol 15:116–125, 1995.

69. Bravo EL, Tarazi RC, Fouad FM, et al.: Clonidine suppression test: A useful aid in the diagnosis of pheochromocytoma. N Engl J Med 305:623–626, 1981.

70. Stewart BH, Bravo EL, Haaga J, et al.: Localization of pheochromocytoma by computed tomography. N Engl J Med 299:460–461, 1978.

71. Series F, Marc I, Cormier Y, et al.: Utility of nocturnal home oximetry for case finding in patients with suspected sleep apnea hypopnea syndrome. Ann Intern Med 119:449–453, 1993.

72. Stamler J, Stamler R, Neaton JD: Blood pressure, systolic and diastolic, and cardiovascular risks: US population data. Arch Intern Med 153:598–615, 1993.

73. SHEP Cooperative Research Group: Prevention of stroke by antihypertensive drug treatment in older persons with isolated systolic hypertension: Final results of the systolic hypertension in the elderly program. JAMA 266:3255–3264, 1991.

74. Curb JD, Pressel SL, Cutler JA, et al.: Effect of diuretic-based antihypertensive treatment on cardiovascular disease risk in older diabetic patients with isolated systolic hypertension. JAMA 276:1886–1892, 1996.

75. Hostetter TH: The case for intrarenal hypertension in the initiation and progression of diabetic and other glomerulopathies. Am J Med 72:375–380, 1982.

76. Mogensen CH: Preazotemic diabetic nephropathy, inhibited by antihypertensive treatment. In Friedman EA, L'Esperance FA, Jr (eds): Diabetic Renal-Retinal Syndrome. New York: Grune & Stratton, 1980, pp. 182–198.

77. Lewis EJ, Hunsicker LG, Bain RP, et al.: The effect of angiotensin converting enzyme inhibition in diabetic nephropathy. N Engl J Med 323:1456–1462, 1993.

78. Ravid M, Savin H, Jutrin I, et al.: Long-term stabilizing effect of angiotensin-converting enzyme inhibition on plasma creatinine and on proteinuria in normotensive type II diabetic patients. Ann Intern Med 118:577–581, 1993.

79. Lebovitz HE, Wiegmann TB, Cnaan A, et al.: Renal protective effects of enalapril in hypertensive NIDDM: Role of baseline albuminuria. Kidney Int 45(Suppl):S150–S155, 1994.

80. National High Blood Pressure Education Program Working Group: National High Blood Pressure Education Program Working Group report on hypertension in diabetes. Hypertension 23:145–158, 1994.

81. American Diabetes Association: American Diabetes Association: Clinical Practice Guidelines 1999. Diabetes Care 22 (Suppl 1):51–5 114, 1999.

82. Kaplan NM, Rosenstock J, Raskin P: A differing view of treatment of hypertension in patients with diabetes mellitus. Arch Intern Med 147:1160–1162, 1987.

83. Bakris GL, Barnhill BW, Sadler R: Treatment of arterial hypertension in diabetic humans; importance of therapeutic selection. Kidney Int 41:912–919, 1992.

84. Dawson KG, McKenzie JK, Ross SA, et al.: Report of the Canadian Hypertension Society consensus conference. 5. Hypertension and diabetes. Can Med Assoc J 149:821–826, 1993.

85. Moser M, Ross H: The treatment of hypertension in diabetic patients. Diabetes Care 16:542–547, 1993.

86. Arky RA, Caro JF, Johnson C, et al.: Treatment of hypertension in diabetes. Diabetes Care 19(Suppl 1):S107–S113, 1996.

87. Fatourechi V, Kennedy FP, Rizza R, et al.: A practical guideline for management of hypertension in patients with diabetes. Mayo Clin Proc 71:53–58, 1996.

88. Hall WD: Management of systolic hypertension in the elderly. Semin Nephrol 16:299–308, 1996.

89. Amery A, Berthaux P, Bulpitt C, et al.: Glucose intolerance during diuretic therapy. Results of trial by the European Working Party on Hypertension in the Elderly. Lancet 1:681–683, 1978.

90. Berglund G, Andersson O: Beta-blockers or diuretics in hypertension? A six-year followup of blood pressure and metabolic side effects. Lancet 1:744–747, 1981.

91. Warram JH, Laffel L, Valsania P, et al.: Excess mortality associated with diuretic therapy in diabetic patients. Arch Intern Med 151:1350–1356, 1991.

92. Murphy MB, Kohner E, Lewis PJ, et al.: Glucose intolerance in hypertensive patients treated with diuretics, a fourteen year followup. Lancet 2:1293–1295, 1982.

93. Gurwitz JH, Bohn RL, Glynn RJ, et al.: Antihypertensive drug therapy and the initiation of treatment for diabetes mellitus. Ann Intern Med 118:273–278, 1992.

94. Breckenridge A, Dollery CT, Welborn TA, et al.: Glucose tolerance in hypertensive patients on long-term diuretic therapy. Lancet 1:61–64, 1967.

95. Fajans SS, Floyd JC Jr, Knopf RF, et al.: Benzothiadiazine suppression of insulin release from normal and abnormal islet tissue in man. J Clin Invest 45:481–492, 1966.

96. McFarland KF, Carr AA: Changes in the fasting blood sugar after hydrochlorothiazide and potassium supplementation. J Clin Pharmacol 17:13–17, 1977.

97. Kaplan NM, Carnegie A, Raskin P, et al.: Potassium supplementation in hypertensive patients with diuretic-induced hypokalemia. N Engl J Med 312:746–749, 1985.

98. Hoes AW, Grobbee DE, Lubsen J, et al.: Diuretics, β-blockers, and the risk of sudden cardiac death in hypertensive patients. Ann Intern Med 123:481–487, 1995.

99. Siegel D, Hulley SB, Black DM, et al.: Diuretics, serum and intracellular electrolyte levels, and ventricular arrhythmias in hypertensive men. JAMA 267:1083–1089, 1992.

100. Materson BJ: Diuretics, potassium, and ventricular ectopy. Am J Hypertens 10(5, Pt 2):68S–72S, 1997.

101. Kasiske BL, Ma JZ, Kalil RSN, et al.: Effects of antihypertensive therapy on serum lipids. Ann Intern Med 122:133–141, 1995.

102. Elliott WJ: Glucose and cholesterol elevations during thiazide therapy: Intention-to-treat versus actual on-therapy experience. Am J Med 99:261–269, 1995.

103. Roux P, Courtois H: Blood sugar regulation during treatment with indapamide in hypertensive diabetics. Postgrad Med J 57:70–72, 1981.

104. Raggi U, Palumbo P, Moro B, et al.: Indapamide in the treatment of hypertension in non-insulin-dependent diabetes. Hypertension 7(Suppl II):II-157–II-160, 1985.

105. Hall WD, Weber MA, Ferdinand K, et al.: Lower dose diuretic therapy in the treatment of patients with mild to moderate hypertension. J Human Hypertens 8:571–575, 1994.

106. Grossman E, Messerli FH: Diabetic and hypertensive heart disease. Ann Intern Med 125:304–310, 1996.

107. Waller BF, Palumbo PJ, Lie JT, et al.: Status of the coronary arteries at necropsy in diabetes mellitus with onset after age 30 years. Analysis of 229 diabetic patients with and without clinical evidence of coronary heart disease and comparison to 183 control subjects. Am J Med 69:498–506, 1980.

108. Nesto RW, Phillips RT, Kett KG, et al.: Angina and exertional myocardial ischemia in diabetic and nondiabetic patients: Assessment by exercise thallium scintigraphy. Ann Intern Med 108:170–175, 1988.

109. Niakan E, Harati Y, Rolak LA, et al.: Silent myocardial infarction and diabetic cardiovascular autonomic neuropathy. Arch Intern Med 146:2229–2230, 1986.

110. Herlitz J, Malmberg K, Karlson BW, et al.: Mortality and morbidity during a five-year follow-up of diabetics with myocardial infarction. Acta Med Scand 224:31–38, 1988.

111. Yusef S, Peto R, Lewis J, et al.: Beta blockade during and after myocardial infarction, an overview of the randomized trials. Prog Cardiovasc Dis 27:335–371, 1985.

112. Kjekshus J, Gilpin E, Cali G, et al.: Diabetic patients and beta-blockers after myocardial infarction. Eur Heart J 11:43–50, 1990.

113. Holm G, Johansson S, Vedin A, et al.: The effect of beta-blockade on glucose intolerance and insulin release in adult diabetes. Acta Med Scand 208:187–191, 1980.

114. Waal-Manning HJ: Metabolic effects of β-adrenoreceptor blockers. Drugs 11(Suppl 1):121–126, 1976.

115. Davidson NM, Carrall RJM, Shaw TRD, et al.: Observations in man of hypoglycemia during selective and nonselective beta-blockade. Scott Med J 22:69–72, 1977.

116. Molnar GW, Read RC: Propranolol enhancement of hypoglycemic sweating. Clin Pharmacol Ther 15:490–496, 1974.

117. Pickles H, Perucca E, Fish A, et al.: Propranolol and sotalol as antagonists of isoproterenol-enhancing physiologic tremor. Clin Pharmacol Ther 30:303–310, 1981.

118. Shorr RI, Ray WA, Daugherty JR, et al.: Antihypertensives and the risk of serious hypoglycemia in older persons using insulin or sulfonylureas. JAMA 278:40–43, 1997.

119. Jain AK, Hiremath A, Michael R, et al.: Clonidine and guanfacine in hypertension. Clin Pharmacol Ther 37:271–276, 1985.

120. Skyler JS, Marks JB, Schneiderman N: Hypertension in patients with diabetes mellitus. Am J Hypertens 81(12, Pt 2):100S–105S, 1995.

121. Giordano M, Matsuda M, Sanders L, et al.: Effects of angiotensin-converting enzyme inhibitors, Ca^{2+} channel antagonists, and α-adrenergic blockers on glucose and lipid metabolism in NIDDM patients with hypertension. Diabetes 44:665–671, 1995.

122. Lithell HO: Hyperinsulinemia, insulin resistance, and the treatment of hypertension. Am J Hypertens 9:150S–154S, 1996.

123. Deger E: Effect of terazosin on serum lipids. Am J Med 80(Suppl 5B):83–85, 1986.

124. Psaty BM, Heckbert SR, Koepsell TD, et al.: The risk of myocardial infarction associated with antihypertensive drug therapies. JAMA 274:620–625, 1995.

125. Furberg CD, Psaty BM, Meyer JV: Nifedipine. Dose-related increase in mortality in patients with coronary heart disease. Circulation 274:620–625, 1995.

126. Grossman E, Messerli FH: Calcium antagonists in cardiovascular disease: A necessary controversy but an unnecessary panic. Am J Med 102:147–149, 1997.

127. Alderman MH, Cohen H, Roque R, et al.: Effect of long-acting and short-acting calcium antagonists on cardiovascular outcomes in hypertensive patients. Lancet 349:594–598, 1997.

128. Staessen JA, Fagard R, Thijs L, et al: Randomized double-blind comparison of placebo and active treatment for older patients with isolated systolic hypertension. Lancet 350:757–764, 1999.

129. Davis BR, Cutler JA, Gordon DJ, et al.: Rationale and design for the antihypertensive and lipid lowering treatment to prevent heart attack trial (ALLHAT). Am J Hypertens 9:342–360, 1996.

130. Demarie BK, Bakris GL: Effects of different calcium antagonists on proteinuria associated with diabetes mellitus. Ann Intern Med 113:987–988, 1990.

131. Bakris GL, Copley JB, Vicknair N, et al.: Calcium channel blockers versus other antihypertensive therapies on the progression of NIDDM associated nephropathy: Results of a six year study. Kidney Int 50:1641–1650, 1996.

132. Bakris GL, Mangrum A, Copley JB, et al.: Effect of calcium channel or β-blockade on the progression of diabetic nephropathy in African Americans. Hypertension 29:744–750, 1997.

133. Bakris GL, Barnhill BW, Sadler R: Treatment of arterial hypertension in diabetic humans; importance of therapeutic selection. Kidney Int 41:912–919, 1992.

134. Ferriere M, Lachkar H, Richard J-L, et al.: Captopril and insulin sensitivity. Ann Intern Med 102:134–135, 1985.

135. Paolisso G, Gambardella A, Verza M, et al.: ACE inhibition improves insulin sensitivity in aged insulin-resistant hypertensive patients. J Human Hypertens 6:175–179, 1992.

136. Taguma Y, Kitamoto YK, Futaki G, et al.: Effect of captopril on heavy proteinuria in azotemic diabetics. N Engl J Med 313:1617–1620, 1985.

137. Parving H-H, Hommel E, Smidt VM: Protection of kidney function and decrease in albuminuria by captopril in insulin dependent diabetics with nephropathy. Br Med J 297:1086–1091, 1988.

138. Hommel E, Parving H-H, Mathiesen E, et al.: Effect of captopril on kidney function in insulin-dependent diabetic patients with nephropathy. Br Med J 293:467–470, 1986.

139. Marre M, Lablanc H, Suarez I, et al.: Converting-enzyme inhibition and kidney function in normotensive diabetic patients with persistent microalbuminuria. Br Med J 294:1448–1452, 1987.

140. Kasiske BL, Kalil RSN, Ma JZ, et al.: Effect of antihypertensive therapy on the kidney in patients with diabetes: A meta-regression analysis. Ann Intern Med 118: 129–138, 1993.

141. Tuck M: Management of hypertension in the patient with diabetes mellitus. Focus on the use of angiotensin-converting enzyme inhibitors. Am J Hypertens 1(Pt 2): 384S–388S, 1988.

142. Bjork S, Nyberg G, Malec H, et al.: Beneficial effects of angiotensin converting enzyme inhibition on renal function in patients with diabetic nephropathy. Br Med J 293:471–474, 1986.

143. Heeg JE, deJong PE, van der Hem GK, et al.: Efficacy and variability of the antiproteinuric effect of ACE inhibition by lisinopril. Kidney Int 36:272–280, 1989.

144. Bakris GL, Weir WR: Salt intake and reductions in arterial pressure and proteinuria. Is there a direct link? Am J Hypertens 9:200S–206S, 1996.

145. Israili ZH, Hall WD: Cough and angioneurotic edema associated with angiotensin-converting enzyme therapy. A review of the literature and pathophysiology. Ann Intern Med 117:234–242, 1992.

146. Os I, Bratland B, Dahlof B, et al.: Female preponderance for lisinopril-induced cough in hypertension. Am J Hypertens 7:1012–1015, 1994.

147. Brown NJ, Ray WA, Snowden M, et al.: Black Americans have an increased rate of angiotensin converting enzyme inhibition-associated angioedema. Clin Pharmacol Ther 60:8–13, 1996.

148. Friedman JR, Norman DC, Yoshikawa TT: Correlation of estimated renal function parameters versus 24-hour creatinine clearance in ambulatory elderly. J Am Geriatr Soc 37:145–149, 1989.

149. Chrischilles EA, Lemke JH, Wallace RB, et al.: Prevalence and characteristics of multiple analgesic drug use in an elderly study group. J Am Geriatr Soc 38:979–984, 1990.

150. Pitt B, Segal R, Martinez FA, et al.: Randomized trial of losartan versus captopril in patients over 65 with heart failure (Evaluation of Losartan in the Elderly Study, ELITE). Lancet 349:747–752, 1997.

151. Gansevoort RT, de Zeeuw D, Shahinfar S, et al.: Effects of the angiotensin II antagonist losartan in hypertensive patients with renal disease. J Hypertens 12(Suppl 2): S37–S42, 1994.

152. Dostal DE, Baker KM: Angiotensin II stimulation of left ventricular hypertrophy in adult rat heart: Mediation by the AT_1 receptor. Am J Hypertens 5:276–280, 1992.

153. Nunez E, Hosoya K, Susic D, et al.: Enalapril and losartan reduced cardiac mass and improved coronary hemodynamics in SHR. Hypertension 29(pt 2):519–524, 1997.

154. Tedesco MA, Ratti G, Aguino D, et al.: Effects of losartan on hypertension and left ventricular mass: A long-term study. J Human Hypertens 12:505-510, 1998.

39

Hyperlipidemia and Atherosclerotic Cardiovascular Disease

George Steiner

Historical Perspective

Atherosclerosis is the most common complication of diabetes in the Western world (see Chapter 28).[1] In 1938 Warren et al.[2] recognized that atherosclerosis occurs both at a younger age and in a more severe form in those with diabetes than in those without diabetes. Before insulin therapy became available in 1922, atherosclerosis was responsible for only 16–23% of the deaths occurring in Joslin Clinic patients. However, since the advent of insulin therapy, diabetics have survived longer and mortality patterns have changed. Today 75–80% of those with diabetes die of the consequences of arteriosclerotic disease, as shown in Table 39–1. This contrasts with nondiabetic North Americans, one-third of whom die of atherosclerosis-related disorders.[1]

Epidemiology

The data from a large prospective study undertaken in Framingham, Massachusetts, underline the magnitude of the problem with respect to both morbidity and mortality.[3] In comparing those with diabetes from the Joslin Clinic population to those in the general population of the Framingham study, it can be seen that the increase

is found both in type 1 and in type 2 diabetes.[4] Figure 39–1 shows that, in diabetics, morbidity due to coronary heart disease is doubled. Morbidity caused by

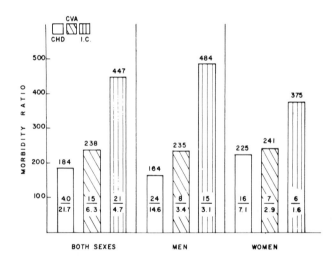

Figure 39–1. Causes of cardiovascular morbidity in diabetics during a 16-year follow-up study in Framingham, Massachusetts. CHD, coronary heart disease; CVA, cerebrovascular accident; IC, intermittent claudication. *Source*: Adapted from Garcia MJ, McNamara PM, Gorden J, et al.: Morbidity and mortality in diabetes in the Framingham population. Diabetes 23:105, 1974. With permission.

TABLE 39–1 Arteriosclerotic Vascular Disease as a Cause of Death—Percent of All Deaths from All Causes[a]

Period	1898–1914	1914–1922	1922–1936	1937–1943	1944–1955	1956–1964
Site of lesion						
Cerebral	3	5	9	12	13	12
Cardiac	6	10	30	41	49	52
Renal[b]	3	4	5	11	15	15
Peripheral	4	4	8	5	2	2
Total arteriosclerotic deaths	16	23	52	63	75	81

[a] Data represent the percentage of deaths in the Joslin Clinic that resulted from arteriosclerotic vascular disease, as this figure has changed since 1898.

[b] Includes arteriolar nephrosclerosis and glomerulosclerosis.

Source: Adapted from Warren S, LeCompte PM, Legg, MA: The Pathology of Diabetes Mellitus, Ed. 4. Philadelphia: Lea & Febiger, 1966, p. 186. With permission.

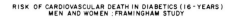

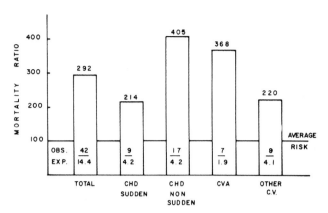

Figure 39–2. Causes of cardiovascular death in diabetic men and women during 16-year follow-up study in Framingham, Massachusetts. CHD, coronary heart disease; CV, cerebrovascular; CVA, cerebrovascular accident; EXP, expected; OBS, observed. *Source:* Adapted from Garcia MJ, McNamara PM, Gorden J, et al.: Morbidity and mortality in diabetes in the Framingham population. Diabetes 23:105, 1974. With permission.

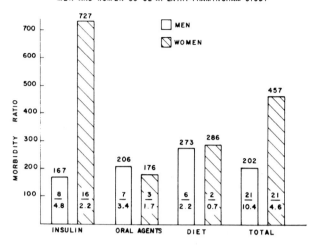

Figure 39–3. Sex distribution of cardiovascular mortality among diabetics on different treatment programs in Framingham study. *Source:* Adapted from Garcia MJ, McNamara PM, Gorden J, et al.: Morbidity and mortality in diabetics in the Framingham population. Diabetes 23:105, 1974. With permission.

cerebrovascular disease is more than doubled, and that due to intermittent claudication is more than quadrupled. Furthermore, with all problems except for peripheral vascular disease, the increase among diabetic women is at least as great as that among diabetic men. Diabetes also increases coronary artery disease mortality (Fig. 39–2). This is partly due to the increased accelerated atherosclerosis seen in diabetes. In addition, it reflects a greater case fatality and a poorer 5-year survival after a heart attack in those with diabetes.[5,6]

Diabetes increases the relative risk for coronary artery disease in women more than it does in men. This is because women without diabetes have a lower risk of coronary artery disease than do men, whereas in diabetes the risk of coronary artery disease is equal in both genders (Fig. 39–3).[7,8]

There are several other interesting and somewhat disturbing aspects of ischemic heart disease (IHD) in those with diabetes. Nearly one-quarter of myocardial infarctions occurring in diabetics are painless, a figure much higher than that in nondiabetics.[9] Some have suggested that the lack of pain is due to autonomic neuropathy.[9,10] However, several questions as to the proximate cause or causes of essentially painless IHD still remain. Furthermore, it is not known whether the neuropathy results from metabolic consequences of diabetes or from neuronal ischemia due to vascular disease.

Epidemiologic data obviously are subject to all the limitations that pertain to the definition of a cause of death, methods of data collection, endpoint identification, and so forth. Furthermore, atherosclerosis is not the only cause of IHD. Even when the endpoint event such as a stroke or myocardial infarct is correctly iden-

tified as the result of ischemia, this is not always the consequence of atherosclerosis. Although some believe that gangrene can only result from atherosclerotic occlusion of major arteries, others believe that it may be the consequence of nonatheromatous microangiopathy.[11] A similar situation may exist with respect to myocardial infarction. IHD may result from either, or both, atherosclerotic or nonatherosclerotic vascular disease. The latter possibility is raised by the observation that in diabetics, the basement membrane of myocardial small vessels may be abnormally thickened.[12]

Another problem in endpoint identification is that some manifestations of cardiac disease may be "labelled" as being due to ischemia when, in fact, they are not. One example of the complexity of this problem is outlined by data from the Framingham study. Diabetics in this population were found to have a high incidence of congestive heart failure. Many studies have used this as an endpoint indicating coronary vascular disease. However, in the Framingham population, it was thought that the cause of the congestive failure was some factor other than coronary atherosclerosis,[13] possibly some form of cardiomyopathy recently identified in diabetics.[14] It has also been suggested that one of the sulfonylureas, tolbutamide, may cause a form of cardiomyopathy (see Chapters 20 and 54).[14]

There is still debate about this and even if true, it is not clear whether this effect would be seen with other members of this class of drugs. However, before completely discounting ischemia as a basis for the increase of heart failure, one must recollect that in diabetics, many ischemic events are silent[9,10] and may therefore be missed. Furthermore, the patchy myocardial fibrosis seen in diabetics[12] may be the result of many small ischemic episodes.

Thus, much of the available epidemiologic data is difficult to interpret. Too often, a clinical endpoint that could result from many different causes has been the only entity recorded, and it has been equated with atherosclerosis. Despite these limitations, there is little doubt that atherosclerosis is the most common complication related to diabetes. It is such a common cause of death in the general population of North America and of Europe that many professionals in Western countries fail to appreciate the role of atherosclerosis in producing mortality and/or morbidity in those with diabetes.

It is fascinating that in contrast to the frequency of heart attacks in Caucasians with diabetes, heart attacks are rare in several other diabetic populations, e.g., the Japanese and certain Native American populations.[15–17] However, in all of these populations the incidence of IHD in those without diabetes is lower than that seen in Caucasians. In fact, in most groups the relative risk of coronary artery disease in those with diabetes is two to four times greater than it is in the comparable nondiabetic population. Thus, absolute rates of atherosclerotic cardiovascular disease between these various populations may be a reflection of incidence of atherosclerosis in the general community. On the other hand, the nature of their diabetes may differ in various groups and this may also be responsible for their differing rates of atherosclerosis.[18]

Hence *the diabetic, in contrast to the nondiabetic, has a much higher risk of IHD, is less likely to have premonitory symptoms, and may have a poorer outcome from any ischemic event.* For these reasons, preventive methods should be developed and implemented to combat this complication of diabetes. To accomplish this, a comprehensive knowledge of the causes of atherosclerosis in the population in general and in diabetes in particular must be developed. Only after the causes have been identified will it be possible to determine whether the incidence of atherosclerosis can be reduced by modifying the causative factors. The treatment of coronary artery disease and other cardiac complications of diabetes is discussed in Chapter 28. The focus of this chapter is directed toward an understanding of both the risk factors that contribute to the development and progression of atherosclerosis to morbidity and mortality and how those risk factors (particularly lipoprotein disorders) can be modified by appropriate preventive measures.

Risk Factors

A risk factor is something that identifies an individual as having an increased likelihood of having a particular phenomenon. It "marks" a person as being at risk and may, but need not, be a causative factor. A number of risk factors for cardiovascular disease have been identified in epidemiologic studies in both the general and diabetic populations. They include some that can be modified, such as hyperlipidemia, hypertension, and smoking. Others, such as age, family history, and gender, are not modifiable. In diabetes the risk factors include those that are generally recognized. Many may be present more frequently or in a more severe form, for example, hypertension and hypertriglyceridemia. Other risk factors are relatively more specific for diabetes. These include insulin resistance and hyperinsulinemia. This is often seen as a part of the constellation called *syndrome X or the insulin-resistance syndrome.*[19–22] It is generally associated with obesity and this obesity tends to be abdominal (android) rather than gluteofemoral (gynoid) in distribution. Another characteristic of diabetes is hyperglycemia. As will be indicated, there is debate both about the risk effect of hyperglycemia and whether increasing glucose levels, even within the normal range, are associated with an increased incidence of coronary artery disease.

Thus, a partial list of demonstrated and potential risk factors for atherosclerosis in diabetes includes a multitude of disorders in addition to the dyslipoproteinemias, the focus of this chapter. Patients with renal disease, either renal failure or proteinuria (including micro-albuminuria), are at greater risk of coronary artery disease. Hypertension, smoking, alterations in soluble clotting factors and in platelet function, age, previous atherosclerotic cardiovascular disease, and possibly hyperglycemia are other risk factors. In addition, pathophysiologic studies suggest other factors that could be atherogenic in diabetes but have either not been examined or examined in as much detail in epidemiologic studies. They include alterations in artery wall metabolism, the accumulation of advanced glycation end-products, and changes in rheology.

Lipoproteins

Hypertriglyceridemia is the most common form of hyperlipidemia found in those with diabetes.[23] Many have thought that it is one of the factors responsible for the accelerated atherosclerosis seen in diabetes. Although there has been considerable controversy, there is now increasing support for the independent coronary risk effect of hypertriglyceridemia.[24] The reasons for this controversy may lie in the heterogeneity of hypertriglyceridemia,[25] in the endpoints used to define coronary disease,[26] and in a failure to distinguish between low-density lipoproteins (LDL) and intermediate density lipoproteins (IDL).[27] Two prospective studies have shown that an increase in plasma triglyceride levels[28] or in triglyceride-rich lipoproteins[29] increase the risk of coronary artery disease in diabetes. The first did not measure high-density lipoprotein

(HDL) cholesterol levels. The second suggested that it may be a combination of increased levels of triglyceride-rich lipoproteins and reduced levels of HDL that is atherogenic. In fact, the very tight inverse association of these two lipoprotein families may make it impossible ever to separate their impact. There is no agreement whether hypertriglyceridemia is atherogenic itself or marks the presence of other atherogenic factors. Such other atherogenic factors, in the case of lipoproteins, would include reduced levels of HDL cholesterol and a shift in LDL characteristics toward particles that are smaller and denser[30-32] and many features of the insulin resistance syndrome. In addition to being a risk factor for the presence or absence of coronary artery disease in diabetes, the triglyceride-rich lipoprotein levels are positively and independently related to the severity of coronary artery disease.[33]

As implied in the preceding paragraph, HDL may also influence the risk of coronary artery disease. However, the influence of HDL differs from that of the other lipoproteins, as increases in HDL diminish the risk of IHD.[34] In diabetes, the pattern of HDL alterations is quite variable. Some have reduced levels of HDL. Others have levels that are no different from that in the nondiabetic population. Finally, HDL levels may actually be increased in some diabetics, particularly those who are treated with insulin. Various epidemiologic studies are summarized[35] and the possible metabolic explanations for these multiple findings are considered later in this chapter.

Most have found that the levels of LDL in a population with diabetes are similar to those in a general population.[23] However, this should not be interpreted as meaning that LDL has no risk effect in diabetes. Indeed, coronary artery disease mortality increases as serum cholesterol rises in those with diabetes. Furthermore, the curve describing the relationship between both is similar in shape to that for the general population. However, at any given cholesterol level the coronary artery disease risk in diabetes is two to four times greater than that in those without diabetes.[36] Three explanations could be given for this greater risk in diabetes. First, serum cholesterol measures not only the cholesterol in LDL, but also that in the triglyceride-rich lipoproteins. Second, diabetes can increase the risk of coronary artery disease through nonlipoprotein mechanisms. Third, the LDL particles in diabetes may be more atherogenic. This may be because they are smaller and denser, because they are nonenzymatically glycated, and/or because they are oxidized.

Lipoprotein Metabolism in Diabetes

The changes in lipoprotein concentrations in those with diabetes have been discussed. It was indicated that the most frequent abnormality is an accumulation of the triglyceride-rich lipoproteins. These may accumulate for either of two reasons, insulin deficiency or hyperinsulinemia. For some years hypertriglyceridemia was attributed exclusively to the first of these. There is no question that insulin deficiency can result in a decrease in the activity of LPL.[37] Since that enzyme limits the removal of circulating triglyceride, it is easy to understand how this would lead to hypertriglyceridemia.

However, most diabetics are not insulin deficient. The majority have type 2 diabetes. They are insulin resistant and have "compensatory" endogenous hyperinsulinemia. Frequently, patients with diabetes treated with insulin are hyperinsulinemic because they are being treated with large doses of exogenous insulin that raises arterial insulin levels. Thus, in the majority, one must examine the relationship between hyperinsulinemia and hypertriglyceridemia. A number of studies have demonstrated a correlation between hypertriglyceridemia and hyperinsulinemia.[38,39] Hyperinsulinemia increases VLDL-triglyceride production. Hence, in the majority of diabetics, hypertriglyceridemia may be caused by overproduction rather than by impaired removal. Because hypertriglyceridemia itself is associated with insulin resistance,[40] the association between hyperinsulinemia and hypertriglyceridemia may establish a vicious circle.[39] This can be intensified by obesity, particularly abdominal obesity. The atherogenic potential of this increase in VLDL production has been described.

The inconsistency of the epidemiologic data with respect to HDL levels in diabetics has been described. The low HDL levels reported by some may reflect the inverse relationship between concentrations of VLDL and HDL levels found in different large population groups. Also, it may reflect the frequent coexistence of obesity, which is associated with a reduced HDL concentration. In some diabetics, the low HDL level may reflect the reduction of activity of LPL. In part, HDL is produced as a product of the lipolytic degradation of triglyceride-rich lipoproteins. Hence, a reduction of the enzyme would decrease the level of HDL. However, as has been noted, hyperinsulinemia may actually increase LPL activity. This could lead to an increase in HDL levels and might account for the elevated HDL concentrations found in insulin-treated diabetics.

Therapeutic Implications

This chapter does not deal with the treatment of end-organ damage (see Chapters 25 through 37) or with vascular bypass surgery in the diabetic (see Chapters 28 and 34). Rather, it is concerned with preventing the atherogenic process.

It is possible that one particular risk factor (e.g., dyslipoproteinemia) brings the patient to a physician's attention. However, in undertaking prevention, all risk factors that potentially can cause atherosclerosis, not only the one in particular, should be addressed. Hence, if they exist, the physician must treat smoking, obesity, hypertension, and so forth. It must be admitted that proof of the efficacy of preventive measures currently rests on data that are often less conclusive than one would wish. However, as long as all indications point toward a causal role for a particular factor and as long as correction of that factor is not harmful, its correction is the only reasonable therapeutic approach. As an example of this uncertainty, there is insufficient current information to permit any dogmatic statement with respect to postmenopausal hormone replacement therapy as a coronary artery disease preventive measure in women with diabetes. In fact, there are some data suggesting that hormone replacement therapy in women with diabetes may have a deleterious effect on lipoproteins.[41] If diabetes reduces the relative protection of women against coronary artery disease, one could ask whether hormone replacement therapy is as useful in reducing the atherosclerosis risk in diabetes as it is in women without diabetes. Against this general background, the rest of this section will deal with treatment of the dyslipoproteinemias of diabetes.

There is strong evidence that reducing LDL cholesterol will decrease the risk of atherosclerotic cardiovascular disease in populations without diabetes. This is so for primary[42–44] and even more so for secondary intervention.[45,46] It also appears that increasing HDL cholesterol will reduce coronary artery disease.[47] However, it is not yet clear whether raising HDL in individuals with no other lipid disorder is or is not beneficial.[48] There is also a suggestion that reducing plasma triglycerides in those who already have coronary disease will reduce angiographic progression of coronary artery disease,[49] new cardiac events, and mortality from IHD.[49,50]

Until recently, lipid intervention studies excluded those with diabetes from their population in order to avoid too many variables being present. Therefore, advice in diabetes was based on extrapolation. In one study, the Helsinki Heart Study, a post hoc analysis of the data in a small group of people who, despite having diabetes, were entered into the study revealed a reduction in coronary artery disease in the group receiving active treatment with *gemfibrozil* for their dyslipoproteinemia.[51] However, the numbers of events were too few for these results to be statistically significant. Two other studies, the 4S study[52] and the CARE study,[46] have conducted post hoc analyses of subpopulations with diabetes. Both showed similar patterns. However, only the 4S study has published sufficient information on this population to permit a more detailed examination.[52] Both studies examined the effects of cholesterol reduction in populations that had known coronary artery disease, mild to moderate hypercholesterolemia, and relatively normal triglyceride levels. Each used a different cholesterol-lowering drug from the group of drugs known as the *HMG CoA*

reductase inhibitors. In both there was a significant reduction in coronary events in the actively treated group. However, drawing conclusions from each is limited by the fact that they were post hoc analyses, they involved secondary intervention, they were targeted at cholesterol rather than triglyceride reduction, and their diabetic populations (at least in the case of the 4S study, where information is available) may not have been a representative sample of similarly aged people with diabetes. There is one other study nearing completion, the *Diabetes Atherosclerosis Intervention Study (DAIS)*, that has been specifically designed to test whether treating the dyslipoproteinemias of type 2 diabetes with a fibrate, micronized fenofibrate, a drug in a different class, will reduce angiographic coronary disease.[53] At the time of this writing, there are two or three other studies in diabetes that are either in their initial or planning phases. Thus, definitive intervention trial information should soon be available. At present, however, recommendations for the treatment of dyslipoproteinemias in diabetes are based on studies such as those described earlier.

Only a small number of individuals with dyslipoproteinemia have well-characterized single gene mutations. Most dyslipoproteinemias are either polygenic or are related to an interaction between environmental factors and genetic susceptibility. Thus, a dyslipoproteinemia may be primary (genetic or familial) or secondary (environmental factors plus genetic susceptibility). A number of dyslipoproteinemias, particularly those associated with an increase in the triglyceride-rich lipoproteins but not an increase in LDL, may be secondary to diabetes. Other diseases or certain drugs may also cause or aggravate dyslipoproteinemias. This is important as, if any of these conditions is present, it should be treated first. Only if the lipoproteins are not normalized with this should more specific therapy be undertaken.

The dyslipoproteinemias can be treated in many patients by methods that are free of side effects (e.g., *improvement of glycemic control, diet, exercise, and weight loss*). Hence, it is appropriate to treat hyperlipidemia where it exists in the diabetic, at least with these methods. The use of *lipid-lowering drugs should be reserved for those who do not respond adequately to such treatment* (Table 39–2).

The "Problem Statement" and "Assessment" sections that follow have utilized contemporarily recommended terminology to minimize confusion in dealing with this complex, heterogenous group of disorders.[54]

Problem Statement

I. Dyslipoproteinemia
   A. Secondary hyperlipoproteinemias
      1. Due to uncontrolled diabetes mellitus

TABLE 39–2   Drugs That May Be Used to Treat Dyslipoproteinemias[a]

Dyslipoproteinemia	Order of preference of drugs
Hypertriglyceridemia	1. Fibrates 2. Nicotinic acid
Hypercholesterolemia	1. HMG CoA reductase inhibitors ("statins") 2. Bile acid binding resins or fibrates 3. Nicotinic acid
Mixed (i.e., hypertriglyceridemia plus hypercholesterolemia)	1. Fibrates 2. HMG CoA reductase inhibitors ("statins") 3. Combined drug therapy 4. Nicotinic acid

[a] These drugs should be used only if the dyslipoproteinemia persists after any underlying disease that may cause or aggravate the dyslipoproteinemia (e.g., uncontrolled diabetes, hypothyroidism) has been treated and adequate dietary control has been established. They should not be used or should be used with caution in individuals in whom there may be a contraindication.

2. Due to other diseases (see Assessment)
3. Due to drugs or alcohol (see Assessment)

B. Primary (genetic) hyperlipoproteinemias (see Assessment items I.B.1–I.B.6)
C. Primary (genetic) hypolipoproteinemia (see Assessment items I.B.7–I.B.9)
D. Primary (genetic) enzyme [lecithin: cholesterol acyltransferase] deficiency (see Assessment item I.B.10)

Subjective

History of abdominal pain; eruptive xanthoma; yellowish discoloration of palmar creases; xanthoma tuberosum of hands, elbows, feet, knees, and buttocks; tendon thickening; arcus corneae; lipemia retinalis; lipemic serum; hypercholesterolemia; hypertriglyceridemia; hyperlipoproteinemia or hypolipoproteinemia; hepatosplenomegaly; atherosclerosis (coronary, peripheral, cerebral, general); family history of lipid disorder; atherosclerosis; NIDDM; or IDDM.

Objective

Physical Examination.   Eruptive xanthoma (see Fig. 45–9); arcus corneae (lipid deposits surrounding the periphery of the corneas); xanthalasmas (lipid deposits in the upper and/or lower eyelids); lipemia retinalis; palmar xanthoma (yellowish discoloration of palmar and digital creases secondary to lipid deposits); tuberous xanthoma; tendonous xanthoma (calcaneal or Achilles tendons, extensor tendons of hands, patellar tendon, elbows, and buttocks); hepatosplenomegaly; atherosclerosis.

Laboratory.   *Screening for dyslipoproteinemias*: 12-hr fasting plasma sample. There are no truly normal values for these parameters. The plasma lipoprotein concentrations in a population generally have a normal distribution and are not bimodal. In addition, there is

no threshold value that is accompanied by an increase in risk. Hence, one can not distinguish "normal" from "abnormal" populations, nor can one say that on one side of a given value the individual is completely free from risk. Therefore, what has been accepted is to refer to target values. These are values, reached by consensus, at which the risk effect becomes much more pronounced: (1) *triglyceride*—the target level recommended by most consensus groups is <2.3 mmol/L; (2) *cholesterol*—most do not use a value for total plasma cholesterol as a target but use values for LDL cholesterol and HDL cholesterol. The target for LDL cholesterol used by most is <3.4 mmol/L; for HDL cholesterol >0.9 mmol/L.

Lipid battery test: Measure cholesterol, TG, and HDLC. May calculate LDLC from the following formula: LDLC (mmol/L) = total cholesterol (mmol/L) − [plasma TG (mmol/L)/2.2] − HDLC (mmol/L). Plasma TG divided by 2.2 represents an estimate of the VLDL cholesterol. There may be considerable error in using this formula to calculate LDLC in anyone with plasma TG levels over 4.5 mmol/L or in anyone with type 3 hyperlipoproteinemia.

Follow-up testing: May include IDL and apoprotein E isoforms (type 3 dyslipoproteinemia), postheparin LPL activity (PHLA), apolipoprotein assays (A-I, B, CII), or, rarely, analytic ultracentrifugation (the reference method). See Chapter 13 for a detailed description of valid methods for initial evaluation and for follow-up monitoring of the dyslipoproteinemias.

Assessment

There are more than 30 causes of dyslipoproteinemia. The presence of two or more of the disorders in an individual may, but does not necessarily, indicate that there is a causal relationship between them. The dyslipoproteinemias are listed in secondary and primary (genetic) forms. The first four of the secondary forms (items I.A.1.a.–I.A.1.d.) are commonly seen in those with diabetes (especially in uncontrolled diabetes), and the next five secondary forms (items I.A.2–I.A.6) are seen more frequently in those with diabetes than in those who do not have diabetes. The other secondary forms and the primary (genetic) forms of dyslipoproteinemia occur with the same frequency in those who have and in those who do not have diabetes.

I. Dyslipoproteinemia
   A. Secondary to:
      1. Uncontrolled diabetes
         a. Hyperchylomicronemia: Markedly elevated chylomicrons (CM) (pronounced hypertriglyceridemia), eruptive xanthomas, lipemia retinalis, pancreatitis, hepatosplenomegaly, low or absent PHLA
         b. Dysbetalipoproteinemia (Type 3 dyslipoproteinemia): Tuberoeruptive xanthomas, palmar xanthoma, overweight (obese), accelerated coronary and peripheral atherosclerosis, elevated CM and cholesterol, abnormal form of VLDL (B-VLDL), absence of apolipoprotein E-3
         c. Endogenous hypertriglyceridemia (hyperprebetalipoproteinemia): Overweight (obese), glucose intolerance, elevated VLDL
      2. Diet high in fat, cholesterol, and calories leading to obesity
      3. Pancreatitis
      4. Alcoholism
      5. Nephrotic syndrome or uremia (may be secondary to diabetic nephropathy)
      6. Drugs: Estrogen and progesterone-containing birth control pills, corticosteroids, diuretics, β-blockers, antibiotics, and other drugs may alter lipoprotein metabolism and elevate lipoprotein levels
      7. Biliary obstruction
      8. Glycogen storage disease
      9. Hypothyroidism
      10. Myeloma
      11. Systemic lupus erythematosus
   B. Primary (genetic):
      1. Hyperchylomicronemia
      2. Familial hypercholesterolemia
      3. Familial dysbetalipoproteinemia (type 3 hyperlipoproteinemia)
      4. Familial hypertriglyceridemia
      5. Familial combined hyperlipidemia: Elevation of either, or both, TG and cholesterol plus demonstration of hypertriglyceridemia in some, and demonstration of hypercholesterolemia in other affected family members; postulated autosomal dominant; may be associated with hyperapobetalipoproteinemia
      7. Familial hyperalphalipoproteinemia: Increased concentrations of HDL, autosomal

dominant trait (associated with longevity), decreased incidence of coronary atherosclerosis
      8. Familial β-lipoprotein deficiency
         a. Recessive abetalipoproteinemia: Absence of lipoproteins that contain apolipoprotein B
         b. Familial hypobetalipoproteinemia: Low but detectable amounts of apolipoprotein B-containing lipoproteins
      9. Familial HDL deficiency
         a. Tangler disease
      10. Familial lecithin: Cholesterol acyltransferase (LCAT) deficiency
         a. Increased cholesterol (most unesterified) and TG, plasma LCAT very low

Plan

Initial. *Diet therapy is the cornerstone of therapy for hyperlipoproteinemia.* In general, one should start by setting the calorie content at a level that reduces and maintains weight at ideal. The distribution of nutrients should be as close as possible to the Step I American Heart Association diet. This is one in which 30% of the calories would be derived from fat, with not more than one-third coming from saturated fat and with less than 300 mg/day of cholesterol. This may have to be modified in those with diabetes to handle the requirements for carbohydrates that are necessitated by the diabetes. Where carbohydrate is given, as much as possible should be complex rather than simple sugars. The rare patient with hyperchylomicronemia may require a diet that has even less fat. Some but not all people increase their levels of triglycerides in response to moderate amounts of alcohol. They may have to have their alcohol intake restricted or eliminated. Those who have an increase in LDL cholesterol should be started on an American Heart Association Step I diet. If that is insufficient to bring their LDL to target levels, they should be advised to consume a Step II diet. That is one in which the amount of fat does not exceed 7% of the total calorie intake and less than 200 mg cholesterol are consumed per day.

Pharmacologic therapy of hyperlipoproteinemias should be approached with caution and should be reserved for those in whom diet therapy has failed. All drugs can cause adverse reactions and are expensive, and no single drug is effective in all forms of hyperlipoproteinemia. A summary of the order of preference of currently available drugs directed at specific lipoprotein fractions is noted in Table 39–2.

Follow-up. In each individual with diabetes, an attempt to attain and maintain ideal body weight, normal or near-normal lipid levels, and normal or near-normal plasma glucose levels should be part of continuing follow-up therapy.

Adherence and Audit

A careful follow-up audit is valuable to monitor patient adherence and to alert the physician to initiate corrective action when control of hyperlipidemia fails.

Research Considerations

A great deal of research has been done to improve the knowledge of the epidemiology, pathophysiology, and treatment of the dyslipoproteinemias in general and in diabetes in particular. At present, one must await the completion of the clinical trials that are specifically designed to test whether correcting the dyslipoproteinemias will reduce the risk of atherosclerosis in those with diabetes, as it does in the general population. That will permit recommendations for therapy and for desirable target levels to be made with greater certainty. In addition, one must still learn what factors other than dyslipoproteinemias increase the risk of atherosclerosis in diabetes. The mechanisms underlying their genesis and their impact need to be understood. Finally, the effect of treating an abnormality in any of these problems needs to be examined.

References

1. Steiner G: Atherosclerosis, the major complication of diabetes. In Vranic M, Hollenberg CH, Steiner G (eds): Comparison of Type I and Type II Diabetes. New York: Plenum, 1985, pp. 277–297.

2. Warren S, LeCompte PM, Legg MA: The Pathology of Diabetes Mellitus, Ed. 4. Philadelphia: Lea & Febiger, 1966, p. 186.

3. Garcia MJ, McNamara PM, Gorden J, et al.: Morbidity and mortality in diabetics in the Framingham population. Diabetes 23:105–111, 1974.

4. Krolewski AS, Kosinski EJ, Warram JH, et al.: Magnitude and determinants of coronary artery disease in juvenile-onset insulin-dependent diabetes mellitus. Am J Cardiol 59:750–755, 1987.

5. Smith JW, Marcus FI, Serokman R, et al.: Prognosis of patients with diabetes mellitus after acute myocardial infarction. Am J Cardiol 54:718–721, 1984.

6. Jaffe AS, Spadaro JJ, Schechtman K, et al.: Increased congestive heart failure after myocardial infarction of modest extent in patients with diabetes mellitus. Am Heart J 108:31–37, 1984.

7. Haffner SM, Stern MP, Rewers M: Diabetes and atherosclerosis: Epidemiological considerations. In Draznin B, Eckel RH (eds): Diabetes and Atherosclerosis. Amsterdam: Elsevier, 1993, pp. 229–254.

8. Barrett-Connor E, Wingard DL: Sex differential in ischemic heart disease mortality in diabetics: A prospective population-based study. Am J Epidemiol 118:489–496, 1983.

9. Faerman I, Faccio E, Milei J, et al.: Autonomic neuropathy and painless myocardial infarction in diabetes patients. Diabetes 26:1147–1158, 1977.

10. Langer A, Freeman MR, Josse RG, et al.: Detection of silent myocardial ischemia in diabetes mellitus. Am J Cardiol 67:1073–1078, 1991.

11. Strandness DE, Priest RE, Gibbons GE: Combined clinical and pathological study of diabetic and non-diabetic peripheral arterial disease. Diabetes 13:366–372, 1964.

12. Silver MD, Huckell VF, Lorber M: Basement membranes of small cardiac vessels in patients with diabetes and myxedema: Preliminary observations. Pathology 9:213, 1977.

13. Kannel WB, Hjortland M, Castelli WP: Role of diabetes in congestive heart failure: The Framingham Study. Am J Cardiol 34:29–34, 1974.

14. Rubler S, Dlugash J, Yuceoglu YZ, et al.: New type of cardiomyopathy associated with diabetic glomerulosclerosis. Am J Cardiol 30:595–602, 1972.

15. Goto Y, Sato S, Masuda M: Causes of death in 3151 diabetic autopsy cases. Tohoku J Exp Med 112:339–353, 1974.

16. Sasaki A, Vehara M, Horiuchi N, Hasegawa: A long-term follow-up study of Japanese diabetic patients: Mortality and causes of death. Diabetologia 25:309–312, 1983.

17. Prosnitz LR, Mandell GL: Diabetes mellitus among Navajo and Hopi Indians: The lack of vascular complications. Am J Med Sci 253:700–705, 1967.

18. Baba S, Goto Y, Fukui I (eds): Diabetes Mellitus in Asia, Proceedings of the Second Symposium. Amsterdam: Excerpta Medica, 1976.

19. Modan M, Halkin H, Almog S, et al.: Hyperinsulinemia: a link between hypertension, obesity and glucose intolerance. J Clin Invest 75:809–817, 1985.

20. Reaven GM: Banting lecture 1988: Role of insulin resistance in human disease. Diabetes 37:1595–1607, 1988.

21. Kaplan NM: The deadly quartet: Upper-body obesity, glucose intolerance, hypertriglyceridemia, and hypertension. Arch Int Med 149:1514–1520, 1989.

22. Crepaldi G, Tiengo A, Manzato E (eds): Diabetes, Obesity and Hyperlipidemias:V. The Plurimetabolic Syndrome. Amsterdam: Excerpta Medica, 1993.

23. Steiner G: The dyslipoproteinemias of diabetes. Atherosclerosis 110:527–533, 1994.

24. Austin MA, Hokanson JE: Epidemiology of triglycerides, small dense low-density lipoprotein, and lipoprotein(a) as risk factors for coronary heart disease. Med Clin N Amer 78:99–115, 1994.

25. Brunzell JD, Schrott HG, Motulsky AG, et al.: Myocardial infarction in the familial forms of hypertriglyceridemia. Metabolism 25:313–320, 1976.

26. Aberg H, Lithell H, Selinus I, Hedstrand H: Serum triglycerides are a risk factor for myocardial infarction but not angina pectoris. Results from a 10–year follow-up of UPPSALA primary preventive study. Atherosclerosis 54:89–97, 1985.

27. Steiner G, Schwartz L, Shumak S, Poapst M: The association of increased levels of intermediate-density lipoproteins with smoking and with coronary artery disease. Circulation 75:124–130, 1987.

28. Fontbonne A, Eschwege E, Cambien F, et al.: Hypertriglyceridemia as a risk factor for coronary heart disease mortality in subjects with impaired glucose tolerance or diabetes. Results from an 11-year follow-up of the Paris Prospective Study. Diabetologia 32:300–304, 1989.

29. Lehto S, Ronnemaa T, Haffner SM, et al.: Dyslipidemia and hyperglycemia predict coronary heart disease events in middle–aged patients with NIDDM. Diabetes 48:1354–1359, 1997.

30. Coresh J, Kwiterovich POJ, Smith HH, Bachorik PS: Association of plasma triglyceride concentration and LDL particle diameter, density, and chemical composition with premature coronary artery disease in men and women. J Lipid Res 34:1687–1697, 1993.

31. Lahdenpera S, Syvanne M, Kahri J, Taskinen MR: Regulation of low-density lipoprotein particle size distribution in NIDDM and coronary disease: Importance of serum triglycerides. Diabetologia 39:453–461, 1996.

32. Feingold KR, Grunfeld C, Pang M, et al.: LDL subclass phenotypes and triglyceride metabolism in non-insulin-dependent diabetes. Arterioscler Thromb 12:1496–1502, 1992.

33. Tkac I, Kimball BP, Lewis G, et al.: The severity of coronary atherosclerosis in type 2 diabetes mellitus is related to the number of circulating triglyceride-rich lipoprotein particles. Atherosclerosis, Thrombosis, Vascular Biol 17:3633–3638, 1997.

34. Miller NE, Forde OH, Thelle DS, et al.: The Tromso heart study. High density lipoprotein and coronary heart disease: a prospective case control study. Lancet 1:965–967, 1977.

35. Nikkila EA: High density lipoproteins in diabetes. Diabetes 30(Suppl 2):82–87, 1981.

36. Stamler J, Vaccaro O, Neaton JD, Wentworth D: Diabetes, other risk factors, and 12–yr cardiovascular mortality for men screened in the Multiple Risk Factor Intervention Trial. Diabetes Care 16:434–444, 1993.

37. Steiner G, Poapst M, Davidson JK: Production of chylomicron-like lipoproteins from endogenous lipid by the intestine and liver of diabetic dogs. Diabetes 24:263–271, 1975.

38. Olefsky JM, Farquhar JW, Reaven GM: Reappraisal of the role of insulin in hypertriglyceridemia. Am J Med 57:551–560, 1974.

39. Steiner G, Vranic M: Hyperinsulinemia and hypertriglyceridemia, a vicious cycle with atherogenic potential. Int J Obesity 6(1):117–124, 1982.

40. Steiner G, Morita S, Vranic M: Resistance to insulin but not to glucagon in lean human hypertriglyceridemics. Diabetes 29:899–910, 1980.

41. Robinson JC, Folsom AR, Nabulsi AA, et al.: Can postmenopausal hormone replacement improve plasma lipids in women with diabetes? The Atherosclerosis Risk in Communities Study Investigators. Diabetes Care 19:480–485, 1996.

42. Lipid Research Clinics Programs: The Lipid Research Clinics Coronary Primary Prevention Trial results. I. Reduction in incidence of coronary heart disease. JAMA 251:351–364, 1984.

43. Lipid Research Clinics Programs: The Lipid Research Clinics Coronary Primary Prevention Trial results. II. The relationship of reduction in incidence of coronary heart disease to cholesterol lowering. JAMA 251:365–374, 1984.

44. Shepherd J, Cobbe SM, Ford I, et al.: Prevention of coronary heart disease with pravastatin in men with hypercholesterolemia. New Engl J Med 333:1301–1307, 1995.

45. Anonymous. Randomised trial of cholesterol lowering in 4444 patients with coronary heart disease: The Scandinavian Simvastatin Survival Study (4S) Lancet. 344: 1383–1389, 1994.

46. Sacks FM, Pfeffer MA, Moye LA, et al.: The effect of pravastatin on coronary events after myocardial infarction in patients with average cholesterol levels. N Engl J Med 335:1001–1009, 1996.

47. Manninen V, Elo MO, Frick MH, et al.: Lipid alterations and decline in the incidence of coronary heart disease in the Helsinki Heart Study. JAMA 260:641–651, 1988.

48. Bloomfield-Rubins H, Robins SJ, Collins D: The Veterans Affairs High-density Lipoprotein Intervention Trial: Baseline characteristics of normocholesterolemic men with coronary artery disease and low levels of high-density lipoprotein cholesterol. Am J Cardiol 78:572–575, 1996.

49. Ericsson C-G, Hamsten A, Nilsson J, Grip L, Asvnae B, de Faire U: Angiographic assessment of effects of bezafibrate on progression of coronary artery disease in young male postinfarction patients. Lancet 347:849–853, 1996.

50. Carlson LA, Rosenhamer G: Reduction of mortality in the Stockholm Ischaemic Heart Diseases Secondary Prevention Study by combined treatment with clofibrate and nicotinic acid. Acta Med Scand 223:405–418, 1988.

51. Koskinen P, Manttari M, Huttunen JK, et al.: Coronary heart disease incidence in the NIDDM patients in the Helsinki Heart Study. Diabetes Care 15:820–825, 1992.

52. Pyorala K, Pedersen TR, Kjekshus J, et al.: Cholesterol lowering with simvastatin improves prognosis of diabetic patients with coronary heart disease. A subgroup analysis of the Scandinavian Simvastatin Survival Study (4S). Diabetes Care 20:614–620, 1997.

53. Steiner G: The Diabetes Atherosclerosis Intervention Study (DAIS), A Study Conducted in Cooperation with the World Health Organization. Diabetologia 39:1655–1661, 1996.

54. Steiner G, Shafrir EA: Primary Hyperlipoproteinemias. New York: McGraw-Hill, 1991.

40

Medical Management of Diabetes in Pregnancy

Lisa P. Purdy and Boyd E. Metzger

In the preinsulin era, the majority of type 1 diabetic women were infertile. On the rare occasions when pregnancy did occur, it was associated with considerable maternal and fetal morbidity and mortality. Maternal morbidity declined with the advent of insulin therapy, but perinatal morbidity and mortality did not fall until the modern era with the development of improved maternal and fetal monitoring and intensive diabetic management.

Pathophysiology

The Diabetogenic Stress in Pregnancy

Peripheral tissue insulin resistance is a normal occurrence in all human pregnancies, but its purpose is appreciated only in the context of maternal and fetal placental weight gain and fetal development. During the first half of normal gestation the increments in total body weight primarily represent tissue accretion in the mother.[1] In the second half, maternal weight levels off as fetal-placental mass increases geometrically. Insulin is the principal anabolic hormone in mammalian pregnancy. Soon after conception, postprandial plasma insulin concentrations begin to rise in the absence of altered carbohydrate tolerance or generalized insulin resistance. In the second trimester, anabolic effects of hyperinsulinemia result in increased subcutaneous fat deposition and enlargement of fat cells. In animal models hepatic glycogen also increases and lean skeletal mass expands, although these insulin-like effects have not been documented in the human being. The stimulus for early maternal hyperinsulinemia is unknown, but numerous investigations suggest that progesterone, acting separately or in concert with estrogens, has a direct betacytotrophic action on pancreatic islets. Moreover, when the two sex steroids are administered in combination in appropriate molar concentration ratios to nonpregnant animals, similar effects on plasma

insulin and fuel storage phenomena in liver and adipose tissue are observed without significantly affecting skeletal muscle sensitivity to insulin.[2] Thus, it appears that these two sex steroids in combination, which dominate the hormonal profile of early gestation, set in motion physiological events that are fundamentally anabolic for the mother.[2] Islet and β-cell hyperplasia during pregnancy have been clearly documented in rodents. Gestational hormones such as placental lactogen, the placental growth hormone variant, and growth factors may facilitate this adaptation to the insulin resistance of pregnancy.

The time course of changing insulin sensitivity during pregnancy is not defined precisely. Serial estimates of insulin sensitivity before and during pregnancy in women with normal carbohydrate metabolism indicate a slight reduction in insulin sensitivity by 12–14 weeks,[3] further decline by the end of the second trimester,[4] and the appearance of marked insulin resistance during the third trimester. In women with gestational diabetes mellitus (GDM), Catalano et al.[3] found a modest improvement in insulin sensitivity at 12–14 weeks compared to their state of insulin resistance prior to pregnancy, followed by progression to severe insulin resistance in late gestation, similar in magnitude to that found in the control subjects with normal glucose tolerance. Women with type 1 diabetes who are in optimal metabolic control before conception have little change in insulin requirement during the first trimester, and may even experience some reduction in dosage because of hypoglycemia around 11–15 weeks of gestation. During the latter half of pregnancy, hormonal profiles change dramatically. In the presence of increasing circulating insulin levels, human placental lactogen, free cortisol, prolactin, and progesterone reach maximal plasma concentrations. Although concentrations of pituitary growth hormone fall,[5,6] this is offset by increasing levels of the placental growth hormone variant.[5,6] The combined effects of these hormones oppose insulin at peripheral (muscle and adipose tissue) and hepatic loci. The intracellular site(s) and molecular mediator(s) of insulin resistance during and outside of pregnancy remain uncertain. Currently, potential roles of tissue necrosis factor-α and the recently discovered hormone of adipose tissue origin, leptin, are being investigated intensively. During the fed state, maximal hyperinsulinemia continues to promote higher rates of maternal fuel storage, but this is now offset by the catabolic effects of hormonal insulin antagonists in the fasted state. The final outcome in late gestation is a rapid turnover of stored nutrients as a consequence of large fed-fasted, anabolic-catabolic undulations in substrate uptake and release.[7]

From these observations, one can conclude that the period of insulin resistance in late gestation coincides with the maternal need to cease net accumulation of fuels and to sustain rapid transfer of stored nutrients during fasting into the maternal plasma compartment for extraction by the fetal-placental unit. Insulin resistance prolongs the containment of nutrients within the plasma compartment after feeding for greater fetal accessibility. The entire process from the early stages of pregnancy to parturition is controlled and modulated by a variety of peptide and steroid hormones. When maternal insulin secretion is inadequate, as it is in DM, this sequence of events is markedly disturbed.

Plasma Fuels in Normal Pregnant Women

In normal women there is a progressive fall in fasting plasma glucose (FPG) concentration despite relatively higher postmeal glucose levels in late gestation. The greatest decline in 10- to 12-hr overnight FPG occurs early in gestation, well before the high rate of glucose turnover in the conceptus can account for an increase in total glucose turnover.[8,9] Basal concentrations of plasma glycerol and free fatty acids (FFA) do not change until late gestation, at which time significant elevations occur and the transition to the metabolic profile characteristic of the fasting state is accelerated[10] in association with mounting lipolysis and insulin resistance. There is also a progressive increase in all major lipid fractions, including triglycerides, cholesterol, and phospholipids.[2] The reasons for prompt establishment of lower total plasma amino acid concentrations in early pregnancy and their persistence throughout gestation[11] are not clear. During early pregnancy, tissue anabolism is extant and heightened insulin action is evident. The suppressive effects of insulin on plasma amino acids are well known and may account for this finding. In later gestation the release of amino acids from skeletal muscle of the pregnant rat is less restrained by insulin, suggesting that the principal cause of hypoaminoacidemia during this time of insulin resistance is increased fetal removal as opposed to impaired muscle release.[12]

Plasma Fuels in Women With GDM

Plasma substrate disturbances have been extensively studied in GDM. After dietary treatment, basal and postprandial levels of glucose, FFA, triglycerides, and amino acids may exceed control values, with the extent of the abnormalities being related to the severity of the diabetes.[13,14] Branched-chain amino acids, which are exquisitely sensitive to insulin, are among the most consistently disturbed.[14] Women with GDM have a predisposition to "accelerated starvation" that is similar to that in women with normal glucose homeostasis.[15]

Plasma Fuels in Women With Pregestational DM

In women with well-controlled type 1 DM, the greatest departures from the norm during pregnancy occur in plasma glucose profiles. This is in contrast to relatively few disturbances in plasma lipids, including FFA, cholesterol, and triglycerides, and the paucity of changes in lipid content of individual lipoprotein fractions.[16] Plasma amino acid concentrations may be markedly disturbed in pregnant women with type 1 DM and there is a poor correlation between these changes and plasma glucose control and hemoglobin A_{1c} levels, especially in late pregnancy.[17] Studies of type 2 diabetes mellitus in pregnancy suggest that total plasma triglycerides and triglyceride content of very low density lipoproteins are increased, and cholesterol content of high density lipoproteins is decreased, as opposed to normal and to pregnant women with type 1 DM.[16] Additional investigations are required to separate the relative roles of obesity and diabetes in the development of these lipid aberrations.

Metabolic Disturbances And Adverse Pregnancy Outcome

It is now generally accepted that metabolic disturbances in the mother mediate virtually all of the adverse effects of DM on the offspring.[18–21] Experimental and clinical support of this premise has been built on the pioneering hypothesis advanced by Pedersen,[22] which stated that maternal hyperglycemia leads to fetal hyperinsulinism which is responsible for macrosomia and neonatal morbidities. The importance of other metabolic fuel alterations was recognized later.[14] Freinkel[18,19] made major contributions in advancing the concept of pregnancy as "a tissue culture experience," emphasizing the importance of the temporal relationships between the metabolic insult and the kind of adverse outcome that could be expected ("fuel-mediated teratogenesis") and postulating that the altered intrauterine enviroment of

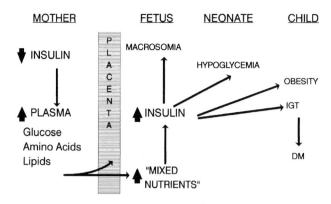

Figure 40–1. Pedersen/Freinkel hypothesis. Effect of maternal fuels on fetal development. The classical "hyperglycemia-hyperinsulinemia" hypothesis of Pedersen[22] has been modified[18] to include the contributions of other maternal fuels besides glucose that are also responsive to maternal insulin. All of these can influence the growth of the fetus and the maturation of fetal insulin secretion. Within this formulation, growth will be disparately greater in insulin-sensitive than in insulin-insensitive tissues in the fetus. Reprinted with permission from Silverman BL, Purdy LP, Metzger BE: The intrauterine environment: Implications for the offspring of diabetic mothers. Diabetes Rev 4:21–35, 1996.

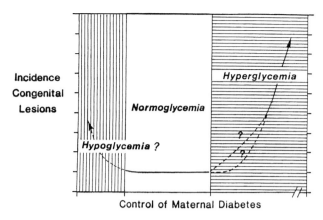

Figure 40–2. Therapeutic dilemma in early diabetic pregnancy. Hypoglycemia during the period of glycolytic dependence in the rodent embryo has been shown to be teratogenic. Whether the human embryo is similarly vulnerable during the corresponding developmental interval (i.e., about day 16–18 to 24–25 postconception) has not been established. Moreover, the thresholds for the various factors in maternal serum that account for teratogenesis of diabetes (broadly designated as "hyperglycemia") have not been ascertained. Thus, the optimal target for metabolic regulation prior to and during the first 4–6 weeks following conception is not yet precisely established. Adapted with permission from Freinkel N: Diabetic embryopathy and fuel-mediated organ teratogenesis: Lessons from animal models. Horm Metab Res 20:463–475, 1988.

diabetes can have life-long as well as perinatal consequences. The key hypotheses of Pedersen and Freinkel and illustrated schematically in Fig. 40–1.

Congenital Malformations and Early Fetal Loss.
Many experimental, clinical, and epidemiological studies indicate that increased risks of congenital malformations and spontaneous abortions in pregnancies complicated by diabetes result from disturbances in maternal metabolism that are present around the time of conception.[18,20,21] The frequency of spontaneous abortions is increased in direct proportion to glycohemoglobin concentration measured in early pregnancy.[23,24] The general relationships between metabolic control and the risk of congenital malformations and fetal loss are illustrated schematically in Fig. 40–2. The Diabetes in Early Pregnancy (DIEP) study found a 4.9% incidence of birth defects in patients recruited within 21 days of conception, a rate approximately twofold that in the nondiabetic control group (2.1%; $p = 0.027$).[25] Most of these subjects were in fair to good control during the first trimester (glycohemoglobin within 7 standard deviations of the mean for controls in 93% of cases). Green et al.[24] reported a prevalence of congenital anomalies of about 5% (almost identical to that of the DIEP Study) until first-trimester glycohemoglobin concentrations exceeded the mean control value by 10–12 standard deviations, beyond which the rate of malformations increased greatly.

Results of in vitro studies (embryo culture) and experiments in animal models indicate that predisposi-

tion to congenital malformations is likely multifactorial rather than the result of exposure to a single toxin or factor.[21] Supplementing embryo culture media with a high concentration of D-glucose, or ketones, or with intermediate concentrations of the two in combination profoundly disrupts the development of rodent embryos.[21] Conversely, hypoglycemia of relatively short duration can also induce teratogenesis in animal models[26] or in rodent embryo culture.[27] However, alterations in the concentrations of metabolic fuels singly or in combination do not appear to directly account for the potent dysmorphic actions of serum from pregnant diabetic women or diabetic animals.[21,28] A number of other factors that might mediate "metabolic teratogenesis" have been described (myoinositol depletion,[29] polyol accumulation,[30] arachidonic acid deficiency,[31] free oxygen radical generation).[32]

Although neither the precise time or duration of exposure to an abnormal metabolic environment necessary for adverse events to develop in the human embryo has been pinpointed, it is clear that they can be prevented. When women enroll for care prior to conception, several groups have found rates of major congenital malformations that are no greater than expected in a general obstetrical population. However, these studies have not included data on rates of malformation in concurrently examined controls.[33,34] In Denmark, where the majority of pregnancies in women with diabetes are now planned, a nationwide decline in the rate of major congenital malformations from 7.4 to 2.7% has been reported.[35] These encouraging trends have stimulated efforts to educate health-care professionals and patients concerning the benefits of preconception care. Unfortunately, the level of compliance in the United States remains substantially below that of the Danish population mentioned above.

Disturbances in Fetal Growth. Macrosomia (traditionally defined as birth weight in excess of 4000 g or above the 90th percentile for gestational age) is a frequent complication of pregestational as well as GDM. Increased adiposity is the primary component of the macrosomia. Infants of diabetic mothers may have almost twice as much body fat as infants of normal mothers.[36] Skinfold measurements have been used to document such adiposity at birth and may correlate with maternal metabolic regulation.[37] Skinfold measurements are difficult to standardize and reference values may differ among ethnic groups. Consequently, this technique is seldom used as a routine clinical assessment. Infants of diabetic mothers tend to have larger amounts of subcutaneous fat around their shoulders,[38] which increases the risk of shoulder dystocia, birth trauma, and cesarean delivery. Other insulin-sensitive tissues such as liver and heart are also often enlarged.[36] Although skeletal growth may not be dependent on insulin action, a modest increase in fetal height (length) is commonly found. Head size, though normal, often appears small because of the concurrent truncal obesity.

The majority of infants classified large for gestational age, based solely upon birth weight, are born to women with normal carbohydrate tolerance.[39] Conversely, heavy neonates born to women with DM do not always represent diabetic macrosomia. Keller et al.[40] observed a subset of infants of diabetic women in whom birth weights exceeded 4000 g, but where biparietal diameter, length, and birth weight were proportionally increased above standard norms and there was no evidence of fetal hyperinsulinism. Excessive increase in abdominal circumference in the presence of normal growth of the head typifies the fetal macrosomia of diabetes mellitus.[41] Fetal humeral soft tissue thickness has recently been shown to be an even more accurate predictor of asymmetrical fetal growth.[42]

We have used Farquhar's simple expression of the relative proportionality between weight and height[43] (designated Symmetry Index [SI]) for clinical evaluation of the disparate growth of "insulin-sensitive" tissues. SI values in offspring of diabetic mothers correlate with increased levels of maternal metabolic fuels in the second as well as the third trimester,[44] and with increased insulin or C-peptide in amniotic fluid and cord blood, consistent with premature activation of fetal islet function.[41,45] Others have also demonstrated correlation between amniotic fluid insulin or C-peptide and macrosomia and neonatal morbidity in diabetic pregnancies.[46,47] Persson et al.[48] and our group[44] have also found correlation between fetal islet function and maternal levels of insulinogenic amino acids as well as glucose.

Increased fetal insulin secretion may already be present during the second trimester. This is suggested from histologic and morphometrical evidence for islet hypertrophy and hyperplasia in the pancreas of fetuses of mothers with diabetes delivered at this time.[49,50] Although excessive deposition of fat develops mainly during the third trimester, we found a stronger association between fetal islet function at or near delivery and metabolic control in the second trimester than in the third trimester.[44]

Studies in monkey fetuses with implanted insulin pumps show that hyperinsulinemia per se can accelerate the growth of insulin-responsive tissues, even without attendant increases in metabolic fuels.[51] Thus, once increased function of the fetal β cells develops, it is possible that hyperinsulinemia and augmented fetal growth may continue in the absence of elevated maternal nutrients.[44] While it is clear that the insulin has direct effects upon fetal tissues, concurrent increases in the availability of insulin-like growth factors and other growth factors may also be contributory.[52,53]

In the past, intrauterine growth retardation (IUGR), the converse of macrosomia, was frequently observed in offspring of type 1 diabetic mothers, and was often attributed to "utero-placental insufficiency" secondary to maternal vascular disease.[22] Recent reports indicate that, except for pregnancies complicated by hypertension and/or diabetic nephropathy, IUGR is now rare[54]; whereas, the occurrence of macrosomia in pregestational diabetic pregnancies has markedly increased (30–40%) as the majority now occur at or near term. Clinical observations[55] and studies in animal models and in rodent embryo cultures[56] suggest that disturbances in maternal metabolism in early pregnancy may retard growth irreparably, with or without associated birth defects. Better control of diabetes in early pregnancy and discontinuation of routine delivery before term, may account for the rarity of IUGR and the high prevalence of macrosomia in the newborns of women with pregestational diabetes noted above.

Long-term Anthropometric and Metabolic Impact. An increase in the prevalence of obesity in the offspring of diabetic mothers has been suggested in a number of early reports.[57] It was also noted that obesity is more frequent in the offspring of diabetic mothers than diabetic fathers. However, none of the early reports provided direct correlations with metabolic status during intrauterine development. Pettitt and coworkers[58] have correlated the 2-hr response of Pima Indian mothers to oral glucose during pregnancy with the occurrence of obesity in their offspring. They have found that at age 15–19 obesity is present in two thirds of the offspring who were exposed to an abnormal intrauterine environment by virtue of their mothers being diabetic during gestation, compared to obesity in 40% of those whose mothers had the genetic propensity to diabetes, but did not become diabetic until after the pregnancy (i.e., "prediabetic mothers"), and in 30% of the offspring whose mothers never became diabetic. Moreover, offspring of diabetic women were heavier than offspring of nondiabetic and prediabetic women regardless of birth weight.[57,59] A report from Italy of greater relative weight/height at age 4 in the offspring of diabetic mothers whose control was "poor" rather than "good" during the index pregnancy provides additional support.[60] In a prospective long-term follow-up study of offspring of diabetic mothers (ODM), we have found that neonatal macrosomia in ODM disappears by one year of age. After 2–3 years of age, the ODM gained weight faster than other children, and by 8 years almost half of the offspring of diabetic mothers had a weight greater than the 90th percentile.[57,61] These studies have also provided evidence that fetal islet function may predict long-term anthropometric development. Relative obesity at ages 6–8 was significantly correlated with insulin secretion in utero (amniotic fluid insulin content at 32–34 weeks' gestation).[61]

Animal models and epidemiological studies suggest that disturbance in islet function during intrauterine and early postnatal life, produced by a variety of mechanisms, predisposes to metabolic disturbances and impaired glucose tolerance in later life. In addition, Rhesus monkeys made hyperinsulinemic, but euglycemic, in utero by infusion of insulin into the fetus, develop abnormal glucose tolerance as pregnant adults.[62] Pettitt et al.[63] have reported that type 2 DM is present by age 20–24 in 45.5% of the offspring of "diabetic mothers," but in only 8.6 and 1.4% of the respective offspring of "prediabetic" or "nondiabetic mothers" (see above for definition of these categories). These differences persisted after taking into account diabetes in the father, age at onset of diabetes in either parent, or obesity in the offspring. Pettitt et al.[63] conclude that "the intrauterine environment is an important determinant of the development of diabetes and that its effect is in addition to effects of genetic factors." The offspring of diabetic mothers enrolled in the Northwestern University Diabetes in Pregnancy center long-term follow-up are demonstrating an increased frequency of impaired glucose tolerance (IGT).[64] The prevalence of IGT increased from 1.2% at ages younger than 5, to 5.4% at 5–9 years of age. At age 12.3 ± 1.7 years, ODM had significantly higher 2-hr glucose concentrations when compared to an age- and sex-matched normal control group, and a

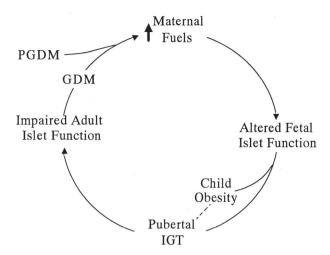

Figure 40–3. Diabetes begets diabetes. The alterations of maternal fuel metabolism lead to altered fetal islet function (hyperinsulinism). This intrauterine event predisposes to childhood obesity and adolescent IGT. Our hypothesis is that it will also lead to impaired adult islet function and IGT and/or GDM. Reprinted with permission from Metzger BE, Cho NH: Epidemiology and genetics. In Reece EA, Coustan DR (eds): Diabetes Mellitus in Pregnancy, 2nd ed. New York: Churchill Livingstone, 1995, pp. 11–26.

much higher prevalence of IGT (19.3 vs. 2.5%). Impaired glucose tolerance has developed at similar rates in offspring of mothers with gestational and pregestational diabetes. Most interestingly, excessive insulin secretion in utero, as assessed by the amniotic fluid insulin concentration, is a strong predictor of impaired glucose tolerance in childhood.[64]

The data summarized above indicate that nature (as embodied by "genetic" propensities) may be modified by nurture (as determined by "congenital" contributions via the intrauterine metabolic environment) in the pathogenesis of obesity and type 2 Diabetes (Fig. 40–3).

Epidemiology

According to data from NHANES III, 1.7% of women age 20–39 and 6.1% of women age 40–49 have DM.[65] A further 5.5 and 11.2%, respectively, have impaired fasting glucose or glucose intolerance. Altogether, 2.9–17.3% of nonpregnant women age 20–49 have some form of abnormal glucose tolerance, which might be associated with maternal or fetal risks should they conceive. Pregestational diabetes occurs in 0.2–0.5% of pregnancies according to statewide vital statistics.[66] GDM, defined as "glucose intolerance with onset or first recognition during pregnancy," has a prevalence of 1.6–15%, based on the population studied and the diagnostic criteria used.[67–69] The National Maternal and Infant Health Survey (NMIHS) found diabetes in 4% of all pregnancies, with GDM in 88%, type 2 DM in 8%, and type 1

DM in 4%.[70] Based on the NHANES data, it has been suggested that the diagnosis of gestational diabetes represents the discovery of women in the reproductive age range who have preexisting glucose intolerance.[71] However, the prevalence of GDM is higher in late gestation than early in pregnancy,[72,73] and the majority of women have normal glucose tolerance tests immediately postpartum. Nevertheless, those with a history of GDM have a high risk of progression to type 2 DM,[74,75] suggesting that the insulin resistance of pregnancy provides a "stress test" that unmasks women at high risk for the development of type 2 diabetes.

Classification

The original White classification[76] was an attempt to identify high-risk pregnancies based on age of onset and duration of maternal diabetes, and the presence of microvascular and/or macrovascular complications. Maternal and fetal risks are now more specifically defined by the degree of metabolic control throughout pregnancy, while the presence of vascular and neurological complications remains an important determinant of perinatal risk.[77,78] Gestational diabetes is also classified based on the severity of the metabolic disturbance,[18,19,45,79] using the fasting plasma glucose as the distinguishing characteristic. Those with a history of GDM in a previous pregnancy, who had no reclassification postpartum, or whose glucose tolerance tests demonstrated impaired glucose tolerance, should not be reclassified as GDM in a subsequent pregnancy. Until a better definition can be determined, they should be noted as "previous GDM." This modified classification is presented in Table 40–1.

GDM

GDM is defined as "carbohydrate intolerance of varying degrees of severity with onset or first recognition during pregnancy."[80,81] This applies regardless of the treatment used during pregnancy, or whether the condition persists postpartum. It does not exclude the possibility that unrecognized diabetes may have predated the pregnancy.

Pathogenesis of GDM

As defined above, GDM is heterogeneous in nature, and the detection process (see below) captures glucose intolerance of any etiology.[82] Some patients exhibit autoimmune phenomenon,[79] with GAD[83] or islet cell antibodies[79,84,85] found with variable prevalence depending on the population studied and the methods used. This is more common in Scandanavian countries where there is greater prevalence of type 1 diabetes.[85] These findings suggest that a small proportion of patients with

TABLE 40–1   Classification of Carbohydrate Intolerance During Pregnancy

I. Pregestational diabetes mellitus	
Type 1 diabetes mellitus	
Uncomplicated	
Complicated*	
Type 2 diabetes mellitus	
Uncomplicated	
Complicated*	
II. Gestational diabetes mellitus (GDM)—(see text)	
GDM—Class A$_1$	Fasting glucose < 105 mg/dL (5.8 mmol/L)
GDM—Class A$_2$	Fasting glucose ≥ 105 mg/dL (5.8 mmol/L)
III. Previous gestational diabetes mellitus	
Prev. GDM—Class A$_1$	Fasting glucose < 105 mg/dL (5.8 mmol/L)
Prev. GDM—Class A$_2$	Fasting glucose ≥ 105 mg/dL (5.8 mmol/L)

*Microvascular and macrovascular complications defined as follows: BDR = background diabetic retinopathy; PDR = proliferative diabetic retinopathy; NEPH = diabetic nephropathy (≥ 0.5 g protein in 24-hr urine collection, and/or serum creatinine consistently ≥ 1.2 mg/dL [106 μmol/L]); NEUR = neuropathy (known gastroparesis when not pregnant, orthostatic hypotension, or sensory abnormalities in lower extremities detected at bedside examination); CAD = coronary artery disease diagnosed by history, ECG, or stress ECG; PVD = diminished pulses, bruits, or symptomatic claudication; HTN = hypertension (BP ≥ 140/90 consistently). Designations are appended to primary diagnosis as appropriate: e.g., diabetes mellitus, type 2—uncomplicated; Diabetes mellitus, type 1—BDR, NEPH.

Adapted and reprinted with permission from Metzger BE, Phelps RL: Diabetes during pregnancy. In Bardin CW (ed): Current Therapy in Endocrinology & Metabolism, 6th ed. St. Louis: Mosby-Year Book, Inc., 1997, pp. 318–324.

GDM may have evolving type 1 diabetes mellitus with first appearance in pregnancy. Efforts to identify the specific cases prospectively may be justified in populations with a higher prevalence of type 1 diabetes.

The majority of the GDM patients display features found in patients with type 2 diabetes. As with type 2 diabetes, the frequency of GDM increases with progressive age and body weight, and in high-risk ethnic populations. Many of the metabolic abnormalities are also consistent with that of type 2 diabetes. As indicated above, insulin sensitivity diminishes throughout gestation in all pregnant women.[3] Those with normal glucose tolerance respond with a compensatory increase in first- and second-phase insulin response.[86] In GDM with mild to moderate elevations in FPG, fasting plasma insulin is elevated in parallel. However, first-phase insulin response as well as subsequent insulin release is generally attenuated in women with GDM, when adjusted for their level of insulin resistance.[86,87]

This insulinopenia is not invariable, as the insulin response to glucose and mixed meals is heterogeneous.

Screening and Detection

Women with gestational diabetes are generally asymptomatic, and identification of those with the condition requires a program of active screening. The diagnosis is made by a glucose tolerance test, but the prevalence of GDM is sufficiently low in most populations that it would not be cost-effective to perform this test in all pregnant women. In several populations it has been well documented that historical screening for the presence of "risk factors" has poor sensitivity and specificity for identifying cases for diagnostic testing.[88] Repeat random measurements of blood or plasma glucose concentration have insufficient sensitivity to be an effective screening procedure.[89,90] Similarly, glycohemoglobin measurements[91,92] and fructosamine levels[93,94] do not adequately separate normals from those with gestational diabetes, even though glycated protein levels diminish in normal pregnancy.[95] Measuring second-trimester amniotic fluid insulin content, while demonstrating reasonable sensitivity for early diagnosis of GDM,[96,97] is costly, invasive, and carries risk.

Current screening recommendations involve the administration of a 50-g oral glucose challenge test between 24 to 28 weeks' gestational age, without regard to the time of day or time of the last meal.[80,81] Women with a 1-hr plasma glucose value ≥ 140 mg/dL (7.8 mmol/L) require definitive evaluation with an oral glucose tolerance test. In the United States, this encompasses approximately 14–18.5% of pregnant women,[68,98] and has a sensitivity of 79% and a specificity of 87%.[99] Decreasing the screening threshold to 130 mg/dL (7.2 mmol/L), increases the need for oral glucose tolerance tests to 20–25% of all pregnant women,[68,88] but also increases the diagnostic yield, probably to more than 90%. In high-risk populations it is justified to use a diagnostic test for all subjects.

Universal blood glucose screening may not be cost-effective in populations or clinics that include a large proportion of subjects at low risk for GDM. Table 40–2 summarizes the strategy for the detection of GDM recommended by the 4th International Workshop Conference on Gestational Diabetes Mellitus.[81] Low-risk subjects are those with all of the following characteristics: member of racial/ethnic group with a low prevalence of GDM; age <25 years; normal weight; no family history of diabetes; no personal history of abnormal glucose metabolism or poor obstetrical outcome. Those at particularly high risk for developing GDM (marked obesity, strong family history of type 2 DM, personal history of GDM, glucose intolerance, or glucosuria) should be screened as soon after enrolling for prenatal care as is feasible to allow early intervention.[81,100]

TABLE 40–2 Screening Strategy for the Detection of GDM

GDM risk assessment—Should be ascertained at the first prenatal visit.

Low risk: Blood glucose testing is not routinely required if all of the following characteristics are present:
- Member of an ethnic group with a low prevalence of GDM
- No known diabetes in first degree relatives
- Age <25 years
- Weight normal before pregnancy (BMI <26 kg/m^2)
- No history of abnormal glucose metabolism
- No history of poor obstetric outcome

Average risk: Defined as a patient outside one or more of the above characteristics.
Perform blood glucose testing at 24–28 weeks using either:
- Two step procedure: 50-g glucose challenge test (GCT)* followed by a diagnostic oral glucose tolerance test in those meeting the threshold value in the GCT.
- One-step procedure: Diagnostic oral glucose tolerance test performed on all subjects.

High risk: Defined as a patient with one or more of the following characteristics:
- marked obesity (BMI >40 kg/m^2)
- strong family history of type 2 diabetes mellitus
- personal history of GDM, glucose intolerance, or glucosuria

Perform blood glucose testing as soon as feasible, using the procedures described above.
- If GDM is not diagnosed, blood glucose testing should be repeated at 24–28 weeks, or at any time a patient has symptoms or signs that are suggestive of hyperglycemia.

*Fifty-gram oral glucose load administered without regard to time of day or time of last meal. Venous plasma glucose is measured 1 hr later. A value of ≥ 140 mg/dL [7.8 mmol/L] indicates the need for a full diagnostic glucose tolerance test.

Adapted and reprinted with permission by Metzger BE: Summary and recommendations of the Fourth International Workshop Conference on Gestational Diabetes Mellitus. Diabetes Care 21(52):B161–B167, 1998.

If GDM is not found, testing should be repeated at 24–28 weeks or at any time the patient develops symptoms suggestive of hyperglycemia. All others should be screened at 24–28 weeks' gestational age. Blood glucose meters are inadequate for the screening process as they carry an intratest variability of 10–15%; they would require such a low glycemic threshold to capture cases that an inordinate number of diagnostic tests would need to be performed.[81,101]

Diagnosis

From an obstetrical perspective, the justification for making a diagnosis of GDM is to detect pregnancies at risk for perinatal morbidity and/or mortality that can be reduced or eliminated by appropriate intervention. The O'Sullivan and Mahan criteria for the diagnosis of GDM were developed originally to identify a population of pregnant women who were at high risk for developing DM postpartum.[74] In the absence of criteria that are based on the specific relationships between hyperglycemia and adverse perinatal outcome, the work of O'Sullivan and Mahan has been used as the basis for the criteria recommended by the National Diabetes Data Group (NDDG),[102] the GDM Workshop Conferences,[103] and the American Diabetes Association[80] because it represents a well-designed, population-based study. The NDDG extrapolated values for AutoAnalyzer measured plasma glucose from the criteria originally derived from whole blood glucose determination,[102] and Carpenter and Coustan[104] later adjusted the values to more closely approximate the values obtained with the glucose oxidase enzymatic assay of plasma or serum glucose (Table 40–3). Use of the criteria of Carpenter and Coustan labels nearly 50% more subjects as GDM than is the case when the NDDG criteria are applied.[68,105] Data from several populations now indicate that the additional cases diagnosed by Carpenter–Coustan criteria have risk of perinatal morbidities similar to those of women diagnosed with the NDDG criteria.[105–108] Thus, the 4th International Workshop Conference on GDM recommended that the Carpenter–Coustan criteria be used for the 100-g oral glucose tolerance test (OGTT).[81]

Values for 75-g oral glucose tolerance tests have been defined in several study populations in the United States of America, Europe, Brazil, and Australia.[81]

The specific values vary from group to group, as is expected from differences in factors known to influence glucose tolerance test values including age, obesity, ethnic group, and the background prevalence of type 2 diabetes in the population. As a general statement, it can be said that the various cutoff values that have been recommended for the 75-g OGTT do not differ greatly from the Carpenter and Coustan criteria for the 100-g OGTT. However, studies in which perinatal outcome has been evaluated in large numbers of pregnancies meeting the 75-g OGTT criteria for GDM are lacking. At this time, we recommend that clinics that have established programs for GDM detection and diagnosis continue to use the diagnostic procedure with which they are familiar, pending the availability of criteria that are based on the relationship between degree of hyperglycemia and risk of adverse perinatal outcome.

Pregestational Diabetes Mellitus

Diabetic Complications

As noted above, perinatal risk may be affected by the presence and severity of maternal microvascular, neurological, and macrovascular complications. Pregnancy may also alter the rapidity of progression of these complications. Preconception assessment of potential complications is important for counseling a patient regarding her risk. This should involve a comprehensive eye examination to determine the risk of progression of any existing diabetic retinopathy and allow prophylactic intervention.[109] Baseline renal function and neurological function should also be determined. We recommend that our patients with type 1 diabetes of greater than 25 years' duration undergo an exercise stress test to rule out occult coronary heart disease. Those patients with identified diabetic complications should be counseled regarding their perinatal risk, and should have intensive monitoring throughout pregnancy and the postpartum period using a team approach of specialists.

TABLE 40–3   Criteria for the Diagnosis of Gestational Diabetes Mellitus Based on Data from O'Sullivan and Mahan

	O'Sullivan–Mahan[74] Whole Blood Somogyi–Nelson (mg/dL [mmol/L])	NDDG[102] Plasma—AutoAnalyzer (mg/dL [mmol/L])	Carpenter–Coustan[104] Plasma—Glucose Oxidase (mg/dL [mmol/L])
Fasting	90 [5.0]	105 [5.8]	95 [5.3]
1 hr	165 [9.2]	190 [10.6]	180 [10.0]
2 hr	145 [8.1]	165 [9.2]	155 [8.6]
3 hr	125 [6.9]	145 [8.1]	140 [7.8]

The 100-g oral glucose tolerance test is performed in the morning after an overnight fast of at least 8 hr, but not more than 14 hr, and after at least 3 days of unrestricted diet ($\geq$ 150 g carbohydrate/day) and physical activity. The subject should remain seated and should not smoke throughout the test. Two or more of the venous plasma concentrations must be met or exceeded for a positive diagnosis.

Microvascular

Retinopathy. Women with pregestational diabetes who have retinopathy may demonstrate progression during pregnancy.[110–112] Progression may be secondary to poor glycemic control prior to pregnancy, rapid improvement in glycemic control during pregnancy,[110–113] and concomitant hypertension or preeclampsia in pregnancy.[113,114] Progression is also influenced by duration of diabetes and the baseline severity of retinopathy.[110,112]

Whether pregnancy per se contributes to the risk of progression remains uncertain.[115] While normal pregnant patients exhibit retinal vessel constriction to protect the retina from the hyperdynamic circulation of pregnancy, diabetics lack this autoregulation, and an increase in retinal blood flow is particularly marked in patients with retinopathy progression.[116] Circulating levels of the potent angiogenic factor, *fibroblast growth factor-2*, are substantially elevated in the second and third trimesters in patients with retinopathy, and correlate with glycohemoglobin levels.[117] Further study is needed to determine if the changes in blood flow or FGF-2 contribute to the progression of retinopathy.

Clinically significant retinopathy may be managed by laser photocoagulation, and does not preclude a successful retinal and pregnancy outcome.[118] Though postpartum regression of diabetic retinopathy has been reported,[119] some patients have aggressive retinopathy that continues to progress in the postpartum period.[120] This is particularly true when macular edema develops during pregnancy.[121] The data that are available suggest that, in general, pregnancy does not have long-term deleterious effects on diabetic retinopathy.[122]

Nephropathy. Historically, 10–40% of individuals with type 1 diabetes developed nephropathy.[123] Microalbuminuria may be seen within 5–10 years of diagnosis, with overt manifestations occurring 10–30 years after the initial diagnosis of diabetes. Diabetic pregnancies are associated with as much as a fourfold increased risk of hypertension or preeclampsia,[124] which may accelerate nephropathy. Normal physiological adaptations of pregnancy include an increased GFR, increased renal plasma flow, and afferent arteriolar vasodilation. These result in glomerular hyperfiltration, which may be maladaptive in patients with preexisting renal disease, and an increased systemic pressure transmitted to the glomerulus in the setting of hypertension. In addition, pregnancy is associated with an increase in urinary tract infections and pyelonephritis secondary to ureteral hypomotility with vesicoureteral reflux, physiological hydronephrosis, and increased urinary nutrient content. Angiotensin-converting enzyme (ACE) inhibitors may not be used in pregnancy because of the risk of fetal anephrism. This combination of factors may predispose to accelerated deterioration of renal function in pregnancy. Observa-

tions of patients with mild diabetic nephropathy (microalbuminuria, proteinuria, or mild renal insufficiency with a creatinine <1.4 mg/dL [124 μmol/L]) suggest that pregnancy does not permanently accelerate their nephropathy, though there may be a transient worsening of proteinuria and creatinine clearance.[77,125] However, studies of patients with moderate or severe renal insufficiency raise concern that pregnancy may accelerate the decline in renal function,[126,127] as seen in patients with moderate renal insufficiency of nondiabetic etiology. Pregnancy in women with more severe degrees of nephropathy may be complicated by exacerbation of hypertension/preeclampsia, acceleration of retinopathy, and fetal/neonatal morbidity (prematurity, IUGR).[77,126,127] Prophylactic measures to preserve renal function include maintaining good glycemic and blood pressure control, frequent urine cultures with antibiotic therapy as necessary, and careful monitoring of maternal renal function and fetal well-being.

Neuropathy

Little is known of the effect of pregnancy on diabetic neuropathy. Neuropathy exists in 7–50% of patients after 1 to 25 years diabetes duration, respectively. The presence of autonomic neuropathy may have a potentially adverse impact on maternal morbidity[128] and pregnancy outcome.[129] Gastroparesis is particularly concerning, as the irregular gastric emptying may result in inadequate nutrition, marked fluctuation in blood glucoses, and maternal aspiration. Genitourinary disturbances with bladder dysfunction may result in recurrent urinary tract infections and worsening renal function in patients with diabetic nephropathy.

Macrovascular

Patients with macrovascular disease have significant risks in pregnancy from maternal and fetal morbidity. Pregnancy may exacerbate preexisting vascular disease. Cholesterol levels increase approximately 50–60%, while triglyceride levels increase two- to three-fold with decreasing hepatic lipase activity.[130,131] The individual particles have not been studied extensively in diabetes, but in nondiabetic pregnant women LDL-C levels increase proportionally to total cholesterol, and a rise in apoB is also seen. HDL_3 levels remain relatively constant, but the more antiatherogenic HDL_2 rise during the first half of gestation, then fall but remain 15% higher than baseline values at term.[131] Systolic blood pressure may increase significantly in type 1 diabetic women, while diastolic blood pressure tends to be higher than in controls at conception and throughout gestation.[132]

Coronary Artery Disease. Myocardial infarction in pregnancy has been associated with a 50% mortality in the limited number of cases reported.[78,133] Since these reports were published more than 3 decades ago, the outcomes should not be generalized to current medical therapy. Women with coronary artery disease are also vulnerable to myocardial infarction and congestive heart failure in the immediate postpartum period. This may be secondary to marked fluid shifts that occur postpartum (autotransfusion of uteroplacental blood, rapid mobilization of extravascular fluid with increased venous return, and release of the venocaval obstruction) resulting in an increase in stroke volume and cardiac output.[134]

Obstetrical Complications

Pregnancy-induced Hypertension.   Diabetes is considered a risk factor for the development of preeclampsia or pregnancy-induced hypertension (PIH).[132,135] Reported rates of PIH in diabetic pregnancies differ substantially, confounded by the lack of unanimity in the definitions of preeclampsia and PIH and the potential existence of chronic hypertension. Whether there is an association between PIH and poor glycemic control is uncertain.[136] Women with GDM also have an increased risk of PIH, perhaps related to the association of GDM with the insulin resistance syndrome.[137]

The etiology of PIH/preeclampsia is unknown, but it appears to involve endothelial dysfunction[138] and maladaptation of the maternal and uteroplacental vasculature in pregnancy. It is postulated that poor glycemic control may contribute to the restriction of normally occurring physiological vascular changes, such as the formation of large sinusoidal vessels. Microvascular disease seen with advancing White class may potentially interfere with the normal autoregulation of the maternal vasculature in pregnancy, contributing to the development of PIH.

Management

Women with a history of GDM need to to have their glucose tolerance status reevaluated prior to pregnancy to see if they require prepregnancy intervention.[81] Women with known type 2 diabetes prior to pregnancy require initiation of insulin therapy. In pregestational and gestational diabetic pregnancies, the goal of therapy is to maintain normal maternal pre- and postprandial blood glucoses to avoid the immediate and long-term risks to the offspring. Whether maintaining euglycemia also normalizes other maternal fuels is uncertain. The trade-off of tight control is an increased risk of hypoglycemia, which is more often observed in type 1 patients, rather than in those with type 2 diabetes or GDM.

Hypoglycemia

Hypoglycemia occurs with increased frequency in patients with type 1 diabetes mellitus who are on intensive insulin therapy. Hypoglycemia during pregnancy is frequent, particularly in the first trimester,[139,140] often during the nocturnal hours. Many episodes of hypoglycemia in pregnancy require second-person assistance to treat.

The increased frequency of hypoglycemia in the first trimester may be secondary to the institution of intensive insulin management,[140] with the secondary effects of diminished counter-regulatory hormonal responses and increased hypoglycemic unawareness.[141] The hormonal changes of pregnancy may increase the risk of hypoglycemia and reduce counter-regulatory responses,[141] though this putative mechanism is speculative. The high frequency of hypoglycemia supports the need for intensive self-glucose monitoring during pregnancy, including occasional nocturnal tests in type 1 diabetics.

Metabolic Monitoring

Patients with GDM or pregestational diabetes should monitor urinary ketones prior to breakfast to assess the adequacy of their carbohydrate intake. Pregestational diabetics should also assess urine ketones when preprandial glucoses exceed 150 mg/dL (8.3 mmol/L) to detect potential metabolic decompensation early in its development. Gestational diabetics on dietary therapy check fasting and 1- or 2-hr postprandial glucoses to monitor the adequacy of dietary therapy and allow intervention should glucose tolerance deteriorate. The accuracy of self-glucose monitoring needs to be assessed by comparing meter results against venous plasma glucose measurements. Patients requiring insulin therapy additionally monitor premeal and bedtime glucoses to guide adjustment of insulin doses. Some centers also recommend that patients monitor capillary blood glucose concentration 1 or 2 hr after meals to guide further adjustments in diet and insulin,[142] as these levels more accurately reflect fuel delivery to the fetus and have better correlation with birth weight than measurements that are limited to premeal intervals.[143] If postprandial hyperglycemia persists despite normal preprandial measurements, meal size and frequency may be adjusted. To date, the safety and utility of lispro insulin for control of postprandial hyperglycemia during pregnancy have not been fully evaluated (see Chapter 18).

In pregestational diabetics and in GDM diagnosed early in pregnancy, first-trimester glycohemoglobin measurements provide an assessment of the risk for congenital malformations.[24] Serial assessments affirm patient efforts to improve glycemic control, while a disparity with self-glucose monitoring may signal an error in monitoring techniques or malfunction of the equipment. In patients with hemoglobinopathies, fructosamine or glycated albumin measurements may need to be substituted. Glycohemoglobin measurements provide little benefit in monitoring patients with GDM with normal fasting glucoses.

Nutrition Therapy

General Guidelines. Diet is the cornerstone of diabetic therapy. Core recommendations are similar for pregnancy complicated by GDM and pregestational diabetes as for normal pregnancy, except that complex carbohydrate replaces simple sugars. Because of the predilection to accelerated starvation,[10,15] intake is spread to avoid fasts greater than 4–5 hr through the day, and a bedtime snack is added. The distribution of carbohydrate through the day may be individualized, but patients generally are intolerant of large amounts of carbohydrate at breakfast. Consistency from day to day must be stressed to attain good control, especially for women who are not skilled in successfully linking variable carbohydrate intake to insulin needs and physical activity.

Dietary prescriptions are individualized for prepregnancy body weight to height, activity level, and ethnic and personal preferences. The Institute of Medicine of the National Academy of Sciences has published guidelines for optimal weight gain in pregnancy,[144] based on reported associations between perinatal morbidity and weight gain during pregnancy. Recommended gestational weight gain is inversely proportional to maternal adiposity prior to conception, and vary from a gain of approximately 7 kg (15 lbs) in the morbidly obese to 18 kg (40 lbs) in those underweight, and are delineated in Table 40–4. In the absence of specific information for women with diabetes, we make the same dietary recommendations for those with pregestational diabetes mellitus or GDM as for nondiabetic subjects.

To attain these weight goals, a diet of 30–32 kcal/kg [125–135 kJ/kg] ideal body weight (IBW) is prescribed in the first trimester. This is increased to 35 to 38 kcal/kg [145–160 kJ/kg] IBW in the second trimester, depending on appetite and weight gain. Variations of up to ±30% in total calories may be necessary to attain the desired weight gain. The calories are distributed as 50–55% carbohydrate, <30% fat, and 1.0–1.5 g/kg IBW protein. Periconception supplementation with folic acid (0.4–0.8 mg/day) is recommended, as it is for women with normal carbohydrate metabolism, to reduce the increased risk of neural tube defects.

Other Considerations. A majority of women with GDM or type 2 diabetes are obese, and hypocaloric diets have been endorsed by some.[145] Accelerated starvation is not more pronounced in obese women with GDM than in normal pregnancy,[15] and moderate caloric restriction (20–25% below standard diets) may reduce hyperglycemia, without increasing ketonemia or ketonuria.[145,146] More significant caloric restrictions may result in elevations in free fatty acids and plasma ketones, despite improvement in glucose, insulin, and triglyceride levels,[146] and are not recommended at this time, except in research.

Utilization of a high fiber diet has not proved beneficial in reducing postprandial glucose levels.[147] "Isocaloric" modifications, such as reducing carbohydrate to 30–40% of total calories, reduces postprandial hyperglycemia.[148] However, the impact of increased fat and protein content on maternal amino acid, ketone, and lipid profiles has not been determined. Postprandial glucose peaks may also be diminished by ingesting more frequent smaller meals[149]; however, data on mean 24-hr glucose level and neonatal adiposity are limited. Further study is necessary to determine the perinatal and long-term impact of these manipulations on the offspring.

Insulin Therapy

Type 1 Diabetes Mellitus. Patients with type 1 diabetes mellitus are predisposed to wide glycemic fluctuations because they lack endogenous insulin and often

TABLE 40–4 Recommended Weight Gain for Pregnant Women by Prepregnancy Body Mass Index (BMI)

Category	BMI (kg/m²)	Recommended Weight Gain kg (lbs)	Weight Gain/Trimester	
			TR1	TR2-3
Underweight	<19.8	12.5–18 [28–40]	2.3 [5]	0.5 [1]/week
Normal weight	19.8–26.0	11.5–16 [25–35]	1.6 [3.5]	0.4 [1]/week
Overweight	26.0–29.0	7–11.5 [15–25]	0.9 [2]	0.3 [0.7]/week
Severely obese	>29.0	~6.8 [15]*	—	—

*The recommended weight gain for morbidly obese women is at least 6.0 kg (accounting for the products of conceptus). This recognizes that many gain less weight with good pregnancy outcomes.

Adapted from the recommendations of the Subcommittee on Nutritional Status and Weight Gain During Pregnancy, Food and Nutrition Board, Institute of Medicine: Nutrition During Pregnancy. Washington, DC: National Academy Press, 1990.

have impaired secretion of counter-regulatory hormones. Application of intensive therapy must be individualized and closely supervised, and involve either basal insulin with multiple premeal injections or insulin pump therapy, though the latter has not proven more effective.[150] Individual algorithms are provided at each meal to deal with the expected variations in glycemia, food intake, and physical activity. Modifications are made every 1 to 2 weeks, or more if needed, based on results of home glucose monitoring. Intensive insulin management in pregnant women with type 1 diabetes has been shown to normalize other maternal fuels that may affect fetal development, such as branched chain amino acids, alanine, and free fatty acids.

Around the end of the first trimester (10–14 weeks' gestation), the insulin requirement may decline and may be associated with a higher risk of severe hypoglycemia. Subsequently, insulin requirements increase substantially to plateau late in the third trimester at total daily doses up to threefold above prepregnant levels. Therapeutic modifications must keep pace with these expected changes in insulin sensitivity. A modest decline in insulin requirements sometimes occurs near term for reasons that are not known. A marked decline in insulin requirements may be seen in the presence of serious obstetrical complications and warrants intensive and ongoing maternal and fetal assessments.

Type 2 Diabetes Mellitus. Patients with type 2 diabetes mellitus should be placed on insulin prior to conception, or at the first prenatal visit should they have an unplanned pregnancy. Generally they will respond well to an insulin regimen as described below for the GDM, as they usually retain significant endogenous insulin secretion. Modifications are made every 1 to 2 weeks based on home glucose monitoring.

Gestational Diabetes Mellitus. No consensus has been reached on the identification of subjects with GDM who should receive insulin therapy. There is little controversy about those who meet current criteria for diabetes mellitus based on the presence of fasting hyperglycemia (fasting plasma glucose ≥ 126 mg/dL [7.0 mmol/L]). These patients require immediate institution of insulin therapy, as the risks to the fetus equal those of pregestational diabetic pregnancies. There is also general agreement that those with fasting plasma glucoses ≥ 105 and <126 mg/dL [5.8–7.0 mmol/L], which persists on two separate occasions after a dietary trial should also receive insulin therapy.[81]

The controversy exists when the fasting glucoses are "normal" (i.e., <105 mg/dL [5.8 mmol/L]), as is the case in the majority of patients with GDM. Indeed, in most populations that have been studied, the upper level of FPG is in the range of 95 to 100 mg/dL [5.3–5.6 mmol/L]. There is little evidence that such pregnancies are at high risk for perinatal loss; however, there is an increased risk of macrosomia, cesarean delivery, and birth trauma,[57,66] and offspring may be at increased risk for obesity and diabetes mellitus in later life.[57,58,63] Furthermore, several studies reported recently indicate an increased risk for these morbidities in pregnancies where maternal glucose intolerance on the OGTT is less severe than that required to meet the diagnostic criteria that are currently used, for example, those with one abnormal value on the OGTT[151,152] rather than two or those that have two or more values exceeding the more conservative thresholds recommended by Carpenter and Coustan.[104–108] In situations where all or a large majority of the GDM population with FPG <105 mg/dL [5.8 mmol/L] has received insulin therapy, the rate of macrosomia has been reduced to that of the general obstetrical population.[81,153]

A benefit/cost advantage has not been established over the short or long term. Others have attempted to define those pregnancies at risk by using amniotic fluid insulin levels as a marker of fetal hyperinsulinism,[98,99] or fetal ultrasound measurements of shoulder soft tissue[154] or abdominal circumference[155] to predict macrosomia. The former method has resulted in good fetal outcomes, but is complex and invasive, and is not likely to be generally accepted. Using ultrasound determinants of macrosomia to target pregnancies for insulin does eliminate the excess macrosomia, but does not necessarily protect against long-term risk of obesity and glucose intolerance in the offspring because the offspring at risk may have normal birth weights.[57,59] A well-designed clinical trial is needed to determine the parameters where intervention is most beneficial. In the meantime, we recommend insulin therapy for our patients whose fasting and/or postprandial glucoses on an appropriate diet *repeatedly exceed* the following target ranges: fasting (laboratory FPG <100 mg/dL [5.6 mmol/L], self-monitored fasting capillary blood glucose <90–94 mg/dL [5.0-5.2 mmol/L]); 1-hr laboratory postprandial glucose <140 mg/dL [7.8 mmol/L], self-monitored postprandial capillary glucose <130–135 mg/dL [7.2–7.5 mmol/L]; 2-hr laboratory postprandial plasma glucose <120 mg/dL [6.7 mmol/L], self-monitored postprandial capillary glucose <110–115 mg/dL [6.1-6.4 mmol/L]. Insulin doses ranging from 0.5 to 2.0 units/kg may be needed to achieve fasting and postprandial glucoses below the thresholds indicated above. Generally, a twice daily "mixed-split" insulin regimen is used, though multiple daily injections may be used when needed to correct specific patterns of hyperglycemia.

Peripartum. For GDM and pregestational diabetic women, the goal of therapy in labor is to maintain glucoses in the physiological range of 70 to 120 mg/dL [3.9–6.7 mmol/L]. To avoid hyperglycemia, oral and intravenous carbohydrate is restricted. Intravenous dextrose in water is administered at rates of 5–8 g/hr using 10% dextrose in water (50–80 cc/hr). All other intravenous fluids are devoid of glucose. Glucose is monitored every 1 to 4 hr, and insulin is administered as necessary either by an intravenous infusion (0.01 to 0.04 U/kg actual body weight/hr)[156] or by subcutaneous injection of short-acting insulin every 3 to 6 hr.[157] The need for glucose and insulin is modified by the prevailing blood glucose, the time and nature of the last insulin injection, and the time of food ingestion prior to the onset of labor. The "exercise" effect of labor may enhance the rate of glucose utilization,[158] but may be modulated by the use of a continuous epidural anesthetic throughout labor. Insulin therapy is rarely required in GDM to maintain intrapartum normoglycemia, and some with type 2 diabetes also do not require insulin in labor.

Insulin requirement declines dramatically immediately postpartum (by as much as 50–90%), and the administered dose may need to be reduced temporarily to 30% or less of the total daily antepartum dose. Failure of this enhanced insulin sensitivity to appear may be an early sign of impending postpartum infection. The effects of intravenous insulin dissipate rapidly. If this method was used to maintain glycemic control in labor in type 1 diabetic patients, subcutaneous insulin must be administered prior to discontinuing the intravenous infusion. After a variable period, insulin requirements generally return to prepregnancy levels.

Other Therapies

Exercise. Exercise improves insulin sensitivity, insulin binding to receptors, recruitment of glucose transporter proteins, and glucose disposal in nonpregnant patients. Concerns have been expressed regarding potential detrimental effects of exercise (including increased uterine contractility, prematurity, IUGR, fetal bradycardia, and ketonuria)[159] in patients who were previously inactive. However, moderate exercise has been safely and effectively initiated in pregnancy using arm ergometry[160] or bicycle[161] and found to improve glycemic control. Other studies have demonstrated no benefit to glycemic control with moderate exercise, but an improvement in cardiovascular fitness.[162]

Oral Agents. None of the oral pharmacological therapies that are approved for the treatment of hyperglycemia has Food and Drug Administration (FDA) approval for use in pregnancy. Though no class of agent has been identified as a teratogen and a considerable number of pregnancies have occurred in women using sulfonylurea or biguanide compounds, it has not been established that any of these drugs is safe to use during organogenesis.[163,164] Thus, we strongly recommend that women with type 2 diabetes receive preconception counseling and therapy as given for women with type 1 diabetes, and that the transfer to insulin therapy be included.

Postpartum Follow-Up and Counseling

Breastfeeding

Breastfeeding increases the caloric requirements by 400–500 kcal/day [1650–2000 kJ/day] above the baseline nonpregnant need of 30–32 kcal/kg IBW [125–135 kJ/kg]. The benefits of breastfeeding are similar for the offspring of nondiabetic and diabetic women and should be encouraged. In addition, the epidemiological study in the Pimas suggests additional long-term benefit in reducing the risk of developing type 2 diabetes in this population.[165]

Women with type 2 diabetes who wish to breastfeed but require pharmacological intervention postpartum are continued on insulin therapy until the child is weaned. Sulfonylureas may be secreted in breast milk and cause hypoglycemia in the infant. The effects of other oral agents on a neonate have not been determined.

Reclassification, Follow-up, and Prevention

GDM is usually a transitory period of glucose intolerance, but may represent the initial stage of type 1 or type 2 diabetes mellitus. Postpartum reclassification is therefore essential (see Table 40-5). A fasting plasma glucose, or if indicated, a glucose tolerance test is performed at approximately 6 weeks postpartum for reclassification, and is followed by postpartum counseling.

Ongoing insulin resistance and β-cell insufficiency of variable degrees have been documented in women with previous GDM who are at high risk for progression to type 2 diabetes mellitus.[88,89] A number of features including severity of hyperglycemia at diagnosis, relative insulinopenia with blunted first-phase insulin response, early gestational age at diagnosis, obesity, family history of diabetes mellitus, and racial/ethnic origin identify those at highest risk for progression.[166–168] Some also have other features of the insulin resistance syndrome (hypertension, elevated triglycerides, low HDL-C).[169] Thus, cardiovascular disease risk factors should also be monitored regularly and treated when present in women with previous GDM.

Women who have or develop type 2 diabetes should receive appropriate counseling and therapy. In those with impaired glucose tolerance or a normal OGTT, counseling should include recommendations for measures that can improve insulin sensitivity, such as diet, exercise, and weight loss in those who are obese. The role of pharmacological agents in the prevention of progression to type 2 diabetes will be ascertained in the

TABLE 40–5   Reclassification of Glucose Tolerance Status Postpartum

	Fasting Plasma Glucose	2-Hour OGTT
Normal	<110 mg/dL [6.1 mmol/L][†]	<140 mg/dL [7.8 mmol/L]
Impaired	110-125 mg/dL [6.1–6.9 mmol/L][*]	140–199 mg/dL [7.8–11.0 mmol/L][**]
Diabetes mellitus[‡]	≥126 mg/dL [7.0 mmol/L]	≥200 mg/dL [11.1 mmol/L]

[†]OGTT indicated to detect impaired glucose tolerance which predicts the risk of progression to diabetes.

[*]Defined as *Impaired fasting glucose.* OGTT indicated to detect those with diabetes.

[**]Defined as *Impaired glucose tolerance.* Warrants routine screening for diabetes, and counseling on diabetes prevention.

[‡]Repeat on a second day to confirm diagnosis.

Adapted from Metzger BE: Summary and recommendations of the Fourth International Workshop Conference on Gestational Diabetes Mellitus. Diabetes Care 21(52):B161–B167, 1998. Expert Committee on the Diagnosis and Classification of Diabetes Mellitus: Report of the Expert Committee on the Diagnosis and Classification of Diabetes Mellitus. Diabetes Care 20:1183–1197, 1997.

ongoing Diabetes Prevention Program, which is actively recruiting women with a history of GDM. Patients should receive continuing follow-up with annual glucose testing, as well as re-evaluation prior to any future pregnancies. Therapy should be initiated preconceptionally as necessary, to avoid an increased risk of congenital anomalies. Those with normal glucose tolerance before pregnancy should also be evaluated early in gestation, and if normal, again at the usual time of 24–28 weeks' gestation. GDM recurs in more than half of subsequent pregnancies,[170,171] though the risk of recurrence might possibly be reduced by interpregnancy intervention.[172]

Contraception

It is important that future pregnancies be planned in women with previous GDM as well as those with type 1 and type 2 diabetes mellitus. Thus, adequate contraception for these women is vital. Most methods used for the general population are available for women with diabetes or prior GDM.[173] Low-dose oral contraceptives provide acceptable protection and have not been found to increase hyperlipidemia or glucose intolerance. However, the studies reported to date have been of limited duration. Preparations containing the progestins norethindrone or desogestrel have also shown minimal metabolic effect. Patients treated with the thiazolidinedione derivatives such as troglitazone need to be aware of possible loss of efficacy of contraception from low-dose oral contraceptives.

Enormous strides have been made in the management of diabetes in pregnancy and in the understanding of its implications for mother and progeny. With optimal care, pregnancy outcome appoaches that of a nondiabetic patient. However, in the United States, preconception care is currently sought in only one third of patients with pregestational diabetes.[174] Interventions must address prevention of unplanned pregnancies, and providers should regard every visit with a diabetic woman of childbearing age as a preconception visit. In addition, further work needs to be done to improve our understanding of the pathophysiology of the adverse effects of diabetes in pregnancy, develop therapeutic measures to further reduce congenital anomalies, lessen macrosomia and the associated risk of a traumatic delivery, and diminish the adverse long-term impact on the offspring. Early diagnosis of GDM with criteria designed to identify the fetus at risk, optimal maternal care, and prevention of diabetes postpartum are also important topics for future research.

References

1. Pitkin RM: Nutritional requirements in normal pregnancy. Diabetes Care 3:472–475, 1980.

2. Kalkhoff RK, Kissebah AH, Kim HJ: Carbohydrate and lipid metabolism during normal pregnancy. Relationship to gestational hormone action. Semin Perinatol 2:291–307, 1978.

3. Catalano PM, Tyzbir ED, Wolfe RR, et al.: Carbohydrate metabolism during pregnancy in control subjects and women with gestational diabetes. Am J Physiol 264: E60–E67, 1993.

4. Cousins L, Rea C, Crawford M: Longitudinal characterization of insulin sensitivity and body fat quantitation in normal and gestational diabetic pregnancies. Diabetes 37(Suppl. 1):251A, 1988.

5. Eriksson L, Frankenne F, Eden S, et al.: Growth hormone 24-h serum profiles during pregnancy: Lack of pulsatility for the secretion of the placental variant. Br J Obstet Gynaecol 96:949–953, 1989.

6. Daughaday WH, Trivedi B, Winn HN, et al.: Hypersomatotropism in pregnant women, as measured by a

human liver radioreceptor assay. J Clin Endocrinol Metab 70:215–221, 1990.

7. Freinkel N, Metzger BE, Nitzan M, et al.: Facilitated anabolism in late pregnancy: Some novel maternal compensations for accelerated starvation. In Malaise WJ, Pirart J (eds): Proceedings of the VIIIth Congress of the International Diabetes Foundation. Excerpta Medica International Congress Series No. 312, Amsterdam, 1974, pp. 474–488.

8. Mills JL, Jovanovic L, Knopp R, et al.: Physiological reduction in fasting plasma glucose concentration in the first trimester of normal pregnancy: The Diabetes in Early Pregnancy Study. Metabolism 47:1140–1144, 1998.

9. Ogata ES, Metzger BE, Freinkel N: Carbohydrate metabolism in pregnancy: XVI. Longitudinal estimates of the effects of pregnancy on D-(6^3H) glucose and D-(6^{14}C) glucose turnovers during fasting in the rat. Metabolism 30:487–492, 1981.

10. Metzger BE, Ravnikar V, Vilesis R, et al.: Accelerated starvation and the skipped breakfast in late normal pregnancy. Lancet 1:588–592, 1982.

11. Shoengold DM, DeFiore RH, Parlett RC: Free amino acids in plasma throughout pregnancy. Am J Obstet Gynecol 131:490–499, 1978.

12. Rushakoff RJ, Kalkhoff RK: Effects of pregnancy and sex steroid administration on skeletal muscle metabolism in the rat. Diabetes 30:545–550, 1981.

13. Persson B, Lunnel NO: Metabolic control in diabetic pregnancy. Variations in plasma concentrations of glucose, free fatty acids, glycerol, ketone bodies, insulin and human chorionic somatomammotropin during the last trimester. Am J Obstet Gynecol 122:737–745, 1975.

14. Metzger BE, Phelps RL, Freinkel N, et al.: Effects of gestational diabetes on diurnal profiles of plasma glucose, lipids and individual amino acids. Diabetes Care 3:402–409, 1980.

15. Buchanan TA, Metzger BE, Freinkel N: Accelerated starvation in late pregnancy: A comparison between obese women with and without gestational diabetes mellitus. Am J Obstet Gynecol 162:1015–1020, 1990.

16. Hollingworth DR, Grundy SM: Pregnancy-associated hypertriglyceridemia in normal and diabetic women. Differences in insulin-dependent and non-insulin dependent, and gestational diabetes. Diabetes 31:1092–1097, 1988.

17. Kalkhoff RK, Kandaraki E, Morrow PG, et al.: Relationship between neonatal birth weight and maternal plasma amino acid profiles in lean and obese nondiabetic women and in type I diabetic women. Metabolism 37:234–239, 1988.

18. Freinkel N: The Banting Lecture 1980: Of Pregnancy and progeny. Diabetes 29:1023–1035, 1980.

19. Freinkel N, Metzger BE: Pregnancy as a tissue culture experience: The critical implications of maternal metabolism for fetal development. *In* Pregnancy Metabolism, Diabetes and the Fetus (CIBA Foundation Symposium No. 63), Amsterdam: Exerpta Medica, 1979, pp. 3–23.

20. Mills JL, Baker L, Goldman AS: Malformations in infants of diabetic mothers occur before the seventh ges-tational week: Implications for treatment. Diabetes 28:292–293, 1979.

21. From research to practice: Diabetes and birth defects: Insights from the 1980s, prevention in the 1990s. Diabetes Spectrum 3:150–184, 1990.

22. Pedersen J: The Pregnant diabetic and her newborn: Problems and management. Baltimore: Williams & Wilkins, 1977.

23. Mills JL, Simpson JL, Driscoll SG, et al.: The NICHHD-Diabetes in Early Pregnancy Study: Incidence of spontaneous abortion among normal women and insulin-dependent diabetic women whose pregnancies were identified within 21 days of conception. N Engl J Med 319:1617–1623, 1988.

24. Greene MF, Hare JW, Cloherty JP, et al.: First trimester hemoglobin A₁ and risk for major malformations and spontaneous abortion in diabetic pregnancy. Teratology 39:225–231, 1989.

25. Mills JL, Knopp RH, Simpson JL, et al.: Lack of relation of increased malformation rates in infants of diabetic mothers to glycemic control during organogenesis. N Engl J Med 318:671–676, 1988.

26. Buchanan T, Schemmer JK, Freinkel N: Embryotoxic effects of brief maternal insulin-hypoglycemia during organogenesis in the rat. J Clin Invest 78:643–649, 1986.

27. Akazawa S, Akazawa M, Hashimoto M, et al.: Effects of hypoglycaemia on early embryogenesis in rat embryo organ culture. Diabetologia 30:791–796, 1987.

28. Buchanan TA, Denno KM, Sipes GF, et al.: Diabetic teratogenesis: In vitro evidence for a multifactorial etiology with little contribution from glucose per se. Diabetes 43:656–660, 1994.

29. Strieleman PJ, Connors MA, Metzger BE: Phosphoinositide metabolism in the developing conceptus: Effects of hyperglycemia and *scyllo*-inositol in rat embryo culture. Diabetes 41:989–997, 1992.

30. Hashimoto M, Akazawa S, Akazawa M, et al.: Effects of hyperglycemia on sorbitol and myo-inositol contents of cultured embryos: Treatment with aldose reductase inhibitor and myo-inositol supplementation. Diabetologia 33:597–602, 1990.

31. Goldman AS, Baker L, Piddington R, et al.: Hyperglycemia-induced teratogenesis is mediated by a functional deficiency in arachidonic acid. Proc Natl Acad Sci USA 82:8227–8231, 1985.

32. Eriksson UJ, Borg LAH: Diabetes and embryonic malformations: Role of substrate-induced free-oxygen radical production for dysmorphogenesis in cultured rat embryos. Diabetes 42:1411–1419, 1993.

33. Fuhrmann K, Reiher H, Semmler K, et al.: Prevention of congenital malformations in infants of insulin-dependent diabetic mothers. Diabetes Care 6:219–223, 1983.

34. Kitzmiller JL, Gavin LA, Gin GD, et al.: Preconception care of diabetes. Glycemic control prevents congenital anomalies. JAMA 265:731–736, 1991.

35. Damm P, Molsted-Pedersen L: Significant decrease in congenital malformations in newborn infants of an unselected population of diabetic women. Am J Obstet Gynecol 161:1163–1167, 1989.

36. Naeye RL: Infants of diabetic mothers: A quantitative, morphologic study. Pediatrics 35:980–988, 1965.

37. Whitelaw A: Subcutaneous fat in newborn infants of diabetic mothers: An indication of quality of diabetic control. Lancet 1:15–18, 1977.

38. Elliot JP, Garite TJ, Freeman RK: Ultrasonic prediction of fetal macrosomia in diabetic patients. Obstet Gynecol 60:159–164, 1982.

39. Larson G, Spjuth J, Ranstam J, et al.: Prognostic significance of birth of large infant for subsequent development of maternal non-insulin-dependent diabetes mellitus: A prospective study over 20–27 years. Diabetes Care 9:359–364, 1986.

40. Keller JD, Metzger BE, Dooley SL, et al.: Infants of diabetic mothers with accelerated fetal growth by ultrasonography: Are they all alike? Am J Obstet Gynecol 163:893–897, 1990.

41. Ogata ES, Sabbagha R, Metzger BE, et al.: Serial ultrasonography to assess evolving fetal macrosomia: Studies in 23 pregnant diabetic women. JAMA 243:2405–2408, 1980.

42. Landon MB, Mintz MC, Gabbe SG: Sonographic evaluation of fetal abdominal growth: Predictor of the large-for-gestational-age infant in pregnancies complicated by diabetes mellitus. Am J Obstet Gynecol 160:115–121, 1989.

43. Farquhar JW: Prognosis for babies born to diabetic mothers in Edinburgh. Arch Dis Child 44:36–47, 1969.

44. Metzger BE: Biphasic effects of maternal metabolism on fetal growth: The quintessential expression of "fuel-mediated teratogenesis." Diabetes 40(Suppl. 2):99–105, 1991.

45. Ogata ES, Freinkel N, Metzger BE, et al.: Perinatal islet function in gestational diabetes: Assessment by cord plasma C-peptide and amniotic fluid insulin. Diabetes Care 3:425–429, 1980.

46. Weiss PAM, Hofman H, Winter R, et al.: Gestational diabetes and screening during pregnancy. Obstet Gynecol 63:776–780, 1984.

47. Fallucca F, Gargiulo P, Troili F, et al.: Amniotic fluid insulin, C-peptide concentrations, and fetal morbidity in infants of diabetic mothers. Am J Obstet Gynecol 153:534–540, 1985.

48. Persson B, Pschera H, Lunnell N-O, et al.: Amino acid concentrations in maternal plasma and amniotic fluid in relation to trimester of pregnancy in gestational and type I diabetic women and women with small-for-gestational-age infants. Am J Perinatol 3:98–103, 1986.

49. Van Assche FA, Aerts L: The fetal endocrine pancreas. *In* Keller PJ (ed): Contributions to Gynecology and Obstetrics. Basel: Karger, 1979, pp. 44–57.

50. Reiher H, Fuhrmann K, Noack S, et al: Age-dependent insulin secretion of the endocrine pancreas in vitro from fetuses of diabetic and nondiabetic patients. Diabetes Care 6:446–451, 1983.

51. Susa JB, Neave C, Sehgal P, et al.: Chronic hyperinsulinemia in the fetal rhesus monkey: Effects of physiologic hyperinsulinemia on fetal growth and composition. Diabetes 33:656–660, 1984.

52. Verhaeghe J, Van Bree R, Van Herck E, et al.: C-peptide, insulin-like growth factors I and II, and insulin-like growth factor binding protein-1 in umbilical serum: Correlations with birth weight. Am J Obstet Gynecol 169:89–97, 1993.

53. Culler FL, Tung RF, Jansons RA, et al.: Growth promoting peptides in diabetic and non-diabetic pregnancy: Interactions with trophoblastic receptors and serum carrier proteins. J Pediatr Endocrinol Metab 9:21–29, 1996.

54. Neiger R: Fetal macrosomia in the diabetic patient. Clin Obstet Gynecol 35:138–150, 1992.

55. Pedersen JL, Molsted-Pedersen L: Early fetal growth delay detected by ultrasound marks increased risk of congenital malformation in diabetic pregnancy. BMJ 283:269–271, 1981.

56. Eriksson UJ, Lewis NJ, Freinkel N: Growth retardation during early organogenesis in embryos of experimentally diabetic rats. Diabetes 33:281–284, 1984.

57. Silverman BL, Purdy LP, Metzger BE: The intrauterine environment: Implications for the offspring of diabetic mothers. Diabetes Rev 4:21–35, 1996.

58. Pettitt DJ, Baird HR, Aleck KA, et al.: Excessive obesity in offspring of Pima Indian women with diabetes during pregnancy. N Engl J Med 308:242–245, 1983.

59. Pettitt DJ, Knowler WC, Bennett PH, et al.: Obesity in offspring of diabetic Pima Indian women despite normal birth weight. Diabetes Care 10:76–80, 1987.

60. Gerlini G, Arachi S, Gori MG, et al.: Developmental aspects of the offspring of diabetic mothers. Acta Endocrinol (Copenhagen) 112(Suppl. 277):150–155, 1986.

61. Silverman BL, Rizzo T, Green OC, et al.: Long-term prospective evaluation of offspring of diabetic mothers. Diabetes 40(Suppl. 2):121–125, 1991.

62. Susa JB, Sehgal P, Schwartz R: Rhesus monkeys made exogenously hyperinsulinemic in utero as fetuses, display abnormal glucose homeostasis as pregnant adults and have macrosomic fetuses. Diabetes 42(Suppl. 1):86A, 1993.

63. Pettitt DJ, Aleck KA, Baird HR, et al.: Congenital susceptibility for NIDDM: Role of intrauterine environment. Diabetes 37:622–628, 1988.

64. Silverman BL, Cho NH, Metzger BE: Impaired glucose tolerance in adolescent offspring of diabetic mothers: Relationship to fetal hyperinsulinism. Diabetes Care 18:611–618, 1995.

65. Harris MI, Flegal KM, Cowie CC, et al.: Prevalence of diabetes, impaired fasting glucose, and impaired glucose tolerance in U.S. adults: The third National Health and Nutrition Examination Survey, 1988–1994. Diabetes Care 21:518–524, 1998.

66. Connell FA, Vadheim, Emanuel I: Diabetes in pregnancy: A population based study of incidence, referral for care and perinatal mortality. Am J Obstet Gynecol 151:598–603, 1985.

67. Beischer NA, Oats JN, Henry OA, et al.: Incidence and severity of gestational diabetes mellitus according to country of birth in women living in Australia. Diabetes 40(Suppl. 2):35–38, 1991.

68. Dooley SL, Metzger BE, Cho NH: Gestational diabetes mellitus: Influence of race on disease prevalence and peri-

natal outcomes in a U.S. population. Diabetes 40(Suppl. 2): 25–29, 1991.

69. Metzger BE, Cho NH: Epidemiology and genetics. *In* Reece EA, Coustan DR (eds): Diabetes Mellitus in Pregnancy, 2nd ed. New York: Churchill Livingstone, 1995, pp. 11–26.

70. Engelgau MM, Herman WH, Smith PJ, et al.: The epidemiology of diabetes and pregnancy in the U.S., 1988. Diabetes Care 18:1029–1033, 1995.

71. Harris M: Gestational diabetes may represent discovery of pre-existing glucose intolerance. Diabetes Care 11:402–411, 1988.

72. Jovanovic L, Peterson CM: Screening for gestational diabetes: Optimum timing and criteria for retesting. Diabetes 34(Suppl. 2):21–23, 1985.

73. Super DM, Edelberg SC, Philipson EH, et al.: Diagnosis of gestational diabetes in early pregnancy. Diabetes Care 14:288–294, 1991.

74. O'Sullivan JB, Mahan CM: Criteria for the oral glucose tolerance test in pregnancy. Diabetes 13:278–285, 1964.

75. Catalano PM, Vargo KM, Bernstein IM, et al.: Incidence and risk factors associated with abnormal postpartum glucose tolerance in women with gestational diabetes. Am J Obstet Gynecol 165:914–919, 1991.

76. White P: Pregnancy complicating diabetes. Am J Med 7:609–616, 1949.

77. Kitzmiller JL, Brown ER, Phillippe M, et al.: Diabetic nephropathy and perinatal outcome. Am J Obstet Gynecol 141:741–751, 1981.

78. Reece EA, Egan JFX, Coustan DR, et al.: Coronary artery disease in diabetic pregnancies. Am J Obstet Gynecol 154:150–151, 1986.

79. Freinkel N, Metzger BE, Phelps RL, et al.: Gestational diabetes mellitus: Heterogeneity of maternal age, weight, insulin secretion, HLA antigens, and islet cell antibodies and the impact of maternal metabolism on pancreatic B-cell and somatic development in the offspring. Diabetes 34(Suppl. 2):1–7, 1985.

80. Kahn R, and the Expert Committee on the Diagnosis and Classification of Diabetes Mellitus: Report of the Expert Committee on the Diagnosis and Classification of Diabetes Mellitus. Diabetes Care 20:1183–1197, 1997.

81. Metzger BE, Coustan DR, and the Organizing Committee: Summary and recommendations of the Fourth International Workshop-Conference on Gestational Diabetes Mellitus. Diabetes Care, 21(S2):B161–B167, 1998.

82. Freinkel N, Metzger BE, Phelps RL, et al.: "Gestational diabetes mellitus": A syndrome with phenotypic and genotypic heterogeneity. Horm Metab Res 18:427–430, 1986.

83. Beischer NA, Wein P, Sheedy MT, et al.: Prevalence of antibodies to glutamic acid decarbosylase in women who have had gestational diabetes. Am J Obstet Gynecol 173:1563–1569, 1995.

84. Catalano PM, Tyzbir ED, Sims EAH: Incidence and significance of islet cell antibodies in women with previous gestational diabetes. Diabetes Care 13:478–482, 1990.

85. Buschard K, Buch I, Molsted-Pedersen L, et al.: Increased incidence of true type I diabetes acquired during pregnancy. BMJ 294:275–279, 1987.

86. Buchanan TA, Metzger BE, Freinkel N, et al.: Insulin sensitivity and B-cell responsiveness to glucose during late pregnancy in lean and moderately obese women with normal glucose tolerance or mild gestational diabetes. Am J Obstet Gynecol 162:1008–1014, 1990.

87. Kautzky-Willer A, Prager R, Waldhausl W, et al.: Pronounced insulin resistance and inadequate β-cell secretion characterize lean gestational diabetes during and after pregnancy. Diabetes Care 20:1717–1723, 1997.

88. Coustan DR, Nelson C, Carpenter MW, et al.: Maternal age and screening for gestational diabetes: A population-based survey. Obstet Gynecol 73:557–561, 1989.

89. Jowett NI, Samanta AK, Burden AC: Screening for diabetes in pregnancy: Is a random blood glucose enough? Diabetic Med 4:160–163, 1987.

90. Nasrat AA, Johnstone FD, Hasan SAM: Is random plasma glucose an efficient screening test for abnormal glucose tolerance in pregnancy? Br J Obstet Gynaecol 95:855–860, 1988.

91. Cousins L, Dattel BJ, Hollingsworth DR, et al.: Glycosylated hemoglobin as a screening test for carbohydrate intolerance in pregnancy. Am J Obstet Gynecol 150:455–460, 1984.

92. Shah BD, Cohen AW, May C, et al.: Comparison of glycohemoglobin deterioration and the one-hour oral glucose screen in the identification of gestational diabetes. Am J Obstet Gynecol 144:774–777, 1982.

93. Vermes I, Zeyen LJJM, van Roon E, et al.: The role of serum fructosamine as a screening test for gestational diabetes mellitus. Horm Metabol Res 21:73–76, 1989.

94. Hughes PF, Agarwal M, Newman P, et al.: An evaluation of fructosamine estimation in screening for gestational diabetes mellitus. Diabetic Med 12:708–712, 1995.

95. Kurishita M, Nakashima K, Kozu H: Glycated hemoglobin of fractionated erythrocytes, glycated albumin, and plasma fructosamine during pregnancy. Am J Obstet Gynecol 167:1372–1378, 1992.

96. Weiss PAM, Hofmann HMH, Kainer F, et al.: Fetal outcome in gestational diabetes with elevated amniotic fluid insulin levels: Dietary versus insulin treatment. Diabetes Res Clin Practice 5:1–7, 1988.

97. Carpenter MW, Canick JA, Star J, et al.: Fetal hyperinsulinism at 14-20 weeks and subsequent gestational diabetes. Obstet Gynecol 87:89–93, 1996.

98. Sermer M, Naylor CD, Gare DJ, et al.: Impact of time since last meal on the gestational glucose challenge test: The Toronto Tri-Hospital Gestational Diabetes Project. Am J Obstet Gynecol 171:607–616, 1994.

99. O'Sullivan JB, Mahan CM, Charles D, et al.: Screening criteria for high-risk gestational diabetic patients. Am J Obstet Gynecol 116:895–900, 1973.

100. Meyer WJ, Carbone J, Gauthier DW, et al.: Early gestational glucose screening and gestational diabetes. J Reprod Med 41:675–679, 1996.

101. Carr S, Coustan DR, Martelly P, et al.: Precision of reflectance meters in screening for gestational diabetes. Obstet Gynecol 73:727–731, 1989.

102. National Diabetes Data Group: Classification and diagnosis of diabetes mellitus and other categories of glucose intolerance. Diabetes 28:1039–1057, 1979.

103. Metzger BE, Organizing Committee: Summary and Recommendations of the Third International Workshop-Conference on Gestational Diabetes Mellitus. Diabetes 40(Suppl. 2):197–201, 1991.

104. Carpenter MW, Coustan DR: Criteria for screening tests for gestational diabetes mellitus. Am J Obstet Gynecol 159:768–773, 1982.

105. Magee MS, Walden CE, Benedetti TJ, et al.: Influence of diagnostic criteria on the incidence of gestational diabetes and perinatal morbidity. JAMA 269:609–615, 1993.

106. Berkus MD, Langer O, Piper JM, Luther MF: Efficiency of lower threshold criteria for the diagnosis of gestational diabetes. Obstet Gynecol 86:892–896, 1995.

107. Rust OA, Bofill JA, Andrew ME, et al.: Lowering the threshold for the diagnosis of gestational diabetes. Am J Obstet Gynecol 175:961–965, 1996.

108. Deerochanawong C, Putiyanun C, Wongsuryrat M, et al.: Comparison of the National Diabetes Data Group and World Health Organization criteria for detecting gestational diabetes mellitus. Diabetologia 39:1070–1073, 1996.

109. American Diabetes Association: Diabetic retinopathy: Position statement. Diabetes Care 21:157–159, 1998.

110. Phelps RL, Sakol P, Metzger BE, et al.: Changes in diabetic retinopathy during pregnancy: Correlations with regulation of hyperglycemia. Arch Ophthalmol 104:1806–1810, 1986.

111. Axer-Siegel R, Hod M, Fink-Cohen S, et al.: Diabetic retinopathy during pregnancy. Ophthalmology 103:1815–1819, 1996.

112. Chew EY, Mills JL, Metzger BE, et al.: Metabolic control and progression of retinopathy: The diabetes in early pregnancy study. Diabetes Care 18:631–637, 1995.

113. Rosenn B, Miodovnik M, Kranias G, et al.: Progression of diabetic retinopathy in pregnancy: Association with hypertension in pregnancy. Am J Obstet Gynecol 166:1214–1218, 1992.

114. Lovestam-Adrian M, Agardh C-D, Aberg A, et al.: Preeclampsia is a potent risk factor for deterioration of retinopathy during pregnancy in type 1 diabetic patients. Diabet Med 14:1059–1065, 1997.

115. Lachin J, Cleary P, Molitch M, et al.: Pregnancy increases the risk of complications in the DCCT. Diabetes, 47(S1):A50, 1998.

116. Chen HC, Newsom RSB, Patel V, et al.: Retinal blood flow changes during pregnancy in women with diabetes. Invest Ophthalmol Vis Sci 35:3199–3208, 1994.

117. Hill DJ, Flyvbjerg A, Arany E, et al.: Increased levels of serum fibroblast growth factor-2 in diabetic pregnant women with retinopathy. J Clin Endocrinol Metab 82:1452–1457, 1997.

118. Reece EA, Lockwood CJ, Tuck S, et al.: Retinal and pregnancy outcomes in the presence of diabetic proliferative retinopathy. J Reprod Med 39:799–804, 1994.

119. Serup L: Influence of pregnancy on diabetic retinopathy. Acta Endocrinol 27(Suppl. 1986):122–124, 1994.

120. Conway M, Baldwin J, Kohner EM, et al.: Postpartum progression of diabetic retinopathy. Diabetes Care 14:1110–1111, 1991.

121. Sinclair SH, Nesler C, Foxman B, et al.: Macular edema and pregnancy in insulin-dependent diabetes. Am J Ophthalmol 97:154–167, 1984.

122. Chaturvedi N, Stephenson JM, Fuller JH, and the EURODIAB IDDM Complications Study Group: The relationship between pregnancy and long-term maternal complications in the EURODIAB IDDM Complications Study. Diabetic Med 12:494–499, 1995.

123. Bojestig M, Arnqvist HJ, Hermansson G, et al.: Declining incidence of nephropathy in insulin-dependent diabetes mellitus. N Engl J Med 330:15–18, 1994.

124. Siddiqi T, Rosenn B, Mimouni F, Khoury J, Miodovnik M: Hypertension during pregnancy in insulin-dependent diabetic women. Obstet Gynecol 77:514–519, 1991.

125. Reece EA, Coustan DR, Hayslett JP, et al.: Diabetic nephropathy: pregnancy performance and fetomaternal outcome. Am J Obstet Gynecol 159:56–66, 1988.

126. Biesenbach G, Stoeger H, Zazgornik J: Influence of pregnancy on progression of diabetic nephropathy and subsequent requirement of renal replacement therapy in female type I diabetic patients with impaired renal function. Nephrol Dial Transplant 7:105–109, 1992.

127. Purdy LP, Hantsch CE, Molitch ME, et al.: Effect of pregnancy on renal function in patients with moderate-to-severe diabetic renal insufficiency. Diabetes Care 19:1067–1074, 1996.

128. Macleod AF, Smith SA, Sonksen PH, Lowy C: The problem of autonomic neuropathy in diabetic pregnancy. Diabetic Med 7:80–82, 1990.

129. Airaksinen KEJ, Anttila LM, Linnaluoto MK, et al.: Autonomic influence on pregnancy outcome in IDDM. Diabetes Care 13:756–761, 1990.

130. Picchota W, Staszewski A: Reference ranges of lipids and apolipoproteins in pregnancy. Eur J Obstet Gynecol Reprod Biol 45:27–35, 1992.

131. Desoye G, Schweditsch M, Pfieffer KP, et al.: Correlations of hormones with lipid and lipoprotein levels during normal pregnancy and postpartum. J Clin Endocrinol Metab 64:704–712, 1987.

132. Siddiqi T, Rosenn B, Mimouni F, et al.: Hypertension during pregnancy in insulin-dependent diabetic women. Obstet Gynecol 77:514–519, 1991.

133. Hare JW, White P: Pregnancy in diabetes complicated by vascular disease. Diabetes 26:953–955, 1977.

134. Ueland K, Metcalfe J: Circulatory changes in pregnancy. Clin Obstet Gynecol 18:41–50, 1975.

135. Cousins L: Pregnancy complications among diabetic women: Review 1965–1985. Obstet Gynecol Surv 42:140–149, 1987.

136. Coustan DR, Berkowitz RL, Hobbins JC: Tight metabolic control of overt diabetes in pregnancy. Am J Med 68:845–852, 1980.

137. Suhonen L, Teramo K: Hypertension and pre-eclampsia in women with gestational glucose intolerance. Acta Obstet Gynecol Scand 72:269–272, 1993.

138. Knock GA, McCarthy AL, Lowy C, et al.: Association of gestational diabetes with abnormal maternal vascular endothelium. Br J Obstet Gynaecol 104:229–234, 1997.

139. Kimmerle R, Heinemann L, Delecki A, et al.: Severe hypoglycemia, incidence and predisposing factors in 85 pregnancies of type I diabetic women. Diabetes Care 15:1034–1037, 1992.

140. Rosenn BM, Miodovnik M, Holcberg G, et al.: Hypoglycemia: The price of intensive insulin therapy in insulin-dependent diabetes mellitus pregnancies. Obstet Gynecol 85:417–422, 1995.

141. Rosenn BM, Miodovnik M, Koury JC, et al.: Counterregulatory responses to hypoglycemia in pregnant women with insulin-dependent diabetes mellitus. Obstet Gynecol 87:568–574, 1996.

142. deVeciana M, Major CA, Morgan MA, et al.: Postprandial versus preprandial blood glucose monitoring in women with gestational diabetes mellitus requiring insulin therapy. N Engl J Med 333:1237–1241, 1995.

143. Jovanovic-Peterson L, Peterson CM, Reed GF, et al.: Maternal postprandial glucose levels and infant birth weight: The Diabetes in Early Pregnancy Study. Am J Obstet Gynecol 164:103–111, 1991.

144. Subcommittee on Nutritional Status and Weight Gain During Pregnancy, Food and Nutrition Board, Institute of Medicine: Nutrition During Pregnancy. Washington, DC: National Academy Press, 1990, pp. 10–13.

145. Algert S, Shragg P, Hollingsworth DR: Moderate caloric restriction in obese women with gestational diabetes. Obstet Gynecol 65:487–491, 1985.

146. Knopp RH, Magee MS, Raisys V, et al.: Metabolic effects of hypocaloric diets in management of gestational diabetes. Diabetes 40(Suppl. 2):165–171, 1991.

147. Reece EA, Hagay Z, Caseria D, et al.: Do fiber-enriched diabetic diets have glucose-lowering effects in pregnancy? Am J Perinatol 10:272–274, 1993.

148. Peterson CM, Jovanovic-Peterson L: Percentage of carbohydrate and glycemic response to breakfast, lunch and dinner in women with gestational diabetes. Diabetes 40(Suppl. 2):172–174, 1991.

149. Jovanovic-Peterson L, Peterson CM: Dietary manipulation as a primary treatment strategy for pregnancies complicated by diabetes. J Am Coll Nutr 9:320–325, 1990.

150. Coustan DR, Reece EA, Sherwin RS, et al.: A randomized clinical trial of the insulin pump vs. intensive conventional therapy in diabetic pregnancies. JAMA 255:631–636, 1986.

151. Lindsay MK, Graves W, Klein L: The relationship of one abnormal glucose tolerance test value and pregnancy complications. Obstet Gynecol 73:103–106, 1989.

152. Sermer M, Naylor CD, Gare DJ, et al.: Impact of increasing carbohydrate intolerance on maternal–fetal outcomes in 3637 women without gestational diabetes. Am J Obstet Gynecol 173:146–156, 1995.

153. Coustan DR, Imarah J: Prophylactic insulin treatment of gestational diabetes reduces the incidence of macrosomia, operative delivery and birth trauma. Am J Obstet Gynecol 150:836–842, 1984.

154. Landon MB, Sonek J, Foy P, et al.: Sonographic measurement of fetal humeral soft tissue thickness in pregnancy complicated by GDM. Diabetes 40(Suppl. 2): 66–70, 1991.

155. Bochner CJ, Medearis AL, Williams J, et al.: Early third trimester ultrasound screening in gestational diabetes to determine the risk of macrosomia and labor dystocia at term. Am J Obstet Gynecol 157:703–708, 1987.

156. Caplan RH, Pagliara AS, Beguin EA, et al.: Constant intravenous insulin infusion during labor and delivery in diabetes mellitus. Diabetes Care 5:6–10, 1982.

157. Haigh SE, Tevaarwerk GJM, Harding PEG, et al.: A method for maintaining normoglycemia during labor and delivery in insulin-dependent diabetic women. Can Med Assoc J 126:487–490, 1982.

158. Jovanovic L, Peterson CM: Insulin and glucose requirements during the first stage of labor in insulin-dependent diabetic women. Am J Med 75:607–612, 1983.

159. Revelli A, Durando A, Massobrio M: Exercise and pregnancy: A review of maternal and fetal effects. Obstet Gynecol Surv 47:355–367, 1992.

160. Jovanovic-Peterson L, Durak EP, Peterson CM: Randomized trial of diet versus diet plus cardiovascular conditioning on glucose levels in gestational diabetes. Am J Obstet Gynecol 161:415–419, 1989.

161. Bung P, Artal R, Khodiguian N, et al.: Exercise in gestational diabetes: An optimal therapeutic approach? Diabetes 40(Suppl. 2):182–185, 1991.

162. Lesser KB, Gruppuso PA, Terry RB, et al.: Exercise fails to improve postprandial glycemic excursion in women with gestational diabetes. J Mat-Fetal Med 5:211–217, 1996.

163. Hellmuth E, Damm P, Molsted-Pedersen L: Congenital malformations in offspring of diabetic women treated with oral hypoglycaemic agents during embryogenesis. Diabetic Med 11:471–474, 1994.

164. Piacquadio K, Hollingsworth DR, Murphy H: Effects of in-utero exposure to oral hypoglycaemic drugs. Lancet 338:866–869, 1991.

165. Pettitt DJ, Forman MR, Hanson RL, Knowler WC, Bennett PH: Breastfeeding and incidence of non-insulin-dependent diabetes mellitus in Pima Indians. Lancet 350:166–168, 1997.

166. Metzger BE, Cho NH, Roston SM, et al.: Prepregnancy weight and antepartum insulin secretion predict glucose tolerance five years after gestational diabetes mellitus. Diabetes Care 16:1598–1605, 1993.

167. Kjos SL, Peters RK, Xiang A, et al.: Predicting future diabetes in Latino women with gestational diabetes: Utility

of early postpartum glucose tolerance testing. Diabetes 44:586–591, 1995.

168. Damm P, Kuhl C, Bertelsen A, et al.: Predictive factors for the development of diabetes in women with previous gestational diabetes. Am J Obstet Gynecol 167:607–616, 1992.

169. Clark Jr CM, Qiu C, Amerman B, et al.: Gestational diabetes: should it be added to the syndrome of insulin resistance? Diabetes Care 20:867–871, 1997.

170. Gaudier FL, Hauth JC, Poist M, et al.: Recurrence of gestational diabetes mellitus. Obstet Gynecol 80:755–758, 1992.

171. Spong CY, Guillermo L, Kuboshige J, et al.: Recurrence of gestational diabetes mellitus: Identification of risk factors. Am J Perinatol 15:29–33, 1998.

172. Moses RG, Shand JL, Tapsell LC: The recurrence of gestational diabetes: Could dietary differences in fat intake be an explanation? Diabetes Care 20:1647–1650, 1997.

173. Kjos SL: Contraception in diabetic women. Obstet Gynecol Clin North Am 23:243–258, 1996.

174. Janz NK, Herman WH, Becker MP, et al.: Diabetes and pregnancy: Factors associated with seeking pre-conception care. Diabetes Care 18:157–165, 1995.

41

Diabetes Mellitus: Obstetrical Management

Mark B. Landon and Steven G. Gabbe

Our understanding of the pathophysiology of diabetes in pregnancy and the development of therapeutic techniques to prevent or improve complications has advanced significantly. Excluding deaths to major congenital malformations, the perinatal mortality rate in diabetic women receiving optimal care is comparable to that observed in normal gestations. This chapter will review contributions that have reduced perinatal morbidity and mortality for pregnant women with diabetes mellitus and their offspring.

Historical Perspective

Preinsulin Era

Before the discovery of insulin, pregnancy in patients with insulin dependent diabetes mellitus (IDDM) was disastrous for the mother and her fetus. Many women failed to ovulate as a consequence of this serious metabolic disorder and were, thus, infertile. For those who did become pregnant, ketoacidosis resulted in a maternal mortality often in excess of 50%. In 1882, a British obstetrician, J. Matthews Duncan, reviewed the outcomes of 22 pregnancies in 15 patients. He described four maternal deaths and reported seven perinatal deaths. Duncan observed that the stillborn infants of the mothers were often "enormous."

1922–1940: Period of Maternal Insulin Therapy

During this 19-year period, the primary concern was maternal survival, for perinatal morality rates remained nearly 30%. Most of the perinatal deaths were due to sudden intrauterine losses in the third trimester. In 1924, H.J. Wiener observed that pregnant women with diabetes mellitus often developed pregnancy-induced hypertension or toxemia.

1941–1970: Period of Team Care

During the next three decades, perinatal mortality rates declined to approximately 20%. During this time, the concept of team care was developed. The best outcomes in the pregnancy complicated by diabetes mellitus were realized when an internist, obstetrician, pediatrician, nurse-specialist, and nutritionist collaborated.

In 1949, Priscilla White[1] proposed her now widely applied clinical classification based primarily on the patient's condition prior to pregnancy. This risk assessment system permitted the estimation of maternal and perinatal risks and the formulation of management protocols. He originally proposed designation by the letters A through F. Class E, which included patients with pelvic calcifications demonstrated on X-ray examination was later dropped. Class R, H, and T describing women with proliferative retinopathy, arteriosclerotic heart disease, and kidney transplantation, respectively, were added later (see Table 41–1).

Women with class A diabetes were those "in whom the diagnosis of diabetes were made upon a glucose tolerance test which deviates but slightly from normal" and are usually included in discussion of gestational diabetes. Class A diabetes has been further subdivided into classes A_1 and A_2.

Class A_1 diabetes mellitus includes those women who have demonstrated carbohydrate intolerance during a 100-g, 3-hr oral glucose tolerance test (GTT); however, their fasting and postprandial glucose levels are <105 mg/dL and 120 mg/dL, respectively. These patients are generally managed by dietary regulation alone. If the fasting value of the GTT is elevated (≥ 105 mg/dL) or 2-hr postprandial levels are >120 g/dL, patients are designated Class A_2. Insulin is most often required for these women. Gestational diabetes compromises approximately 90% of all diabetes in pregnancy and may occur in approximately 100,000 women each year in the United States.[2]

TABLE 41–1 Modified White Classification of Pregnant Diabetic Women

Class	Diabetes Onset Age (Year)		Duration (Year)	Vascular Disease	Insulin Need
Gestational diabetes					
A₁	Any		Any	0	0
A₂	Any		Any	0	+
Pregestational diabetes					
B	>20		<10	0	+
C	10–19	or	10–19	0	+
D	<10	or	>20	+	+
F	Any		Any	+	+
R	Any		Any	+	+
T	Any		Any	+	+
H	Any		Any	+	+

Patients requiring insulin were designated by White as classes B, C, D, F, and R. Class B patents are those whose disease had its onset after age 20 and has been present for less than 10 years.

Class C women are those whose diabetes is of 10–19 years duration and in whom the onset of their disease occurred between 10 and 19 years of age.

Class D applies to those whose diabetes is of 20 or more years duration or whose onset of the disease occurred before the age of 10 or who have benign retinopathy. Class F designated those women with diabetic nephropathy who demonstrate proteinuria in excess of 400 mg in 24 hr in their urine prior to 20 weeks' gestation or those who have reduced creatinine clearance.

During this period, stillbirth rates of 10 to 30% were common. These losses were most often observed after the 36th week of pregnancy in patients having vasculopathy, poor control of diabetes, hydramnios, fetal macrosomia, or pregnancy-induced hypertension. In an effort to prevent such deaths, a schedule of preterm delivery was established. It was accepted practice to terminate Class D, F, and R pregnancies at 35 to 36 weeks' gestation while permitting Class B and C patients to deliver at 37 to 38 weeks' gestation. However, errors in the estimation of fetal size and gestational age as well as the functional immaturity characteristic of the infant of the diabetic mother contributed to many deaths from prematurity. Almost 60% of this neonatal mortality could be attributed to hyaline membrane disease.

In 1954, the Danish internist, Jorgen Pederson, et al.[3] proposed the hyperglycemia-hyperinsulinemia theory to explain much of the perinatal morbidity and mortality in pregnancies complicated by diabetes. Glucose crosses the placenta by carrier-mediated facilitated diffusion. Insulin does not cross the placenta, however, although the fetus receives a continuous supply of maternal glucose, it will not be affected by maternal insulin. During pregnancy, periods of maternal hyperglycemia will produce fetal hyperglycemia. Elevated levels of glucose in the fetus stimulate the fetal pancreas resulting in fetal β-cell hyperplasia and hyperinsulinemia. Fetal hyperinsulinemia has been cited as responsible for much of the morbidity and mortality observed in the infant of the diabetic mother.

1971–1976: Period of Fetal Surveillance

During the early 1970s techniques become available to assess accurately fetal well-being and pulmonary maturation. The application of these methods led to a decline in perinatal mortality rates to approximately 10%. The development of these specialized procedures for antepartum fetal evaluation also demanded that care be centralized and, in many cases, required hospitalization of the patient for several weeks prior to delivery. Important advances in fetal evaluation included antepartum surveillance with the use of biochemical assay of estriol, antepartum fetal heart rate testing, and maternal assessment of fetal activity, continuous intrapartum fetal heart rate monitoring during labor, the determination of fetal pulmonary maturity with the lecithin/sphingomyelin (LS) ratio and lung profile, and the evaluation of fetal growth by ultrasound. In addition, advances in neonatology decreased the postnatal morbidity of the infant of the diabetic mother. See Chapter 42.

1976–present: Period of Metabolic Normalization

During the past 20 years, perinatal mortality rates have continued to fall in pregnancies complicated by diabetes mellitus. Excluding deaths due to major congenital malformations, the perinatal mortality rate in diabetic women receiving optimal care is as low as that observed in normal gestations. This reduction in mortality can be attributed to greater familiarity with the antepartum assessment techniques that have been described. However, perhaps the most striking change

TABLE 41–2 Target Plasma Glucose Levels in Pregnancy

Time	mg/dL
Before breakfast	60–90
Before lunch, supper, bedtime snack	60–105
Two hours after meals	≤ 120
2 to 6 a.m.	> 60

in recent years has been the aggressive efforts to achieve normal or near-normal glucose levels in insulin-dependent patients. Careful assessment of control through self blood glucose monitoring, the application of multiple-dose insulin regimens and better understanding of the dietary needs of pregnant diabetic women have proven important in improving outcome.[4]

In 1982, Mills[5] pointed out the likely relationship between poor maternal control in early pregnancy and the major congenital malformations that are now the leading cause of perinatal mortality in pregnancies complicated by IDDM. Miller and colleagues[6] observed that women who had an elevated hemoglobin A_{1c} level in the first trimester of pregnancy were more likely to delivery infants with major malformations. Several studies have now confirmed that meticulous control of maternal diabetes during organogenesis can prevent many congenital defects. Therefore, emphasis has been placed on normalization of maternal control during the prepregnancy period and the weeks of embryogenesis as well as later in pregnancy (see Table 41–2).

Epidemiology

Gestational diabetes has been estimated to occur in 3 to 12% of the obstetrical population, depending on the patients screened and the diagnostic criteria utilized.[2] The overall incidence of pregestational diabetes (or IDDM) has been found to be approximately 0.1 to 0.5%. It is certainly higher in centers specializing in the care of these women.

Pathophysiology

Maternal Metabolism

During gestation, significant metabolic changes occur that must be understood for the successful management of the pregnancy complicated by diabetes. The fetus depends on the maternal compartment for an uninterrupted supply of fuel. Several maternal adaptations are normally made to meet these fetal needs. Pregnancy is characterized by maternal hyperinsulinemia associated with insulin resistance, changes that are most marked late in gestation. There is also an increased likelihood of ketosis developing during

maternal food deprivation, a state of "accelerated starvation" related to the limited availability of gluconeogenic precursors. After meals, a state of "facilitated anabolism" characterized by prolonged glucose excursions, greater carbohydrate-induced hypertriglyceridemia, and enhanced suppression of glucagon has been described. The placental syncytiotrophoblast is the source of human placental lactogen (hPL), a growth hormone-like protein, which produces insulin resistance and augments maternal lipolysis. With increased maternal utilization of fats for energy, glucose is spared for fetal consumption. Fasting hypoglycemia may appear more rapidly in late pregnancy as the conceptus increases its glucose utilization coupled with a reduction in maternal gluconeogenic substrates and hepatic glucose production.

Levels of hPL are directly related to placental mass, increasing as pregnancy progresses and heightening the "diabetogenic stress." However, absolute levels of hPL do not necessarily correlate with glucose intolerance. Other hormones that also provide this state of insulin resistance include free cortisol and possibly prolactin. In normal pregnant women, glucose homeostasis is maintained by an exaggerated rate and amount of insulin release, which accompanies decreased sensitivity to insulin. Resistance to insulin action during pregnancy has been documented by a reduction in glucose required to maintain euglycemia with insulin infusion (clamp technique)[7] as well as with intravenous glucose tolerance testing with frequent sampling and simultaneous determination of insulin and glucose levels (minimal model technique).[8]

Effects of Maternal Hyperglycemia

During pregnancy, periods of maternal hyperglycemia will produce fetal hyperglycemia and hyperinsulinemia. Insulin is an important fetal growth hormone. Cord blood and amniotic fluid levels of C-peptide have been correlated with infant birth weight. The combination of excess glucose plus excess insulin can lead to excessive fetal growth. A birth weight in excess of 4000 g is two to three times more likely to result in pregnancies complicated by diabetes mellitus. Such fetal macrosomia may be associated with an increased risk for shoulder dystocia during vaginal delivery. If shoulder dystocia results, perinatal asphyxia as well as injuries to the brachial plexus may occur. Other consequences of macrosomia include an increased risk for obesity and diabetes in later life.

After 36 weeks' gestation, the frequency of fetal deaths in pregnancies complicated by diabetes is increased. Patients who are poorly controlled who have had a prior stillbirth, or who have pregnancy-induced hypertension or vasculopathy are at a greater risk for an intrauterine death. Although the etiology for these intrauterine deaths remains unknown, data from the animal laboratory indicate that fetal hyperglycemia and hyperinsulinemia play important roles. Insulin infusions in fetal sheep increase the oxidative metabolism of glucose and reduce fetal arterial oxygen content. Recent studies of fetal umbilical cord blood samples *in utero* have demonstrated relative fetal erythremia and lactic acidemia.[8]

It remains a common practice to terminate pregnancies complicated by diabetes at term to prevent intrauterine fetal deaths. In the past, premature delivery was undertaken, which often resulted in increased morbidity and mortality from respiratory distress syndrome. There is controversy as to whether diabetes in pregnancy as currently managed is a risk factor for the development of respiratory distress syndrome. Yet, cesarean section not preceded by labor and prematurity, both of which are increased in diabetic pregnancies, clearly increase the likelihood of neonatal respiratory disease.[9]

Improved understanding of maternal metabolism and the need to regulate carefully maternal glycemia as well as reliable techniques for fetal surveillance and improved neonatal care have markedly reduced perinatal mortality arising form intrauterine deaths, trauma, and respiratory distress syndrome. At the present time, the most devastating perinatal complication in pregnancies complicated by insulin-dependent diabetes may be attributed to congenital malformations.[5] Infants of diabetic mothers have a two- to threefold greater frequency of severe malformations involving many organ systems. The incidence of major malformations in normal pregnancies may be 2 to 3%, but the frequency observed in the offspring of patients with IDDM is 6 to 10%. The caudal regression syndrome, cardiac, renal, and central nervous system anomalies, especially anencephaly, are most common. Such anomalies must result during the first 7 weeks of development, long before most diabetic patients seek prenatal care. In addition to previously mentioned maternal hyperglycemia, hyperketonemia, hypoglycemia, somatomedin inhibitor excess, arachidonic acid deficiency as well as excess free oxygen radicals have all been proposed as teratogenic factors.

After delivery, considerable neonatal morbidity has been reported in the offspring of diabetic women. The characteristic triad of hypoglycemia, hypocalcemia, and hyperbilirubinemia may be seen in as many as 25% of these offspring. The incidence of macrosomia and hypoglycemia can be related to cord C-peptide levels, thus, reflecting in utero hyperinsulinemia.[10] Infants of diabetic mothers have been observed to demonstrate a cardiomyopathy associated with septal hypertrophy.

Polycythemia with hyperviscosity may be observed as a result of *in utero* hypoxia and hyperinsulinemia.

Effects of Pregnancy on Maternal Morbidity

Women with vascular complications and/or unstable diabetes are at greater risk for morbidity and mortality during pregnancy. There is no evidence that pregnancy shortens the life expectancy of women with diabetes and maternal mortality is rare. Women with diabetes who have coronary artery disease (Class H) may have increased mortality during pregnancy.[11] Pregnancy does not produce a permanent deterioration of renal function in women with diabetic nephropathy (Class F) yet controlled studies are lacking in this regard[12]. Women with diabetic nephropathy cannot be treated with angiotensin-converting enzyme (ACE), inhibitors during pregnancy as these agents impair fetal urine production. No difference has been found in the prevalence of severity of retinopathy, nephropathy, or neuropathy in patients who had been pregnant compared to those who had never been pregnant. However, there is concern that diabetic retinopathy may worsen during gestation. Benign retinopathy may worsen as the pregnancy advances, but will usually regress after delivery. Women who demonstrate neovascularization that has not been treated with laser therapy before pregnancy are at great risk for deterioration of their vision.[13] In contrast, women with proliferative changes who have been treated prior to pregnancy with laser therapy will most often remain stable. See Chapter 26.

Much of the maternal morbidity observed in pregnancies complicated by diabetes can be attributed to the changes in maternal metabolism that cause deterioration of glycemia control. A review of maternal mortality in diabetic patients noted that 7 to 24 deaths could be directly attributed to the metabolic complications of diabetes.[14] Before the utilization of self blood glucose monitoring techniques, severe hypoglycemic reactions requiring hospitalization occurred in approximately 10% of insulin-dependent patients. Nausea and vomiting, common problems early in pregnancy, may necessitate a reduction in insulin dosage. After delivery, the contrainsulin effects of hPL are lost and hypoglycemia may again result. Insulin-dependent diabetics will usually require a small dose of insulin or need no insulin replacement during the first days after delivery.

Ketoacidosis most often occurs during the second and third trimester when the "diabetogenic stress" of pregnancy is greatest. The recently diagnosed diabetic is most likely to develop ketoacidosis in pregnancy because she fails to appreciate its cause and symptoms. Ketoacidosis presents a risk for maternal mortality and perinatal mortality, which fortunately is less common with this complication than in the past.

Problem Statement

Risk Assessment

A program of patient care may be developed if the risks to the patient and her infant are first considered. Pregnancies complicated by diabetes mellitus may be divided into two groups; women with pregestational diabetes (usually IDDM), including patients with vascular complications, and women with gestational diabetes mellitus (GDM).

The most widely applied risk assessment system, that of Dr. Priscilla White, has been described before. She observed that the age of onset of diabetes, its duration , and the presence of maternal vascular disease, factors that could be determined in the prepregnant state, would all have an important impact on pregnancy outcomes[1] (see Table 41–1). In general, the earlier the onset of diabetes, the longer its duration and the greater the degree of vasculopathy, the worse the prognosis in pregnancy. Of course, the quality of maternal glucose control must also be considered in assessing perinatal risk. Women who have gestational diabetes, but maintain a normal fasting glucose level will rarely experience an intrauterine death.

Pedersen et al.[15] noted that prognostically bad signs of pregnancy, specifically ketoacidosis, pyelonephritis, pregnancy-induced hypertension, and poor clinic attendance or neglect were more often associated with unfavorable outcomes.

Maternal Assessment

Evaluation of the reproductive age women with IDDM should begin prior to gestation. The patient must be assessed as to her suitability for pregnancy.[16] Ophthalmological evaluation, electrocardiography, and a 24-hr urine collection for creatinine clearance and protein excretion should be performed.

With increasing evidence indicating that congenital malformations and spontaneous abortions are related to hyperglycemia during early embryogenesis, insulin dependent patients should be in optimum control at the time of conception and throughout the first trimester of pregnancy. In normal pregnancies, maternal plasma glucose levels rarely exceed 100 mg/dL, with excursions between fasting levels of 60 mg/dL and postprandial levels of 120 mg/dL. Mean plasma glucose concentrations during the third trimester are 86 mg/dL.[17]

The benefits of careful regulation have been recognized for many years. More than 20 years ago, Karlsson and Kjellmer[18] observed a perinatal mortality of 38/1000 when mean maternal blood glucose levels were maintained below 100 mg/dL during the third trimester. If mean glucose levels exceeded 150 mg/dL, perinatal mortality rose almost sixfold.

Diabetic control must be assessed regularly. Table 41–2 documents the authors goals for capillary blood glucose control. This surveillance should be achieved at home using blood glucose oxidase reagent strips. The physiological glycosuria of pregnancy limits the value of urine tests. Patients should, therefore, be instructed to use glucose oxidase-impregnated strips with a glucose reflectance meter. In this way, they may assess their control prior to and following meals while maintaining their usual diet and program of exercise. When maternal mean capillary glucose levels are maintained below 110 mg/dL, the incidence of neonatal morbidity is significantly lower.[19]

Hemoglobin A_{1c} determination may provide an overview of maternal control in the management of the pregnant patient with IDDM. This determination may be made at the patient's first prenatal visit to provide rapid assessment of prior diabetic regulation and to assess the risk for malformations. Second- and third-trimester determinations may aid in validating the level of control achieved.

Early in gestation, hospitalization may be required to assess diabetic management and help educate patients who have not had regular health care prior to pregnancy. The initial hospitalization also provides an opportunity to assess the patient's vascular status.

Insulin therapy must be individualized with dosage determinations tailored to diet and exercise. Beef and pork insulin have largely been replaced by synthetic human insulin preparations. Because human insulin is far less immunogenic than animal insulin, it is preferred for pregnant women and especially for those receiving insulin for the first time. Human insulin may have a more rapid onset and shorter duration of action, factors that must be considered when changing patients to these preparations.

Insulin is generally administered in two or three injections. We prefer a three-injection regimen, although most patients present taking a combination of intermediate-acting and regular insulin before dinner and breakfast. As a general rule, the amount of intermediate-acting insulin will exceed the regular component by a two-to-one ratio. Patients usually receive two thirds of their total dose with breakfast and the remaining third in the evening as a combined dose with dinner or split into components with regular insulin at dinner time and then intermediate acting insulin at bedtime in an effort to minimize periods of nocturnal hypoglycemia. These episodes frequently occur when the mother is in a relative fasting state while placental and fetal glucose consumptions continue. Finally, some women may require a small dose of regular insulin before lunch, thus constituting a four-injection daily regimen.

Most patients with IDDM are followed with outpatient visits at 1- to 2-week intervals. At each visit, control is assessed and adjustments in insulin dosage are made. However, patients should be instructed to call at any time if periods of hypoglycemia (<50 mg/dL) or hyperglycemia (>200 mg/dL) occur. The increased risk of hypoglycemia in pregnant individuals may be related to defective glucose counterregulatory hormone mechanisms. Both epinephrine and glucagon appear to be suppressed in pregnant diabetic women during hypoglycemia. For these reasons, family members should be instructed on the technique of glucagon injection for the treatment of severe reactions.

Fetal Assessment

Screening for fetal neural tube defects by maternal serum α-fetoprotein should be performed at 15–20 weeks' gestation. Ultrasound studies have permitted the assessment of fetal growth as well as detection of anomalies. A detailed sonogram should be performed at 18 to 22 weeks' gestation as a baseline and then repeated at 4 to 6 week intervals to assess fetal growth. In addition, one may detect fetal structural anomalies such as anencephaly. Fetal echocardiography should be performed at 20–22 weeks to detect cardiac anomalies. Such anomalies comprise 50% of all defects found in the offspring of IDDM women.

During the third trimester, when sudden intrauterine deaths are most likely to occur, a program of daily fetal surveillance should be initiated.[20] The primary value of these tests has been to allow the perinatologist to delay delivery safely and gain further fetal maturity, for it has been well accepted that normal tests are rarely associated with intrauterine fetal death.

A major advance in the management of the pregnancy complicated by diabetes mellitus has been the application of antepartum fetal heart rate testing to determine fetal status.

The nonstress test (NST) has been utilized in the assessment of the diabetic pregnancy. This test of fetal well-being examines the reactivity of the fetal heart rate. Accelerations of the fetal heart rate demonstrate intact function of the fetal autonomic nervous system and reflect a well oxygenated fetus. The NST does not require an i.v. infusion, can be performed in a physician's office, requires no more than 15 min to perform in most patients, and can be easily interpreted. A reactive NST or one that shows fetal heart rate accelerations has a similar predictive value to the negative contraction stress test (CST). However, the NST does have a significant false-positive rate. If the initial NST fails to demonstrate fetal heart rate accelerations, a biophysical profile (BPP) or CST is then undertaken.

A simple and practical approach in the evaluation of fetal condition has been maternal assessment of fetal activity. Patients are asked to monitor fetal activity each day for several periods of time. Although many testing protocols have been utilized, all have shown that a consistent pattern of fetal activity is associated with good fetal outcome. Like other antepartum fetal tests, maternal assessment of fetal activity does have a high false-positive rate. Therefore, with an apparent reduction in fetal activity, further antepartum testing must be used.

As mentioned previously, clinicians have utilized the fetal biophysical profile (BPP) to assess fetal well-being after a nonreactive NST. Real-time ultrasound is used to monitor four parameters—fetal breathing movements, fetal body movements, fetal tone, and amniotic fluid volume. The fetus is awarded 2 points for each variable found to be normal during a 30-min observation period. A score of 8 has been associated with a false-negative rate as low as that found with a negative CST. A score of 5 or less may lead to delivery.

It is important not only to include the results of antepartum fetal testing, but also to consider all the clinical features involving mother and fetus before a decision is made to intervene for suspected fetal distress, especially if the decision is made to proceed with preterm delivery. In reviewing nine series involving nearly 1000 IDDM pregnancies, an abnormal test of fetal condition led to delivery in 5% of cases.[21]

In the past, much emphasis was placed on a decreasing insulin requirement as an indication of fetal distress. It was presumed that reduced insulin needs reflected placental failure and a decrease in production of the contrainsulin hormones of pregnancy. However, recent evidence has indicated that decreasing insulin requirements are generally not an indication of fetal compromise.

If the patient has been maintained in excellent glycemic control and all parameters of antepartum surveillance have remained normal, delivery may be safely delayed until fetal maturation has been achieved. Elective delivery should be considered at term if amniotic fluid analysis reveals evidence of completed pulmonary maturation.[22] For the highest risk patients, those who have been in poor control, who have had a previous stillbirth, or who have not been compliant, delivery should be accomplished at 38 weeks or sooner if fetal pulmonary maturation can be confirmed. As stated earlier, when antepartum testing suggests fetal compromise, delivery must be considered. Other indications for preterm delivery include significant preeclampsia, worsening renal function, or deteriorating vision secondary to proliferative retinopathy.

If an immature L/S ratio and the absence of PG are noted on amniotic fluid evaluation, betamethasone or dexamethasone may be used to induce pulmonary maturation. Corticosteroids will cause hyperglycemia and may precipitate ketoacidosis. Therefore, if steroids are given prior to delivery, glycemic control must be carefully assessed by obtaining blood sugar levels every 2 to 4 hr. Intravenous insulin infusion and continuous fetal monitoring is often required to follow such a patient.

Premature labor may occasionally occur in pregnancy complicated by diabetes. Combined therapy with corticosteroids and beta-sympathomimetic drugs has been used to accelerate fetal lung maturation and halt uterine contractions. However, such treatment may lead to rapid decompensation of diabetic control and also requires intensive glucose monitoring.

Plan

Objectives and Strategy

The pregnancy complicated by diabetes mellitus must be managed by skilled and experienced individuals. A team approach involving the diabetologist, specialist in maternal-fetal medicine, teaching nurse, dietitian, and a neonatologist is essential. The timing of any delivery must be coordinated with the neonatologist who is to be present. If adequate neonatal care cannot be provided, the pregnant women with diabetes should be transferred to a center with a specialized neonatal care unit.

During pregnancy, abnormal carbohydrate metabolism must be detected and precisely defined. Gestational diabetes has been characterized as a state restricted to pregnant women in whom the onset or recognition of diabetes or impaired glucose tolerance occurs during pregnancy and is, therefore, most often encouraged in late pregnancy. These patients are diagnosed using a 100-g oral glucose tolerance test (See Table 41–3).

A well-organized screening program must be established to detect this abnormality. In the past, screening was based on recognized historical or clinical clues,

including a family history of diabetes, delivery of a macrosomic infant, an infant with a malformation, or an unexplained stillborn; or the presence of obesity, hypertension, or glycosuria. Screening patients by risk factors is inadequate, because up to 50% of women who go on to develop GDM fail to manifest these clues.[23] Furthermore, glycosuria is extremely common in pregnancy as a result of the physiological increase in glomerular filtration rate. Whether all pregnant women should be screened for GDM remains controversial, yet it is the practice of most obstetricians in the United States. Screening is performed using a 50-g oral glucose load followed by a glucose determination 1 hr later.[23] Using a plasma cut-off of 135–140 mg/dL, this screening test has a sensitivity of 90% when compared with subsequent glucose tolerance test results. If one uses this approach, the estimated cost per patient screened and per case of GDM detected are approximately $5.00 and $222.00, respectively.

Delivery produces a rapid change in the hormonal milieu that has produced the "diabetogenic stress" of pregnancy. The fall in hPL after the placenta has been removed causes a marked decrease in the insulin replacement required to maintain glycemic control. Thus, management of the patient's glucose homeostasis during labor, delivery, and postpartum is most challenging. The incidence of neonatal hypoglycemia can be related to the level of maternal glycemia maintained during labor as well as the degree of antepartum control.

Several approaches have been employed to maintain normal maternal blood sugar levels in insulin-dependent women during labor while preventing hypoglycemia after delivery.

A continuous i.v. infusion of insulin and glucose is generally used during labor and delivery. Ten units of regular insulin may be added to 1000 mL of a dextrose containing solution. The mixture is given at an infusion rate of 100 mL/hr. In most patients, regardless of their antepartum insulin requirements, this combination infused at 100 mL/hr will usually result in good glycemic control. Insulin may also be infused from a syringe pump at a dose of 0.25 to 2.0 units/hr and adjusted to maintain normal glucose levels.

With techniques now available for antepartum fetal surveillance, unexpected intrauterine deaths, deaths due to trauma, and perinatal morbidity and mortality arising from iatrogenic prematurity are uncommon. As already noted, if antepartum fetal testing reflects fetal well-being, elective delivery is planned at approximately 38 weeks' gestation or beyond. However, when fetal distress is suggested by antepartum testing, immediate delivery must be considered. If acute distress is not present, consideration is given to performing an amniocentesis to assess fetal lung maturity. If the findings suggest immaturity, then clinical management

TABLE 41–3 Detection of Gestational Diabetes—Upper Limits of Normal

Screening Test (50 g) 1 hr Oral GTT*	Plasma (mg/dL)(130–140)	
	NDDG	Carpenter and Coustan
Fasting	105	95
1 hr	190	180
2 hr	165	155
3 hr	145	140

* Diagnosis of gestational diabetes is made when any two values are met or exceeded.

must be individualized. If fetal activity has declined significantly, but the antepartum heart rate test remains reassuring, the patient can be allowed to continue her pregnancy. If, however, the NST, CST, BPP, and fetal activity determinations all indicate fetal jeopardy, delivery should be undertaken. In this circumstance, delaying delivery to permit corticosteroid treatment is rarely warranted.

In approximately 50% of cases, the infants of women with IDDM will be delivered by cesarean section. If antepartum testing suggests intrauterine fetal distress, cesarean section is indicated. In patients at 38 weeks' gestation with documented fetal lung maturation who are suspected to be at increased risk for an intrauterine death because of poor control or a history of a previous stillbirth, elective section should be considered if the cervix is not favorable for induction. If labor is induced, electronic fetal heart rate monitoring is mandatory.

Patients with GDM may be safely followed until 40 weeks as long as glucose levels remain normal.[24] If they cannot be induced at 40 weeks, fetal surveillance should be initiated with twice weekly NSTs. The risk of intrauterine deaths is greater in those gestational diabetics who have had a prior stillbirth or who develop pregnancy-induced hypertension. In these patients, as well as those requiring insulin, therefore, a program of fetal surveillance should be initiated at 32–34 weeks' gestation.

Patient Adherence and Education

Most women with diabetes mellitus are highly motivated and comply with the rigorous regimen required to achieve a successful pregnancy. The patients learn that their ability to regulate their blood glucose levels will have a direct effect on fetal outcome.

In recent years, larger and teaching centers have developed specialized units to meet the needs of these high-risk obstetrical patients. Ideally, care should be initiated prior to conception so that optimal glycemic control may be attained and maternal vasculopathy evaluated. In the past, the diabetic gravida approaching the final month of gestation was frequently hospitalized. Such a policy was considered an important part of a successful treatment program. Women who cannot maintain reasonable glycemic control may require hospitalization, despite physicians being comfortable treating most diabetic gravidas as outpatients. The assessment of a maternal glycemia using the glucose reflectance meter at home and the use of outpatient fetal testing has reduced the need for hospitalization.

As the time of delivery approaches, the patient's anxiety level will increase. Frequently, there is uncertainty regarding the method of delivery. Because all of these patients may require an operative delivery, child-birth classes should place equal emphasis on vaginal delivery and cesarean section. It is often reassuring for the patient and her support person to visit the labor and delivery suite and nursery facilities prior to delivery.

Family planning and contraception must be reviewed with the patient in the postpartum period. In the insulin-dependent gravida, the increased risk of thromboembolic disease has raised concerns about the use of combined estrogen/progesterone oral contraceptive preparations.[25] However, in women without vasculopathy or hypertension, a low-dose oral contraceptive or progestin-only pill appears to be safe. These patients may also be offered mechanical methods. Sterilization should be discussed after the diabetic woman has completed her family. In the past, patients diagnosed as gestational diabetics did not subsequently receive oral contraceptive agents because these hormones may produce the derangement in carbohydrate metabolism observed during pregnancy. In recent studies, however, no significant changes in glucose tolerance were observed in women with a history of gestational diabetes treated with a low-dose oral contraceptive.

Audits of Data

Marked improvements in perinatal survival for pregnancies complicated by diabetes mellitus have been documented. However, both immediate perinatal morbidity and long-term effects of the altered intrauterine environment created by maternal diabetes mellitus must be evaluated. As emphasized by Freinkel,[26] "concepts of teratogenesis should be expanded to include alterations occurring subsequent to organogenesis. Such changes could cause long-range effects on behavior, anthropometric, and metabolic functions."[26]

Using a rat model, Aerts and Van Assche[27] have observed that the female offspring of rats made mildly diabetic during pregnancy are at an increased risk to develop gestational diabetes when they become pregnant. They have suggested that gestational diabetes is an inherited disorder. The incidence of subsequent insulin-dependent diabetes in the infants of those women who themselves have insulin-dependent diabetes is approximately 2.1%. Infants of diabetic mothers are also more likely to be obese later in life and are at risk for impaired glucose tolerance.

Pregnancy may have a deleterious effect on maternal retinopathy, as already noted. More information is needed to assess this risk and identify women likely to experience progression of such vasculopathy during gestation.

As many as 50% of patients who exhibit GDM will show further deterioration of carbohydrate metabolism during the next 15 years of life. Diabetes is most likely to occur in the obese woman or those who have required insulin therapy during pregnancy. These patients may also be a greatest risk for mortality due to atherosclerotic cardiovascular disease.

Research Considerations

Research efforts have focused on the teratogenic effects of maternal diabetes and its influence on fetal growth and development.

Several multicenter studies have explored the association between alterations in maternal metabolism and congenital anomalies. A reduction in the incidence of congenital malformations by optimizing maternal control before pregnancy and during the early weeks of embryogenesis has been achieved in various centers. Further strategies to reduce the frequency of malformations may include vitamin supplementation including vitamin E.

Studies in animal models, especially primates and sheep, have yielded valuable data in our understanding of the fetal risks associated with hyperglycemia and hyperinsulinemia. Infusing fetal sheep with insulin or glucose will produce fetal hypoxemia. Fetal rhesus monkeys made chronically hyperinsulinemic demonstrate excessive growth. Such research has confirming the important principle that meticulous control of maternal diabetes is essential for normal fetal growth and development.

Finally, the spectrum of gestational diabetes has been confirmed as an independent risk for fetal macrosomia, yet establishing optimal criteria for screening and diagnosis remain research concerns for the future.

References

1. White P: Pregnancy complicating diabetes. Am J Med 7:609–616, 1949.

2. Freinkel N: Gestational diabetes 1979: Philosophical and practical aspects of a major health problem. Diabetes Care 3:399–401, 1989.

3. Pederson J, Bojsen-Moller B, Poulson H: Blood sugar in newborn infants of diabetic mothers. Acta Endocrinol (Copenh) 15:33–52, 1954.

4. Jovanovic L, Druzin M, Peterson CM: Effect of euglycemia on the outcome of pregnancy in insulin-dependent diabetic women as compared with normal control subjects. Am J Med 71:921–927, 1981.

5. Mills JL: Malformations in infants of diabetic mothers. Teratology 25:385–394, 1982.

6. Miller E, Hare JW, Cloherty JP, et al.: Elevated maternal hemoglobin A_{1c} in early pregnancy and major congenital anomalies in infants of diabetic mothers. N Engl J Med 304:1331–1334, 1981.

7. Catalano P, Tyzbir E, Roman NW, et al.: Longitudinal changes in insulin release and insulin resistance in non-obese pregnant woman. Am J Obstet Gynecol 165:1667–1671, 1991.

8. Salvesen DR, Brudenell MJ, Nicolaides KH: Fetal polycythemia and thrombobocytopenia in pregnancies complicated by maternal diabetes Am J Obstet Gynecol 166:1987–1991, 1992.

9. Robert MF, Neff RK, Hubbell JP, et al.: Maternal diabetes and the respiratory distress syndrome. N Engl J Med 294:357–360, 1976.

10. Sosenko IR, Kitzmiller JL, Loo SW, et al.: The infant of the diabetic mother. Correlation of increased cord C-peptide levels with macrosomia and hypoglycemia. N Engl J Med 301:859–862, 1979.

11. Gordon MC, Landon MB, Boyle J, et al.: Coronary artery disease in insulin-dependent diabetes mellitus of pregnancy (Class H): A review of the literature. Obstet Gynecol Surv 51:437–444, 1996.

12. Gordon M, Landon MB, Samuels P, et al.: Perinatal outcome and long-term follow-up associated with modern management of diabetic nephropathy (Class F). Obstet Gynecol 87:401–409, 1996.

13. Klein BEK, Moss Klein P: Effect of pregnancy on the progression of diabetic retinopathy. Diabetes Care 13:34–40, 1990.

14. Gabbe SG, Mestman JH, Hibbard LT: Maternal mortality in diabetes mellitus. Obstet Gynecol 48:549–551, 1976.

15. Pederson J, Pederson LM, Anderson B: Assessors of fetal perinatal mortality in diabetic pregnancy. Diabetes 23:302–305, 1974.

16. Steel JM, Duncan JP, Clarke BF: Letter Br Med J 1:1536, 1977.

17. Cousins L, Rigg L, Hollingsworth D, et al.: The 24–hour excursion and diurnal rhythm of glucose, insulin, and C-peptide in normal pregnancy. Am J Obstet Gynecol 136:483–488, 1980.

18. Karlsson K, Kjellmer I: The outcome of diabetic pregnancies in relation to the mother's blood sugar level. Am J Obstet Gynecol 112:213–220, 1972.

19. Landon MB, Gabbe SG, Piana R, et al.: Neonatal morbidity in pregnancy complicated by diabetes mellitus: predictive value of maternal glycemia profiles. Am J Obstet Gynecol 156:1089, 1987.

20. Landon MB, Langer O, Gabbe SG: Fetal surveillance in pregnancies complicated by insulin-dependent diabetes mellitus. Am J Obstet Gynecol 167:617–621, 1992.

21. Landon MB, Gabbe SG: Fetal surveillance in the pregnancy complicated by diabetes mellitus. Clin Perinatol 20:549–557, 1993.

22. Kjos SL, Walther F: Prevalence and etiology of respiratory distress in infants of diabetic mothers: Predictive

value of lung maturation tests. Am J Obstet Gynecol 163:898–902, 1990.

23. Coustan DR, Nelson C, Carpenter M, et al.: Maternal age and screening for gestation diabetes: A population-based study. Obstet Gynecol 73:557, 1989.

24. Gabbe SG, Mestman JH, Freeman RK, et al.: Management and outcome of Class A diabetes mellitus. Am J Obstet Gynecol 127:465–469, 1977.

25. Steel JM, Duncan LJP: Contraception for the insulin-dependent diabetic woman: The view from one clinic. Diabetes Care 3:557–560, 1980.

26. Freinkel N: Banting Lecture 1989. Of pregnancy and progeny. Diabetes 29:1023, 1980.

27. Aerts L, Van Assche FA: Is gestational diabetes an acquired condition? J Dev Physiol 1:219, 1979.

Supplementary Readings

American Diabetes Association: Summary of recommendations of the Second International Workshop-Conference on Gestational Diabetes Mellitus. Diabetes 34 (Suppl. 2): 123–126, 1985.

Cartensen LL, Frost-Larsen K, Fugleberg S, et al.: Does pregnancy influence the prognosis of uncomplicated insulin dependent diabetes mellitus? Diabetes Care 5:1–5, 1982.

Cohen AW, Gabbe SG: Intrapartum management of the diabetic patient. Clin Perinatol 8:165–172, 1981.

Datta S, Kitzmiller JL: Anesthetic and obstetric management of diabetic pregnant women. Clin Perinatol 9:153–166, 1982.

Fuhrmann K, Reiher H, Semmler K, et al.: Prevention of congenital malformations in infants of insulin-dependent diabetic mothers. Diabetes Care 6:219, 1983.

Mills JL, Knopp RH, Simpson JL, et al.: Lack of relation of increased malformation rates in infants of diabetic mothers to glycemic control during organogenesis. N Engl J Med 318:671, 1988.

Mills JL, Simpson JL, Driscoll SG, et al.: Incidence of spontaneous abortion among normal women and insulin dependent diabetic women whose pregnancies were identified within 21 days of conception. N Engl J Med 319:1617, 1988.

Ney D, Hollingsworth DR: Nutritional management of pregnancy complicated by diabetes: Historical perspective. Diabetes Care 4:647–655, 1981.

Warram JH, Krolewski AS, Kahn CR: Determinants of IDDM and perinatal mortality of children of diabetic mothers. Diabetes 37:1328, 1988.

42

The Infant of the Diabetic Mother

Robert Schwartz

Although most infants of diabetic mothers (IDMs) have an uneventful perinatal course, there is an increased risk for untoward complications in infants of pregnant women either previously identified as diabetics as well as those with undiagnosed diabetes (gestational diabetes). Appropriate medical and obstetrical intervention can minimize many of the problems; nevertheless, the physician should be knowledgeable regarding the complications which may develop. Ideally, a pediatrician should be familiar with the mother's prenatal course; indeed, he should participate in her care during the pre- and intrapartum phases. Because several of the infant's problems may not initially be associated with clinical signs, appropriate laboratory studies may be needed to detect them.

Historical Perspective

Since the discovery of insulin in 1921, three contributions have been of particular importance to improving maternal and neonatal outcomes in diabetes associated with pregnancy. White developed a classification based on age, duration of insulin dependency, and complications, which resulted in more individualized care of the mother. Pedersen[1] emphasized the pathogenetic mechanisms that related maternal glucose control to fetal hyperinsulinism. He also developed a classification which emphasized the status of the current pregnancy. O'Sullivan defined the criteria for the diagnosis of gestational diabetes and emphasized the high frequency compared to known insulin-dependent pregnant women (see Chapter 40).

The macrosomia, so well recognized in the first half of this century, was originally considered to be nonpitting edema. In the 1960s total body water studies by Osler and Pedersen as well as whole-body direct analysis for fat by Fee and Weil definitively established that increased fat was present. H.C. Miller and associates recognized symptomatic hypoglycemia, cardiac hypertrophy, erythroblastosis, and hyperplasia of the islands

of Langerhans in the early 1940s. The latter had been first recognized by Dubreuil and Anderodias in 1920. The advent of specific histochemical and subsequently immunocytochemical techniques established that pancreatic β-cell hyperplasia was associated with increased insulin storage.

Pedersen's[1] classic report in 1954 related neonatal hypoglycemia to maternal hyperglycemia. Eight years later, Baird and Farquhar demonstrated increased insulin-like material using the rat diaphragm bioassay of umbilical (portal) vein plasma following a glucose stimulus. Subsequently, Isles and Farquhar found increased immunoreactive insulin (IRI) in plasma of infants whose mothers had no insulin antibodies because they had not received exogenous insulin (i.e., gestational diabetics). The presence of hyperinsulinemia has been confirmed by many investigators since, including those who found elevated plasma C-peptide levels.

The period from 1960 to 1980 has been remarkable for the scientific advances in understanding and management of infants of diabetic mothers. These may be attributed to improved obstetrical care, improved neonatal care, and the ability to study the fetus and infant by newer methodologies.

The high neonatal mortality and morbidity associated with respiratory distress syndrome (RDS) rapidly decreased following the identification of surfactant by Avery and Mead in 1959. The subsequent role of various phospholipid components in amniotic fluid by Gluck and associates led to improved obstetrical prediction of at-risk infants. Liggins noted the induction of surfactant following betamethazone administration to the mother. The detailed retrospective analysis by Robert and colleagues in 1975 indicated that RDS was five- to sixfold greater in IDM compared to appropriate control infants of nondiabetic mothers. With improved management of the mother and infant, RDS no longer is the major risk factor.

As noted in Chapters 40 and 41, congenital anomalies have been recognized as important risk factors since detailed statistics have accumulated in major centers. They were noted in the 1930s, but only in the past decade have they emerged as the major problem of these infants.

The etiologies of the secondary erythroblastosis, polycythemia, and hyperbilirubinemia have only recently emerged. While in utero hypoxia was suspected, in 1981 Widness and colleagues demonstrated increased plasma erythropoietin levels in infants of diabetic mothers as well as in rhesus fetuses with experimental in utero primary hyperinsulinemia.

With the advent of microchemical techniques in the 1940s and 1950s, symptomatic hypocalcemia was recognized as a significant cause of morbidity. Tsang and colleagues demonstrated the interrelationships of calcium, phosphorus, parathormone, and vitamin D metabolites.

Epidemiology

Perinatal Mortality and Morbidity[1-5]

IDMs have greater morbidity than infants of nondiabetic women. Many infants of insulin-dependent diabetic women experience an uneventful clinical course and even more infants of gestationally (chemically) diabetic women do well. The more closely metabolically controlled the diabetic pregnant patient, the greater the potential for a subsequently normal infant. In recent series, perinatal mortality, except for congenital anomalies, approached that for infants of nondiabetic mothers.

In 1974, Pedersen and colleagues[1] published a review of their experiences over a 26-year period with an analysis of 1332 diabetic pregnancies. Perinatal mortality varied directly with maternal severity of diabetes as judged by two commonly used maternal classification schema: White's original classification of diabetes in pregnancy and Pedersen's Prognostically Bad Signs in Pregnancy (PBSP) classification. The risk to the fetus was increased when the PBSP classification was "added" to the White classification. While these investigators noted an improvement in nondiabetic pregnancy outcome during this same period, they emphasized that the improved classification schema combined with increased experience were the major reasons for the improved results in the diabetic pregnancies. Although the frequency of macrosomia (Fig. 42–1) has decreased, the rate is still higher than that in infants born to nondiabetic women. The gestational diabetic with glucose intolerance during late pregnancy often remains undiagnosed and may have an infant at greater risk for perinatal complications compared with normal infants.

An evaluation of perinatal mortality from Helsinki compared two time periods: 1970–1971 and 1975–1977. The review focused on the differences, after 1974, resulting from changes in management, which involved

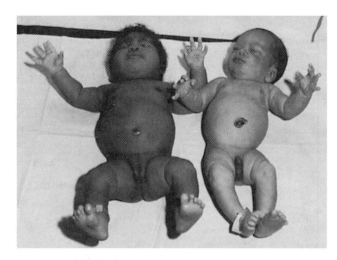

Figure 42–1. Two infants born at term from diabetic mothers. The appropriate-sized infant on the right was born to a White class C mother who was rigidly controlled during pregnancy. The macrosomic infant on the left was born to a woman diagnosed as gestationally diabetic late in pregnancy and whose management was inadequate.

increased monitoring and more frequent hospitalization for metabolic control, especially in the third trimester. During the period 1975–1977 all diabetic patients were hospitalized from the 32nd week of pregnancy until delivery. Strict maintenance of normoglycemia (blood glucose <120 mg/dL [6.67 mM]) was the goal of management, and, in the latter years, a permanent interdisciplinary team was in charge of the treatment of the patient. Gestational age of the infants was increased significantly; however, mean birth weights were unchanged. The perinatal mortality rate fell markedly as did neonatal morbidity. The authors concluded that while advances were obvious, the final answers were far from apparent because of the significant percentage of neonatal morbidities still present. Because the long-term effects of many of the neonatal morbidities remain to be defined, further efforts must be directed to minimize their incidence.

Thus, the maintenance of a normal metabolic state, including euglycemia, should diminish the increased perinatal and neonatal mortalities and morbidities noted in the diabetic pregnancy.

Pathogenesis of the Effects of Maternal Diabetes on the Fetus[1,3-10]

As yet, no single pathogenic mechanism has been clearly defined to explain the diverse problems observed in IDMs. Nevertheless, many of the effects can be attributed to maternal metabolic (glucose) control. Pedersen emphasized the relationship between maternal glucose concentration and neonatal hyperglycemia. His simplified hypothesis recognized that maternal hyperglycemia was paralleled by fetal hyperglycemia, which stimulated the fetal pancreas, resulting in B-cell hypertrophy and hyperplasia with increased insulin content. Hyperinsulinemia in utero has recently been demonstrated by cordocentesis. On separation of the fetus from the mother, the former no longer is supported by placental glucose transfer, resulting in neonatal hypoglycemia.

Hyperinsulinemia in utero affects diverse organ systems including the placenta. Insulin acts as the primary anabolic hormone of fetal growth and development resulting in visceromegaly (especially heart and liver) and macrosomia. In the presence of excess substrate (glucose), increased fat synthesis and deposition occur during the third trimester. Fetal macrosomia (see Fig. 42–1) is reflected by increased body fat, muscle mass, and organomegaly but not in increased size of the brain. After delivery there is a rapid fall in plasma glucose with persistently low concentrations of plasma free fatty acids (FFA), glycerol, and betahydroxybutyrate. In response to an i.v. glucose stimulus, plasma insulin-like activity is increased as are plasma IRI (determined in the absence of maternal insulin antibodies) and plasma C-peptide. The insulin response to i.v. arginine is also exaggerated in infants of gestationally diabetic mothers.

The response to an oral glucose load results in an earlier plasma insulin rise compared to normal infants, although the area under the insulin curve is similar. During the initial hours after birth, the response to an acute i.v. bolus of glucose in IDMs compared to normal subjects is a rapid rate of glucose disappearance from the plasma. In contrast, the rise in plasma glucose concentration following stepwise hourly increases in the rate of continuously infused glucose results in elevations even at normal rates, that is, 4 to 6 mg/kg/min. The latter may be attributed to a persistence of hepatic glucose output which differs from the normal infant. In fact, kinetic studies with D(1–13C) glucose in the initial 2 hr after delivery in infants of insulin-dependent mothers indicate a hepatic glucose production of approximately half that observed in normal infants. Studies with D(u-13C) glucose, however, have revealed a heterogeneous hepatic response so that suppression of hepatic glucose output in response to exogenous glucose is not a consistent occurrence. This effect may reflect the prior maternal metabolic condition.

On the basis of animal and in vitro studies of the isolated pancreas, the simplified hyperglycemia-hyperinsulinemia hypothesis has been expanded by Freinkel and later Milner to include maternal "mixed nutrients" as controlling factors (Fig. 42–2). Of the major maternal nutrients (glucose, fatty acids, ketones, and amino acids), it is likely that, in addition to glucose, amino acids are important to maturation of the fetal B cell and release of insulin, although the evidence is not definitive. Ketones readily cross the placenta and may provide substrate, but they do not

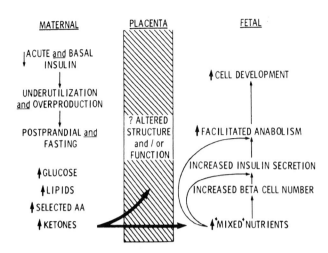

Figure 42–2. Freinkel's modified Pedersen schema as proposed by Milner. [Source: Merkatz IRE, Adam PAJ (eds): The Diabetic Pregnancy. A Perinatal Perspective. New York: Grune & Stratton, 1979. With permission.]

affect insulin secretion. With the exception of essential fatty acids, long chain fatty acids probably do not cross the placenta in sufficient quantities to influence growth and development *in utero.*

Alterations of plasma glucocorticoids and growth hormones have not been significant in IDMs. Definitive studies of the somatomedins (IGF-I, IGF—II) have not been found to be increased in umbilical plasma of infants of diabetic mothers nor of the rhesus with primary fetal hyperinsulinemia. In contrast, urinary excretion of catecholamines is diminished, especially in infants with low plasma glucose concentrations, In addition, plasma glucagon levels are less elevated after delivery in comparison to normal infants.

Studies of insulin receptors on fetal monocytes isolated from placental blood of infants of gestationally diabetic mothers (IGDM) at delivery indicated that IGDMs had more receptor sites per monocyte than normal adults or normal infants. Monocytes from both normal infants and IGDMs showed greater affinity for insulin than did those from adults. Furthermore, in the presence of increased ambient levels of plasma insulin, monocytes of the IGDM seem to develop increased (not decreased) concentrations of insulin receptors as well as increased affinity for the hormone. The significance of these observations for the physiological effects of insulin are unclear. However, there are implications for competition of insulin and its antibodies for receptor sites and resultant cell metabolism in insulin-sensitive tissues.

Congenital Anomalies in IDMs[5–11]

While most of the morbidities and mortality data for the IDM have shown definite improvement in the past two decades, congenital anomalies remain as the major unexplained problem. The three- to fourfold increase in the incidence of congenital anomalies in the offspring of diabetic women has continued to be noted in most centers and remains the most frequent contributor to perinatal mortality. This comes at a time when centers are reporting perinatal mortalities in offspring of insulin-dependent diabetic women that are no different from nondiabetic after correction for deaths due to congenital anomalies (Fig. 42–3).

The pathogenesis of this increase in congenital anomalies among IDMs has remained obscure, although several etiologies have been proposed to account for these, including: (1) hyperglycemia, either preconceptional or postconceptional, (2) hypoglycemia, (3) fetal hyperinsulinemia, (4) uteroplacental vascular disease, and/or (5) genetic predisposition. Although there are data to support each of these, currently the evidence is best for the postconceptional hyperglycemia etiology.

If a preconceptional influence of hyper- or hypoglycemia or a genetic predisposition for congenital anomalies were operative, than one might anticipate that offspring of diabetic fathers and nondiabetic mothers would have an increased incidence of anomalies. This assumes, of course, that the sperm and egg would be equally affected by the physiological and biochemical permutations of the diabetes. In a careful hospital chart review by Neave of 1262 offspring of diabetic fathers, only a slight increase in anomalies of questionable sig-

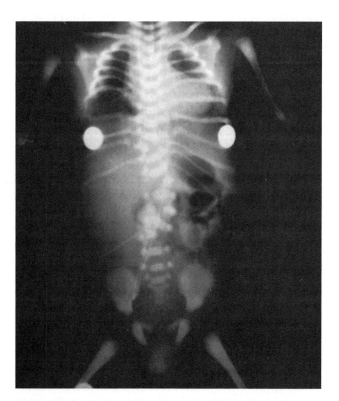

Figure 42–3. Fatal malformations in an infant of an insulin-dependent diabetic whose maternal control was suboptimal in the first trimester. There were cardiac and skeletal malformations.

nificance was found when compared to matched-control subjects. In this same study, however, a marked increase in anomalies was found in the offspring of diabetic mothers compared to either the offspring of the diabetic fathers or to an independent control group.

Few studies of normalization of blood glucose concentration before conception in diabetic women have been reported. One large European (Karlsburg, German Democratic Republic) diabetic population, which included nonpregnant women that were cared for in an ongoing diabetic outpatient program whose objectives included normalization of blood glucose concentration, had a 50% lower incidence of congenital anomalies compared to a simultaneously studied group of women who had no such therapeutic diabetic regimen applied before they knew they were pregnant.

There are scant human data on the association of hyperglycemia and anomalies. This may be due in part to the fact that organogenesis is taking place at a time during pregnancy when many diabetic women are not usually carefully evaluated for hyperglycemia. HbA_{1c}, which reflects ambient plasma glucose concentrations over the previous 4 to 6 weeks, has the potential advantage of offering one indicator of integrated "chronic" blood glucose control. Maternal HbA_{1c} values obtained during the initial visit of the first trimester in a group of insulin-dependent subjects were higher in those diabetic women subsequently giving birth to babies with anomalies compared to women with normal infants.

In 1988, a multicenter prospective, controlled collaborative study (National Institute of Child Health and Human Development: Diabetes in Early Pregnancy Study) enrolled 347 diabetic and 389 control women within 21 days of conception.[11] An additional 279 diabetic women were entered later. Significantly different frequencies were found in major malformation detection among the three groups (4.9, 2.1, and 9.0%, respectively). In contrast to previous studies, no correlation between hyperglycemia and glycosylated hemoglobin and malformation rates was found. Patient selection may have been a critical factor to explain the differences. Nevertheless, the study group supported the concept of normalization of metabolic control before and during pregnancy.

A significant analysis of the relationship of maternal hyperglycemia to fetal congenital anomalies has recently been reported.[12] The multicenter trial of rigid versus standard glucose control of 1440 subjects over 9 years included 270 pregnant subjects in both groups. As soon as pregnancy was diagnosed, all subjects irrespective of their randomization assignment were placed on the intensive control program. Thus, this study will compare preconception and periconception rigid control with early standard control. Because normalization was not always achieved, a spectrum of glucose control as manifest in glycohemoglobin will be available for analysis. This study differs from the

NICHHD multicenter study in timing and magnitude of glucose control. The results should contribute significantly to our understanding of the pathogenesis of congenital anomalies in the diabetic pregnancy. Although the glycosylated hemoglobin level was significantly lower in the intensively treated group at conception, rapid institution of intensive therapy in all patients abolished this difference. Thus, timely institution of intensive therapy resulted in rates of spontaneous abortion and of congenital anomalies similar to those in the nondiabetic population.

Hypoglycemia may also play a teratogenic role in the diabetic pregnancy. Symptomatic hypoglycemia during the first trimester is a frequently observed symptom in insulin-dependent diabetics although quantification has been difficult. Moreover, animal studies in pregnant rats made hypoglycemic by insulin injections suggest a significant association with increased anomalies. These data also raise the etiological possibility of the transplacental passage of exogenous maternal insulin. The question of whether or not insulin can cross during the critical period of organogenesis remains to be answered.

The increase in anomalies with increasing duration and severity of diabetes (i.e., White's classification) has been interpreted to indicate that the degree of maternal vascular disease may play a role. Hypoxia, as might be expected to occur with uterine vascular compromise, has been shown to cause anomalies in murine species after exposure periods as short as 5 hr.

Although anomalies in offspring of diabetic mothers tend to encompass a spectrum of organ systems rather than a specific, discrete syndrome, some individual patterns tend to occur more frequently. Thus, major congenital heart disease, musculoskeletal deformities (anencephaly, spina bifida, hydrocephalus) have been reported. Based on these findings, the critical period of teratogenesis for the pregnant diabetic has been inferred to take place before the seventh week following conception.

One rare congenital defect that is increased in IDMs is the small left colon syndrome. The etiology of this deformity is obscure. With conservative medical management, the condition usually resolves spontaneously within the neonatal period.

Although cardiac hypertrophy apart from congenital heart disease has been recognized in autopsies of IDMs for the past three decades, it has only been in the last 10 years that attention has been directed to a peculiar form of subaortic stenosis similar to the idiopathic hypertrophic subaortic stenosis found in adults. This particular entity may be associated with symptomatic congestive heart failure. As with the adult variant, in these infants, therapy with digoxin is contraindicated because the resultant increased myocardial contractility has been reported to be deleterious. Propranolol appears to be the therapeutic drug of choice, as in the adult. Although the pathogenesis remains controver-

sial at present, fetal hyperinsulinism, and, hence, the degree of maternal hyperglycemia, may be the major stimulus. Primary fetal hyperinsulinemia in the rhesus fetus has been found by Susa and colleagues to be associated with significant cardiac muscular hypertrophy and cardiomegaly. Clinically, this disorder resolves spontaneously over a period of weeks to months with correction of the echocardiographic features as well.

Macrosomia, Birth Injury, and Asphyxia[3,4,13,14]

The obstetrical and pediatric literature is confusing because of lack of agreement as to the definition of macrosomia. The multiplicity of factors that affect fetal growth may be ignored when a weight of 4000 alone is the reference standard. The best current definition is two standard deviations above the mean weight for gestational age corrected for sex in an appropriate population (ethnic at defined altitude). However, this will not characterize the selective organomegaly seen in the infant of the diabetic mother.

At birth, the infant of the poorly controlled diabetic woman will often appear macrosomic in contrast to infants born to well-controlled diabetic and nondiabetic, nonobese mothers. One consequence of undetected fetal macrosomia may be a difficult vaginal delivery due to shoulder dystocia with resultant birth injury and/or asphyxia. Potential birth injuries include: cephalohematoma, subdural hemorrhage, facial palsy, ocular hemorrhage, clavicular fracture, and brachial plexus injuries. Because of the associated organomegaly in IDMs, hemorrhage in the abdominal organs is possible, specifically liver and adrenals. Hemorrhage into the external genitalia of these large infants has also been reported.

Because the subjects are at high risk, intrapartum monitoring is essential to minimize potential complications. At delivery, the physician evaluating the infant should assign Apgar scores to document the presence or absence of asphyxia. While the specific etiology of asphyxia may be unclear, it may be due to difficulty in the intrapartum period because of relative macrosomia.

Asphyxia may have diverse consequences for the infant. Acutely, it may affect respiratory, renal, and central nervous system functions. Thus, decreased fluid intake is usually recommended until the degree of injury to the renal and central nervous systems can be ascertained. An important complication of asphyxia in the newborn may be later respiratory difficulties.

Current management of the pregnant diabetic includes determining the degree of pulmonary maturity from amniotic fluid study by the lecithin/sphingomyelin (L/S) ratio, the presence of phosphatidylglycerol (PG), and/or foam stability test (FST) prior to delivery. A false-positive L/S ratio may be associated with asphyxia. In one study in 150 women who had had an amniocentesis within 72 hr of delivery with an L/S ratio $\geq$ 2:1, the incidence of RDS was significantly increased in infants who had low Apgar scores at 1 and 5 min, respectively. This was independent of whether or not the mother had diabetes mellitus.

Identification of maternal diabetes and maintenance of good metabolic control in the pregnant diabetic should diminish the frequency and magnitude of macrosomia and its attendant complications; careful obstetrical management should prevent birth injury and asphyxia.

The precise growth factor basis for macrosomia is unproven, although most evidence (direct and inferential) supports increased insulin action as the major responsible factor.

In one large study, fetal macrosomia (>2 SD above the mean weight) was correlated significantly with fetal umbilical plasma insulin concentrations or fetal C-peptide concentrations but not with maternal glycosylated hemoglobin.[13] Thus, the simplified Pedersen hypothesis does not adequately explain the pathogenesis of macrosomia in the diabetic pregnancy. Similar results have been found with *in utero* hyperinsulinemia found at cordocentesis.[15]

RDS and Transient Tachypnea[3–6]

Respiratory distress, including RDS, is a frequent and potentially severe complication in the infant of the diabetic mother. While the clinical association has been long recognized, recent investigations have increased our understanding of the pathophysiological interrelationships. Neonatal RDS, a pathological correlate of hyaline membrane disease, develops because of lung immaturity in the newborn and remains a major cause of mortality in the newborn.[3–6]

RDS has a typical course that is manifest by increasing oxygen requirements due to progressive respiratory compromise. Tachypnea, intercostal and subcostal retractions, nasal flaring, and expiratory grunting, appearing in the first few minutes to hours of life, are the cardinal signs of the disease. In uncomplicated cases, the disease peaks by 74 hr of age. Complications commonly associated with the disease include the presence of a persistent patent ductus arteriosus in the very small (>1500-g) infant and bronchopulmonary dysplasia in neonates requiring prolonged ventilatory support and high ambient oxygen concentrations. Both of these conditions may significantly lengthen the clinical course of an otherwise self-limited disease.

Surfactant is produced in the type 11 pneumocyte and is composed of protein and phospholipids. It normally functions to diminish surface tension at the air-alveolar interface. Absence of this material results in pulmonary atelectasis and the clinically characteristic picture. On roentgenographic examination of the chest,

a diffuse reticulogranular pattern and air bronchograms are observed. The phospholipid components of surfactant progressively increase with advancing gestational age and are the basis for utilization of specific laboratory tests of pulmonary maturity, that is, L/S ratio, PG determination, and the FST.

While the increased susceptibility to RDS has been suspected in the infant of the diabetic mother, a definitive retrospective analysis by Robert and colleagues evaluated the relative risk of RDS in the IDM in a large series of diabetic pregnancies from the Joslin Clinic and the Boston Hospital for Women. The relative risk of RDS in IDMs was higher in comparison to infants of nondiabetic mothers. If specific confounding variables were excluded, including gestational age, delivery by cesarean section, presence of labor, birth weight, sex, Apgar score at 5 min, antepartum hemorrhage, presence of hydramnios, maternal anemia, and maternal age, the relative risk was 5.6 times higher in the IDM. This effect was primarily confined to infants whose gestational age was 38 weeks or less. Present obstetrical management, however, has been noted to reduce the frequency of RDS.

In 1973, 2 years after initially reporting on the value of the L/S ratio in normal pregnancies, Gluck and Kulovich noted that diabetes mellitus was associated with a delay in maturation of the ratio for White classes A, B, and C, while an acceleration was found for classes D, E, and F diabetic pregnancies evaluated at specific gestational ages. There may be an increased frequency of "false positives" in all diabetic classes when L/S ratio equals 2:0. Further advance in the assessment of fetal lung maturation has been due to analysis of PG, the absence of which has been correlated with increased incidence of RDS even with an L/S ratio of $\geq$ 2:1. The presence of PG in amniotic fluid increases the probability that an infant can be delivered without signs of respiratory distress due to surfactant deficiency.

Currently there is considerable research on early lung development. Heber and associates[16] are studying the effects of EGF and TGFβ on embryonic lung in culture. They have described morphogenetic aspects as well as the effect on epithelial proliferation and differentiation. They are characterizing the role of homeobox genes in the process of branching morphogenesis. These observations precede but may set the stage for later surfactant development. In contrast, Hacklett et al[17] have studied members of the winged helix/forkhead family of transcription factors believed to play a role in cell-specific gene expression. They have found a unique temporal and spatial pattern of HFH-4 gene expression in the developing lung which defines the protein marker for the initiation of bronchial epithelial cell differentiation and suggests that it may play an important role in cell fate determination during lung development. These studies have important implications for understanding pulmonary disease in later development.

Pulmonary surfactant production increases near term and probably results from the activation of the pathway for dipalmitoyl lecithin, which in turn may be mediated through increases in fetal plasma cortisol levels. While plasma cortisol production rates are normal in the IDM, it has been shown that insulin can interfere with incorporation of choline into lecithin even when cortisol is present. Incorporation of labeled glucose and fatty acid residues into saturated PG is reduced in fetal rabbit lung slices in the presence of insulin. Thus, endogenous insulin, known to be increased in the fetus of the poorly controlled pregnant diabetic, may play a role in delaying pulmonary maturation. While the specific biochemical mechanisms are unclear, these studies correlate with the clinical situation in which pulmonary maturation is not only delayed in the IDM, but RDS is noted with L/S ratios $\geq 2:1$. The protein components of surfactant have been isolated, characterized, and synthesized. Surfactant from bovine lungs, human amniotic fluid, or synthetic has now been used to treat infants with respiratory distress syndrome successfully. This has been particularly important for very small, preterm infants.

The trend to deliver diabetic patients later in gestation rather than earlier is increasing. Previously, early delivery was advised to diminish the risk of intrauterine fetal death, but increasing assessment of fetal well-being (estriols, ultrasound, stress and nonstress testing of fetal heart rate, and so forth) affords the obstetrician the opportunity of delivering the patient at the optimal time. RDS must be managed with particular attention to fluid administration, oxygen, correction of acidosis, and ventilator support when necessary.

Hypoglycemia[3–8,10]

A rapid fall in plasma glucose concentration following delivery is characteristic of the IDM. Values <35 mg/dL (1.94 mM) in term infants and <25 mg/dL (1.39 mM) in preterm infants are abnormal and may occur within 30 min after clamping the umbilical vessels. Factors that are known to influence the degree of hypoglycemia include: prior maternal glucose homeostasis and maternal glycemia during delivery. An inadequately controlled pregnant diabetic will have stimulated the fetal pancreas to synthesize excessive insulin, which may be readily released. Administration of i.v. dextrose during the intrapartum period, which results in maternal hyperglycemia (>125 mg/dL [6.94 mM]), will be reflected in the fetus and will exaggerate the infant's normal postdelivery fall in plasma glucose concentration. In addition, hypoglycemia may persist for 48 hr or may develop after 24 hr.

As noted previously, fetal hyperinsulinemia is associated with suppressed levels of plasma FFA and/or

diminished hepatic glucose output. Other factors that may contribute to the development of hypoglycemia include defective counter-regulation by catecholamines and/or glucagon.

Most infants of diabetic mothers are asymptomatic with very low plasma glucose levels. This may be due to the initial brain stores of glycogen; however, the exact biochemistry is as yet undefined. Signs and symptoms that may be observed are nonspecific and include tachypnea, apnea, tremulousness, sweating, irritability, and seizures. Asymptomatic infants do not require parenteral treatment. Early administration of food at 3 to 4 hr of age may, however, be beneficial if plasma glucose levels are not markedly depressed.

Rigid maternal control of blood glucose levels during pregnancy and delivery minimizes the risk of *neonatal hypoglycemia*. Plasma glucose values should be obtained at delivery from the umbilical vein. Subsequently, the infant should be screened by a rapid bedside technique at 1/2, 2, and 4 hr and then prior to feeding until stable. Abnormal glucose values require verification by chemical analysis.

The symptomatic infant should be treated i.v. with 0.25 g/kg of 25% dextrose as a bolus administered during 2 to 4 min and must be followed by a continuous infusion at 4 to 6 mg/kg/min. Bolus injections alone without subsequent infusion will only exaggerate the hypoglycemia by a rebound mechanism and are contraindicated. Once the plasma glucose stabilizes above 45 mg/dL (2.50 mM), the infusion may be slowly decreased while oral feeds are initiated and advanced. If hypoglycemia persists, higher glucose rates of 8 to 12 mg/kg/min or more may be necessary.

Glucagon has been administered within 15 min after delivery to prevent hypoglycemia. Because the majority of infants are asymptomatic, this does not appear warranted. Furthermore, glucagon may stimulate insulin release, which may exaggerate the tendency to hypoglycemia.

Prompt recognition and treatment of symptomatic infants has minimized sequelae. No specific late central nervous system complications have been attributed to neonatal hypoglycemia per se in IDMs. Whether the occasional delayed motor development or psychological dysfunction observed after 5 years is related to early hypoglycemia is unclear.

Hypocalcemia and Hypomagnesemia[6]

Besides hypoglycemia, hypocalcemia ranks as one of the major metabolic derangements observed in the IDM. Normally, serum calcium is elevated following a rise in parathyroid hormone (PTH) levels by three mechanisms: mobilization of bone calcium, reabsorption of calcium in the kidney, and increased absorption of calcium in the intestine through action of vitamin D.

In opposition, serum calcium is decreased following a rise in calcitonin, which antagonizes the action of PTH. Serum calcium may also be elevated by vitamin D (1,25 dihydroxy vitamin D), which improves absorption of calcium in the intestine after feeding as well as reabsorption from bone.

During pregnancy, calcium is transferred from mother to fetus, concomitant with an increasing hyperparathyroid state in the mother. Plasma calcium concentrations are higher in the fetus than in the mother. This hyperparathyroid state may function as a homeostatic compensation to restore the maternal calcium that is diverted to the fetus. Neither calcitonin nor parathyroid hormone crosses the placenta. At birth, because of the levels of calcitonin, PTH, and 1,25 dihydroxy vitamin D, serum calcium falls, subsequent to interruption of materno-fetal calcium transfer. Elevations in PTH and 1,25 dihydroxy vitamin D as early as 24 hr of age ensure correction of the low serum calcium concentration.

Tsang has shown that there are a number of neonates who are prone to hypocalcemia, particularly the prematurely born, the infant who is asphyxiated, and the infant of the diabetic mother. Approximately 50% of infants born to insulin-dependent diabetic women develop hypocalcemia (7 mg/dL [<1.75 mM]) during the first 3 days of life. This high incidence of hypocalcemia is not seen in infants of gestationally diabetic women when compared to control subjects. Evaluation of the mechanism(s) has failed to establish prematurity or asphyxia per se (both of which may be present in IDMs) as associated factors. However, the frequency and severity of serum hypocalcemia is directly related to the severity of the diabetes and potentiated if birth asphyxia is superimposed on the clinical state. It has been postulated that the mechanism at least partially responsible for hypocalcemia is hyperphosphatemia, which is present during the initial 48 hr after birth.

In the infant of the insulin-dependent diabetic, failure of an appropriate rise in PTH concentration in response to hypocalcemia has been reported in contrast to infants of gestational diabetics and nondiabetics. The PTH response in the normal infant, which occurs on the second to third day, does not occur in the IDM until 48 hr or later on the third or fourth day.

Hypomagnesemia (<1.5 mg/dL [0.02 mM]) has been found in as many as 33% of IDMs. As with hypocalcemia, the frequency and severity of clinical symptoms is correlated with the maternal status. Neonatal magnesium concentration has been correlated with that in the mother, as well as with the maternal insulin requirements, and the concentration of i.v. glucose administered to the infant. Hypomagnesemia may suppress parathyroid activity and thus produce hypocalcemia.

Hypocalcemia and hypomagnesemia, which have similar clinical manifestations to hypoglycemia, must be considered and treated appropriately. The long-term potential deleterious effects of either hypocalcemia or hypomagnesemia are unknown.

Hyperbilirubinemia and Polycythemia[3,18]

Hyperbilirubinemia is observed more frequently in the IDM than in the normal infant.[3,18] Although a number of hypotheses have been suggested, the pathogenesis remains uncertain. Prematurity (biochemical immaturity), which is present in many IDMs, was one explanation that was rejected after gestationally age-matched comparisons with non-IDMs showed the IDM to be more jaundiced. There is no increased incidence of Coombs-positive ABO incompatibility. Red cell lifespan, osmotic fragility, and deformability have not been found to be appreciably different in IDMs compared to normal infants, neither has an increased umbilical cord bilirubin nor an increased postnatal rate of hemoglobin decline been demonstrated. In one evaluation, only macrosomic IDMs were noted to be at risk for hyperbilirubinemia; increased heme turnover was postulated to be a significant factor in the pathogenesis. However, Stevenson and colleagues suggested that delayed clearance of the bilirubin load was a factor as measured by pulmonary excretion of carbon monoxide as an index of bilirubin production.

Indirect evidence for fetal hypoxia in IDMs may explain the neonatal polycythemia and hyperbilirubinemia. Umbilical cord erythropoietin levels measured by Widness[18] at birth using a highly sensitive and specific radioimmunoassay for this hormone, which is stimulated by hypoxemia, have been found to be above the narrow range for control subjects in one third of a group of 61 IDMs. Moreover, there was an association with relative hyperinsulinemia at birth. Fetal rhesus monkeys made hyperinsulinemic in the last third of gestation in the absence of maternal diabetes have been shown to have markedly elevated plasma erythropoietin levels as well as other evidence of increased fetal erythropoiesis such as elevated reticulocyte counts. In addition, chronically catheterized fetal sheep who have been infused with insulin have been found to have increased oxygen consumption and decreased distal aortic arterial oxygen content. Furthermore, Philipps and colleagues have observed elevation of erythropoietin in chronically catheterized fetal lambs made hyperglycemia by infusion. Teramo et al.[19] studied insulin-dependent diabetic women delivered by elective cesarean section who were shown to have a strong correlation of amniotic fluid and umbilical plasma erythropoietin ($r = 0.90$) at delivery. The previously reported increased erythropoietin levels were confirmed.

A final consideration is the concept of ineffective erythropoiesis in IDMs. Further support for this comes from a study of gestationally age-matched controls and IDMs; the latter had increased carbon monoxide excretion derived from heme metabolism. Hemoglobin levels were not significantly higher in the IDM. Hemolysis was not evident by evaluation of Coombs-positive blood group incompatibilities. Increased ineffective erythropoiesis, defined as erythroid precursors harbored in body organs such as the liver and spleen and not released into the peripheral circulation, was postulated as an etiology for the observed increased bilirubin levels in the IDMs.

The polycythemia frequently observed in IDMs may well be the most important factor associated with hyperbilirubinemia. Venous hematocrits 65% or more have been observed in 20 to 40% of IDMs during the first days of life and have sometimes been associated with signs and symptoms of neonatal polycythemia such as jitteriness, seizures, tachypnea, priapism, and oliguria. Therapy with the use of a partial exchange transfusion (10 to 15% of total blood volume) through the umbilical vein using plasmanate or 5% albumin has been associated with a rapid resolution of symptoms. Careful studies examining the relationship of neonatal polycythemia to maternal blood glucose control and/or other perinatal factors associated with the diabetic pregnancy have not been done as yet.

Renal Vein Thrombosis[3]

Renal vein thrombosis is a severe, life-threatening, but very rare occurrence in the perinatal period. Its occurrence is more frequently associated with maternal diabetes mellitus than in the normal population. Although Pedersen[1] failed to mention this condition in his monograph, in one postmortem survey of 16 cases of neonatal renal vein thrombosis, 5 were found in IDMs. Seven other infants in this report were born to mothers without known diabetes but with fetal macrosomia and pancreatic β-cell hypertrophy and hyperplasia.

The pathogenesis of this lesion remains obscure although most speculation has centered around the possible etiologic role of polycythemia (see before). Sludging of blood combined with a further reduction in cardiac output as a result of diabetic cardiomyopathy may be a contributing factor. Because platelet endoperoxides are increased in the IDM, the normal balance between proaggregatory platelets and anti-aggregatory vascular prostaglandins may be disrupted in the IDM, thus favoring the development of thrombosis. Why this lesion shows selectivity for the kidneys and not other organs is obscure. Birth trauma is an unlikely initiating factor because this lesion has been observed in stillborns and IDMs delivered by cesarean section.

In the liveborn infant, the diagnosis is usually made in the first hours or days of life with the findings of hematuria and flank mass(es). Therapy is aimed at careful fluid and electrolyte management and correction of polycythemia with a plasma exchange. A pediatric surgical consultation is indicated for evaluation of possible nephrectomy. The role of heparinization in the therapy of this entity remains controversial.

Long-term Prognosis and Follow-up[3,5,19–21]

There is concern not only for the problems found in the immediate neonatal period, but also for the long-term effects of maternal diabetes and neonatal complications on growth and development, on psychosocial intellectual capabilities, and finally on the risk to the infant of subsequently developing diabetes. One of the important factors influencing long-term prognosis is the improvement in management of the pregnant diabetic and her infant. Assuming that many of the deleterious effects of the diabetic pregnancy are being modified by normalization of metabolic status in both the pregnant woman and her conceptus, the poor prognoses that have been reported in previous retrospective studies should be ameliorated in future prospective evaluations.[3,5,19,20]

There are a few prospective studies of growth and development of the IDM. Farquhar's analysis of 231 of a group of 320 infants is significant in that more children up to 15 years of age fell below the 3d percentile for height than exceeded the 97th percentile (21 vs. 5). Weight, in contrast, seemed to be equally divided above and below the normal range. This was confirmed by evaluating the weight and height index of each child expressed as a percentage of the 50th percentile for age and sex. Evaluation by these parameters suggested that excessive weight is almost 10 times more common than unusually low weight. Farquhar suggests that this may represent a potential "return to obesity" noted at birth in this group of infants. In another study, Bibergeil noted that height was elevated in 16.7%, but below normal in 9.3%. Newborns >4 kg had significant elevations of height and weight at time of entrance to school.

In consideration of neuropsychological development, it is important to note that the high frequency of congenital malformations may be directly or indirectly associated with neuropsychological handicaps. In a large series, Yssing found that 36% (265 children) had evidence of cerebral dysfunction or related conditions. Cerebral palsy and epilepsy were found to be three to five times higher in comparison to the normal population, but mental retardation was not noted to be different. When present, the difficulties seemed to be related to extremes of maternal age, severity of diabetes, low birth weight for gestational age, or complications during pregnancy.

The outcome of children at 1, 3, and 5 years of age was evaluated by Stehbens and coworkers. Psychological evaluations suggested that at 3 and 5 years of age the IDM is more vulnerable to intellectual impairment, especially if children were born small for gestational age or if their mother's pregnancy was complicated by acetonuria.

The Diabetes in Early Pregnancy Study allowed for a 3-year follow-up study of 109 IDMs and 90 control infants.[21] Seventy-one percent of subjects completed the serial follow-up evaluations. Neurodevelopment of early entry subjects were similar to that of control subjects, whereas late entry subjects scored less well on language measures. Less optimal intellectual development was associated with reduced head circumference. The investigators concluded that mothers with insulin-dependent diabetes who maintain good control during pregnancy can expect to have infants who are neurodevelopmentally normal, whereas mothers whose diabetes is less well controlled may have infants with less optimal neurodevelopment.

The presence of hypoglycemia per se has not been related to later neuropsychological defects. Persson and Gentz found no evidence that asymptomatic hypoglycemia leads to intellectual impairment by 5 years of age.

The question of whether the IDM has an increased likelihood of becoming diabetic is important and has been the subject of a number of studies and a recent review. Previous data have indicated that 4 to 6% of siblings of diabetic individuals developed diabetes. While family aggregates do exist, transmitted through and within generations, a simple mode of inheritance is inconsistent with the reported data. Some investigators have suggested that a polygenic multifactorial model best explains the reported observations. From recent studies of IDMs, the prevalence of insulin-dependent diabetes mellitus (IDDM) among offspring of diabetic mothers was approximately 1.0%. Thus, it appears that the infant born to a mother with diabetes is at increased risk for developing the disease in comparison to the normal population.

Warram and associates[22] have reported on the extensive series from the Joslin Clinic (1940 to 1984). In 1391 offspring who survived the perinatal period, the net cumulative risk of IDDM by age 20 years was only 2.1 ± 0.5% (mean ± SE), which was one third that reported for the offspring of men with IDDM: 6.1 ± 1.8%. Although the risk of diabetes in the off-spring of diabetic mothers was increased significantly in young mothers, it was otherwise independent of risk factors for perinatal mortality. From a careful analysis of early fetal or perinatal loss, no evidence was found for selective loss of diabetes susceptible fetuses. They speculated that exposure *in utero* to an affected mother can protect a fetus from developing IDDM later in life.

Research Considerations

While there has been continued improvement in outcome for IDM, such infants remain at high risk. Optimal results are obtained when meticulous medical-obstetrical care during pregnancy is combined with expert neonatal supervision. Thus, these high-risk patients should be delivered in tertiary care centers where those infants requiring specialized management may be best treated. Many of the risks previously identified are now less frequent; however, congenital anomalies remain an unresolved and major problem.

Physician and patient education for those with IDDM and the role of preconception metabolic control require study and implementation in the prevention or minimization of the incidence of congenital anomalies. Parallel animal or tissue (organ) studies to define specific teratogenic agents are equally important.

As noted previously, screening for and treatment of gestational diabetes remains a high priority, which can prevent significant neonatal morbidity.

As yet, no unifying hypothesis has related all neonatal morbidities to maternal–fetal metabolic control. Although the expanded Pedersen hypothesis is predominant, further studies of hypoxemia and polycythemia as well as of the hypocalcemia-hypomagnesemia problems are indicated.

Finally, the risk for subsequent IDDM in infants born to mothers with IDDM as well as those with gestational diabetes requires further definition. Equally important are long-term studies of the effects of neonatal morbidities on subsequent neuropsychosocial development.

References

1. Pedersen J (ed): The Pregnant Diabetic and Her Newborn, Ed. 2. Baltimore: Williams & Wilkins, 1977.

2. Teramo K, Kuusisto AN, Raivio KO: Perinatal outcome of insulin-dependent diabetic pregnancies. Ann Clin Res 11:146–155, 1979.

3. Cornblath M, Schwartz R (eds): Disorders of Carbohydrate Metabolism in Infancy, Ed. 3. Cambridge: Blackwell Scientific Publications Inc., 1991.

4. Sutherland HW, Stowers JM, Pearson DWM (eds): Carbohydrate Metabolism in Pregnancy and the Newborn, IV. New York: Springer-Verlag, 1989.

5. Gabbe SG, Oh W (eds): Infant of the Diabetic Mother. Report of the 93rd Ross Conference on Pediatric Research, 1987.

6. Merkatz IR, Adam PAJ (eds): The Diabetic Pregnancy. A Perinatal Perspective. New York: Grune & Stratton, 1979.

7. Ciba Foundation Symposium 63: Pregnancy Metabolism, Diabetes and the Fetus. New York: Excerpta Medica, 1979.

8. Persson B, Gentz J, Lunell NO: Diabetes in pregnancy. *In* Scarpelli EM, Cosmi EV (eds): Reviews in Perinatal Medicine, Vol. 2. New York: Raven Press, 1978.

9. Reece EA, Coustan DR (eds): Diabetes Mellitus in Pregnancy, Ed. 2. New York: Churchill Livingstone, 1995.

10. Cowett RM (ed): The infant of the diabetic mothers: *In* Nestle Nutrition Workshop Series #35. New York: Raven Press Ltd., 1995, pp. 149–170.

11. Mills JL, Knopp RH, Simpson JL, et al.: Lack of relation of increased malformation rates in infants of diabetic mothers to glycemic control during organogenesis. N Engl J Med 318:671–676, 1988.

12. DCCT Research Group: Pregnancy outcomes in the Diabetes Control and Complications Trial. Am J Obstet Gynecol 174:1343–1353, 1996.

13. Schwartz R, Gruppuso PA, Petzold K, et al.: Hyperinsulinemia and macrosomia in the fetus of the diabetic mother. Diabetes Care 17:640–648, 1994.

14. Schwartz R, Teramo KA: What is macrosomia? J Perinatol Diabetes Care (in press).

15. Salvesen DR, Brudenell JM, Proudler AJ, et al.: Fetal pancreatic β-cell function in pregnancies complicated by maternal diabetes mellitus: Relationship to fetal acidemia and macrosomia. Am J Obstet Gynecol 168: 1363–1369, 1993.

16. Vosatka RJ, Volpa MA, Nielsen HC: Alternations of branching morphogenesis in embryonic lung by EGF and TGFβ analyzed by interpolated cinephotomicrography. Pediatr Res 37:72A, 1995.

17. Hackett BP, Brody SL, Liang M, et al.: Primary structure of hepatocyte nuclear factor/forkhead homologue 4 and characterization of gene expression in the developing respiratory and reproductive epithelium. Proc Natl Acad Sci 92:4249–4253, 1995.

18. Widness JA, Susa JB, Garcia JF, et al.: Increased erythropoiesis and elevated erythropoietin in infants born to diabetic mothers and in hyperinsulinemic rhesus fetuses. J Clin Invest 67:637–642, 1981.

19. Teramo KA, Widness JA, Clemons GK, et al.: Amniotic fluid erythropoietin correlates with umbilical plasma erythropoietin in normal and abnormal pregnancy. Obstet Gynecol 69:710–716, 1987.

20. Camerini-Davalos RA, Cole HS (eds): Early diabetes in early Life. New York: Raven Press, 1975.

21. Sells CJ, Robinson NM, Brown Z, et al.: Long-term developmental follow-up of infants of diabetic mothers. J Pediatr 125:S9–S17, 1994.

22. Warram JH, Krolewski AS, Kahn CR: Determinants of IDDM and perinatal mortality in children of diabetic mothers. Diabetes 37:1324–1328, 1988.

Acknowledgment

This work was supported in part by the National Institutes of Health (NIH)-National Institute of Child Health and Human Development (NICHHD) and the Rhode island Hospital Research Fund.

43

Anesthesia for the Diabetic Patient

Joseph M. Webb and William D. Hammonds

Historical Perspective

In 1966, Root[1] estimated that diabetic patients will have a 50% chance of undergoing surgery at some point during their life. Not only were they at higher risk of having surgery in 1998, surgical options have multiplied, including surgical treatments for retinopathy, cataract removal, penile prosthesis implantation, peripheral vascular disease, coronary artery disease, as well as the increasing use of corneal, renal, and pancreatic transplantation. As the understanding of the metabolic and biochemical basis of diabetes increased in recent years, morbidity and mortality rates related to surgery in these patients significantly improved. A study from the 1960s showed mortality rates to be 3.6 to 13.2%.[2,3] In 1983 Hortrup et al.[4] compared the morbidity and mortality between diabetics and nondiabetics having vascular surgery and found no deaths in either group and no differences in morbidity. It is reasonable to speculate that this improvement is related to the better perioperative care of these patients over the last 20 years.

The Preoperative Visit

Recent changes in the economics of the medical environment rendered the preoperative evaluation and management of the diabetic patient problematic. Restrictions by third-party payers to admitting patients preoperatively has resulted in the majority of these patients being admitted to the hospital on the day of surgery. The preoperative evaluation may take place the day of surgery, or days or weeks prior to elective surgery. Nevertheless, a careful preoperative evaluation of the diabetic patient is mandatory. It is during this preoperative interval that coordinated efforts are needed among all physician consultants. The patient's medical evaluation should include thorough assessment of the cardiovascular status. A careful history of angina or myocardial infarction must be taken. Painless angina and silent myocardial infarction occur more commonly in diabetic patients than in the general population. The presence of atypical symptoms increases the difficulty of obtaining a history of cardiovascular disease. The presence of heart disease has important implications for any patient who is to have anesthesia. If the patient has had a myocardial infarction in the past 3 months, the risk of reinfarction at the time of anesthesia and surgery is 27%, whereas, if 4 to 6 months have elapsed, the risk of reinfarction is 11%. The overall mortality of patients with a previous myocardial infarction who have a reinfarction in the intraoperative or postoperative period is 69%.[5] Rao et al.[6] have shown reinfarction rates of 5.7 and 2.3%, when the time elapsed from prior infarction was up to 3 months and 4 to 6 months, respectively. Myocardial infarction is a serious complication in any patient, but the poorly controlled diabetic patient with fluid and electrolyte disturbances and altered metabolism is a poor candidate for anesthesia and surgery. Solar and colleagues[7] have shown that diabetic patients who have a myocardial infarction have a poorer outcome than do their nondiabetic peers. Other facts contributing to the poor outcome in the patient who has a perioperative myocardial infarction are that three quarters or more of diabetic patients who have surgery are over the age of 50 years. Obesity is common in this group, and there is an increased incidence of peripheral vascular and myocardial disease as well as renal impairment. Many of the patients who have had diabetes for several years have multisystem disease. Cardiac autonomic neuropathy has become a well-recognized syndrome in the diabetic patient, which may serve as a predictor of poor prognosis in the long term and as a cardiorespiratory hazard in the short term. Several studies[8–10] have demonstrated impaired cardiovascular responses to induction of anesthesia and tracheal intubation, which correlate with abnormal responses to preoperative autonomic testing. Components of these tests include heart rate responses to Valsalva maneuvers, heart rate and diastolic blood pressure changes associated with changes in posture. These studies suggest that the diabetic population undergoing surgery may be at increased risk for undesirable cardiovascular events compared to the general population. These events include bradycardia and hypotension unrelated to blood loss and unexplained cardiorespiratory arrest in the perioperative period.[11-13] See Chapters 27, 28, 35, 36, and 38.)

Rao and coworkers[6] have presented evidence that preoperative optimization of the patient's physiological status, use of recently introduced cardioactive and vasoactive drugs, invasive hemodynamic monitoring postoperatively, and treatment of any hemodynamic aberration with appropriate drugs immediately after its onset were associated with a significantly lower reinfarction rate and mortality following anesthesia and surgery in patients at risk because of recent myocardial infarction. It is therefore a prudent approach to identify patients with recent myocardial infarction or ischemia, aggressively monitor them, and plan to have them spend the first part of their postoperative time in the intensive care unit.

In addition to the routine preanesthetic evaluation, some special points regarding anesthesia for the diabetic patient should be discussed at the time of the preoperative visit. A route for sampling blood for glucose and potassium determinations will be required. An arterial line is usually the optimal sampling port so that blood samples for glucose determination can be obtained frequently. The cannulation of the radial artery is a safe procedure if careful technique is used. Slogoff and colleagues[14] found no serious ischemic complications in 1699 nondiabetic patients after radial artery cannulation. These investigations also concluded that an abnormal Allen's test, which is found in many diabetic patients with peripheral vascular disease, was not predictive of ischemic damage after cannulation. Though arterial cannulation may be optimal, a more practical way is the use of capillary blood glucose monitors, which have proven to be compact and easy to use in the operating room.

During the preoperative evaluation, the customary careful airway examination to evaluate for potential difficulties in mask fit, endotracheal intubation, or any other factors that might interfere with ventilation should be made. Numerous case reports and studies[15] have demonstrated an increased incidence of difficult intubation in the diabetic population. Though controversy may exist as to its impact, the existence of limited joint mobility syndrome, or stiff joint syndrome, occurs in 30 to 40% of insulin-dependent diabetics and is thought to be due to glycosylation of tissue proteins in patients with chronic hyperglycemia.[16] A predictor of limited joint mobility is the "prayer sign," caused by the inability of the patient to straighten the interphalangeal joints of the forth and fifth fingers.[17] (See Chapter 37.) A retrospective study by Hogan et al.[15] demonstrated a 32% incidence of difficult laryngoscopy in diabetic renal transplant patients. Controversy exists as to the exact incidence of difficult laryngoscopy, and points to the need of a prospective study for a more accurate determination.

Maintenance of the airway can present serious problems in the diabetic patient with autonomic neuropathy. One insidious consequence of autonomic neuropathy is gastroparesis. The patient with gastroparesis will have weak or absent esophageal motility. When the patient is supine, food and liquid pool in the esophagus, and the stomach empties slowly. This set of circumstances is a concern for the anesthesiologist because of the increased risk of aspiration of stomach contents during induction or maintenance of anesthesia. Vomiting and aspiration have also been reported in the postoperative interval.[18] The aspiration of gastric contents, known as *Mendelson's syndrome*,[19] is associated with serious complications, including pneumonitis, lung abscess, myocardial infarction, and renal failure.[20] The overall mortality rate is approximately 30%.[21] Poor gastric emptying occurs in approximately 30% of diabetic patients. Gastroparesis is not always symptomatic, but may be associated with epigastric fullness, or early satiety following eating. A history of gustatory sweating or vomiting food eaten hours or days before may be obtained. These symptoms are vague and nonspecific; better ways to detect patients with gastroparesis are needed. Tests of sympathetic integrity will identify the group at high risk for this condition. Burgos et al.,[22] in a comparison of tests for autonomic neuropathy in patients with and without diabetes, showed that diabetic patients had less tachycardia in response to the Valsalva strain and head-up tilt. They also demonstrated that the diastolic blood pressure of diabetic patients decreased during head-up tilt, whereas nondiabetic patients had increases in diastolic pressure. (See Chapter 36.)

The consequences of the aspiration of gastric contents are grave, but there are treatment methods that will help prevent this complication. Placing the patient in a nil per os status after midnight is a long tradition in preparing the patient for surgery. Because of slow gastric emptying in the patient with gastroparesis, the traditional 6- to 12-hr fast might not be long enough. A longer fast will not ensure an empty stomach, but it will help to prevent the aspiration of food mixed with gastric secretions, which is the most serious kind of aspiration. Cimetidine is an antagonist of histamine-2 receptors. It is through these receptors that the secretion of hydrochloric acid is mediated. Weber and Hirshman[23] found that 300 mg of cimetidine orally the night before surgery and 300 mg intramuscularly 1 hr before anesthesia raised the pH of the gastric contents above 2.5, which is believed to be the value below which patients are at risk. Ranitidine 150 mg orally the night before and the morning of surgery, or 50 mg i.v.

at least 15 minutes prior to the induction of anesthesia is a reasonable alternative.

Metoclopromide acts centrally and peripherally to stimulate gastric emptying in the diabetic patient[24] and has been used to decrease gastric volume before the induction of anesthesia.

Capan et al.[25] reported that a combination of cimetidine and metoclopromide was more effective in reducing volume and pH of gastric contents than either drug alone. This combination of drugs administered the night before, and the other premedicants administered the morning of surgery, has a very low incidence of side effects and should reduce the incidence of aspiration pneumonitis by decreasing the pH and volume of gastric contents.

In patients with evidence of autonomic neuropathy, we recommend a rapid sequence induction to further reduce the risk of aspiration. The endotracheal tube should be placed while an assistant maintains cricoid pressure (Sellick maneuver). Burgos et al.[22] studied cardiovascular morbidity in diabetics undergoing general anesthesia and determined that diabetic autonomic neuropathy is associated with an increased risk of perioperative cardiovascular instability. They noted bradycardia and hypotension in 35% of diabetic patients with autonomic neuropathy. These cardiovascular events occurred most frequently following induction and intubation. Because diabetic patients have a high incidence of hypertension and peripheral vascular disease, they are at risk for ischemic injury to the heart, kidney, and brain during hypotensive or bradycardiac episodes. Careful monitoring of the cardiovascular system is warranted in all patients, but especially in the diabetic patient with autonomic neuropathy. The anesthesiologist should be prepared to treat aggressively either hypotension or bradycardia and should be especially vigilant in the interval following induction and intubation.

The internist or diabetologist should have the diabetic patient in the best possible control prior to elective surgery. Oxygen-carrying capacity of the blood is influenced by the long-term blood glucose control. Factors that influence oxygenation should be optimized prior to anesthesia. These factors are of increased importance during anesthesia. An increase in hemoglobin A_{1c} causes a shift of the oxyhemoglobin dissociation curve to the left, so that oxygen is more tightly bound to the hemoglobin. This shift is similar to that which occurs with alkalosis, hypothermia, and decreased levels of 2,3 diphosphoglycerate. Such shifts cause hemoglobin to give up its bound oxygen less readily and lead to a decline in tissue oxygenation. The fraction of hemoglobin that has been converted to glycosylated hemoglobin reflects what the blood glucose level has been in the 2 to 3 months preceding the measurement. *The anesthe-*

siologist should encourage his medical and surgical colleagues to maintain careful control of the blood glucose level for months before planned surgery.

Choice of Anesthetic Technique

There is no "best" anesthetic for the diabetic patient. Each anesthetic must be a mixture of medicines, techniques, and monitoring that is suited to the patient's physiological reserve and the planned anatomical trespass. The modern inhalation anesthetics are widely used and they modify carbohydrate metabolism. The inhalation anesthetics cause insulin secretion to be decreased, secondary to increased sympathetic activity and increased norepinephrine levels. The increase in levels of norepinephrine as well as increases in cortisol and growth hormone levels contribute to elevated intraoperative blood glucose levels. (See Chapter 17.) Decreased insulin release has been reported as an effect of halothane[26] and enflurane.[27] The effects on carbohydrate metabolism of isoflurane have been studied more closely by Diltoer and Camu.[28] They studied glucose tolerance in three groups of human subjects: awake, anesthetized with isoflurane, and anesthetized with isoflurane during surgery. They found that isoflurane anesthesia resulted in impaired insulin secretion. The expected glucose intolerance during anesthesia resulted. In the patients that they studied who underwent anesthesia and surgery, there was an increased plasma level of cortisol and growth hormone. The end result in this group was increased glucose intolerance, even though insulin secretion was not reduced further than in the group with anesthesia alone. The authors of this study speculated that increased glucose intolerance was due to peripheral tissue effects. Saho et al.[29] demonstrated that sevoflurane has a rapidly reversible inhibitory effect on basal and glucose-stimulated insulin secretion in pigs. Controversy has existed for many years about whether general anesthesia or regional anesthesia offers more advantages for the surgical patient.[30] The same controversy has existed about the best anesthetic technique for the diabetic patient. Objections to spinal and epidural anesthesia in the diabetic have been made on medicolegal grounds. Many, possibly all, diabetic patients have some degree of diabetic neuropathy. Therefore, the reasoning goes, regional anesthesia is contraindicated because, if the patient develops postoperative neurological deficit from any cause, the patient might later blame the neurological deficit on the regional anesthetic. There is, however, no convincing evidence regional anesthesia makes diabetic neuropathy worse.

Regional anesthesia, especially spinal and epidural, is associated with less hyperglycemia than is general anesthesia in the nondiabetic patient. Afferent blockade of painful operative stimuli and blockade of sympathetic input from the operative site help prevent the hyperglycemia.[31] There is a strong clinical impression that there is less hyperglycemia in the diabetic patient who has a high-level epidural blockade. This impression is attributed to splanchnic blockade and draws on the work of Griffiths,[32] who showed that sympathetic blockade with hexamethonium decreased the hyperglycemic response to surgery in diabetic patients who have general anesthesia. Epidural or spinal anesthesia of an appropriate level would cause a local anesthetic block of the sympathetic fibers to the splanchnic plexus. In a 1980 report, Romano and Gullo[33] described a diabetic patient who became hypoglycemic following the institution of epidural blockade for a surgical procedure. The hypoglycemia was believed to be caused by splanchnic blockade and resulting abolishment of adrenal release of catecholamines and inhibition of hepatic glycogenolysis.

An advantage of regional anesthesia is that the physician is dealing with an awake patient who will become aware of hypoglycemia if his or her blood sugar becomes low enough to cause him or her to be symptomatic. There is less pain in the immediate postoperative interval, often enabling the patient to return to a normal diet earlier. The use of regional anesthesia enables the patient to avoid narcotics that can promote nausea and vomiting; and, of course, this method has an unexcelled safety record. The final choice of anesthetic technique should be made only after careful evaluation of the patient's preoperative medical condition.

Rationale for Close Control of the Blood Glucose During Anesthesia

It is increasingly common for intraoperative hyperglycemia to be treated aggressively. This approach is relatively new in the intraoperative management of the diabetic patient. Cahill and colleagues,[34] in 1976, stressed the importance of close control of the blood glucose in preventing or delaying the development of late complications such as nephropathy and retinopathy. Their editorial summarized the belief of many physicians that careful control of the blood glucose over the long term is desirable to prevent later complications. However, the value of close control of the blood glucose for the short duration of a surgical procedure is less clear. Despite the technical ability to normalize the blood glucose, prospective data comparing surgical outcomes following improved glycemic control during the perioperative period are not available.[34] The fear of hypoglycemia is one factor that makes physicians reluctant to maintain normal blood glucose levels in anesthetized diabetic patients. It is true that more than customary care must be exercised because the unconscious patient cannot detect the symptoms of early hypoglycemia. Also, the external signs are subtle, such as a slight increase in pulse rate and decreased urinary output. Understandably, these signs are difficult to detect and interpret clinically during anesthesia.

The rationale for maintaining the blood sugar in a normal range is that the physiological changes resulting from hyperglycemia increase the risk of, and thus delay recovery from, surgery.

The most common causes of morbidity and mortality in the diabetic surgical patient are infection and myocardial infarction. The sequelae of intraoperative hyperglycemia contribute directly or indirectly to these two complications. Hyperglycemia leads to glycosuria, which leads to polyuria, which yields a patient dehydrated by osmotic diuresis. (See Chapter 24.) Such a patient can be hemodynamically unstable during anesthesia when drugs that cause vasodilation, such as the inhalation anesthetics or propofol, an intravenous anesthetic, are administered. Hyperglycemia renders the patient less able to resist infection.[35] Intraoperative hyperglycemia has also been shown to decrease tensile strength and healing of the wound,[36] to impair phagocytosis by neutrophilic leukocytes,[37] and to increase circulating free fatty acids. The utilization of free fatty acids in myocardial metabolism requires a higher oxygen consumption than does glucose utilization.[38] When oxygen is being consumed at a higher rate, and the patient has borderline oxygenation because of increased pulmonary shunt or other problems seen in the anesthetized patient, increased tissue oxygen consumption can have grave consequences. Though there are no controlled prospective studies showing that close control of the blood glucose in the relatively brief intraoperative period lowers morbidity in the diabetic patient, much is known about the body's metabolic response to surgery and how that response is altered by insulin. This knowledge reinforces the clinical impression that close control of the blood glucose in the perioperative period has advantages for the patient that outweigh possible disadvantages. In the normal state, when the body is fed, there is increased insulin release, which promotes anabolism. Food is stored in the form of glycogen and triglycerides; protein synthesis is also promoted. In the fasting state, as in the perioperative period, the blood glucose drops and the body begins to utilize the food stores. First, the liver glycogen is used; then, if the fast is prolonged, protein is used. Even in the fasting state, there is a low basal level of insulin available. This low level of insulin protects the body because insulin is a totally anabolic hormone. It promotes glycogenesis, lipogenesis, and protein synthesis. It retards glycogenolysis, gluconeogenesis, lipolysis, ketogenesis, and proteolysis. It is this function of acting as a brake on the tearing down of the body's stores that makes its presence necessary. (See Chapter 7.)

In the surgical patient who is diabetic, there should be adequate insulin present. It is possible for a patient with insulin-dependent diabetes to develop DKA with a blood glucose that is only moderately elevated. Seventeen percent of all diagnosed diabetic ketoacidosis is in patients with blood glucose concentrations <300 mg/dL and values <100 mg/dL have been reported.[39–41] (See Chapter 24.) The insulin brake on catabolic processes is needed, for surgery might well be termed "maximum starvation." Caloric and nutritive intake is down at a time when substrate needs are at their highest. In addition, the catabolic hormones cortisol, catecholamines, and glucagon are present at high levels. The insulin-dependent diabetic, then, unless provided with exogenous insulin, has impaired defenses against the accelerated catabolism of surgery. (See Chapter 17.)

Administration of Insulin on the Day of Surgery

There was a time when great emphasis was placed on making sure that the diabetic patient was first on the surgical schedule. In the past, more often than not, no insulin was given until surgery was over. Today, the complexities of a busy operating room schedule as well as the reality that many, if not most patients, will arrive at the hospital on the day of surgery, do not allow diabetic patients always to be first on the surgical schedule. All these uncertainties not withstanding, a patient *should not be without fluids and insulin* until the hour of surgery arrives. A reasonable approach is to begin intravenous fluids containing glucose at an appropriate rate to keep the patient hydrated and to administer a continuous low-dose infusion of regular or lispro insulin. Blood glucose levels should be monitored through this interval of insulin administration, and appropriate changes in administration rates made, to keep the blood glucose near the normal range. The patient treated in such a way will arrive in the operating room hydrated and in an anabolic state. *The practice of giving no insulin before or during surgery is mentioned only to condemn it.* The only rationale for this outdated practice is that it avoids the threat of hypoglycemia. Today's technology has provides a simple, expedient, and low-cost means to avoid hypoglycemia by intermittent monitoring of the blood glucose.

A popular method of administering insulin on the day of surgery is to give one half or two thirds of the patient's usual dose of intermediate-acting insulin subcutaneously in the morning.

One of the *major disadvantages of this method involves the lack of predictability of absorption from the subcutaneous tissue* in surgical patients. During anesthesia, shivering is abolished, and patients are exposed in cold operating rooms while they are painted with cold antiseptic solutions. A significant amount of heat is lost from the body during induction, positioning, and preparation. The heat loss continues during surgery, at a slower rate. The cold patient develops peripheral vasoconstriction, which impedes uniform predictable absorption of drugs from the subcutaneous tissue. When the patient rewarms in the recovery room, long-delayed insulin absorption begins and unexpected hypoglycemia can occur.

A study of the "partial-dose" treatment method was carried out by Walts et al.[42] They compared the intraoperative plasma glucose levels in patients who received no insulin and who served as control subjects, with patients who received a partial dose, one fourth to one half of their usual dose, subcutaneously. The group receiving a partial dose of insulin did not differ significantly in blood glucose levels from the control group that received no insulin. In both groups, during surgery, blood glucose values increased during surgery by at least 75% of baseline values. The "partial-dose" method of administration insulin might perform a useful function, such as providing sufficient insulin to promote anabolism, but it does not contribute to improved control of the blood glucose.

The third method of insulin administration is continuous intravenous infusion before and during surgery. This method was prompted by reports that appeared in the mid-1970s of the successful treatment of diabetic ketoacidosis with low-dose continuous insulin infusions. A few years later, Taitelman and colleagues,[43] in a prospective, randomized study, showed that they could achieve better intraoperative control of the blood sugar with a continuous infusion of regular insulin at 2 U/hr than by using two thirds the daily dose of intermediate-acting insulin given subcutaneously in the preoperative interval.

Intravenous administration of insulin during surgery is a practical way to meet the intraoperative insulin needs. Various protocols have been presented for the control of hyperglycemia during surgery.[44] Instead of rigid protocols, flexibility in intraoperative insulin administration is desirable. This flexibility should be based on frequent, reliable, and readily available blood glucose determinations. The insulin administration rate should be changed as often as necessary to achieve the target blood glucose values. A reasonable goal for the intraoperative blood glucose is 80 to 180 mg/dL.

Two generally accepted methods of continuous glucose administration are the (1) GIK infusion wherein glucose, insulin, and potassium are contained in the same bag, and (2) a protocol whereby glucose, insulin, and potassium are infused separately. The GIK infusion has the disadvantage in that the whole bag must be changed each time the blood glucose in outside the target range.[42,45] One must keep in mind that it is not always neccessary to infuse potassium along with glucose and insulin, though it is prudent to be aware of serum potassium levels as long as insulin is infused.

The practice of administering insulin by injecting large intravenous doses is controversial and should be considered dangerous and unphysiological. This "roller coaster" approach can ultimately lead to a greater rate of lipolysis and ketogenesis as well as dangerous hypoglycemia.

In the postoperative interval, when the physician is not continuously present, an algorithm for insulin administration is recommended. Watts et al.[46] compared blood glucose control in two groups of patients, one in which a "glucose-feedback" formula was used to maintain the plasma glucose between 120 and 180 mg/dL, and a control group of routinely managed diabetic patients, during the first 24 hr after surgery. They showed that better control of the blood glucose was achieved with the algorithm than in the control group. This algorithm was well accepted by the nursing staff and produced no dangerously high or low blood glucose values.

Insulin is absorbed by intravenous bags, bottles, and tubing. The amount of insulin that the patient actually receives has been reported over a wide range of values. Petty and Cunningham[47] showed a 52.5% rate of absorption by the fluid bottle or bag, with an additional 55.4% of the remaining drug absorbed by the tubing, for a total of 78.8% that remains on the plastic and glass containers. The wide range of reported absorption probably means that every combination of container and tubing absorbs a different amount of insulin. There are steps that can be taken to moderate this phenomenon. The addition of 1 mL of 25% human albumin to each liter of fluid will decrease absorption by one half or more. The insulin binds to receptor-like sites on the glass and plastic containers. These sites can be saturated by allowing the first portion of the fluid to run freely through the system. This serves to fill the available sites, and less insulin will be lost from the subsequent flow to the patient.[48]

Insulin is not the only factor of importance in the control of the blood glucose. Intravenous fluids must be given in a considered way. Glucose should be given at a constant rate, and 100 mg/kg/hr will provide enough glucose to spare glycogen stores. Rapid fluid administration is often needed during anesthesia to replenish the intravascular volume at the time of hemorrhage or to fill the vascular system after vasodilating inhalation anesthetic agents are given. Therefore, a fluid that does not contain glucose must be used as the primary intravenous fluid for rapid administration when needed, and the glucose-containing fluid is con-

tinued as a piggyback administration. The primary intravenous fluid should not be lactated Ringer's solution. Lactate is a glycogenic precursor, and the rate of gluconeogenesis may be enhanced by lactate in diabetic patients, especially in the stressful surgical setting. Thomas and Alberti[49] compared the blood glucose concentrations of patients with noninsulin-dependent diabetes who received lactated Ringer's solution during surgery, with the blood glucose concentrations of similar patients who did not receive intravenous fluids. The patients receiving lactated Ringer's solution had significantly higher blood glucose concentrations than the comparison group. Their study suggests that solutions containing lactate may be metabolically disadvantageous in the diabetic patient.

Monitoring Glucose and Electrolytes

If the patient is to receive insulin intraoperatively, the blood glucose must be monitored. It is equally important that frequent measurements of electrolyte levels be made. Multiple samples of blood that are not contaminated by intravenous fluids are necessary during longer cases. An intra-arterial catheter is one practical approach to access. Many operating room suites now have on-site laboratories where glucose, electrolyte, and other laboratory studies can be done. It is *important to have laboratory tests performed rapidly and returned within minutes* to the operating room, so that frequent changes in the rate of insulin administration can be made.

The reflectance photometer [One Touch®, (Johnson & Johnson) Milpitas, California; Accu-Check® (The Roche Group) Basel, Switzerland] is another way to obtain rapid blood glucose determinations in the operating room. The reflectance photometer has been shown to provide accurate blood glucose values when compared with traditional laboratory measurements.[50]

Some medicines commonly given to anesthetized patients have an effect on laboratory glucose determinations. This phenomenon has not been thoroughly studied, but it has been reported that dopamine inhibits the chemical reaction in glucose reagent strips used in reflectance photometers.[51] In general, however, the reflectance photometer provides glucose determinations of satisfactory reliability in the operating room.

Positioning the Diabetic Patient for Surgery

There is an *increased risk of nerve injury in the diabetic patient during anesthesia*. In the unconscious, analgesic, and immobile anesthetized patient, the protective shifts and turns of normal sleep are abolished. If such a patient is then positioned so that the weight of the body compresses the brachial plexus or other nerves, nerve damage can occur. In addition, stretching of trunks and plexuses produces a similar injury. One of the most common ways that this happens is when the patient's arm is elevated more than 90° from the trunk, especially if it is allowed to sag below the midplane of the body in the supine patient. Turning the patient's head severely away from the outstretched arm can also promote nerve damage. This produces nerve injury because the brachial plexus is stretched around the head of the humerus. Injury also occurs when surgeons and assistants lean on, or hyperextend, the patient's outstretched arms in their efforts to gain access to the surgical field.

In a report published during the 1950s, the authors reported that awake volunteers would tolerate hyperabduction of the arms and a steep Trendelenburg position for only a few minutes, and that the radial pulse disappeared in 83% of the volunteers so positioned.[52] The promise that the procedure is to be brief often lulls the anesthesiologist into a false sense of security and causes clinicians not to pad or position the patients as carefully as they do for longer procedures. Britt and colleagues[53] claim that only 30 to 40 min of anesthesia in an unfavorable position is sufficient to result in nerve palsy. The vast majority of nerve injuries, however, occur in procedures that last longer than 6 hr. A 1989 study of closed malpractice claims between 1961 and 1984, related to anesthetic care showed 15% of all claims were related to nerve injuries, a rate second only to death as an outcome.[54]

Gilliatt and Willison[55] have suggested from information gained in a study of peripheral nerve conduction in diabetic patients that mononeuritic lesions are common and often follow even minor trauma. Studies such as these have reinforced the commonly held belief that neuropathies following surgery are more common in the diabetic patient.

The mechanism of nerve injury is compromise of small-caliber vascular beds in the nerve, resulting in ischemic damage. The most common way that this occurs is by stretching the nerve. It also occurs from compression, but less often. Positioning must be done carefully and padding must be generous in those patients with a propensity to neural injury.

The outlook for nondiabetic patients who have nerve injuries is good; for the patient with diabetes mellitus, it is not so favorable. Patients with grade 1 injuries, that is, those with no axonal degeneration, will recover in a matter of weeks and should have no motor or sensory deficit. In patients with grade 2 injuries there is damage to the axon but the nerve sheath remains intact. This type of injury is less common but heals spontaneously in weeks or months. Nerve regeneration can be expected to progress at the rate of approximately 1 mm/day.

In Parks[56] retrospective study of postoperative peripheral neuropathies, 72 patients who developed neuropathies out of 50,000 patients who had surgery were identified, for an incidence of 1.5/1000 individuals. Eight of those 72 patients had diabetes. This represents 11% of those affected and is higher than the 5% prevalence of diabetes mellitus in the general population.

The Diabetic Patient in the Recovery Room

Insulin infusion, regulation of glucose-containing fluids, and frequent monitoring of the blood glucose and electrolytes should continue during the recovery room stay. Patients with autonomic neuropathy should have especially close cardiorespiratory monitoring. Page and Watkins[57] reported on 12 cardiorespiratory arrests that occurred in eight young diabetics with severe autonomic neuropathy. Five of the episodes occurred during or immediately after anesthesia. These authors suggested that the mechanism of the arrests involved defective respiratory rather than cardiovascular reflexes. They further speculated that the administration of respiratory depressant drugs during anesthesia, and for postoperative pain, was the precipitating event. It is known that, in animals, the ventilatory response to hypoxia is decreased by vagal blockade[58] or by carotid body denervation.[59] *Patients with autonomic neuropathy are very vulnerable to the anesthesia and analgesic drugs that they are given.* More intensive monitoring and observation in the postoperative interval are warranted.

Research Considerations

A large-scale audit of the outcome of surgery in diabetic patients needs to be done. Drugs used for anesthesia, techniques, and monitoring procedures have changed dramatically in the past few years. There has not been an investigation of morbidity and mortality in the diabetic surgical patient since these changes occurred. *Comparisons need to be made of the morbidity and mortality in well-controlled and poorly controlled diabetic patients.* The incidence of morbidity and mortality for each anesthetic technique and agent should be tabulated. Optimal strategies for managing the diabetic patient can be formulated from this information. Such a study would more clearly delineate the risk that poor or good control of the blood glucose conferred on the surgery patient. Basic science and clinical studies into the nature and significance of the hyperglycemic response to trauma and surgery need to be done. More than 100 years ago, Claude Bernard observed that hyperglycemia followed head injury. The significance of this phenomenon is still incompletely understood. The hyperglycemic response has been said to be protective for the organism. Investigations need to be done to evaluate whether or not hyperglycemia during surgery is indeed protective in humans and to determine at what point it ceases to be protective and when measures to lower the blood glucose level should be initiated in the diabetic patient.

Conclusion

The anesthesiologist is in a unique position to intervene positively in the diabetic surgical patient's care. By monitoring the blood glucose during surgery, in addition to the other physiological variables monitored routinely, and by using insulin to limit hyperglycemia, the surgical experience can become a metabolically stable interval for the patient with diabetes.

References

1. Root HF: Pre-operative care of the diabetic patient. Post grad Med 40:439–444, 1966.

2. Galloway JA, Shuman CR: Diabetes and surgery. A study of 667 cases. Am J Med 34:177–192, 1963.

3. Wheelock FC Jr, Marble A: Surgery and diabetes. In Marble A, White P, Bradley RF, Krall LP (eds): Joslin's Diabetes Mellitus, Ed. 11. Philadelphia: Lea & Febiger, 1971, pp. 599–620.

4. Hjortrup A, Rasmussen B, Kehlet H: Morbidity in diabetic and non-diabetic patients after major vascular surgery. Br Med J 257:1107–1108, 1983.

5. Steen PA, Tinker JH, Tarhan S: Myocardial reinfarction after anesthesia and surgery. JAMA 239:2566–2570, 1978.

6. Rao TLK, Jacobs KH, El-Etr AA: Reinfarction following anesthesia in patients with myocardial infarction. Anesthesiology 59:499–505, 1983.

7. Solar NG, Pentecost BL, Bennett MA, et al.: Coronary care for myocardial infarction in diabetics. Lancet 1:475, 1974.

8. Burgos LG, Ebert JE, Asiddao C, et al.: Increased intraoperative morbidity in diabetics with autonomic neuropathy. Anesthesiology 70:591–597, 1989.

9. Latson TW, Ashmore TH, Reinhart DJ, et al.: Autonomic dysfunction in patients presenting for elective surgery is associated with hypotension after anesthesia induction. Anesthesiology 80:326–337, 1994.

10. Vohra A, Kumar S, Charlton AJ, et al.: Effect of diabetes mellitus on the cardiovascular responses to induction of anaesthesia and tracheal intubation. Br J Anaesth 71:258–261, 1993.

11. Triantafillou AN, Tseuda K, Berg J, et al.: Refractory bradycardia after reversal of muscle relaxant in a diabetic with vagal neuropathy. Anesth Analg 65:1237–1241, 1986.

12. Page MM, Watkins PJ: Cardiorespiratoy arrests and diabetic autonomic neuropathy. Lancet 1:14–16, 1978.

13. Ciccarelli LL, Ford CM, Tseuda K: Autonomic neuropathy in a diabetic patient with renal failure. Anesthesiology 64:283–287, 1986.

14. Slogoff S, Keats A, Arlund C: On the safety of radial artery cannulation. Anesthesiology 59:42–47, 1983.

15. Hogan K, Rusy D, Springman SR: Difficult laryngoscopy and diabetes mellitus. Anesth Analg 67:1162–1165, 1988.

16. Salzarulo HH, Taylor LA: Diabetic "stiff joint syndrome" as a cause of difficult endotracheal intubation. Anesthesiology 64:366, 1986.

17. Finucane BT, Santora AH: Principles of Airway Management, 2nd Ed., Mosby, 1996, pp. 109–110. St. Louis, MO.

18. Mulhall BP, O'Fearghail M: Diabetic gastroparesis. Anaesthesia 39:468–469, 1984.

19. Mendelson CL: The aspiration of stomach contents into the lungs during obstetric anesthesia. Am J Obstet Gynecol 52:191, 1946.

20. Gibbs CP, Modell JH: Aspiration pneumonitis. In Miller RD (ed): Anesthesia, Ed. 2. New York: Churchill Livingstone, 1986, pp. 2023–2050.

21. Cameron JL, Mitchell WH, Zuidema GD: Aspiration pneumonia anesthetic: Clinical outcome following documented aspiration. Arch Surg 106:49, 1973.

22. Burgos LG, Ebert TJ, Caridad A, et al.: Increased intraoperative cardiovascular morbidity in diabetics with autonomic neuropathy. Anesthesiology 70:591–597, 1989.

23. Weber L, Hirshman CA: Cimetidine for prophylaxis of aspiration pneumonitis: Comparison of intramuscular and oral dose schedules. Anesth Analg 58:427, 1979.

24. Snape WJ, Battle WM, Schwartz SS, et al.: Metoclopramide treatment of gastroparesis due to diabetes mellitus, a double-blind controlled trial. Ann Intern Med 96:444–446, 1982.

25. Capan LM, Rosenberg AD, Carni A, et al.: Effect of cimetidine-metoclopramide combination on gastric fluid volume and acidity. Anesthesiology 59:A402, 1983.

26. Camu F: Carbohydrate intolerance during halothane anesthesia in dogs. Acta Anaesthesiol Belg 24:177–188, 1973.

27. Camu F: Impaired early insulin response to glycemic stimulus during enflurane anesthesia in dogs. Acta Anaesthesiol Belg 27:S267–S271, 1976.

28. Diltoer M, Camu F: Glucose homeostasis and insulin secretion during isoflurane anesthesia in humans. Anesthesiology 68:880–886, 1988.

29. Saho S, Kadota Y, Sameshima T, et al.: The effects of sevoflurane anesthesia on insulin secretion and glucose metabolism in pigs. Anesth Analg 84:1359–1365, 1997.

30. Hammonds W, Freniere S, O'Brien D, et al.: A retrospective comparison of spinal and general anesthesia for

transurethral resection of the prostate. Reg Anesth 4:8–10, 1979.

31. Bromage PR, Shibata HR, Willoughby HW: Influence of prolonged epidural blockage on blood sugar and cortisol responses to operation upon the upper part of the abdomen and the thorax. Surg Gynecol Obstet 132: 1051–1056, 1971.

32. Griffiths IA: The effects of general anaesthesia and Hexamethonium on the blood sugar in non-diabetic and diabetic surgical patients. Q J Med 22:405–418, 1953.

33. Romano E, Gullo A: Hypoglycaemic coma following epidural analgesia. Anaesthesia 35:1084–1086, 1980.

34. Cahill GF Jr, Etzwiler DD, Frienkel N: "Control" and diabetes. N Engl J Med 294:1004–1010, 1976.

35. Cruse PJ, Foord R: A 5–year prospective study of 23,649 surgical wounds. Arch Surg 107:206–210, 1973.

36. Goodson WH, Hunt TK: Studies of wound healing in experimental diabetes mellitus. J Surg Res 22:221–227, 1977.

37. Bagdade JD: Phagocytic and microbiological function in diabetes mellitus. Acta Endocrinol (Copenh) 83:27–31, 1976.

38. Wahlquist ML, Kayser L, Lassers BW: Fatty acids as a determinant of myocardial substrate and oxygen metabolism in man at rest and during prolonged exercise. Acta Med Scand 193:83–96, 1973.

39. Monro JF, Campbell IW, McGuish AG, et al.: Euglycemic diabetic ketoacidosis. Br Med J 2:578–580, 1973.

40. Bradley RF: Diabetic ketoacidosis and coma. *In* (eds): Joslins's Diabetes Mellitus, 11th. Philadelphia: Lea & Febiger, 1971, p. 380.

41. Hirsch IB, McGill JB, Cryer PE, et al.: Perioperative management of surgical patients with diabetes mellitus. Anesthesiology 74:346–359, 1991.

42. Walts LF, Miller JD, Mayer B, et al.: Perioperative management of diabetes mellitus. Anesthesiology 55:106–109, 1981.

43. Taitelman U, Reece E, Bessman A: Insulin in the management of the diabetic surgical patient. JAMA 237: 658–660, 1977.

44. Woodruff RD, Lewis SE, McLeskey MD, et al.: Avoidance of surgical hyperglycemia in diabetic patients. JAMA 244:166–168, 1980.

45. Alberti KGMM, Gill GV, Elliot MJ: Insulin delivery during surgery in the diabetic patient. Diabetes Care 5(Suppl.):65–77, 1982.

46. Watts NE, Gebhart SSP, Clark RV, et al.: Postoperative management of diabetes mellitus: Steady-state glucose control with bedside algorithm for insulin adjustment. Diabetes Care 10:722–728, 1987.

47. Petty C, Cunningham NL: Insulin absorption by glass infusion bottles, polyvinylchloride infusion containers and intravenous tubing. Anesthesiology 40:400–404, 1974.

48. Peterson L, Caldwell J, Hoffman J: Insulin adsorbance to polyvinylchloride surfaces with implications for constant infusion therapy. Diabetes 25:72–74, 1976.

49. Thomas DJB, Alberti KGMM: The hyperglycemic effects of Hartmann's solution in maturity-onset diabetics during surgery. Br J Anaesthesiol 50:185–188, 1978.

50. Peterson CM: Quality control for glucose monitoring programs. Diabetes Educ 11:19–21, 1985.

51. Keeling AB, Schmidt P: Dopamine influence on whole blood glucose reagent strips. Diabetes Care 10:532, 1987.

52. Westin B: Prevention of upper limb nerve injuries in Trendelenburg position. Acta Clin Scand 108:61–69, 1954.

53. Britt BA, Joy N, Mackay MB: Positioning trauma. *In* Orkin FK, Cooperman LH (eds): Complications in Anesthesiology. Philadelphia: J.B. Lippincott, 1983, pp. 646–670.

54. Cheney FW, Posner MA, Caplan RA, et al.: Standard of care and anesthesia liability: JAMA 261:1599–1603, 1989.

55. Gilliatt RW, Willison RG: Peripheral nerve conduction in diabetic neuropathy. JNeurol Neurosurg Psychiatry 25:11–18,1962.

56. Parks BJ: Postoperative peripheral neuropathies. Surgery 74:348–357, 1973.

57. Page M, Watkins PJ: Cardiorespiratory arrest and diabetic autonomic neuropathy. Lancet 1(8054):14–16, 1978.

58. Phillipson EA, Hickey RF, Bainton CR: Effect of vagal blockade on regulation of breathing in conscious dogs. J Appl Physiol 29:475–479, 1970.

59. Bisgard GE, Forster HV, Orr J: Hypoventilation in ponies after carotid body denervation. J Appl Physiol 40: 184–190, 1976.

44

Infections in Diabetes Mellitus

Kathryn E. Arnold and John E. McGowan, Jr.

Historical Perspective

The relationship between diabetes and infection has been important to clinicians for many centuries. Before the advent of insulin therapy and availability of antimicrobial agents, infection was a major cause of death for diabetic patients and occurred frequently in the short life span expected for those with this disease. In developed countries today, mortality among patients with diabetes is largely attributed to associated cardiovascular and renal problems, but infection is a major cause of excess morbidity.[1,2] Infection continues to be a principal cause of death among diabetics in developing countries. Recent work has questioned the concept of a generalized susceptibility to infection, but has confirmed that diabetic patients are at increased risk for infection at specific sites and due to certain organisms.[3]

Epidemiology

Infection is a leading cause of hospitalization among diabetic patients, with foot infection alone accounting for more than one in four hospital admissions.[4,5] Diabetes is associated with increased severity of infection and prolonged hospital stays.[6,7] Diabetics are overrepresented among patients in many studies of common infections such as urinary tract infection, soft-tissue infection, pneumonia, and osteomyelitis. However, it has been difficult to document that diabetics have an increased frequency of these infections because large prospective studies are lacking. A recent review of the existing data concludes that diabetic patients are at higher risk than nondiabetics for asymptomatic bacteriuria, lower extremity infections, surgical wound infections, group B streptococcal infections, and reactivation of tuberculosis.[3] Rates of influenza and pneumonia may be similar among diabetic and control populations, but mortality rates are higher for diabetic patients with these diagnoses. Although definitive data are lacking, dia-

betes may also be associated with increased prevalence of cystitis, pyelonephritis, candida vulvovaginitis and cystitis, bacteremia, primary tuberculosis, mucormycosis, malignant otitis externa, Fournier's gangrene, periodontal disease, salmonella infections, pneumonia, influenza, and chronic bronchitis.[3,8] Although they are rare even among diabetics, clinicians should be mindful of uncommon severe infections such as rhinocerebral mucormycosis, necrotizing soft-tissue infections, malignant otitis externa, endophthalmitis and emphysematous cholecystitis or pyelonephritis in order to allow for early recognition and intervention (see Problem Statements).

Effect of Diabetes Control on Occurrence of Infection

The Diabetes Control and Complications Trial (DCCT) did not study infection as an outcome of glycemic control, but *in vitro* data and clinical studies support the hypothesis that near-normoglycemia may lower risk for infection. Rayfield and colleagues[9] demonstrated a strong association between outpatient plasma glucose measurements and incidence of infection requiring hospitalization or emergency room attention. In this study of 261 diabetic patients, the incidence of infection doubled among patients with baseline glucose measurements of 12 to 16.2 mM, demonstrating that hyperglycemia need not be extreme to increase susceptibility to infection.[9] Among surgical patients with diabetes, better perioperative glucose control is associated with fewer wound infections,[10,11] and lower risk for bacteremia and pneumonia.[10] Catheter-related infections are five times more common among diabetic patients on total parenteral nutrition (TPN) than among the general population receiving TPN (17 vs. 2.8–3.5%).[12] Elevated glycosylated hemoglobin levels are associated with higher mortality rates in diabetics hospitalized for suspected acute infection.[13]

Effect of Infection on Management of Diabetes

Infection may impair glycemic control by increasing insulin resistance. Medical stressors such as infection result in a marked increase in plasma levels of counter-regulatory hormones, which increase glucose release from the liver. Rayfield demonstrated that experimental administration of bacterial endotoxin to juvenile diabetics caused significant increases in plasma glucagon, growth hormone, cortisol and adrenocorticotropic hormone (ACTH), necessitating administration of 30% more insulin than at baseline.[14] Cytokines that alter carbohydrate metabolism such as interleukin-1 (IL-1) and tumor necrosis factor (TNF) are increased in plasma during infection, and may also stimulate the release of counter-regulatory hormones.[15] Infection is frequently a precipitating factor for diabetic ketoacidosis.[16,17]

Pathophysiology

The altered milieux of hyperglycemia and/or ketoacidosis impair host defenses. In addition, diabetic complications of neuropathy (autonomic, sensory, and motor) and vascular abnormalities compromise defenses against infection. Colonization and overgrowth of organisms may predispose to infection with specific pathogens. Vascular abnormalities may impair healing and delivery of medications (see below).

Altered Host Defenses

Polymorphonuclear leukocytes (also called neutrophils, granulocytes, or PMNs) are phagocytic cells that ingest and kill opsonized (antibody- and complement-coated) bacteria. Many studies document abnormalities of PMN function in diabetic patients. However, abnormal PMN adherence,[18,19] chemotaxis,[20,21] phagocytosis,[22] respiratory burst,[23–26] and microbicidal ability,[9,25,27] all can improve with tighter glycemic control. A recent in vitro study also suggests that granulocyte-colony stimulating factor (G-CSF) can improve respiratory burst in neutrophils from poorly controlled diabetics.[28] Hyperglycemia and acidemia may both affect PMN function.[15] Several authors have found that in poorly controlled diabetics, PMN respiratory burst is increased at baseline[25,29] and impaired with stimulation.[25,26,30,31] This counterproductive state could predispose to tissue damage as well as poor bacterial killing.

Antibody production and complement levels are normal in diabetics. Cell-mediated immunity relies on the interaction of T lymphocytes and mononuclear phagocytes (monocytes), to control intracellular pathogens such as viruses, fungi, and tuberculosis.[32,33] Impaired monocyte chemotaxis is reported in diabetic patients.[34]

Vascular Abnormalities

Medium and smaller blood vessels may be insufficient in diabetic patients, resulting in poor circulation to tissues, with hypoxemia. These conditions favor microorganisms that can survive anaerobically, predisposing to necrotizing soft tissue infections, abscess formation, and emphysematous complications. Diminished blood flow also slows the local inflammatory response and delivery of antimicrobial agents.

Role of Procedures

There is an increased likelihood that invasive medical procedures will be performed in diabetics; many of these precedures may increase risk of infection. Examples include postoperative wound infection after cardiac surgery and catheter-associated urinary tract infections. A recent report of hepatitis B transmission in a hospital setting associated with a reusable multipatient autolet serves as a reminder that meticulous care is needed to ensure patient safety where percutaneous procedures are common, as they are in diabetics.[35] Hepatitis serum markers are two to four times more prevalent among diabetic patients than among the general population, possibly as a result of nosocomial exposures.[36–38]

Neurological Abnormalities

Diabetic patients with peripheral motor neuropathy are prone to the development of neuropathic ulcers through anatomic deformities and altered weight-bearing surfaces. Lack of sensation associated with peripheral sensory neuropathy leads to delayed recognition of soft-tissue injury. Autonomic neuropathy causes diminished perspiration, and leads to dry, cracked skin. These changes allow microorganisms to penetrate the skin barrier.

Autonomic cystopathy predisposes to urinary retention and bacteriuria, and gastroparesis may result in malnutrition, dehydration and/or delayed absorption of oral antimicrobial drugs. Emphysematous complications of infections in the urinary and gastrointestinal tracts may result from local stasis and tissue hypoxia.

Organisms

Staphylococcus aureus

Staphylococcus aureus is the principal cause of skin and soft-tissue infections and osteomyelitis in diabetic patients as well as normal hosts. Despite prevailing belief, no controlled studies document that diabetic patients in general are at increased risk for staphylococcal bacteremia. However, it has been shown that diabetic hemodialysis patients are at increased risk of *S. aureus* infections. Higher mortality rates occur among diabetics with *S. aureus* bacteremia than among nondiabetics, and diabetics may be at higher risk for endocarditis when bacteremia is found. Cooper and Platt[39] compared the presentation and course of 27 episodes of *S. aureus* bacteremia in diabetic patients with 34 episodes in nondiabetic patients. Endocarditis was diagnosed in 30% of diabetics and 12% of nondiabetics. Of the diabetic patients with infective endocarditis, 88% were community-acquired, compared with 100% of endocarditis infections in nondiabetics. One of three diabetics with a primary focus of infection (foot ulcer, osteomyelitis, surgical wound, i.v. catheter, dialysis shunt, or pneumonia) had infective endocarditis, compared with none of the 22 nondiabetics. This suggests that short-course therapy for *S. aureus* bacteremia may not be appropriate for diabetics, even for those with a primary focus of infection. Most diabetics with endocarditis and a primary focus had chronic infections involving soft tissue or bone.[39]

Studies of staphylococcal carriage have yielded conflicting results. Some studies have shown that diabetics who inject insulin have higher carriage rates of *S. aureus* than either those who use oral hypoglycemic therapy or nondiabetics.[40,41] One study showed that skin and nasal carriage of *S. aureus* was greater among diabetic outpatients, whether insulin-using or noninsulin-dependent diabetes mellitus (NIDDM), than among nondiabetics.[42] It is not clear whether needle use[43,44] or glycemic control[41,42] may contribute to this finding. One study showed that better glycemic control was associated with *increased* carriage of *S. aureus*.[41]

Candida albicans *and other fungi*

Fungal infections (especially with Candida) are common in the general population. At least at skin and vaginal sites, the occurrence of infections due to these organisms is thought to be more common in diabetics with poor metabolic control. Mucocutaneous candidiasis is relatively frequent and often follows periods in which the patient is glycosuric, but not necessarily hyperglycemic. Candidal growth is enhanced by glucose concentrations of the magnitude found in uncontrolled diabetics.[45] The fungi responsible for mucormycosis (e.g., *Rhizopus*) are favored in conditions of acidosis, possibly as a result of altered iron metabolism. These infections appear to be more frequent in diabetic patients and others (such as dialysis patients) at risk for acidosis, as well as in those with deficient phagocytic cell function.[46]

Group B streptococci

Greater likelihood of group B streptococcal infection has been described in adult diabetics, especially when severe peripheral vascular disease is present. This is most often manifest as soft-tissue infection or osteomyelitis.[47,48]

Tuberculosis

For diabetics the risk of reactivation tuberculosis is as much as four times that of the general population, emphasizing the need for skin testing with purified protein derivative (PPD) antigen. Diabetic patients with positive skin tests should receive isoniazid (INH) chemoprophylaxis, regardless of age.[49]

Problem Statements

Problem 1: Increased Susceptibility to Urinary Tract Infection (UTI)

Statement   The prevalence of asymptomatic bacteriuria is threefold higher among diabetic than nondiabetic women, and when present is more likely to be associated with upper urinary tract disease.[50] Symptomatic pyelonephritis is four to five times more common among diabetic than non-diabetic patients, probably due to secondary structural or functional abnormalities of the urinary tract. Long-term effects of diabetes on the genitourinary system include nephropathy, renal papillary necrosis, renal artery stenosis, neurogenic bladder, and vas deferens calcification. Diabetic women have an increased prevalence of urinary tract structural abnormalities such as cystocele, cystourethrocele, and rectocele, possibly resulting from vascular disease and recurrent vaginitis.[51]

Diabetic patients are also at higher risk for complicated urinary tract infections, which include renal abscess and, rarely, emphysematous infection or xanthogranulomatous pyelonephritis. Severe necrosis with parenchymal gas formation is rare, and requires three prerequisite conditions: (1) the presence of gas-forming bacteria, (2) high tissue glucose levels, and (3) local ischemia.[52] A rare lesion known as xanthogranulomatous pyelonephritis is thought to arise from partially treated chronic urosepsis, renal ischemia, and obstruction. It involves extensive scarring, inflammation, and sequestered infectious foci. These topics are expertly reviewed by Patterson and Andriole.[51]

Clinical Assessment

Although symptoms may be absent or mild, patients with cystitis generally report dysuria, frequency, and urgency. Patients with acute pyelonephritis may have the same symptoms, as well as flank pain or tenderness, fever, chills, nausea, and vomiting. Fever, chills, and flank pain are common to several pathological diagnoses, including renal abscess, renal carbuncle, perinephric abscess, papillary necrosis, infected renal cyst, and renal carcinoma. Most upper UTIs result from ascending infection, and are more frequent among women. An exception is the renal carbuncle, which is derived from a hematogenous source and is more common among men. *S. aureus* is the likely pathogen in renal carbuncle, and bacteremia may antedate renal symptoms by many weeks. Patients with renal carbuncle generally do not have bladder symptoms or abnormal urine, and blood cultures are often negative at the time of presentation.

Urinalysis and culture should be obtained in all patients with suspected UTI. Blood cultures are also recommended for patients with high fever or sepsis syndrome. Because diabetic patients are at risk for emphysematous complications, some experts recommend a screening abdominal radiograph for those with pyelonephritis, but the cost-effectiveness of this is unclear.[51,52] Gas may be localized to the kidney (emphysematous pyelonephritis), the collecting system (pyelitis), or the bladder (cystitis). If gas is seen on the abdominal film, a computed tomography (CT) scan should be performed to accurately determine the location of gas because approach to treatment differs according to infection site.

Ultrasound is warranted for patients in whom obstruction is a concern and is preferred to intravenous pyelography to avoid contrast-associated renal toxicity. Retrograde pyelography is useful if postrenal obstruction is suspected. Contrast-enhanced CT or the more expensive magnetic resonance imaging (MRI) is recommended for patients with suspected abscess formation.

Therapy

Asymptomatic Bacteriuria and Uncomplicated Cystitis   Many experts believe that asymptomatic bacteriuria should be treated in diabetic patients because of the high likelihood (>50%) of concurrent upper urinary tract involvement.[51] Excepted are patients with anatomic abnormalities of the genitourinary tract (such as cystocele/rectocele), who may not benefit from treatment because of difficulty in eradicating bacteriuria. Sequelae of asymptomatic bacteriuria in this population and benefits of eradication have not been demonstrated. When treated, asymptomatic bacteriuria and uncomplicated UTI require 7 to 14 days of oral therapy because of the risk of upper tract involvement.

Common pathogens include *Escherichia coli*, *Klebsiella pneumoniae*, and *Proteus mirabilis*. For patients with recent hospitalization or urological instrumentation, *Enterobacter*, *Enterococcus*, and *Pseudomonas* should be considered. Empiric therapy with trimethoprim/sulfamethoxazole (TMP/SMZ) is recommended, but should be used cautiously for patients taking oral hypoglycemic agents because of the risk for potentiation of the hypoglycemic effect. Fluoroquinolones are also effective but should be used as second-line agents to prevent the selection of resistant organisms. Ampicillin and amoxicillin are less likely to be effective due to antimicrobial resistance among common pathogens.

Therapy should be modified if indicated by culture result or clinical response.

Acute Pyelonephritis   Prompt parenteral antibiotic therapy and intravenous hydration may prevent later complications. Empiric therapy with extended spectrum beta-lactam antibiotics, TMP/SMZ, fluoroquinolones, or the combination of ampicillin with gentamicin is suggested. However, intravenous TMP/SMZ may cause severe hypoglycemia when used in combination with oral hypoglycemics and should be used with great caution in such patients. Fever and discomfort should respond within 72 hr, at which time oral antibiotics may be substituted to complete a 14-day course of therapy. Follow-up culture is recommended. For patients with delayed response to therapy, further studies are warranted to evaluate for abscess, obstruction, or other complications.

Complicated UTI   Patients with renal carbuncle and small renal abscess generally respond to parenteral antibiotics within 1 week, then complete oral antibiotics for another 2 weeks, and have no chronic sequelae. Radiological follow-up is recommended. Large abscesses, persistent fever, and persistent symptoms after 1 week are indications for drainage. For patients with obstructive uropathy, percutaneous nephrostomy should be promptly requested. Nephrectomy is rarely needed, except for xanthogranulomatous pyelonephritis, emphysematous complications, life-threatening sepsis, or for extensive perinephric abscess.

Emphysematous Complications   When gas is limited to the bladder wall, the disease is managed in the same manner as other UTIs and usually responds to antimicrobial therapy. Emphysematous changes in the kidney are much more severe; in this case, surgical removal of an emphysematous kidney lowers mortality from approximately 60 to 20%.[51,52]

Perinephric Abscess   Drainage is the principal treatment of perinephric abscess, and prognosis is guarded even with therapy. Until culture results are available, empiric antibiotics are directed toward common Gramnegative uropathogens and *S. aureus*. Perinephric abscess may result from rupture of a renal abscess through the capsule, direct extension from an intraabdominal source, or hematogenous spread. Thus, a variety of other organisms may be found, including anaerobes, fungi, or *Mycobacterium tuberculosis*.

Fungal UTI   Fungal UTIs are not uncommon in diabetic patients, particularly those with perineal candidiasis and recent use of antibacterials. Most patients with candiduria have indwelling urinary catheters or urinary obstruction. The presence of yeast in urine may signify benign colonization of the catheter and lower urinary tract or may result from invasive disease. Fungal organisms will often be eliminated from the bladder if catheters are removed, antibacterial therapy is discontinued, and metabolic control is achieved.

Distinguishing patients with renal candidiasis is important because this condition requires parenteral therapy and is usually associated with hematogenous spread. Blood cultures, urinalysis and quantitative urine cultures are recommended. Urinalysis demonstrating renal tubular casts containing pseudohyphae is diagnostic of renal candidiasis. Blood cultures will be positive in only half of renal candidiasis patients. In the absence of a urinary catheter, a midstream urine specimen with $>10^4$ CFU/mL of yeast is predictive of renal infection.[53] When these methods are inconclusive, consider treatment, which also serves as a diagnostic test, by bladder irrigation with amphotericin B (50 μg/mL) for 3 to 5 days. If candiduria persists, a retrograde pyelogram is indicated to evaluate for obstruction, and renal candidiasis is likely. Treatment with parenteral amphotericin B or fluconazole is then recommended.[53,54]

Prevention/Education   Avoid bladder catheterization as much as possible in the diabetic. Educate the patient with neuropathy about the importance of frequent voiding, complete emptying of the bladder, and seeking care immediately when even minor symptoms develop. For women with frequent recurrences, consider prophylactic antibiotic regimens.

Problem 2: Increased Susceptibility to Complications of Respiratory Infection

Statement   Diabetic patients are at increased risk for certain types of pneumonia, and have more severe and longer illnesses when pneumonia occurs. Pathogens affecting diabetic patients disproportionately include *M. tuberculosis*,[55,56] *S. aureus*, *Klebsiella* (and other enteric Gram-negative bacteria), and certain fungi (mucormycosis, coccidioidomycosis, and cryptococcosis). Despite frequent skin and mucous membrane colonization, Candida is a rare cause of pneumonia. *Burkholderia (Pseudomonas) pseudomallei* is a bacterium that causes disease in India, Southeast Asia, and Australia, and affects diabetic patients disproportionately. Because of unique drug-susceptibilities, this pathogen should be borne in mind if a patient has been to these endemic areas.[57] This pathogen may cause sepsis, lobar pneumonia, or a cavitary apical pneumonia resembling tuberculosis.

Pneumonia due to the most common bacterial cause, the pneumococcus, is not more frequent in diabetic patients. However, when it does occur, pneumococcal pneumonia in a diabetic is more likely to be associated with bacteremia, and to be rapidly fatal.[58–60] Similarly, influenza virus and legionella are thought to cause dis-

proportionate morbidity and mortality among diabetic patients.[61,62] Diabetic patients with pneumonia are more likely to die than age- and sex-matched nondiabetic controls ($RR = 7.6$ for those less than age 30).[1] The reasons for these associations are only partly understood. Possible reasons for pulmonary complications in diabetes include diabetic gastroparesis, which may increase the risk of aspiration, microangiopathic changes in the lung, pulmonary edema associated with cardiovascular disease, altered mental status with metabolic imbalances, and immune deficiencies. Function of pulmonary macrophages is essential to control of infection with intracellular organisms such as *M. tuberculosis* and legionella; tissue macrophages are derived from circulating monocytes, which demonstrate *in vitro* defects in diabetics.[34] Immune dysfunction associated with diabetic nephropathy may further compromise some patients.

Clinical Assessment

In many cases, pneumonia will present with cough, fever, dyspnea, and pulmonary infiltrates. The diagnosis is more difficult in patients with ketoacidosis, associated hyperpnea and dehydration, and inapparent pulmonary infiltrates. Pneumonia may also be difficult to distinguish from pulmonary edema. Laboratory testing, including chest radiographs, WBC and differential, chemistries, and blood gas assessment may be essential to management. Gram-stained sputum and cultures of sputum and blood should be obtained before antimicrobial therapy whenever possible. Bronchoscopy, diagnostic thoracentesis in patients with pleural effusion, urine for legionella antigen testing, and sputum AFB smears and cultures may be useful for guiding therapy. Serologic testing for atypical pneumonia pathogens may provide a diagnosis after therapy is completed, but is rarely useful for management decisions. Purified protein derivative (PPD) skin-testing is indicated for patients previously tuberculin-negative.[49] Patients with cavitary pneumonia or hemoptysis should be evaluated for fungal pneumonia or tuberculosis. If tuberculosis is a possibility, respiratory isolation should be maintained.

Therapy

Even where extensive testing for pathogens has been done, the etiology of pneumonia is determined in only about half of all cases.[63] In keeping with the guidelines of the American Thoracic Society, empiric therapy is based on the severity of illness at presentation and likelihood of given etiologic agents. Less ill patients may be treated with a second generation cephalosporin, TMP/SMX, a β-lactam/β-lactamase inhibitor combination with or without a macrolide, or a newer fluoroquinolone with expanded spectrum. A macrolide alone would not be the drug of choice because of the relative importance of aerobic Gram-negative pathogens in diabetic patients with pneumonia. Patients requiring hospitalization might be treated with a second- or third-generation cephalosporin, a β-lactam/β-lactamase inhibitor combination, with or without a macrolide, or a newer fluoroquinolone. Severely ill patients should be hospitalized and receive a macrolide sufficient to treat legionellosis as well a broad-spectrum antipseudomonal agent such as an antipseudomonal third-generation cephalosporin or imipenem/cilastin or fluoroquinolone.[63] When tuberculosis is likely, three or four empiric anti-tuberculous drugs are indicated, depending upon local prevalence of drug-resistant tuberculosis.[63,64] In considering the choice of drugs for treatment of nosocomial pneumonia, it is wise to consider the susceptibility patterns of isolates from the setting where pneumonia was acquired.

During outbreaks of influenza A, amantadine or rimantadine should be considered for patients with symptoms of influenza who present within 48 hr of onset.[65] Fungal pneumonia often requires surgical resection in addition to systemic therapy.

Prevention/Education

After the 23-valent pneumococcal polysaccharide vaccine is given to diabetic adults, antibody production is normal, and studies have estimated pneumococcal vaccine efficacy to be 84 to 90% in this population.[66,67] Pneumococcal vaccination is recommended for diabetic patients, and assumes greater importance as the prevalence of drug-resistant pneumococcal disease increases.[68,69] Although revaccination is not routine, if earlier vaccination status is unknown, patients should be offered pneumococcal vaccine.[68] Conjugate pneumococcal vaccines are in development, but their role for prevention of pneumococcal disease in adults is as yet undefined.[70]

Yearly influenza vaccine is also highly effective and cost saving.[71-73] If the patient is immunized late in the season, amantadine may be given adjunctively for 2 weeks following vaccination.[65]

Diabetes increases the risk of progression to active tuberculosis if primary infection occurs. Because of this, PPD skin-testing is recommended for diabetic patients.[49] The PPD skin test is considered positive if more than 10 mm of induration occurs in a diabetic, and evaluation for active tuberculosis in those with positive PPD tests should then include a chest radiograph. If the radiograph is normal, the patient should be considered a candidate for preventive therapy with isoniazid *regardless of age*. Treatment with isoniazid (INH) 300 mg a day for 6 months is standard, with close follow-up. Pyridoxine (vitamin B6), 25 to 50 mg a day, should always be provided to diabetic patients taking INH because of increased risk of neuropathy.[49,64]

Problem 3: Increased Likelihood of Soft Tissue Infection (see Chapters 31–33, 45 and 46) (Including Surgical Wound Infection, Pyomyositis, Necrotizing Fasciitis, Fourniere's Gangrene)

Statement Localized soft-tissue infections caused by *Staphylococcus aureus* and β-hemolytic streptococci are common in diabetic patients, including impetigo, cellulitis, carbuncles, and furuncles. Secondary infections of cutaneous ulcers resulting from peripheral vascular disease, autonomic and sensory neuropathy also occur frequently (discussed in the section on diabetic foot infection). Surgical wound infections are more frequent among diabetics.[11] Some of these involve foreign bodies; for example, up to one in three men undergoing penile implant procedures for therapy of impotence is diabetic. Postoperative infection rate averages 2 to 3%, usually occurring within the first year.[74,75] *Staphylococcus epidermidis* is the primary pathogen, but mixed infections are common, and severe gangrenous infections have been reported.

Although no population-based studies have been done to prove that deep soft-tissue infections are more frequent among diabetics, recent reviews suggest as many as one of four patients with necrotizing fasciitis or pyomyositis is diabetic.[74-78] Pyomyositis, a bacterial infection of skeletal muscle, is usually caused by *S. aureus*, and may progress to abscess formation. Necrotizing fasciitis is an aggressive, destructive bacterial infection that spreads rapidly along tissue planes. Most such infections are synergistic mixed infections, although *Streptococcus pyogenes* (group A streptococcus) is capable of such destruction even when present alone.[78] A subcategory of necrotizing fasciitis is Fourniere's gangrene, where perineal, perianal, or ureteral lesions provide an entry for bacteria to reach deeper tissues from whence they spread in defined anatomic planes to the thighs and abdomen.[79] Fungi of the order *Mucorales* are also capable of causing gangrenous soft-tissue infections (discussed in the section on mucormycosis).

Clinical Assessment

The presentation of abscess, carbuncle, or surgical wound infection is similar to that of nondiabetic patients. Pyomyositis characteristically causes pain, fever, and "woody" induration of the deep soft tissues. Patients with necrotizing fasciitis may present initially with unimpressive physical findings. Pain out of proportion to visible inflammation is an early sign, but is often accompanied by marked systemic toxicity, which may progress to multisystem organ dysfunction. The infection passes unimpeded along deep fascial planes, and tissue damage may be widespread over a matter of hours. Later, signs of gangrene, ulceration, bullae, and discoloration (as well as anaesthesia with nerve destruction) may occur. Crepitus is present in half of patients, and radiographic gas is found in more. This infection results in a high mortality rate, even under optimal treatment, and requires urgent surgical intervention to assess extent of spread and to limit further tissue destruction. Operative cultures may guide therapy, but empiric treatment with broad-spectrum antimicrobials is needed urgently, especially to cover anaerobes, aerobic Gram negatives, streptococci, and staphylococci.

Therapy

Incision and drainage and local care of the affected area are the cornerstones of therapy for carbuncle or furuncle. Antistaphylococcal antibacterials are adjunctive and help keep the infection from seeding elsewhere in the body. Surgical wound infections in diabetics usually are due to *S. aureus* or aerobic Gram-negative bacilli. Appropriate antimicrobial choice for these pathogens depends on local patterns of susceptibility in the hospital where the surgery took place. Treatment of penile implant infection generally requires removal of the device, and subsequent attempts at implantation have a much higher risk of infection.[75] Initial antimicrobial choice should include vancomycin for coverage of coagulase-negative staphylococci as well as antibiotic coverage for aerobic gram-negative pathogens. Treatment of soft-tissue infection involving the extremity is discussed in the section on diabetic foot infection.

Pyomyositis requires anti-staphylococcal antibacterials, and surgical drainage if abscess is demonstrated on MRI or CT scan.[77] For life-threatening deep soft-tissue infections such as necrotizing fasciitis, surgical exploration, and wide debridement are urgent, and hemodynamic support, control of hyperglycemia, and broad-spectrum antimicrobial therapy are essential. Use of growth factors to facilitate healing is being evaluated.[80]

Consultation with Other Professionals

The surgeon is an essential consultant for patients with serious soft-tissue infections that require debridement and exploration.

Prevention/Education

Preoperative blood sugar control appears to decrease risk of postoperative infection, and should be optimized for elective procedures such as penile implantation.[10,11,81] Patients should be instructed to seek medical attention for early signs of infection.

Problem 4: Increased Likelihood of Osteomyelitis (with Special Reference to the Diabetic Foot)

Pathophysiology and Conservative Treatment of the Diabetic Foot are also Covered in Chapters 31–33

Statement Diabetic foot infections are very common, and a leading cause of hospitalization.[4,5] The majority are associated with peripheral neuropathy, which alters sensation, weight bearing, and skin integrity. Vascular insufficiency may also be contributory. Prevention and early intervention is the goal, as amputation is a too common result of these infections. However, most diabetic patients who present with previously untreated foot infections have nonlimb-threatening infections and can be managed as outpatients with oral antimicrobial therapy.[82] These milder infections include acute cellulitis, acute infection of a chronic ulcer, paronychia, and superficial abscess. Uncomplicated infections are commonly caused by aerobic Gram-positive cocci such as *Staphylococcus aureus*, *Staphylococcus epidermidis*, *Streptococcus* sp., and enterococci. Lipsky et al.[82] reported a 90% cure rate among these patients using oral clindamycin or cephalexin for 2 weeks. It is important to carefully examine and probe ulcers that may underly crusted material to avoid overlooking a deeper and more severe infection.

Complicated infections include severe cellulitis, necrotic or deep soft-tissue infection, and osteomyelitis. These infections are more commonly polymicrobial, with a mean of 4.1 to 5.8 bacterial species per culture, including the above aerobic Gram-positive cocci, aerobic Gram-negative bacilli, and anaerobes including *Peptostreptococcus* and *Bacteroides* sp.[83,84] Broad-spectrum antimicrobial therapy is recommended for at least 6 weeks and should initially be parenteral (see Table 44–1). Devascularized tissue should be carefully debrided, and multiple limb sparing procedures are preferable to primary major amputation.[85–87]

Clinical Assessment

Most patients with diabetic foot infection are not febrile, leukocytosis may be absent, and the foot ulcer may not appear inflamed.[88] Because the patient may be unaware of the problem, careful inspection of both feet should be routine when examining a diabetic patient. Signs of infection include sinus tract formation, seepage, foul odor, purulent discharge, crepitus, and local inflammation with edema and erythema. A flu-like illness and impaired glucose control also suggest infection.[88]

About one in three patients who present with foot infections is found to have osteomyelitis. Distinguishing osteomyelitis from noninfectious neuropathic bony abnormalities can be challenging. For example, erythema, swelling, and warmth in a nonulcerated foot may indicate Charcot's osteopathy rather than infection.[88] Osteomyelitis is likely in patients with skin ulcer or soft-tissue infection that has been present for more than one or 2 weeks, especially if located over a bony prominence. A past history of osteomyelitis is also a risk for recurrent bony involvement. Clinical findings associated with the presence of osteomyelitis include larger, deeper ulceration and elevated erythrocyte sedimentation rate (ESR). Clinicians at The Joslin Clinic diagnose osteomyelitis by clinical assessment that includes unroofing of the ulcer and probing of the wound with a blunt needle.[89] If bone or joint can be contacted with a gently advanced sterile surgical blunt probe, the positive predictive value for bone or joint involvement is 89%, although this technique is insensitive, with a negative predictive value of 56%.[89] To avoid missing osteomyelitis, Lipsky advocates[111] Indium-labelled WBC scan for patients with suspected osteomyelitis when probing to bone is not possible.[87] Radiographic studies should never delay debridement and drainage of severe infections. Failure to debride necrotic tissue and drain infections increases the risk of amputation.

Radiological evaluation for the presence of osteomyelitis is problematic. Plain radiographs lack sensitivity and specificity for osteomyelitis, and are negative until 10 to 20 days after infection. Although sensitive,[99m] technetium bone scans are too expensive for screening tests and lack specificity unless other causes for bone remodelling can be ruled out. For most patients,[111] Indium-labelled leukocyte scans are the most accurate of currently available radionucleide studies, although they are also expensive and difficult to interpret in the presence of local soft tissue infection.[87] MRI scans, also expensive, may show marrow abnormalities in osteomyelitis, but are insensitive for cortical changes. Diabetic bone infection typically affects the cortex first and may affect small bones of the foot which do not contain marrow. Similar marrow changes may also be seen in osteoarthropathy.[87]

The definitive test to diagnose osteomyelitis is bone biopsy and culture, which should be performed either percutaneously through uninfected tissues or at surgery. An alternative way to obtain specimens involves curettage of the base of the ulcer after debridement. Superficial swabs are not helpful because they often recover colonizing organisms, and may miss the actual pathogen. Recovery of anaerobic bacteria requires special media and handling.

Therapy

Immediately after debridement and obtaining appropriate cultures, empirically chosen antibiotics should be administered based on suspected pathogens and severity of infection (see Table 44–1) and modifications later made based on culture results. A team approach is necessary, including surgical debridement and bone biopsy as indicated, vascular evaluation with testing of transcutaneous pO_2, and angiography if pulses are weak, and for some patients, vascular surgery intervention. In addition, attention is needed to metabolic control, antimicrobial therapy, and minimizing edema. Avoidance of weight bearing is essential to prompt healing. Adjunctive use of hyperbaric oxygen remains controversial.[90] A randomized, double-blind, placebo-controlled study recently demonstrated improved outcome when foot infection in diabetic patients was treated with adjunctive granulocyte-colony stimulating factor (G-CSF).[91] In this series, G-CSF use was associated with earlier eradication of pathogens from the infected ulcer, more rapid resolution of cellulitis, and earlier hospital discharge.

TABLE 44–1   Antimicrobial Therapy for Diabetic Foot Infections

	Oral	Parenteral
Nonlimb-threatening (superficial, no osteomyelitis)	Cephalexin Clindamycin Amoxicillin-clavulanic acid Dicloxacillin	Cefazolin Clindamycin Oxacillin Nafcillin
Limb-threatening (deep ulcer, osteomyelitis, necrosis, fetid)	Fluoroquinolone and clindamycin (after initial parenteral therapy)	Ampicillin-sulbactam Ticarcillin-clavulanic acid Piperacillin-tazobactam Cefoxitin Cefotetan Fluoroquinolone and clindamycin
Life-threatening		Imipenem-cilastin Ampicillin-sulbactam and aminoglycoside Vancomycin, metronidazole, and aztreonam

Multiple appropriate antimicrobial regimens could be used for treatment in each classification of infection severity (see Table 44–1). Newer fluoroquinolones may be used to treat diabetic foot infections, but ciprofloxacin or ofloxacin should not be used alone because of limited activity. Aminoglycosides should be avoided if less nephrotoxic alternatives are available. Antimicrobials should be modified based on clinical response and results of culture and susceptibility testing. Broadening therapy to cover resistant isolates is not necessary if the infection is responding to initial therapy, but therapy that is broader than necessary may be simplified if a good response is observed. Doses should be adjusted based on the severity of the infection and for renal dysfunction when indicated. Traditional therapy for osteomyelitis includes 4 to 6 weeks of parenteral antimicrobials, though some continue therapy for 10 weeks total, using oral antimicrobials later in the course. If the infected bone is completely removed, antimicrobial treatment for 2 to 3 weeks is usually sufficient.

Prevention/Education

Health-care providers must educate patients to care for and examine their feet daily, including attention to skin and nails, to always wear proper shoes, to avoid smoking, and to seek medical attention promptly should signs of infection begin. The diabetic must be taught that no infection of an extremity is trivial.

Problem 5: Malignant External Otitis

Statement This severe, necrotizing infection of the external auditory canal, associated with invasive complications, was originally described in elderly diabetics. It is usually caused by *Pseudomonas aeruginosa*.[92,93] A similar syndrome may rarely be seen in nondiabetic patients, but some physicians require that the patient have diabetes before they will make this diagnosis. This makes the relative risk for diabetic patients difficult to infer. Microangiopathy may be a predisposing condition. *P. aeruginosa* may colonize the ear without causing infection, and is a common cause of external otitis in conditions of maceration and wetness (swimmers' ear), so an ear culture positive for this organism does not, by itself, establish the diagnosis.

Clinical Assessment

Diagnosis of malignant external otitis requires evidence of tissue invasion. As infection spreads from the external ear canal through natural fissures traversing cartilage to the temporal bone, an intensely painful ear results, with purulent discharge and granulation tissue at the junction of bone and cartilage in the affected posteroinferior ear canal. Inflammation may be present in

the pinna, periauricular, and mastoid areas. Complications may may be life-threatening, and include cranial nerve paralysis (usually involving the facial nerve), mastoiditis, osteomyelitis of the temporal bone, cranial sinus thrombosis, or meningitis. Of special note is that fever is *not* a prominent sign of the illness, and the peripheral WBC may remain normal.[94] The erythrocyte sedimentation rate (ESR) is often markedly elevated.[93] MRI and CT scans can be used to evaluate spread of infection to adjacent soft tissue and bone.[93,95]

Therapy

Standard therapy includes a combination of antipseudomonal β-lactam agent with an aminoglycoside for a minimum of 4 weeks in limited disease, and up to 8 weeks if cranial nerve involvement is present. Single agent therapy with fluoroquinolones has been used successfully in limited disease.[96] The ear canal should be cleansed, debrided, and antipseudomonal eardrops combined with steroid instilled.[97]

Prevention/Education

The patient must be made aware of the existence of this syndrome, and taught to consider all ear infections as potentially serious, requiring medical evaluation rather than self-therapy.

Consultation with Other Professionals

The otolaryngologist should be consulted to provide local debridement and drainage. Neurosurgical assistance may also be required for extensive invasive disease.

Follow-up

Because recurrence is possible due to sequestered foci of infection, follow-up should extend well beyond the period of acute care and antimicrobial therapy.

Problem 6: Dermatitis, Vaginitis, and Vulvitis

Statement Vulvovaginal candidiasis is common in diabetic and nondiabetic women, with an estimated 75% of women experiencing an episode of *Candida* vaginitis in their lifetime.[98] Poorly controlled diabetic patients may be at higher risk, because *Candida* overgrowth is promoted by hyperglycemia. Other conditions that favor vulvovaginal candidiasis include high-estrogen states such as pregnancy, and contraceptive or hormone replacement therapy, as well as use of antimicrobials or systemic glucocorticoids. Invasive candidiasis is neither more common nor more deadly when it occurs in diabetic patients.[53]

Clinical Assessment:

Itching is the major symptom of candidal vulvovaginitis, and increased vaginal discharge (often described as a "cheesy" white exudate) may be present. Vulvar edema or excoriation may be seen. *Candida* can cause dermatitis in moist areas where skin is macerated; this is a common superinfection of diaper dermatitis in babies, and may be seen in adult intertriginous areas as well. It is characterized by a salmon-pink color with satellite lesions. Potassium hydroxide preparation of skin scrapings or vaginal secretions reveals the characteristic fungal pseudohyphae.

Therapy

Oral fluconazole is a convenient and inexpensive treatment for nonpregnant women with vulvovaginal candidiasis; most patients will be cured after a single 150-mg dose of fluconazole, orally.[99] Systemic therapy may also decrease gastrointestinal carriage of Candida and thus prevent recurrences. Mycolog® cream, which combines nystatin with steroid provides symptomatic relief when applied to the vulva. Other treatment options include clotrimazole or nystatin suppositories, and miconazole or clotrimazole creams.

Prevention/Education

Avoidance of unnecessary antimicrobial and steroid use, and optimal metabolic control may prevent some cases of Candida infection. Wearing cotton undergarments, and avoidance of tight clothes such as pantyhose may also prevent candidal overgrowth.

Problem 7: Increased Susceptibility to Mucormycosis

Statement Mucormycosis is a rare infection caused by environmental fungi (*Rhizopus, Mucor, Absidia*), which are common in decaying organic matter such as moldy bread. These organisms are ubiquitous, making frequent exposures likely, and they are clearly of low virulence under ordinary circumstances. Spores gain entry through inhalation or direct skin inoculation, and if not contained, undergo germination to a hyphal or mold form. Their predilection to invade blood vessel walls leads to necrosis and characteristic black pus. Rhinocerebral mucormycosis is a devastating infection involving the nose and soft palate that may eventually progress to involve brain. Mucormycosis may also involve the lung, causing massive hemoptysis, or the skin and soft tissues resulting in life-threatening gangrene.[92,100,101]

Patients at risk for mucormycosis include diabetics, patients with neutropenia, and those on dialysis, especially when treated with deferoxamine. In addition to phagocytic cell function, iron availability, which is altered by acidosis and deferoxamine, appears to be important for containment of fungal growth.[102]

Clinical Assessment

When mucormycosis occurs in diabetics, it is usually in patients with poorly controlled metabolism and acidosis. The most common site is rhinocerebral, beginning in the soft palate, nasal mucosa, or sinuses. Orbital cellulitis or sinusitis may be the initial manifestation. The patient typically develops sudden periorbital or perinasal pain and congestion. A bloody, dark-colored nasal discharge may develop, and the turbinates may become necrotic. The infection causes thrombosis and necrosis as it spreads, leading to facial swelling, proptosis, cranial nerve deficits, and cranial sinus thrombosis. Neurological signs may progress quickly leading to coma and death. Diagnosis is usually made by biopsy of mucosal tissue. Culture is less reliable and takes a number of days to become positive.

Therapy

Surgical debridement, metabolic control, and administration of amphotericin B are required. With aggressive application of these measures, cure is often possible. Liposomal amphotericin B has been used to deliver higher doses of antifungal with lower renal toxicity.[103–105] Granulocyte colony-stimulating factor is useful in neutropenic patients with mucormycosis, but has not been evaluated in diabetic patients for this indication, despite theoretical benefits.[28,105]

Prevention/Education:

Because of the difficulty in avoiding exposure to these ubiquitous organisms, the only means to avoid mucormycosis appears to be maintaining optimal metabolic control.

Consultation with Other Professionals

Otolaryngology and/or neurosurgical referrals can assist in establishing the diagnosis early in a case, and in debridement of necrotic tissues.

Follow-up

If the infection is eradicated, further visits may be necessary for reconstructive surgery and other rehabilitative processes.

Problem 8: Increased Frequency of Periodontal Infection

Statement Infection of periodontal tissue and dental calculus formation can be more frequent in diabetics who have poor metabolic control or long-standing disease. Such involvement correlates with duration of diabetes, presence of complications and elevated blood glucose levels.[106,107] In addition to concerns over tooth loss, studies have demonstrated that metabolic control can be improved by decreasing periodontal inflammation.[107]

Prevention/Education

Regular dental visits, including professional calculus removal is important for diabetic patients.

Referral to Other Professionals

This problem should be referred to a competent dental practitioner or oral surgeon, depending on the degree of involvement at the time of recognition (see Chapter 46).

Problem 9: Infection in Diabetic Patients Undergoing Dialysis

Statement At least one of four insulin-dependent diabetic patients eventually requires dialysis for chronic renal failure due to diabetic nephropathy. Patients on dialysis, whether hemodialysis or peritoneal dialysis, tend to develop infections with endogenously carried strains of *S. aureus*. The risk is higher in hemodialysis patients with diabetes than in nondiabetic hemodialysis patients.[108] This is a group of patients for whom attempted eradication of staphylococcal carriage with intranasal mupirocin may be warranted.[109,110]

Hemodialysis may be conducted through subclavian or femoral transcutaneous catheters or arterial-venous fistulae (AVF), which in turn may be formed of native vessels or prosthetic materials. Each of these is associated with infection, however, rates of infection vary greatly. Native AVF are infected at a rate of less than 1% per year, compared with 11% of polytetrafluoroethylene (PTFE) and 26% of bovine carotid artery heterografts (BCAH).[111] Graft infection, usually caused by *S. aureus* or coagulase-negative staphylococci, is the leading cause of graft failure or excision. Graft infection occurring immediately after graft placement is usually caused by skin organisms, is external to the graft (not involving lumen or endothelium) and seldom requires removal, although it may delay graft maturation.[108]

Treatment of dialysis-related infections (local or bacteremic) may be attempted with antibiotics alone, and some authors continue dialysis via the infected access during the course of treatment. Observation for metastatic complications is necessary and prolonged parenteral antibiotics may be needed. If aneurysm occurs, removal of the graft is required.

Chronic ambulatory peritoneal dialysis (CAPD) infections commonly include exit-site infection, tunnel infection, and peritonitis. There is a higher risk of peritonitis for diabetics on CAPD than for nondiabetics.[112] Most exit-site and tunnel infections are caused by *S. aureus*. Treatment of peritonitis should include coverage for *S. aureus* and aerobic Gram-negative bacilli. Peritonitis associated with tunnel or exit-site infection necessitates catheter removal.[112]

Problem 10: Infection in Diabetic Transplant Patients

The complex issues of infection in diabetic patients further compromised by transplantation and its requisite immunosuppression are beyond the scope of this chapter. The interested reader is referred to the Chapters 21 and 27, or the following resources[113,114]:

(1) Tolkoff-Rubin NE, Rubin RH: The infectious disease problems of the diabetic renal transplant recipient. Infect Dis Clin North Am 9:117–129, 1995.

(2) Hibberd PL, Rubin RH: Renal transplantation and related infections. Semin Resp Infect 8:216–224, 1993.

Research Considerations

Diabetes mellitus includes a spectrum of diseases with complex pathophysiology. Interest in the potential role of infectious agents such as enteroviruses in the etiology of IDDM and NIDDM continues to foster research and speculation.[115–118] Studies of the treatment of infections listed above are continually appearing in the literature. Progress in infectious diseases also includes evaluation of the clinical utility of newer antimicrobial agents, and of adjunctive therapies such as G-CSF and hyperbaric oxygen. Finally, prevention of infection through improved metabolic conditions, eradication of pathogen carriage, and use of newer vaccines warrants epidemiological study.

References

1. Moss SE, Klein R, Klein BEK: Cause-specific mortality in a population-based study of diabetes. J Public Health 81:1158–1162, 1991.
2. Swerdlow AJ, Jones ME: Mortality during 25 years of follow-up of a cohort with diabetes. Int J Epidemiol 25:1250–1261, 1996.
3. Boyko EJ, Lipsky BA: Infection and diabetes. In National Diabetes Group (eds): Diabetes in America, Bethesda, MD: National Institutes of Health, 1995, pp. 485–499.
4. Brodsky JW, Schneidler C: Diabetic foot infections. Orthopedic Clin North Am 22: 473–489, 1991.

5. Lipsky BA: Osteomyelitis of the foot in diabetic patients. Clin Infect Dis 25:1318–1326, 1997.

6. Ray NF, Thamer M, Taylor T, et al.: Hospitalization and expenditures for the treatment of general medical conditions among the U.S. diabetic population in 1991. J Clin Endocrinol Metab 81:3671–3679, 1996.

7. Aro S, Salinto M, Kangas T, et al.: Hospital use among diabetic patients and the general population. Diabetes Care 17:1320–1329, 1994.

8. Currie BP, Casey JI: Host defense and infections in diabetes mellitus. *In* Porte D, Sherwin RS (eds): Ellenberg and Rifkin's Diabetes Mellitus. Stamford, CT: Appleton and Lange, 1997, pp. 861–874.

9. Rayfield EJ, Ault MJ, Keush GT, et al.: Infection and diabetes: The case for glucose control. Am J Med 72:439–450, 1982.

10. Baxter JK, Babineau TJ, Apovian CM, et al.: Perioperative glucose control predicts increased nosocomial infection in diabetics. Crit Care Med 18:S207, 1990.

11. Zerr KJ, Furnary AP, Grunkemeier GL: Glucose control lowers the risk of wound infection in diabetics after open heart operations. Ann Thorac Surg 63:356–361, 1997.

12. Overett TK, Bistrian BR, Lowry SF, et al.: Total parenteral nutrition in patients with insulin-requiring diabetes mellitus. J Am Coll Nutr 5:79–89, 1986.

13. Leibovici L, Yehezkelli Y, Porter A, et al.: Influence of diabetes mellitus and glycaemic control on the characteristics and outcome of common infections. Diabetic Medicine 13:457–463, 1996.

14. Rayfield EJ, Curnow RT, Reinhard D, et al.: Effects of acute endotoxemia on glucoregulation in normal and diabetic subjects. J Clin Endocrinol Metab 45:513, 1977.

15. McMahon MM, Bistrian BR: Host defenses and susceptibility to infection in patients with diabetes mellitus. Infect Dis Clin North Am 9:1–9, 1995.

16. Soler NG, Bennett MA, FitzGerald MG, et al.: Intensive care in the management of diabetic ketoacidosis. Lancet 1:951–954, 1973.

17. Muller WA, Faloona GR, Unger RH: Hyperglucagonemia in diabetic ketoacidosis: Its prevalence and significance. Am J Med 54:52–57, 1973.

18. Bagdade JD, Root RK, Bulger RJ: Impaired leukocyte function in patients with poorly controlled diabetes. Diabetes 23:9–15, 1974.

19. Bagdade JD, Stewart M, Walters E: Impaired granulocyte adherence: a reversible defect in host defense in patients with poorly controlled diabetes. Diabetes 27:677–681, 1978.

20. Mowat AG, Baum J: Chemotaxis of polymorphonuclear leukocytes from patients with diabetes mellitus. N Engl J Med 284:621–627, 1971.

21. Hill HR, Sauls HS, Dettloffand JL, et al.: Impaired leukotactic responsiveness in patients with juvenile diabetes mellitus. Clin Immunol Immunopathol 2:395–403, 1974.

22. MacRury SM, Gemmell CG, Paterson KR, et al.: Changes in phagocytic function with glycaemic control in diabetic patients. J Clin Pathol 42:1143–1147, 1989.

23. Nielson CP, Hindson DA: Inhibition of polymorphonuclear leukocyte respiratory burst by elevated glucose concentrations in vitro. Diabetes 38:1031–1035, 1989.

24. Ortmeyer J, Mohsenin V: Glucose suppresses superoxide generation in normal neutrophils: Interference in phospholipase D activation . Am J Physiol 264:C402–C410, 1993.

25. Shah SV, Wallin JD, Eilen SD: Chemiluminescence and superoxide anion production by leukocytes from diabetic patients. J Clin Endocrinol Metab 57:402–409, 1983.

26. Marhoffer W, Stein M, Maeser E, et al.: Impairment of polymorphonuclear leukocyte function and metabolic control of diabetes. Diabetes Care 15:256–260, 1992.

27. Nolan CM, Beaty HN, Bagdade JD: Further characterization of the impaired bactericidal function of granulocytes in patients with poorly controlled diabetes. Diabetes 27:889–894, 1978.

28. Sato N, Kashima K, Tanaka Y, et al.: Effect of granulocyte-colony stimulating factor on generation of oxygen-derived free radicals and myeloperoxidase activity in neutrophils from poorly controlled NIDDM patients. Diabetes 46:133–137, 1997.

29. Kantar A, Wilkins G, Swoboda B, et al.: Alterations of the respiratory burst of polymorphonuclear leukocytes from diabetic children. Acta Paediatr Scand 79:535–541, 1990.

30. Delamaire M, Maugendre D, Moreno M, et al.: Impaired leucocyte functions in diabetic patients. Diabetic Med 14:29–34, 1997.

31. Tater D, Tepaut B, Bercovici JP, et al.: Polymorphonuclear cell derangements in type 1 diabetes. Horm Metab Res 19:542–647, 1987.

32. MacCuish AC, Urbaniak SJ, Campbell CJ: Phytohemagglutinin transformation and circulating lymphocyte subpopulation in insulin-dependent diabetic patients. Diabetes 23:708, 1974.

33. Casey JI, Heeter BJ, Klyshevich KA: Impaired response of lymphocytes of diabetic subjects to antigen on Staphylococcus aureus. J Infect Dis 136:495, 1977.

34. Hill HR, Augustine NH, Rallison ML, et al.: Defective monocyte chemotactic responses in diabetes mellitus. J Clin Immunol 3:70–77, 1983.

35. Centers for Disease Control and Prevention: Nosocomial hepatitis B virus infection associated with reusable fingerstick blood sampling. JAMA 277:1106–1107, 1997.

36. Falchuk KR, Conlin D: The intestinal and liver complications of diabetes mellitus. Adv Intern Med 38:269–286, 1993.

37. Khuri KG, Shamma'a MH, Abourizk N: Hepatitis B virus markers in diabetes mellitus. Diabetes Care 8:250–253, 1985.

38. Grimbert S, Valensi P, Levy-Marchal C, et al.: High prevalence of diabetes mellitus in patients with chronic hepatitis C: A case-control study. Gastroenterologie Clinique et Biologique 20:544–548, 1996.

39. Cooper G, Platt R: Staphylococcus aureus bacteremia in diabetic patients: Endocarditis and mortality. Am J Med 73:658, 1982.

40. Smith JA, O'Connor JJ, Willis AT: Nasal carriage of Staphylococcus aureus in diabetes mellitus. Lancet 2:776, 1966.

41. Chandler PT, Chandler SD: Pathogenic carrier rate in diabetes mellitus. Am J Med Sci 273:259, 1977.

42. Lipsky BA, Pecoraro RE, Chen MS, et al.: Factors affecting staphylococcal colonization among NIDDM outpatients. Diabetes Care 10:483, 1987.

43. Tuazon CU, Perez A, Kishaba T, et al.: Staphylococcus aureus among insulin-injecting diabetic patients. JAMA 231:1272, 1975.

44. Berman DS, Schaefler S, Simberkoff MS, et al.: Staphylococcus aureus colonization in intravenous drug abusers, dialysis patients, and diabetics. J Infect Dis 155:829, 1987.

45. Garcia-Caballero J, Herruzo-Cabrera H, Vera-Cortes ML, et al.: The growth of micro-organisms in intravenous fluids. J Hosp Infect 6:154–157, 1985.

46. Rinaldi MG: Zygomycosis. Infect Dis Clin North Am 3:19–341, 1989.

47. Bayer AS, Chow AW, Anthony BF, et al.: Serious infections in adults due to group B streptococci. Clinical and serotypic characterization. Am J Med 61:498–503, 1976.

48. Farley MM, Harvey C, Stull T, et al.: A population-based assessment of invasive disease due to group B streptococcus in nonpregnant adults. N Engl J Med 328:1807–1811, 1993.

49. CDC: Recommendations of the Advisory Committee for Elimination of Tuberculosis. Screening for tuberculosis and tuberculosis infection in high-risk populations, and the use of preventive therapy for tuberculous infection in the United States. MMWR 39(RR-8):1–12, 1990.

50. Zhanel GG, Harding GK, Nicolle LE: Asymptomatic bacteriuria in patients with diabetes mellitus. Rev Infect Dis 13:150–154, 1991.

51. Patterson JE, Andriole VT: Bacterial urinary tract infections in diabetes. Infect Dis Clin North Am 9:25–51, 1995.

52. Evanoff GV, Thompson CS, Foley R, et al.: Spectrum of gas within the kidney. Emphysematous pyelonephritis and emphysematous pyelitis. Am J Med 83:149–154, 1987.

53. Vasquez JA, Sobel JD: Fungal infections in diabetes. Infect Dis Clin North Am 9:97–115, 1995.

54. Fan-Havard P, O'Donovan C, Smith SM, et al.: Oral fluconazole vs. amphotericin B bladder irrigation for treatment of candidal funguria. Clin Infect Dis 21:960–965, 1995.

55. Morris JT, Seaworth BT, McAllister CK: Pulmonary tuberculosis in diabetics. Chest 102:539–541, 1992.

56. Wheat LJ: Infection and diabetes mellitus. Diabetes Care 3:187–195, 1980.

57. Ip M, Osterberg LG, Chau PY, et al.: Pulmonary melioidosis. Chest 108:1420–1424, 1995.

58. Marrie TJ: Bacteraemic pneumococcal pneumonia: A continuously evolving disease. J Infect 24:247, 1992.

59. Watanakunakorn C, Greifenstein A, Stroh K, et al.: Pneumococcal bacteremia in three community teaching hospitals from 1980 to 1989. Chest 103:1152, 1993.

60. Mufson MA, Kreiss DM, Wasil RE, et al.: Capsular types and outcome of bacteremic pneumococcal disease in the antibiotic era. Arch Int Med 134:505–510, 1974.

61. Bouter KP, Diepersloot RJA, van-Romunde LKJ, et al.: Effect of epidemic influenza on ketoacidosis, pneumonia and death in diabetes mellitus: a hospital register survey of 1976–1979 in The Netherlands. Diabetes Res Clin Pract 12:61, 1991.

62. Koziel H, Koziel MJ: Pulmonary complications of diabetes mellitus—pneumonia. Infect Dis Clin North Am 9:65–97, 1995.

63. American Thoracic Society: Guidelines for the initial management of adults with community-acquired pneumonia: diagnosis, assessment of severity, and initial antimicrobial therapy. Am Rev Respir Dis 148:1418–1426, 1993.

64. American Thoracic Society: Treatment of tuberculosis and tuberculosis infection in adults and children: The official statement of the American Thoracic Society. Am J Respir Crit Care Med 149:1359–1374, 1994.

65. Centers for Disease Control and Prevention: Prevention and control of influenza: Recommendations of the Immunization Practices Advisory Committee (ACIP). MMWR Morb Mortal Wkly Rep 46(RR-9):1–25, 1997.

66. Bolan G, Broome CV, Facklam RR, et al.: Pneumococcal vaccine efficacy in selected populations in the United States. Annals Int Med 104:1–6, 1986.

67. Butler JC, Breiman RF, Campbell JF, et al.: Pneumococcal polysaccharide vaccine efficacy—An evaluation of current recommendations. JAMA 270:1826–1830, 1993.

68. Centers for Disease Control and Prevention. Recommendations of the Immunization Practices Advisory Committee: pneumococcal polysaccharide vaccine. MMWR Morb Mortal Wkly Rep 46(RR-8):1–24, 1997.

69. Jernigan DB, Cetron MS, Breiman RF: Minimizing the impact of drug-resistant Streptococcus pneumoniae (DRSP). JAMA 275:206–209, 1996.

70. Baltimore RS: New challenges in the development of a conjugate pneumococal vaccine [Editorial]. JAMA 268:3366–3367, 1992.

71. Pozzilli P, Gale WAM, Visalli N, et al.: The immune response to influenza vaccination in diabetic patients. Diabetologia 29:850–854, 1986.

72. Diepersloot RJA, Bouter KP, Beyer WEP, et al.: Humoral immune response and delayed type hypersensitivity to influenza vaccine in patients with diabetes mellitus. Diabetologia 30:397–401, 1987.

73. Diepersloot RJA, Bouter KP, Hoekstra JBL: Influenza infection and diabetes mellitus. Case for annual vaccination. Diabetes Care 13:876–882, 1990.

74. Sentochnik DE: Deep soft-tissue infections in diabetic patients. Infect Dis Clin North Am 9:53–63, 1995.

75. Blum M: Infections of genitourinary prosthesis. Infect Dis Clin North Am 3:259–274, 1989.

76. Francis KR, Lamaute HR, Davis JM, et al.: Implications of risk factors in necrotizing fasciitis. Am Surg 59:304–308, 1993.

77. Patel SR, Olenginski TP, Perruquet JL, et al.: Pyomyositis: Clinical features and predisposing conditions. J Rheumatol 24:1734–1738, 1997.

78. Sutherland ME, Meyer AA: Necrotizing soft-tissue infections. Surg Clin North Am 74:591–605, 1994.

79. Anzai AK. Fourniere's gangrene: A urologic emergency. Am Fam Physician 52:1821–1825, 1995.

80. Knighton DR, Fiegel VD: Growth factors and comprehensive surgical care of diabetic wounds. Curr Opin Gen Surg 32–39, 1993.

81. Bishop JR, Moul JW, Sihelnik SA, et al.: Use of glycosylated hemoglobin to identify diabetics at high risk for penile periprosthetic infections. J Urol 147:386, 1992.

82. Lipsky BA, Pecoraro RE, Larson SA: Outpatient management of uncomplicated lower-extremity infections in diabetic patients. Arch Intern Med 150:790–797, 1990.

83. Gerding DN: Foot infections in diabetic patients: The role of anaerobes. Clin Infect Dis 20(Suppl. 2):S283–S288, 1995.

84. Wheat LJ, Allen SD, Henry M, et al.: Diabetic foot infections: Bacteriologic analysis. Arch Intern Med 146: 1935–1940, 1986.

85. Lipsky BA, Baker PD, Landon GC, et al.: Antibiotic therapy for diabetic foot infections: comparison of two parenteral-to-oral regimens. Clin Infect Dis 24:643–648, 1997.

86. Grayson ML, Gibbons GW, Habershaw GM, et al.: Use of ampicillin/sulbactam vs. imipenem/cilastin in treatment of limb-threatening foot infections in diabetic patients. Clin Infect Dis 18:683–693, 1994.

87. Lipsky BA: Osteomyelitis of the foot in diabetic patients. Clin Infect Dis 25:1318–1326, 1997.

88. Caputo GM, Cavanagh PR, Ulbrecht JS, et al.: Assessment and management of foot disease in patients with diabetes. N Engl J Med 331:854–860, 1994.

89. Grayson ML, Gibbons GW, Balogh K, et al.: Probing to bone in infected pedal ulcers: A clinical sign of underlying osteomyelitis in diabetic patients. JAMA 273:721–723, 1995.

90. Brakora MJ, Sheffield PJ: Hyperbaric oxygen therapy for diabetic wounds. Clin Podiatr Med Surg 12:105–117, 1995.

91. Gough A, Clapperton M, Rolando N, et al.: Randomised placebo-controlled trial of granulocyte-colony stimulating factor in diabetic foot infection. Lancet 350:855–859, 1997.

92. Tierney MR, Baker AS: Infections of the head and neck in diabetes mellitus. Infect Dis Clin North Am 9:195–216, 1995.

93. Rubin J, Yu VL: Malignant external otitis: insights into pathogenesis, clinical manifestations, diagnosis and therapy. Am J Med 85:391, 1988.

94. Sen P, Louria DB: Infectious complications in the elderly diabetic patient. Geriatrics 38:63–66, 71–72, 1983.

95. Klein JO: Otitis externa, otitis media, mastoiditis. In Mandell GL, Bennett JE, Dolin R (eds): Mandell, Douglas and Bennett's Principles and Practice of Infectious Diseases. New York: Churchill Livingstone Inc., 1995, pp. 579–585.

96. Sadé J, Lang R, Goshen S, et al.: Ciprofloxacin treatment of malignant external otitis. Am J Med 87:S138–S139, 1989.

97. Pollack M: Pseudomonas aeruginosa. In Mandell GL, Bennett JE, Dolin R (eds): Mandell, Douglas and Bennett's Principles and Practice of Infectious Diseases. New York: Churchill Livingstone Inc., 1995, pp. 1980–2003.

98. Fidel PL, Sobel JD: Immunopathogenesis of recurrent vulvovaginal candidiasis. Clin Microbiol Rev 9:335–348, 1996.

99. Desai PC, Johnson BA: Oral fluconazole for vaginal candidiasis. Am Fam Physician 54:1337–1340, 1996.

100. Sugar AM: Mucormycosis. Clin Infect Dis 14(suppl. 1): S126, 1992.

101. Sugar AM: Agents of mucormycosis and related species. In Mandell GL, Bennett JE, Dolin R (eds): Mandell, Douglas and Bennett's Principles and Practice of Infectious Diseases. New York: Churchill Livingstone Inc., 1995, pp. 2311–2321.

102. Artis WM, Fountain JA, Delcher HK, et al.: A mechanism of susceptibility to mucormycosis in diabetic ketoacidosis: Transferrin and iron availability. Diabetes 31:1109–1114, 1982.

103. Ericsson M, Anniko M, Gustafsson H, et al.: A case of chronic progressive rhinocerebral mucormycosis treated with liposomal amphotericin B and surgery [letter]. Clin Infect Dis 16:585–586, 1993.

104. Strasser MD, Kennedy RJ, Adam RD: Rhinocerebral mucormycosis. Therapy with amphotericin B lipid complex. Arch Intern Med 156:337–339, 1996.

105. Gonzalez CE, Couriel DR, Walsh TJ: Disseminated zygomycosis in a neutropenic patient: Successful treatment with amphotericin B lipid complex and granulocyte colony-stimulating factor. Clin Infect Dis 24:192–196, 1997.

106. Tervonen T, Oliver RC: Long-term control of diabetes mellitus and periodontitis. J Clin Periodontol 20:431–435, 1993.

107. Oliver RC, Tervonen T: Diabetes—A risk factor for periodontitis in adults? J Periodontol 65:530–538, 1994.

108. Breen JD, Karchmer AW: Staphylococcus aureus infections in diabetic patients. Infect Dis Clin North Am 9:11–24, 1995.

109. Boelaert JR, DeSmedt RA, DeBaere YA, et al.: The influence of calcium mupirocin nasal ointment on the incidence of Staphylococcus aureus infections in haemodialysis patients. Nephrol Dial Transplant 4:278–281, 1989.

110. Doebbeling BN, Breneman DL, Neu HC, et al.: Elimination of Staphylococcus aureus nasal carriage in health care workers: Analysis of six clinical trials with calcium mupirocin ointment. The Mupirocin Collaborative Study Group. Clin Infect Dis 17:466–474, 1993.

111. Winsett OE, Wolma FJ: Complications of vascular access for hemodialysis. South Med J 78:513–517, 1985.

112. Lye WC, Leong WC, Leong SO, et al.: A prospective study of peritoneal dialysis—related infections in CAPD

patients with diabetes mellitus. Adv Peritoneal Dialysis 9:195–197, 1993.

113. Tolkoff-Rubin NE, Rubin RH: The infectious disease problems of the diabetic renal transplant recipient. Infect Dis Clin North Am 9:117–130, 1995.

114. Hibberd PL, Rubin RH: Renal transplantation and related infections. Semin Resp Infect 8:216–224, 1993.

115. Graves PM, Norris JM, Pallansch MA, et al.: The role of enteroviral infections in the development of IDDM— limitations of current approaches. Diabetes 46:161–168, 1997.

116. Signore A, Procaccini E, Chianelli M, et al.: Retroviruses and diabetes in animal models: Hypotheses for the induction of the disease. Diabete Et Metabolisme 21:147–155, 1995.

117. Helfand RF, Gary HE, Freeman CY, et al.: Serologic evidence of an association between enteroviruses and the onset of type 1 diabetes mellitus. J Infect Dis 172:1206–1211, 1995.

118. Rayfield EJ, Mento SJ: Viruses may be etiologic agents for non-insulin-dependent (type II) diabetes. Rev Infect Dis 5:341–345, 1983.

45

Cutaneous Manifestations of Diabetes Mellitus

Shobana Sood and William D. James

The manifestations of diabetes mellitus (DM) in the skin are varied and numerous. Approximately 30% of patients with diabetes present with skin disease and the number of patients who will have cutaneous manifestation of diabetes during their lifetime approaches 100%. Dermatological disorders associated with diabetes generally appear after the primary disease has developed; however, they may appear at the onset of diabetes or even precede the disease by years. Skin findings in diabetes can be classified into five categories: (1) skin manifestations with strong association with diabetes; (2) diseases of the blood vessels; (3) skin disease with a possible association; (4) infection; and (5) skin reactions to diabetic treatment (Table 45–1). The purpose of this chapter is to provide an approach to diagnosis and treatment of skin diseases associated with diabetes mellitus.

Cutaneous Diseases Associated with Diabetes Mellitus

Diabetic Dermopathy

This condition, also called shin spots, is the most common cutaneous manifestation of diabetes. It begins as small, dull-red, scaly papules and plaques that progress to multiple, bilateral, well-circumscribed, round to oval, atrophic, hyperpigmented lesions on the shins and lateral calves (Fig. 45–1). It is asymptomatic, present mainly in adults and is twice as common in men. Patients tend to have a long history of diabetes.

The pathogenesis is unclear. Some authors describe a preceding papular eruption, which is independent of trauma. However, Lithner[1] was able to duplicate these lesions with local thermal trauma. Dermopathy appears

TABLE 45–I   Spectrum of Skin Disease in Diabetes Mellitus

I. Cutaneous manifestations associated with diabetes:
  A. Diabetic dermopathy
  B. Necrobiosis lipoidica diabeticorum
  C. Diabetic thick skin
    1. Scleredema
    2. Subclinical thickening
    3. Finger pebbles
    4. Limited joint mobility and waxy skin
  D. Bullous diabeticorum
  E. Perforating disease
  F. Insulin resistance syndromes (Acanthosis nigricans)
  G. Lipodystrophy
  H. Eruptive xanthomas
II. Diseases of the blood vessels:
  A. Macroangiopathy
  B. Microangiopathy
    1. Rubeosis facei
    2. Erysipelas-like erythema
    3. Pigmented purpura

III. Cutaneous manifestations with possible association with diabetes:
  A. Bullous pemphigoid
  B. Granuloma annulare
  C. Yellow skin/nails (carotenemia)
  D. Pruritus
IV. Infections in diabetics:
  A. Bacterial
    1. Pseudomonas
  B. Fungal
    1. Candida
    2. Phycomycetes (Mucor)
V. Cutaneous reactions to diabetic treatment:
  A. Oral hypoglycemics; complications of
    1. Photosensitivity reactions
    2. Sulfa cross reactions
  B. Insulin; complications of
    1. Allergic reactions
    2. Lipoatrophy
VI. Miscellaneous

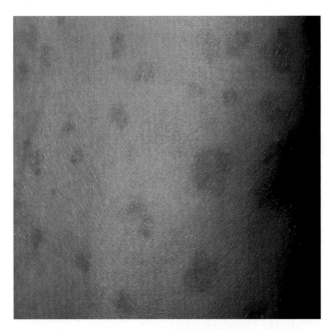

Figure 45–1. Diabetic dermopathy: hyperpigmented oval atrophic macules.

to be posttraumatic atrophy and postinflammatory hyperpigmentation in poorly vascularized skin.[2]

Pathology of acute lesions include edema of the epidermis and papillary dermis, extravasated erythrocytes, and a lymphohistiocytic infiltrate. Older lesions have thickening of the capillary walls and deposition of a periodic acid-schiff PAS-positive, diastase-resistant material in the basement membrane representing neutral mucopolysaccharides. While not specific, these are characteristic findings in diabetic microangiopathy.

Hyperpigmented atrophic patches on the shins are not limited to diabetics; 20% of persons without diabetes in comparable age groups have similar lesions as compared to 30 to 60% of patients with diabetes.[3]

However, when diabetic dermopathy is defined as four or more lesions, lesions were absent in nondiabetics and present in 14% of diabetics.[4] The multilesional definition also had a high correlation with retinovascular disease. Because these lesions are asymptomatic, treatment is not indicated.

Necrobiosis Lipoidica Diabetocorum (NLD)

NLD is present in 0.3 to 0.7% of diabetics. Conversely, 60% of 171 patients with NLD were found to have DM on presentation. Another 20% had glucose intolerance and or a family history of DM. NLD has been reported prior to the onset of diabetes in approximately 15% of patients by an average of 2 years. It is three times more common in females and is associated with both type 1 and type 2 diabetes. Patients with NLD tend to have more severe diabetes than patients without this skin lesion. Although it may appear at any age, the mean age of onset is 34 years. In the insulin-dependent

group, onset is at an earlier age (mean age of 22) than in noninsulin users (mean age of 49).[5] There is spontaneous resolution in 13–19% of cases after 1 to 34 years. Residual scarring and atrophy remain.[6]

The primary lesion is an erythematous papule or plaque (Fig. 45–2). These evolve radially into sharply defined, erythematous plaques with a depressed, waxy, yellow-brown, atrophic and telangiectatic center that can cover the entire pretibial area (Fig. 45–3). In the active lesion, the periphery may be reddish blue and indurated. Ulceration is reported in about one third of lesions after minor trauma.[7] It correlates with sensory impairment and occurs mainly in diabetics. In areas of chronic ulceration, squamous cell carcinoma has been reported in 6 cases. In 15% of cases, lesions are present in other areas, especially on the hands, fingers, forearms, face, and scalp. However, NLD exclusively in areas other than the legs occurs in less than 2% of patients.[8] Such lesions may have a different clinical appearance; they may be raised and firm and have a papular, nodular or plaque-like appearance, which resembles granuloma annulare.

On histologic examination, there is degeneration of collagen throughout the dermis, histiocytes in a palisaded arrangement around the degenerated collagen and vascular changes. Quimby et al.[9] biopsied 12 female patients with NLD and found vasculopathy in all patients with endothelial swelling and thickening and hyalinization often leading to vascular occlusion. Immunoreactants were also found in vessels of involved skin in 11 of 12 patients; most commonly fibrin, C3, and

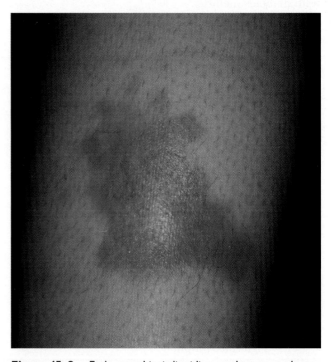

Figure 45–2. Early necrobiosis lipoidica: erythematous plaque on anterior shin.

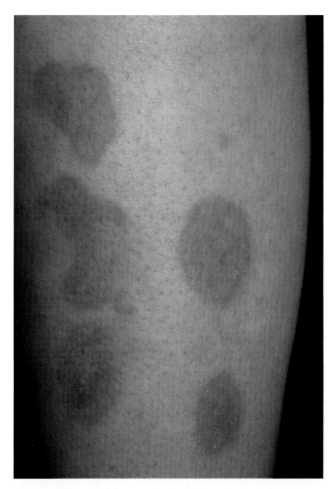

Figure 45–3. Late necrobiosis lipoidica: waxy, atrophic, yellow-brown plaque.

IgM. This is strong evidence for the role of vascular alterations as primary events in the pathogenesis of NLD.[9] In general, however, the diagnosis may be made on clinical grounds alone and it is advisable to avoid surgical procedures on the lower legs in diabetics.

There are a number of treatment options for NLD; none of which have a high success rate. Topical corticosteroids have been shown to be beneficial and high potency topical steroids under occlusion may be used for a few weeks.[10] Intralesional corticosteroids may be helpful. Because atrophy is a feature of the disease itself, it is best to limit topical and intralesional steroids to symptomatic or advancing lesions. Biopsies of uninvolved skin reveal an inflammatory infiltrate extending into normal skin and it may therefore be useful to inject intralesional steroids into clinically normal skin in an attempt to halt progression.[11] Aspirin and dipyridamole modify aggregation of platelets and have been used, alone and in combination with success.[12,13] Pentoxyfylline has been reported to be useful in healing ulcers.[14] Petzelbauer et al.[15] reported that a 5-week course of systemic corticosteroids was given to six patients, four of whom were diabetic with complete res-

olution of NLD lesions. Glycemic control was acheived by increasing either the oral hypogycemic or insulin dose. This approach is useful in early stages of disease because atrophy is not a problem with a short course of systemic steroids. Hyperbaric oxygen was successful in healing ulcerated NLD of 7 years duration.[16]

Diabetic Thick Skin

There are four categories of diabetes associated thick skin as defined by Huntley[2]: (1) scleredema adultorum of Buschke; (2) subclinical but measurable increased skin thickness; (3) finger pebbles; and (4) scleroderma-like skin changes with stiff joints and limited mobility.

Scleredema. Scleredema is a connective tissue disease of unknown etiology. There are two major subtypes of scleredema; diabetes associated, and juvenile onset scleredema. Scleredema diabeticorum most commonly is associated with long-standing, poorly controlled, insulin-dependent diabetes. It typically occurs in middle-aged, overweight men. Scleredema is present in 3% of patients with NIDDM.[17–19] Scleredema adultorum of Buschke, despite its name has been noted primarily in children following a febrile illness. Rarely scleredema has been reported without either of these conditions.[20]

Clinically, scleredema diabeticorum is characterized by diffuse and symmetric induration of the upper posterior neck and back (Fig. 45–4). The skin is hard and shiny with absent superficial markings. It cannot be wrinkled or pressed together into folds. The febrile illness associated subset generally resolves spontaneously in about 18 months. Scleredema diabeticorum does not spontaneously remit and can affect larger areas of the trunk and occasionally the arms and legs.[21]

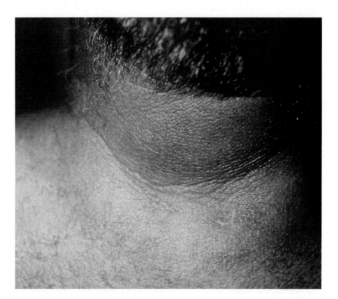

Figure 45–4. Scleredema diabeticorum: indurated, thickened skin of upper back.

Histologic findings are of a thickened dermis with large wide clear spaces between collagen bundles and increased amounts of glycosaminoglycans and collagen.[22,23] Treatment is generally ineffective; however, because pathogenesis may be due to nonenzymatic glycosylation of proteins, tight glucose control may be beneficial. Some reports support this idea.[24]

Subclinical Skin Thickening. Huntley[2] believes there is a continuum in degree of skin thickening; diabetes is generally associated with measurably thickened skin. Collier demonstrated thickened forearm skin in diabetics using pulsed ultrasound. This thickening of skin may be clinically inapparent, but measurable.

Finger Pebbles. Finger pebbles, also known as knuckle pebbles, were described by Huntley[25] as another manifestation of thickening in diabetic skin. In a study of 60 diabetics, 45 (75%) had a visual marker for skin thickening; a pebbly appearance of knuckle and distal finger skin as compared to 21% of control subjects. The lesions are multiple, grouped, minute papules on the extensor surface of the fingers on or near the knuckle or periungual area. They are less extensive than those of acanthosis nigricans. Finger pebbles do not appear to be a marker for microvascular or renal complications.

Limited Joint Mobility and Waxy Skin. Rosenbloom[26] initially described this condition in three teenagers with insulin-dependent diabetes in the mid 1970s. These patients had striking limitations of their fingers and large joints in association with short stature, waxy tight skin, delayed sexual maturation, and early microvascular complications. Rosenbloom et al.[27] reported a 30% prevalence rate of joint limitation in a study of 309 patients; most of whom had juvenile diabetes. One third of these patients also had tight, waxy skin which the examiner could not tent. Limited joint mobility (LJM) has also been found in noninsulin-dependent diabetics and in all age groups.[28] Limited joint mobility in older patients is hard to differentiate from age and occupation-related changes as well as other chronic diseases.[29] This is reflected in the high frequencies of LJM in older control populations.[30] Prevalence of limited joint mobility is approximately 30–35%.

LJM begins in the fifth finger at the metacarpophalangeal and proximal interphalangeal joints and may progress radially to involve other fingers. It is bilateral, symmetric, and painless. Testing of joint limitation is best accomplished by having the examiner individually extend the proximal and distal interphalangeal and metacarpophalangeal joints. Normal extension is 180 degrees for the proximal interphalangeal (PIP) and distal interphalangeal (DIP) joints and 60 degrees for the metacarpophalangeal (MCP). The wrist should be passively extended to at least 70 degrees and the elbow to 180 degrees. Even if range-of-motion is normal, there may be a gritty resistance to movement and an inability to tent the skin; referred to as sclerodermatous changes in the literature. Another easy method of examining for LJM is the use of the "prayer sign." This maneuver revealed a prevalence rate of abnormality of only 7% as compared to 31% when the above more extensive method was used. None of the control group demonstrated abnormalities with the prayer sign.[31]

LJM is important to diagnose because it is associated with microvascular complications of diabetes such as retinopathy and nephropathy. Among patients who had diabetes for more than 4.5 years, 82 of 169 had joint limitation. Fifty percent (41 patients) of those with joint limitation also had microvascular complications while only 10 patients without joint limitation had complications. Life table analysis showed an 83% risk of microvascular complications after 16 years of diabetes if joint limitation was present compared to a 25% risk if joint limitation was absent. These findings are confirmed by other authors. Beacom et al.[32] reported that patients with long-standing diabetes were 2.5 times more likely to have proliferative retinopathy, decreased nerve conduction velocity, and decreased vibration perception if joint limitation was present than if it was absent.

The pathogenesis of LJM is unclear. Early collagen glycosylation products are increased in diabetes but have not been found to correlate with LJM. Lyons et al.[33] purified collagen from forearm biopsies in control patients and diabetics with and without joint limitation. The level of collagen glycosylation in diabetics was significantly greater than that of control patients, but diabetic patients with LJM had a level of collagen glycosylation similar to that of diabetics with normal joints. Thus, there must be some additional mechanism at work in diabetics who develop limited joint mobility and skin thickening.

There are two mechanisms by which hyperglycemia may lead to irreversible tissue damage. A major consequence of hyperglycemia is nonenzymatic glycosylation of proteins.[34] These advanced glycosylation products, as opposed to early glycosylation products, are responsible for increased cross linkage of collagen, decreased susceptibility to proteolysis, and increased stiffness.[35] Monnier et al.[36,37] showed increases with age and that 95% of insulin-dependent diabetes mellitus (IDDM) patients had abnormal increases for age. It correlates with retinopathy, neuropathy and LJM. Another possible mechanism of stiffening of connective tissue is oxidative stress.[38]

Improved glycemic control may result in improvement in skin stiffness. Lieberman et al.[39] showed reduced skin thickness with pump administration of insulin in three patients. Lyons measured levels of advanced glycosylation, products in skin collagen of 14 diabetic patients before and after 4 months of intensive glycemic control. There was a statistically significant fall in mean blood glucose and mean glycated hemoglobin. This correlated with a fall in glycated collagen levels, however, the advanced glycosylation products did not decrease. This suggests that the glycation of long-lived proteins can be decreased by improved glycemic control, but suggests that once cumulative damage to collagen has occurred, it may not readily reverse.

Bullous Diabeticorum

Bullous diabeticorum is an infrequent, but characteristic eruption of diabetes mellitus. It was first reported in 1930 by Kramer. Fewer than 100 cases have been reported to date. Bullous diabeticorum is characterized by painless, spontaneous blisters occurring on the feet and legs, which heal spontaneously in 2 to 5 weeks with minimal scarring. Rarely, it is reported on the hands and forearms. The bullae are on a nonerythematous base and contain a sterile clear fluid (Fig. 45–5). Some patients may have hemorrhagic blisters that heal with slight atrophy.[40] The patient population affected is varied; age ranges are from 17–79 years of age and it occurs in men and women. Most patients have longstanding diabetes with complications of peripheral neuropathy, retinopathy, or nephropathy.[41]

Histologic examination is variable. There are nonacantholytic blisters with separation either in the

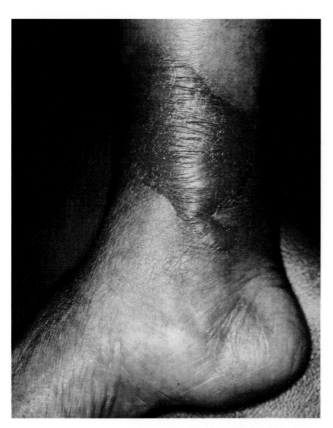

Figure 45–5. Bullous diabeticorum: tense bullous lesion on nonerythematous base.

intraepidermal or subepidermal level. In the dermis, there is thickening of blood vessel walls and minimal inflammation. Direct and indirect immunoflourescence are generally negative; however, James et al.[42] reported a case with positive direct immunofluorescence; with positive staining for IgM, complement and fibrinogen in dermal blood vessels.

Pathogenesis of the eruption is unknown. One theory is that the changes associated with microangiopathy predisposes diabetics to blister formation from even minor trauma. Bernstein et al.[43] showed that insulin-dependent diabetics have a significantly reduced threshold to suction blister development compared to age-matched normal controls. This theory does not explain why most diabetics, even those with microangiopathy do not get bullous lesions. It also does not explain why lesions spontaneously heal and do not recur.

This is a diagnosis of exclusion; appropriate cultures, histopathology, and immunofluorescence is important to rule out other bullous diseases. Because bullous diabeticorum spontaneously resolves, treatment is not indicated.[44]

Perforating Disorders

The perforating disorders encompass four entities based on the nature of the material extruded through the epidermis. These are reactive perforating collagenosis (collagen), Kryle's disease (keratin), perforating folliculitis (infundibulum of the hair follicle), and elastosis perforans serpiginosa (elastin). Clinically, these are umbilicated hyperpigmented papules that contain a central adherent keratotic plug located on the extensor surfaces of the extremities in men and women (Fig. 45–6). There is a predominance in African American patients. Koebner's phenomenon may occur, as evidenced by appearance of new lesions in sites of trauma. Pruritus is the major symptom. Histologically these show transepithelial extrusion of material.[45]

Over the past 15 years, reactive perforating collagenosis (RPC), Kryle's disease, and perforating folliculitis (PF) have all been reported to occur with chronic renal failure most commonly the result of diabetic nephropathy. This otherwise rare phenomenon is reported in a striking number of patients undergoing dialysis (10% Hurwitz et al.; 6% Poliak et al.; and 4.5% Hood et al.).[46–48] Hood et al.[47] reported 9 cases of Kryle's disease in 200 patients; 7 of these patients had IDDM. Poliak[48] reported that of 100 patients studied, all six with reactive perforating collagenosis had severe diabetes mellitus and 5 had chronic renal insufficiency. Though usually occuring in patients on dialysis, perforating disorders have been reported in patients before onset of dialysis[49] and in the absence of dialysis. Successful treatments include topical tretinoin 0.1%[50] and ultraviolet light.[51]

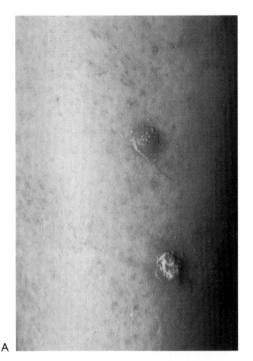
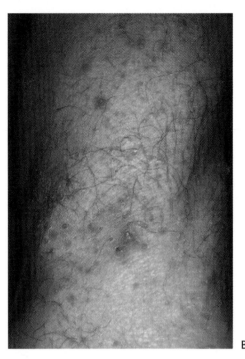

Figure 45–6. Perforating disease: papules with central keratotic plug.

Acanthosis Nigricans

Acanthosis nigricans is characterized by brown, velvety to verrucous, papillomatous, plaques that are most often localized to the axillae but also occur on the neck, under the breasts and in other intertriginous areas (Fig. 45–7). Frequently, they are associated with papillomatous outgrowths, referred to as skin tags.[52] Acanthosis nigricans may be associated with a number of metabolic and endocrinological disorders including DM, obesity, hypothyroidism, Cushing's syndrome, acromegaly, estrogen therapy, androgen excess, and polycystic ovary disease.[53]

Sudden and extensive acanthosis nigricans has been associated with malignancy, most commonly of the gastrointestinal tract, particularly the stomach. It is postulated that the tumor secretes a factor that leads to acanthosis nigricans. Other nonfamilial congenital anomalies, such as Lawrence–Seip syndrome (total lipodystrophy), Bloom syndrome, and the Prader–Willi

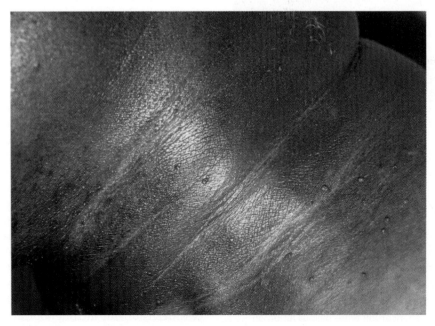

Figure 45–7. Acanthosis nigricans: brown, velvety, verrucous plaques on neck.

syndrome, have been associated with acanthosis nigricans.[54] Drugs such as nicotinic acid, niacinamide, diethylstilbestrol, oral contraceptives, and glucocorticoids have also been causally related to acanthosis nigricans.[55-57] In addition, there is a rare autosomal dominant transmission of the disease.

In recent years, the pathogenesis of acanthosis nigricans and its association with DM has been elucidated. In 1976 Kahn et al.[58] classified two groups of patients based on insulin receptors; type A, patients in whom a receptor abnormality is the result of a genetic defect, and type B patients in whom there are circulating antibodies to the insulin receptor. Type A patients are predominantly African American females with onset of severe, generalized acanthosis nigricans during infancy or childhood. They have hyperandrogenic manifestations such as hirsutism, clitoromegaly, and a masculine habitus. Insulin resistance in type A patients is a genetic deficiency of insulin receptors; leading to a state of hyperinsulinemia. Type B patients are also predominantly African American female patients but acanthosis nigricans tends to present at a later age, with a mean of 39 years. Acanthosis nigricans in these patients is less severe and less extensive and is associated with various chronic diseases; autoimmune disease, scleroderma, Sjogren's, and rheumatoid arthritis. Insulin resistance in type B patients is due to blocking antibodies to the insulin receptor causing hyperinsulinemia which fluctuates in parallel with level of antireceptor antibodies.

The proposed pathogenesis of acanthosis nigricans is as follows: tissue resistance to insulin causes the pancreas to produce more insulin, resulting in hyperinsulinemia. At normal concentrations, insulin binds preferentially to its classic receptor, which mediates glucose metabolism. At high concentrations, insulin acquires greater affinity for insulin-like growth factor receptors which have been cultured from human fibroblasts and keratinocytes and may stimulate keratinocytes to proliferate and form acanthosis nigricans. Also insulin-like growth factors may stimulate the stroma granulosa and increase androgen production and virilization.[59]

Lipodystrophy

Total lipodystrophy, also known as lipoatrophic diabetes was first described by Lawrence in 1946. This syndrome was characterized by loss of subcutaneous tissue in late childhood and early adulthood, followed by insulin-resistant hyperglycemia, hyperlipemia, and fatty enlargement of the liver. Seip described a congenital syndrome similar to that of Lawrence but without diabetes and with rapid growth, advanced bone age, hypermusculature, hepatomegaly, and hyperpigmentation. Since these original descriptions, the syndromes have been further delineated.[60]

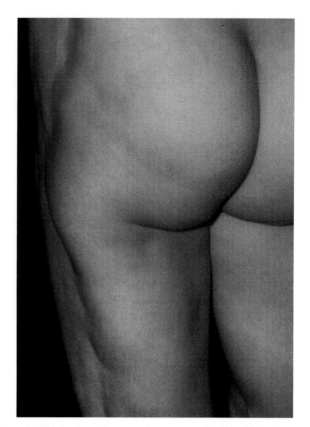

Figure 45–8. Lipodystrophy: loss of subcutaneous adipose tissue.

Total lipodystrophy is characterized by complete absence of subcutaneous adipose tissue (Fig. 45–8) and NIDDM. It can be divided into congenital and acquired lipodystrophy. Congenital lipoatrophic diabetes is more common and accounts for 60% of the cases. Transmission is autosomal recessive and there is often consanguinity. Congenital total lipodystrophy shows a predominance of females with increased stature, advanced bone age, hirsutism, muscular hypertrophy, hepatomegaly with abdominal protuberance, hyperpigmentaion, and hypertriglyceridemia. Women have clitoral enlargement and men have penile enlargement; gonadotropin and androgen levels are normal. Though hyperglycemia is considered a constant component of total lipodystrophy, several children initially did not present with elevated serum glucose. However, they did develop hyperglycemia over time. Other features include nephromegaly, central nervous system abnormalities, and cardiomegaly.[61] Oseid et al.[62] described patients with insulin resistance, acanthosis nigricans, hyperlipemia, and lipodystrophy and suggested that in total lipodystrophy there is an insulin receptor defect in adipose tissue. Although patients with total lipodystrophy and diabetes have shown marked insulin resistance, there is no evidence of insulin antibodies, or antireceptor antibodies.[62] Acquired total lipodystrophy and partial lipodystrophy variants exist. These are not clearly associated with DM.

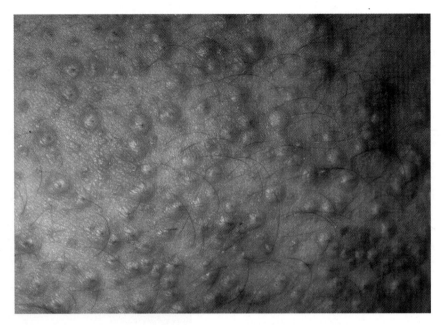

Figure 45–9. Eruptive xanthomas: multiple closely set yellow papules.

Eruptive Xanthomas

Eruptive xanthomas are so named because they are 1- to 4-mm, red-yellow dermal nodules that occur rapidly in crops or showers on the exensor surfaces of hands, arms, knees, and buttocks (Fig. 45–9). They may also arise in areas of trauma (Koebner phenomenon). In the acute stage they have an erythematous halo around the base and can be pruritic and tender. With correction of the lipid abnormalities, they heal spontaneously after a few weeks; first becoming noninflammatory yellow papules and then healing with hyperpigmented scars. The biochemical defect in patients with eruptive xanthomas is an elevated plasma level of chylomicrons. The most common causes of chylomicronemia are the secondary forms of hyperlipoproteinemia: uncontrolled DM, alcohol ingestion, or exogenous estrogens. Less commonly, the primary hyperlipoproteinemias can cause eruptive xanthomas; lipoprotein lipase deficiency manifests in children as eruptive xanthomas, lipemia retinalis, and pancreatitis. Type 5, familial hyperlipoproteinemia occurs in adulthood and may be associated with DM, hypertension, and polyneuropathy.[63]

Blood Vessel Disease in Diabetics

Macroangiopathy

Diabetics have a higher prevalence of large vessel disease. Arterial disease in the legs manifests as pallor on elevation, mottling on elevation, coldness of the toes, skin atrophy, hair loss, and diminished pulses.[64] A reliable sign of large vessel disease is dependent rubor with delayed return of color (>15 sec) after pressure is applied to the skin.

Microangiopathy

The role of diabetic microangiopathy is not completely understood. Capillary basement membrane thickening, deposition of PAS + material, elastic fiber clumping, and increased deposition of type 4 collagen lead to structural changes in the microcirculation.[65] As well, there is functional microangiopathy; most likely secondary to glycosylation of erythrocyte membranes, hemoglobin, fibronectin, fibrinogen, and platelets. Glycosylation decreases red blood cell pliability and leads to sluggish blood flow.[66] There are several excellent references to review the topic in greater detail.[2,66]

Skin signs of microangiopathy include rubeosis facei, erysipelas-like erythema, the pigmented purpuras, diabetic dermopathy, NLD and the diabetic foot.[66] Rubeosis facei, is a manifestation of functional microangiopathy, which is evident by venous engorgement. In a prospective study of 50 patients that compared facial redness, 59% of patients with diabetes had markedly red faces.[67] Erysipelas-like erythema is a well-demarcated erythema on the lower leg or foot that may be evidence of bone destruction and incipient gangrene. Pigmented purpura is characterized by orange pigmented spots on the shins and are secondary to blood vessel extravasation in the superficial vascular plexus. Pigmented purpura has been described in older diabetics who also had a history of cardiac decompensation and diabetic dermopathy.[68] The diabetic foot is covered in Chapters 30–34.

Cutaneous Disease with Possible Association with Diabetes Mellitus

Bullous Pemphigoid

Two reports have demonstrated an increased prevalence of bullous pemphigoid (BP) in patients with diabetes. Chuang and colleagues[69] showed an occurrence rate of 20% of primary diabetes in patients with bullous pemphigoid. Published age-specific prevalence rates of diabetes are significantly lower than those seen in this study.[70] Downham and Chapel[71] found a 41% prevalence of diabetes in patients with bullous pemphigoid.

The mechanism of coexistent BP and DM is unknown. As stated earlier, diabetics have a lower threshold to suction blister formation. Autoimmune mechanisms may play a role in both diseases. Bassiouny et al.[72] reported that glycosylated collagen is antigenic; it is capable of inducing production of autoantibodies against this modified collagen. Similarly, nonenzymatic glycosylation of basement membrane proteins may become targets for autoantibody production in diabetics leading to blister formation.

Treatment of diabetes-associated BP is similar to conventional BP therapy. Therapy with tetracycline and niacinamide is an excellent initial choice that may avoid systemic steroids. If prednisone is necessary, it is desirable to taper off it rapidly and to use steroid sparing agents such as azathioprine whenever feasible. Downham and Chapel[71] found that widespread BP was harder to control in patients with DM. Diabetics required higher initial doses of Prednisone and had more complications of therapy and higher mortality rates than non diabetics with similar extent of disease.

Granuloma Annulare

The typical lesion of localized granuloma annulare (GA) is an annular collection of flesh colored papules with a flat center most often located on the hands and feet of children and young adults (Fig. 45–10). Females are affected two to one. The lesions remit spontaneously without scarring. Other, less common forms of GA are: generalized, macular, nodular, and perforating. Generalized GA consists of numerous disseminated flesh-colored papules in sun exposed areas on the chest, the "V" of the neck and the forearms (Fig. 45–11). It is most common in middle-aged women. The cause of GA is not known. All forms of GA share the same histopathology; the dermis contains palisading granulomas with abundant mucin. Because of the histologic similarity to necrobiosis lipoidica diabeticorum, the relationship of GA to diabetes has been explored for evidence of an association.[73–77]

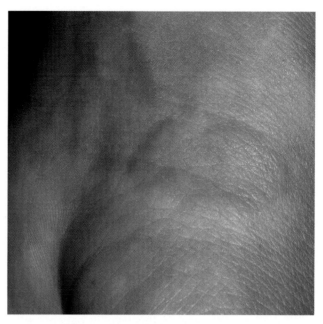

Figure 45–10. Annular collection of papules with flat center.

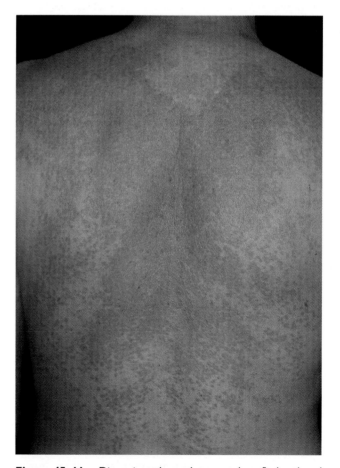

Figure 45–11. Disseminated granuloma annulare: flesh-colored papules in sun exposed distribution.

The reports showing a positive relationship to diabetes share a common theme; it is the generalized, atypical, and perforating types that have shown an increased incidence of diabetes. One series by Muhlemann and Williams[74] shows a higher than expected incidence of diabetes in localized GA. Some reports have failed to show an association,[78,79] while others have shown an association. Dabski and Winkelmann,[73] in a series of 1350 patients, found an incidence of DM in 21% of patients with generalized GA and 9.7% incidence in patients with localized GA. However, the authors state that their study is affected by referral bias. Kidd et al. performed oral and intravenous glucose tolerance tests and found consistently high serum glucose and serum insulin levels in patients with localized and generalized forms of GA. They proposed that was indicative of a state of mild insulin resistance. Conversely, Dandona et al. and Gannon[78,79] measured glycosylated hemoglobin levels and found no difference in this level in patients with and without GA. This, they claim is a better measure of glucose control since it measures long term carbohydrate control. In summary, there may be a greater than expected incidence of abnormal carbohydrate metabolism in patients with the disseminated and perforating forms of GA.

Yellow Nails and Yellow Skin

Lithner noted that 18 of 36 diabetics had yellow nails. Nine control patients did not have this discoloration.[80] This may occur on any nail but it is most evident on the distal aspect of the nail of the hallux. Until recently, it was thought that the yellow hue of diabetics was due to carotenemia, however, this now known to be false. The likely mechanism is glycosylation of long lived proteins such as collagen.[81]

Pruritus

The association between diabetes and generalized pruritus is often cited but poorly documented. In a survey of 500 patients, approximately 3% reported generalized pruritus at some point after the diagnosis of their diabetes.[82] Kantor and Lookingbill[83] did a retrospective study of 44 patients with generalized pruritus to determine the prevalence of systemic disease. They compared the group with 44 age- and sex-matched psoriatic controls. Thirteen of 44 patients were found to have systemic disease as compared to 10 of 44 psoriatic controls. When diabetes and hypothyroidism were excluded, the pruritus group had a statistically significant incidence of systemic disease. Diabetes was more common in the control group.

Infections in Diabetics

This subject is extensively covered in Chapter 44. However, certain points are worth emphasizing. Three types of infection are especially prevalent in diabetics: bacterial, Candidal, and Phycomycetes infections.

Of bacterial infections, malignant otitis externa is of particular concern. It is an uncommon but serious infection caused by *Pseudomonas aeruginosa*. It presents with severe pain and purulent discharge from the external ear. It begins as cellulitis and may progress to chondritis, osteomyelitis, and infectious cerebritis.[66] Treatment is debridement and systemic antibiotics; despite this it often has a fatal outcome.[84]

Candidal infections may be the first sign of diabetes. They occur in poorly controlled disease and can be widespread. Candidal infection can present as stomatitis in children, paronychia, pruritus vulvae, balanitis, and between the third and fourth finger as erosio interdigitale blastomycetica (Fig. 45–12). Control of these lesions requires good glucose control and topical and, occasionly, oral, antifungal treatment. Dermatophytosis does not appear to be more frequent in diabetics.[85]

Patients with uncontrolled DM and ketosis may be predisposed to deep fungal infections or rhinocerebral mucormycoses of the nose and sinuses. Opportunistic infections with phycomycetes can also establish infection in traumatized skin, such as chronic ulcers that may lead to gangrene. Treatment is aggressive: debridement and intravenous antifungal treatment.[66]

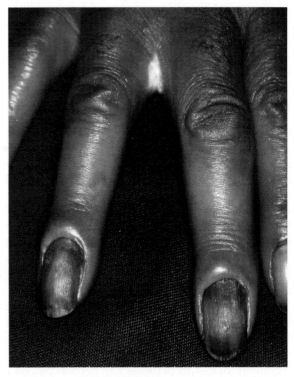

Figure 45–12. Erosio interdigitale blastomycetica: chronic candidal paronychia (nail fold infection).

Cutaneous Reactions to Diabetic Treatment

Allergic reactions occur in 1–5% of patients taking sulfonylureas. Most commonly this is an exanthematous morbilliform, eruption that appears within the first month of therapy[66] (Fig. 45–13). Urticaria, angioedema, pruritus, and generalized erythema can also be seen. Sulfonylureas can also cause photosensitive reactions, usually of the photoallergic type as well as lichenoid and rosacea-like eruptions.[86]

The chlopropamide-alcohol flush is similar to the disulfiram-alcohol reaction. It may occur in 10–30% of patients and begins 15 min after alcohol ingestion. There is flushing, headache, tachycardia, and shortness of breath that lasts about 1 hr. It is a dominantly inherited trait that is seen mainly in NIDDM patients. Pathogenesis is thought to be due to an increased sensitivity to endogenous opioids.[87]

Allergic reactions to insulin were much more common before the availability of recombinant human insulin (see Chapter 18). In the past, allergic reactions to animal insulins occurred in as many as 10–56% of all diabetics. About 8–12% required modification in their insulin regimen. Although far fewer patients use pork and beef insulin, it is still available (Eli Lilly and Co.

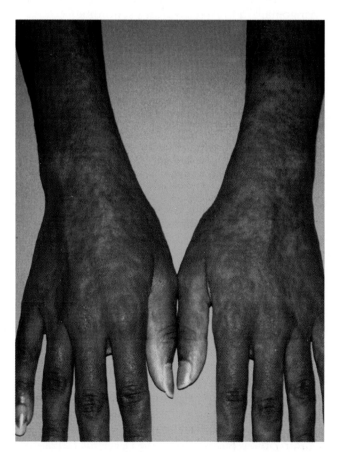

Figure 45–13. Allergic reaction to sulfonylurea.

Indianapolis, IN) and still in use in select patients. Approximately 25% of those with insulin allergy had a concomitant history of penicillin allergy. Clinically, reactions of the local delayed type are localized to the site of injecton and the surrounding skin. They peak at 24 to 48 hr and present with itching or burning erythema followed by indurated papule or nodule formation. They occur about 1 month after starting therapy and usually resolve with continued injections. These reactions are due to cell-mediated immunity. Immediate reactions to insulin can either be localized or generalized; local reactions are far more common. Localized immediate allergy is pruritic erythema at the injection site, which leads to urticaria and sometimes vesiculation. Reaction begins 20 min after injection and disappears in the next 6–18 hr without residua. This reaction is seen soon after starting therapy or after years of uncomplicated treatment.

IgG antibody mediates this reaction.[88] Changing to a more purified form, or human recombinant insulin is the treatment of choice; beef insulin has been shown to be more allergenic than pork.[89] Human insulin is the least allergenic though there have been reports of allergy to that as well.[90,91] Generalized insulin reactions are rare; less than 1% of patients with insulin allergy have generalized reactions. They present with widespread erythema or urticaria with or without angioedema with severe pruritus and are usually preceded by a local reaciton. Anaphylaxis may occur. This type of reaction is mediated by IgE.[88] Some patients have been reported with a delayed, serum sickness-like reaction following the immediate allergic reaction.[92,93]

Insulin-induced lipoatrophy is loss of subcutaneous fat at sites of insulin injection. It occurs 6 to 24 months after injections are started. It may be due to lipolytic components of some insulin preparations or secondary to the immune complex mediated inflammatory response.[94] Spontaneous resolution of the site is rare. In some children, painless nodules can occur at sites of repeated injection; these may resemble a lipoma.[66]

Diabetes Caused by Systemic Disease

Hemochromatosis is characterized by cutaneous hyperpigmentation, cirrhosis, and diabetes mellitus. The bronze color of the skin is due to excess melanin production not to increased iron stores. (Fig. 45–14).

The glucagonoma syndrome is caused by tumors of the alpha cell glucagon secreting portion of the pancreas; it is characterized by hypersecretin of glucagon, mild diabetes without ketosis, weight loss, and necrolytic migratory erythema. The latter is a chronic, fluctuating dermatitis with an annular and figurate erythema that forms bullae and erosions. It is pronounced

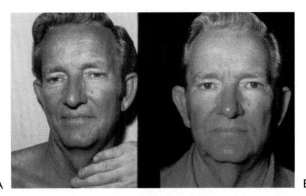

Figure 45–14. A. Classic bronze pigmentation of primary hemochromatosis. Note marked difference in color of nurse's hand. B. Decreased bronzing of skin after 196 phlebotomies (each 500 mL blood) over a 2-year follow-up period.

A   B

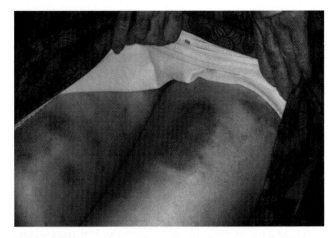

Figure 45–15. Patches of necrolytic, migratory erythema typical of glucagonoma syndrome.

in the intertriginous and periorificial areas (Fig. 45–15). The rash improves after removal of the glucagon secreting tumor.[21]

Miscellaneous

Other conditions that have a reported higher incidence in diabetics will be briefly mentioned. Dermatitis herpetiformis has been reported with increased frequency; of 18 Finnish patients who had both diseases, 9 had the HLADR3 DRW2 genotype.[21] Thus, the HLA association of DM and IDDM may be an explanation for the concomitant existence of these diseases.[95]

A higher than expected incidence of vitiligo has been seen in diabetics; in both maturity onset (4.8% of diabetics had vitiligo)[96] and in juvenile onset diabetes (1.6%.)[97,98] This may be because both are autoimmune disorders.[99]

Other diseases with reported association with diabetes are erosive oral lichen planus,[100–102] clear cell syringoma,[103] and Alezzandrini's syndrome.[104]

References

1. Lithner F: Cutaneous reactions of the extremities of diabetics to local thermal trauma. Acta Med Scand 198:319–325, 1975.

2. Huntley AC: Cutaneous manifestations of diabetes mellitus. Dermatol Clin 7:531–546, 1989.

3. Feingold KR, Elias PM: Endocrine-skin interactions. J Am Acad Dermatol 17:921–940, 1987.

4. Murphy R: Skin lesion in diabetic patients: The "spotted leg" syndrome. Lahey Clin Found Bull 14:10–14, 1965.

5. Shall L, Millard LG, et al.: Necrobiosis lipoidica: "The footprint not the footstep." Br J Dermatol 123:47, 1990.

6. Lowitt MH, Dover JS: Necrobiosis lipoidica. J Am Acad Dermatol 25:735–748, 1991.

7. Meurer M, Szeimies RM: Diabetes mellitus and skin disease. Curr Probl 20:11–23, 1991.

8. Muller SA, Winkelman RK: Necrobiosis lipoidica diabeticorum: A clinical and pathological investigation of 171 cases. Arch Dermatol 93:272–281, 1966.

9. Quimby SR, Muller SA, Schroeter AL: The cutaneous immunopathology of Necrobiosis lipoidica diabeticorum. Arch Dermatol 124:1364–1371, 1988.

10. Goette K: Resolution of necrobiosis lipoidica with occlusive clobetasol propionate treatment. J Am Acad Dermatol 22:855–856, 1990.

11. Boulton AJM, Cutfield RG, et al.: Necrobiosis lipoidica diabeticorum: A clinicopathologic study. J Am Acad Dermatol 18:530–537, 1988.

12. Heng MCY, Song MK, Heng MK: Healing of necrobiotic ulcers with antiplatelet therapy correlation with plasma thromboxane levels. Int J Dermatol 28:195–197, 1989.

13. Quimby SR, Muller SA, Schroeter AL, et al.: Necrobiosis lipoidica diabeticorum: Platelet survival and response to platelet inhibitors. Cutis 43:213–215, 1989.

14. Noz KC, Korstanje MJ, Vermeer BJ: Ulcerating necrobiosis lipoidica effectively treated with pentoxifylline. Clin Exp Dermatol 18:78–79, 1993.

15. Petzelbauer P, Wolff K, Tappeiner G: Necrobiosis lipoidica: Treatment with systemic corticosteroids. Br J Dermatol 126:542–545, 1992.

16. Weisz G, Ramon Y, Waisman D, et al.: Treatment of necrobiosis lipoidica diabeticorum by hyperbaric oxygen. Acta Derm Venereol 73:447–448, 1993.

17. Cohn BA, Wheeler CE, Briggamon RA: Scleredema adultorum of Buschke and diabetes mellitus. Arch Dermatol 101:27–35, 1970.

18. Venencie PY, Powell FC, et al.: Scleredema: A review of thirty-three cases. J Am Acad Dermatol 11:128–134, 1984.

19. Cole GW, Headley J, Skowsky R: Scleredema diabeticorum: A common and distinct cutaneous manifestation of diabetes mellitus. Diabetes Care 6:189–192, 1983.

20. Varga J, Gotta S, et al.: Scleredema adultorum: Case report and demonstration of abnormal expression of extracellular matrix genes in skin fibroblasts in vivo and in vitro. Br J Dermatol 132:992–999, 1995.

21. Jelinek JE: Cutaneous manifestations of Diabetes mellitus. Int J Derm 33:605–617, 1994.

22. Fleischmajer R, Perlish JS: Glycosaminoglycans in scleroderma and scleredema. J Invest Dermatol 58:129–132, 1972.

23. Roupe G, Laurent TC, et al.: Biochemical characterization and tissue distribution of the Scleredema in a case of Buschke's disease. Acta Derm Venereol 67:193–198, 1987.

24. Lieberman LS, Rosenbloom AL, Riley WJ, et al.: Reduced skin thickness with pump administration of insulin. N Engl J Med 303:940–941, 1980.

25. Huntley AC: Finger pebbles: A common finding in diabetes mellitus. J Am Acad Dermatol 14:612–617, 1986.

26. Rosenbloom AL, Frias JL: Diabetes, short stature and joint stiffness- a new syndrome. Clin Res 22:92A, 1974.

27. Rosenbloom AL, Silverstein JH, et al.: Limited joint mobility in childhood diabetes mellitus indicates increased risk for microvascular disease. N Engl J Med 305:191–194, 1981.

28. Lawson PM, Maneschi F, Kohner EM: The relationship of hand abnormalities to diabetes and diabetic retinopathy. Diabetes Care 6:140–143, 1983.

29. Larkin JG, Frier BM: Limited joint mobility and Dupuytren's contracture in diabetic, hypertensive, and normal populations. Br Med J 292:1494, 1986.

30. Rosenbloom AL: Limited joint mobility in insulin dependent childhood diabetes. Eur J Pediatr 149:380–388, 1990.

31. Clarke CF, Piesowicz AT, Spathis GS: Limited joint mobility in children and adolescents with insulin dependent diabetes mellitus. Ann Rheumatic Dis 49:236–237, 1990.

32. Beacom R, Gillespie EL, et al.: Limited joint mobility in Insulin-dependent Diabetes: Relationship to retinopathy, peripheral nerve function and HLA status. Q J Med 219:337–344, 1985.

33. Lyons TJ, Kennedy L: Non-enzymatic glycosylation of skin collagen in patients with type I diabetes mellitus and limited joint mobility. Diabetologia 28:2–5, 1985.

34. Lyons TJ, Bailie KE, et al.: Decrease in skin collagen glycation with Improved glycemic control in patients with insulin-dependent diabetes mellitus. J Clin Invest 87:1910–1915, 1991.

35. Collier, A, Patrick AW, et al.: Relationship of skin thickness to duration of diabetes, glycemic control, and diabetic complications of male IDDM patients. Diabetes Care 12:309–312, 1989.

36. Monnier VM, Vishwanath V, et al.: Relation between complications of type I diabetes mellitus and collagen linked fluorescence. N Engl J Med 314:403–408, 1986.

37. Monnier VM, Kohn RR, Cerami A: Accelerated age related browning of human collagen in diabetes mellitus. Proc Natl Acad Sci USA 81:583–587, 1984.

38. Aoki Y, Yazaki K, et al.: Stiffening of connective tissue in elderly diabetic patients: Relevance to diabetic nephropathy and oxidative stress. Diabetologia; 36:76–83, 1993.

39. Lieberman LS, Rosenbloom AL, et al.: Reduced skin thickness with pump administration of Insulin. NEJM 303:940–941, 1980.

40. Toonstra J: Bullous diabeticorum. J Am Acad Dermatol 13:799, 1985.

41. Allen GE, Hadden DR: Bullous lesion of the skin in diabetes. Br J Dermatol 82:216–220, 1970.

42. James WD, Odom, RB, Goette K: Bullous eruption of Diabetes mellitus. A case with positive immunofluorescence findings. Arch Dermatol 116:1191–1192, 1980.

43. Bernstein, JE, Levine LE, et al.: Reduced threshold to suction-induced blister formation in insulin-dependent diabetics. JAAD 8:790–791, 1983.

44. Oursler JR, Goldblum OM: Blistering eruption in a diabetic. Arch Derm 127:217, 1991.

45. Patterson JW: The perforating disorders. J Am Acad Derm 10:561–581, 1984.

46. Chang P, Fernandez V: Acquired perforating disease: report of nine cases. Int J Dermatol 32:874–876, 1993.

47. Hood, AF, Hardegan GL, Zarate AR, et al.: Kryle's disease in patients with chronic renal failure. Arch Dermatol 118:85–88, 1982.

48. Poliak SC, Lebwohl MG, Parris A, et al.: Reactive perforating collagenosis associated with diabetes mellitus. N Engl J Med 306:81–84, 1982.

49. Hudson RD, Apisarnthanarax P: Renal failure and perforating folliculitis. JAMA 247:1936, 1982.

50. Brand A, Brody N: Keratotic papules in chronic renal disease. Cutis 28:637–639, 1981.

51. Cochran RJ, Tucker SB, Wilkin JK: Reactive perforating collagenosis of diabetes mellitus and renal failure. Cutis 31:55–58, 1983.

52. Brown J, Winkelmann RK: Acanthosis nigricans: A study of 90 cases. Medicine 47:33–51, 1968.

53. Feingold KR, Elias PM: Endocrine-skin interactions. JAAD 19:1–20, 1988.

54. Rendon MI, Cruz PD, et al.: Acanthosis nigricans: A cutaneous marker of tissue resistance to insulin. JAAD 21:461–469, 1989.

55. Tromovitch TA, Jacobs PH, Kern S: Acanthosis-like lesions from nicotinic acid. Arch Dermatol 89:222–223, 1964.

56. Katzenellenbogen I: Dermatoendrocrinologic syndrome due to diethylstilbestrol. JAMA 101:1695–1696, 1956.

57. Randle HW, Winkelmann RK: Steroid-induced acanthosis nigricans in dermatomyositis. Arch Dermatol 115:587–588, 1979.

58. Kahn CR, Flier JS, et al.: The syndromes of insulin resistance and acanthosis nigricans: Insulin receptor disorders in man. N Engl J Med 294:739–745, 1976.

59. Cruz PD, Hud JA: Excess Insulin binding to Insulin-like growth factor receptors: Proposed mechanism for acanthosis nigricans. J Invest Dermatol 98:82S–85S, 1992.

60. Arnold HL, Odom RB, James WD: Andrew's Diseases of the Skin, Clinical Dermatology. Philadelphia: W.B. Saunders Company, 1990, p. 575.

61. Senior B, Gellis SS: The syndromes of total lipodystrophy and of partial lipodystrophy. Pediatrics 33:593–612, 1964.

62. Oseid S, Beck-Nielsen H, Pederson O, et al.: Decreased binding of insulin to its receptor in patients with generalized lipodystrophy. N Engl J Med 296:245–248, 1977.

63. Cruz PD, East C, Bergstresser PR: Dermal, subcutaneous, and tendon xanthomas: Diagnostic markers for specific lipoprotein disorders. J Am Acad Dermatol 19:95–111, 1988.

64. Feingold KR, Siperstein MD: Diabetic vascular disease. Adv Intern Med 31:309–340, 1986.

65. LoGerfo FW, Coffman JD: Vascular and microvascular disease of the foot in diabetes: Implications for foot care. N Engl J Med 311:1615–1619, 1984.

66. Perez MI, Kohn SR: Cutaneous manifestations of diabetes mellitus. J Am Acad Dermatol 30:519–531, 1994.

67. Gitelson S, Wertheimer-Kaplinski N: Color of the face in diabetes mellitus. Observations on a group of patients in Jerusalem. Diabetes 14:201–208, 1965.

68. Lithner F: Purpura, pigmentation and yellow nails of the lower extremities in diabetics. Acta Med Scand 199:203–208, 1976.

69. Chuang TY, Korkji W, et al.: Increased frequency of diabetes mellitus in patients with bullous pemphigoid: A case control study. JAAD 11:1099–1102, 1984.

70. Palumbo PJ, Elveback LR, et al.: Diabetes mellitus: Incidence, prevalence, survivorship and causes of death in Rochester, Minnesota, 1945–1970. Diabetes 25:566–573, 1976.

71. Downham TF, Chapel TA, et al.: Bullous Pemphigoid: Therapy in patients with and without diabetes mellitus. Arch Dermatol 114:1639–1642, 1978.

72. Bassiouny AR, Rosenberg H, McDonald TL: Glycosylated collagen is antigenic. Diabetes 32:1182–1184, 1983.

73. Dabski K, Winkelmann RK: Generalized granuloma annulare: Clinical and laboratory findings in 100 patients. J Am Acad Dermatol 20:39–47, 1989.

74. Muhlemann MF, Williams DRR: Localized granuloma annulare is associated with insulin-dependent diabetes mellitus. Br J Dermatol 111:325–329, 1984.

75. Binazzi M, Simonetti V: Granuloma annulare, Necrobiosis lipoidica and diabetic disease. Int J Dermatol 27:576–579, 1988.

76. Shimizu H, Harada T, Baba E, et al.: Perforating granuloma annulare. Int J Dermatol 24:581–583, 1985.

77. Kidd GS, Graff GE, Davies BF, et. al.: Glucose tolerance in granuloma annulare. Diabetes Care 8:380–384, 1985.

78. Gannon TF, Lynch PJ: Absence of carbohydrate intolerance in granuloma annulare. J Am Acad Dermatol 30:662–663, 1994.

79. Dandona P, Freedman D, Barter S, et al.: Glycosylated haemoglobin in patients with necrobiosis lipoidica and granuloma annulare. Clin Exp Dermatol 6:299–302, 1981.

80. Lithner F: Purpura, pigmentation and yellow nails of the lower extremities in diabetics. Acta Med Scand 199:203–208, 1976.

81. Oimomi M, Maeda Y, Hata F, et al.: Glycosylation levels of nail proteins in diabetic patients with retinopathy and neuropathy. Kobe J Med Sci 31:183–188, 1985.

82. Gilchrest BA: Pruritus. Arch Intern Med 142:101–105, 1982.

83. Kantor GR, Lookingbill DP: Generalized pruritus and systemic disease. J Am Acad Dermatol 9:375–382, 1983.

84. Petrozzi JW, Warthan TL: Malignant external otitis. Arch Dermatol 110:258–260, 1974.

85. Lugo-Somolinos A, Sanchez JL: Prevalence of dermatophytosis in patients with diabetes. J Am Acad Dermatol 26:408–410, 1992.

86. Stern RS, Wintroub BU: Adverse cutaneous reactions to medication. Adv Dermatol 2:3–17, 1987.

87. Wilkin JK: Flushing reactions: Consequences and mechanisms. Ann Intern Med 95:468–476, 1981.

88. Jegasothy BV: Allergic reactions to insulin. Int J Dermatol 19:139–141, 1980.

89. Schernthaner G: Immunogenicity and allergenic potential of animal and human insulins. Diabetes Care 16(Suppl. 3):155–165, 1993.

90. Small P, Lerman S: Human insulin allergy. Ann Allergy 53:39–41, 1984.

91. Grammer LC, Metzger BE, Patterson R: Cutaneous allergy to human insulin. JAMA 251: 1459–1460, 1984.

92. DeShazo RD, Levinson AI, Boehm T, et al.: Severe persistent biphasic local (immediate and late) skin reactions to insulin. J Allergy Clin Immunol 59:161–164, 1977.

93. Galloway J, DeShazo RD: Insulin chemistry and pharmacology; insulin allergy, resistance, and lipodystrophy. In Ellenberg and Rifkin's Diabetes Mellitus, 4th ed. 1990, p. 504.

94. Edidin DV: Cutaneous manifestations of diabetes mellitus in children. Pediatr Dermatol 2:161–179, 1985.

95. Reunala T, Maki H: Dermatitis herpetiformis: A genetic disease. Eur J Dermatol 3:519–526, 1993.

96. Dawber RPR: Vitiligo in mature onset diabetes mellitus. Br J Dermatol 80:275–278, 1968.

97. Macaron C, Winter RJ, et al.: Vitiligo and juvenile diabetes mellitus. Arch Dermatol 113:1515–1517, 1977.

98. Gould IM, Gray RS, Urbaniak SJ, et al.: Vitiligo in diabetes mellitus. Br J Dermatol 113:153–155, 1985.

99. Abraham Z, Lahat N, et al.: Psoriasis, necrobiosis lipoidica, granuloma annulare, vitiligo and skin infections in the same diabetic patient. J Dermatol 17:440–447, 1990.

100. Nigam PK, Singh G, Agrawal JK: Plasma insulin response to oral glycemic stimulus in lichen planus. Br J Dermatol 19:128–129, 1988.

101. Lundstrom IM: Incidence of diabetes mellitus in patients with oral lichen planus. Int J Oral Surg 12:147–152, 1983.

102. Lozada-Nur F, Luangjarmekorn I, Silverman S, et al.: Assessment of plasma glucose in 99 patients with oral lichen planus. J Oral Med 40:60–61, 1985.

103. Kudo H, Yonezawa I, Ieki A, et al.: Generalized eruptive clear cell syringoma. Arch Dermatol 125:1716–1717, 1989.

104. Hoffman MD, Dudley C: Suspected Alezzandrini's syndrome in a diabetic patient with unilateral retinal detachment and ipsilateral vitiligo and poliosis. J Am Acad Dermatol 26:496–497, 1992.

46

Oral Disorders in Diabetes Mellitus

Sara G. Grossi, Steven Offenbacher, and Michael Edward Fritz

The periodontal diseases are a group of chronic, progressive bacterial infections resulting in inflammation and destruction of tooth supporting tissues. They include two distinct groups: gingivitis, which is a reversible inflammatory response of the gingiva to bacterial plaque; and periodontitis, which is an irreversible extension of the inflammatory process into the surrounding periodontal tissues. The periodontitis group includes the early-onset and adult-onset forms. These forms are distinguished from each other by the age of onset, the clinical picture and the etiological agents involved in the infectious process (Table 46–1). Usually, in the disease process, bacteria colonize the teeth, forming an adherent plaque that progressively becomes more Gram-negative, anaerobic, and virulent in composition as it matures. All forms of periodontitis include the common feature of destruction of connective tissue attachment and alveolar bone loss. Clinically this is manifested as deepening of periodontal pockets, gingival recession, increased tooth mobility, and ultimately tooth loss. It would appear from recent literature that all of the periodontal diseases are episodic in

nature, generally characterized by long periods of remission and short terms of exacerbation. The prevalence of the periodontal diseases in the general population is second only to caries and it is, therefore, not surprising that they represent the principal oral complications associated with diabetes mellitus: both insulin-dependent diabetes mellitus (IDDM) and non-insulin-dependent diabetes mellitus (NIDDM). Prevention of periodontal diseases is therefore essential in people with diabetes, in whom these diseases pose a dual clinical management problem. First, they are more prevalent, more severe, and progress more rapidly in diabetics and second, the concomitant chronic Gram-negative periodontal infection may complicate the metabolic control of diabetes.

Historical Perspective

Periodontal Disease

The relationship between diabetes mellitus and periodontal disease has been extensively studied. As early

TABLE 46–1 Types of Periodontal Diseases

Disease	Found in	Clinical Appearance	Etiological Agents
Gingivitis	Children Adults	Red, swollen, bleeding gingiva	*Actinomyces viscosus* certain cocci

Periodontitis
Early-onset
Periodontitis
  Juvenile
  periodontitis
	Young adults
	  (<20 years old)
		May show normal or swollen gingiva
		Severe bone loss localized to few teeth only
			Actinobacillus
			Actinomycetemcomitans

Prepubertal
  periodontitis
	Children
	  (<10 years old)
		Same as "Juvenile periodontitis" above	?

Periodontitis	Adults	May show normal or swollen gingiva; Generalized pocketing and radiographic evidence of bone loss	*Porphyromonas gingivalis* *Bacteroides forsythus* *Prevotella intermedia*

as 1862, Sieffert[1] described an association between diabetes and pathological changes in the oral cavity. Prior to 1920, investigators reported that almost all diabetics had severe periodontal inflammation, often with resorption of the alveolar process, with pus formation (pyorrhea or periodontoclasia). In the 1920s to the 1940s the acceptable profile for a definite clinical entity called *diabetic periodontopathy* was established. Changes were observed in the periodontium, with tendencies toward periodontal abscesses and rapid alveolar bone destruction.[2–6]

Belting and co-workers,[7] in a well-defined study, demonstrated that the severity of periodontal disease was significantly greater among persons with diabetes than in normal subjects. Glavind and colleagues,[8] utilizing detailed analysis of 51 diabetics and 51 control subjects, concluded that diabetics less than 30 years of age have an accelerated rate of periodontal destruction. Patients with diabetes of 10 or more years duration had greater alveolar bone loss than those with less than 10 years duration. Other longitudinal studies in humans have documented the fact that there is not only more severe periodontal disease in diabetics but that periodontal disease progresses more rapidly.[9]

Several groups of investigators have recently discussed the relationship between periodontal disease and diabetes. Bacic et al.[10] found significantly more missing teeth among diabetics than nondiabetics. Hugoson et al.[11] and Thortensson et al.[12] showed that long-duration diabetes (>18 years) was associated with more severe periodontal disease compared to short-duration (<5 years), especially in diabetics aged 40 to 49 years. This is consistent with trends seen in other complications of diabetes such as retinopathy and nephropathy, in that the longer the duration of diabetes, the greater the prevalence and severity of the complications. Conclusive evidence of the relationship between diabetes mellitus and periodontal disease came from the studies conducted in Pima Indians. Researchers at State University of New York at Buffalo, studying 3300 Pima Indians, showed that periodontal disease is more prevalent and severe among diabetic compared to nondiabetic Pimas.[13] In this same population, Nelson et al.[14] reported that the incidence of periodontitis was 2.6 times greater in Pimas with diabetes compared to nondiabetics. Fritz and coworkers[15] examined diabetic patients in ambulatory diabetic clinics and found that controlled diabetics had a higher incidence of periodontal disease than age- and sex-matched controls without the disease. These studies concluded that diabetes mellitus increased the risk for developing periodontitis in a manner that could not be explained on the basis of age, sex, or amount of dental plaque or calculus. Accordingly, periodontal disease has been recognized as the sixth complication of diabetes mellitus.[16] Increased susceptibility to periodontal

infections, impaired host response, and excessive collagenolytic activity have been proposed as possible mechanisms.

The environment of the ginigival sulcus in patients with diabetes may be significantly different compared with nondiabetics. Urea glucose levels have been found to be elevated in gingival crevicular fluids. Studies by Golub and coworkers[17] have demonstrated a greater tissue collagenase activity in diabetic rats. It is now speculated that local alterations of the crevicular environment, as well as microvascular changes, could cause changes in the subgingival flora that affect periodontal health.

It is well known that diabetics have an increased risk for bacterial infections. Several studies demonstrate chemotactic functional defects in leukocytes in patients with diabetes.[18–21] Studies by Van Dyke and coworkers[21] have suggested a reduction in the number of surface receptors on neutrophils of juvenile diabetics and a decrease in neutrophil locomotion. Recently, hyperglycemia and more specifically nonenzymatic glycation of extracellular matrix components and intracellular proteins have been identified as the common basis for diabetic complications such as retinopathy, nephropathy, and neuropathy. The biochemical basis whereby hyperglycemia may lead to the microvascular complications seen in diabetes is increased accumulation of advance glycosylation end products (AGE). AGEs accumulate in diabetic plasma and tissues and recently have been demonstrated also in gingiva of diabetic patients.[22] Macrophages and endothelial cells have specific receptors for common structural elements in AGEs. Interaction of mononuclear phagocytes with AGE-modified proteins induces up regulation of cytokine expression, especially secretion of TNF-α and IL-1 and induction of oxidative stress. Interestingly, the most destructive mechanism operative in the pathogenesis of periodontal disease includes the interaction of bacterial products (mostly LPS) with mononuclear phagocytic cells and fibroblasts resulting in activation and production of catabolic inflammatory mediators including primarily IL-1β, PGE$_2$, TNF-α, and IL-6. These cytokines mediate the secretion of matrix metalloproteinases and ultimately the ensuing tissue destruction. The combination of these two pathways of cytokine upregulation, namely "infection and AGE-mediated" may explain the increase in tissue destruction seen in diabetic periodontitis, and how periodontal infection may in turn complicate the severity of diabetes and the degree of metabolic control.

Caries

In 1947, Cohen[2] could find no difference in caries susceptibility in diabetic patients. However, Sterky and associates[23] demonstrated in a Swedish population that the caries frequency was higher in healthy subjects than in diabetics. This finding was confirmed in 1975 in a study of Matsson and Koch,[24] which compared 33 controlled diabetic children with age- and sex-matched nondiabetic classmates. Both studies suggested that the low refined carbohydrate intake of diabetics may explain the lower frequency of caries in the diabetic patients.[23,24] However, two recent and independent studies have demonstrated that children with IDDM and poor glycemic control have a higher caries index compared to children with IDDM and good metabolic control.[25,26] Therefore, it appears that degree of metabolic control is of importance in the relationship between diabetes mellitus and dental caries. One may speculate that poor control of diabetes is likely associated with differences in bacterial composition in dental plaque, which may in turn be associated with greater caries experience.

Developmental Defects

An influence on the eruption and exfoliation of the teeth has been observed in diabetic children. Accelerated dental development has been described in diabetic children under age $11\frac{1}{2}$ years, whereas there was a delayed dental development in older children.[27]

In addition to eruption and exfoliation of teeth, some data have described a higher tendency of cleft palate development in the offspring of insulin-dependent mothers.

Oral-Vesicular Lesions in the Diabetic

Patients with diabetes have a higher incidence of lichen planus. A syndrome or oral lichen planus, diabetes mellitus, and hypertension was described by Grinspan and colleagues.[28] In addition, atrophic changes of the tongue have been reported, often associated with candidal infection.[29]

Epidemiology

Early limited studies by Sheppard[5] and Rutledge[4] had shown that the prevalence of IDDM was approximately 10% of all periodontitis patients seen. A more recent study[8] demonstrated that patients with a history of diabetes of 10 or more years' duration were much more susceptible to periodontal disease, possibly due to deficiency in host periodontal resistance when confronted with bacterial burden. Szpunar et al.[30] analyzed data from the HANES I and HANES II reporting a substantially higher prevalence of periodontal disease among people with diabetes (33 vs. 14% in diabetics vs. nondiabetics in HANES 1 and 36 vs. 10% in HANES II). Grossi et al.[31] reported in a survey of 1426 adults from Erie County that 45% of diabetics showed severe periodontal disease compared to only 18% of nondiabetics. Diabetes mellitus was the

only systemic disease from a total of 31 diseases examined, that increased the risk for severe periodontitis with an odds ratio of 2.3.

A well-controlled study of 263 patients was done at the State University of New York at Buffalo to determine the prevalence of periodontal disease in diabetics and to assess the relationship of periodontal disease to age and to onset and duration of diabetes.[18] This study demonstrated that periodontitis is more prevalent in IDDM patients than nondiabetic control subjects. In diabetic patients between 10 and 19 years of age or older, the prevalence of overt periodontitis was found to be 9.8%, whereas in those 19 years of age, the prevalence of overt periodontitis was found to be 9.8%, whereas in those 19 years of age or older, the prevalence rose to 39%. Although severe gingivitis was found in diabetic children 11 to 12 years of age, no periodontitis was found before age 12. The prevalence of periodontal disease ranged from 0.1 to 13.3% in the nondiabetic, age-matched control groups.

The studies previously noted from diabetic clinics in Atlanta, Georgia, and in Yugoslavia reported increased periodontal disease and tooth loss when compared with control populations.[10,15] Thus, it is clear that most current studies agree that periodontal disease is more prevalent and severe in patients with IDDM compared with age and oral hygiene status of matched nondiabetic control subjects.

Pathophysiology

The microangiopathies associated with the periodontal tissues of diabetic patients are well-documented in the dental literature.[32] It has been postulated that the decrease in luminal size and vascular perfusion may reduce oxygen consumption in the tissues, thereby providing conditions for growth of anaerobic microorganisms. Furthermore, decreased perfusion has been suggested to depress polymorphonuclear leukocyte mobilization and the availability of plasma antibody and complement to the tissues. No direct evidence has been provided to substantiate any of these concepts. Changes in perfusion are not needed for colonization of anaerobes, because they are consistently found in diseased periodontal pockets of nondiabetic patients.

Several lines of evidence have recently suggested that the function of the neutrophil may be compromised in the diabetic. Because the neutrophil represents the host's first line of defense against bacterial infection, the concept of depressed neutrophil function in the diabetic has enticing implications. Thus, it appears that the diabetic patient may have two problems: first, because of impaired neutrophil function, the possibility exists that periodontal disease may become rampant; and second, chronic Gram-negative periodontal infections may exacerbate the metabolic imbalances of diabetes, causing more frequent acute complications. The latter statement is supported in a study by Taylor et al.,[33] which showed that history of periodontal disease at baseline, that is, chronic bacterial infection, adversely affects control of diabetes at a 3-year follow-up examination, thus suggesting that periodontal infections may indeed, as other infections, complicate diabetes status.

According to Zambon et al.,[34] "the effect of impaired host immune responses as may exist in patients with NIDDM (non-insulin-dependent diabetes mellitus) is apparently not reflected in the subgingival microflora." These authors reported that subgingival microflora in severe periodontitis patients with NIDDM is similar to nondiabetic patients with severe periodontitis. The subgingival microflora of juveniles with IDDM is predominantly composed of *Actinobacillus actinomycetemcomitans* and Capnocytophaga species, resembling that found in juvenile periodontitis.[35] Other studies in IDDM patients[36,37] have found the black-pigmented bacteroides species in higher proportions. These studies suggest that the subgingival microflora of periodontal lesions in diabetic and nondiabetic patients may harbor some of the same periodontal pathogens.

Problem Statement I

Undiagnosed Severe Periodontal Disease in a Patient with Diabetes. Uncontrolled diabetes often coexists with severe periodontal disease. More importantly, undiagnosed periodontal disease may be a source of infection, previously unrecognized, which makes control of diabetes more difficult or nearly impossible. Therefore, patients with diabetes should receive as part of their physical exam for monitoring of diabetic infections and ulcers, oral examination as well. If signs of gingival inflammation are detected or the patient reports occasional gingival bleeding, gum boils or other dental symptoms, the patient should be referred to a periodontist for complete periodontal evaluation, diagnosis, and appropriate treatment.

Generalized severe periodontitis with multiple recurrent periodontal abscess formation occurs in the marginally controlled diabetic. Figures 46–1 through 46–3 show the ranges of periodontal destruction in

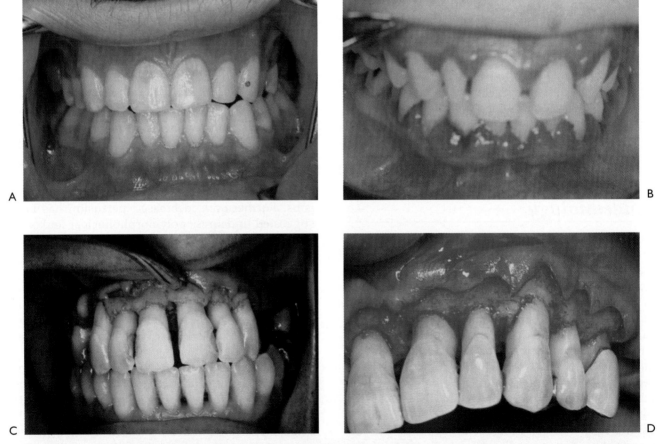

Figure 46–1. A. A 24-year-old diabetic patient with incipient gingivitis. Scaling and home care should reverse this condition. B. A 38-year-old diabetic with severe gingival inflammation and abscess formation. In addition to triage, this patient will probably need soft tissue surgical intervention. C, D. Reflected gingival flaps showing typical bone destruction (*left*) and loss (*right*) in diabetic patients.

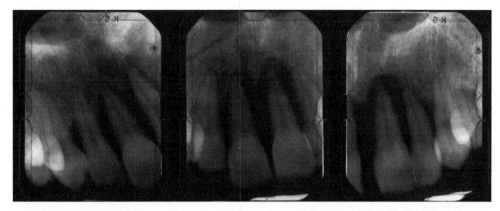

Figure 46–2.   Radiograph of 14-year-old diabetic patient with extensive tooth loss and bone destruction.

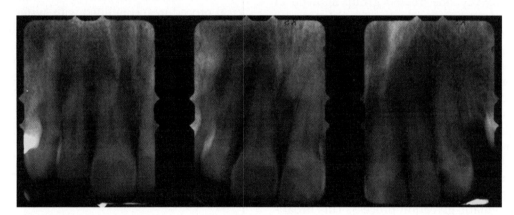

Figure 46–3.   Radiograph of 58-year-old patient with NIDDM showing tooth loss and bone destruction.

patients with diabetes. Dental history usually reveals previous formations of painful gum abscesses, which rapidly swell and drain, becoming asymptomatic. The abscess formation results in a localized, rapid resorption of the alveolar bone.

The extraoral examination of the patient is usually unremarkable, although there may be submaxillary and submental lymphadenopathy and fever, if there is a state of acute infection present. The intraoral examination will reveal erythematous, exophytic, edematous gingiva with moderate plaque and calculus deposits, generalized moderate to severe periodontal pockets ranging from 5 to 10 mm in depth with bleeding on probing, and tooth mobility. Gingival suppuration is usually apparent on gentle palpation. Radiographic evidence of generalized 50 to 70% alveolar bone loss is common. Microbial tests of subgingival plaque will be positive for periodontal pathogens in high numbers.

Problem Statement II

Undiagnosed Diabetes in a Patient Presenting with Severe Periodontal Disease.   Diabetes mellitus could be an undiagnosed systemic factor complicating the severity of periodontal disease. Patients who present with repeated intraoral infections, a slow healing pos-

textraction socket, severe periodontal disease with extensive alveolar bone loss or who do not respond favorably to standard periodontal therapy, including mechanical debridement and/or periodontal surgery, should be screened for diabetes. There have been recent studies that have discussed the pattern of alveolar bone breakdown in some of the periodontally involved diabetics seen in a hospital-based population.[18,19] Although this was variable, bone loss was much more severe in the first molar and incisor regions than in other areas. The molar/incisor distribution of alveolar bone loss is found in juvenile periodontitis (periodontosis) and in periodontitis seen in the trisomy 21 patient. Both of these diseases have been associated with leukocytes with depressed chemotactic function. The overall clinical presentation is so characteristic that any patient who presents with only moderate plaque and calculus, with an exaggerated alveolar bone loss, or with frequent periodontal abscess formation should be screened for diabetes (see Chapters 11 and 12).

Definitive Treatment Plan

Treatment of periodontal disease in a diabetic patient should be targeted at arresting the periodontal infection and controlling the inflammatory destructive process. Control of the Gram-negative periodontal infection and the ensuing inflammation will in turn benefit the overall diabetic status and degree of metabolic control. Two lines of evidence support this observation. A small pilot study by Williams and Mahan,[38] showed that seven of nine patients with diabetes mellitus had a significant reduction in insulin requirement following successful treatment of the periodontal disease. Recently Grossi et al.[39] conducted a large randomized clinical trial including 85 diabetic Pima Indians. Treatment of periodontal disease included ultrasonic subgingival debridement and systemic doxycycline (100 mg/day for 14 days), compared to ultrasonic debridement alone (control group). The doxycycline-treated group showed at 3 months after treatment a reduction in pocket depth, subgingival *Porphyromonas gingivalis* and a 9.0% reduction in HbA_{1c}. The changes were significantly better ($p \leq 0.04$) compared to the control group. This study concluded that effective treatment of periodontal infection and reduction of periodontal inflammation resulted in a significant short-term reduction in level of HbA_{1c}. Thus control of periodontal disease should be part of the overall management of the diabetic patient. The reduction in HbA_{1c} in the doxycycline-treated group likely was the result of the antimicrobial effect combined with a possible doxycycline-mediated inhibition of the nonenzymatic glycation process. This broadspectrum antibiotic is concentrated seven- to tenfold in the gingival fluid over serum levels, thus providing an important adjunct in the reduction of periodontal pathogens. In addition, a reduction in level of glycosylated hemoglobin and collagen degradation has been reported in diabetic rats following administration of doxycycline and other tetracyclines.[40] A body of evidence supports the anti-collagenolytic and inhibition of activation of matrix metalloproteinases properties of tetracyclines. Therefore, diabetic patients suffering periodontal disease benefit from systemic administration of tetracycline derivatives in two ways: first, as a potent antimicrobial agent effective in elimination of most periodontal pathogens, and second, as a potent modulator of the diabetic patient's host response to the periodontal infection.

Although it is not practical to run specific laboratory tests on all individuals, many patients with diabetes may benefit from microbiological culturing, sensitivity testing, and leukocyte function tests. The results obtained by these studies may shed light on why some of these individuals present with advanced periodontal disease.

Local anesthesia can be tolerated well. Periodontal surgical procedures can be utilized to further debride the area if bone destruction is apparent. Uniformity of opinion regarding the medical regimen prior to dental surgery does not exist. Nonstressful early morning appointments following insulin therapy and breakfast are recommended to minimize the possibility of insulin-induced hypoglycemia. Surgery can be done with either a local or general anesthetic. It should be noted that insulin-induced hypoglycemia and diabetic coma are possibilities in the dental environment, and the dentist should be aware of their signs and symptoms, and be ready to institute emergency care. Patients who go into hypoglycemic coma cannot take anything by mouth; the most effective treatment is the injection of glucagon or intravenous glucose.

Outcomes

Following successful arrest of the periodontal infection by mechanical debridement (either scaling and/or surgical procedures) combined with systemic antibiotics, periodic (3-month interval) supportive therapy should be instituted to prevent recurrence of the infection and further periodontal destruction. Therefore, the standard professional tooth cleaning and reinstruction in bacterial plaque removal should be combined with possible administration of systemic antibiotic therapy in the case of a positive microbiological test result. During any type of periodontal therapy, the insulin requirement should be carefully monitored because this may change as periodontal infection is brought under control.

The other common alterations of diabetes that have been noted earlier in this chapter, such as oral vesicular lesions, are usually brought under control with the control of the diabetes. Residual candidiasis infections may be controlled with oral suspension or lozenges of nystatin.

Patient Education and Follow-up

The importance of oral health in the diabetic patient must be constantly reinforced. In addition, there should be cooperation with the physician to monitor, and with the patient for periodic recall, of disease-control procedures and prevention of periodontal infection. It is recommended that 3-month recall examination, professional tooth cleaning, and periodic microbiological testing for periodontal pathogens, should be routinely done in the diabetic patient. In addition, full mouth radiographs every 2 years to determine if there has been any progression of bone loss are a requisite part of dental therapy. After therapy, if further periodontal problems arise, patient nonadherence to oral hygiene, systemic antibiotic, and/or insulin therapy is suspected.

Audits of Data

Periodontal status should be evaluated every 3 months for signs of subgingival infection, attachment loss, and inflammation. If a well-controlled diabetic maintains excellent oral hygiene and still develops periodontal abscesses, the predominant microbiological composition of the plaque should be determined. Anaerobic culture and antibiotic sensitivity testing should be considered for these patients. Appropriate antibiotic therapy such as doxycycline, tetracycline HCl, or minocycline should be considered as an important adjunct to standard treatment regimes.

Research Considerations

The bacterial plaque within the periodontal pocket interposed at the tooth-tissue interface represents a significant biological burden to the host. The periodontal pocket is anaerobic and rich in nutrients. Crevicular fluid, which is a serum transudate, continually bathes the subgingival microflora. This fluid is an excellent source of nitrogenous nutrients such as amino acids and proteins for the growth of many asaccharolytic or fastidious microorganisms. The saliva, by comparison, has a relatively high oxygen concentration and only contains one eighth of the nitrogenous substrates that are present in the gingival crevice. The subgingival environment is also conducive to colonization because it is isolated from the cleansing effects of saliva and the mechanical disruptive forces of the tongue and cheeks. Thus, it is not surprising that many fastidious organisms are found virtually exclusively in the periodontal pocket. Subgingival plaque organisms can mature and flourish to reach an extremeely high density of about 10^{11} bacteria/g of plaque. This bacterial density approximates that found in feces. In the lower gastrointestinal tract, the host protects itself from this bacterial burden, in part, by having an elevated rate of epithelial desquamation in direct apposition to the feces. The adherence, colonization, and invasion of the gastrointestinal flora are thus controlled, in part, by epithelial sloughing. However, the tooth is a nondesquamating surface that presents a continual host challenge. The analogous protective mechanism would be destruction of bone and ligamentous attachment, leading to tooth exfoliation. For these reasons, the host's defense mechanisms are particularly important in maintaining host–pathogen homeostasis in the disease process. Many of the organisms that are associated with periodontitits are virulent pathogens, including *Porphyromonas*, *Bacteroides*, *Capnocytophaga*, *Campylobacter*, *Eikenella*, *Treponema*, and

Fusobacterium. The inability of the compromised diabetic host to resist the bacterial assault is the principal modifier leading to the increased severity of disease expression in the diabetic with periodontitis.

The neutrophil is an important phagocytic cell in bacterial clearance and serves as the first line of defense against bacterial infection. Molenaar and coworkers[41] demonstrated that neutrophils from diabetic patients have a significantly decreased chemotactic response. The increased severity of periodontitis in patients with neutrophil abnormalities associated with diseases such as juvenile periodontitis, cyclic neutrophenia, Chediak–Higashi syndrome, and Papillon–LeFevre syndrome has been extensively reviewed.[42] The mechanism of tissue destruction that results from leukocyte dysfunction is unknown but represents a current research interest. Metabolic imbalances in the uncontrolled diabetic, such as hyperglycemia or ketoacidosis, have been demonstrated to decrease neutrophil chemotaxis and phagocytosis. It is conceivable that the sluggish neutrophils may undergo premature degranulation within the tissue, causing severe destruction, rather than within the gingival crevice adjacent to the target microorganisms. Decreased phagocytic function may permit direct tissue invasion of the organisms and further destruction. Irrespective of pathogenic mechanism, it appears likely that neutrophil impairment plays an important role in the pathogenesis of periodontitis in the insulin-dependent patient.

Recent studies by Molvig et al.[43] suggest that macrophage responses to bacterial endotoxins are genetically determined in humans and may therefore reflect susceptibility to Gram-negative bacterial infections. These investigators suggest that the amount of prostaglandin E_2, interleukin-1β, and tumor necrosis factor that is released by macrophages in response to endotoxin challenge is an important host-specific trait that determines the expression of the severity of Gram-negative infections. These studies further suggested that individuals with a "diabetes-resistant" human lymphocyte antigen haplotype also express decreased penetrance of endotoxin response genes. In this context, the susceptibility of diabetic patients to Gram-negative infections may well be a phenotypic representtion of the co-penetrance of exaggerated endotoxin response genes.

References

1. Seiffert A: Der Zahnaszt als Diagnostiker. Dtsch Wehn Zahnheil 3:153, 1862.
2. Cohen MM: Clinical studies of dental caries susceptibility in young diabetics. J Am Dent Assoc 34:239–243, 1947.
3. Hirschfeld L: Periodontal symptoms associated with diabetes. J Periodontol 5:37–46, 1934.
4. Rutledge C: Oral and roentgenographic aspect of the teeth and jaw of juvenile diabetics. J Am Dent Assoc 27:1740–1750, 1940.
5. Sheppard IM: Alveolar resorption in diabetes mellitus. Dental Cosmos 78:1075–1079, 1936.
6. Sheppard IM: Oral manifestations of diabetes mellitus: A study of 100 cases. J Am Dent Assoc 29:1188–1192, 1942.
7. Belting CM, Hiniker JJ, Dummett CO: Influence of diabetes mellitus on the severity of periodontal disease. J Periodontol 35:476–480, 1964.

8. Glavind I, Land B, Loe H: The relationship between periodontal state and diabetes duration, insulin dosage, and retinal changes. J Periodontol 39:341–347, 1968.

9. Cohen DW, Friedman LA, Shapiro J, et al.: Diabetes mellitus and periodontal disease: Two-year longitudinal observations. Part I. J Periodontol 41:709–712, 1970.

10. Bacic M, Plancak D, Granic: CPITN assessment of periodontal disease in diabetic patients. J Periodontol 59:816–822, 1988.

11. Hugoson A, Thortensson H, Falk H, Kuylenstierna J: Periodontal conditions in insulin dependent diabetics. J Clin Periodontol 16:215–223, 1989.

12. Thortensson H, Hugoson A: Periodontal disease experience in adult long-duration insulin-dependent diabetics. J Clin Periodontol 20:352–358, 1993.

13. Shlossman M, Knowler WC, Pettitt DJ, et al.: Type 2 diabetes mellitus and periodontal disease. J Am Dent Assoc 121:532–536, 1990.

14. Nelson RG, Shlossman M, Budding L, et al.: Periodontal disease and NIDDM in Pima Indians. Diabetes Care 13:836–840, 1990.

15. Fritz ME, Zinney W, Hameroff J, Offenbacher S, Van Dyke T: Periodontal attachment loss in an ambulatory diabetic center population. J Dent Res 67:2275, 1988.

16. Löe H: Periodontal disease. The sixth complication of diabetes mellitus. Diabetes Care 16:329–334, 1993.

17. Golub LM, Goodson JM, Lee HM, Vidac AM, McNamara TF, Ramamunthy NS: Tetracyclines inhibit tissue collagenase. In new approaches to the diagnosis and chemotherapeutic management of the periodontal diseases. J Periodontol 56:93–97, 1984.

18. Cianciola LJ, Park BH, Bruck E, et al.: Prevalence, of periodontal disease in insulin-dependent diabetes mellitus. J Am Dent Assoc 104:653–660, 1982.

19. Genco RJ, McMullen JA: The oral complications of diabetes. In Brodoff BN, Bleicher S (eds): Diabetes Mellitus and Obesity. Baltimore: Williams and Wilkins, pp 40–650, 1982.

20. McMullen JA, Van Dyke TE, Horoszewicz H, et al.: Neutrophil chemotaxis in individuals with advanced periodontal disease and a genetic predisposition to diabetes mellitus. J Periodontol 52:167–173, 1981.

21. Van Dyke TE, Horoszewicz H, Cianciola L, et al.: Neutrophil chemotaxis dysfunction in human periodontitis. Infect Immun 27:124–132, 1980.

22. Schmidt AM, Weidman E, Lalla E, et al.: Advanced glycosylation endproducts (AGEs) induce oxidant stress in the gingiva: A potential mechanism underlying accelerated periodontal disease associated with diabetes. J Periodont Res 31:508–515, 1996.

23. Sterky G, Kjellman O, Hogberg O, et al.: Dietary composition and dental disease in adolescent diabetics. A pilot study. Acta Paediatr Scand 60:461–464, 1971.

24. Mattson L, Koch G: Caries frequency in children with controlled diabetes. Scand J Dent Res 83:327, 1975.

25. Canepari P, Zerman N, Cavalleri G: Lack of correlation between salivary Streptococcus mutans and lactobacilli counts and caries in IDDM children. Minerva Stomatologica 43:501–505, 1994.

26. Karjalainen KM, Knuttila ML, Kaar ML: Relationship between caries and level of metabolic balance in children and adolescents with insulin-dependent diabetes mellitus. Caries Res 31:13–18, 1997.

27. Bohatka L, Adler P, Wegner H: Influence of age and duration of diabetes on dental development in diabetic children. J Dent Res 52:535–537, 1973.

28. Grinspan D, Diza J, Villapol LO, et al.: Lichen ruper planus de la muqueuse buccale. Son Association a un diabete. Bull Soc Fr Dermatol Syphiligr 73:898–899, 1966.

29. Farman AG: Atrophic lesions of the tongue: A prevalence study among 175 diabetic patients. J Oral Pathol 5:255–264, 1976.

30. Szpunar SM, Ismail AI, Eklund SA: Diabetes and periodontal disease: Analyses of NHANES I and HHANES. J Dent Res 68:382, 1989.

31. Grossi SG, Zambon JJ, Ho AW, et al.: Assessment of risk for periodontal disease I. Risk indicators for attachment loss. J Periodontol 65:260–267, 1994.

32. Listgarten MA, Ricker FH Jr, Laster I, et al.: Vascular basement lamina thickness in the normal and inflamed gingiva of diabetics and non-diabetics. J Periodontol 45:676–684, 1974.

33. Taylor GW, Burt BA, Becker MP, et al.: Severe periodontitis and risk for poor glycemic control in subjects with non-insulin-dependent diabetes mellitus. J Periodontol 67:1085–1093, 1996.

34. Zambon JJ, Reynolds HS, Fisher JG, et al.: Microbiological and immunological studies of adult patients with non-insulin-dependent diabetes mellitus. J Periodontol 59:23–31, 1988.

35. Mashimo PA, Yamamoto Y, Slots J, et al.: The periodontal microflora of juvenile diabetes. Culture, immunofluorescence and serum antibody levels. J Periodontol 54:420, 1983.

36. Mandell RL, Dirienzo J, Kent R, et al.: Microbiology of healthy and diseased sites in poorly controlled insulin dependent diabetics. J Periodontol 63:274–279, 1992.

37. Sastrowijoto SH, Hillemans P, van Steenberg TJM, et al.: Periodontal condition and microbiology of healthy and diseased periodontal pockets in type 1 diabetes mellitus patients. J Clin Periodontol 16:316–322, 1989.

38. Williams RC, Mahan CJ: Periodontal disease and diabetes in young adults. J Am Med Assoc 172:776–778, 1960.

39. Grossi SG, Skrepcinski FB, DeCaro T, et al.: Response to periodontal therapy in diabetics and smokers. J Periodontol 67:1094–1102, 1996.

40. Ryan M, Ramamurthy N, Golub LM: Six CMT's modulate MMPs and non-enzymatic glycosylation in diabetic rats. J Dent Res 74(Abs.), 1995.

41. Molenaar DM, Palumbo P, Wilson WR, et al.: Leukocyte chemotaxis in diabetic patients and their non-diabetic first degree relatives. Diabetes 25:880–883, 1976.

42. Van Dyke TE: The role of the neutrophil in oral disease-receptor deficiency in leukocytes from patients with juvenile periodontitis. Rev Infect Dis 7:419–425, 1985.

43. Molvig J, Baek L, Christensen P, et al.: Endotoxin-stimulated human monocyte secretion of interleukin 1, tumor necrosis factor alpha, and prostaglandin E2 shows stable interindividual differences. Scand J Immunol 27:705, 1988.

Section VI.
Socioeconomic Problems

47

Living with Type 1 Diabetes Mellitus

Psychosocial Ramifications

Michael D. Harris and Ruchi Mathur

The psychosocial ramifications of diabetes are far-reaching and often overwhelming. Any chronic medical disorder will result in a need for emotional adjustment and the development of new coping mechanisms. Diabetes is unique in that the patient and his or her family assumes daily responsibility for regimentation of meals, multiple self-injections of insulin, frequent self-monitoring of capillary blood glucoses, and integration of daily exercise. This is superimposed on the constant fear of hypoglycemic symptoms, hyperglycemic swings, and long-term sequelae.

A unique study performed by Welborn and Duncan[1] uncovered some of the unforeseen pitfalls in the practical aspects of daily living with diabetes. Eleven health-care providers (including four physicians) were asked to comply with a simulated diabetic lifestyle for 1 week, including twice daily injections, urine testing, and dietary regimentation. Despite the high level of education in these participants, dietary noncompliance and "errors" in insulin administration were common. The difficulty of lifestyle modification and the large time commitment required for self-care were commented on by a majority of the participants. Insight was gained into the practical aspects of living with diabetes, including difficulties with the storage of diabetic supplies, lack of spontaneity in social activities, and subsequent intramarital conflicts.

There is an expansive literature dealing with the impact of psychosocial stress and the onset of diabetes, the role of stress in glycemic stability, and the influence of diabetes on the psychosocial stability of the individual and his or her family. Diabetes can emerge at any age. The impact of the illness on an individual's perception of themselves, his or her emotional development, and ego development are greatly influenced by the stage of psychosocial development at the time of onset of the disorder.

My daughter, Erin Harris, is a 13-year-old who was diagnosed as having type 1 diabetes mellitus at the age of 4. Not only did Erin have to adjust to numerous lifestyle changes, including twice daily insulin injections, frequent fingersticks for capillary blood sugar monitoring, and dietary restrictions, but it was also suggested that she not attend her best friend's birthday party because the other parents felt uncomfortable about assuming the responsibility for enforcing dietary restrictions and a common concern that the disease may be "contagious."

A 30-year-old attorney with a 15-year history of poorly controlled diabetes was interested in becoming pregnant and was placed on an insulin infusion open-loop pump to optimize her diabetic control prior to conception. Despite meticulous attention to capillary blood sugar monitoring, pump maintenance, and dietary compliance, she was plagued by recurrent symptomatic hypoglycemic episodes, making it impossible for her to function at work.

These two brief case examples illustrate the diverse psychosocial influence that diabetes has on the individual throughout life. The psychosocial impact of the disorder affects not only the individual with diabetes, but also the individual's family, spouse, friends, and business associates. A comprehensive approach to diabetes management obviously demands an understanding of the mind as well as the body. Despite an increased understanding of the genetic basis of diabetes, and the pharmaceutical progression in the treatment of the disease, there has been little advance in the appreciation and management of the psychosocial aspects of diabetes.

In this chapter, the data regarding a unique personality type associated with diabetes, the impact of psychosocial stresses on glycemic stability and family harmony, and the psychological disruption of the fear of long-term sequelae will be reviewed. Emphasis will be placed on means of optimizing coping mechanisms and stress reduction, improving self-esteem, ego development, and maximizing therapeutic compliance and ultimately blood glucose control.

The Fallacy of the "Diabetic Personality"

William Menninger,[2] in 1935, systematically looked at the psychological makeup of diabetic individuals and described a "diabetic personality." He stipulated that diminished alertness, indifference, hypochondriacal complaints, anxiety, and depression were characteristic of the "diabetic personality" pattern. Psychological factors have been postulated to be important etiological triggers in the onset of diabetes in predisposed individuals,[3] important factors in glycemic lability,[4-13] and important influences on subsequent maturation and psychosocial developments.[14] More recent reviews have emphasized that methodological problems in the literature, such as a lack of representativeness of the population studied, absence of controls, and a lack of experimental reproducibility invalidated the generalization of specific findings from these studies to the diabetic population as a whole.[15,16] Therefore, no set of personality traits or emotional characteristics have been consistantly described in patients with diabetes.

Impact of Emotional Stress on the Metabolic Control of Diabetes Mellitus

Several studies have looked at the correlation between psychological and emotional stress and glycemic control in individuals with diabetes. The earliest work of this kind was performed by Hinkle and Wolf.[4] They studied blood glucose changes resulting from stresses induced by interviews focusing on personal problems and conflicts identified during prior psychotherapy sessions. Blood glucose changes seemed to vary with the type of emotion elicited. Experiences of anxiety and tension during these interviews were associated with decreases in blood glucose, whereas anger or resentment were associated with increases in blood glucose.

These authors postulate that different emotional stresses result in the release of different combinations of stress-related hormones (catecholamines, cortisol, glucagon, free fatty acids, and growth hormone) resulting in different effects on glucose homeostasis. Baker et al.[17] documented that children with diabetes were more sensitive to the lipolytic and glycogenolytic effect of exogenous catecholamines compared with nondiabetic individuals. Beta-adrenergic blockade significantly decreased the glycemic and ketogenic effect of the infused epinephrine. In a subsequent study, these authors studied two diabetic preadolescent girls who were hospitalized every 3 to 4 weeks secondary to recurrent ketoacidosis usually related to emotional arousal.[18] A specific stress interview with one child pro-

TABLE 47-1 Causes of Brittle Diabetes

	No.	%
Noncompliance/psychosocial	15	53.0
Defective absorption/excessive degradation	7	25.0
Overinsulinization (Somogyi effect)	4	14.3
Recurrent infection (pharyngitis)	3	10.7
Cellular resistance	2	7.1
Insulin antibodies	1	3.5
Underinsulinization	1	3.5

*Some subjects were thought to have more than one etiology.
[Source: Modified from White NH, Santiago JV: Clinical features and natural history of brittle diabetes in children. In Pickup JC (ed): Brittle Diabetes. London: Blackwell Scientific, 1985, pp. 19–28. With permission.]

duced marked changes in blood glucose, plasma free fatty acid levels, and concentrations of epinephrine, cortisol, and growth hormone. This effect was diminished by β-adrenergic blockade. A therapeutic trial with β-adrenergic blockade over a 12-month period markedly diminished the need for subsequent hospitalization of these children. White and Santiago[19] studied the clinical features and etiology of brittle diabetes (Table 47–1). The term "brittle diabetes" was arbitrarily defined as the state where an individual's life is constantly being disrupted by recurrent, unpredictable episodes of hypoglycemia or hyperglycemia independent of their cause. In 53% of the brittle subjects, poor compliance and psychosocial maladjustment were believed to be the primary problems. Examples of the maladapted behaviors included gross dietary excesses, giving extra insulin, omitting injections, interference with infusion pumps, and dilution of infusion fluids with tap water. In some patients, this behavior secured or prolonged hospital admissions to avoid intolerable domestic circumstances, but there was not always such as obvious motive. It is unclear, however, whether these emotional problems are a consequence rather than the cause of the brittle state. Stenstrom[20] found that in males, poor metabolic control, as measured by HbA_{1c} correlated with the presence of more negative life events by questionnaire, while in women, a greater number of positive events correlated with improved glycemic control.

The above examples illustrate that stress can exert an impact on glycemic control. However, does poor glycemic control result in changes in an individual's psychological profile? Lustman et al.[21] suggested that certain psychological problems may result from glycemic instability. They studied the effect of elevated plasma glucose levels on counter-regulatory hormone responses and psychological indices. Hyperglycemia resulted in increases in cortisol, glucagon, heart rate, and skin conductance levels. These authors suggested that hyperglycemia-induced nervous system arousal may make an individual more susceptible to environmental stress and result in an increased frequency of anxiety, depression, and interpersonal conflict. One can, therefore, postulate a vicious cycle between hyperglycemia and emotional duress.

Several studies have investigated the relationship between the psychological makeup of the individual and subsequent control. These studies are often conflicting in their conclusions. Even when psychosocial problems are found to be associated with poor metabolic control, it is unclear whether these problems are causal, consequential, or merely coincidental. The impact of the "locus of control" (the extent to which the individual feels able to influence the course of the illness) on compliance with the diabetic regimen and on subsequent metabolic control has been extensively evaluated. Simonds et al.[22] found no difference in the locus of controlled adolescent subjects with IDDM. Hamburg et al.[23] related an internal (individual does have control over disease outcome) locus of control to good metabolic control in girls but to poor metabolic control in boys. Peyrot et al.[24] found that specific components within this heading of internality (such as autonomy) were associated with good outcomes. However, other components of internality such as self-blame were associated with poor outcomes. Consistency in the measurement of locus of control has not been found between the various scales used in its assessment.[23] The relevance of locus of control to diabetic control therefore remains controversial.

A possible link between psychological disturbance and poor metabolic control is noncompliance. Diabetic management might be deliberately sabotaged for several possible reasons. A person may not believe that he or she has a chronic, permanent metabolic imbalance and thus uses noncompliance as a diagnostic tool. There is also the perception that bad tests may be associated with "bad disease."

During a 6-week summer camp session, 6% of 198 children consistently presented false reports of urine tests.[25] Ernould et al.[26] followed 77 patients for a mean of 6 years and found that the prevalence of false reporting of urine tests to be approximately 45%. It has been estimated that up to 30% of patients falsify their blood glucose records.[26] Negative urine tests may be associated with a decrease in insulin dose and an assumed improvement in the condition. Cheating may be a form of acting out by an angry or depressed child. It is a powerful weapon with which to manipulate family members. Children soon learn that illness attracts attention, sympathy, and affection. Additionally, diabetic management might be deliberately disrupted by the patient to remove himself from an uncaring or hostile environment at home or work to the protective environment of the hospital.

As already discussed, the effect of psychological stress in patients with type 1 diabetes mellitus may have a variable impact on blood glucose levels. However, the effect of a stressful stimuli in a given individual appears to be reproducible.[27] Blood glucose response to stress may depend on the nature of the stress and the specific emotions activated,[3] the degree of anxiety present,[28] the degree of baseline glycemic control,[29] the extent of autonomic neuropathy present,[29] and the amount of muscular tension or activity elicited by the stressful stimuli. Several studies have attempted to evaluate the impact of relaxation training, biofeedback therapy, and support group interaction on improving glycemic control in patients with diabetes. One may postulate that these behavioral modalities may facilitate improved glycemic control by reducing sympathetic and adrenal cortical overactivity. Landis et al.[29] found that relaxation training in five well-controlled subjects resulted in a clinically meaningful reduction in the daily range of blood glucose excursions, thereby improving metabolic stability. Surwit et al.[30] showed that progressive muscle relaxation techniques can improve glucose tolerance in subjects with type 2 diabetes mellitus who had a history of stress-induced hyperglycemia. These investigators were unable to reproduce these results in a group of poorly controlled type 1 diabetic subjects.[27] Further studies will have to be done to assess the effect of more prolonged administration of stress reduction techniques on glycemic control and whether certain subpopulations of type 1 diabetes subjects can be identified to maximize the efficacy of this intervention.

Group therapy has been used to maximize coping strategies and subsequently improve glycemic control. The group therapy process has been promoted to provide insight into an individual's behavior, provide feedback from others living with diabetes, improve socialization skills, provide role models, and impart information.[31] A pilot study by Warren–Boulton et al.[32] looked at the efficacy of group therapy in improving metabolic control in seven inner city African American women with diabetes over an 18-month period. Following group therapy intervention, there was a significant improvement in glycemic control, decrease in serum cholesterol levels, and improved psychosocial adjustment to diabetes. A recent study performed in our office by Holvey evaluated the psychological makeup, coping strategies, and glycemic control in 40 type 1 diabetes mellitus female patients before and after 6 months of psychosocial group interactions.[33] Participation in a psychosocial support group was associated with improved self-esteem, decrease in depression, increase in knowledge of diabetes, an increase in the range of adaptive coping styles, and improved glycemic control. Because, in most patients diabetes is associated with alteration in body image, self-perception and self-esteem, psychosocial group therapy should be considered as a potential therapeutic modality.

It is difficult enough to achieve initial compliance with an intensive regimen, but it is even more difficult to maintain that compliance over a long period of time. Few, if any, studies have studied ways of maintaining motivation and compliance over the long term. Rosenstock[34] suggested that the relapse prevention model that involves the patient's identifying high-risk situations for relapse and learning coping skills to deal with these situations *a priori*, may be a means of achieving long-term motivation.

Diabetes and Depression

Another psychological parameter that has been extensively evaluated in patients with diabetes is depression. The triggers for the development of depression in this patient population are likely mutifactorial. Various physical, psychological, and genetic factors may contribute to the onset of depression, and the makeup of these etiological variables will differ between individuals. Data on depression in patients with diabetes appear to indicate an increased prevalence and incidence over the general population.[35,36] However, the relationship between depression and glycemic control remains controversial. The diagnosis of depression in this population may be a difficult one because symptoms of physical and cognitive dysfunction may be common in true depression and in a poorly controlled glycemic state.[37,38] Several authors have identified depression as the most common disturbance in the psychological state associated with diabetes. Sullivan[39] found that adolescent girls with diabetes displayed significantly more depression on psychological testing than did girls without diabetes. Depression in this group with diabetes was expressed through physiological symptoms as measured by vital depression scores. Vital depression scores measure the extent of difficulty with parameters such as sleep, appetite, libido, fatigue, and somatic preoccupation. Lustman et al.[40] reported a 32.5% prevalence of a prior major depressive episode in 114 adults with diabetes mellitus and follow-up revealed an increased risk of recurrence.[41] Unlike Sullivan's findings, the symptomatic expression of depression was statistically similar in depressed patients with and without diabetes. These investigators found no difference in the prevalence of diabetic neuropathy, retinopathy, or nephropathy in the depressed relative to the nondepressed subjects. This observation has been challenged by other authors who report a notable increase in retinopathy among depressed patients with resulting poor glycemic control.[42] Further fueling the debate, Robinson et al.[43] reported a 17.7% prevalence of depression in subjects with diabetes studied in the United Kingdom, which was comparable to the control group without diabetes. In this study, blood glucose control (as assessed by glycosylated hemoglobin levels) did not statistically differ in the depressed diabetic patients and those who were not depressed. However, depressed subjects had significantly more vascular complications than did nondepressed controls. From the above data, the prevalence of depression and its relationship to glycemic control and development of complications remain inconclusive. This may be due to differences in means of assessing depression and a lack of standardization of subjects studied.

When depression is identified, it should be treated appropriately. Along with the various forms of therapy discussed in the previous section, pharmacological therapy may be an option. Antidepressive agents may have an effect on glycemic control, further compounding the situation. Alterations in appetite may be seen, resulting in a relative anorexia (such as with serotonin reuptake inhibitors) or increased hunger (as with tricyclic antidepressants) thereby predisposing the patient to increased hypoglycemia or hyperglycemia, respectively. If therapy is successful, a subsequent change in daily lifestyle may require further adjustments in insulin therapy as energy levels improve and activity increases.

Impact of Diabetes on Family Stability

The diagnosis and course of diabetes in a child will have an impact on the family. Individuals within that family structure will be affected in various ways. The presence of a child with diabetes places the family unit as a whole under strain. Mothers tend to be more depressed and anxious,[44] parents show more marital conflict,[31] and the child's diabetes, while strengthening the relationship between child and mother, may adversely affect the mother's relationship with her other children.[31,45] Kovacs et al.[44] performed a prospective, longitudinal study of young children with newly diagnosed type 1 diabetes mellitus, looking at parental coping strategies. These authors failed to confirm reports of high rates of mental disturbances or maladjustment among parents of children with diabetes within the first year of diagnosis. The initial strain of living with diabetes elicited mild and subclinical depression, anxiety, and overall stress primarily in the mothers. The initial emotional disruption resolved in 6 months. This study failed to document any increase in intramarital difficulties in these families. Mothers of younger diabetic children viewed them as adaptable, happy, active, but more demanding than nondiabetic children. When this data is examined carefully, more than half of the children with diabetes were noted to have more negative moods and possessed other characteristics that were seen as less acceptable and reinforcing to their mothers, conceivably resulting in a more strained mother–child relationship. These mothers reported less attachment to their children, less spousal support, and poorer health compared with mothers of children without diabetes. It is generally accepted that mothers are more involved in the daily management of their child's diabetes than are fathers.[46,47] In a study by Standen et al.,[47] fathers thought the worst part of diabetes for their child was diet, whereas mothers considered it to be the injections. Both parents thought the worst aspects for themselves were the possibility of future complications, avoidance of hypoglycemia, and achievement of metabolic control[47,48] (Fig. 47–1). Although maternal and paternal evaluations reveal differences in disease interpretation and child rearing roles, behavioral patterns used by both groups to aid in coping were quite similar.[49] Maintaining family integration and optimism was considered the most important coping pattern by 47% of fathers and 65% of mothers. Understanding the medical situation was deemed imperative by 36% of fathers and 61% of mothers. Believing that the child is getting the best possible care was the most important coping behavior a parent could have according to 80% of fathers and 95% of mothers, while trusting in a spouse for support was important to 80% of men and 95% of women with diabetic children.[49]

Several family characteristics have been correlated with good glycemic control (Table 47–2). Characteristics such as good self-esteem in both parents and chil-

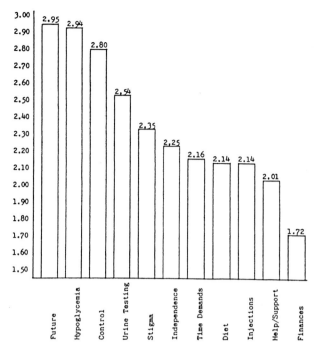

Figure 47–1. Maternal apprehension and diabetes: Maternal concern on 11 aspects of diabetes management, including dietary management, urine testing, insulin injections, diabetes control, future concerns, hypoglycemic episodes, finances, regularity of daily activities/time demands, social support, and psychological stigma. The ratings were scored from "no problems" (1) to "a very big problem" (5). The possibility of future complications, avoidance of hypoglycemia, and achievement of diabetes control were the items of most significant concern. (*Source:* Banion CR, Miles MS, Catter MC: Problems of mothers in management of children with diabetes. Diabetes Care 6:548–551,1983. With permission.)

TABLE 47–2   Familily Influences That Have Been Shown to Impact on Metabolic Control

Good Control	Poor Control
Parent and child characteristics 1. Good parental and child self-esteem[51] 2. Parents are involved in management and share responsibilities[53] 3. Encouraging child's independence	1. Poor parental and child self-esteem[51] 2. Child carries all the responsibility for care[53] 3. Parental overprotection[54]
Family relationships 1. Low family conflict[55,56] 2. High family cohesion[51,56]	1. Marital conflict[55,56] 2. Child using diabetes as a weapon[51] 1. Parental blame and guilt 2. Family eating pattern deviates from child's[55]
Adaptation 1. Perceiving the child as a normal child[54]	1. Isolated families[55] 2. Reliance on peers without diabetes for support[55]
Relationship with the Community: 1. Relationship with community social support 2. Reliance on parents for social support[55]	

[*Source:* Newbrough JR, Simpkins CG, Maurer N: A family development approach to studying factors in the management and control of childhood diabetes. Diabetes Care 8:83–92, 1985. With permission.]

dren have been associated with better blood glucose control.[50,51] Positive family relations (high family cohesion and low family conflict) also correlated with improved metabolic control,[52] as did situations in which parents were actively involved in management and shared responsibilities for diabetes care with their children. Poor control was found in children who had to shoulder all responsibility for their management.[53] Poorer control has also been found in children with anxious or overprotecting parents.[54] Stable family structure and a lack of family conflict has also been associated with good glycemic control.[55,56] In addition, the better a family adapts to having a child with diabetes and adjusts its own eating habits and meal schedule to that of the child's, the better the glycemic control.[55]

The actual family structure has been shown to have an influence on a child's blood sugar control. Of 30 children admitted for DKA, White et al.[57] found that twice as many lived in single parent or step-parent homes. Similarly, HbA_{1c} measurements in children living with both biological parents were lower than children from single parent homes.[58]

Because of the inherited nature of the predisposition to diabetes, parental guilt, especially if one or both of the parents also have diabetes, may be overwhelming. The idea of parental fault or blame may be severely destructive to the integrity of the family. Hostile feelings may develop in the unaffected spouse toward the spouse with diabetes.[45]

Sibling rivalry and attention-seeking behavior may be anticipated responses from unaffected children in the family given the amount of parental attention and time required to care for the child with diabetes. Some siblings have an overwhelming concern over their risk for developing the disorder in the future. Some develop a parental role in protecting and helping to care for the affected child. The potential adverse psychological effect of a child with diabetes on an unaffected sibling may be greater in lower socioeconomic groups.[59]

From the data just presented, one can conclude that there is considerable interplay between child, family, community support structures, and ultimate development of a healthy psychosocial adaptation to diabetes. These variables may also be extremely important in optimizing metabolic control. Once the factors having the greatest impact on family stability and psychosocial adaptation to diabetes are realized, then individual and parental support systems can be formulated that may result in improved psychosocial development and familial adaptation. Family counseling may not be necessary, but family education is imperative. Specifically addressing issues such as parental guilt, spousal blame, financial concerns, disease education, and sibling rivalry will help to provide a stronger family support system for the patient as well as other family members, and ultimately result in improved glycemic control.

Predictable Crises of Diabetes

The time of diagnosis, developmental issues, dealing with daily management issues, and the development of complications all represent predictable crises, presenting unique stresses for the individual with diabetes. The particular psychosocial issues surrounding each of these crises will now be considered.

Diagnosis of Type 1 Diabetes Mellitus

The diagnosis of diabetes has a traumatic effect on the child and parents. The patient and the family are placed in a new and unfamiliar situation full of challenges. The initial period of adjustment is a difficult one during which maladaptive coping mechanisms can be developed. The shock and pain of the diagnosis is followed by anger, guilt, mourning, and hopefully acceptance. The following areas are sources of potential distress for the patient and family:[56]

1. uncertainty about the outcome of the immediate situation;

2. guilt or anger about the occurrence of diabetes;

3. feelings of incompetence and helplessness over the responsibility for management of the disorder;

4. fears about future complications and shortened life span;

5. concerns about life goals and aspirations;

6. and recognition of the need for a permanent change in lifestyle. Family problems and maladjustments early in the course of the disease often herald future problems with glycemic control.[60]

The parental perceptions of obstacles to their child's care may be different from that of the health-care team, and be a source of conflict and uncertainty. Warzak et al.[61] surveyed parents and professionals and explored their concerns about the management of children with diabetes. The primary parental concern was whether their child would monitor blood sugars without prompting, followed closely by concerns for consumption of balanced meals. The health professionals perceived obstacles as more common and difficult than the family members who experienced them. In addition, health-care professionals place more emphasis on being able to decide if a child's behavior resulted from complications of diabetes or everyday anger and frustration. Thus, health-care members must recognize the parents concerns and tailor their interactions accordingly.

The psychological impact of the initial hospitalization for diabetes can be devastating. The forced confinement, the discomfort of repeated phlebotomies, the separation from one's family and familiar surroundings, and the helplessness exemplified by an indwelling intravenous line can have long-term negative effects on the young patient with type 1 diabetes mellitus. Recurrent nightmares involving segments of the initial hospitalization are often experienced years after the onset of the disorder. As long as the patient is not dehydrated or ketonemic, initiation of insulin therapy and diabetic education can be started on an outpatient basis.

Galatzer et al.[62] attempted to treat patients with new type 1 diabetes mellitus with a multidisciplinary team consisting of an endocrinologist, nurse, dietitian, social worker, psychologist, and psychiatrist. Hospitalization was avoided. Emphasis was placed on the development of positive defense mechanisms and coping strategies. These individuals, when compared with historical controls treated conventionally, were subsequently found to develop better compliance, better familial relationships, and better social skills.

The behavioral and emotional impact of diabetes at the time of diagnosis on the preadolescent child is less disrupting than it is on the adolescent individual. The preadolescent is usually able to reintegrate into school and other social activities quickly and without major alteration in performance. Grey et al.[63] looked at a cohort of newly diagnosed children with diabetes and their healthy peers. All were between the ages of 8 and 16 years old and had similar socioeconomic and educational backgrounds and family supports. There was no significant difference between self-perceived confidence, adjustment, or psychological status. However, coping mechanisms differed in that children with diabetes reported that they vented their feelings more often in the form of yelling and complaining.

It has also been emphasized that secondary to the stress and anxiety associated with the initial diagnosis of diabetes, information processing is often impaired.[56] Instructions and explanations should be simple, specific, and when possible, written out in detail to avoid misunderstanding and lack of recall.

Developmental Issues

Diabetes has a major impact on the psychosocial makeup of any individual; however, the particular stresses and obstacles vary with the developmental stage of the individual. Infancy (birth to 1 year), preschool (1 year to 5 years), school-aged (5 years to 9 years), and adolescence are all associated with developmental milestones that can be altered by diabetes.

Little formal data are available on the psychosocial impact of diabetes during infancy. Most developmentalists believe that the emotional well-being of the individual stems from the infant's development of a basic sense of trust that his or her needs can and will be met.[64] Object permanence (the awareness that objects and people continue to exist even when they are out of sight) develops by approximately 9 months, making parental separation for a hospitalization even more traumatic. Hatton et al.[65] documented a number of specific experiences that parents of diabetic infants fear. The demands of complex management, social isolation, an inability to rely on others for child-care support, anticipated future worries, and plans for other children all weigh heavily in a parents' mind during this crucial time. Inflicting the pain of injections and blood testing on the child may arouse extreme anxiety in the parent. Breast-feeding or bottle-feeding on a set schedule rather than on demand becomes extremely important if significant glycemic lability is to be avoided. The difficulty of correlating hyperglycemia or hypoglycemia with behavioral changes in this age group can be appreciated.

During the preschool years, the major developmental changes include increasing motor skills, developing psychological autonomy, and developing social skills. This tendency toward enhanced independence may obviously be suppressed by the presence of diabetes. The diagnosis of diabetes at this stage may result in a decrease in self-esteem, emotional insecurity, and less positive relations with parents, which may result in a regression in behavioral patterns, thereby leading to behaviors such as clinging, bed-wetting, or tantrums.[64] The preschool years are associated with Erikson's third stage of development.[66] During the third stage, the child has a limited capacity to understand the nature of chronic illness. As a result, discomfort may be seen as a form of punishment. In addition, children at this stage of cognitive development often perceive that an adult has "magical powers," and feelings of resentment and confusion can arise when a caregiver does not "cure" the disease. The development of language skills may help in correlating certain behavior patterns and symptoms with glycemic peaks and valleys. There is a fine line between providing appropriate, but not excessive, protection for the child and thereby promoting feelings of self-competence and self-esteem rather than overdependence.

During the school-age years, the child is ready to start to absorb the world beyond that of his or her family. School and peer groups start to play an increasingly important role and there is a sense of growing independence However, if frequent absences from school occur, the acquisition of new skills and adaptive social behaviors may be delayed.[66] Most children at this stage gradually become involved with the management of their diabetes. Their level of responsibility varies with experience and maturity. McNabb et al.[67] demonstrated that children in this age group can be educated to manage their diabetes without a deterioration in HbA$_{1c}$ levels. A major concern at this stage of development is a child's ability to accept the fact that he or she has a disease, while still being able to interact with their peer group. Grey et al.[68] performed a study to look at the adjustment patterns of children recently diagnosed with diabetes and a cohort of peer selected children without diabetes. These children were between the ages of 8 and 14 years old. The investigators concluded that after an initial period of adjustment, both groups had equivalent psychosocial status, with the exception that the children with type 1 diabetes mellitus experienced more depression and anxiety. The early school years may also be a stressful period for parents of children with type 1 diabetes mellitus. Commonly, parents may become overwhelmed by the amount of information they have to consume as well as experiencing intense grief, resentment, and anxiety over the diagnosis. Insecurity about leaving the young child at school results in multiple daily visits to the school for blood glucose monitoring and verification of dietary compliance to avoid the fear of hypoglycemia. Parents may obtain enormous benefit from talking with other parents who have children with diabetes. This provides reassurance, stimulates confidence, and decreases isolation. Through play, stories, drawings, and games, the child with diabetes can express his/her fears, hidden feelings, and concerns.[64]

It has been stated that the child enters adolescence as a dependent, unthinking, sexually and physically immature being and leaves as a mature and independent adult.[69] Adolescence has been termed a period of "storm and stress," referring to the changes youngsters undergo in their social, personal, and physical development.[64] Increasing production of hormones results in physical growth, secondary sexual characteristics, and increasing sexual drives. Thought processes become more abstract. Diabetes obviously adds to the burden of this difficult period and it is a sharp blow to developing sexual identity and body image perception. Unpredictable hypoglycemia can be viewed as a loss of self-control. Many adolescents maintain high blood glucose levels in a conscious effort to avoid even mild hypoglycemia in the presence of their peers. It is at this age that an understanding of the management of diabetes and its importance starts to develop. The desire to be responsible in the management of this chronic illness is often in conflict with feelings of anger and resentment. Diabetes is thought of as a limiting factor to freedom and independence, and can be viewed as a threat to physical, emotional, and social well-being.[70]

Several studies have shown lower self-esteem and ego development in adolescents with diabetes relative to controls without diabetes.[71,72] A study performed by Kellerman et al.[73] assessed the impact of several chronic illnesses (including diabetes) on anxiety and self-esteem relative to healthy controls. No difference in anxiety or self-esteem was found between healthy and ill groups. Stability and prognosis were related to low anxiety, as was length of time since diagnosis. A follow-up study revealed that restriction of freedom and disruption of relationships with peers, siblings, and parents were the major consequences of chronic illness.[74] Adolescents often are in the position to direct their anger or depression toward themselves by not taking care of their diabetes properly.[64,75] Omitting an insulin dose is a common occurrence whether due to forgetfulness, a purposeful gesture of rebellion, or as an attempt to reign supreme over the disease process. In the same manner, nutrition may suffer and subsequently lead to worsening glycemic control. Sex, alcohol, and employment opportunities are major concerns of many adolescents.

Contraception should be openly discussed with both sexes. Issues regarding sexuality in the presence of a chronic illness should be dealt with by reassurance and understanding. Adolescents should be educated about alcohol and told that alcohol is a major source of calories and also augments the hypoglycemic effects of insulin by inhibiting gluconeogenesis. Because independence is a significant goal at this age, employment opportunities may become a concern. Prejudice in the job market may be another source of anxiety and frustration. Most adolescents start to realize the implications of diabetes as a chronic disease for the first time. Concerns and questions about long-term complications and shortened life span need to be addressed and discussed at a level tailored to each individual.

Marriage is another milestone that poses special concern to the individual with diabetes. The possibility of shortened life span, the added economic stresses imposed by diabetes, concerns about the danger of pregnancy, and the transfer of the genetic predisposition for diabetes to one's offspring are all areas of potential concern. Specific issues regarding women and diabetes are discussed later.

With advancing age, diabetes tends to emphasize one's mortality. Escalating health-care costs and a fixed income become a major concern. Employment concerns are carried over into adulthood. Petrides et al.[76] found that approximately 10% of people with type 1 diabetes reported discrimination in the work place. Specifically, these subjects felt that discrimination was related to job application and positional advancement. The issue of lifestyle modifications, such as time to check blood sugars, or scheduled snacking may add to difficulties in an already intolerant workplace. Fears about forced retirement and future disability, are commonly faced concerns in this age group.

Specific Concerns In Women with Diabetes

Although the prevalence of diabetes does not differ significantly between males and females, the disease process does carry with it specific concerns for women. These issues vary depending on the age group—however, some of the more common women's concerns revolve around pubertal development, reproduction, eating disorders, and the management of general women's health issues in the face of diabetes.

As previously discussed, adolescence is a difficult time for all teens, and perhaps more so if a chronic disease is present. Women with diabetes may face delays in development of breasts and onset of menarche, particularly if their diabetes is poorly controlled.[77] This may add to an already fragile body image. Concerns over sexuality may also arise during this age. In the United States, approximately 80% of teenage girls have had intercourse before the age of 18[78] while, alarmingly, only 53% of 19-year-olds use contraception.[79] Although specific statistics are not available, it is thought that sexual practices are similar in teenage girls with diabetes. Given the increased risks involved with pregnancy in this subgroup, education and counseling are essential.

Women also face many issues involving reproduction. There may be an underlying concern over potential genetic transmission that should be addressed. In 1988 the DIEP (Diabetes in Early Pregnancy) study[80] showed that there was little relationship between fetal malformations and glycemic control (as defined by glycated hemoglobin) during organogenesis. However the study design and methodology has been widely criticized. Despite this publication, it is a prevailing belief that congenital malformation rates decrease with preconception counseling and glycemic control, and that overall a favorable cost–benefit ratio exists when preconception counseling is used. The American Diabetes Association has published a position paper on preconception care of women with diabetes[81] in which a multidisciplinary approach is recommended. Although the concept of good glycemic control in the peripartum state cannot be overemphasized, the pregnant woman with diabetes should be encouraged to maintain a tight level of glycemic control beyond her pregnancy.

Although eating disorders are not exclusive to women, the majority of patients suffering from these conditions are female. The *DSM-IV*[82] defines three disorders: Anorexia nervosa, bulemia nervosa, and eating disorders not otherwise specified. Subclinical eating disorders are also being recognized with increasing frequency. The prevalence of eating disorders in the general population has been estimated at between 5 and 10%; however, the prevalence of eating disorders in patients with diabetes has not been quantitated. Because treatment of diabetes focuses heavily on dietary intake and weight control, it has been postulated that these factors may contribute to abnormal eating patterns in young women with diabetes.[83] Neumark-Sztainer et al.[84] found that 27% of adolescent females with type 1 diabetes purged and 24% dieted, compared to 9 and 14% of their peers, respectively. La Greca et al.[85] studied eating behavior in female adolescents with type 1 diabetes. Subjects were divided into good, fair, and poor control groups on the basis of HbA_{1c} levels. Fifty percent of the women in the fair control group and 70% in the poor control group indicated that they coped with overeating by reducing or omitting their insulin. Diabetes, therefore, provides a unique way of purging in a bulimic personality. These individuals produce self-induced glycosuria by avoiding their insulin injections.[86] This may result in ketogenesis and dangerous electrolyte imbalances. In addition, diabetic patients may find that weight gain, due to water retention from reinstituting insulin is so upsetting that the patient reenters a purgative phase (avoidance of insulin to induce glycosuria) without binging. It has been suggested that because bulimia is common and is often unrecognized, it should be suspected in young women with unexplained poor blood glucose control.[86] Bulimia in diabetic patients may be extremely difficult to treat. Some researchers suggest that many bulimics have a primary affective disorder and, as a consequence, antidepressants may be helpful in combination with psychotherapeutic intervention.[87] Unfortunately, disordered eating patterns have been linked not only to worsening glycemic parameters, but also to accelerated progression of end-organ involvement such as retinopathy.[88] In addition, although the DCCT trial[89] has shown significant benefits of an intensive insulin regimen in delaying the onset and slowing the progression of end-organ damage, the increase in insulin dosage may be associated with weight gain, thus further discouraging women from optimizing glycemic control.

Women with type 1 diabetes share the same general concerns about overall health as does the general female population. Areas of concern may include issues dealing with hormone replacement, osteoporosis, and depression. Postmenopausal osteoporosis is a major cause of morbidity and subsequent mortality in aging women. Unlike women with type 2 diabetes, women with type 1 diabetes have lower bone mineral densities than their age-matched nondiabetic cohorts.[90] No studies specifically looking at bone mineral density response to estrogens in type 1 diabetic females has been performed at this time. Similarly, there is no specific data to address the role of hormone replacement therapy and adverse events in women with type 1 diabetes. As with all women, the role of estrogen replacement must be assessed on an individual basis taking into account family history, risk factors for breast cancer, and the patient's preference. If hypertriglyceridemia is present, care must be taken as hormone replacement may increase the risk for pancreatitis.[91] The impact of estrogen on increasing peripheral insulin resistance is a theoretical concern.

Although depression has been discussed elsewhere in this chapter, there are a few issues surrounding women specifically. In general, women experience more depressive episodes than men. In subjects with diabetes, the overall prevalence is approximately 20%, or three to four times that of the nondiabetic population.[35] Specifically, women with diabetes were found to have a greater risk of depression than healthy women and men without diabetes.[36] Depression in females with type 1 diabetes may be associated with disordered eating behaviors and a distorted body image. It may also manifest with pregnancy and postpartum states,[92] and may contribute to poor metabolic control.

Psychosocial Issues Associated with the Development of Complications

All patients with diabetes mellitus live in fear and anticipation of the development of complications. Multiple reports emphasize that anxiety about the future is a major concern for parents and children with diabetes.[47,48] With the recent trend toward early identification and treatment of complications, often the first indication of a problem is an abnormal lab value in an asymptomatic individual, and may therefore come as an unanticipated shock. When complications arise, the patient may react with extreme anger and depression that appears out of proportion to the severity of the complication diagnosed. The initial identification of complications of diabetes reinforces the patient's sense of vulnerability and lack of control over the future. For patients who have neglected their disease in the past, the appearance of complications may bring out feelings of intense guilt. Those who have maintained good glycemic control, in the belief that good control would prevent future complications, often feel betrayed and angry. Some overreact and live in constant fear of future hyperglycemia. Many individuals cope with their diabetes through the use of denial. With the occurrence of complications, the defense mechanism of denial breaks down, resulting in severe depression and emotional distress. Anger toward the caregiver may occur, and often heralds deeper emotions such as fear and guilt. Patients should be acquainted with the possibility of complica-

tions early in the disease, in an attempt to prepare emotionally for a possible future diagnosis.

The evolution of complications to levels of severity where function is compromised leads to feelings of increased dependency, increased depression, and chronic emotional duress. Gafvels et al.[93] showed that in general, men worried less about possible long-term complications than women. Blindness is one of the most feared complications of diabetes because it results in major lifestyle alterations, further loss of independence, financial concerns, and depression over the loss of one's profession. Therefore, even the diagnosis of minor background retinopathy may result in overwhelming anxiety and fear. In a study measuring quality of life in adults with type 1 diabetes, those with nephropathy were 3.8 times more likely to have a poorer perception of their health then their non-nephropathic cohorts. D'elia et al.[94] studied the psychological adjustment of patients with diabetes and end-stage renal disease. They found that objective psychological testing was a poor indicator of adjustment to hemodialysis or subsequent rehabilitation. Rehabilitation potential was correlated inversely with the presence of other complications, specifically the degree of visual impairment. Kidney transplantation represents a last chance for independence and an improved quality of life. Failure of the transplant often results in severe depression and suicidal ideation. A severe chronic painful neuropathy can be incapacitating, and subsequently may result in increased dependence, anger, anxiety, depression, and fear.

Special Psychosocial Issues Related to Diabetes

Provider Burnout. Caregivers of patients with chronic diseases such as diabetes may suffer from chronic job stress and subsequent physician burnout. Unrealistic demands and expectations may lead to a loss of idealism and energy. Provider burnout may manifest as chronic exhaustion and depersonalization when confronted by patient, staff and coworkers. There is a sense of being defeated and the provider may unknowingly harbor anger toward the patient for poor glucose control. Provider burnout may be seen when unrealistic patient and caregiver goals are set, and when too much responsibility for continued support falls on the provider, instead of a support network. Strategies to prevent provider burnout will depend on the underlying trigger. It is important for the caregiver to remain sensitive to his/her own feelings and that of the patient and family. Setting realistic goals may also help minimize the pressure on the provider. Taking advantage of available support and referral services may help to take the onus off a single individual, while providing a team approach to patient management.

Patient Burnout. The burden of coping with a chronic disease can take a toll on patients with type 1 diabetes. The vigilance required to maintain optimal glycemic control can be exhausting, resulting in fatigue and a sense of being overextended. Further compounding this situation may be feelings of guilt and helplessness. Patients experiencing burnout are more likely to have an increased HbA$_{1c}$ level, become discouraged, and spiral down into noncompliance and worsening control. Often this group of patients becomes more despondent and less likely to seek medical attention. It is imperative for health-care providers to constantly monitor their patient's coping mechanisms and openly address any concerns that the patient may have. Feelings of isolation and loss of control are common in patients dealing with chronic disease states. If patient burnout is identified, the caregiver must set attainable goals and provide a referral base for social support. Whenever possible, family involvement through counseling and education should be attempted to provide the family with specific goals and responsibilities. This will help furnish the patient with a familiar network of social support.

Neurobehavioral Impact of Diabetes

There is increasing data to suggest that diabetes mellitus may be associated with neurobehavioral or cognitive dysfunction, including difficulties with learning and memory, visuospatial processes, general intelligence, and mental and motor speed.[95,96] Four risk factors for the development of cognitive dysfunction have been discovered:[97]

1. Several studies have shown that children who develop diabetes before the age of 5 years had lower IQ scores, learned new information less efficiently, made more errors on visuospatial tests, and were slower on tasks that required dexterity than either individuals with age of onset greater than 5 years or than controls without diabetes.[95–97] This has been postulated to occur secondary to the increased vulnerability of the brain of the young child to metabolic imbalances, such as hypoglycemia or ketonemia. Duration of disease did not appear to have a significant impact on these neurobehavioral skills. Studies in children and adolescents have failed to show any correlation between neurobehavioral test scores and recent metabolic control.[96]

2. In adults, however, poor metabolic control has been associated with subtle changes on measures of mental efficiency.[96]

3. Some workers have found an association between patients' estimates of previous hypoglycemic episodes and neuropsychological test performance.

4. Finally, increased school absences have been correlated with lower verbal IQ scores and academic achievement test scores.[96] Draelos et al.[98] showed that cognitive function in adults with type 1 diabetes was well preserved even at significantly elevated glucose levels, but cognitive defects were seen during hypoglycemic episodes, and the degree of impairment was more significant in men.[98] The DCCT research group looked at neuropsychological assessments at baseline and years 2, 5, and 7 of their study. They found no significant cognitive impairment of the intensively treated group, even though their risk for hypoglycemia was increased over their conventionally treated cohort.[99]

Psychosocial Aspects of Insulin Therapy and Intensive Insulin Management

Because the current goal of therapy for diabetes is to achieve euglycemia with an acceptable frequency of hypoglycemia in order to delay the onset or slow the progression of long-term complications, more and more patients are being treated with either a mechanical insulin infusion pump or multiple injections of insulin. Because these regimens require frequent monitoring of blood glucose levels (four to seven times daily) and possibly the adjustment to wearing a mechanical device continuously, it is appropriate to question the psychosocial impact of these modes of therapy. Wearing an insulin infusion pump is a declaration of having diabetes. It stimulates the curiosity of others. Denial and concealment are no longer possible coping mechanisms. After a 2-month study period, Skyler and colleagues[100] noted that both multiple injection therapy and insulin pump therapy resulted in lower ratings on standardized depression and anxiety scores and in the case of insulin pump therapy to higher self-esteem. There were no appreciable adverse psychological effects of wearing an insulin infusion pump. In fact, there was an improvement in psychosocial functioning. There was no evidence that asking a patient to monitor blood glucose levels four to seven times a day was psychologically harmful. These authors also found a consistent relationship between glycosylated hemoglobin level and the degree of satisfaction with the treatment regimen used and suggested that patient preference for a particular insulin regimen may be an important factor in promoting good glycemic control. In a prospective study to identify risk factors for the discontinuation of the pump, Floyd et al.[101] found that a high baseline hemoglobin A$_{1c}$ correlated with an increased rate of pump discontinuation. In addition, this study showed that a low estimation by the patient of their own ability to manage their disease also predicted problems with pump therapy. One of the problems we have experienced with insulin pump therapy is a waning of motivation with time. To sustain long-term motivation, patients on pump therapy have been encouraged to keep a journal of pump-related experiences.[102] Support groups offer an opportunity for sharing experiences, providing technical updates, permitting physician–patient contact, and instructing new pump wearers. These groups may thereby promote adaptive coping mechanisms while helping to sustain motivation. Follow-up on the DCCT trial revealed that under close medical treatment, patients undergoing intensive therapy of their diabetes do not have a subjective decrease in their quality of life, even though their management demands more attention.[103]

Conclusions and the Authors' Assessment of Needed Future Research

Appreciating the psychosocial ramifications of diabetes is of key importance in understanding patient compliance, glycemic lability, stability within the family structure, and contentment within the individual. There appear to be no psychological characteristics inherent to the diabetic state. Many factors may influence the individual's ability to cope in an adaptive way with his or her diabetes, including family response, social support, developmental level, age of onset, premorbid personality, and the interaction with a supportive, well-rounded medical team. Emotional and psychological stress is part of living with any chronic illness, especially with one in which the future remains unknown. Data have been presented to show that the physiological consequence of this stress can result in glycemic instability. In attempts to achieve near euglycemic blood glucose control in a majority of patients with diabetes, the importance of psychosocial stresses and their modification cannot be overemphasized. More extensive use of relaxation techniques, stress reduction, focused imagery, psychosocial support, and possibly pharmaceutical manipulation of counterregulatory responses may be useful in improving glycemic control in certain subpopulations of patients. Extensive psychosocial evaluation continues to be important in assessing appropriate patient selection for insulin pump therapy and possibly for pancreatic transplantation in the future. Future research considerations should include discovering individual and family characteristics predictive of later maladaptive coping mechanisms, longitudinal studies of the neurobehavioral implications of long-term recurrent hypoglycemic episodes, and longitudinal studies of the impact of intensive psychosocial intervention at the onset of diabetes on future psychological adjustments and glycemic control.

References

1. Welborn TA, Duncan N: Diabetic staff simulation of insulin dependent diabetic life. Diabetes Care 3:679–681, 1980.

2. Menninger WC: Psychological factors in the etiology of diabetes. J Nerv Ment Dis 81:1–13, 1935.

3. Slawson DF, Flynn WR, Kollar EJ: Psychological factors associated with the onset of diabetes mellitus. JAMA 185:166–170, 1963.

4. Hinkle LE, Wolf S: Experimental study of life situations, emotions and the occurrence of acidosis in a juvenile diabetic. Am J Med Sci 217:130–136, 1949.

5. Simmonds JF: Psychiatric status of diabetic youth matched with a control group. Diabetes 26:921–925, 1977.

6. Schafer LC, Glasgow RE, McCaul KD, et al.: Adherence to IDDM regimens: Relationship to psychosocial variables and metabolic control. Diabetes Care 6:493–498, 1988.

7. Fonagy D, Morgan GS, Lindsay MK, et al.: Psychological adjustment and diabetic control. Arch Dis Child 62:1009–1013, 1987.

8. Lane JD, Stabler B, Ross SL, et al.: Psychological predictors of glucose control in patients with IDDM. Diabetes Care 11:798–800, 1988.

9. Rovet JF, Ehrlich RM: Effect of temperament on metabolic control in children with diabetes mellitus. Diabetes Care 11:77–82, 1988.

10. Mazze RS, Lucido D, Shamoon H: Psychological and social correlations of glycemic control. Diabetes Care 7:360–366, 1984.

11. Surwit RS, Scovern AW, Feinglos MN: The Role of behavior in diabetes care. Diabetes Care 5:337–342, 1982.

12. Kaplan RM, Chadwick MW, Schimmel LE: Social learning intervention to promote metabolic control in type I diabetes mellitus: Pilot experimental results. Diabetes Care 8:152–155, 1985.

13. Glasgow RE, Toobert DJ: Social, environment and regimen adherence among type II diabetes patients. Diabetes Care 11:377–386, 1988.

14. Pless IB, Heller A, Belmonte M, et al.: Expected diabetic control in childhood and psychosocial functioning in early adult life. Diabetes Care 11:387–392, 1988.

15. Dunn SM, Turtle JR: The myth of the diabetic personality. Diabetes Care 4:640–646, 1981.

16. Jacobson AM, Havier ST: Behavioral and psychological aspects of diabetes. *In* Ellenberg M, Rifkin H (eds): Diabetes Mellitus: Theory and Practice, Ed. 3. New York: Medical Examination Publishing, 1983, pp. 1037–1052.

17. Baker L, Kaye R, Hague N: Studies on metabolic homeostasis in juvenile diabetes mellitus. Role of catecholamines. Diabetes 16:504A, 1964.

18. Baker L, Barcagi A, Kaye R, et al.: Beta adrenergic blockade and juvenile diabetes: Acute studies and long term therapeutic trial. J Pediatr 75:19–29, 1969.

19. White NH, Santiago JV: Clinical features and natural history of brittle diabetes in children. *In* Pickup JC (ed): Brittle Diabetes. London: Blackwell Scientific, 1985, pp. 19–28.

20. Stenstrom U, Wikby A, Hornquist JO, et al.: Recent life events, gender and the control of diabetes mellitus. Gen Hosp Psychiatry 15:82–88, 1993.

21. Lustman PJ, Skor DA, Carney RM, et al.: Stress and diabetic control. Lancet 2:588, 1988.

22. Simonds J, Goldstein D, Walker B, et al.: The relationship between psychological factors and blood glucose regulation in insulin-dependent diabetic adolescents. Diabetes Care 4:610–615, 1981.

23. Hamburg BA, Lipsett LF, Drash AL, et al.: Behavioral and psychosocial issues in diabetes: Summary of proceedings of the national conference. Diabetes Care 3:379–381, 1980.

24. Peyrot M, Rubin RR: Structure and correlates of diabetes-specific locus of control. Diabetes Care 17:994–1001, 1994.

25. Belmonte MM, Gunn T, Gonthier M: The problem of "cheating" in the diabetic child and adolescent. Diabetes Care 4:116–120, 1981.

26. Ernould C, Graff MP, Bourguigon JP: Incidence of `cheating' in diabetic children and adolescents. Pediatr Adolesc Endocrinol 10:43–46, 1982.

27. Feinglos MN, Hastedt P, Surwit RS: Effects of relaxation therapy on patients with type 1 diabetes mellitus. Diabetes Care 10:72–75, 1987.

28. Turkat ID: Glycosylated hemoglobin levels in anxious and nonanxious diabetic patients. Psychosomatics 23:1056–1058, 1982.

29. Landis B, Jovanovic L, Landis E, et al.: Effect of stress reduction on daily glucose range in previously stabilized insulin-dependent diabetic patients. Diabetes Care 8:624–626, 1985.

30. Surwit RS, Feinglos MN: The effects of relaxation on glucose tolerance in non-insulin dependent diabetes mellitus. Diabetes Care 6:176–179, 1983.

31. Tatterall RB, McCulloch DK, Aveline M: Group therapy in the treatment of diabetes. Diabetes Care 8:180–188, 1985.

32. Warren-Boulton E, Anderson BJ, Schwartz NL, et al.: A group approach to the management of diabetes in adolescents and young adults. Diabetes Care 4:620–623, 1981.

33. Holvey EL: The effect of a psychosocial support group on adaptation and coping strategies of women with insulin-dependent diabetes mellitus. USC, Dissertation, 1989.

34. Rosenstock IM: Understanding and enhancing patient compliance with diabetic regimens. Diabetes Care 8:610–616, 1985.

35. Gavard JA, Lustman PJ, Clouse RE: Prevalence of depression in adults with diabetes: And epidemiological evaluation. Diabetes Care 16:1167–1178, 1993.

36. Popkin MK, Callies AL, Lenta RD, et al.: Prevalence of major depression, simple phobia, and other psychiatric disorders in patients with long-standing type 1 diabetes mellitus. Arch Gen Psychiatry 45:64–68, 1988.

37. Lustman PJ, Freedland KE, Carney RM, et al.: Similarity of depression in diabetic and psychiatric patients. Psychosom Med 54:602–611, 1992.

38. Goodnik PJ, Henry JH, Buki VMV: Treatment of depression in patients with diabetes mellitus. J Clin Psychiatry 56:128–136, 1995.

39. Sullivan BJ: Self-esteem and depression in adolescent diabetic girls. Diabetes Care 1:18–22, 1978.

40. Lustman PJ, Griffith LS, Clouse RE, et al.: Psychiatric illness in diabetes mellitus: Relationship to symptoms and glucose control. J Nerv Ment Dis 174:736–742, 1986.

41. Lustman PJ, Griffith LS, Clouse RE: Depression in adults with diabetes. Diabetes Care 11:605–612, 1988.

42. Cohen T, Welch G, Jacobson AM, et al.: The association of psychiatric illness and increased prevalence of retinopathy in patients with type 1 diabetes mellitus. Psychosomatics 38:98–108, 1997.

43. Robinson N, Fuller JH, Edmeades SP: Depression and diabetes. Diabetic Med 5:269–274, 1988.

44. Kovacs M, Finkelstein R, Feinberg TL, et al.: Initial psychologic responses of parents to the diagnosis of insulin-dependent diabetes mellitus in their children. Diabetes Care 8:568–575, 1985.

45. Pond H: Parental attitudes toward children with a chronic medical disorder: Special reference to diabetes mellitus. Diabetes Care 2:431–435, 1979.

46. Hauenstein EJ, Marvin RS, Snyder AL, et al.: Stress in parents of children with diabetes mellitus. Diabetes Care 12:18–23, 1989.

47. Standen PJ, Hinde RJ, Lee PJ: Family involvement and metabolic control of childhood diabetes. Diabetic Med 2:137–140, 1985.

48. Banion CR, Miles MS, Catter MC: Problems of mothers in management of children with diabetes. Diabetes Care 6:548–551, 1983.

49. Auslander WF, Bubb J, Rogge M, et al.: Family stress and resources: Potential areas of intervention in children recently diagnosed with diabetes. Health Soc Work 18:101–113, 1993.

50. Hanson CL, Henggler SW: Metabolic control in adolescents with diabetes: An examination of systemic variables. Fam Syst Med 2:5–16, 1984.

51. Anderson BJ, Miller JP, Auslander W, et al.: Family characteristics of diabetic adolescents: relationship to metabolic control. Diabetes Care 4:586–591, 1981.

52. Hanson CL, De Guire MJ, Schinkel AM, et al.: Empirical validation for a family-centered model of care. Diabetes Care 18:1347–1356, 1995.

53. La Greca AM: Behavioral aspects of diabetes management in children and adolescents. Diabetes 31:12A, 1982.

54. La Hood BS: Parental attitudes and their influence on the medical management of diabetic adolescents. Clin Pediatr 9:468–471, 1970.

55. Newbrough JR, Simpkins CG, Maurer N: A family development approach to studying factors in the management and control of childhood diabetes. Diabetes Care 8:83–92, 1985.

56. Hambug BA, Inoff GE: Coping with predictable crisis of diabetes. Diabetes Care 6:409–416, 1983.

57. White K, Kolman ML, Wexler P, et al.: Unstable diabetes and unstable families: A psychosocial evaluation of diabetic control. J Child Psychol Psychiatry 28:923–833, 1987.

58. McKelvey J, Waller DA, North AJ, et al.: Reliability and validity of the Diabetes Family Behavior Scale. Diabetes Educator 19:125–132, 1993.

59. Lavigne JV, Traisman HS, Marr TJ, et al.: Parental perceptions of the psychological adjustment of children and their siblings. Diabetes Care 5:420–426, 1982.

60. Jacobson AM, Hauser S, Lavori P: Family environment and glycemic control: Four-year prospective study of children and adolescents with insulin-dependent diabetes mellitus. Psychosom Med 56:401–409, 1994.

61. Warzak W, Majors CT, Ayllon T, et al.: Parental versus professional perceptions of obstacles to pediatric diabetes care. Diabetes Educator 19:121–124, 1993.

62. Galatzer A, Amir S, Gill R, et al.: Crisis intervention program in newly diagnosed diabetic children. Diabetes Care 5:414–419, 1982.

63. Grey M, Cameron ME, Lipman TH, et al.: Initial adaptation in children with newly diagnosed diabetes and healthy children. Pediatr Nursing 20:17–22, 1994.

64. Norman DK: Psychological commentary on insulin-dependent diabetes mellitus: Infancy to age 5 years. In Brink SJ (ed): Pediatric and Adolescent Diabetes Mellitus. Chicago: Year Book Medical Publishers, 1987, pp. 33–43.

65. Hatton DL, Canam C, Thorne S, et al.: Parents perceptions of caring for an infant or toddler with diabetes. J Adv Nurs 22:569–577, 1995.

66. Pond JS, Peters ML, Pannell DL, et al.: Psychosocial challenges for children with insulin-dependent diabetes mellitus. Diabetes Educator 21:297–299, 1995.

67. McNabb WL, Quinn MT, Murphy DM, et al.: Increasing children's responsibility for diabetes self care: The In Control Study. Diabetes Educator 20:121–124, 1994.

68. Grey M, Cameron ME, Lipman TH, et al.: Psychosocial status of children with diabetes in the first 2 years after diagnosis. Diabetes Care 18:1330–1336, 1995.

69. Tattersall RB, Lowe J: Diabetes in adolescence. Diabetologia 20:517–523, 1981.

70. Kyngas H, Barlow J: Diabetes: An adolescent's perspective. J Adv Nurs 22:941–947, 1995.

71. Hauser ST, Pollers D, Turner BL, et al.: Ego development and self-esteem in diabetic adolescents. Diabetes Care 2:465–471, 1979.

72. Orr DP, Golden MP, Myers G, et al.: Characteristics of adolscents with poorly controlled diabetes referred to a tertiary care center. Diabetes Care 6:170–175, 1983.

73. Kellerman J, Zeitzer L, Ellenberg L, et al.: Psychological effects of illness in adolescence. I. Anxiety, self-esteem and perception of control. J Pediatr 97:126–131, 1980.

74. Zeitzer L, Kellerman J, Ellenberg L, et al.: Psychologic effects of illness in adolescence. Impact of illness in adolescents—crucial issues and coping styles. J Pediatr 97:132–138, 1980.

75. Orr DP, Eccles T, Lawlor R, et al.: Surreptitious insulin administration in adolescents with insulin-dependent diabetes mellitus. JAMA 256:3227–3230, 1986.

76. Petrides P, Petermann F, Henrichs HR, et al.: Coping with employment discrimination against diabetics: Trends in social medicine and social psychology. Patient Educ. Couns. 26:203–208, 1995.

77. Travis L, Brouhard B, Schreiner BJ: Diabetes mellitus in children and adults. Philadelphia: W.B. Saunders Co., 1987.

78. Zelnik M, Shah F: First intercourse among young Americans. Fam Plan Perspec 15:64–70, 1983.

79. Zelnik M, Kantuer J: Sexual activity, contraceptive use and pregnancy among metropolitan area teenagers. Fam Plann Perspec 12:230–231, 1980.

80. Mills JL, Knopp RH, Simpson JL, et al.: Lack of relation of increased malformation rates in infants of diabetic mothers to glycemic control during organogenesis. N Engl J Med 318:671–676, 1988.

81. American Diabetes Association: Position statement: Preconception care of women with diabetes. Diabetes Care 20(Suppl. 2):s40–43, 1997.

82. American Psychiatric Association: Diagnostic and Statistical Manual of Mental Disorders, 4th ed. Washington DC: Author, 1994.

83. Rodin GM, Johnson LE, Garfinkel PE, et al.: Eating disordersin female adolescents with insulin dependent diabetes mellitus. Int J Psychiatr Med 16:49–57, 1987.

84. Neumark-Sztainer D, Story M, Toporoff E, et al.: Psychosocial predictors of binge eating and purging behaviors among adolescents with and without diabetes mellitus. J Adolesc Health 19:289–296, 1996.

85. La Greca AM, Schwarz LT, Satin W: Eating patterns in young women with IDDM: Another look. Diabetes Care 10:659–660, 1987.

86. Hudson JI, Hudson MS, Wentworth SM: Self-induced glycosuria, a novel method of purging in bulimia. JAMA 249:2501, 1983.

87. Jacobson AM, Leibovich J: Diabetes mellitus: Psychosocial issues in patient management. In Olefsky JM, Sherwin RS (eds): Diabetes Mellitus: Management and Complication. New York: Churchill Livingstone, 1985, pp. 353–377.

88. Rydall AC, Rodin GM, Olmsted MP, et al.: Disordered eating behavior and microvascular complications in young women with insulin-dependent diabetes mellitus. N Engl J Med 336:1849–1854, 1997.

89. The DCCT Research Group: The effect of intensive treatment of diabetes on the development of long term complications in insulin-dependent diabetes mellitus. N Engl J Med 329:977–986, 1993.

90. Forst T, Pfutzner A, Kann P, et al.: Peripheral osteopenia in adult patients with insulin-dependent diabetes mellitus. Diabetic Med 12:874–879, 1995.

91. Glueck CJ, Lang J, Hamer TY, et al.: Severe hypertriglyceridemia and pancreatitis when estrogen replacement therapy is given to hypertriglyceridemic women. J Lab Clin Med 123:59–64, 1994.

92. York R, Volpicelli J, Brooten D, et al.: Anxiety, depression and hostility during pregnancy and postpartum. J Perinat Ed 1:10–13, 1992.

93. Gafvels C, Lithner B, Borjeson B: Living with diabetes: Relationship to gender, duration and complications. A survey in northern Sweden. Diabetic Med 10:768–773, 1993.

94. D'elia JQ, Piening S, Kaleany A, et al.: Psychosocial crisis in diabetic renal failure. Diabetes Care 4:99–103, 1981.

95. Rovet JF, Ehrlich RM, Hoppe M: Intellectual deficits associatedwith early onset of insulin-dependent diabetes mellitus in children. Diabetes Care 10:510–515, 1987.

96. Ryan CM: Neurobehavioral complications of type I diabetes. Diabetes Care 11:86–93, 1988.

97. Ryan CM, Vega A, Drash A: Cognitive deficits in adolescents who developed diabetes early in life. Pediatrics 75:921–927, 1985.

98. Draelos MT, Jacobson AM, Weinger K, et al.: Cognitive function in patients with insulin-dependent diabetes mellitus during hyperglycemia and hypoglycemia. Am J Med 98:135–144, 1995.

99. The Diabetes Control and Complications Trial Research Group: Effects of intensive diabetes therapy on neuropsychological function in adults in the diabetes control and complications trial. Ann Intern Med 124:379–388, 1996.

100. Siegler DE, La Green A, Citrin WS, et al.: Psychological effects of intensification of diabetic control. Diabetes Care 5:19–23, 1982.

101. Floyd JC, Cornell RG, Jacober SJ, et al.: A prospective study identifying risk factors for discontinuance of insulin pump therapy. Diabetes Care 16:1470–1478, 1993.

102. Stein C: Psychological reactions to insulin infusion pumps. Med Clin North Am 66:1285–1293, 1982.

103. The Diabetes Control and Complications Trial Research Group: Influence of intensive treatment on quality of life outcomes in the Diabetes Control and Complications Trial. Diabetes Care 19:195–203, 1996.

48

Electronic Medical Records for Diabetes

Peter C. Butler, John McKnight, and Jean-Pierre Sorensen

Introduction

Diabetes mellitus (DM) is a chronic disease with complications that can be postponed and/or prevented with appropriate monitoring and treatment. Although the Diabetes Control and Complications Trial (DCCT) has established the importance of tight glucose control and regular monitoring, it is difficult to translate these into clinical practice.[1–3] One difficulty is the usual poor quality of patients' records. As with most chronic diseases, patients with diabetes commonly make multiple visits to different physicians and paramedical staff each year over many years. Conventional paper records usually become unmanageable under these circumstances because (1) usually the record is divided into several volumes, (2) finding the trend of disease progression can be time consuming or impossible, (3) illegibility of hand-written entries, and (4) important data may not be available because of misfiling or recent use by another caregiver. In theory, an electronic medical record (EMR) would overcome most of these problems.[4–6] See Chapter 19.

Potential Benefits of an EMR

Patient Management

The most important potential benefit of an EMR is improved patient care. The optimal management of diabetes requires regular collection of various clinical parameters (e.g., glycosylated hemoglobin, blood pressure, lipids).[7] Appropriate decisions are required by the clinician in response to these data, and an EMR can provide prompts for data that lie outside acceptable limits and require a clinical management decision. Under these circumstances, the EMR facilitates the clinician by both providing easy access to the relevant data (otherwise buried in a large paper record) and stimulating a management change that may have otherwise been overlooked. Therefore, an EMR facilitates adher-

ence to established national/local guidelines for best clinical practice.[8]

Complication Screening

In addition, optimal diabetes management requires screening for early (and therefore reversible) complications and the appropriate action when these are identified, for example, the detection of micro-albuminuria and institution of an angiotensin-converting enzyme inhibitor.[9] A well-designed EMR will prompt care providers when such screening events are required and when results require action.[8]

Clinic Costs/Billing

An EMR will ensure that all required processes are carried out, documented, and, where relevant, billed. By improving the efficiency of health care delivery they should also reduce costs of care.[10]

Audit

When patient data are collected into an EMR, they can then be readily analyzed for the purpose of tracking the progress of individual patients over time as well as the performance of the caregivers in meeting the established targets. These data can be used to obtain an overview of the overall performance of the clinic (audits) and to examine the outcome of efforts to enhance shortcomings identified in previous audits.[8,10] Shortcomings related to patient compliance, clinic organization, and individual care provider performance are much more readily identifiable in the setting of an EMR.[11] Audit by use of an EMR should also allow for better characterization of at-risk patients and targeting of resources to them.[12]

Shared Care

There is an increasing emphasis on shared care by primary, secondary, and tertiary care of patients with chronic diseases.[13] An EMR provides the potential for a shared record in which care events by multiple caregivers (nurses, dietitians, physicians) are recorded and become immediately available to all involved care providers in different locations.

Education

Another important benefit when an EMR is used for management of diabetes is enhanced education. For example, the relationship between trends in important clinical parameters (e.g., blood pressure, lipids, glycosylated hemoglobin) and compliance with treatment can readily be shown to patients, allowing for their active participation in care management.[14] An EMR may also provide information for health care providers (and patients) through a linked information system (e.g., CD-ROM, textbook, Internet). Prompts that show clinical data that lie outside acceptable limits and require a management decision are also important for the education of trainees.[8]

Research

The benefits of an EMR also include enhanced possibilities for research. For example, a clinic population can rapidly be screened for appropriate volunteers for research studies. An EMR will also greatly facilitate epidemiologic outcome, benefit, and cost studies.

Existing Systems

Given the obvious advantages of an EMR, it is hard to understand at first sight why these are not already extensively in use for diabetes management. However, there are relatively few systems in place, and the merits and pitfalls of some of these have been discussed.[15-18] To understand why there are so few existing systems, it is worth considering the difficulties of implementing an EMR.

Obstacles to Establishing an EMR for Diabetes Management

The obstacles in successful implementation of an EMR are not trivial.[4-6,19] Most EMRs falter after considerable effort has already been expended in their development. Clearly, this is a great waste of human resource and money. It is therefore important to consider the following obstacles that must be overcome to successfully introduce an EMR into clinical practice before embarking on such a project.[20-22]

Doctors and Other Care Provider Resistance.

1. A paper medical record is the conventional clinical document and therefore is familiar to practicing physicians. All medical training has been geared toward the completion of a standard written history and physical examination. Over their careers, individual physicians evolve personal abbreviated formats for collecting patient information and develop their own sense of what points of information are important. Abandoning this familiar personal system for an EMR, which is initially unfamiliar, will naturally be met with resistance.

2. Many diabetes clinics have trainee physicians spending relatively short periods of time attached to the clinic. Use of the system must be immediately obvious; otherwise it will be met with resistance by rotating staff.

3. In nondiabetes clinics (e.g., general practice), the management of diabetes and screening for diabetes is usually one of many activities undertaken by the caregivers. Unless a caregiver spends a minimum period per week using the EMR, familiarity with the system will be hard to achieve and maintain. If visits from diabetic patients are interspersed with those of other patients, logging in and out of the system for single patients may be perceived as too time consuming.

4. Some physicians may be troubled by the privacy of their clinical practice when documented by an EMR,[11] as access to individual clinicians' performance in meeting targets for screening and treatment can readily be compared to other individuals, both within the practice and nationally. This information could be perceived as a threat in the hands of medical insurance companies, peers, and national accreditation bodies, although the evidence that this is the case in practice is to the contrary.[11]

Technical Obstacles.

1. Hardware is often underpowered and insufficiently flexible for renewal and amendments. If the system is underpowered, waiting times for screen retrieval will be unacceptably long. The configuration of the hardware is rarely appropriate to the physician–patient environment. A large personal computer occupying much of the physician's desk and providing an obstacle between the physician and the patient is likely to be perceived as intrusive by both parties. There already exist systems that can be built into desks and occupy minimal space between patient and physician. Another simple issue often overlooked is the need for a quiet computer for such an environment. Systems that were developed in isolation from those in other units of the medical center result in fragmentation of patient records.

2. Software that is too slow or not user-friendly (but inexpensive) has often been used. High-quality professional development is usually required to design

good systems. The combination of computer and medical expertise is crucial. The most common problem is insufficient investment in software development. If the system is only designed to collect outcome data and provides extra work for no immediate advantage to the health care provider, it will not succeed.

3. One perceived problem with EMRs is the potential loss of patient confidentiality. In practice, this is no more of a problem than with paper records.

4. All systems are completely dependent on the quality of data entered. Very often it is difficult to prove the quality of the data. Qualitative data is difficult to record in a standardized fashion that is easily retrievable. If more than one laboratory is providing data, the ranges of results may be different.

Successful Implementation of an EMR: Overcoming the Obstacles

Successful establishment of an EMR requires a clear plan of the purposes of the EMR before it is developed. Thus, it must be established if it will be a system that will be shared with primary care, and, if so, the pri-

mary caregivers must be involved in the design of the record. The system must be built on a sufficiently robust platform that all the potential uses of the system can be readily met. The system must also be sufficiently adaptable that it can be modified with time and converted from obsolete hardware. In Table 48–1, we offer solutions to the most common obstacles that need to be overcome to successfully establish an EMR.

In conclusion, an EMR appears to be a logical asset in the management of care of patients with DM, as indeed it would be with other patients with chronic disease. The most appealing aspects of an EMR include (1) the improved storage and access to information for the team of care providers and (2) feedback to both care providers and patients on the need for changes in behavior and/or practice to ensure the most effective care. The challenges for implementation of an EMR are, however, considerable and require an appropriate investment of both time and money to be overcome. Nonetheless, it is likely that data will become increasingly available that will indicate that the use of an EMR enhances patient care and reduces costs of care delivery, at which point the onus will be on care providers to ensure that such a system is in place within their institutions.

TABLE 48–1   Common Obstacles, and Proposed Solutions, for Installation of an EMR.

Obstacle	Solutions
Lack of clear goals	It is very important that the potential users (doctors, nurses, dietitians, ophthalmologists) and stakeholders (local IT organization, administration, etc.) are involved in the specification process of an EMR from the very beginning and that they all understand what is in it for them and their responsibilities.
Payers and policy makers uncertain of advantage	An EMR must be able to document quality of care and the most rational use of resources, including time consumption. Tailormade reports must be available from the system. An EMR must be able to provide an overview very quickly and with use of few resources (standard reports, etc.).
Patient concerns	In clinical use, patients must feel included in the activities going on on the screen rather than having it come between them and the care provider. The screen must be used actively to show trends in relevant data and the response to treatments. Patients must be assured that data confidentiality is the same or better than standard paper records.
Resistance from doctors and other health care providers	It must be realized up front that the implementation of an EMR in the daily clinical work for many users will provoke both fear and resistance.
Computer illiteracy	This demands a thorough communication and structured change management program before the system is installed. Many professionals are more or less computer illiterate, and a training course both in basic computer use and the EMR is mandatory.
Time consumption	Many professionals will claim that, as a result of the EMR, time consumption will increase. The system must therefore document time utilization. Time saving should be observed from the automatic generation of diagnosis, ICD9 codes, reports, billing codes, referrals, and electronic prescriptions. The fast overview delivered by the EMR should quickly begin to save the user's time.
Accessibility of data	Many health care providers are nervous that the accessibility of the data will be used against them. To address this, it is advisable to develop a structured bench-marking system for each caregiver to review their own performance, which allows for comparison to other providers anonymously.

(continued)

TABLE 48–1 *(continued)*

Obstacle	Solutions
Restriction of clinical choice	The ability of the EMR to impose guidelines and check follow-up is perceived by many physicians as a reduction of their clinical freedom. An EMR must always suggest, and never demand, clinical actions. The spirit of the team should clearly emphasize that complex clinical situations may need very individualized solutions. To implement these are clearly the responsibility of the caregiver, not the system.
Shared care versus hospital-based specialist	The EMR allows for a fast or even on-line clinical support of GPs from specialists. This requires agreed transfer and return guidelines and a revenue structure to cover the time spent by specialists. It allows patients to stay longer in GP care, rationalizes the use of specialist time, and clearly improves consistency of care in a region.
Goals unrealistic	It is very important to build systems in a stepwise manner. The first step must be sufficiently sophisticated to support the daily clinic routine or it will not be used. The first step might include a system for data collection that makes it possible to run a quality of care circle. In the second step, the EMR can then be guideline driven, i.e., the EMR will keep track of all data and treatment and suggest change in treatment when necessary. In the final step, shared care (between primary care and specialist clinics) can be integrated.
Inadequate investment	Physicians planning to develop an EMR should first look for existing systems that can be used or modified.
Hardware	A professional IT company must be consulted to provide estimates of resources needed and time lines.
Software	The care group must, early in the progress, thoroughly specify performance indicators such as screen turnaround time, opening time, printout time, and integration with other IT systems, such as laboratory systems, billing, prescriptions, etc.

Data issues
  Selection of data set
  Definition and standardization
  Data quality
  Data security
	In the selection of a data set, it is very important to distinguish between a mandatory minimum and an optional data set. The minimal data set must include all necessary information to ensure a rational use of the data set for analysis and, at the same time, secure that data collection is not too ambitious, leading to difficulty in daily use of the EMR. The optional data set should be easily available for special projects. These data must not interfere with the daily work flow. As much data as possible must be entered in a numerical fashion or using pick lists. There must be a written definition of data, including ranges, wherever possible. If data are to be used in quality circles between a number of centers, the data definitions must be agreed upon and standardized. Procedures for quantitative data-quality evaluation must be established to ensure data validity.

Data Security	As EMRs are production systems, professional IT expertise is required for issues such as mirrored hard disks, automated backup, and encryption. Long-term data storage is necessary. In daily use, protection can be enhanced by implementation of differentiated levels of password access. The critical database access should be restricted to a small number of certified persons.
Insufficient education and training of users	Training and education of all users are extremely important. Structured education modules must be a part of the EMR development/modification process. Education must start before implementation as part of the start-up phase, and a running maintenance program in which program updates can be included must exist. Education must be structured at the user, super-user, and database administrator levels.

References

1. The DCCT Research Group: The effect of intensive treatment of diabetes on the development and progression of long-term complications in insulin-dependent diabetes mellitus. New Engl J Med 329:977–986, 1993.

2. The DCCT Research Group: Implementation of conventional and intensive treatment in the Diabetes Control and Complications Trial. Diabetes Care 18:361–376, 1995.

3. The DCCT Research Group: Adverse events and their association with treatment regimens in the Diabetes Control and Complications Trial. Diabetes Care 18:1415–1427, 1995.

4. Wyatt JC: Clinical-data systems. 1. Data and medical records. Lancet 344(8936):1543–1547, 1994.

5. Wyatt JC: Clinical-data systems. 2. Components and techniques. Lancet 344(8937):1609–1614, 1994.

6. Wyatt JC: Clinical-data systems. 3. Development and evaluation. Lancet 344(8938):1682–1688, 1994.

7. American Diabetes Association: Clinical Practice Recommendations 1997. Diabetes Care 20(S1):S1–S70, 1997.

8. Lobach DF, Hammond WE: Computerized decision support based on a clinical practice guideline improves compliance with care standards. Am J Med 102:89–98, 1997.

9. Viberti GC, Wiseman MJ: The kidney in early diabetes; significance of the early abnormalities. J Clin Endocrinol Metab 15:753–782, 1986.

10. Tierney WM, Overhage JM, McDonald CJ: Demonstrating the effects of an IAIMS on health care quality and cost. J Am Med Informatics Assoc 4(2SS):S41–S46, 1997.

11. Chassin MR, Hannan EL, Debuono BA: Benefits and hazards of reporting medical outcomes publicly. New Engl J Med 334(6):394–398, 1996.

12. Tierney WM, Takesue BY, Vargo DL, Zhou XH: Using electronic medical records to predict mortality in primary-care patients with heart-disease—prognostic power and pathophysiologic implications. J Gen Intern Med 11(2):83–91, 1996.

13. Hirsch IB: Who is best suited to manage patients with diabetes? Int Diabetes Monitor 8(3):1–4, 1996.

14. Golin CE, DiMatteo MR, Gelberg L: The role of patient participation in the doctor visit. Diabetes Care 19(10): 1153–1164, 1996.

15. Lehmann ED, Deutsch T: Application of computers in diabetes care—a review. 2. Computers for decision-support and education. Med Informatics 20(4):303–329, 1995.

16. Lehmann ED, Deutsch T: Application of computers in diabetes care—a review. 1. Computers for data-collection and interpretation. Med Informatics 20(4):281–302, 1995.

17. Weng C, Coppini DV, Sonksen PH: Linking a hospital diabetes database and the national health service central register: a way to establish accurate mortality and movement data. Diabetic Med 14(10):877–883, 1997.

18. Gorman C, Looker J, Fisk T, et al.: A clinically useful diabetes electronic medical record—lessons from the past—pointers toward the future. Eur J Endocrinol 134(1):31–42, 1996.

19. Heller EE: The computer-based patient record vision contrasted with HIS/MIS. Int J Bio med Comput 39(1):19–23, 1995.

20. Wyatt JC: Hospital information management—the need for clinical leadership. Br Med J 311(6998):175–178, 1995.

21. Carpenter PC: The electronic medical record—perspective from Mayo Clinic. Int J Bio med Comput 34(1–4):159–171, 1994.

22. Cushman R: Serious technology assessment for health care information technology. J Am Med Informatics Assoc 4(4):259–265, 1997.

49

From Metabolic Crisis
to Long-Term Diabetes Control

A Plea for More Efficient Therapy

Jean-Philippe Assal

Therapeutic efficiency, particularly in the treatment of chronic diseases, is often disappointing and far from optimal, despite outstanding scientific equipment for diagnostic procedures and drugs with remarkable pharmacologic properties. There are several difficulties related to the therapeutic attitudes of the doctor and patient and the characteristics of a silent disease, as well as the attitude of society toward medicine, disease, and the patient. All these factors may create important barriers that interfere with long-term diabetes control.

To improve long-term therapeutic efficiency, *it is therefore important that health care providers integrate the biomedical characteristics of the disease and its treatment into a much more global perspective.* This focuses on the individual bearer of the disease, the patient, while simultaneously embracing the biomedical, psychological, and sociological consequences of disease and its treatment (the biopsychosocial model of Engel, also known as the "holistic" approach[1]). This approach is a working process, but so far it has mostly been described as a theoretical model. It now has to be integrated into medical practice. However, this three-dimensional approach is not enough; the efficiency of diabetes control, like for many other chronic diseases, is strongly dependent on how the patient has *learned* the daily management of his or her disease. Therefore, a fourth educational dimension is mandatory. Physicians have to take these four dimensions actively and *simultaneously* into account at the time of the medical visit with the patient.

Diabetes is the model of a four-dimensional approach, *biopsychosocial and educational.* This is why the World Health Organization (WHO) has fully recognized and promoted the concept of integrated therapeutic patient education.[2,3]

Concern for the global approach to disease and the patient has long existed. The holistic approach is therefore not a new concept. What is nevertheless new is that there is increasing awareness among health care providers that such integration does not happen spontaneously, that many of its aspects have to be learned, and that specific skills have to be developed. Daily medical routine most often disturbs the equilibrium (psychological, educational, sociological), favoring one dimension (usually the biological) at the expense of the others. Therefore, it is not enough for physicians to rely on good sense, human warmth, and intuition. Educating physicians and other health care personnel in the field of doctor–patient relationships, interpersonal communication, educational strategies, health beliefs, locus of control, coping with the disease, and relapse prevention are essential in the therapeutic approach to chronic diseases. This requires training in the field of patient psychology and therapeutic patient education, as well as understanding problems facing the social dimensions of disease.

The Case of Mr. John B.

The following case illustrates both the efficiency and the limitations of the biomedical approach to diabetes and shows the need for a more global, integrated, simultaneous approach of diagnosis, treatment, and follow-up.

Mr. John B., a 52-year-old white male accountant, a widower with two children, was admitted to our hospital for reequilibration of his diabetes because of sustained hyperglycemia (12 to 15 mm/L), hypertriglyceridemia, and 10 kg excess weight.

Mr. B.'s past revealed no family history of diabetes. He had enjoyed good health until the age of 48, when he began to lose weight (a total of 12 kg); weight loss was accompanied by polydipsia and polyuria, and Mr. B. was first admitted to the hospital in severe ketoacidosis [blood glucose (BG) = 25 mm/L; pH = 7.01]. Treatment of this acute situation was successful and the patient left the hospital with almost normal blood glucose profiles, on insulin therapy, and with a meal plan consisting of 280 g carbohydrate (CHO) and 2,400 calories/day. Upon leaving the hospital, he was referred to the family doctor who had cared for his wife. The latter had died of cancer of the pancreas 1 year before Mr. B.'s diabetes had been diagnosed. The patient had an excellent relationship with his doctor, whom he described as "a very friendly man and a warm human being." One year after the initial ketoacidosis, Mr. B. was referred to us a second time. This second hospitalization became necessary due to poor control of diabetes, despite a marked increase in insulin dosage of about 40%. In addition, the patient had been having difficulty following his diet. No organic reason was found to explain this poor control of diabetes. Questions concerning the patient's professional life revealed that Mr. B. had recently been promoted to an important position in his company. His private life was also satisfactory: He had a good relationship with the woman with whom he had been living for 2 years, and his children, a boy of 19 at college and a girl of 22 who worked as a nurse, were both successful.

At the end of the second hospitalization, Mr. B.'s diabetes was under satisfactory control, due mainly to the patient's stricter adherence to his diet. However, this therapeutic effectiveness did not last long. After only a few months, his diabetes was as poorly controlled as before, despite the fact that he had been taught about his disease and how to manage it correctly.

The general practitioner asked us for a follow-up, and Mr. B. began to visit our outpatient unit. It was only then that more careful interviews with different members of the medical team concerning his personal and professional life revealed the main reason for Mr. B.'s inability to maintain good control over his diabetes. The death of his wife from cancer had left Mr. B. with an unconscious anxiety: Having seen the one he loved "waste away," he had developed a hidden, morbid fear of weight loss. In addition, his professional promotion to chief manager forced him into a hyperactive life into which he refused to allow his diabetes to interfere.

As discussed further in this chapter, the case of Mr. B. shows that even in specialized centers problems can easily be overlooked, particularly when the patient may have strong defense mechanisms. However, this example also illustrates the beneficial effect of better interviewing skills, improved medical interdisciplinary teamwork, and time needed for adaptation to a chronic condition. This example will now be analyzed according to several aspects involved in medical care.

Historic Phases in the Treatment of Diabetes

Therapeutic efficiency in diabetes has passed through distinct phases (Fig. 49–1), each of which is characterized by a particular medical approach.

Insulin

The most dramatic and specific phase began in 1921 with the introduction of insulin (Fig. 49–2). However, despite the remarkable metabolic improvement with insulin, periods of lack of diabetes control remained a severe problem particularly at the time of infections.

Antibiotics

The introduction of antibiotics in 1946 (which marks the beginning of the second phase of our model) was responsible for a marked reduction in infections and consequent diabetic decompensations. This coupling of insulin and antibiotics exemplifies the fundamental role of biomedical research and its clinical applications. As far as oral hypoglycemic agents are concerned, these medications, used since 1956, have in no way contributed to the drop in acute diabetic episodes or long-term complications.

Patient Education

The third phase of our model could be centered around 1972, when the effect of patient education was quantified on a large scale. That year saw the publication of articles on two important studies, one by Miller and Goldstein[4] and the other by Davidson.[5] The study by Miller and Goldstein was based on a 2-year study of a population of 8,000 diabetics in Los Angeles, all of whom had undergone an educational program on diabetes, self-management, and prevention of complications. Although the therapeutic role of patient education had been advocated for many years,[6,7] the publication of Miller and Goldstein's and Davidson's studies marked for the first time significant, large-scale benefits of patient education in the treatment of diabetes and its long-term complications. Not only did the diabetics, having been educated, suffer markedly fewer acute episodes (80% decrease of comas—Davidson), but, thanks to education aimed at better control of their diabetes, the annual rate of hospitalization for these patients plummeted from 5.4 to 1.7 days. Thus diabetics who had followed a training program were hospitalized nearly three times less than those who did not. This annual hospitalization rate of 1.7 days is all the more impressive when compared to the average rate for the nondiabetic population (1.2 days), which was statistically not different (Table 49–1 and Fig. 49–1). For the first time on a large scale, improvement in diabetic control was *not* directly related to drugs (biomedical therapy) but to a much wider medical approach that considered not only the disease but the role of its *bearer*, the patient, who had to learn and master the skills for daily control. In Geneva, Switzerland, patient education and training in foot

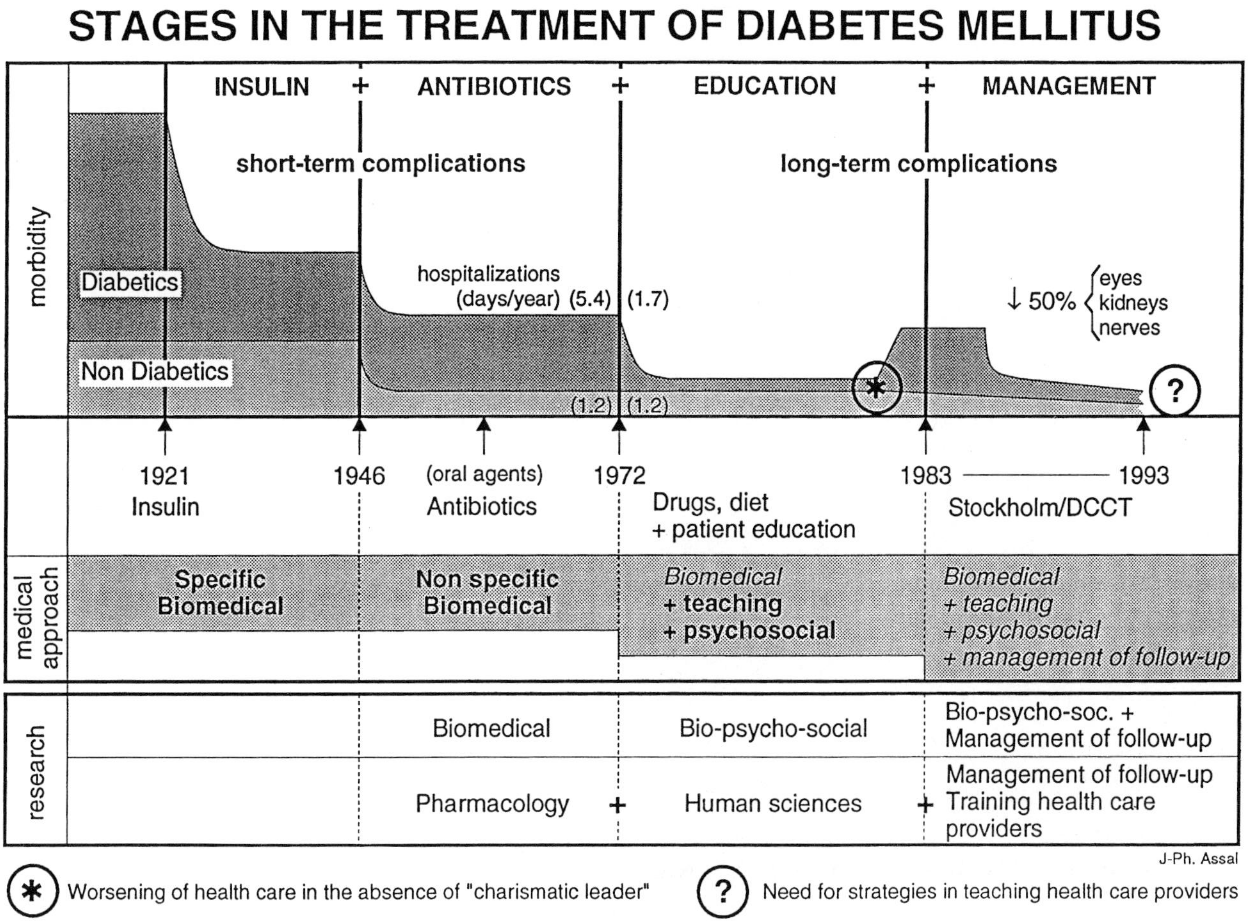

STAGES IN THE TREATMENT OF DIABETES MELLITUS

Figure 49–1. The four stages in the history of the treatment of diabetes. From Ref. 4, with permission. See also Ref. 10.

care has brought about a dramatic 82% reduction in amputations over a 10-year survey. (Fig. 49–3).[8,9]

Long-term Management and Control

Two major studies have shown, over a 7- to 10-year follow-up, that metabolic control could decrease the incidence or the progression of long-term complications by about 50%. The DCCT Study and the study of Reichard illustrated this in 1993.[10,11] Those studies are two remarkable examples of a systematic, strict organization of long-term follow-up of patients with many weekly evaluations of the quality of care. This fourth phase (see Fig. 49–1) illustrates that education in itself is not sufficient and has to be coupled with the strict systematic organization of long-term follow-up strategies. This is also a sector of management that is not sufficiently integrated in the medical training of doctors and nurses. Quality of care for patients with chronic diseases also strongly depends on managerial skills.

Diagnosis, Choice, and Application of Treatment and Long-Term Follow-up: A Therapeutic Process that Requires an Integrated Approach to the Patient

The history of the treatment of diabetes, considered outside the framework of this specific disease, illustrates the development of a medical model that has moved through the strict biomedical phase to include a psychosocial and educational approach as well as a managerial dimension for long-term follow-up. Although life-saving (see Fig. 49–2), the biomedical approach could not encompass all the therapeutic aspects of the disease in its chronic phase. While patient education in itself is no warranty for the holistic approach, it might still help the physician arrive at a more comprehensive

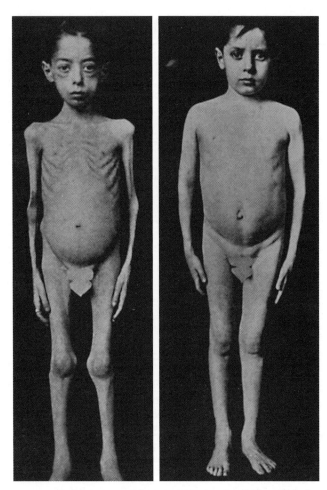

Figure 49–2. Insulin treatment. One of the first children treated with insulin (1922). (Left) The day of the first injection. (Right) 2 months later.

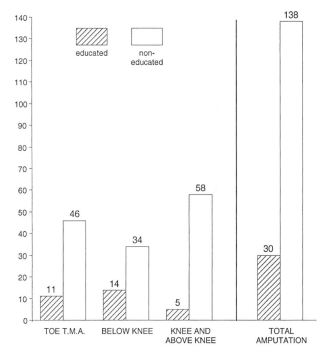

Figure 49–3. Diabetic patient education for foot care and level of amputation; t.m.a., transmetatarsal amputation. Source: University Hospital, Geneva.

global therapy for the disease and its complications. Thus the treatment of diabetes presents an exemplary model to which historians of medicine may refer when considering the ways in which the dimensions (biomedical, psychosocial, educational, and managerial) of a disease are complementary rather than separate, or even opposed entities. Regardless of the efficiency of combining the aforementioned four dimensions, this wider approach is, as yet, an integral part of treatment programs in only a few medical centers. Among these centres this approach is usually due to the efforts of a single highly skilled and primarily intuitive physician

who knows exactly how to do things but has difficulties in teaching and training his collaborators to do them on their own. Examples show that, should this physician leave the medical center, the holistic system immediately breaks down and the health care system returns to the traditional, biomedical model: Once again, doctors concern themselves mainly with organic and pathophysiological check-ups and begin once more to chase after BG levels mechanically, while doctor–patient relationships, patient education, and the inevitable psychosocial problems present in the lives of diabetic persons are considered of secondary importance and pushed aside.

Reality shows how easy it is for physicians to fall back on the biomedical model only. Several reasons can explain this shortcoming. We do not know how to integrate the psychosocial and educational dimensions of diseases with the biomedical one. There is no systematic practical training of doctors, nurses, or dietitians in this field. A system that cannot be taught

TABLE 49–1 Effect of patient education on acute episodes in diabetes[a]

	Hospital Days/Year	DM comas (n/year)	Foot problems (n/week)	Phone calls (n/day)	Savings ($US)
Without patient education	5.6	300	320	1	
With patient education	1.7	100	40	20	2,000,000

[a] Los Angeles County Hospital (8,000 diabetics, 1971). From Ref. 4, with permission.

can only rely on the good sense and intuition of some skilled health care providers and therefore cannot be easily transmitted.

The following sections of this chapter will attempt to compensate for this shortcoming by providing an analyses of physicians' (often unconscious) resistance to an integrated approach to disease. Some suggestions will also be made on how an integrated approach toward the disease and its bearer can be planned and realized. It is significant that WHO-Euro has published the report of an international Working Group on Therapeutic Patient Education (TPE) for health care providers who treat patients with chronic diseases in the management of long-term follow-up.[2] Among others, there is a request that medical schools and schools of nursing deliver a systematic teaching program for health care providers at the pre-, post- and continuing education levels with official certification. It is only through approaches of this kind that quality of care for chronic diseases may be improved.

The Difficulties of Practicing the Integrated Approach

Medical School: Training in Reductionism

The long training that medical students undergo often modifies their attitude toward their future patients. At the beginning of their studies, one frequently hears medical students express a desire "to help suffering people." However, by the end of their training their point of view has been modified by their medical identity. Rather than *helping people*, they come to see themselves as *fighters of disease*.

One of a student's first contacts with the human being in medical school is the *dissection of a dead human body*, which fragments the spontaneous, original, holistic approach the young student favors (Fig. 49–4). Thus, from the beginning the medical school fosters a reductive approach toward the human being through analysis of his anatomic, organic, and biochemical subsystems. Moreover, the organism is never studied as a functioning whole but as a successive series of smaller and smaller units seen in isolation—body parts, organs, tissues, cells, and, finally, subcellular components. As Engel has pointed out: "The bio-medical model embraces both reductionism, the philosophic view that complex phenomena are ultimately derived from a single principle, and mind–body dualism that separates the mind from the somatic."[1]

This is illustrated in the case of Mr. B., where we all expressed our reductionist approach in thinking that problems with his diabetes were solved as soon as his blood sugar was under control in the hospital, both at the time of the first ketoacidosis and when he was later

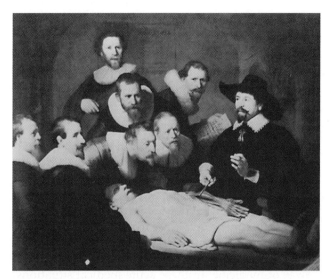

Figure 49–4. Rembrandt van Rijn (1606–1669): "The Anatomy Lesson of Professor Tulp," 1632. A representation of the biomedical model: from the anatomical to the biological understanding of human beings. Photograph courtesy of Mauritshuis, The Hague, The Netherlands.

admitted for an imbalance in his diabetes. In the biomedical, analytical reductionist approach, there is little or no room given to the psychological, sociological, and educational aspects of the patient or to his or her consequential behavior when encountering problems in these areas.

Hospital Training: Training for Crises

After medical school, the next step in the doctor's training is classically internship and residency in a hospital. There the young physician, who has already acquired medical knowledge through segmentation of the body, is geared toward diagnosis and treatment for acute or subacute diseases that also represent rather specific, segmental deviations from either good health or chronic diseases. In the case of diabetes, physicians have been remarkably well trained to treat acute decompensations (such as ketoacidosis, hyperosmolar comas, acute foot problems, kidney insufficiencies, and so on). At the time of these acute metabolic and organic decompensations, diagnosis and treatment follow very standardized procedures that can be learned and applied through algorithms. In fact, as soon as Mr. B.'s biochemical abnormalities were corrected, he was discharged from the hospital. We doctors had fulfilled our biomedical role. The crisis was over.

The situation, for physicians and patients alike, changes when both have to face the chronic phases of diabetes. In this situation the physician's linear intervention (as in the hospital) plays only a small part toward the patient's general health. Other innovative medical approaches to patients and their diseases are therefore needed, but, unfortunately for the majority of patients, they have yet to be learned and practiced in existing medical systems.

The Physician's Operative Thought: Immediate, Effective, and Identifiable Results

Medicine in acute conditions requires a high grade of efficiency that can only be evaluated by looking at palpable, objective results that deal with "rubor", "dolor", "tumor", and "calor"; improvement of biochemical data; electrocardiograms (ECGs); X-ray films; and so forth. The immediately objectifiable results of a patient's treatment in a life-threatening situation profoundly mark the physician concerning his own efficiency and deeply convince him of his role and of the power of medicine. In these acute medical situations, the physician comes close to the concept found in physics: Action equals reaction. It is difficult for a physician, who has been trained in such a system, to later be efficient enough when the patient's problems require not only a purely medico-technical approach but a more global one including psychological and educational support.

The Doctor as a Prisoner of His Training

Taking the case of Mr. B. as an example, it becomes evident that the patient was saved at the time of his initial ketoacidosis (ph = 7.01), specifically through the usual biomedical approach. However, for *long-term control* of his disease, this approach proved deficient. It was only when Mr. B. was able to take advantage of the outpatient facilities run by personnel trained in patient education and psychology that the ongoing problems of his diabetes were brought to light. These finally clarified the reasons for his excess weight, which was associated with his protection against death (the pancreatic cancer of his wife), and his refusal to accept his diabetes, which was due to his fear that doing so would interfere with his family and professional life.

Technical and Psychological Help

Acute Medical Conditions

When Mr. B. was hospitalized the first time for ketoacidosis and the second time for persistent hyperglycemia, medical knowledge translated these high BG values into technical solutions: The first time, rehydration, insulin, potassium, and so forth were administered; the second time he was hospitalized, insulin doses were changed and the dietary program was renewed. In these situations medical knowledge conferred the physician with power over the disease that only the physician, not the patient, could have. The

effects of this power could be rapidly evaluated by both doctor and patient alike.

Impact of the Psychological and Social Dimensions of the Disease

When Mr. B., despite the efficacy of the treatment, needed to be followed more carefully as an outpatient due to his recurrent high blood sugar, there was an indication that our previous medical approach had been inadequate for long-lasting diabetes control. Although it was obvious to all of us that Mr. B. had not been following his diet, the patient could not spontaneously explain the root of his problem. However, after several discussions with a physician and a psychologist, Mr. B. was gradually able to clarify the problem for himself. Firstly, he discovered to what extent he did not want the "sick person" role to interfere with his private life. It was very important to him that his female companion perceive him as healthy and not be reminded of his diabetes in any way. Secondly, he sought to hide his diabetes from his professional colleagues, for fear—probably well founded—that being a diabetic would interfere with his image as a leader in his company. Furthermore, Mr. B. perceived the role of a "leader" as being one who "did more" than others: as a result, he not only worked more but also behaved as the "leader" at meal times. And, as stated previously, he finally described the morbid fear he had of cancer of the pancreas and its devastating weight loss. Given these concerns, it is obvious that prescribing a new diet would make little sense compared to an integrated approach, which would help the patient clarify the many reasons behind this dietary behavior.

Characteristics of Psychological Support

The purpose of psychological support is to lead the patient to a point where he or she can cope better with the disease and the management of the treatment. This can be achieved after personal, psychological problems are clarified.

The *unease* of the patient is much less specific than the organic *disease* handled through the biomedical approach. The doctor–patient relationship in psychological aid is *fundamentally* different from that of technical support, for in psychological help the biomedical knowledge of the physician bears little weight compared to the crucial role of listening attentively to the patient. There is a real need to take time to listen to patients because they are restricted in easily and quickly explaining their feelings when encountering difficulties with their disease. When given the time to explain to the health care providers, the patient may gradually clarify for *himself* the various problems involved in his personal behavior. The doctor's sole power in the psychological relationship consists in helping the patient clarify his or her problems: He cannot impose the same sort of solutions that he does in the sector of biomedical intervention.

So, although psychological help may bring the patient to find his or her own solutions, it is usually a gradual one. Even if the solution may appear suddenly, most of the time it is after a period of step-by-step maturation. Thus, it is not as easy to evaluate the efficacy of this psychological approach as it is to evaluate, for example, the effect of laser therapy on the development of new vessels on the retina.

Need for Psychological Training

To identify underlying personal conflicts, specific knowledge and the use of psychological *techniques* are required.

Technical and psychological help are so fundamentally different that it is almost impossible to imagine a given physician having equal skill in both areas if no specific training has been acquired. Although we physicians involved in organic medicine agree that technical help must be learned, we do not realize that the ability to give psychological help also requires as much or even more training. Among practitioners, psychological help is too often currently based on, or confused with, human warmth and good sense. This was the case with the general practitioner whom Mr. B. greatly appreciated. Despite this doctor's warmth and good will, his lack of a structured psychological approach rendered him incapable of helping Mr. B. understand what was going on inside himself and find his own solutions regarding how to cope with his diabetes control.

Of course, one of the difficulties for physicians is the constant interference of the need for psychological skills while dealing with the biomedical aspect of the disease. These two interrelated dimensions are simultaneously present in all cases of human disease and require the physician to oscillate between them.

A physician who has no clear understanding of the nature of psychological help may spontaneously, and even unconsciously, apply the biomedical model with its decision-making strategies to the psychological problems of the patient. His attitude may be: " I know, therefore I can decide for you." Such a physician could have said to Mr. B., "I know why you do not eat properly at home or at the office: It is because you don't accept your diabetes, and therefore I am going to tell you what to do in order to cope with your disease. Here is a list of advice…." Such a doctor is trying to give what he cannot give to a patient who may not even want it.

In the field of psychological help and the doctor–patient relationship, we have experienced positive results with our medical residents after providing training in the fields of "active listening," "nondirective interviews," and "Balint groups."[12,13]

The Disease and Its Bearer

Diagnosis and Treatment: The Patient's and the Doctor's Perspective

Particularly when dealing with chronicity, the broadest possible definition of "disease" is needed. It appears mandatory that physicians with their biomedical approach learn more about what *patients* think about their disease and its treatment. Indeed, patients often have a definition that may be quite different to the biological-anatomical definition of the physician. This observation might play an important role in the efficacy of therapeutic programs described by Fabrega.[14]

To encourage the patient's compliance with the treatment, it is important for health care providers to familiarize themselves with the patient's health beliefs and experience, as well as those of his peers and of the society in which he lives. For instance, there is a common belief found among the general public that diabetics inevitably go blind. How, therefore, can a physician really motivate a patient toward more efficient metabolic control of his diabetes and regular eye checkups if this patient, although remaining silent on the subject, is convinced that he will go blind in any case? *Seen globally, there is more than one diagnosis and treatment for any given disease*: the "official," bioanatomic one (that of the medical faculty) and the subjective one (that of the patient) (Figs. 49–5 and 49–6). These two diagnoses do not always coincide with each other, and the patient's subjective diagnosis, as a result, may interfere with the treatment the doctor's diagnosis requires. The less these two diagnoses coincide, the more difficult it will be for the physician to obtain the patient's adherence to treatment.

The Example of Mr. B.

Let us return to the case of Mr. B. Open discussions with the patient revealed that he had decided to wait a long time before entering the hospital the first time (in almost final stage ketoacidosis), because the 12 kg he had lost were for him the sign of cancer. This attitude was understandable: His wife had been diagnosed as having cancer at the time of investigation for weight loss. Therefore, weight loss was equal to the definition of cancer. This resulted in the following health belief: "If I gain weight, I am sure I *don't* have cancer; if I lose weight, I *may well* have cancer; if my weight is stable, I *can't know* either way."

Although Mr. B.'s health belief might have been logical consequence, he was nevertheless so concerned with the possibility of having cancer that he did not take

THE PATIENT - DOCTOR CIRCLE OF COMMUNICATION FOR DIAGNOSIS AND TREATMENT

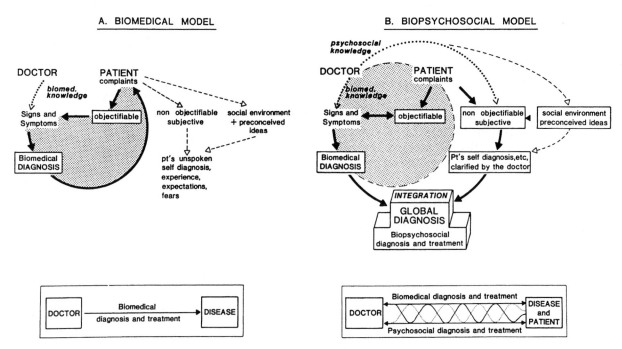

Figure 49–5. The patient–doctor circle of communication for diagnosis and treatment. (A) The biomedical model. (B) The biopsychosocial/medical model.

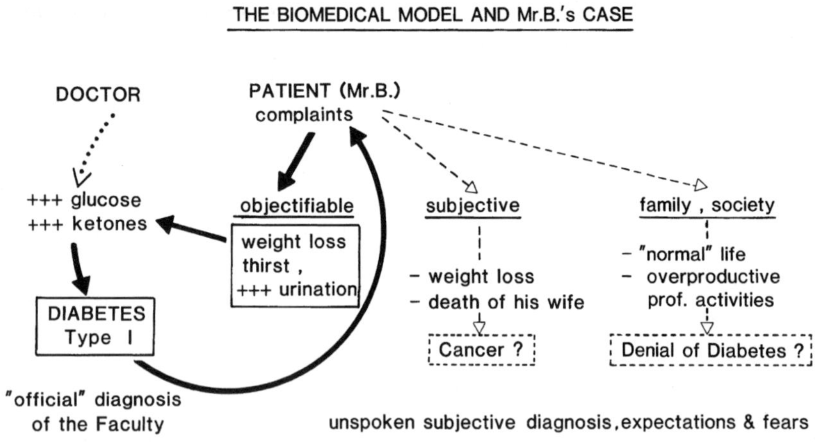

THE BIOMEDICAL MODEL AND Mr.B.'s CASE

Figure 49–6. The chronic diabetes of Mr. B.: short-circuiting his personal problems through the reductionism of the biomedical approach.

into consideration that his wife had not had the intense thirst and polyuria he experienced. In the hospital, although remarkably improved by insulin treatment and aware that he had diabetes, Mr. B. nevertheless was certain that the doctors were hiding the news that he also had cancer of the pancreas. The patient never spoke of these problems. It was only in the family history that our resident briefly mentioned that Mr. B.'s wife had died from cancer of the pancreas 2 years prior to his *second* hospitalization. Therefore, because we did not take into account the necessity of discovering the patient's own subjective personal diagnosis, we chose the bio-

medical path and continued to prescribe new weight-reduction diets that evidently did not work.

The Biomedical and Bio-psychological Medical Model

The case of this patient forces us to consider the two dimensions of diagnosis and treatment: one restricted to the disease itself (the bio-medical model) and the other in which both the disease and its bearer, the patient, are actively taken into account (the bio-psycho-social medical model as described by Engel).[1,15]

The doctor–patient relationship starts with the patient's request for help. In the bio-medical model (see Fig 49–5A) the patient's complaints present rapidly identifiable signs (in the case of Mr. B., thirst, excess urination, weight loss, high blood and urine glucose). In this biomedical model (see Fig. 49–6) the doctor does not take into account the patient's subjective impressions and fears, which are neither immediately identifiable nor spontaneously voiced. The doctor's professional training has provided him with knowledge and skill to take into account mainly physical symptoms and signs. He interprets these to arrive at a diagnosis that will allow him to select the appropriate treatment. Although this anatomical and biochemical approach plays a fundamental role in acute situations, it does not take into account the patient's subjective experience of the disease and its treatment, which is so important in chronic diseases.

In the case of Mr. B. such a globally integrated approach would have helped us rid the patient of the false ideas he had regarding his disease because of the death of his wife. If we had discovered the patient's very important self-diagnosis, it would have been easier to obtain compliance with dietary advice (see Figs. 49–5B and 49–6).

Patient's Subjective Preconceived Ideas

To take into account the psychological burden the patient has to face with the disease is neither evident nor easy. Patients do not spontaneously describe their personal problems if they are not invited to do so, mainly because these problems are not always easy to articulate, especially during a doctor's appointment, which may last only a few minutes.

Another problem arises because patients often tend to speak of their illnesses in terms of their physician's bio-medical expertise and language. They do this because, at first, it seems to be the easiest path for the patient to follow in the doctor–patient relationship. They see in their diabetologist a professional who mainly deals with BG levels, insulin doses, diet programs, calories, grams, and so forth. In these cases patients see their doctors as the incarnation of the bio-medical model and intuitively try to respond mainly in those terms. Thus, they are unconsciously trapped in a vicious circle by censoring themselves and never speaking of their beliefs and fears of the disease and its long-term complications.

Patients also do not speak about their fears because they are worried that the physician may actually confirm them. It is fundamental for therapeutic efficiency that physicians be aware of patients' beliefs and fears about diabetes and its complications.

Many patients refuse insulin at bedtime because they are convinced that one may die during a nocturnal hypoglycemia. Many patients refuse to see a dietitian because they think a diabetic diet is practically no different from slow starvation.

Regarding long-term complications, many patients are convinced that they are doomed to blindness and/or leg amputation. This myth is so prevalent that, at the time they were diagnosed as being diabetic, about one-third of our patients associated diabetes with blindness and amputation, although they were ignorant of the characteristics of the disease. The same is true of the myth of male impotence. In one case, a young man, aged 26, who had just been diagnosed as diabetic, wanted to have children that same year because he was convinced that within a short time he would become impotent. Young diabetic females are often so certain that they will give birth to a diabetic child that they decide never to marry and/or to remain childless. Others use no contraceptives because they believe they cannot become pregnant. For the reasons discussed earlier, these and other fears are rarely spoken of spontaneously in the doctor's office unless the doctor broaches, or otherwise encourages, their discussion.

The Role of Peers and Society

It is not within the scope of this chapter to discuss the various origins of preconceived ideas about diabetes, but certainly many of them are prevalent in society at large and vary from one subgroup of people to another. Although medical information given via the newspapers, television programs, or by health care providers tends to be fairly objective and simple, it cannot be objectively received by patients. This once-objective information will be distorted by preconceived notions, subjective personal concerns, and the degree of coping with the disease. Consequently, this information may easily be minimized or appear threatening.[16]

Coping with the Disease

As many personal experiences with diabetes exist as there are individuals, but a number of common attitudes in coping with the disease can be observed. For a patient to accept his or her chronic disease implies an acceptance of the loss of his/her biological and psychological normality. In other words, coping with the disease is tantamount to mourning the death of previous good health.

Freud described the three stages of normal mourning: denial of reality, depression, and adapation to the new reality.[17] In *On Death and Dying*, Kübler-Ross went into even greater detail.[18] She distinguished five stages of mourning: (1) shock and denial ("No, not me"), (2) revolt ("Why me? "), (3) "bargaining" ("Yes, but…"), (4) depression accompanied by hope, and

(5) acceptance. Analysis of tape recordings of 500 round-table discussions with patients in our division shows that acceptance of diabetes is a continuum in which certain stages are very close to those described by Freud and Kübler-Ross.

These stages are somewhat artificially focused, as they are only labels to help understand certain key aspects of this continuing dynamic process. It normally occurs as an individual progresses through the difficult periods of disease acceptance. Reality shows that the developmental stages of acceptance of a disease are never entered into in isolation, one at a time, but rather in relationship to the stage before and after. For example, a person in the stage of revolt might, at the same time, be partially in the stage of denial while also exhibiting characteristics of bargaining, the stage that follows revolt.

The speed at which one passes from one stage to another varies greatly from one individual to another, depending on the individual, the personal surroundings, and the doctor–patient relationship experienced. Indeed, many factors favor the acceptance or inhibit its evolution.

To accept one's own disease is a process that progresses with oscillations back and forth. The general movement goes forward toward active acceptance with intermittent backward movements at the time of setbacks. A chronic illness always presents a series of painful situations that the patient must surmount. In the case of diabetes there are several constraints, such as diet, insulin injections, and daily glucose monitoring. Much later, at the time of occurrence of long-term complications, acceptance of those new handicaps will be necessary and will start the processes of acceptance again. These difficult phases of coping with the disease seem necessary and normal. What is abnormal is for a given patient to remain in one or the other intermediary stage, e.g., permanent denial or revolt. Active communication with the patient, patient education, and training for self-care monitoring have quite positive effects on the evolution of the patient's acceptance.

A global approach, both biologically and psychosocially, to the patient requires the *recognition* of these dynamic stages of acceptance and their *adequate support* by the medical team.

The Human Being as an Integrated System

What Is the Meaning of System?

As Mr. B.'s case showed convincingly, the biological, psychological, and sociological dimensions of his diabetes were intimately interdependent, yet taken on their own and considered separately, none of these aspects can explain in itself what happened to this

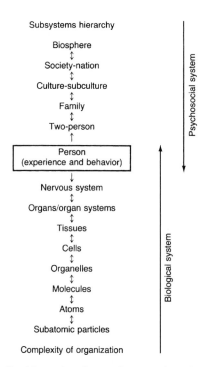

Figure 49–7. Hierarchy of natural systems based on the degree of complexity of subsystems. From Refs. 19 and 20, with permission.

patient. In his fundamental article, "The System of Nature and the Nature of Systems," Weiss stresses two essential aspects of nature that are particularly valid for medicine.[19] First, a human being is composed of different subsystems ranging from the intracellular level to that of society (Fig. 49–7). Each of these subsystems has its own internal regulation. A specialist who adopts an analytical, reductionist approach that attempts to understand only single subsystems (such as only the cell or only the family subsystem) tends "to know more and more about less and less."

The increase in knowledge limited to the structure and function of a single subsystem alone will not automatically help the physician better understand the whole. To attain global understanding, a second task is indispensable. Each subsystem of nature is in a *hierarchical* order, and each of the subsystems in the hierarchy enters into relation with all of the others and is part of the general system of nature (Fig. 49–8). For example, the subsystem "person" (the individual) is simultaneously at the highest level of the biological hierarchy and at the lowest level of the social hierarchy, thus introducing a fundamental characteristic: The "lower subsystems" are constantly integrated into the "higher" ones. In other words, the concept of a "system" can be defined as

the existence of a stable configuration in time and space, a configuration that is maintained not only by the

THE SYSTEM OF NATURE

From the PART to the WHOLE
Each system being a PART and a WHOLE

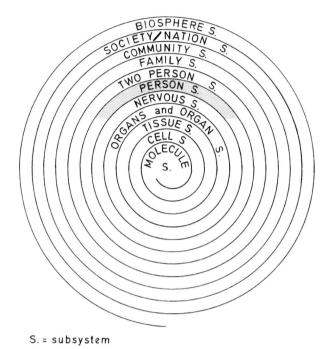

S. = subsystem

Figure 49–8. The interconnection of subsystems in nature: a fade-in/fade-out process. Adapted from Figure 49–7.

coordination of component parts in some kind of internal dynamic network but also by the characteristics of the larger system of which it is a component part. Stable configuration also implies the existence of boundaries between organized systems across which material and information flow.[19,20]

Homeostasis, a term familiar to physicians, which expresses internal body regulation, is yet another expression of this general concept of systems.

Scientific study attempts to analyze each subsystem as an independent entity. As in biology, psychology, and sociology, humans have developed different analytical approaches, each specific to a single subsystem and each characterized by its own specialized language and its specific methods of evaluation. Due to these specialized languages, integration between the various subsystems has become extremely problematic. However, the integration between these artificially isolated subsystems remains an absolute necessity. This integration is not easy to achieve in medicine. Acute situations, such a ketoacidosis, technical diagnostic procedures, and treatment, impose a reductionist approach with an artificial separation of the subsystem: the biochemical, metabolic

crisis of the patient. Although it is self evident that the holistic approach is more important in chronic diseases, such an approach should also be present in the management of acute medical situations.

To return to Weiss, the holistic system in nature is such that unit and whole cannot be separated:[19]

> Nature itself does not know the distinction at all, but it is we who, in our view of nature, have introduced it in accordance with our preference and profit. The study of parts—analytical information about parts—paid off magnificently as long as we indulged primarily in learning more and more about less and less, relying on the ingrained conviction that from the pieces of that diminutive knowledge, we would be able to reconstruct—"synthesize" (at least in our minds)—the typically patterned order of the phenomenon that we had deliberately disordered in our analytical procedure, as if we could resurrect the phoenix from its ashes.

Integrating the Subsystems Hierarchy in the Therapeutic Process

Let us now visualize, using Figures 49–9 and 49–10, the involvement of various subsystems at two different moments in the life of Mr. B. as a diabetic. Figure 49–9 reveals the various subsystems involved at the time of the acute initial diabetic ketoacidosis. Figure 49–10 illustrates the systems involved at the time of the second hospitalization for treatment of chronic hyperglycemia. Both figures exemplify that the initial insulin lack had general consequences in nearly all other subsystems, whether in acute or chronic situations. The use of the biopsychosocial medical model therefore reflects the need to analyze and give support to all the subsystems involved.

Figures 49–9 and 49–10 illustrate the hierarchical classification of the subsystems and represent a more precise and analytical graphic description of the biopsychosocial model previously seen in Figure 49–5B. Presenting the subsystems in their hierarchical order and describing some changes that characterize each subsystem have the advantage of helping the physician clarify the interactions of those various subsystems. This represents a kind of global "mapping" of the problems encountered by the patient. Such a "map" may help physicians reintegrate the bioanatomical markers of disease into a more global perspective that also includes the patient and the society in which he lives. This process is essential since the medical approach is directed at the subsystem person—the patient—who is the *nexus* of the biological and psychosocial hierarchical systems. Therefore, for any given patient, global diagnosis and treatment imply that the physician master widely different areas of knowledge and skill with the corresponding approaches of therapy specific to each subsystem.

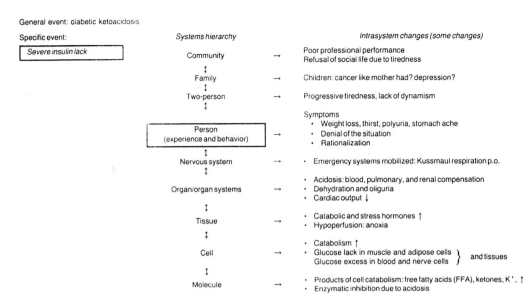

Figure 49–9.   The biopsychosocial medical model and Mr. B.'s case: the event of diabetic ketoacidosis. From Ref. 20, with permission.

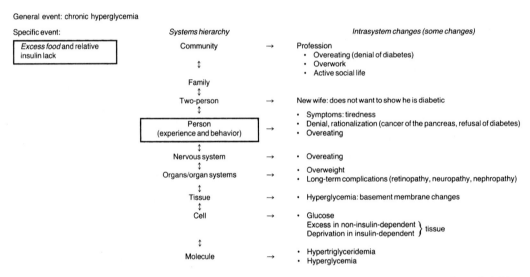

Figure 49–10.   The biopsychosocial medical model and Mr. B.'s case: the event of chronic hyperglycemia. From Ref. 20, with permission.

The Integration of the Psychosocial Dimensions of Disease

It is essential to understand that the bio-*psychosocial* approach is not opposed to the biomedical approach but that is an opening, an enlargement of the biomedical model (see Fig. 49–5B). The latter remains unaltered, since it covers the clinical signs and symptoms and the anatomical and biochemical markers of disease. It is, however, *integrated* into a larger system taking into account the bearer of the disease and society. The psychosocial dimensions cannot stand on their own. Therefore, if the diagnostic and therapeutic global approach to disease is to be efficient, in addition to

acquiring sound biomedical knowledge, the physician must be educated to master the psychosocial dimension of the disease (see Fig. 49–5B). Thus, the biopsychosocial medical model necessitates a double education (e.g., in internal medicine and psychology, psychiatry and/or sociology). Such a double education of the physician is rare but appears to be more and more mandatory.

An interdisciplinary team of health care providers can have a holistic approach, even if some of its members might not be capable individually of treating a patient on a holistic basis. The various members of the team specialized in different subsystems will only be able to develop an integrated holistic approach to the disease and the patient when they systematically, day after day, share their experiences and approaches. To promote an integrated approach implies that group dynamic techniques be actively developed in the management of the health care team. It is essential therefore that members of the team have acquired the necessary skills in the field of group dynamics.

What Do Physicians Need?

Following a series of 50 workshops held in Geneva and attended by some 2,000 physicians, nurses, and dietitians, there emerged the following questions constantly posed by physicians:[21]

- How to listen to patients?

- How can we motivate patients to follow their treatment?

- Which strategies should be developed for relapse prevention?

- How can we help patients better cope with the disease?

- Which methodologies are appropriate for therapeutic patient education?

- How should group discussions with patients be run?

- How do we improve group dynamic techniques and communication among health care workers?

Taking into account the subsystem hierarchy (see Figs. 49–7, 49–8), we can see that the majority of these requests belong to the psychosocial subsystems. For example, listening to and motivating the patient is part of the two-person subsystem. Group discussions with patients and group dynamics between health care workers take into consideration the family, the community, the culture, and the subculture subsystems. Each of those subsystems is one sector of human sciences and has its own body of knowledge and scientific approach. The aim is that specialists from each of those subsystems should participate in the professional training of physicians and other health care providers. Therefore, in the treatment of chronic diseases in general, and diabetes in particular, postgraduate training and continuing education can no longer be limited to physicians teaching physicians: It requires interconnection with nonmedical specialists coming from the fields of psychology, sociology, and education.

Practical Training for the Therapeutic Education of Patients

At the request of WHO-Euro, a group of experts have prepared a special report ("Therapeutic Patient Education: Continuing Education for Healthcare Providers in the Management of Chronic Diseases") indicating the need of the medical community for more specific training of health care providers in the management and long-term follow-up of chronic diseases. One key con-

cept emerged from this expert group: Patient education should be replaced by *therapeutic* patient education.

When health care providers teach patients, they tend to spend more time and energy speaking about the disease than providing the patient with the appropriate skills for the daily management of his or her condition. Therapeutic patient education therefore focuses on the skills for effective self-management of the treatment adaptation to a chronic disease and coping processes and skills, while also taking into consideration the cost to the patient and society.

Therapeutic patient education is an essential component for the efficient self-management and quality of care of all long-term diseases and conditions. However, patients with acute diseases should not be excluded from its benefit.[16,22–26]

The Need for Educational Programmes in Therapeutic Patient Education.   Description of these various needs is beyond the scope of this chapter, but the following is a list of topics that are now part of a postgraduate and continuing education curriculum given at the Faculty of Medicine of the University of Geneva. It leads to a diploma in the field of therapeutic education of patients with chronic diseases. (See also the Appendix at the end of this book.)

- The characteristics of chronic diseases compared to the acute medical situations (how to adapt the behavior of physicians to the specificity of chronic diseases).

- Understanding how the patient with a chronic disease functions with regard to his treatment and daily management of the control of his illness.

- Taking into account the patient's coping strategies with the disease (Which counterattitude do physicians develop in front of a patient who is in revolt or in the bargaining stage with his treatment?).

- Communicating with the patient and mastering the "active listening" technique (Which strategies should be used to facilitate the communication?).

- Giving therapeutic instructions to the patient (Which approach should help the physician deal with the health beliefs of the patient? How can the physician evaluate if the patient's locus of control is external or internal?).

- Assisting a patient in coping with his illness and its treatment (mastering the various barriers that interfere with the patient's adherence to the treatment, developing specific attitudes that would reinforce the process of coping).

- Integrating the patient's own experience in his therapeutic educational program (Which educational strategies are recommended to help the patient acquire the skills for self-management?).

- Evaluation of a learning process and methods used (methodologies for the evaluation of courses given to patients and the evaluation of the impact of the courses on the patients).

- Long-term follow-up of patients (Which strategies are needed to integrate patients' relapse prevention, therapeutic education, and psychosocial support into the biomedical activity of the physician?).

Conclusions

The physician's identity has been molded during medical school and years of hospital training into a way of thinking about specific subsystems dealing with anatomopathology, biochemistry, and organic and laboratory diagnostic procedures—each of these representing a subsystem, a speciality in itself, a rather "closed" entity. Management of chronic diseases forces the physician, whether he likes it or not, to face other subsystems that deal with the entire person, two persons, the family, the community, and society. In this perspective, professional specialities (endocrinology, diabetology, etc.) always fall short of the need to simultaneously handle the various problems and requirements of the patient as the bearer of the disease and his family.

A professional who accepts this interrelatedness will eventually face an identity crisis, discovering that his subspeciality is only part of the whole. Although it is not within the scope of this chapter to address the problematic issue of professional identity, it is important here to note, at least, that this broadening of professional orientation is often initially experienced by the physician as a loss of his specialized medical power.

Due to the (often unspoken) underlying assumptions of the importance of the biomedical field, physicians who also concern themselves with the psychosocial dimensions of disease develop a feeling of uncertainty. This feeling of uncertainty, which often results in a feeling of insecurity, leads to the development of defense mechanisms that draw the physician back to the biomedical approach. For instance, for a patient with uncontrolled diabetes whose poor control is the result of psychosocial problems, how many physicians constantly repeat a complete laboratory investigation to evaluate if there is *still* not a biological cause of this poor control? The initial professional identity is thus one of the greatest barriers to achieving a holistic approach, for it causes the physician to restrict his attention to the subsystems that his training in medical school and in the hospital has led him to master.

Integration of the various subsystems from the subcell to the individual and from the individual to the society can only be achieved with difficulty, if at all. The artificially opposed, pejorative labels "hard" and "soft"

sciences indirectly indicate this situation. These labels have in fact been created by scientists belonging only to basic science. This testifies to the fundamental misunderstanding between biological and human sciences. "Hard" for the bioscientists, is a positive term, signaling the reliability of testable facts obtained through the almost mechanical—but highly effective—bimodal analytical approach. These scientists are extremely skeptical of the facts specific to the human sciences as they are delineated only with extreme difficulty and involve a large number of variables. Yet not only do the members of the various scientific communities misunderstand each other, but the self–imposed segregation of science into different "camps" also illustrates that scientists of all sorts fail to comprehend that the system of nature itself is a *continuum* (as illustrated by the spiral shown in Figure 49–8).

Diabetic ketoacidosis can be taken as a case in point, as it can be analyzed through several clearly delineated biochemical sequences resulting in hard facts. However, such a metabolic decompensation can also be influenced by many other variables that pertain to the patient's psychological problems. The psychological approach can effectively clarify these problems, as the case of Mr. B. illustrates. These "soft" facts are therefore as much a part of the reality of the patient and his disease as are the "hard" data with which the biomedical sciences deal.

To treat the individual (who simultaneously finds himself at the highest of the biomedical systems and at the lowest of the psychosocial systems) remains one of the most difficult challenges in the treatment of chronic diseases in general and diabetic therapy in general. A systematic, structured training of health care providers is mandatory for a holistic medical approach to patients with chronic diseases.

Medical training is slowly, but surely, improving. The fact that WHO is now strongly recommending training in therapeutic patient education and that some medical schools already have developed specific training programs into their medical curricula is a major step forward for the quality of care. This training is also an answer to what patients and patients' associations have asked for for so many years.

Note: See Appendix XI.

Acknowledgments

The author wishes to thank Mrs. M. Käser for expert editorial assistance as well as the collaboration of Dr. A. Golay, M.D.; Drs. R. Gfeller and C. Chollet, psychiatrists; Mrs. A. Lacroix, psychologist; and Mr. S. Jacquemet, specialist in adult education, as well as the nursing staff of the Division of Therapeutic Education for Chronic Diseases, University Hospital, Geneva, Switzerland.

References

1. Engel GL: The need for a new medical model: a challenge for biomedicine. Science 196:129–136, 1977.

2. WHO Expert Document. Report of a WHO-EURO Working Group: Therapeutic Patient Education. Continuing education for healthcare providers in the management of chronic diseases, 1998.

3. Diabetes mellitus in Europe: A problem at all ages in all countries. A model for prevention and self care. The Saint Vincent Declaration. Issued by the WHO and IDF in Europe on Diabetes Care and Research in Europe, 10–12 October, 1989.

4. Miller LV, Goldstein J: More efficient care of diabetic patients in a county hospital setting. New Engl J Med 286:1388–1391, 1972.

5. Davidson JK, Alogna M, Goldsmith M, et al.: Assessment of programme effectiveness at Grady Memorial Hospital. In Steiner G, Lawrence PA (eds): Educating Diabetic Patients, New York: Springer, 1981, pp. 239–248.

6. Joslin EP: A Diabetic Manual, Ed. 2. New York: Lea & Febiger, 1919.

7. Lawrence RD: The Diabetic Life. London: Churchill, 1925.

8. Assal J-Ph, Ekoe J-M, Lacroix A.: L'enseignement au malade sur sa maladie et son traitement. Un succes thérapeutique—un echec du corps médical. Journées de Diabétologie 1984, p. 193–207.

9. Assal, J-Ph, Albeanu A, Peter Riesch B, Vaucher J: Coût de la formation du patient atteint d'un diabète sucré. Effets sur la prévention des amputations. Diabetes Metab 19:491–495, 1993.

10. Diabetes Control and Complications Trial Research Group: The effect of intensive treatment of diabetes on the development and progression of long-term complications in insulin-dependent diabetes mellitus. New Eng J Med 329(14): 977–986, 1993.

11. Reichard P, Nilsson BY, Rosenqvist U: The effect of long-term intensified insulin treatment on the development of microvascular complications of diabetes mellitus. New Eng J Med 329(5):304–309, 1993.

12. Rogers C: On Becoming a Person, a Therapist's View of Psychotherapy. Boston: Houghton Mifflin, 1961.

13. Balint M: The Doctor, His Patient and the Illness. 2nd Edition. London: Churchill Livingstone, 1995.

14. Fabrega H: The need for an ethnomedical science. Science 189:969–975, 1975.

15. Assal J-Ph: The Treatment of Long-Term Illness: Transition from the Acute to the Chronic State. A Different Management of Illness, a New Approach. (Translated from the French: Traitement des maladies de longue durée: de la phase aïgue au stade de la chronicité.) Encycl. Med. Chir. (Paris Elsevier), Thérapeutique, 25-005-A-10, 1997.

16. Gfeller R, Assal J-Ph: Developmental stages of patient acceptance in diabetes. In Assal J-Ph, Berger M, Gay N, Cavinet J (eds): Diabetes Education: How to Improve Patient Education. New York: Exerpta Medica, 1983, pp. 207–218.

17. Freud S: Trauer und Melancholie. Gesammelte Werke, Vol. 10. 1977.

18. Kübler-Ross E: On Death and Dying. New York: Macmillan, 1969.

19. Weiss PA: The system of nature and the nature of systems: Empirical holism and practical reductionism harmonized. In Schaefer KE, Brody R (eds): Toward a Man-Centered Medical Science. Mount Kisco, NY: Futura, 1977.

20. Engel GL: The clinical application of the biopsychosocial model. Am J Psychiatry 137:535–544, 1980.

21. Assal J-Ph, Lion S: Difficulties encountered with patient education in European diabetic centers. In Assal J-Ph, Berger M, Gay N, Cavinet J (eds): Diabetes Education: How to Improve Patient Education. New York: Excerpta Medica, 1983, pp. 78–89.

22. Lacroix A, Assal J-Ph: Active listening: How to make sure that what we heard was what the patient really meant. In Assal J-Ph, Berger M, Gay N, Cavinet J (eds): Diabetes Education: How to Improve Patient Education. New York: Excerpta Medica, 1983, pp. 236–238.

23. Hopper R, Whitehead JL: Communications Concepts and Skills. New York: Harper & Row, 1979.

24. Bloom BS, Hastings J-Th, Madans GF: Handbook on Formative and Summative Evaluation of Student Learning. New York: McGraw Hill, 1971.

25. Sund RB: Piaget for Educators. Colombus, OH: Charles E. Merrill, 1976.

26. Haynal A, Schulz P: Compliance: One aspect of the doctor-patient relationship. An overview. In Assal J-Ph, Berger M, Gay N, Cavinet J (eds): Diabetes Education: How to Improve Patient Education. New York: Excerpta Medica, 1983, pp. 259–271.

Selected Readings

Assal J-Ph, Berger M, Gay N, Cavinet J (eds): Diabetes Education: How to Improve Patient Education. New York: Excerpta Medica, 1983.

Engel GL: Physician-scientists and scientific physicians. Resolving the humanism-science dichotomy. Am J Med 82:107, 1987.

Foss L, Rothenberg K: The Second Medical Revolution. From Biomedicine to Infomedicine. Boston: New Science Library, Shambhala, 1987.

Steiner G, Lawrence P: Educating Diabetic Patients. New York: Springer, 1980.

Von Bartalanffy L: General System Theory. New York: Braziller, 1980.

White KL: The Task of Medicine. Dialogue at Wickenburg. The Henry J. Kaiser Family Foundation, 1987.

50

The Economics of Diabetes Mellitus

William H. Herman

Between 1970 and 1993, health expenditures in the United States grew from $74 billion to $884 billion.[1] In 1970, health expenditures represented 7% of the gross domestic product, and by 1993 they represented nearly 14%.[1] This increase occurred because health care expenditures grew at a faster pace than the economy as a whole. The cost of diabetes also increased. Economic analyses performed in the early 1970s suggested that the direct medical cost of diabetes in the United States was $1–$2 billion.[2] Studies performed in 1992 estimated the direct costs of diabetes to be $45 billion and the direct costs of medical care for people with diabetes to be over $100 billion.[2]

There has been considerable public concern about the rapidly increasing costs of health care, and many have sought to explain and control costs.[3] Explanations have included inflation, changes in birth and death rates, changes in the age and sex composition of the population, availability and utilization of health resources, new technologies, and reimbursement mechanisms. Attempts to control the costs have focused on government regulations, the search for new methods of health care delivery, and preventive medicine. There is no reason to expect the costs of the treatment of diabetes to be any more predictable or easier to control than those of other health care. Although new drugs, treatments, and technologies have proven to be both effective and cost effective, they will likely increase the short-term costs of diabetes.

In this chapter, we review some of the methodological issues in estimating the costs of disease and the cost-effectiveness of new therapies, temporal trends in the cost of diabetes, the current costs of diabetes, per capita annual health care expenditures for people with and without diabetes in the United States, and the cost-effectiveness of interventions in diabetes.

Methodological Issues

In general, there are two types of economic studies: descriptive and analytic (Table 50–1).[4] Descriptive studies include cost of illness and cost identification studies. They ask the question, "What is the cost?" Because such studies do not evaluate what expenditures bring in terms of health outcomes, they cannot be used to directly compare alternative health programs that produce different health outcomes. Such studies can be used to describe costs, plan for costs, and assess costs as barriers.

Analytic studies include cost-benefit, cost-effectiveness, and cost-utility analyses. Analytic studies compare a new treatment with an explicitly defined alternative and assess both costs and outcomes. The primary outcome of interest in analytical studies is the cost-effectiveness ratio.[5] In the cost-effectiveness ratio, the numerator is calculated as the difference in cost between a candidate intervention and the alternative to which it is being compared. The denominator is calculated as the difference in health outcomes between the two interventions. The ratio reflects the incremental cost/unit gain in health. In cost-benefit analyses, the gain in health is expressed in financial terms (dollars); in cost-effectiveness analyses, it is expressed in conventional clinical terms (cases of disease prevented or life

TABLE 50–1 Types of Economic Analyses

Descriptive
    Cost of illness
    Cost identification
Analytic
    Cost-benefit
    Cost-effectiveness
    Cost-utility

TABLE 50–2   Critical Issues in Economic Analyses

Perspective
    Payer
    Health system
    Society
Types of costs
    Direct medical
    Direct nonmedical
    Indirect
Choice of comparator
Definition of costs and benefits
Identification, measurement, and valuation of costs
    and benefits
Discounting
Sensitivity analyses

gained); and in cost-utility analyses, it is expressed in quality-adjusted life-years (QALYs) or a similar measure that weighs years of life by quality of life.[4]

Economic analyses must address several critical issues (Table 50–2). In any economic analysis, the perspective selected for the analysis must be identified and the types of costs considered must be specified.[4–6] Typical perspectives are those of the payer, the health system, and society. Types of costs include direct medical costs, direct nonmedical costs, and indirect costs. Direct medical costs reflect resources used for inpatient care, outpatient care, self-management, medications, laboratory tests, procedures, supplies, and durable medical equipment. Direct nonmedical costs arise as a result of illness but do not involve purchasing medical services. They include costs of transportation, lodging, house-keeping, clothing, and food incurred as a result of illness. Indirect costs arise from being absent from work, having decreased earning ability when working because of long-term disability, or having lost earnings because of premature mortality. From the perspective of a payer or health system, direct medical costs are relevant. From the societal perspective, direct medical, direct nonmedical, and indirect costs may be relevant.

Economic analyses must also clearly define the new treatment and the alternative treatment or comparator.[5,7] Ideally, a new treatment should be compared with all relevant alternative treatments, recognizing that the latter will vary among health systems, regions, and countries. If a new treatment is not compared with multiple alternatives, it should be compared with the treatment option it is most likely to replace. Comparing a new treatment with a third-line alternative or placebo will result in a more favorable cost-effectiveness picture than if the alternative were stronger.

In economic analyses, the strategy for defining costs and benefits must be explicit.[5,6] The inclusion or exclusion of comorbid clinical conditions such as cardiovascular disease as a cost of diabetes or benefit of diabetes treatment may result in considerable differences in the estimated economic impact of a treatment. An overly broad attribution of comorbidities to specific diseases may lead to double counting and overestimation of the cost of a disease or benefit of treatment and an overly restrictive attribution may underestimate the true economic impact.

Defining costs involves identifying resources, measuring resources, and valuing resources.[5] It is most important that all areas of relevant health care utilization be identified and measured. Subsequently, resources can be valued by applying unit cost information. In health care, charges may not be a valid estimate of cost.[8] Charges are essentially list prices and are adjusted to allow for expansion of facilities and replacement of equipment, bad debt, courtesy care, disallowed costs, and profit. In economic analyses that adopt a societal perspective, resources should be valued according to their opportunity cost, the value of the resources in their next best alternative use.[5] The opportunity cost reflects the real cost of a given resource to society.

There are many alternative clinical approaches to the treatment of diabetes. These include both secondary interventions to prevent the development of adverse outcomes of pregnancy, microvascular, neuropathic, and cardiovascular complications and tertiary interventions to prevent the development of blindness, end-stage renal disease, amputations, and death in persons with early complications. In some instances, the cost-effectiveness of interventions has been assessed in the context of clinical trials and observational studies. In general, however, no single clinical trial or observational study can address the relative effectiveness and cost-effectiveness of all alternative strategies over a lifetime.

In such instances, economic modeling is necessary.[5] Economic models synthesize information from diverse sources of varying quality to estimate patient outcomes and cost-effectiveness. In economic modeling, the issues of perspective, types of cost, choice of comparator, defining costs and benefits, and identifying, measuring, and valuing resources must be addressed. If costs and benefits accrue during different periods, then discounting must be used to adjust for the time value of money.[5,6] Since uncertainty regarding underlying assumptions is inherent in analytic studies, sensitivity analyses should also be performed to test the robustness of conclusions to variations in underlying assumptions.[5,6]

Analytic analyses raise the question of how attractive a new therapy must be to warrant its adoption and utilization.[9] Laupacis and colleagues have proposed a system to rate economic analyses according to the magnitude of the benefit associated with their application (Fig. 50–1). A grade A therapy is both more effective and cheaper than the existing one, and a grade E therapy is less effective and more costly. Grade A and

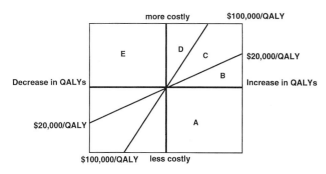

Figure 50–1. How attractive does a new technology have to be to warrant adoption and utilization? (Adapted from Ref. 9.)

Grade E therapies present no difficulties with respect to policy implications. Grade A therapies should be rapidly implemented and Grade E therapies should be abandoned. Grades B, C, and D therapies are both more effective and more costly than existing therapies, with progressive increases in cost/unit gain in health. The decision to adopt such therapies depends on available resources and considerations, including ethics and politics.

A recent review of the cost-effectiveness of over 300 life-saving interventions in medicine demonstrated a range of cost-effectiveness from cost-saving to $34 billion/year of life gained.[10] The median cost/year of life gained was $19,000. Only about 15% of interventions were cost saving, and they were generally in the areas of prenatal care, childhood immunizations, venous thromboembolism prevention, and drug and alcohol treatment. Most interventions in areas such as cholesterol, blood pressure, cardiovascular disease, and cancer screening and treatment were associated with net resource costs.

Temporal Trends in the Costs of Diabetes in the United States

Table 50–3 summarizes the temporal trend in the direct, indirect, and total costs of diabetes in the United States over the past quarter century.[2] The results clearly demonstrate increasing costs. Over the period between approximately 1969 and 1992, the total cost of diabetes in the United States rose from about $3 billion to $100 billion. The reasons for this increase are growth of the U.S. population (from 210 million in 1972 to 255 million in 1992), increased prevalence of diabetes (from <4 million in 1972 to nearly 8 million in 1992), and general inflation ($1 in 1972 was equivalent to $3.20 in 1992). There remains, however, a tendency for a more rapid rate of increase in direct costs in recent years. This is probably multifactorial, due to the increase in health care costs above the rate of inflation; the development of new tests and medications, such as glycosylated hemoglobin, self-monitoring of blood glucose, ACE-inhibitors, and HMG-CoA reductase inhibitors; and the broader application of costly new technologies such as insulin infusion pumps, laser photocoagulation, dialysis, transplantation, percutaneous transluminal angioplasty, and coronary artery bypass surgery.

The ratio of indirect to direct costs in most industrialized countries is fairly constant, with a mean of approximately 120% and a range from between 70%

TABLE 50–3 Temporal trends in the cost of diabetes mellitus, United States[a]

Study	Year	Direct Cost (US$)	Indirect Cost (US$)	Total Cost (US$)
Metropolitan Life[42]	1969	1.0 billion	1.6 billion	2.6 billion
Metropolitan Life[42]	1973	1.7 billion	2.3 billion	4.0 billion
Metropolitan Life[42]	1975	2.5 billion	2.8 billion	5.3 billion
Metropolitan Life[42]	1977	3.4 billion	3.4 billion	6.8 billion
Nat Med Care Expend[42]	1977	6.9 billion	N/A[b]	N/A
Policy Analysis Inc.[43]	1977	3.7 billion	7.1 billion	10.8 billion
Platt, Sudovar[44]	1977	5.6 billion	10.1 billion	15.7 billion
Miller[45]	1979	7.4 billion	5.0 billion	12.4 billion
Metropolitan Life[42]	1980	4.8 billion	4.9 billion	9.7 billion
Smeeding, Booton[46]	1980	5.7 billion	10.0 billion	18.9 billion
Carter Center[47]	1980	7.9 billion	N/A[a]	N/A
Metropolitan Life[42]	1984	7.4 billion	6.3 billion	13.8 billion
Huse (type 2 diabetes only)[48]	1986	11.6 billion	8.2 billion	19.8 billion
Fox, Jacobs[49]	1987	9.6 billion	10.8 billion	20.4 billion
Fox-Ray et al.[11]	1992	45.2 billion	46.6 billion	91.8 billion
Rubin et al.[12]	1992	105.2 billion	N/A	N/A

[a] Adapted from Ref. 2.

[b] N/A, not assessed.

and 180%.[2] Over the past quarter century, the indirect costs of diabetes have risen in parallel to the direct costs.

Current Costs of Diabetes in the United States

Two recent studies estimated the costs of diabetes mellitus in the United States in 1992. The study by Fox-Ray et al. for the American Diabetes Association (ADA) estimated the cost to be $91.8 billion,[11] and that by Rubin et al. for the Diabetes Treatment Centers of America (DTC) estimated the cost to be $105.2 billion.[12]

Because of methodological differences in these studies, their estimates are not directly comparable. The ADA study estimated both direct and indirect costs, while the DTC study estimated only direct costs. The estimates of direct costs were also substantially different. This was largely because the ADA study estimated direct costs *attributable to diabetes*, whereas the DTC study estimated direct costs *among people with diabetes*. Costs attributable to diabetes are a subset of all costs incurred by people with diabetes; health care costs incurred by people with diabetes include nondiabetes-related costs. In addition, while the ADA study limited itself to people with a confirmed diagnosis of diabetes, the DTC study included 3.4 million people for whom the diagnosis of diabetes was not confirmed but who used diabetes-related services and bought drugs and devices specifically needed for this disease. Table 50–4 summarizes the costs of diabetes derived from these studies.

Another explanation for the differences in direct costs between the two studies relates to more complete capture of costs in the DTC study.[11,12] The DTC study used a single survey to identify people with diabetes and to estimate costs (the 1987 National Medical Expenditure Survey), whereas the ADA study relied on

TABLE 50–5　Indirect Costs of Diabetes Mellitus in the United States, 1992 ($ billion)[a]

Short-term morbidity	$8.5
Long-term morbidity	$11.2
Mortality	$27.0
Total[b]	$46.6

[a] Adapted from Ref. 11.
[b] Does not equal sum of costs due to rounding.

the recording of diabetes in health care utilization and claims data to estimate costs. For example, in the ADA study hospitalizations among people with diabetes were only identified and counted when discharge abstracts listed diabetes as a discharge diagnosis. It is well recognized that diabetes is underreported in medical care encounters. As a result, the ADA study tended to underestimate direct medical costs. There were a number of additional differences between the studies. Whereas the ADA study included nursing home costs ($1.8 billion) as a direct cost of diabetes, the DCT study did not. Whereas the DTC study included the costs of dental care ($1.4 billion) as a direct cost of diabetes, the ADA study did not. Other important direct costs not estimated by either study include these associated with inpatient and outpatient care by federal, military, and veterans administration providers and the direct costs of nonprescription drugs.

Only the ADA study estimated the indirect costs of diabetes.[11] These are summarized in Table 50–5. Total indirect costs, including short-term and long-term morbidity as well as mortality, were estimated at $46.6 billion, approximately 51% of the total economic burden of diabetes mellitus in the United States in 1992.

Per Capita Annual Health Care Expenditures for People with and without Diabetes

The DTC study also estimated per capita annual health care expenditures in 1992 for people with and without diabetes by type of service.[12] Per capita health care expenditures for people with diabetes averaged $9,493 in 1992 compared with $2,604 for people without diabetes. People with diabetes incurred annual health care expenditures 3.6 fold higher, on average, than people without diabetes. The difference in both absolute and relative expenditures were generally greatest in the inpatient setting (Table 50–6).

As people with diabetes are on average older than the general population, part of the results in Table 50–6 are accounted for by the older age distribution of persons with diabetes, as older people use more health ser-

TABLE 50–4　Direct Costs of Diabetes Mellitus in the United States by setting, 1992 ($ billion)

Setting	Fox-Ray (ADA)[11]	Rubin (DTC)[12]
Hospital	37.2	65.2
Nursing home	1.8	—
Office	1.1	11.0
Outpatient	2.9	12.5
Emergency room	0.2	1.3
Drugs and DME	1.7	9.9
Home health	0.0	4.0
Dental	—	1.4
Total[a]	45.2	105.2

[a] Does not equal sum of costs due to rounding.
DME = Durable Medical Equipment.

TABLE 50–6   Per capita annual health care expenditures for people with and without diabetes by setting, 1992[a]

Setting	Diabetes	Nondiabetes	Ratio of diabetes to nondiabetes
Hospital	$5,885	$1,222	4.8
Office	989	554	1.8
Outpatient	1,127	330	3.4
Emergency room	115	84	1.4
Drugs and DME	891	201	4.4
Home health	357	67	5.3
Dental	130	145	0.9
Total	$9,493	$2,604	3.6

[a] Adapted from Ref. 12. All differences between diabetes and nondiabetes are statistically significant at $p < 0.01$, except for dental costs.

DME = Durable Medical Equipment.

TABLE 50–7   Per capita annual health care expenditures for people with and without diabetes by age, 1992[a]

Age	Diabetes	Nondiabetes	Ratio of diabetes to nondiabetes
0–17	2,342	1,181	2.0
18–24	2,809	1,923	1.5
25–34	6,531	2,416	2.7
35–44	6,946	2,087	3.3
45–54	11,102	3,695	3.0
55–64	9,337	3,603	2.6
65–74	10,669	5,112	2.1
75+	10,346	7,103	1.5

[a] Adapted from Ref. 12. Differences between diabetes and nondiabetes are statistically significant at $p < 0.01$.

vices than younger people. Table 50–7 shows the relative health care expenditures of people with and without diabetes controlling for age. Differences between people with and without diabetes were statistically significant in all age categories except 0–34 years. When adjusted for age, per capita expenditures for people with diabetes remained approximately 2.5-fold higher than for people without diabetes ($6,425/person/year vs. $2,604/person/year).[12]

The Cost-Effectiveness of Interventions in Diabetes

In this final section, we review the cost-effectiveness of secondary and tertiary intervention strategies in the treatment of diabetes. Many but not all studies are described. Table 50–8 summarizes the published studies that have adopted a payer's perspective, considered direct medical costs, assessed years of life or QALYs as outcomes, and discounted both costs and outcomes.

Preconception Care for Women with Established Diabetes

Two groups have addressed the cost-benefit of preconception care by weighing the costs of preconception care against the potential savings resulting from adverse maternal and neonatal outcomes averted. Both demonstrated that preconception care for women with established diabetes is cost saving.

Cost-benefit studies by Elixhauser et al. used consensus development, surveys of medical care personnel, and literature review to develop a model to determine whether the additional costs of preconception care are balanced by the savings from complications averted.[13,14] The analyses adopted the perspective of a third-party payer and considered direct medical costs. Results were expressed in 1989 dollars. Discounting was not employed. Preconception care cost $2,638/enrollee and $4,092/delivery (recognizing that more women receive preconception care than go on to deliver). The additional cost associated with preconception care was offset by the cost savings associated with adverse maternal outcomes averted ($1,990 for women who received preconception care vs. $3,191 for those who received prenatal care only, cost saving = $1,201) and adverse neonatal outcomes averted ($7,665 for infants of mothers who received preconception care vs. $10,181 for infants of mothers who received prenatal care only, cost saving = $2,516). When the direct medical costs of preconception care, prenatal care, delivery, and adverse maternal and neonatal outcomes were considered, the benefits of preconception care for women with established diabetes were $1,720 per enrollee. The benefit-cost ratio was 1.86; for every dollar spent on the preconception care program, $1.86 was gained.[13] When costs associated with postneonatal intensive care and long-term care were excluded, the cost-benefit ratio was 1.24.[14]

TABLE 50–8 Economic Analyses of Diabetes Treatment that have Adopted a Payer Perspective, Considered Direct Medical Costs, Assessed Years of Life and QALYs as Outcomes, and Discounted both Costs and Outcomes

Treatments (Ref.)	Population	$	Discount Rate	Type 1 Diabetes		Type 2 Diabetes	
				$/YOL[a]	$/QALY	$/YOL	$/QALY
DCCT intensive vs conventional[18]	Prevalent type 1 diabetes	1994	3%	$29,000	$20,000	–	–
Comprehensive vs community[22]	Incident type 2 diabetes	1994	3%	–	–	$26,000	$16,000
AAO preferred vs community[29]	Incident diabetes	1990	5%	–	$2,000	–	$3,000
ACE inhibitor vs. blood pressure control[33]	Incident nephropathy	1994	5%	($15,000)[b]	–	($10,000)[b]	–
CABG vs. angioplasty[38]	Diabetes and prevalent CAD	1995	3%	two vessel disease three vessel disease		$26,000[b] ($19,000)[b]	– –

[a] YOL, year of life; QALY, quality-adjusted life-year.   AAO = American Academy of Ophthalmology.
[b] Amounts in parentheses indicate cost-saving.   ACE = Angiotensin Converting Enzyme.
DCCT = Diabetes Control and Complications Trial.   CABG = Coronary Artery Bypass.

Thus, even from the short-term third-party payer perspective, preconception care was cost saving.

A second study by Scheffler et al. assessed the cost-benefit of preconception care by estimating the costs of a preconception care program using a "time-motion" methodology and analyzing actual hospital charges and length of stay data for women enrolled in the California Diabetes and Pregnancy Program and for matched women with diabetes drawn from control hospitals outside the program's catchment area.[15] The researchers examined two groups of enrollees—those enrolled before 8 weeks of gestation and those enrolled after 8 weeks of gestation—and compared them with women who did not enroll in the program. The analysis adopted the perspective of a third-party payer and considered only direct medical costs. Costs were expressed in 1988 dollars and were discounted to the time of delivery using an 8% discount rate. Not unexpectedly, the costs of preconception care were greatest for early enrollers ($1,300), lower for late enrollers ($800), and lowest for nonenrollers ($0). In contrast, both maternal and neonatal charges increased from early enrollers to late enrollers to nonenrollers. The charges for maternal care increased from $8,936 for early enrollers to $9,516 for late enrollees to $11,025 for nonenrollers. The charges for neonatal care increased dramatically from $2,263 for infants of early enrollers to $6,599 for infants of late enrollers to $10,674 for infants of nonenrollers. Compared with nonenrollers, early enrollers experienced a savings of $7,253 per enrollee, and late enrollers experienced a savings of $5,715 per enrollee. The benefit-cost ratio for this program was 5.19, suggesting that for every dollar spent on the program, $5.19 was recovered in charges averted.

Intensive Therapy for Type 1 Diabetes

Intensive therapy for persons with type 1 diabetes uses more resources and is more expensive than conventional therapy.[16] On the other hand, intensive therapy is associated with a lower incidence of costly chronic complications.[17] The Diabetes Control and Complications Trial (DCCT) Research Group described resource utilization and costs associated with intensive and conventional therapy and estimated the lifetime costs and benefits of intensive therapy relative to conventional therapy.[16,18] Although more expensive than conventional therapy, intensive therapy is cost effective relative to conventional therapy.

The analysis adopted the perspective of the health system and described the direct medical costs associated with the treatment, side effects of treatment, and microvascular and neuropathic complications of type 1 diabetes.[16] Intensive therapy with multiple daily injections (MDI) was 2.4 times as expensive as conventional therapy ($4,014/patient/year vs. $1,666/patient/year). The difference in cost between MDI and conventional therapy was approximately $2,300/patient/year. Three-quarters of the difference in cost was due to the greater use of outpatient services (difference = $730 per year) and self-care (difference = $977 per year) by MDI patients. Monthly as opposed to quarterly clinic visits accounted for most of the difference in the cost of outpatient services between MDI and conventional therapy patients, and the increased frequency of self-monitoring of blood glucose (1460 tests per year vs. 267 tests per year) accounted for most of the difference in the cost of self-care. The ongoing costs of intensive therapy with CSII ($5,784/patient/year) were 44% higher than those of

MDI. The difference in cost was $1,770/patient/year. Essentially all of the difference in cost was due to the greater costs of the insulin infusion pump and pump supplies.

The DCCT did not continue long enough nor was it designed to demonstrate reductions in the costly, end-stage complications of diabetes such as blindness, end-stage renal disease, and lower extremity amputation. These complications are clearly expensive. It is estimated that the direct medical cost of blindness is $1,900/patient/year, that of ESRD is $45,000/patient/year, and that of lower extremity amputation is $29,500/episode.[18] Since the incidence of all levels of diabetic complications studied in the DCCT was reduced by intensive therapy, it is likely that preventing the early complications of type 1 diabetes with intensive therapy delays or prevents the expensive end-stage complications.

Using a simulation model, the DCCT Research Group determined that intensive therapy would reduce the lifetime cumulative incidence of all of the microvascular and neuropathic complications of type 1 diabetes and that such benefits would translate into improvements in survival.[18] Intensive therapy was associated with a 41% reduction in the cumulative incidence of blindness, a 71% reduction in end-stage renal disease, a 43% reduction in amputations, and a 5.1 year increase in survival (without discounting). The expected lifetime costs associated with intensive therapy, including the costs of treatment, the side effects of treatment, and complications, were more than the expected lifetime costs associated with conventional therapy.[18] Using a 3% discount rate and 1994 dollars, the expected lifetime cost/patient was $99,822 for intensive therapy and $66,076 for conventional therapy. On average, intensive therapy cost $33,746 more than conventional therapy/patient over a lifetime. If, however, the additional benefits measured in terms of length of life are compared to the incremental costs of intensive therapy and both benefits and costs are discounted at 3%/year, then intensive therapy costs $28,661/year of life gained.[18] When length of life is adjusted for quality of life, the incremental cost/QALY gained is $19,987.[18]

Medical Nutrition Therapy for Type 2 Diabetes

Franz and colleagues conducted a cost-effectiveness analysis of medical nutrition therapy for type 2 diabetes based on a randomized clinical trial comparing basic nutrition care and practice guidelines nutrition care provided by dietitians in outpatient clinics.[19] The analyses show that individualized nutrition interventions can be delivered by experienced dietitians with a reasonable investment of resources and that practice guidelines nutrition care is more cost-effective than basic nutrition care.

The clinical trial lasted 6 months. Basic nutrition care consisted of one visit with a dietitian during which data from the patient and referring physician were used to develop a nutrition care plan. Practice guidelines care consisted of a minimum of three visits with the dietitian. The dietitian assumed responsibility for selecting the appropriate nutrition prescription and educational interventions and for evaluating therapy. Cost was calculated from the perspective of the health care organization. The analysis considered costs of nutritional counseling, laboratory evaluations, changes in medical therapy, and changes in fasting plasma glucose levels. Results were expressed in 1993 dollars. Discounting was not employed.

Practice guidelines care cost more than basic care: $112 vs. $42/patient/year. Practice guidelines care was, however, associated with greater costs savings than basic care due to changes in medical therapy ($31 vs. $3 cost saving/patient/year) and was associated with a greater improvement in fasting plasma glucose level (1.1 vs. 0.4 mmol/l reduction). A one millimolar decrease in fasting plasma glucose level cost $4.20 for practice guidelines nutrition care and $5.32 for basic nutrition care, assuming the medical changes in therapy were maintained for 12 months. Thus, practice guidelines nutrition care cost $1.12 less than basic nutrition care/1 millimolar decrement in fasting plasma glucose.

Comprehensive Therapy for Type 2 Diabetes

Eastman and colleagues developed a simulation model using data from health surveys, population-based epidemiologic studies, and clinical trials to assess the long-term impact of comprehensive and community therapy when applied to incident cases of clinically diagnosed type 2 diabetes in the U.S. population 25–74 years of age.[20–22] They found that comprehensive therapy is cost effective compared to community therapy.

Comprehensive therapy included annual retinal screening and employed intensified pharmacologic therapy to achieve HbA_{1c} levels of 7.2%. Community therapy represented usual clinical care for type 2 diabetes in the United States. With community therapy, approximately 50% of patients had annual retinal exams. With community therapy glycemic management used pharmacologic therapies as described in the National Health Interview Survey, and therapy achieved HbA_{1c} levels of 9.2%. The analysis assessed the direct costs associated with treatment, side effects of treatment, and microvascular, neuropathic, and cardiovascular complications of type 2 diabetes. Results were expressed in 1994 dollars and discounting was employed.

Comprehensive therapy for type 2 diabetes was predicted to reduce the cumulative incidence of blindness, end-stage renal disease, and lower extremity amputation by 76%, 88%, and 67%, respectively. Cardiovascular disease risk increased by 3%. Life expectancy increased 1.4 years (undiscounted). The lifetime cost of treatment increased by almost two-fold, from approximately $32,000 to $58,000 (discounted at 3%/year), which was partially offset by reductions in the cost of complications. When both costs and benefits were discounted at 3%/year, the incremental cost/QALY gained was approximately $16,000. In sensitivity analyses, the treatment was more cost effective for those with longer glycemic exposure (earlier diagnosis of diabetes), in minorities, and in subjects with higher glycosylated hemoglobin levels at baseline.

Detecting and Treating Diabetic Retinopathy

A number of groups have assessed the cost-effectiveness of different approaches to screening for diabetic retinopathy. In general, both primary-care-based and more sophisticated approaches have shown reasonable cost-effectiveness.

Sculpher and colleagues estimated the cost of screening/true positive case of sight-threatening retinopathy detected based on estimates of sensitivity, specificity, and prevalence generated in the screening of over 3,000 diabetic patients in three centers in the United Kingdom.[23] In general, there was substantial overlap in the cost/true positive case detected. Relative cost-effectiveness varied according to whether the screening could take place without an additional patient visit and was strongly related to the sensitivity of the screening method and the prevalence of retinopathy in the diabetic population.

Lairson and colleagues evaluated the relative cost of four methods of screening for nonproliferative and proliferative diabetic retinopathy among 352 diabetic patients seen at Veterans Administration (VA) and Department of Defense facilities in Texas.[24] The reference standard was seven-field stereoscopic fundus photography interpreted by trained readers at the University of Wisconsin Fundus Photograph Reading Center. Costs and effectiveness were presented from the perspective of the VA Health Care System. Medical care cost/true positive case detected was lower for the 45° camera with dilation ($295) compared with the 45° camera without dilation ($378), the standard ophthalmologic examination ($390), and direct funduscopic examination by a physician's assistant or nurse practitioner ($794).

Dasbach and colleagues used data from epidemiologic studies and clinical trials to develop a simulation model to evaluate the impact of annual and biannual screening programs using ophthalmoscopy, fundus photography with a nonmydriatic camera, and fundus photography with a mydriatic camera on blindness due to proliferative diabetic retinopathy over a lifetime.[25] The analyses did not deal with other frequent or potentially remedial causes of blindness, including macular edema, cataract, and glaucoma. The analyses compared screening and treatment to no care. Computations were performed for three subpopulations representing patients with type 1 diabetes of 5 years or more duration, those with type 2 diabetes taking insulin, and those with type 2 diabetes not taking insulin. The authors adopted a third-party payer perspective and considered both direct medical costs and rehabilitative costs. Costs were discounted at 5%/year and were expressed in 1989 dollars.

Annual screening with fundus photography using a mydriatic camera was the most effective program; however, the incremental gain in effectiveness was small compared to nonmydriatic photography and ophthalmoscopy. In general, the costs of the screening programs were covered by avoided costs of blindness in the population subgroups taking insulin. In patients with type 1 diabetes of 5 years or more duration, biannual and annual screening with ophthalmoscopy, nonmydriatic photography, and mydriatic photography were all cost saving. Among patients with type 2 diabetes taking insulin, all forms of biannual screening and annual ophthalmoscopic screening were cost saving. Among patients with type 2 diabetes not taking insulin, only biannual ophthalmoscopic screening was cost saving.

Javitt and colleagues also developed a simulation model to estimate the current and potential federal savings resulting from the screening and treatment of retinopathy in patients with type 1 diabetes and type 2 diabetes based on cross-sectional and longitudinal epidemiologic studies and clinical trials that have assessed the efficacy of treating both macular edema and proliferative diabetic retinopathy.[26–28] Javitt and colleagues considered both the direct medical costs of screening, treatment, and blindness and the indirect costs associated with social security disability insurance, social security payments, and lost tax revenues. They did not include costs associated with rehabilitation, welfare, and other state or local expenses. Costs were discounted and expressed in 1990 dollars.

As a base case analysis, the authors modeled care as recommended by the American Academy of Ophthalmology (AAO), which suggests dilated ophthalmoscopy annually for patients with no retinopathy and every 6 months for those with retinopathy. They compared no screening with prevailing implementation of appropriate eye care in patients with type 2 diabetes (60% screening) and recommended care (100% screening). When costs were discounted at 5%, they estimated that current care, as opposed to no care, saved $4,600/year of sight gained. If all patients with type 2 diabetes received recommended care (100% screening) as opposed to no care, the predicted savings were approximately $5,000/year of sight gained. The authors concluded that enrolling each additional person with type 2 diabetes into currently recommended ophthalmologic care results in an average net savings of $975/person, even if all costs were borne by the federal government.

More recently, Javitt and Aiello have revised these analyses to determine the cost of preventing vision loss in patients with diabetes mellitus from the health insurers' perspective.[29] In the analysis, the authors compared screening under an ideal program done according to the Preferred Practice Pattern for Diabetic Retinopathy published by the AAO with current ophthalmic screening of patients with diabetes as determined from regional and national surveys. The model was applied to persons with incident type 1 diabetes and type 2 diabetes treated with insulin and not treated with insulin in the United States. Unlike the earlier analyses that included social security payments and lost tax revenues, this analysis included only direct medical costs. Screening and treatment costs were derived from the average Medicare charges in 1990. All costs were expressed in 1990 dollars using a discount rate of 5%. QALYs were also discounted at 5%.

Screening and treatment of eye disease in patients with diabetes mellitus cost $3,190/QALY gained. This cost was a weighted average of the cost-effectiveness of detecting and treating diabetic eye disease in people with type 1 diabetes ($1,996/QALY gained), those with type 2 diabetes who used insulin ($2,933/QALY gained), and those with type 2 diabetes who did not use insulin ($3,530/QALY gained). Thus, prevention programs aimed at improving eye care for diabetic persons compared to current clinical practice are cost effective, though not cost saving, investments from the health insurers' perspective.

Screening and Early Treatment for Diabetic Nephropathy

Several groups have assessed the cost-effectiveness of screening and early treatment for nephropathy in patients with diabetes. Diabetic end-stage renal disease is associated with reduced quality of life and length of life and with enormous cost. Thus, it is not suprising that interventions at the stage of clinical nephropathy are cost saving. Indeed, ACE-inhibitor therapy, if administered to patients with diabetes and overt nephropathy, provides a savings in direct cost and thus would reduce total health care expenditures for treatment of end-stage renal disease.

Borch-Johnsen and colleagues analyzed the cost-effectiveness of screening for and antihypertensive treatment of early renal disease indicated by microalbuminuria in patients with type 1 diabetes.[30] Previously published data were used to estimate transition probabilities for each step from normal albuminuria until death. The effect of antihypertensive treatment on urinary albumin excretion rate was arbitrarily set at three different levels. All direct costs (screening, anti-

hypertensive treatment, treatment of end-stage renal failure) were included in the economic analysis. Results were expressed in 1991 U.S. dollars and discounting was performed using a 2.5% rate.

Assuming treatment effects of 33% and 67%, median life expectancy increased by 4 to 14 years, respectively, and the need for dialysis or transplantation decreased by 21% to 63%. Costs and savings would balance if the annual rate of increase of albuminuria was decreased from 20% to 18% a year. The authors concluded that screening and intervention programs are likely to have life saving effects and lead to considerable economic savings.

Siegel and colleagues simulated the natural history of nephropathy in a hypothetical cohort of subjects with type 1 diabetes from the time of diabetes diagnosis, assumed to be age 15 years, until the time of death.[31] Transition probabilities between disease states were derived from epidemiologic studies. The effectiveness of ACE-inhibitor treatment in retarding the progression of nephropathy was estimated from the literature though the study was performed before the publication of the results of major clinical trials of ACE-inhibitor treatment and diabetic nephropathy. Mortality from renal failure and coronary artery disease were estimated from prior studies in diabetic populations, and life tables were used to estimate mortality from other causes. Costs were estimated from the perspective of a third-party payer on the basis of resources used. Costs were discounted at 5%/year. Results were expressed in 1991 dollars.

Dipstick screening for proteinuria and ACE-inhibitor treatment at diagnosis of proteinuria was associated with increased survival and decreased cost relative to no screening for proteinuria and ACE-inhibitor treatment only at the diagnosis of hypertension. Compared to urine dipstick screening for proteinuria and ACE-inhibitor treatment at diagnosis of proteinuria, screening and ACE-inhibitor treatment at the stage of microalbuminuria had a cost-effectiveness ratio of approximately $8,000–$17,000/year of life saved. The authors concluded that urine dipstick protein screening followed by treatment at the stage of proteinuria was cost saving and that screening and treatment at the stage of microalbuminuria compare favorably to other life-saving interventions.

Kiberd and Jindal adapted the models of Borch-Johnsen and Siegel to further evaluate screening for microalbuminuria in patients with type 1 diabetes.[32] Two strategies were compared: The first consisted of screening for microalbuminuria in patients with more than 5 years of diabetes and treatment with an ACE inhibitor if two out of three tests were positive, and the second consisted of treating patients with hypertension or macroproteinuria or both. In the analyses, direct costs from the perspective of the third-party payer and government were included. Costs and outcomes were discounted and utilities were used to calculate QALYs. In addition, extensive sensitivity analyses were performed on the effect of false-positive rates of microalbuminuria screening, efficacy rates of treatment, and incidence rates of diabetic nephropathy.

As demonstrated in the previous studies, initiation of ACE-inhibitor treatment at the start of hypertension or macroproteinuria not only increased QALYs but also reduced costs compared with no treatment. In the base case analysis, the incremental cost/QALY gained for screening for microalbuminuria and treatment with an ACE-inhibitor if two out of three tests were positive compared to treating patients with hypertension or macroproteinuria or both was approximately $27,000. In sensitivity analyses, when the positive predictive value of the screening test was reduced, the incremental cost/QALY gained increased. If the effect of early drug treatment to delay transition from microalbuminuria to macroproteinuria was reduced, the incremental cost/QALY gained also increased dramatically. Likewise, if the cumulative lifetime incidence of diabetic nephropathy fell below 20%, the incremental cost of screening for microalbuminuria would increase to greater than $75,000/QALY gained. The authors concluded that although initiation of ACE-inhibitor therapy at the start of hypertension or macroproteinuria is cost saving and screening for microalbuminuria is cost effective if baseline values and assumptions are correct, screening for microalbuminuria may not be cost effective if these values and assumptions deviate substantially from baseline.

Recently, Rodby and associates performed an economic analysis of the multicenter clinical trial studying the effect of ACE inhibition on nephropathy in type 1 diabetes.[33] The trial was a randomized placebo-controlled trial comparing captopril with placebo to determine whether captopril had kidney-protecting properties independent of its effect on blood pressure. The endpoints of the trial were doubling of serum creatinine, dialysis, transplantation, and death. Captopril reduced the risk of these endpoints by approximately 50% in patients with type 1 diabetes. Using data from the clinical trial, the authors developed a model of medical treatment for patients with type 1 diabetes from the time they developed overt diabetic nephropathy until they developed end-stage renal disease. To model the course of illness after patients developed the disease and to extend the model to patients with type 2 diabetes, they used data from the published literature and from the U.S. Renal Data System.

The model was comprehensive. It captured medical events both before and after the onset of the disease and took into account comorbid conditions and complications at all stages of disease including death. Medical resource cost data were based predominately on Medicare reimbursement rates, published wholesale drug prices, and surveys of health care providers. The economic model adopted a payer perspective to estimate direct costs. The cost to society (indirect costs) associated with lost productivity due to the disease was also estimated. Direct and indirect costs were expressed in 1994 dollars, and a discount rate of 5%/year was used for costs as well as life-year saved.

For patients with type 1 diabetes, the model was extended to as many years as were required for all the patients in the captopril group to die (31 years). The type 2 diabetes model was extended similarly, to 12 years. When both cohorts were followed until everyone had died, a savings of $32,550 for each patient with type 1 diabetes treated with captopril and $9,900 for each patient with type 2 diabetes treated with captopril was realized. In addition, the captopril type 1 diabetes group saved an average of 2.15 years of life over the 31 year follow-up, and the captopril type 2 diabetes group saved an average of 1.04 years of life over the 12 years of follow-up. Because, on average, life was extended with captopril therapy for both patients with type 1 diabetes and type 2 diabetes, this translated into a negative cost (or savings) to prolong life. Indirect cost savings/patient with captopril therapy were even more dramatic: $84,390 for type 1 diabetes patients over 31 years and $45,730 for type 2 diabetes patients over 12 years.

Foot Care and Lower Extremity Amputation

Two groups have addressed the cost-effectiveness of alternative approaches to the prevention of diabetic amputations. In general, treatment of diabetic foot ulcers by a multidisciplinary team, surgical debridement, and long-term antibiotic therapy are cost saving compared to amputation.

In a series of reports, Apelqvist and colleagues retrospectively assessed the costs associated with primary healing and healing with amputation for diabetic patients with foot ulcers treated in a multidisciplinary setting.[34-36] In a prospective observational study of 314 consecutive patients with foot ulcers referred to the Department of Internal Medicine at the University of Lund, 197 patients healed primarily, 77 patients healed after minor or major amputation, and 40 patients died before healing occurred. Patients who healed primarily or with amputation were included in a retrospective economic analysis. The general treatment goals were to achieve primary healing, avoid any unnecessary amputation, and when necessary, amputate as distal as possible and maintain ambulation. All patients were treated by a combined foot care team as both inpatients and outpatients. Inpatient treatment was used only when surgery was required, in septic conditions, or because of incurrent diseases. Direct costs for inpatient care, antibiotics, surgery, outpatient care, staff attendance, drugs, orthopedic appliances, and prostheses were calculated from the date when the patient with the ulcer was first seen by the foot care team until healing was achieved. Indirect costs were not included. Costs were converted to 1990 dollars and future costs were discounted to present value with a 5% discount rate.

Total present value cost/patient during 3 years of observation was $16,100 for primarily healed patients without critical ischemia, $26,700 for primarily healed patients with critical ischemia, $43,100 for patients who healed with a minor amputation, and $63,100 for patients who healed with a major amputation. The expected average long-term costs/patient during the first 3 years after healing ranged from $5,200 to $11,200 for primarily healed patients and $14,000 to $32,200 for patients who healed with amputation. The long-term cost for patients with primary healing was explained mainly by the frequency of new ulcerations. The long-term costs for patients with amputation corresponded to increased inpatient care, home care, and social services. Although not a randomized clinical trial, these findings indicate the potential cost-savings of preventive foot care compared to amputation.

Eckman and colleagues performed decision and cost-effectiveness analyses using a Markov model to examine the cost-effectiveness of alternative approaches to the diagnosis and treatment of patients with type 2 diabetes with foot infections and suspected osteomyelitis.[37] Costs included direct medical costs at an urban Massachusetts teaching hospital and were expressed in 1993 dollars. In general, initial hospitalization for surgical debridement followed by a long course of antibiotic therapy was the least expensive strategy, with an average lifetime cost of roughly $31,000. Performing noninvasive tests to select patients for long-term antibiotic therapy cost from $31,000 to $34,000, depending on the testing sequence. Immediate amputation was the most expensive strategy, costing approximately $47,000.

The authors concluded that in a primary care setting, noninvasive testing adds expense to the treatment of patients with type 2 diabetes in whom pedal osteomyelitis is suspected and may result in little improvement in health outcomes. Similarly, bone biopsy to determine the presence of osteomyelitis affords no advantage over empiric treatment with a long course of a culture-guided antibiotics. Even when osteomyelitis is known to be present, antibiotic treatment is preferred to early amputations, as currently available oral antibiotics have both high efficacy and minimal toxicity. The authors conclude that the empiric therapy, within limited clinical settings, produces outcomes equivalent to those of more aggressive and expensive approaches. Although strategies that decrease uncertainty are intu-

itively more comfortable for physicians, they may expose patients to additional risks and may engender unnecessary costs. In patients who show no signs of systemic infection and have adequate perfusion, surgical debridement followed by a 10-week course of culture-guided oral antibiotics may be as effective as and less costly than other approaches.

Cardiovascular Risk Factor Detection and Intervention

Although cardiovascular risk factor detection and intervention trials have published economic analyses and post hoc diabetic subgroup analyses, none has published economic analyses of cardiovascular risk factor detection and treatment in diabetic populations. In nondiabetic populations, targeted cardiovascular risk factor detection and treatment strategies have been demonstrated to be cost effective although generally not cost saving.

Economic analyses of medical therapy for hypertension in the general population have demonstrated a range of cost-effectiveness from approximately $1,000 to $93,000/life-year gained with a median of approximately $15,000.[10] In general, intervention is more cost effective in populations at higher risk, that is, individuals with higher blood pressure levels who are at greater risk for cardiovascular events.

Studies of cholesterol treatment in the general population have showed a range of cost-effectiveness from cost-savings to $1.8 million/life-year gained with a median of $154,000.[10] In general, secondary intervention programs in populations with angina pectoris or history of myocardial infarction are more cost effective than primary interventions in patients without known cardiovascular disease. In addition, interventions in older population with very high cholesterol levels are more cost effective than those in younger populations with moderately elevated cholesterol levels.

In the general population, smoking cessation interventions have been demonstrated to be quite cost effective.[10] Both medical counseling and counseling with adjacent pharmacologic therapy have been shown to cost approximately $3,000/life-year gained.

Coronary Angioplasty and Coronary Bypass Surgery for Multivessel Coronary Disease

Studies of percutaneous transluminal coronary angioplasty and bypass surgery for coronary artery disease in the general population have showed a range of cost-effectiveness from approximately $2,000 to $429,000/life-year gained with a median of approximately $25,000.[10] A recent economic analysis of the Bypass Angioplasty Revascularization Investigation

(BARI) demonstrated that bypass surgery compared to angioplasty is quite cost effective in diabetic patients because of their significantly better survival with bypass.[38]

BARI was a 5-year randomized prospective clinical trial of angioplasty and bypass surgery in patients with multivessel coronary disease.[38] Patients' use of medical services, including hospitalizations, visits to physicians and other health care providers, and outpatient cardiac tests and procedures, were documented quarterly. Charges were converted to costs from the perspective of Medicare and were adjusted to 1995 dollars. Future costs were adjusted to present value at a rate of 3%/year after the date of randomization. Among patients with diabetes, surgery lead to lower costs and longer life expectancy than did angioplasty. Among diabetic patients with two vessel disease, surgery cost $70,830 and resulted in 4.4 years of added life and angioplasty cost $60,445 and resulted in 4 years of added life. Among diabetic patients with three vessel disease, surgery cost $72,837 and resulted in 4.3 years of added life and angioplasty cost $95,376 and resulted in 3.5 years of added life.

Summary

Over the past 20 years, health care expenditures and diabetes care expenditures have grown dramatically in the United States. In part, this growth has reflected growth in the U.S. population, aging of the population, and general inflation. It is clear, however, that health care costs have increased above the rate of inflation and the costs of health care for people with diabetes are substantially greater than those for people without diabetes. Expressed in terms of per capita annual health care expenditures, people with diabetes incur health care costs 3.6-fold higher than those without diabetes ($9,493 vs. $2,604/person/year). Even after adjusting for differences in age, per capita expenditures for people with diabetes remain approximately 2.5-fold higher than for people without diabetes ($6,425 vs. $2,604/person/year). In 1992, it was estimated that the direct and indirect costs of diabetes in the United States were over $45 billion and $46 billion, respectively, and the direct costs of medical care for people with diabetes was over $100 billion.

It is unclear whether these expenditures represent good value for money. Descriptive cost analyses have demonstrated that the major proportion of health care expenditures for diabetes, approximately 75% of direct medical costs, are spent for hospital care and are associated with treatment of the late, end-stage, microvascular, neuropathic, and cardiovascular complications of diabetes.

Well-designed and conducted clinical trials and economic analyses have now demonstrated that interventions to prevent and treat the complications of diabetes are both effective and cost effective. Preconception care for women with pregestational diabetes is cost saving—the incremental cost of such care is overshadowed by savings resulting from adverse maternal and neonatal outcomes averted. Intensive therapy for both type 1 and type 2 diabetes is cost effective compared to conventional therapy. With a cost/QALY gained of <$20,000, such care is on a par with antihypertensive therapy for high-risk individuals and represents good value for the money. Screening for and laser treatment of diabetic retinopathy is also extremely cost effective, and screening for and ACE-inhibitor treatment of diabetic nephropathy is cost saving. In people with diabetic foot ulcers, treatment by a multidisciplinary team, surgical debridement, and long-term antibiotic therapy are cost saving compared to amputation. Data from analysis in the general population suggest that antihypertensive therapy and lipid lowering therapy should be cost effective in diabetic populations, and interventions to achieve smoking cessation should be extremely cost effective or even cost saving. Finally, a recent analysis suggests that bypass surgery compared to angioplasty is cost effective in diabetic patients with two vessel coronary artery disease and is cost saving in diabetic patients with three vessel disease.

Unfortunately, despite the proven effectiveness and cost-effectiveness of these interventions, patient and provider surveys and medical record audits have demonstrated that such preventive services and preferred treatments are not being routinely applied to patients with diabetes.[39–41] Over the long-term, systematic support for and application of such interventions have the potential to improve outcomes and control costs and improve the value achieved by such substantial investments of resources.

References

1. Levit KR, Cowan CA, Lazenby HC, et al.: National Health Spending Trends, 1960–1993. Health Aff 13:14–31, 1994.
2. Gruber W, Lander T, Leese B, Songer T, Williams R (eds.): The Economics of Diabetes and Diabetes care. A Report of the Diabetes Health Economics Study Group. Brussels, Belgium: International Diabetes Federation, and Geneva, Switzerland: World Health Organization, Division of Noncommunicable Diseases, 1997.
3. Zwaag RV, Connor M, Dickson HD, et al.: Cost of diabetes care. In Davidson JK (ed.): Clinical Diabetes Mellitus. New York: Thieme, 1991, pp. 717–722.
4. Eisenberg JM: Clinical economics: a guide to the economic analysis of clinical practices. JAMA 262:2879–2886, 1989.

5. Gold MR, Siegel JE, Russell LB, Weinstein MC (eds.): Cost-Effectiveness in Health and Medicine. New York: Oxford University Press, 1996.

6. Udvarhelyi IS, Colditz GA, Rai A, et al.: Cost-effectiveness and cost-benefit analyses in the medical literature. Are the methods being used correctly? Ann Int Med 116:238–244, 1992.

7. Taylor TN, Chrischilles EA: Economic evaluation of interventions in endocrinology. Endocrinol Metab Clin North Am 26:67–87, 1997.

8. Finkler SA. The distinction between cost and charges. Ann Int Med 96:102–109, 1982.

9. Laupacis A, Feeny D, Detsky AS, et al.: How attractive does a new technology have to warrant adoption and utilization? Tentative guidelines for using clinical and economic evaluations. Can Med Assoc J 146:473–481, 1992.

10. Tengs TO, Adams ME, Pliskin JS, et al.: Five-hundred life-saving interventions and their cost-effectiveness. Risk Anal 15:369–390, 1995.

11. Fox-Ray N, Wills S, Thamer M: Direct and Indirect Costs of Diabetes in the United States in 1992. Alexandria, VA: American Diabetes Association, 1993, pp. 1–27.

12. Rubin RJ, Altman WM, Mendelson DN: Health care expenditures for people with diabetes mellitus, 1992. J Clin Endocrinol Metabl 78:809A–809F, 1994.

13. Elixhauser A, Weschler JM, Kitzmiller JL, et al.: Cost-benefit analysis of preconception care for women with established diabetes mellitus. Diabetes Care 16:1146–1157, 1993.

14. Elixhauser A, Kitzmiller, JL, Weschler JM: Short-term cost benefit of pre-conception care for diabetes. Diabetes Care 19:384–385, 1996.

15. Scheffler RM, Feuchtbaum LB, Phibbs CS: Prevention: The cost-effectiveness of the California diabetes and pregnancy program. Am J Public Health 82:168–175, 1992.

16. The Diabetes Control and Complications Trial Research Group: Resource utilization and costs of care in the Diabetes Control and Complications Trial. Diabetes Care 18:361–376, 1995.

17. The Diabetes Control and Complications Trial Research Group: The effect of intensive treatment of diabetes on the development and progression of long-term complications in insulin-dependent diabetes mellitus. New Engl J Med 329:977–986, 1993.

18. The Diabetes Control and Complications Trial Research Group: Lifetime benefits and costs of intensive therapy as practiced in the Diabetes Control and Complications Trial. JAMA 276:1409–1415, 1996.

19. Franz MJ, Splett PL, Mond K, et al.: Cost-effectiveness of medical nutrition therapy provided by dietitians for persons with non-insulin-dependent diabetes mellitus. J Am Diet Assoc 95:1018–1024, 1995.

20. Eastman RC, Javitt JC, Herman WH, et al.: Prevention strategies for non-insulin-dependent diabetes mellitus: an economic perspective. In LeRoith D, Taylor SL, Olefsky JM (eds.): Diabetes Mellitus. Philadelphia: Lipincott-Raven, 1996, pp. 621–630.

21. Eastman RC, Javitt JC, Herman WH, et al.: Model of complications of NIDDM. I. Model construction and assumptions. Diabetes Care 20:725–734, 1997.

22. Eastman RC, Javitt JC, Herman WH, et al.: Model of complications of NIDDM. II. Analysis of the health benefits and cost-effectiveness of treating NIDDM with the goal of normoglycemia. Diabetes Care 20:735–744, 1997.

23. Sculpher MJ, Buxton MJ, Ferguson BA, et al.: A relative cost-effectiveness analysis of different methods of screening for diabetic retinopathy. Diabetic Med 8:644–650, 1991.

24. Lairson DR, Pugh JA, Kapadia AS, et al.: Cost-effectiveness of alternative methods for diabetic retinopathy screening. Diabetes Care 15:1369–1377, 1992.

25. Dasbach EJ, Fryback DG, Newcomb PA, et al.: Cost-effectiveness of strategies for detecting diabetic retinopathy. Medical Care 29:20–39, 1991.

26. Javitt JC, Canner JK, Sommer A: Cost effectiveness of current approaches to the control of retinopathy in type I diabetes. Ophthalmology 96:255–264, 1989.

27. Javitt JC, Aiello LP, Bassi LJ, et al.: Detecting and treating retinopathy in patients with type I diabetes mellitus. Ophthalmology 98:1565–1574, 1991.

28. Javitt JC, Aiello LP, Chiang Y, et al.: Prevention eye care in people with diabetes is cost-saving to the federal government. Implications for health-care reform. Diabetes Care 17:909–917, 1994.

29. Javitt JC, Aiello LP: Cost-effectiveness of detecting and treating diabetic retinopathy. Ann Intern Med 124:164–169, 1996.

30. Borch-Johnsen K, Wenzel H, Viberti GC, et al.: Is screening and intervention for microalbuminuria worthwhile in patients with insulin dependent diabetes? Br Med J 306:1722–1723, 1993.

31. Siegel JE, Krolewski AS, Warram JH, et al.: Cost-effectiveness of screening and early treatment of nephropathy in patients with insulin-dependent diabetes mellitus. J Am Soc Nephrol 3:S111–S119, 1992.

32. Kiberd BA, Jindal KK: Screening to prevent renal failure in insulin dependent diabetic patients: an economic evaluation. Br Med J 311:1595–1599, 1995.

33. Rodby RA, Firth LM, Lewis EF, The Collaborative Study Group: An economic analysis of captopril in the treatment of diabetic nephropathy. Diabetes Care 19:1051–1061, 1996.

34. Larsson J, Apelqvist J: Towards less amputations in diabetic patients. Incidence, causes, cost, treatment, and prevention—a review. Acta Orthop Scand 66:181–192, 1995.

35. Apelqvist J, Ragnarson-Tennvall G, Persson U, et al.: Diabetic foot ulcers in a multidisciplinary setting. An economic analysis of primary healing and healing with amputation. J Int Med 235:463–471, 1994.

36. Apelqvist J, Ragnarson-Tennvall G, Larsson J, et al.: Long-term costs for foot ulcers in diabetic patients in a multidisciplinary setting. Foot Ankle Int 16:388–394, 1995.

37. Eckman MH, Greenfield S, Mackey WC, et al.: Foot infections in diabetic patients. Decision and cost-effectiveness analyses. JAMA 278:712–720, 1995.

38. Hlatky MA, Rogers WJ, Johnstone I, et al.: Medical care costs and quality of life after randomization to coronary angioplasty or coronary bypass surgery. New Engl J Med 336:92–99, 1997.

39. Bechner RJ, Cowie CC, Howie J, et al.: Ophthalmic examination among adults with diagnosed diabetes mellitus. JAMA 270:1714–1718, 1993.

40. Kenny SJ, Smith PJ, Goldschmid MG, et al.: Survey of physician practice behaviors related to diabetes mellitus in the U.S. Diabetes Care 16:1507–1510, 1993.

41. Peters AL, Legorreta AP, Ossorio RC, et al.: Quality of outpatient care provided to diabetic patients. Diabetes Care 19:601–606, 1996.

42. Entmacher PS, Sinnock P, Bostic E, Harris MI: Economic impact of diabetes. In National Diabetes Data Group (ed.): Diabetes in America (NIH Pub. No 85-1468). Washington, DC: US Government Printing Office, 1985.

43. Policy Analysis Inc.: The incidence-based economic costs of diabetes mellitus. In National Center for Health Statistics (ed.): Evaluation of Cost of Illness Methodology. Part II: Applications of Methodology to Ascertain Lifetime Economic Costs of Illness in an Incidence Cohort (Final report on a research project under contract to the Department of Health and Human Services). Hyattsville, MD: 1981.

44. Platt WG, Sudovar SG: The Social and Economic Costs of Diabetes: An Estimate for 1979. Elkhart, IN: Home Health Care Group, Ames Division, Miles Laboratories Inc, 1983, p. 120.

45. Miller LV: Socioeconomic impact of diabetes mellitus. In Brodoff BN, Bleicher SJ (eds.): Diabetes Mellitus and Obesity. Baltimore: Waverly Press, 1982.

46. Smeeding TM, Booton LA: Measuring and valuing the economic benefits of diabetes control. 19th National Meeting of the Public Health Conference on Records and Statistics, 23–24 August, 1983, pp. 80–85.

47. The Carter Center of Emory University: Closing the gap: the problem of diabetes mellitus in the United States. Diabetes Care 8:391–406, 1985.

48. Huse DM, Oster G, Killen AR, et al.: The economic costs of non-insulin-dependent diabetes mellitus. JAMA 262:2708–2713, 1989.

49. Fox NA, Jacobs J: Direct and Indirect Costs of Diabetes in the United States in 1987. Alexandria, VA: American Diabetes Association, 1988.

51

Employment, Health Insurance, and Diabetes Mellitus

Joe V. Selby and Bix E. Swain

Persons with chronic disorders such as diabetes face many socioeconomic challenges. Among these are the medical expenses of treating the illness and its complications and barriers to finding and maintaining employment. Because health insurance is generally obtained through employment in this country, the problems are linked. This chapter examines the employment and insurance status of Americans with diabetes. To obtain recent information, we have analyzed representative U.S. data obtained from the National Health Interview Survey (NHIS) for the years 1992 through 1994.

Employment for Persons with Diabetes

When considered as a group, employed persons with diabetes have higher rates of illness-related absenteeism than nondiabetics as well as higher mortality;[1–3] for these reasons diabetes has historically been considered a disqualifying condition for employment. However, the observed differences in absenteeism rates are due largely to a rather small proportion of diabetic employees with severe disease. For most persons with the disorder, absenteeism is similar to that of their nondiabetic coworkers. Thus, disqualification for employment solely on the basis of having diabetes is equivalent to other forms of unlawful discrimination.

In the past 20 years, social legislation in the United States and elsewhere has aimed at eliminating employment discrimination. In the United States, the Rehabilitation Act of 1973 prohibited discrimination in the employment and advancement of workers with handicaps.[4] This act applied to the executive branch of the federal government, to companies that contract with the federal government, and to institutions receiving federal grants. In 1988, the Americans with Disabilities Act[5] extended this prohibition on employment discrimination against qualified individuals with disabil-

ities to cover all employers of 15 or more persons. The act also requires that employers make reasonable accommodations to enable workers with disabilities to perform their job functions.

In the years before this legislation, some evidence of employment discrimination against persons with diabetes had been reported for persons with type 1 diabetes. In a matched sample of young persons with diabetes and their nondiabetic siblings living in the Pittsburgh, Pennsylvania, area,[6] siblings with diabetes were significantly less likely to be employed full-time than their nondiabetic siblings (55% vs. 73%, $p = 0.001$). The lower employment rate appeared to be due principally to greater frequency of work disability associated with diabetes. However, diabetic siblings also reported a higher frequency of previous job refusals (64% vs. 42%, $p = 0.02$), but only if they had reported their diabetes at the time of the job interview. In this study, there were no differences in reported absenteeism between diabetic and nondiabetic siblings among those working. In surveys conducted in the late 1980s in the United Kingdom,[7] young patients with insulin-dependent diabetes mellitus (IDDM) were more likely to report being unemployed, having difficulties finding a job, having lost a job due to their diabetes, and being unable to perform the job they preferred.

To update these reports and generalize them to the larger U.S. adult population with diabetes, we obtained data from the NHIS[8] for the years 1992 through 1994, the first 3 years after enactment of the Americans with Disabilities Act. In each of these years, the survey included a supplement to assess health insurance status. Persons with diabetes were identified on the basis of responses to a chronic conditions checklist. Those who indicated that diabetes mellitus was present were compared with respondents who denied having diabetes. Employment status was assessed from questions contained in the core survey. One question asked whether respondents had worked within the past 2 weeks. A second question asked about "activity limitations" that prevented or restricted their ability to work. Employment trends among nondiabetic respondents were examined for the same period to check for possible secular trends in employment related to an improving economy.

Among respondents aged 18–64 years, persons with diabetes were much less likely to be employed during the past 2 weeks than those without diabetes in each year (Fig. 51–1a). This gap was still apparent after stratification on age within the working population (data not

shown). For persons with diabetes, employment rose slightly from 1992 to 1994 (from 51.5% to 55.1%). Increases among nondiabetic patients during the same time period were smaller (from 74.6% to 75.7%).

The difference between those with and without diabetes was attributable almost entirely to larger proportions of those with diabetes who responded that they were "out of the workforce." After excluding persons who stated that they were presently unable to work because of activity limitations (Fig. 51–1b), differences

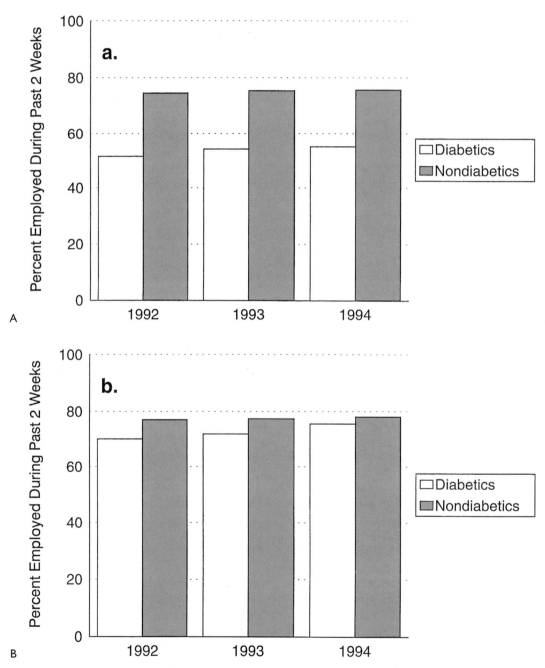

Figure 51–1. Percent of adults ages 18–64 years who report being currently employed and having worked during the past 2 weeks (a) among all respondents and (b) after excluding respondents reporting that they are unable to work because of activity limitations, by diabetes status. From NHIS 1992–1994.

between diabetic and nondiabetic respondents were much smaller. The temporal increase in employment rates for those with diabetes was also somewhat greater. Thus, during the first 3 years following enactment of the Americans with Disabilities Act, the employment status of working-age persons with diabetes appears to have improved slightly compared to that of nondiabetics.

Health Insurance and Diabetes

Health Insurance Coverage for Persons with Diabetes

Most diabetic patients in the United States have some form of health insurance.[9,10] In the 1989 NHIS, 86.5% of diabetic persons below 65 years of age and 98.8% of those above age 65 were covered by at least one form of private, military, or government (Medicare, Medicaid) health insurance.[10] These percentages did not differ from those for nondiabetics. However, compared with nondiabetics, persons with diabetes were less likely to have private insurance both before age 65 (69.3% vs. 78.5%) and for ages 65 and above (69.2% vs. 79.9%), were more likely to have Medicare before age 65 (10.3% vs. 1.6%), and were nearly three times as likely as nondiabetics to have Medicaid coverage at any age. These differences reflect the greater likelihood of both disability and unemployment among persons with diabetes and the higher prevalence of diabetes among low-income, non-white populations.

Based on data from the Health Insurance Supplement of the NHIS for the years 1992–1994, the proportion of diabetic persons less than 65 years of age who report having any form of health insurance is slightly higher than for nondiabetics of similar age. Moreover, the proportion of diabetic persons with coverage rose modestly (from 84% to 90%) from 1992 to 1994 (Fig. 51–2). For persons without diabetes, this proportion was essentially constant over the same period. Most of the increase in insurance coverage for persons with diabetes appeared to be due to increases in the proportion with private insurance (Fig. 51–3), with a modest increase in the proportion with Medicaid and no change in the proportion with Medicare. The magnitude of the increase in private insurance is consistent with the rise in employment for persons with diabetes during the same period. For those age 65 years and above, insurance coverage was reported by nearly 100% of both diabetic and nondiabetic respondents in each year, primarily because of Medicare coverage.

Effects of Lack of Insurance in Diabetes

Diabetes is among the most complex of chronic illnesses. Optimal care usually requires lifelong use of medication, periodic preventive screening, medical supplies such as syringes and glucose testing strips, and health education. Considering the costs of each of these services, it is reasonable to expect that those with health insurance should have higher rates of compliance with each service and, consequently, better medical outcomes.

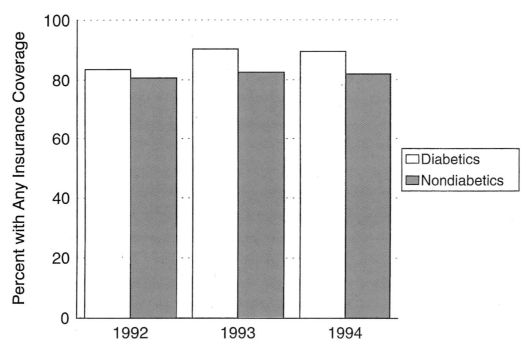

Figure 51–2. Percent of adults ages 18–64 years who report having health insurance coverage of any type (private, medicare, medicaid), by diabetes status. From NHIS 1992–1994.

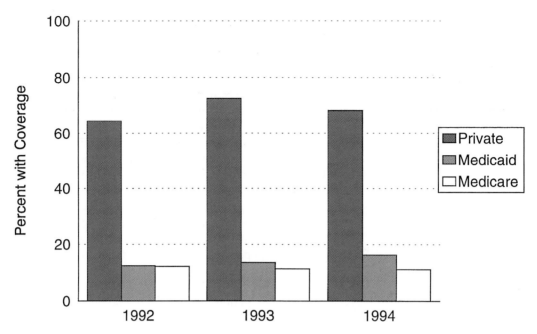

Figure 51–3. Types of health insurance coverage among adults ages 18–64 years with diabetes. From NHIS 1992–1994.

Three reports from the 1989 NHIS[11–13] found, at best, weak evidence for associations of having health insurance with higher rates of receiving health education, a dilated eye examination within the past year, and self-monitoring of blood glucose. These surprising findings may be misleading for several reasons. First, because more than 90% of persons with diabetes in the United States have some form of health insurance, it may be difficult to isolate and study the effects of a lack of insurance using cross-sectional comparisons. The small minority without insurance may differ in many other ways from the majority. For example, given the high costs of health insurance when purchased individually, healthy self-employed persons may opt to go without insurance for a period of years knowing that their risk for complications is low. This could confound the association of health insurance with self-care practices as well as with outcomes. Secondly, other factors may sometimes override any effects of health insurance. For example, Brechner et al.[12] found that receipt of a dilated eye examination during the past year was quite low (about 50%) regardless of health insurance status, duration of diabetes, or the number of visits to a primary care physician. In this case, physician compliance with referral guidelines for preventive examinations may have been the principal determinant of whether individuals received the examination. Third, health insurance has historically not covered preventive care, including health education, screening, and some medical supplies. That self-monitoring of blood glucose was not significantly higher among persons with health insurance in this 1989 survey[13] may not be surprising, given that most insurance did not cover glu-

cose testing strips or health education (a necessary prerequisite and important determinant of self-monitoring) during the 1980s.

Third-party reimbursement for diabetes-related health education services has increased dramatically in recent years.[14] Most private insurers now cover at least part of the costs of outpatient health education. As part of the Budget Reconciliation Act of 1998, Medicare has extended coverage for blood glucose monitoring supplies to all diabetic patients who have either Medicare part B coverage or are enrolled in Medicare managed care plans, regardless of how their diabetes is treated. Previously, these supplies were covered only for insulin-using patients. Expanded Medicare coverage of health education services is due to begin in early 1999. The coverage policies of private insurers often follow those of medicare.

Physician awareness of the importance of glycemic control and of preventive measures has also increased, in part due to publication of the Diabetes Control and Complications Trial[15] in 1993. Interestingly, two more recent surveys now find stronger associations of health insurance with various self-care practices. Ruggiero et al.[16] in studying a large, nationally representative sample obtained through a marketing company, found that diabetic persons with Medicare/Medicaid reported higher levels of self-monitoring than those with private or HMO insurance, who were in turn somewhat higher than persons with no insurance. In an analysis of the CDC-sponsored Behavioral Risk Factor Surveillance System data from 22 states in 1994, Beckles et al.[17] found health insurance to be among the strongest predictors of self-monitoring of blood glucose and of having received a dilated eye exam and a foot examination.

The importance of health insurance is somewhat clearer in studies among the poor. In a follow-up study of adult diabetic patients from an inner-city diabetes clinic, Nordberg et al.[18] found that persons with no insurance coverage used fewer services and appeared to experience an increase in Hb A_{1c} during the follow-up compared to those who were insured. Similarly, Lurie et al.[19] studied the impact of withdrawal of Medicaid coverage from medically indigent adults in a university-based ambulatory care center in California in 1982. Diabetic individuals whose Medicaid was terminated showed a 1.5% mean increase in Hb A_{1c} during 6 months follow-up, compared with only a 0.4% rise in the group continuing Medicaid. Blood pressure control also deteriorated significantly among hypertensive patients who lost their Medicaid compared with those who did not.

Another approach to measuring the effect of insurance on receipt of needed health care is to compare persons receiving free care with persons who are compelled to pay out-of-pocket for a portion of that care. The Health Insurance Experiment[20,21] randomized individuals to entirely free health care or to varying levels of cost-sharing. Persons with any degree of cost-sharing reduced use of health care services for a wide variety of conditions and problems compared to those receiving free care. Reductions in use increased in relation to the level of costs paid by the patient, and, at all levels, reductions were greater among the poor. Diabetes control was not specifically studied. However, blood pressure control was shown to deteriorate in those who were required to pay for a part of their care.[21] Other studies of copayment[22,23] confirm that use of health care services is highly sensitive to even modest levels of cost-sharing. It is unclear from these studies whether patients can differentially decrease use of less effective forms of care.

A second form of underinsurance is the failure of plans to cover the costs of important elements of diabetes care such as preventive care, health education, medications, or supplies such as glucose testing strips. Although families with a child who has type 1 diabetes are as likely to have health insurance as those without a diabetic child, families with a diabetic child pay substantially larger amounts out-of-pocket than those without diabetes,[24] primarily because of copayments and uncovered services such as glucose strips. Not surprisingly, the relative impact of these expenses was greatest among the poor. Recent legislation extending Medicare coverage to glucose monitoring strips and outpatient education raises the hope that insurers may finally be aligning their coverage policies with knowledge about the effectiveness of preventive therapy.

Conclusions

Recent legislation has attempted to protect Americans with diabetes from discrimination in employment. Data from the years immediately following implementation of this legislation now suggest that employment and private health insurance coverage have risen modestly for persons with diabetes. Continued monitoring of these trends will be important, particularly as the next economic downturn approaches. Discriminatory pressures often increase as economic circumstances worsen.

A substantial body of evidence supports the notion that health insurance coverage can help guarantee receipt and practice of important preventive and self-care measures by persons with diabetes. For measures that have been proven to effectively lower complication rates, it is prudent to eliminate financial barriers through comprehensive insurance, particularly for the poor, who are most sensitive to financial barriers and are disproportionately represented among persons with diabetes.

References

1. Nasr ANM, Block DL, Magnusen JH: Absenteeism experience in a group of employed diabetics. J Occup Med 3:621–625, 1966.

2. Pell S, D'Alonzo CA: Sickness absenteeism experience in a group of employed diabetics. Am J Public Health 57:253–260, 1967.

3. Moore RH, Buschborn RL: Work absenteeism in diabetes. Diabetes 23:425–453, 1974.

4. Goldstone RL, Entmacher PS: Employment and insurance for those with diabetes. In Davidson JK (ed.): Clinical Diabetes Mellitus: A Problem-oriented Approach, Ed. 2. New York: Thieme, 1991; pp. 723–726.

5. Equal Employment Opportunity Commission: A Technical Assistance Manual on the Employment Provisions (Title 1) of the Americans with Disabilities Act. Pittsburgh, PA: Superintendent of Documents, 1992.

6. Songer TJ, LaPorte RE, Dorman JS, et al.: Employment spectrum of IDDM. Diabetes Care 12:615–622, 1989.

7. Robinson N, Yateman NA, Protopapa LE, et al.: Unemployment and diabetes. Diabetic Med 6:797–803, 1989.

8. National Center for Health Statistics: Current Estimates from the National Health Interview Survey, 1994. Vital and Health Statistics, Series 10: No. 193, pp. 1–8.

9. Drury TF, Montgomery LE, Cohen BB: Health insurance and health care coverage of adult diabetics. In Diabetes in America.

10. Harris MI, Cowie CC, Eastman R: Health-insurance coverage for adults with diabetes in the U.S. population. Diabetes Care 17:585–591, 1994.

11. Coonrod BA, Betschart J: Frequency and determinants of diabetes patient education among adults in the U.S. population. Diabetes Care 17:852–858, 1994.

12. Brechner RJ, Cowie CC, Howie J, et al.: Ophthalmic examination among adults with diagnosed diabetes mellitus. JAMA 270:1714–1718, 1993.

13. Harris MI, Cowie CC, Howie LJ: Self-monitoring of blood glucose by adults with diabetes in the United States population. Diabetes Care 16:1116–1123, 1993.

14. Tobin CT: Health care policy, finance, and law. Report on the AADE survey for third-party reimbursement. Diabetes Educator 19:62–68, 1993.

15. The Diabetes Control and Complications Trial Research Group: The effect of intensive treatment of diabetes on the development and progression of long-term complications in insulin-dependent diabetes mellitus. New Engl J Med 329(14):977–986, 1993.

16. Ruggiero L, Glasgow RE, Dryfoos JM, et al.: Diabetes self-management. Self-reported recommendations and patterns in a large population. Diabetes Care 20:568–576, 1997.

17. Beckles GLA, Engelgau MM, Venkat Narayan KM, et al.: Population-based assessment of the level of care among adults with diabetes in the U.S. Diabetes Care 21:1432–438, 1998.

18. Nordberg BJ, Barlow MS, Chalew SA, McCarter RJ: Effect of third-party reimbursement on use of services and indexes of management among indigent diabetic patients. Diabetes Care 16:1076–1080, 1993.

19. Lurie N, Ward NB, Shapiro NF, et al.: Termination from Medi-Cal B: Does it affect health? New Engl J Med 311:480–484, 1984.

20. Brook RH, Ware JE Jr, Rogers WH, et al.: Does free care improve adults' health? Results from a randomized controlled trial. New Engl J Med 309:1426–1434, 1983.

21. Lohr KN, Brook RH, Kamberg CJ, et al.: Use of medical care in the Rand Health Insurance Experiment. Med Care 24(Sept/suppl.):S1–S87, 1986.

22. Cherkin DC, Grothaus L, Wagner EH: The effect of office visit copayments on preventive care services in an HMO. Inquiry 27(1):24–38, 1990.

23. Selby JV: Cost sharing in the emergency department—is it safe? Is it needed? New Engl J Med 336(24):1750–1751, 1997.

24. Songer TJ, LaPorte RE, Lave JR, et al.: Health insurance and the financial impact of IDDM in families with a child with IDDM. Diabetes Care 20:577–584, 1997.

Section VII.
Development and Evaluation of Diabetes Care Programs

52

A Public Health Response to Diabetes Mellitus

Diabetes Prevention and Control Programs at the Centers for Disease Control and Prevention

Frank Vinicor, Michael Engelgau,
Dara Murphy, and Russell Swiegowski

Diabetes Mellitus: Current Status

Presently, two statements characterize the status of diabetes mellitus (DM) in the United States: (1) It is a "big problem" for both individuals and society in general—DM is common, serious and costly, (2) the problems of diabetes do *not* have to be so big—scientifically and economically validated prevention strategies exist that could significantly reduce, delay, or even prevent the large and growing diabetes disease burden (see Chapters 10, 14, and 50).

Regarding the magnitude and dimension of the diabetes problem, almost 16 million persons, or about 5.9% of the population, have DM, although about one-third (5.4 million individuals) have not had the condition formally diagnosed. Each year, about 800,000 persons are diagnosed with diabetes in the United States—over 2000 people/day, or 90/hr.[1] Particularly in individuals over 45 years of age as well as in ethnic/minority populations, these trends and realities are even more disturbing.[2]

DM is the single greatest cause of nontraumatic amputations, visual impairment and blindness in working-age adults, and end-stage renal disease in the United States.[3] Even though DM is underreported on death certificates,[4] it is the seventh leading cause of death in this country (primarily from coronary artery disease) and a major contributor to disability and impaired quality of life.[1]

Given how common diabetes is and the serious nature of associated complications, it should not be surprising that DM is very costly, both from a societal and an individual perspective. In 1997, a careful study of the direct and indirect costs of just diabetes care indicated an economic burden to the United States of $98 billion.[5] From an individual perspective, having diabetes results in health costs from three to four times that of nondiabetic individuals.[5,6]

Perhaps even more distressing than the present burden of diabetes is the fact that the prevalence of diabetes and its associated complications and cost will likely worsen in the near future.[7,8] Finally, this large and growing burden of diabetes is "wasteful"; efficacious and cost-effective programs exist today that, if widely applied, could substantially mitigate diabetes-related problems.

Three general preventive strategies exist to reduce the problems of diabetes: primary, secondary, and tertiary prevention (Table 52–1) (see Chapter 14). Scientific investigations validating primary prevention programs to decrease or even delay the onset of either type 1 or 2 DM are presently in progress.[9,10] Currently, however, there exist convincing efficacy and economic studies[11] that support benefits to society as a whole as well as individuals in terms of both improved glucose, blood pressure, and lipid control—i.e., secondary prevention[12,13]—and early diabetes complication detection and treatment—i.e., tertiary prevention.[3]

Thus, there is *not* a lack of efficacious programs (interventions validated under ideal circumstances) to control and reduce the burden of DM; rather, for a variety of reasons, these prevention programs are not being widely and routinely applied in regular clinical and public health practice, i.e., effectiveness.[14,15] Hence, while the quest for new and better ways to both prevent and control DM—"science"—must continue, simultaneously, additional efforts must be made to implement those interventions already demonstrated to be efficacious and cost-effective.[16,17] It is primarily

TABLE 52–1 Strategies to Reduce the Burden of Diabetes

Level of Prevention	Example
Primary	Decreasing the incidence of type 2 DM
Secondary	Controlling glucose to prevent complications
Tertiary	Detecting complications early and treating early

this latter challenge—"translating science into practice"—toward which the Centers for Disease Control and Prevention (CDC) directs much of its effort.

Diabetes as a Public Health Problem

Since the discovery of insulin,[18] DM has primarily been viewed as a "clinical disorder"—one that would be addressed by the individual patient and the doctor alone, either in the office or the hospital bed.[19] However, as noninfectious diseases are now emerging as *the* dominant causes of morbidity, mortality, and costs, not only in the United States[20] but throughout the world,[21] concerns have been expressed about the persistence of an "acute medical care" model in a "chronic disease world."[22,23] Further, it is evident that for noninfectious disorders, e.g., chronic diseases, injuries, and so forth, public health dimensions must be integrated into a medical and managed care system if the burden of these noninfectious conditions is to be controlled and reduced.[22–24]

The magnitude of the present and future burden of DM—the number of people affected, the seriousness of complications, cost, and so on—would itself justify a complimentary public health approach. In addition, the fact that DM is particularly devastating to "vulnerable populations," e.g., the elderly and minority communities, further justifies additional "community" and "environmental" considerations beyond just medical-based interventions. Finally, because efficacious and "economical" prevention strategies are not yet widely and consistently applied, a need exists for public health programs in DM to increase the likelihood of access to high-quality and efficient diabetes management.[14–16,24,25]

For chronic diseases like DM, persons other than the patient and his or her health care professional—e.g., family, employers, fellow workers, and church leaders—influence individual decisions.[26] Further, policy issues, e.g., reimbursement strategies, availability of diabetes education programs and community/school physical activity projects, guidelines for effective diabetes management, and diabetes outcome assessment, have a substantial impact on individual clinical diabetes practices.[27] Finally, surveillance data increase awareness of the entire burden of DM (not just of those diabetic persons who visit the clinic or office) and effectiveness of intervention strategies.[28]

Centers for Disease Control and Prevention

The vision of the CDC is "Healthy People in a Healthy World—Through Prevention." Within this vision is a commitment to "promote health and quality of life by

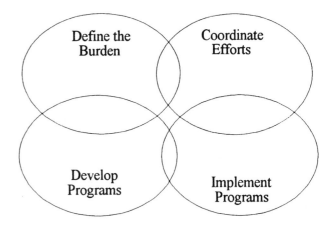

Figure 52–1.   Division of diabetes translation activities.

preventing and controlling disease, injury and disability."[29] While in the past, CDC has focused on infectious diseases, at present chronic diseases, injuries, and the environment are also being addressed from a public health perspective. Particularly relevant to chronic diseases such as DM, quality of life and disability are now viewed as important indicators of "health." Finally, all aspects of prevention—primary, secondary and tertiary (Table 52–1)—are legitimate public health dimensions being addressed in CDC programs.[29]

Within the Division of Diabetes Translation (DDT) at CDC's National Center for Chronic Disease Prevention and Health Promotion, four closely interrelated public health activities have been established: (1) defining the burden of diabetes, (2) developing public health programs, (3) implementing public health programs, and (4) coordinating programs with the greater diabetes community (Fig. 52–1).

Defining the Burden

The 1986 Institute of Medicine's Report from the Committee for the Study of the Future of Public Health outlined the role of the government in public health as "assessment, policy development, and assurance."[30] The committee further recommended that every public health agency: (1) perform assessment by regular and systematic collection, assembly, and analysis of health information; (2) use this information for public policy health decisions; and (3) assure that agreed-upon health goals are being achieved. DDT scientific efforts have thus focused on: (1) assessing the burden through diabetes public health surveillance and epidemiologic studies, (2) developing a comprehensive science base for policy decisions through diabetes translation research, and (3) assuring delivery of effective diabetes-related preventive care through use of "quality indicators" relevant to health care systems, providers, and persons with diabetes.

TABLE 52–2 National Surveillance Systems

Type of Information	Source
NHIS data tape (raw data), research reports, or methodological information	Data Dissemination Branch National Center for Health Statistics Centers for Disease Control and Prevention 6525 Belcrest Road, Room 1064 Hyattsville, MD 20782 (303) 436-8500 http://www.cdc.gov/nchs www/nchshome.htm nchsquery @ nch 10a.em.cdc.gov
BRFSS data tape (raw data), research reports, or methodological information	BRFSS/Division of Adult and Community Health National Center for Chronic Disease and Health Promotion Centers for Disease Control and Prevention 4770 Buford Highway, NE Atlanta, GA 30341 http://www.cdc.gov
NHANES III data tape (raw data), research reports, or methodological information	Data Dissemination Branch National Center for Health Statistics Centers for Disease Control and Prevention 6525 Belcrest Road, Room 1064 Hyattsville, MD 20782 (303) 436-8500 http://www.cdc.gov/nchs www/nchshome.htm nchsquery @ nch 10a.em.cdc.gov
State Specific Surveillance Data, including BRFSS	State Diabetes Control Program (located within each state's health department) or CDC Diabetes Home Page http://www.cdc.gov/diabetes
National Diabetes Fact Sheet: national estimates and general information on diabetes in the United States	Division of Diabetes Translation National Center for Chronic Disease and Health Promotion Centers for Disease Control and Prevention 4770 Buford Highway, NE Atlanta, GA 30341 http://www.cdc.gov/diabetes

DDT utilizes a comprehensive and dynamic public health surveillance system that assesses the past and current burden of diabetes in the U.S. population[31] and facilitates projection of future trends. National surveys and various vital record data systems used are listed in Table 52–2. In some areas, national surveys do not collect important surveillance data, and, if available, state-based or regional information is assessed and used to describe national trends.[32]

Gaining a comprehensive understanding of the burden of diabetes requires consideration of several types of epidemiologic measurements and several individual and population "dimensions" (Table 52–3). Estimates of incidence and prevalence, e.g., the number and type of persons developing or currently affected by diabetes, as well as the nature and extent of diabetic complications, permit description of the current magnitude of the burden—information necessary to formulate public health responses, determine resource needs, plan programs, coordinate implementation efforts, and evaluate impact.

These national incidence and prevalence estimates of diabetes reflect population size and systems/structure changes that, over time, give important insights into secular trends. These trends describe the evolution of diabetes—its rate of growth or reduction—and lend insight into what may occur in the future. Understanding trends (especially among those at higher risks of diabetes and associated complications such as minority populations and the elderly) is of particular relevance and importance to public health programs.

Tracking complications of diabetes more directly and clearly conveys the devastation of diabetes. Surveillance of diabetes as the underlying or contributing cause of death describes the substantial magnitude of mortality, even when considering the underreporting of diabetes on death certificates.[4] Efforts also focus on the major diabetes-specific, related complications such as eye disease,[32] amputations, end-stage renal disease diabetic ketoacidosis,[31] and cardiovascular morbidity/mortality.[33] Finally, information on utilization of services, e.g., hospital admissions and outpatient clinic

TABLE 52–3   Dimensions of the National Diabetes Burden

Number of affected persons
Incidence
Prevalence
Major complications
    Mortality
    Lower extremity amputations
    End-stage renal failure
    Blindness
    Diabetic ketoacidosis
    Cardiovascular disease
Disability
Utilization of health services
    Hospital admissions
    Outpatient visits
    Emergency room visits
Preventive health and care behaviors
    Persons at risk for diabetes
    Persons with diabetes
Diabetes in pregnancy
    Gestational diabetes
    Existing type 1 and 2 diabetes
Secular trends for all dimensions

TABLE 52–4   BRFSS Diabetes Module—Questions

1. How old were you when you were told you have diabetes?
2. Are you now taking insulin?
3. Currently, about how often do you use insulin?
4. About how often do you check your blood for glucose or sugar?
5. Have you ever heard of glycosylated hemoglobin or hemoglobin A_{1c}?
6. About how many times in the last year have you seen a doctor, nurse, or other health professional for your diabetes?
7. About how may times in the last year has a doctor, nurse, or other health professional checked you for glycosylated hemoglobin or hemoglobin A_{1c}?
8. About how many times in the last year has a health professional checked your feet for any sores or irritation?
9. When was the last time you had an eye exam in which the pupils were dilated? (This would have made you temporarily sensitive to bright light.)
10. How much of the time does your vision limit you in recognizing people or objects across the street?
11. How much of the time does your vision limit you in reading print in a newspaper, magazine, recipe, menu, or numbers on the telephone?
12. How much of the time does your vision limit you in watching television?

and emergency room visits, help describe the challenges of diabetes for the health care delivery system.[5]

Disability related to diabetes is another important dimension of the "diabetes burden." Either limitation in or inability to perform major daily activities can have a tremendous impact on the quality of life. While population-based tools to quantify disability and quality of life are presently limited, current data indicate that the burden of diabetes-related disability is substantial and much greater compared to the nondiabetic population.[31]

Monitoring health-related behaviors is an important surveillance dimension to identify not only who might be at risk for diabetes and associated complications but also what steps need to be taken to sustain health among persons currently living with this condition. For example, among persons with diabetes, the importance of self-care, lifestyle (e.g., diet and physical activity), and comprehensive preventive care is now more fully appreciated.[34] CDC has developed and implemented a state-base Behavioral Risk Factor Surveillance System (BRFSS).[35] The BRFSS is a population-base telephone survey that includes a diabetes-specific module (Table 52–4). As of 1996, 43 states have implemented this module. This unique information provides great insights into areas where interventions are most urgently needed and also provides a means to monitor population-based preventative behavioral trends.

In a world of "limits," where decisions among several important programs must be made,[36,37] understanding the economic burden of diabetes is another important area for surveillance. Describing "economics"

requires consideration of several perspectives including that of individuals with diabetes, health care providers, the health care system (e.g., managed care organizations), governments, and society in general. While it is certain that the cost burden of diabetes is substantial,[5,38] this economic information has different meaning from each perspective. Because it is clear that diabetes consumes a disproportionate amount of health care resources, given its prevalence,[6,38–40] economics can be a critical element in making decisions among various interventions. Of more practical importance, however, is understanding the portion of this economic burden of diabetes that can be prevented, the cost of preventing it, and the value of intervention strategies in terms of cost/unit of benefit. DDT's current efforts in the economic arena of diabetes are to complete cost-effectiveness (cost/event prevented) and cost-utility (cost/year of life gained or cost/quality-adjusted year of life gained) evaluations that can show the relative value of various diabetes intervention strategies (Table 52–5). (see Chapters 10, 50, and 51).

Minority populations, including African Americans, Hispanics, American Indians, Asians, and Pacific Islanders, all suffer disproportionately from diabetes and associated complications compared to the white, non-Hispanic population.[41–44] National surveys, however, typically do not result in sufficient numbers of

TABLE 52–5 Examples of Economic Evaluations
of Cost-Effectiveness and Cost-Utility Studies

Intensive glycemic control
Screening for undiagnosed diabetes
Screening and early detection and treatment of diabetic
  kidney disease
Primary prevention of type 2 diabetes
Economics of diabetes in individuals 65 years old or older.

study subjects to make burden estimates for some minority populations. Thus, special studies and surveys are often required to characterize the impact of diabetes for these groups, such as the Hispanic Health and Nutritional Examination Survey[45] and Project DIRECT, a community diabetes demonstration project for African Americans in Raleigh, North Carolina.[46] The impact of diabetes on the elderly, poor and underserved, women, and pregnant women[47] appropriately is gaining attention and is being included in strategies for improving surveillance efforts to "define the burden of DM."

Finally, the substantial increase in managed care organizations providing health care to a growing portion of the population has lead DDT to coordinate development of a "managed care surveillance system for diabetes." This system identifies the diabetes population that is being served, the level of preventive care delivered, and the prevalence of diabetic complications and other comorbidities.[48] Surveillance systems for other large health care delivery systems such as Medicare and Medicaid programs are currently under development.[48]

The need to establish useful and cost-effective interventions has never been greater.[49] DDT is conducting "translation" or applied research and economic studies to address this need. A goal is to transform efficacious treatments developed in experimental and clinical trials into routine clinical and public health practice that results in improving the processes, quality, and outcomes of care at all three levels of prevention (see Table 52–1). To assess current levels of preventive health care for secondary and tertiary prevention, DDT has thus far primarily used the BRFSS.[35] *Unfortunately, but consistent with most other investigations,[50] the level of preventive diabetes care for diabetes is uniformly quite low.[51,52]* Subsequently, determining the impact and cost-effectiveness of diabetes care delivery and identifying the factors that account for variations in diabetes health care delivery are also important challenges for CDC.

Translation research and development of a science base for a public health response, however, span beyond health care delivery. For example, early detection of undiagnosed diabetes with "screening" presently has a limited science base. DDT's strategy has been to assess the burden of undiagnosed diabetes, compare the appropriateness of screening for undiagnosed diabetes to screening for other chronic conditions, quantitatively determine screening test performance, and determining effectiveness and cost-effectiveness of various screening strategies through computer model simulation (see Chapters 11 and 12).[53,54]

Primary prevention of diabetes, especially type 2 DM, requires additional investigation before public health decisions can occur.[10,55] While observational studies have found lifestyle important in the apparent prevention of type 2 DM, DDT's present strategy is to support additional rigorous control trials,[10] assess the burden of persons at risk for DM who may experience maximum benefit, determine potential detection and implementation strategies if interventions are found efficacious, and estimate the cost-effectiveness of primary prevention interventions.

Communities, each possessing unique qualities, strengths, and challenges,[56] also may play important roles for diabetes prevention and control. Project DIRECT is a community diabetes demonstration project examining multilevel community-based strategies targeting persons at risk for diabetes, affected persons and their families, health care providers, health care delivery systems, and the community environment.[46,57]

Ensuring that quality diabetes care is being delivered within the managed care system is important to individuals with diabetes, as well as employers and the nation.[58,59] DDT has supported the National Committee for Quality Assurance (NCQA) and their efforts to develop and refine the Healthplan and Employer Data Information Set (HEDIS).[58] HEDIS is used to determine uniformly and systematically the quality of care being delivered across the entire managed care industry. DDT has developed and submitted indicators for measuring quality of care and is consulting with NCQA as HEDIS is revised and updated. This "system-level approach" has a great potential to broadly influence and improve the level of preventive diabetes care.[59]

Developing Public Health Programs

Many factors influence decisions by individuals, including persons with DM and health care professionals, as well as groups and organizations. Certainly knowledge—knowing what to do—is important, but it is often not sufficient to result in improved decisions.[60] Support systems at home or work,[61] reimbursement and coverage practices,[62] policies and laws,[63] standards or guidelines,[64] time,[65] reminder systems,[66] review of practice decisions,[67] community support,[68] media,[69] and more are all approaches that together can substantially influence individual practitioner and patient behaviors and decisions.

Recognizing the importance of all of the aforementioned approaches and opportunities, DDT significantly altered the direction of its programs in 1994. Past efforts involved increased awareness and application of diabetes education as well as programs specific to the prevention and/or treatment of complications of diabetes, including eye disease, lower extremity disease, cardiovascular disorders, and pregnancy complicated by diabetes.[70]

These experiences allowed DDT to embark on its current programmatic directions. Recognizing that (1) CDC and DDT was actually influencing diabetes care of only a very small percentage of persons the United States, (2) most persons with diabetes were receiving care in health systems with which CDC did not then interact, and (3) evolving science now indicated the benefits of glucose, blood pressure, and lipid control in persons with DM,[12,13] the focus of the programs of DDT changed to address the "environment" or "system" in which *all* persons with DM live, work, and receive preventative care from a variety of practitioners.

Programmatic efforts became directed at (1) employers who purchase health care insurance for workers; (2) communities with cultural uniqueness wherein many people with diabetes live; (3) public agencies and organizations at the federal and state level that determine policies, e.g., reimbursement for preventative diabetes care; (4) managed care systems; (5) media as a source of information and behavior change; and (6) policies that would encourage and facilitate active coordination among other private, public, academic, voluntary, professional, and commercial organizations within the greater diabetes community.

While these new directions meant that it would be challenging to objectively document impact and that direct clinical care would no longer be supported by CDC, it was concluded that improving the "larger and ever-present diabetes environment" would result in a substantially greater likelihood of better diabetes preventative care for more people. This decision, however, also required new health professionals, e.g., behavioral scientists, economists, and sociologists, who would need to help shape the diabetes public health programs at CDC.

Implementing Programs

The relationships between CDC and state health departments, from both a constitutional and historical perspective, have always been important, wherein the states themselves most often implement actual public health programs. Thus, the activities of the CDC, as delineated in the previous editions of this textbook,[70] will continue to depend upon the experiences, expertise, and commitment of state and territorial health departments.

Several permutations in the "programmatic implementation" strategies of DDT, however, have occurred. First, the directions of the state-based Diabetes Control Programs (DCPs) now reflects the philosophy and approaches described earlier and are administered through cooperative agreements between states/territories and CDC.[71] Second, DCPs now exist in *all* states and territories. "Core" DCPs provide a basic foundation for public health diabetes activities—a specific "diabetes presence" in health departments, a Diabetes Advisory Board with broad statewide membership, explicit state diabetes prevention and control plans, limited diabetes surveillance activities, and local diabetes program activities, e.g., church-based diabetes information programs.

This beginning infrastructure that the state-based core programs provide has, in large measure, enabled the DCPs to successfully define the burden of diabetes at the state level and maximize the reach and impact of the program through coordination within the larger statewide diabetes community.

Resources within the "core" DCPs mechanisms are, however, limited. To expand the influence and interactions of the state health departments in diabetes, "comprehensive" DCPs are being established in several jurisdictions. Beyond public health programs in every state and territory and programs that focus on improving the environment wherein diabetes prevention and control activities occur, comprehensive DCPs thus represent a third evolutionary diabetes activity of CDC. Comprehensive DCPs are characterized by a substantial presence in state health departments, e.g., two to four professional personnel; multiple surveillance and epidemiologic activities, e.g., within managed care organizations and minority communities using the state-based BRFSS,[35] statewide diabetes prevention and control programs such as media campaigns regarding influenza vaccination in persons with DM, and so on; and coordination among all other important partners with the state diabetes community, e.g., the American Diabetes Association, Medicaid, and Medicare, etc. It is anticipated that approximately 15 comprehensive DCPs will exist in 1999.

Finally, DDT, in addition to greater and improved support to all state and territorial health departments, has now established direct relationships with various agencies/organizations from the private sector, including managed care organizations, academic centers, national and community minority organizations, professional societies, and international diabetes programs. These activities represent efforts to further broaden the diabetes public health link between CDC and important private-sector organizations involved with diabetes prevention and control.[72]

Coordination

In large part, because of the prevalence, seriousness, and cost of diabetes, as well as the "preventability" of a large component of this disease burden, DM has received increasing attention from public, private, academic, voluntary, commercial, and political interests and organizations in the United States.[73] Each of these many organizations focuses on specific components of the overall diabetes challenge, and while considerable interaction naturally occurs, additional explicit, systematic, and structured coordination has been an important leadership challenge for the diabetes public health mission at CDC.

State and territorial DCPs must establish broad-based "diabetes advisory committees" for each geographical area. Further, at a national level, the need for prospective coordination among diabetes organizations remains substantial. Three examples of such efforts include (1) the Diabetes Mellitus Interagency Coordinating Committee, chaired by the National Institute of Diabetes, Digestive and Kidney Diseases (NIDDK), which serves as a venue for coordination among all federal agencies and organizations involved in diabetes research, prevention, and control[74]; (2) the Translation Advisory Committee for Diabetes Prevention and Control Programs, a congressionally mandated committee comprised of representatives from various diabetes communities whose responsibilities include advising CDC on important public health activities in DM[75]; and the National Diabetes Education Program (NDEP).[76] The NDEP, cochaired by NIDDK and CDC, coordinates emerging national education efforts in diabetes to the public, patients, health professionals, policy-makers, and purchasers of diabetes care.

At the international level, diabetes is also now viewed as a major public health challenge.[77–79] CDC has been designated a World Health Organization Diabetes Collaborating Center for Primary Care Programs in Diabetes.[80] In addition, the DDT is an active partner with such organizations as the International Diabetes Federation and the Pan American Health Organization,[81] and has provided consultation with specific countries facing the epidemic of DM.[82] Coordination within the international community facilitates an open sharing of programs and preventive strategies, and CDC has learned greatly from the experiences of other approaches to reducing the growing burden of DM (see Appendixes I, II, and V).

While it is often difficult to quantitatively document the precise impact and benefit of "coordination," CDC remains committed to both leading and participating in such efforts, with the strong perspective that in public health, involving the "many" will ultimately result in great progress and accomplishment.[83]

Future

It is clear that as large as the burden of diabetes is in the United States today, it will likely get worse before it gets better.[7,8,21,84] With "Westernization" and its associated obesity and diminishing physical activity, this prediction will also be true internationally.[7,84,85] Given the traditions and leadership responsibilities of CDC, it is imperative that a public health perspective be further developed and made complimentary to the important clinical approach to controlling preventable illness associated with DM. This "imperative" means that CDC must (1) expand its surveillance and epidemiologic activities, including economic, health services, and behavioral science programs[86]; (2) develop and implement public health strategies that will ensure an optimal "environment" for improved decision making by persons with diabetes as well as health professionals who provide care for these individuals; (3) understand and eliminate the bases for disparities in diabetes and associated complications and care among various populations groups in the United States[87]; (4) interact with purchasers of care and policy-makers at the local, state, and federal levels, as well as managed care organizations[25,88]; and (5) establish a cooperative and coordinated atmosphere to maximize the productive interactions among the many members and member organizations of the greater diabetes communities in the United States and globally.

These approaches reflect the past history, present activities, and future opportunities for CDC's diabetes programs and can contribute to better understanding, prevention, and control of the personal and societal burden associated with DM.

References

1. Centers for Disease Control and Prevention: National Diabetes Fact Sheet: National Estimates and General Information on Diabetes in the United States. Atlanta, GA: U.S. Department of Health and Human Services, Centers for Disease Control and Prevention, 1997.

2. Centers for Disease Control and Prevention: Trends in the prevalence and incidence of self-reported diabetes mellitus—United States, 1980–1994. Morbid Mortal Wkly Rep 46:1014–1018, 1997.

3. Clark C, Lee D: Prevention and treatment of the complications of diabetes mellitus. New Engl J Med 332:1210–1217, 1995.

4. Bild D, Stevenson J: Frequency of recording of diabetes on U.S. death certificates: Analysis of the 1986 National Mortality Followback Survey. J Clin Epidemiol 45:275–281, 1992.

5. American Diabetes Association: Economic consequences of diabetes mellitus in the U.S. in 1997. Diabetes Care 21:296–309, 1998.

6. Selby J, Ray G, Zhang D, Colby C: Excess costs of medical care for patients with diabetes in a managed care population. Diabetes Care 20:1396–1402, 1997.

7. Aubert R: Trends in the global burden of diabetes, 1995–2025. Diabetes 46(Suppl 1):139A, 1997.

8. Kelly D: Our future society: a global challenge. Circulation 95;2459–2464, 1997.

9. The DPT 1 Study Group: The diabetes prevention trial: Type 1 diabetes (DPT-1): Implementation of screening and staging of relatives. Transplant Proc 27:3377, 1995.

10. National Institutes of Health: Non-insulin dependent diabetes primary prevention trial. NIH Guide Grants Contracts 22:1–20, 1993.

11. Eastman R, Javitt J, Herman W, et al.: Prevention strategies for non-insulin-dependent diabetes mellitus: an economic perspective. In LeRoith D, Taylor S, Olefsky J (eds): Diabetes Mellitus. Philadelphia: Lippincott-Raven, 1996, 621–630.

12. The Diabetes Control and Complications Trial Research Group: The effect of intensive treatment of diabetes on the development and progression of long-term complications in insulin-dependent diabetes mellitus. New Engl J Med 329:977–986, 1993.

13. Gotto, A: Cholesterol management in theory and practice. Circulation 96:4424–4430, 1997.

14. McDonald R: The evolving care of diabetes: Models, managed care and public health. Ann Intern Med 20:685–686, 1997.

15. Vinicor, F: Challenges to the translation of the DCCT. Diabetes Rev 2:371–383, 1994.

16. Detsky A, Naglie, I: A clinician's guide to cost-effectiveness analysis. Ann Intern Med 113:147–154, 1990.

17. Miller N, Hill M, Kottke T, Ockene I: The multilevel compliance challenge: recommendations for a call to action. A statement for healthcare professionals. Circulation 95:1085–1090, 1997.

18. Bliss, M: The Discovery of Insulin. Toronto: McClelland and Stewart, 1982.

19. Peters A, Davidson M, Schriger D, et al.: A clinical approach for the diagnosis of diabetes mellitus. JAMA 276:1246–1252, 1996.

20. McGinnis M, Foege, W: Actual causes of death in the United States. JAMA 270:2207–2212, 1993.

21. Murray C, Lopez A: Alternative projections of mortality and disability by cause 1990–2020: Global burden of disease study. Lancet 349:1498–1504, 1997.

22. Wagner E, Austin B, von Korff, M: Organizing care for patients with chronic illness. Milbank Q 4:511–544, 1996.

23. Etzwiler, D: Chronic care: a need in search of a system. Diab Educator 23:569–573, 1997.

24. Vinicor, F: Is diabetes a public-health disorder? Diabetes Care 17(Suppl 1):22–27, 1994.

25. Fairfield G, Hunter D, Mechanic D, Roseleff, F: Managed care: Origins, principles and evolution. Br Med J 314:1823–1826, 1997.

26. Kendrick T, Hilton S: Broader team work in primary care. Br Med J 314:672–675, 1997.

27. Cohen S, Halvorson H, Gosselink, C: Changing physician behavior to improve disease prevention. Prev Med 23:284–291, 1994.

28. Pearce N: Traditional epidemiology, modern epidemiology, and public health. Am J Pub Health 86:678–683, 1996.

29. Etheridge E: Sentinel for Health: A History of the Centers for Disease Control. Berkeley: University of California Press, 1992.

30. Committee for the Study of the Future of Public Health: The Future of Public Health. Washington, DC: National Academy Press, 1988.

31. Centers for Disease Control and Prevention: Diabetes Surveillance, 1997. Atlanta, GA: U.S. Department of Health and Human Services, 1997.

32. Centers for Disease Control and Prevention: Blindness caused by diabetes—Massachusetts, 1987–1994. Morbid Mortal Wkly Rep 45:937–940, 1996.

33. Ochi J, Melton L, Palumbo P, Chu-Pin C: A population-based study of diabetes mortality. Diabetes Care 8:224–229, 1985.

34. Wender R: Preventive health care for diabetics: a realistic vision. Arch Fam Med 6:38–41, 1997.

35. Powell-Griner E, Anderson J, Murphy W: State and sex-specific prevalence of selected characteristics—behavioral risk factor surveillance system, 1994, 1995. Morbid Mortal Wkly Rep 46:1–31, 1997.

36. Eddy D: Principles for making difficult decisions in difficult times. JAMA 271:1792–1798, 1994.

37. Vinicor F: The public health burden of diabetes and the reality of limits. Diabetes Care 21(S3):5–8, 1998.

38. Rubin R, Altman W, Medelson D: Health care expenditures for people with diabetes mellitus. J Clin Endocrinol Metab 78:809A–809F, 1992.

39. The Diabetes Control and Complications Trial Research Group: Lifetime benefits and costs of intensive therapy as practiced in the Diabetes Control and Complications Trial. JAMA 276:1409–1415, 1996.

40. Vijan S, Hofer T, Hayward R: Estimated benefits of glycemic control in microvascular complications in type 2 diabetes. Ann Intern Med 127:788–795, 1997.

41. Tull E, Roseman J: Diabetes in African Americans. In Harris M (ed): Diabetes in America Ed. 2. Washington, DC: National Institutes of Health, National Institutes of Diabetes and Digestive and Kidney Diseases (NIH Pub. No. 95-1468), 1995, pp. 613–630.

42. Stern M, Mitchell B: Diabetes in Hispanic Americans. In Harris M (ed): Diabetes in America, Ed. 2. Washington, DC. National Institutes of Health, National Institutes of Diabetes and Digestive and Kidney Diseases (NIH Pub. No. 95-1468), 1995, pp. 613–630.

43. Gohdes D: Diabetes in North American Indians and Alaska Natives. In Harris M (ed): Diabetes in America Ed. 2. Washington, DC: National Institutes of Health, National Institutes of Diabetes and Digestive and Kidney Diseases (NIH Pub. No. 95-1468), 1995, pp. 613–630.

44. Fujimoto W: Diabetes in Asian and Pacific Islander Americans. In Harris M (ed): Diabetes in America, Ed. 2. Washington, DC: National Institutes of Health, National

Institutes of Diabetes and Digestive and Kidney Diseases (NIH Pub. No. 95-1468), 1995, pp. 613–630.

45. Flegal K, Ezzati T, Harris M, et al.: Prevalence of diabetes in Mexican Americans, Cubans and Puerto Ricans from the Hispanic Health and Nutritional Examination Survey, 1982–1984. Diabetes Care 14:628–638, 1991.

46. Herman W, Thompson T, Visscher W, et al.: Diabetes mellitus and its complications in an African American community: Project DIRECT. J Nat Med Assoc, 147–156, 1998.

47. Lesser K, Carpenter M: Metabolic changes associated with normal pregnancy and pregnancy complicated by diabetes mellitus. Seminars Perinat 18:399–406, 1994.

48. Yox S: Diabetes care: an opportunity for collaboration. HMO Practice 11:164–167, 1997.

49. Asch D, Ubel P: Rationing by any other name. New Engl J Med 336:1668–1671, 1997.

50. Peters A, Legorreta A, Ossorio R, Davidson M: Quality of outpatient care provided to diabetic patients: a health maintenance organization experience. Diabetes Care 19:601–606, 1996.

51. Centers for Disease Control and Prevention: Diabetes specific preventive-care practices among persons with diabetes mellitus—Colorado, Behavior Risk Factor Surveillance System, 1995. Morbid Mortal Wkly Rep 46:1018–1023, 1997.

52. Centers for Disease Control and Prevention: Preventive-care knowledge and practices among persons with diabetes mellitus—North Carolina, Behavior Risk Factor Surveillance System, 1995–1995. Morbid Mortal Wkly Rep 46:1023–1027, 1997.

53. Englegau M, Aubert R, Thompson T, Herman W: Screening for NIDDM in nonpregnant adults. A review of principles, screening tests, and recommendations. Diabetes Care 18:1606–1618, 1995.

54. The screening muddle. Lancet 351:459, 1998.

55. Vinicor F: Primary prevention of type 2 diabetes mellitus. In Dyck P, Thomas P (eds): Diabetic Neuropathy. Philadelphia: W.B. Saunders, 1998.

56. Feinlieb M: New directions for community interventions studies. Am J Pub Health 86:1696–1698, 1996.

57. Engelgau M, Narayan V, Geiss L, et al.: A project to reduce the burden of diabetes in the African-American community: Project DIRECT. J Nat Med Assoc, 90:605–613, 1998.

58. Thompson J, Bost J, Ahmed F, et al.: The NCQA's quality compass: Evaluating managed care in the United States. Health Affairs 17:152–158, 1998.

59. Nolan T: Understanding medical systems. Ann Intern Med 128:293–298, 1998.

60. Glasgow R, Osteen V: Evaluating diabetes education— are we measuring the most important outcomes? Diabetes Care 15:1423–1432, 1992.

61. Berwick D: A primer on leading the improvement of systems. Br Med J 312:619–622, 1996.

62. Bodenheimer T, Grumbach K: Capitation or decapitation: Keeping your heads in changing times. JAMA 276:1025–1034, 1996.

63. Brown E, Viscoli C, Horwitz R: Preventive health strategies and the policy-makers paradox. Ann Intern Med 116:593–597, 1992.

64. Smallwood R, Lapsley H: Clinical practice guidelines: To what end. Med J Austral 166:592–595, 1997.

65. Walker R, Adam J. Time-sensitive clinical management: a case study of acute asthma care. Soc Sci Med 46:539–547, 1998.

66. Overage J, Tierney W, McDonald C: Computer reminders to implement preventive care guidelines for hospitalized patients. Arch Intern Med 156:1551–1556, 1996.

67. Rundall T, Schauffler H: Health promotion and disease prevention in integrated delivery systems: the role of market forces. Am J Prev Med 13:244–250, 1997.

68. Sussman L: Socio-cultural concerns of diabetes care. In Haire-Joshua D (ed): Management of Diabetes Mellitus: Perspectives of Care across the Life Span, Ed. 2. St. Louis, MO: Mosby, 1996, pp. 473–512.

69. Wallack L, Dorfman L: Media advocacy: a strategy for advancing policy and promoting health. Health Ed Q 23:293–317, 1996.

70. Ring A, DeStefano F, Geiss L, et al.: Centers for Disease Control community-based diabetes control programs and the diabetes translation center. In Davidson J (ed): Clinical Diabetes Mellitus, Ed. 2. New York: Thieme, 1991, pp. 728–737.

71. Anderson L, Bruner L, Satterfield D: Diabetes control programs: New directions. Diabetes Educator 21:432–438, 1995.

72. Lasker R (ed): Medicine and Public Health: The Power of Collaboration. New York Academy of Medicine, 1997.

73. Molotsky, I. Clinton unveils plan to battle diabetes. NY Times 9 Aug 1997, p. 10.

74. National Diabetes Advisory Board: The National Long-Range Plan to Combat Diabetes 1987. U.S. Department of Health and Human Services, Public Health Service, National Institutes of Health (NIH Pub. No. 871587), Washington, DC, 1987.

75. National Commission on Diabetes: Report of the National Commission on Diabetes to the Congress of the United States: The Long-Range Plan to Combat Diabetes. U.S. Department of Health, Education, and Welfare, Public Health Service, National Institutes of Health (DEW Pub. No. (NIH) 76-1018), Washington, DC, 1976.

76. Leontos C, Wong F, Gallivan J, Lising M: National diabetes education program: Opportunities and challenges. J Am Diet Assoc 98:73–75, 1998.

77. Amos A, McCarty D, Zimmet P: The rising global burden of diabetes and its complications: Estimates and projections to the year 2010. Diabetic Med 14(Suppl. 5):1–85, 1997.

78. Home P: The Lisbon statement. Diabetic Med 14:517–518, 1997.

79. White F: Declaration of the Americas on diabetes: Overview. IDF Bull 42:10–11, 1997.

80. King H: Diabetes and the World Health Organization: Progress towards prevention and control. Diabetes Care 16:387–390, 1993.

81. Diaz-Kenney R, Liburd L, Murphy D, Vinicor F: Hispanic/Latino diabetes initiative for action. IDF Bull 42:26–29, 1997.

82. Thompson T, Engelgau M, Hegazy M, et al.: The onset of NIDDM and its relationship to clinical diagnosis in Egyptian adults. Diabetic Med 13:337–340, 1996.

83. Goldhager J, Chiu T: A view from the horizon: Strategic partnerships of public health, academic medical centers, and managed care. J Pub Health Management 4:29–35, 1998.

84. Alwan A, King H: Diabetes in the Eastern Mediterranean (Middle East) region: the World Health Organization responds to a major public health challenge. Diabetic Med 12:1057–1058, 1995.

85. Martensen R, Jones D: Diabetes mellitus as a "disease of civilization." JAMA 278:345, 1997.

86. Glasgow R: A practical model of diabetes management and education. Diabetes Care 18:117–126, 1995.

87. Calman K: Equity, poverty and health for all. Br Med J 314:1187–1191, 1997.

88. Quickel K: Diabetes in a managed care system. Ann Intern Med 124:160–163, 1996.

53

Diabetes and Minorities

Lessons from the American Indians

Dorothy Gohdes

Controlling the epidemic of non-insulin-dependent diabetes mellitus (NIDDM) in minority communities around the world is a major public health imperative. Chronic diseases like infectious diseases are more efficiently controlled by prevention than by treatment. But the prevention of diseases like NIDDM and atherosclerotic heart disease is challenging because of the complex interaction of the risk factors. The World Health Organization (WHO) has defined stages of diabetes prevention.[1] Primary prevention includes activities aimed at preventing the development of NIDDM; secondary prevention is detecting and stopping the progression of diabetes; and tertiary prevention is preventing the development, progression, and/or disability from complications. Each stage of prevention, as shown in Table 53–1, involves individuals, communities, and the health care system. Successful tertiary prevention is a partnership between individual patients and their health care system, while primary prevention depends largely on individual behavior and community lifestyle. The scientific basis underlying secondary and tertiary prevention is well developed and growing.[2–4] Modifying the health care system to deliver preventive diabetes care in a cost-effective manner has now become a major focus.

The best strategies for primary prevention in high-risk individuals and in communities remain to be determined prospectively.[5] Data from a large study in China show that simple lifestyle changes can decrease the risk of developing diabetes in high-risk individuals.[6] The scientific documentation for primary prevention rests upon the epidemiologic research suggesting that lifestyle can alter the risk factors for NIDDM. People who are fit, physically active, and slender appear to have a decreased risk for developing NIDDM.[7]

In minority communities, primary prevention holds an exciting promise. Health promotion efforts in the United States, including Healthy People 2000, target obesity and physical inactivity in specific communities.[8] Among American Indians, preliminary data from a comprehensive school health program show that children exposed to a school health curriculum adapted to their culture, Growing Healthy, gain weight more slowly over the school year than their schoolmates who were not given this health curriculum in their classrooms.[9] The revival of traditional long-distance running and other activities focused on wellness have emphasized fitness as part of overall health in the American Indian community of Zuni.[10] The primary prevention of diabetes in many minority communities

TABLE 53–1 World Health Organization Stages of Diabetes Prevention

Stage	Goal	Examples	Location	Target
Primary	Preventing the development of disease	Weight loss programs Wellness centers	Community	Community-at-large Family High-risk individuals
Secondary	Detecting diabetes Reversing or stopping progression	Routine blood sugar screening Exercise programs Diet classes	Community Health care system	High-risk communities Prenatal patients Overweight individuals with family history
Tertiary	Development of complications, progression, or disability	Eye screening and referral Foot care programs Lipid lowering therapy	Health care system	Diagnosed diabetic patients

TABLE 53–2   Selected Measures of Diabetes Prevention Reported by Health Care Systems

Patient Characteristics	Process of Care	Indicators of Adverse Outcomes	Metabolic Outcomes
Age	Setting (frequency, practitioner)	Retinopathy stage	Glycosylated hemoglobin
Sex	Eye screening	Proteinuria/creat level	Blood glucose levels
Duration of diabetes	Foot examination	Foot ulcer/amputation	Cholesterol levels
Obesity	Renal screening	Hypertension	Triglyceride levels
Mode of therapy	Diet therapy	Smoking status	Creatinine levels
	Education/selfmonitoring	Cardiovascular disease	

will also address the prevention of coronary heart disease by decreasing obesity and promoting fitness.

Secondary diabetes prevention in minority communities must address screening for diabetes. In many minority communities, the high rates of gestational diabetes warrant routine screening of all prenatal patients.[11] In such high-risk communities, women may already have NIDDM but not be aware of the condition; early screening can thus detect pregnant diabetic women who were not known to be diabetic previously. For most adults, the necessity for screening programs and their effectiveness depend on the prevalence of diabetes in particular communities and the resources in the health care system.[12] In communities where diabetes rates are high, access to health care is readily available, and providers are oriented to NIDDM, the reservoir of undiagnosed diabetes may be relatively small. The Strong Heart Study examining cardiovascular risk factors among American Indian populations aged 45–74 found a relatively small ratio (4:1) of known to unknown cases.[13] Among other minority populations in the United States, however, the ratio of new to unknown showed a larger reservoir of undiagnosed diabetes with one undiagnosed case for every known one.[14,15] Therefore, screening and follow-up are major concerns in most minority communities. The strategies to attract participants vary by community, but appropriate follow-up must be organized as an integral part of screening.

Tertiary prevention in minority communities depends on the availability of basic health care. Because of the high rates of diabetes, community-oriented primary care is essentially diabetes care in many communities. Organizing and implementing educational programs to inform patients and their families about diabetes self-care and ongoing monitoring of patients for complications make up a complex package of services. Organizing these preventive services challenges health care organizations to deliver more than urgent care. Indian Health Service, along with many other large systems, has begun defining and tracking preventive health services provided to diabetic patients. Such measures include rates of complication screening as well as tracking levels of metabolic and hypertension control.[16–18] Table 53–2 presents categories of measures and examples of each measure that appear commonly in the growing literature. Studies reporting the implementation of tertiary prevention are increasing, but the categorization and definition of measures are not yet standard. When the tertiary prevention measures are standard, variations in care affecting minorities can be evaluated and improvements effectively made.

In summary, the emergence of chronic disease, primarily diabetes and heart disease, challenges minority communities worldwide to implement comprehensive diabetes prevention programs involving individuals, families, communities, and their health care systems. The surveillance systems to measure the extent and success of implementation are under development across many communities. The need for specific public health emphasis on diabetes is acute in the many minority communities struggling with chronic disease.

References

1. World Health Organization: Prevention of Diabetes Mellitus. WHO Technical Report Series #844. Geneva: WHO, 1994.
2. The Diabetes Control and Complications Trial Research Group: The effect of intensive treatment of diabetes on the development and progression of long-term complications in insulin dependent diabetes mellitus. New Engl J Med 339:977–986, 1993.
3. Lasker RD: The Diabetes Control and Complications Trial: Implications for policy and practice New Engl J Med 329:1035–1036, 1993.
4. Clark CM Jr, Lee DA: Drug therapy: Prevention and treatment of the complications of diabetes mellitus. New Engl J Med 322:1210–1217, 1995.
5. Knowler WC, Narayan KMV: Prevention of non-insulin-dependent diabetes mellitus. Preventive Med 23:701–703, 1994.
6. Pan X, Li G, Hu Y, Bennett PH, Howard BV et al.: Effects of diet and exercise in Diabetes Care Preventing NIDDM in people with impaired glucose tolerance 20:537–544, 1997.

7. Knowler WC, Narayan KMV, Hanson RL, et al.: Preventing non-insulin-dependent diabetes. Diabetes 44:483–488, 1995.

8. Healthy People 2000: National Health Promotion and Disease Prevention Objectives. Public Health Service DHHS Pub. No. PHS 91-50212. Washington, DC: U.S. Department of Health and Human Services, 1991.

9. Broussard B, Sugarman J, Bachman-Carter K, et al.: Toward comprehensive obesity prevention programs in Native American communities. Obesity Res 3(Suppl 2):289–297, 1995.

10. Benjamin EM: Community-based exercise programs. In Ruderman N, Devlin JT (eds.): The Health Care Professional's Guide to Diabetes and Exercise. American Diabetes Association Clinical Education Series, American Diabetes Association 1995, pp. 259–264.

11. American College of Obstetricians and Gynecologists: Diabetes and Pregnancy (Technical Bull. #200). Washington, DC: ACOG, 1994.

12. Engelgau MM, Aubert RE, Thompson TJ, Herman WH: Screening for NIDDM in non-pregnant adults: A review of principles, screening tests and recommendations. Diabetes Care 18:1606–1618, 1995.

13. Lee ET, Howard BV, Savage PJ, et al.: Diabetes and impaired glucose tolerance in three American Indian populations aged 45-74 years: The Strong Heart Study. Diabetes Care 18:599–610, 1995.

14. Flegal KM, Ezzati TM, Harris MI, et al.: Prevalence of Diabetes and impaired glucose tolerance in Mexican Americans, Cubans, and Puerto Ricans ages 20–74 in the Hispanic Health and Nutrition Examination Survey, 1982–1984. Diabetes Care 14 (Suppl 3) 628–638, 1991.

15. Kenny SJ, Aubert RE, Geiss LS: Prevalence and incidence of non-insulin-dependent diabetes. In: National Diabetes Data Group (eds.): Diabetes in America, Ed. 2 NIH Pub. No. 95-1468. Washington, DC: National Institutes of Health, National Institutes of Diabetes and Digestive and Kidney Diseases; 1995, pp. 47–67.

16. Mayfield JA, Rith-Najarian SJ, Acton KA, et al.: Assessment of diabetes care by medical record review: The Indian Health Service model. Diabetes Care 17:918–923, 1994.

17. Gohdes D, Rith-Najarian S, Acton K, Shields R: Improving diabetes care in the primary health setting: The Indian Health Service experience. Ann Internal Med 124(1 pt. 2):149–152, 1996.

18. Wilson AE: Home PD for the Diabetes Audit Working Group of the Research Unit of the Royal College of Physicians and the British Diabetic Association. A dataset to allow exchange of information for monitoring continuing diabetes care. Diabetic Med 10:378–390, 1993.

54

Controlled Clinical Trials in the Study of Diabetes

Thaddeus E. Prout, M.D.

Historic Perspective

In the Book of Daniel[1] is found the first recorded evidence of a clinical trial. When the child, Daniel, was brought to the court of Nebuchadnezzar, the king decided that four selected children of Israel should be treated as children of the prince and fed meat and wine from the king's table so that they would later be of service to the kingdom. The child, Daniel, persuaded the king's eunuch, Melzar, to allow the children of Israel to have meal and water rather than the king's meat and wine which would have defiled the Israelites. Melzar, concerned over disobeying the king's instructions, was further persuaded by Daniel to allow the children to undergo a dietary trial of ten days' duration. After ten days, finding that their "countenances appeared fairer and fatter in flesh than all the children which did eat the portions of the king's meat," Daniel's request was granted. After three years all of the children were brought before Nebuchadnezzar and he found the children of Israel to be "ten times better than all the magicians and astrologers were in his realm."

Some prefer to trace the origins of clinical trials to the observation by James Lynd[2]:

"On the 20th of May, 1774, I took 12 patients with scurvy aboard the Salisbury at sea. Their cases were similar as I could have them. Two of these were ordered a quart of cider a day. Two others took twenty gutts of Elixir of Vitriol. Two others two spoonfuls of vinegar. Two were put under a course of sea water. Two others had each two oranges and one lemon given them each day. The two remaining took the bigness of a nutmeg. The consequences was the most sudden and visible good were perceived from the use of oranges and lemons."

Lynd had chosen cases of similar severity, treated them in a similar environment, allocated different treatments to each pair in his series, and personally observed the patients for a sufficient follow-up period as to warrant his conclusions. Yet, following this seminal observation, Lynd's observations were rejected for half a century before they were implemented. In 1803, the Royal Navy introduced lime juice into the diet of officers and men, and decreased the number of patients with scurvy at the Royal Naval Hospital in Portsmouth from nearly 1,500 in 1780 to 2 in 1806.[3]

Most of the advances in medicine at the end of the 18th Century came from the astute observations that were confirmed to be of benefit in the treatment of human illness, but many traditional and established "treatments" were continued without demonstration of either their safety or efficacy. Drawing large quantities of blood from patients for treating a fever was still widely used and had a strong advocate in Benjamin Rush of Philadelphia, who wrote in 1794[4] as follows:

"I began by drawing a small quantity [of blood]... The appearance of the blood and the effect upon the system satisfied me as to its safety and efficacy."

This procedure, based only on personal conviction, was the first to be challenged and shown to be without merit by Pierre Charles-Alexandre Louis, utilizing a new method that was later called the "numerical system." This new scientific concept was expressed in unequivocal and uncompromising terms:[5]

"Let those who engage... in the study of therapeutics... demonstrate the influence [of treatment]... on the duration, progress and termination of a particular disease. Nothing is more difficult... it can be effected only by... an extensive series of observations collected with extreme care."

This confrontation of undocumented personal conviction by demonstrable and reproducible facts was aptly heralded by Bartlett in a review of Louis' works:[6]

"With Louis' adaptation of what is called the numerical system has commenced a new era in our science. The true light has at last shown. The safe and straight path has at last been entered upon."

Although "true light... had shown" on the "safe and straight path," over 100 years would pass before the power and relevance of *controlled clinical trials* (CCT) would be recognized and put into practice. These studies began to gain ascendancy when in 1946 the British Medical Research Council, faced with an overwhelming burden of human tuberculosis, published a systematic study to determine the best way to use their limited supply of newly discovered streptomycin.[7] Much of the modern methodology of this experimental approach was written at this early stage and required only minor alterations with further experience.[8]

In spite of the clear demonstrations of the clinical usefulness of the many successful studies that have followed, questions continue to be raised as to the need for random allocation of patients to treatment groups to be tested, as well as the methods of analysis. In all CCT, these questions must be answered in carefully reasoned and clearly stated terms.[9] Opinions that would lead us back to clinical impressions as the final arbiter in deciding the safety and efficacy of therapies are still supported in the marketplace.[10]

Studies of Diabetes Mellitus

It was into this dichotomous world of science that the methodology of CCT was first introduced in the study of diabetes. Therapies that in the past had been shown to be uniquely successful required no further proof of efficacy for acceptance. The introduction of insulin in the treatment of the acute complications of Insulin-dependent diabetes mellitus (IDDM) was an excellent example of this, but the degree to which chronic complications of diabetes might be prevented in diabetic patients by control of blood glucose had never been critically studied.

The University Group Diabetes Program (UGDP)[11]

The first long-term perspective clinical trial in diabetes to address this question in non-insulin-dependent diabetes (NIDDM) was organized by university-based investigators who set themselves the task in 1958 to design a study to assess the effects of then current methods of therapy on the complications of diabetes. This study, the University Group Diabetes Program (UGDP), was funded by the National Institutes of Health (NIH). The details of design and methodology as well as the mortality results of the study have been given in detail elsewhere[11] and summarized in previous editions of this text.[12] Important lasting contributions of this study will be summarized briefly.

Since the first step in the training of all patients with newly diagnosed NIDDM is instruction in an appropriate diet to control their diabetes, this became the uniform basis of therapy to which all other forms of treatment could be compared. Patients could then be assigned by random allocation to one of four treatment groups as follows: The use of a variable insulin dosage IVAR) to normalize blood glucose; a fixed standard dose of insulin (ISTD) to prevent symptoms of hyperglycemia; a fixed dose of the most commonly used sulfonylurea, Tolbutamide (TOLB) and diet alone with a placebo (PLBO) of the oral agent. A second study was added 18 months later and randomized separately utilizing the only available biguanide, Phenformin (PHEN), and a matching placebo (PLBO).

This design made UGDP the first classical placebo controlled cooperative clinical trial utilizing random allocations of available therapies for the long-term study of NIDDM among 12 university centers [Exhibit 54–1].

EXHIBIT 54–1   Methods and Design: UGDP

Design Features

Sample size: 200 patients in each treatment group needed for cooperative study

Random allocation: assignment to treatment group with balanced distribution

Double-blind study: nature of oral agents unknown to both patients and physicians

Standard technique: examinations by objective methods. All tests performed in same manner

Criteria for Entry

Diabetes diagnosed within 12 months

Diagnosis confirmed by glucose tolerance test

Patient nonketotic on diet alone

Life expectancy estimated to be at least 5 years

Patient willing to participate in study and capable of intelligent cooperation

Informed consent

Treatment Groups	
Definition	**Abbreviation**
1. Insulin variable: dose adjusted in attempt to normalize blood glucose concentration	IVAR
2. Insulin standard: dosage not related to blood glucose concentration. Daily dose of 10 to 16 U, according to body surface area	ISTD
3. Tolbutamide: 1.5 g/day in divided dosage	TOLB
4. Phenformin[a]: 100 mg/day in divided dosage	PHEN
5. Placebo (lactose): number of pills corresponding to oral agent	PLBO

[a] This group added 18 months later.

[*Source:* Adapted from University Group Diabetes Program: VIII. Evaluation of insulin therapy: final report. Diabetes 31(Suppl. 5, Part 2): 1–81, 1982. With permission.]

The second important aspect of the UGDP was the impact that this study had in refocusing the attention of primary care physicians and other health advocates on the fundamentals of diabetes care. In practice current management had become complacent and poorly focused. The introduction of the oral hypoglycemic agents had threatened to shorten the important dialogue between patient and physician and to reduce the treatment of this complex disease to a printed diet sheet and a drug prescription with little instruction on behavioral change or lifestyle. This suggested to patients that this new mode of treatment had nullified the threat of future complications. Following the first report of the UGDP,[11] these concerns focused attention to the fundamental principles of treatment for patients with diabetes. This is best represented by the work of Davidson et al [13] which re-emphasized dietary indoctrination and glucose control as the basic principles upon which successful therapy of diabetes must rest.

The third important aspect of the UGPD was the careful documentation of baseline characteristics of the newly diagnosed patients with NIDDM on entrance and the progression of their complications from baseline to 14 years. Only the PLBO, IVAR, and ISTD groups were combined for the tabulations of these observations. The TOLB group was excluded because of an adverse incidence of cardiovascular death requiring discontinuation of this treatment group prematurely. These data will provide the benchmark for the comparison of new modes of therapy in future years.

A fourth contribution of this seminal study was to pose questions to be tested at a future time. In the UGDP experience there was evidence that total patient mortality did not differ by treatment group in the incidence of death due to all causes, and death from all causes correlated well with expected mortality in all treatment groups (Table 54–1). On the other hand, patients achieving good control had a lower incidence of both fatal and nonfatal events than did patients with fair or poor control. (Table 54–2). Since these comparisons were based on selected comparable levels of blood glucose control among the treatment groups, rather than by selection by randomization, there was no test of comparability among patients and no definite conclusions can be drawn. *This observation sets up the hypothesis, however, that the use of insulin may well provide additional therapeutic advantages to the total health of diabetic patients not produced by blood glucose changes alone.*

Finally, the investigators found NIDDM to be a more benign disease than expected. Physicians with experience only of hospital-based patients are frequently surprised to find that among middle-aged NIDDM patients all of whom were followed from a period of 12 to 14 years, 1.9% had an amputation, 1.5%

TABLE 54–1 UGDP: Number and Percentage of Patients Dead by Level of Glucose Control

	PLBO	ISTD	IVAR
Good			
No. patients at risk	46	61	78
% dead			
CV causes	23.9	9.8	11.5
Cancer	10.9	6.6	2.6
All causes	34.8	21.3	16.7
(expected)	(32.0)	(32.0)	(28.0)
Fair/Poor			
No. patients at risk	158	144	120
% dead			
CV causes	12.7	18.1	17.5
Cancer	7.6	4.9	5.0
All causes	28.0	26.4	31.7
(expected)	(28.5)	(31.3)	(29.4)

Abbreviations: PBLO, placebo; ISTD, insulin standard; IVAR, insulin variable; CV, cardiovascular.

[*Source:* Adapted from: University Group Diabetes Program: VIII. Evaluation of insulin therapy: final report. Diabetes 31 (Suppl. 5, Part 2):1–81, 1982.][14]

TABLE 54–2 Occurrence of Fatal and Nonfatal Events in Non-Insulin-Dependent Diabetes Based on the Class of Blood Glucose Control (0–14 Years)[ab]

	Good (183)	Fair (239)	Poor (185)
Retinopathy (−exudates)	38.5	48.2	57.3
Serum creatinine ≥ 1.5 mg/dL	11.6	14.0	14.4
Calcification, any	7.0	13.6	13.5
Hypertension, WHO	52.3	71.3	75.4
Death CV causes			
% of dead	27.4	32.1	40.5
% of total	12.6	11.3	18.3
Death—all causes			
% of dead	25.3	38.0	36.7
% of total	20.8	23.8	29.7

[a] Deaths: Baseline to December 31, 1971.

[b] No. subjects = 607.

Abbreviations as in Table 54–1.

[*Source:* Adapted from UGDP Data Book: UGDP Coordinating Center. 600 Wyndhurst Ave., Baltimore, MD, 21210. With permission.][15]

had retinal neovascular lesions, and 6% had abnormal ECGs with major Q-wave abnormalities (Table 54–3).

The clinical changes tabulated in Table 54–3 were of such subtle degree that the majority of the patients remained free from concerns about their health. It is the latency of the pathophysiologic changes that convinces most diabetic patients that lifestyle changes at these times are unnecessary. The benign early course of the

TABLE 54–3 The Progression of Complications in Patients with Non-Insulin-Dependent Diabetes (0–14 years)

	Percent of Patients	
	Baseline	0–14 Years
Hospitalized with CV disease	4.7	13.3
Angina pectoris	5.4	21.3
Abnormal ECG, major Q wave	0.5	6.0
Cardiac arrhythmias	3.3	17.1
Hypertension (WHO)	31.8	68.0
Hospitalized, renal disease	3.5	8.0
Serum creatinine ≥ 1.5 mg/dL	2.2	13.7
Urine protein ≥ 1 g/L	0.3	4.1
Amputation, any	0.8	1.9
Calcification, any	6.4	28.2
Claudication	4.6	22.1
Hospitalized, eye disease	4.4	14.5
Opacities, either eye	3.3	16.9
Microaneurysm	13.5	45.3
Preretinal hemorrhage	0.2	5.6
Venous pathology eye	2.7	6.8
Arterial pathology eye	0.9	1.4
Neovascular lesions	0.5	1.5
VA $\leq 20/200$	5.4	16.6

Abbreviations: CV, cardiovascular; VA, visual acuity; WHO, World Health Organization (Tech. Rep. Series No. 231, 1962).

[*Source:* Adapted Data Book UGDP, 8/31/75. With permission.]

majority, unlike those patients needing regular care as well as hospitalization for serious complications, is unfortunately only an illusion of normalcy. On the contrary, the data accumulated in Table 54–3 clearly demonstrates that there were many significant changes in both microvascular and macrovascular pathology that had occurred in the 14-year time span. For example, there has been a threefold increase in coronary artery disease and peripheral vascular disease with concomitant physical evidence in visual impairment, angina, claudication, cardiac arrhythmias, and subtle but clear evidence of early renal failure. Other comparative data have been documented in the final monograph of the UGDP.[14]

A complete reference of change over time is on file for intensive review and represents a unique store of basic clinical information for future comparisons as therapy becomes more effective over time.[15]

Fortunately, new evidence on the benefits of normalization of hyperglycemia, hyperlipidemia and blood pressure are now well documented by controlled clinical trials to be described here as sequels to the UGDP as well as in the individual chapters on management elsewhere in this text. See Chapters 2, 3, 10, 14, 15, 16, 17, 18, 19, 20, 21, 24, 38, 39, 49, 50, and 52, and Appendix I.

Diabetes Control and Complication Trial (DCCT)[16]

The second long-term clinical trial funded by NIH was the Diabetes Control and Complication Trial (DCCT).[16] The feasibility trial of the protocol which was prepared in 1982 and begun in 1983 was completed in 1985. The original 278 subjects of the feasibility study were then joined by 1, 163 recruits over the next four years to a total number of 1,441 insulin-dependent individuals. The trial, originally planned to be completed in 1994, was terminated a year in advance of schedule.

The most important aspect of the study was the test of the relative benefit of "intensive care" versus "conventional care" with levels of control in the intensive group such as to create a mean difference in the levels of hemoglobin AIC (Hgb AIC) between the two different cohorts of approximately 2% over the period of study. The details of this study have been reported elsewhere.[16]

The conclusions of the DCCT were significant. With intense therapy there was an average decrease in Hgb AIC of approximately 2% to an overall average of 7.2% or an estimated average blood glucose of 155 mg per deciliter in the intensive therapy group compared to 232 mg per deciliter in the conventional therapy group.

Reduction in the progression of retinopathy in both the Primary Prevention group (PP) and the Secondary Prevention group (SP) began in each group at about the third year into the program. After an average follow-up period of 6.5 years, the reduction of mean risk by intensive therapy (IT) over conventional therapy (CT), in PP was 76% while in SP it was 54%. Similar reduction in proliferative or severe nonproliferative retinopathy was 47% in the two cohorts combined.

Microalbuminuria excretion was down by 39%, urinary albumin excretion by 54%, and clinical neuropathy by 60%. In light of the ages of the participants and the short duration of study, more surprising and gratifying was the reduction of low density lipoproteins by 34% and macrovascular disease by 41%.

The price for these reductions in pathologic changes were not surprising. *Weight was above 120% of ideal body weight—1.6 times more often in IC than in CC and significant hypoglycemia was increased two to threefold by intensive therapy.*

Discussion continues as to the extent to which these findings can be translated to the care of patients with NIDDM, and caution is advised based on the evidence that hyperinsulinemia itself may be a risk factor for atheromatous changes over time in an aging population of diabetic patients.[17]

Genuth[18] has added a well focused analysis of cardiovascular risks in NIDDM and IDDM as seen through the results of UGDP and DCCT. For well stated reasons he finds that "neither trial provides a definitive answer to the questions about the effects of intensive insulin therapy. A better designed clinical trial is needed to determine whether Insulin treatment has beneficial or adverse effects... on the risk of cardiovascular disease in NIDDM and IDDM." He also cautions future critics of controlled clinical trials against "pruning" the results of controlled clinical trials to those portions of interlocking and complicated results that support an effect of one regimen over another and points out, for reasons already discussed, that it is not reasonable to use "tailored post hoc subgroup analyses" to produce "evidence" in support of a personal conviction. It is an appropriate paradox that the crossfire of "inappropriate data analysis" aimed at the UGDP is, in fact, a precise description of the actions taken by the authors themselves.[19] On the contrary, analysis of treatment affects utilizing the full database on all groups, as noted in Table 54–3, is consistent with the hypothesis that insulin is protective of cardiovascular events as shown by the better survival in insulin-treated patients over placebo-treated patients at similar levels of glucose control. The impact of insulin treatment of NIDDM on cardiovascular and peripheral vascular morbidity is perhaps the most important remaining therapeutic opportunity still to be properly studied in order to test the hypothesis that insulin therapy is superior to other hypoglycemic agents for prevention of complications of diabetes even at the same level of glucose control.[14]

United Kingdom Prospective Diabetes Study

The purpose of the United Kingdom Prospective Diabetes Study (UKPDS) has been to determine whether improved glucose control for patients with newly diagnosed type 2 diabetes will be successful in reducing the incidence of diabetes-related complications and diabetes-related deaths[20] (Fig. 54–1). The efforts of this brief review will be to highlight and critique the conclusions of the study group and to add other comments that may aid in understanding this monumental work. Many excellent and comprehensive reviews of the recent publications are now available. Foremost among these is "Implications of UKPDS Studies"[23] a prepared statement by the American Diabetes Association.

UKPDS-33[21]

Background: This paper must be reviewed in some detail, since it is fundamental to understanding other papers in this series. Over 3,800 newly diagnosed patients with type 2 diabetes enrolled in a randomized controlled clinical trial to study the effects of intensive treatment of diabetes using both sulfonylureas and insulin compared to the conventional treatment on diet alone on the risk of development of micro- and macrovascular complications. For the intensive treatment group, the aim of therapy was to achieve fasting plasma glucose levels (FPG) to less than 6 mmol/L. For the conventional treatment group, the aim is to get "the best achievable FPG with diet alone" with the additional safeguard that drug therapy may be used to prevent hyperglycemic symptoms or an FPG of more than 15.

Three aggregate endpoints related to diabetes are designated: (1) Diabetes-related endpoints (D-RE), (2) Diabetes-related mortality (D-RM), and (3) All-Cause Mortality (A-CM).

Findings: Over a 10-year observation period, significant differences in average FPG and Hgb AIC were maintained with a reduction of 11% by the Intensive

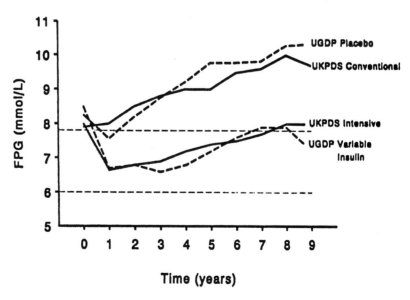

Figure 54–1.   A 9-year comparison of fasting plasma glucose (FPG) levels in the patients of the University Group Diabetes Program (UGDP) (15) who were taking either placebo or variable-insulin doses and in the cohorts of the conventional and insulin therapy groups of the United Kingdom Prospective Diabetes Study (UKPDS) studied for 9 years (20), both analyzed by assignment to therapy. The UGDP measured blood glucose levels and a correction of ×1.1 was used to give equivalent fasting plasma glucose values. The two studies have shown similar deterioration of blood glucose control over 9 years.

Therapy Group (ITG) over that of the Conventional Treatment Group (CTG). Similarly, risk for diabetes-related endpoint (D-RE) in ITG were reduced by 12%, diabetes-related mortality (D-RM) by 12%, and all cause mortality (A-CM) by 10%. There were no significant therapeutic differences between the effects of the sulfonylurea (S) and insulin (I). Hypoglycemia was more frequent as was weight gain in the ITG.

Summary: Intensive glucose control significantly decreased the risk of microvascular but not macrovascular disease. None of the individual drugs had an adverse effect on cardiovascular outcome.

Comment: The last conclusion delivered two messages. First, cardiovascular events were not decreased by intensive therapy, and second, the specific, well-documented and highly significant incidence of diabetes-related and all-cause related mortality, like that found to be related to the sulfonylurea Tolbutamide in the UGDP, was not found in this study. Unfortunately, the opportunity to restudy this problem in the UKPDS was lost for this comparison, since unlike UGDP, patients with evidence of significant cardiac disease were excluded from the study by the UKPDS. The implication that the results from the UKPDS would be able to negate the results of the UGDP regarding the use of sulfonylureas in treatment of diabetes is repeated or implied in several other areas of the UKPDS report but is obviated by their exclusion of the appropriate population. Fortunately, following subsequent research, it was found that the first and second generation sulfonylureas could cause myocardial ischemia[30-35] and the controversy was closed. Sulfonylureas released since that time require further documentation in basic research laboratories to prove their safety.

UKPDS-34[22]

Background: This study investigates whether intensive glucose control with Metformin (M) has specific advantages or disadvantages. 1,704 overweight patients with newly diagnosed type 2 diabetes were allocated for treatment as follows: CTG N = 411; M N = 342; ITG N = 951 with components CHLOR N = 265; GLIB N = 277, 1 N = 409. As stated in UKPDS-33, comparisons of endpoints are: Diabetes-related endpoints (D-RE), diabetes-related mortality (D-RM), and all-cause mortality (A-CM). A supplemental trial will be described following the results for the main allocation here.

Findings: Patients allocated to M had a reduction of risk for aggravated endpoint reduction compared to CTG as follows: (1) D-RE = 30%, (2) D-RM = 42%, and (3) A-CM = 36%. Among patients allocated to the components of ITG, M had greater effect than CHLOR, GLIB and I combined with D-RE, P = 0.034,

and only marginal benefit reduction for D-RM and A-CM (P = 0.021).

Summary: Control of blood levels of FPG at baseline were within normal limits for all drugs. Average elevations of FPG above normal became evident for most drugs after three years. After six years the average level of FPG for Metformin was above that of insulin. After nine years the average level of FPG for Metformin was equivalent to that of patients on diet alone (CTG).

Comment: For patients with type 2 diabetes, evidence that Metformin was superior to other oral agents and insulin in the long term control of fasting blood glucose levels (FPG) was not demonstrated in this study, as has been claimed in the text. FPG levels were comparable at baseline for all patient groups assigned to study medications (Insulin, Metformin, Chlorpramide, Glibenclamide) with levels of 8.0 to 8.2 mmo/L (Table 54-1, ref. 22). However, after a six-year follow-up periods, all patients on oral medications including Metformin were shown to be above baseline, and after nine years to be clustered at 10.0 mmol/L, or 25 percent above their baseline, the same level of "control" found in the Conventional Treatment Groups on "diet alone". Only the Insulin Treated Group maintained FPG at the baseline level over a 12 to 15 year period[22] (Fig. 54-3, ref. 22).

UKPDS-34, Supplemental Study

Background: An effective early lowering of FPG in both nonoverweight and overweight subjects had been demonstrated by Metformin in the main study of UKPDS-34. Most patients on maximum doses of

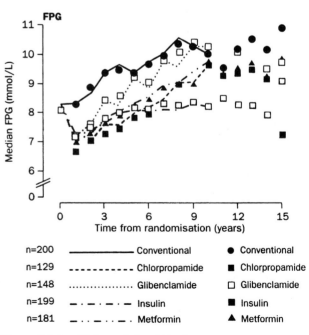

n=200	——————— Conventional	● Conventional
n=129	– – – – – – – Chlorpropamide	■ Chlorpropamide
n=148	·················· Glibenclamide	□ Glibenclamide
n=199	– · – · – · – Insulin	■ Insulin
n=181	– · · – · · – Metformin	▲ Metformin

Figure 54–2. Diabetes-Related Death.

sulfonylureas were found to have uncontrolled glucose levels. This was seen as an opportunity to test the efficacy of Metformin as a possible solution to this problem. Accordingly, 537 nonoverweight and overweight patients already on maximum sulfonylurea treatment were allocated to either continue alone on Chlorpropamide or Glibenclamide, (N = 69) or to continue on the sulfonylureas with the addition of Metformin, (N = 268).

Findings: In a surprising, unexpected and unexplained finding, there was an increase in mortality of the patients enrolled in the Metformin plus sulfonylurea group compared both to the group treated with sulfonylureas alone and, more dramatically, to the Conventional Therapy Group on diet alone. *In comparison to the latter study, there was an increase of 96% for diabetes-related mortality and a 60% increase for all-cause mortality*[21]. In an effort to determine the cause for this dramatic event, additional investigative studies were done without finding an answer. A meta-analysis was performed without identifying the source or the composition of the patient group to which they were compared. An epidemiological comparison was also made on 4,417 patients treated simultaneously with sulfonylurea and Metformin combined but lacked details as to the dosage and duration for the two medications used.

Comment: The difference in diabetes-related mortality between the cohorts of patients treated with Metformin plus sulfonylureas and sulfonylureas alone is too large to be discounted as an aberrant chance event and ignored as if this event never took place. So long as the cause of death remains unknown, there can be no justification for continuing the potential risk of using Metformin with sulfonylureas since other treatment regimens of proven safety can be readily substituted. It is therefore of some concern that the American Diabetes Association has concluded that they will not recommend any changes in current guidelines "for use of Metformin... in combination with sulfonylurea drugs." They further expressed the opinion that a "new appropriately designed... trial" can determine if there is "some specific mechanism of adverse interaction between Metformin and sulfonylurea drugs"[23] ("Question 6"). Any trial design to answer this question as a "new study" would require a full and explicit disclosure of risks in language understood at the fifth grade level to be ethically acceptable. More importantly, one must question the actual basis of conducting such a study designed primarily to determine if a drug combination is "not harmful." It is the function of Phase 1 and 2 studies, appropriately designed to test for harm, not randomized placebo controlled trials.

Before Metformin is offered as "the pharmaceutical therapy of choice" in patients with type 2 diabetes as recommended by the UKPDS group, these deaths must first be understood. This "choice" would certainly involve the decision as to whether the simultaneous use of Metformin is condoned under this "offer". One would hope, rather, that the American Diabetes Association will now, if belatedly, take a more responsible course of action on the use of Metformin and sulfonylureas together.

Conclusion: A medical disaster of this magnitude must be researched in every possible way to give some understanding as to how and why it occurred. Before meta-analysis and the examination of proxy epidemiological material are allowed to be considered as the only appropriate methods of investigation for those deaths, it must be recognized that the pertinent inquiry rests with the data generated by the patients over the nine-year duration of this study. What clinical information was available through the five-year period of observation during which these deaths occurred? On admission to hospital with their fatal last illness, these patients must have had a thorough workup of cardiac and respiratory function, as well as routine blood studies, lactic acid and drug levels, and since most were receiving maximum or near maximum doses of Metformin, blood levels would have been appropriate. Patients on Metformin and sulfonylureas began to separate themselves through diabetes-related deaths from the sulfonylurea only group at an acute upward angle immediately after randomization, as shown on the Diabetes Related Mortality graph which continued to climb throughout the remaining period (Fig. 54–2).

Data are shown for five study groups in UKPDS-34 supplemental group over a period of 16 years. The Sulfonylurea-Metformin vs. Sulfonylurea alone represent a special study added later and demonstrate their remarkable difference in mortality over the final six years of follow-up observation. Sulfonylureas, Clibenclamide, and Chlorpropamide among other potassium blocking agents, have been shown to cause cardiac death in diabetic.[31–33] Has this possibility been entirely ruled out?

Finally, how was it possible that patients placed on Metformin-Sulfonylurea vs. Sulfonylurea alone could be allowed to experience a 96% difference in their mortality compared to the conventional therapy group over a six-year period without discontinuation of the study. Was there no monitoring of these crucial data?

It cannot be repeated too often that the covenant of the medical profession with its patients in conducting randomized controlled trials is that the trial will be discontinued as soon as it is clearly shown that one therapy is either more effective or the other is less safe.

That's the other lesson that the UGDP taught a quarter of a century ago. It should never be forgotten.

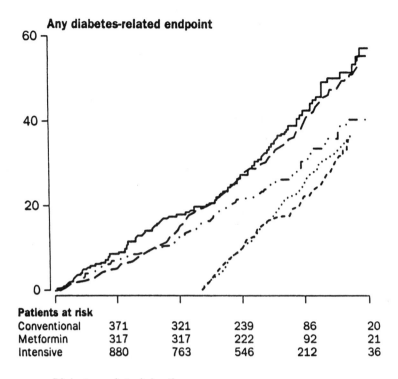

Patients at risk

Conventional	371	321	239	86	20
Metformin	317	317	222	92	21
Intensive	880	763	546	212	36

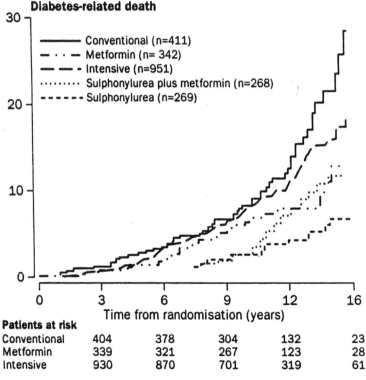

Patients at risk

Conventional	404	378	304	132	23
Metformin	339	321	267	123	28
Intensive	930	870	701	319	61

Figure 54–3. Kaplan-Meler plots in diet/metformin study for any diabetes-related clinical endpoint and diabetes-related death intensive, in this figure, indicates chlorpropamide, glibenclamide, and insulin groups. Similar plots of data for sulphonylurea/metformin study are superimposed showing relative time of commencement.

Diabetes and Ophthalmology

The importance of CCT on the practice of ophthalmology has far exceeded that in most other branches of medicine. The first such trial, the Diabetic Retinopathy Study (DRS)[24] set the standard for excellence in design and management that was followed in rapid succession by the Early Treatment Diabetic Retinopathy Study

(ETDRS)[25] which was designed to establish guidelines for the initiation of therapy before the stage of deterioration investigated in DRS. This in turn was followed by the Diabetic Vitrectomy Study (DVS)[26] to set up a study for the safety and efficacy or further use of this therapy before it proliferated into widespread practice. This is an excellent example of the impression of many that clinical trials should start with the "first case". The footnote of particular interest in this chronology is the reduction by DRS of potential candidates for DVS which precipitated an early termination of recruitment for lack of available candidates.

These important new studies in ophthalmology have now been chronicled in this volume in Chapter 26, Diabetic Eye Disease. A tribute to the work of CCT in ophthalmology cannot be better stated than that recorded in the abstract of "Ten years after the Diabetic Retinopathy Study"[27] as follows:

> "The Diabetic Retinopathy Study (DRS) demonstrated that prompt argo laser photocoagulation, in comparison to... delay in treatment, could reduce by more than 50% the risk of severe visual loss from proliferative diabetic retinopathy. The DRS also enlightened two generations of ophthalmologists about the value of random controlled clinical trials as a way of assessing new and existing treatments for unsolved therapeutic problems.... Clinical practice has benefitted enormously from these studies, all of which owe their existence at least in part to the prototypical clinical trial, the DRS."

Epilogue of the UGDP

The decision of the UGDP to discontinue treatment assigned to Tolbutamide in the original protocol, as mentioned earlier, needs further explanation and a brief follow up of more recent experimental data.

This unusual decision was dictated by the fact that one group of the four named allocations was experiencing a significant difference in mortality in reference to the other three groups under study in the UGDP, and it became ethically essential at this stage in the evolution of the trial to determine the cause of this difference. The data for this unexpected finding was then carefully analyzed and found to be related to an increased incidence of cardiovascular death in the patients receiving Tolbutamide. These results became part of the subject of the first report of this study at the American Diabetes Association meeting, June 14, 1970, as published later.[11]

The obvious need for immediate and independent examination of the data on which the decision was made led to the authorization of two independent blue ribbon audits by the FDA, one by the International Biometrics Society, and a second in-house audit by the FDA itself. Both of these groups agreed with the decision of the UGDP to discontinue the use of Tolbutamide in the study and found no reason for rejecting this conclusion. For further details, this entire process and the sequelae are clearly documented in "Clinical Trials: Design, Conduct and Analysis" by Meinert and Tonascia.[28]

No clear physiologic reason for these deaths could be ascribed to Tolbutamide, and the very fact that this fundamental question could not be given a positive answer led to concern and skepticism at that time as to the validity of the results reported.

Recently, new studies have been published on the effects of sulfonylureas on myocardial function. These studies provide a physiologic mechanism by which the unexpected mortality associated with the sulfonylureas had occurred.[29,30] Under normal physiologic circumstances, normal coronary arteries dilate when intravascular oxygen tension falls. In studies of perfused guinea pig hearts[29], it has been demonstrated that vasodilation of coronary arteries by hypoxia is mediated through potassium sensitive channels (KSC). Vasodilation can also be caused by Cromakalim, an antihypertensive drug that opens KSC. Interestingly, vasodilation of myocardial vessels caused by both hypoxia and Cromakalim are blocked by Glibenclamide, a sulfonylurea currently in use as a hypoglycemic medication. Glibenclamide can also cause a negative inotropic effect on the myocardium with reduction of the left ventricular pressure by 5 to 20%. The effect of Glibenclamide on coronary perfusion in vivo continues for one hour or longer from a single perfusion but left ventricular pressure gradients do not recover completely in a similar period of time.[32] Confirmatory studies have also been done in other laboratory animals.[30] This is the first demonstration of the physiologic basis for the increase in cardiovascular deaths in patients treated with Tolbutamide as reported by the UGDP over a quarter century ago.[11]

An elegant and carefully documented editorial by Bell[31] has brought these observations up to date and back to their original clinical setting. The demonstrations in laboratory animals of the cardiovascular effects for both first and second generation of sulfonylureas have now been demonstrated in human subjects in studies of Tolbutamide,[29] Glibenclamide,[33] and Glyburide.[30]

The editorial not only documents their negative inotropic effect on cardiac function, but more importantly, the blocking of normal coronary dilatation and ischemic reconditioning initiated by both angina[34] and angioplasty[35]. The risk of death caused by the use of these sulfonylureas can be easily avoided in diabetics known to have coronary artery disease or failure by substitution of other oral hypoglycemic agents without these adverse effects, or more positively, to move directly to the use of insulin that has already been shown to give a better immediate and long-term prognosis for life.[36] To exclude the risk inherent in the use of sulfonylureas in the 28% of diabetic patients who have advanced coronary artery disease without symptoms or signs[37], it will be necessary to avoid the use of the first and second generation sulfonylurea drugs entirely.

It will be recalled that a similar but separate CCT was also conducted on the biguanide, Phenformin[38], started 18 months after the initiation of the original group of the UGDP and separately analyzed. Concern was also aroused by adverse events due to Phenformin, leading to discontinuation of the study. Later an unacceptable incidence of lactic acidosis in clinical practice led to the withdrawal of Phenformin from further use in the United States. Metformin, also a biguanide and used in Europe for over the past 25 years, has recently been introduced into the United States and is receiving wide acceptance as a hypoglycemic agent. It is prudent to remember that the safety and efficacy of biguanides and sulfonylureas in combination, now being used widely, has yet to be proven by a well designed CCT.

Conclusion

The most impressive conclusion that can be made concerning the importance of controlled clinical trials is the recognition that most of the therapeutic advances for the past quarter century have been thoroughly evaluated and proven to be safe and effective by as a result of funding of these studies by NIH and more recently by premarketing studies paid for by industry while being supervised and required by FDA.

Unfortunately post marketing surveillance is much less actively pursued than studies of premarketing side effects and for the most part is based only on voluntary reporting. Since post marketing reporting of side effects is neither required nor considered imperative, it receives only dilatory attention from both the practicing physician and the recipient of the reports of the adverse health risks. The patient is usually unaware of the potential problem with medications until they have become significant enough to cause alarm in the news media. The public curiously is inherently suspicious of the pharmaceutical industry, in spite of careful surveillance by the FDA, but paradoxically unconcerned about the purity, adulterations or other side effects of "natural products" which are widely touted with unproven claims of success and exaggerated boasts that such products can't be harmful because "they are natural!"

Patients with diabetes are especially vulnerable to lack of information of the potential side effects and the hazards of their unsupervised use of health products. These two challenges may be destined to become the problems of growing concern in the next quarter century.

References

1. Book of Daniel, Holy Bible, The Authorized King James Version, Chapter 1, Verse 3–30.
2. Lynn, J: The treatise on the scurvy, Edinborough, Sands, Murray and Chocaran, 1753.
3. Lillenfeld, MA. Ceteris parabus: The evolution of the clinical trial. Bull. Hist. Med. 56:1–18, 1982.
4. Rush, B. An account of the bilious remitting yellow fever as it appeared in the City of Philadelphia. 1793. Philadelphia: Dobson, 1794.
5. Louis, P. Ch.A. Researches on the effects of blood letting in some inflammatory diseases and on the influence of tartolized antimony and vesication and pneumonitides, Putnam C.G., trans. Boston, Hilliard, Gray and Company 1836, 96–98.
6. Bartlett, E. Review of research by then P. Ch. A. Louis (translated by C.G. Putnam). Am J Med Sci 18:102–111, 1836.
7. Medical Research Council (1946). Streptomycin treatment of pulmonary tuberculosis. Brit Med J 2:769–782, 1948.
8. Hill, AB. Medical ethics of controlled trials. Br Med J 1:1043–1049, 1963.
9. Byar, DP et al. Randomization of clinical trials: Perspective on some recent ideas. N. Engl. J Med 295:74–80, 1976.
10. Lasagna, L. The practitioners clinical trial. N Engl J Med 307:1339–1340, 1992.
11. University Group Diabetes Program. I. Design, methods and baseline characteristics. II. Mortality results. Diabetes 19 (Suppl 2): 747–830, 1970.
12. Clinical Trials in the Study of Diabetes, T.E. Prout in Clinical Diabetes Mellitus. Ed. J.K. Davidson. Thieme Med Pub Inc., New York, First Edition, 1986; Second Edition 1991.
13. Davidson, JK. Controlling diabetes with diet therapy, Postgrad. Med 59:114–122, 1976.
14. University Group Diabetes Program: VIII. Evaluation of insulin therapy: Final report, Diabetes 31, (Suppl 5, Part 11) 1–81, 1982.
15. University Group Diabetes Program: Data book. Maryland Metabolic Institute Coordinating Center, Baltimore, MD 21210, 1971.
16. The Diabetes Control and Complications Trial Research Group. The effect of intensive treatment of diabetes on the development and progression of long-term complications in insulin-dependent diabetes mellitus. N Engl J Med 1993; 329:977–986.
17. Colwell, JA. DCCT Finding: Applicability and implications for NIDDM, Diabetes Reviews 2:277–291.
18. Genuth, S. Exogenous insulin administration and cardiovascular risk in NIDDM and IDDM. Ann Intern Med 124:1 (Part 2) 104–109, 1996.
19. Kilo, C, Williamson, J. The crux of the UGDP, Spurious results and biologically inappropriate data analysis. Diabetologia, 18:179–185, 1980.
20. UKPDS Group: UKPDS-17 A 9-year update of a randomized controlled trial on the effect of improved metabolic control on complications in NIDDM. Ann Intern Med 124:1 (Part 2) 136–145, 1996.
21. Intensive blood glucose control with sulphonylureas or insulin compared with conventional treatment and risk of conventional treatment and risk of complications in patients with type 2 diabetes (UKPDS-33) Lancet 352: 832–853, 1998.
22. Effect of intensive blood-glucose control with Metformin on complications in overweight patients with type 2 diabetes. (UKPDS 34) Lancet 352:854–865, 1998.

23. Implication of the United Kingdom Prospective Diabetes Study: American Diabetes Association. Diabetes Care 21:2180–84, 1998.

24. The Diabetic Retinopathy Study Research Group: Preliminary report on effects of protocoagulation therapy. Am J Ophthalmol 81:383–396, 1976.

25. Early Treatment Diabetic Study Group: Study report number 1. Arch Ophthalmol 103:1796–1806, 1985.

26. Diabetic Vitrectomy Study Research Group: Study report 4. Ophthalmol 95: 1321–1334, 1986.

27. Fine, SL and Patz, A. Ten years after the Diabetic Retinopathy Study. Ophthalmol 94:739–740, 1987.

28. Clinical Trials: Design, Conduct and Analysis, Curt L. Meinert, PhD and Susan Tonacia, MSC, Ch 6, Oxford University Press 1986, N.Y.

29. Hypoxic dilation of coronary arteries is mediated by ATP-sensitive potassium channels. J. Daut et al. Science 247: 1341–1344, 1990.

30. Anti-ischemic effects of potassium channel activators Pinacidil and Cromakalim and the reversal of these effects with the potassium channel blocker Glyburide. GJ Grover et al. J. Pharmacol Exp Ther: 251:98–104, 1989.

31. Bell, David SH, University Group Diabetes Program - "Deja vu all over again". Endocrine Practice, 48:64–65, 1998.

32. Bijistra, PJ, Lutterman, JA, Russel, FGM, Thien, T, Smits, P. Effects of Tolbutamide on vascular ATP-sensitive potassium channels in humans: Comparison with literature data on Glibenclamide and Glimepiride. Horm Metab Res 28:512–516, 1996.

33. Bijistra, PJ, Lutterman, JA, Russel, FGM, Thien, T, Smits, P. Interaction of sulfonylurea derivatives with vascular ATP-sensitive potassium channels in humans. Diabetologia, 39:1083–1090, 1996.

34. Andreotti, F, Pascerl, V, Halkett, DP, Davies, GJ, Haider, AW, Maseri, A. Preinfarction angina as a predictor of more rapid coronary thrombolysis in patients with acute myocardial infarction. N Engl J Med 334:7–12, 1956.

35. Tomi, F, Crea, F, Gaspardoni, A. Ischemic preconditioning during angioplasty is prevented by Glibenclamide, a selective APT-sensitive K+ channel blocker. Circulation, 90:700–705, 1994.

36. Malmberg, K, for the DIGAMI (Diabetes Mellitus Insulin Glucose Infusion in Acute Myocardial Infarction) Study Group. Prospective randomized study of intensive treatment on long term survival after acute myocardial infarction in patients with diabetes mellitus. BMJ 314: 1512–1515, 1997.

37. Waller, BF, Palumbo, PJ, Lie, TT et al. Status of the coronary arteries at necropsy in diabetes mellitus with onset after age 30 years. Am J Med 69:498–506, 1980.

38. Knatterud, GL et al. University Group Diabetes Program: A study of the effect of hypoglycemic agents on vascular complications in patients with adult-onset diabetes: V. Evaluation of Phenformin therapy. Diabetes 24(Suppl): 65–84, 1975.

55

Analysis and Interpretation of Results from Clinical Trials

Curtis L Meinert

This chapter focuses on issues concerning the analysis and interpretation of results of trials. The bibliography supporting this chapter and the supplementary readings and references listed at the end of this chapter are for persons desiring more in-depth treatment of this subject.

Design Issues Affecting Data Analysis and Interpretation

The foundation for any analytic effort is laid when the trial is designed. Decisions in such matters as the treatments to be evaluated, patient selection criteria, and choice of the outcome measures for assessing treatment are basic to subsequent analysis. The clinical relevance of the trial will be determined, in large measure, by the decisions made.

The best outcome measure is a clinical event that can be reliably observed and recorded. Obviously, the clinical relevance of a trial demonstrating a difference in mortality, or in some morbidity measure, is greater than for one showing a difference in a surrogate measure considered to be a predictor of clinical outcome.

The choice of the outcome and its characteristics have direct bearing on the number of patients needed in a trial. Trials involving outcome events that occur at low frequencies will require larger numbers of patients or longer periods of follow-up than those involving outcome events occurring at higher frequencies.

The importance of sample size and power calculations has been discussed by various authors.[1–3] It should be obvious that trials should not be undertaken in the absence of plans to achieve an adequate sample size, typically as produced by a traditional sample size calculation.[4] The calculation serves two needs: first, the need to define the outcome measure that will be used for assessment of treatment effects and, second, the need to establish a recruitment goal for the trial.

The majority of trials reported involve samples sizes in the 10s and 100s when they should be in the 100s and 1000s, are single-center when they should be multicenter, and involve short courses of treatment and follow-up when both of these factors should be long. Hence, the approach to sample size should be to determine what is required to answer a question, rather than rationalizing what is possible and affordable.

The evaluation of the test treatment requires a comparable group of control-treated patients. In an ideal world one would select control-treated patients matched to test-treated patients with regard to important predictive characteristics. Usually, however, such matching is out of the question. It is difficult enough to find suitable patients for a trial, let alone matched pairs of patients, even if the matching is for only just a few variables.

A few treatments can be evaluated without the concurrent enrollment and follow-up of a control-treated group of patients. The effect achieved with a new miracle treatment (e.g., when insulin was discovered by Banting and Best, see Chapter 1) contrasted with experience in the absence of the treatment may be sufficient to demonstrate its virtue without a designed experiment. Unfortunately, the additive effects of most new treatments are modest, so they must be assessed against control-treated groups enrolled and followed over the same time frame as that for the test treatments.

All designed trials rest on the assumption that the test and control study groups are created using assignment processes that are free of patient and physician selection biases. Systematic methods of assignment, such as those where every other patient is assigned to the test treatment, are not acceptable because of the potential for selection biases. The same is true for self-administered schemes involving the use of numbered envelopes unless there are adequate safeguards to ensure that the envelopes are used in the proper order.

The best procedures are those in which a patient is assigned to the test or control treatment using a formal randomization process and where that assignment remains unknown to both the physician and patient until the patient has agreed to be enrolled and is ready to start treatment. Even then, the assignment may not be revealed if the trial is masked (blind). The choice of test and control treatments will determine whether or not masked administration is possible. It is not in most surgical trials but is in drug trials where it is ethical to use a placebo as a control treatment or where the different study drugs can be packaged and administered in identical fashion.

Masking is usually out of the question in trials where drug dosage is titrated on a per-patient basis. Furthermore, even when masking is done, it is rarely 100% effective. Side effects that are unique to the test or control treatment may unmask.

A trial does not have to be masked to be valid. Unmasked trials can yield perfectly valid results if the outcome measures can be observed and reported free of treatment-related biases.

Analysis Philosophies and Mistakes

Responsible investigators will establish the ground rules by which they plan to carry out their data analyses before any data are collected. Those ground rules will indicate:

1. The point at which a patient is considered enrolled into the trial (generally when the treatment assignment is issued)

2. The outcome to be used for primary evaluation of the treatment groups

3. How data for patients who did not or could not follow the treatment protocol will be handled

Defining ground rules from the outset will help avoid mistakes later on when results are analyzed.

A practice to be avoided is "data dredging" (ad hoc analyses done during or at the end of the trial without benefit of prior hypotheses that are performed simply to identify differences of note). The medical literature is replete with reports arising from such dredging. The reanalysis of the University Group Diabetes Program (UGDP) tolbutamide results by Kilo and coworkers[5] is a case in point. The authors performed dozens of treatment subgroup analyses and used p values of 0.05 or less as indicators of "significance." They failed to recognize that the frequentist's approach to data analysis and hypothesis testing must be performed under specified constructs if it is to produce useful information. A subgroup identified via a series of ad hoc analyses yielding a given appropriately small p value is far more likely to be due to chance than is one identified a priori yielding the same size p value.

The likelihood of finding some comparison that yields a p value beyond the magical 5% level approaches

unity with the number of ad hoc comparisons done. The work of Canner[6] in the Coronary Drug Project (CDP)[7] indicates that one must achieve conventional p values beyond the 0.01 level before they should be given any real credence.

A second practice to be shunned stems from the desire of investigators, once the trial is finished, to restrict their analyses to the subset of patients who received the "appropriate" treatment or who had the "proper" response to it. The elimination of patients for analysis purposes, for whatever reason, is fraught with difficulties. The UGDP was criticized because investigators from the study based their conclusions on treatment comparisons formed using the original treatment assignment. The analysis approach meant that some patients, while being counted as members of the treatment group to which they had been assigned at the outset, received little or none of that treatment or, worse yet, received one of the other study treatments. Some critics of the study would have had investigators exclude some patients from all data analyses done or retain them but place them in treatment groups dictated by the treatments actually administered.[8–12] The treatment assignment process in any randomized trial is designed to eliminate opportunity for patient or physician selection biases. The risks of such biases coming into play at the time of data analysis are enormous with any rearrangement of patients across treatment groups based on data collected after randomization.

The standard analysis approach espoused by virtually all card-carrying biostatistician-trialists is to perform key analyses by counting patients in the treatment groups to which they were originally assigned, even if some patients received little or none of the assigned treatment. This approach may obscure differences between the treatment groups if there were departures from the treatment protocol. There is a risk of missing differences that might have emerged if there had been perfect treatment adherence. One might do additional analyses that take account of treatment adherence (e.g., as done in the UGDP), but they must be interpreted with caution because of the potential for selection biases.

A third practice to be avoided is counting and reporting only selected outcomes in published reports of trials. The Anturane Reinfarction Trial (ART) serves as a case in point. Investigators based their primary analyses on counts of deaths that excluded those that occurred in patients within the first 7 days of treatment.[13,14] They made the exclusions on the assumption that it would take a minimum of 7 days for Anturane to reach its full therapeutic effect. Much of the furor created over the study could have been avoided had primary analyses been based on all deaths, rather than on the subset used. The investigators could have presented a second set of analyses using the 7-day rule if they so desired. Incidentally, subsequent analyses with all deaths did not alter the interpretation of the study findings.[15]

A fourth and related practice to be avoided has to do with analyses that focus on deaths due to a certain cause to the exclusion of deaths from other causes. That approach is always troublesome, especially when certain kinds of deaths are ignored because they are believed to be unrelated to treatment. If the assumption is correct, there is no harm in including them since the numbers added should be about the same across treatment groups. If it is not correct, one runs the risk of reaching an erroneous conclusion by eliminating them. For example, one cannot interpret the meaning of a treatment difference in cardiovascular mortality without first looking at comparisons involving all-cause mortality.

A fifth practice to be avoided is undue reliance on hypothesis testing and p values as a vehicle for data analysis. The tendency of authors publishing in medical journals simply to categorize results as significant or nonsignificant, depending on whether or not the observed p values reach some magical level (usually 0.05), represents a naive approach to analysis and interpretation of data. The medical literature remains cluttered with far too many articles in which treatment differences are labeled as "S" or "NS" depending on whether or not they reached a specified level of significance. Statistically sophisticated investigators will rely on p values primarily as data descriptors. They will avoid using them as absolute indicators of truth and will pay more attention to the trend of the observed differences over time and to the internal consistency of the results than to the fact of whether or not differences exceed a specified p level.

Reporting Requirements

Exhibit 55–1 lists items of information that should be covered in published manuscripts (see also References).[4,16,17] The results of the analyses and the authors' interpretation of those results should be published in peer-reviewed, indexed journals.

Information on the design and methods used for creating the study groups and for data collection is essential if readers are to understand the results presented. The absence of details on fundamental points such as the method of randomization will, of necessity, leave readers in doubt as to whether or not patient or physician selection biases operated when the treatment groups were created or analyzed. Those details should be supplemented with data on the comparability of the study groups with regard to important demographic and baseline characteristics. In addition, the report should contain sufficient details to allow readers to determine whether or not questionable practices such as those discussed earlier were followed. It should give the actual numbers of patients enrolled in the various treatment groups. Any discrepancies between these numbers and those used for comparisons of the treatment groups should be explained.

The report should contain information on patient and physician compliance to the treatment protocol. As noted in the previous section, it may include results for the subgroup of patients with good compliance, but only if they are accompanied by other more basic *analyses, absent exclusions.*

The report should indicate if only a portion of the results are being reported and, if so, the reasons for this. As noted, explanations are required for any exclusions from the study population occurring after

---

EXHIBIT 55–1   Reporting Recommendations

Descriptive title	Level of treatment masking
Indication of key words for use by the National Library of	Method of data analysis
Medicine indexers	Participating personnel, clinics, and other support centers
Informative abstract that indicates	Organizational structure, especially in multicenter trials
Purpose of study	Results section that indicates
Size of study	Number of patients enrolled per treatment group
Treatments used	Number of dropouts and exclusions during the trial
Primary outcome measure	Baseline comparability of the treatment groups
Key findings and conclusion	Level of adherence to the treatment protocol
Background information that indicates	Conclusions that indicate
Motivation for trial	Main findings and presumed relevance of the findings
Funding sources	Limits on inferences from the trial
Review of pertinent background literature	Literature references
Design and methods information that indicates	Appendices or instructions for how readers may obtain
Rationale for sample size	Manual of operations
Rationale for choice of treatments	Study forms
Outcome measures and rationale	Detailed data listings
Method of treatment assignment	

randomization as well as for exclusions related to the outcome measures used for treatment comparisons.

The report should indicate the source of funding for the trial and the geographic location of the centers in the study. Investigators engaged in studies involving proprietary products have a responsibility to disclose conflicts of interest in relation to the study. Readers have a right to know the role of the vendor of the product being tested and the amount of funding and other perquisites provided to investigators by the firm. The National Cooperative Gallstone Study (NCGS)—a government-funded trial involving an evaluation of a commercial product—required all study investigators, including members of the policy-review and data-monitoring committees, to file disclosure statements regarding potential conflicts of interest.[18,19] The Persantine Aspirin Reinfarction Trial—a study funded by the manufacturer of Persantine—precluded members of the study from receiving funds from the manufacturer during the course of the trial (other than those needed to carry out the trial).[20,21]

Interpretation and Generalizations

Clinical trials, by definition, deal with select groups of patients. The selection occurs because of the consent process required and because of the need to homogenize the study population with regard to selected demographic and disease characteristics. Investigators often find themselves on the horns of a dilemma when specifying patient selection criteria for the trial. On the one hand, they know that the more homogeneous the study population, the smaller the sample size needed to detect a difference of a given size. On the other hand, they also recognize that the more restrictive they are, the more difficult it will be to meet the patient recruitment goal set for the trial.

People often confuse validity and generalizability. A trial with an assignment process that is free of selection bias and with data-collection procedures free of treatment-related observer error has validity. Those who would summarily dismiss the results of a trial because of the select nature of the population studied overlook this fundamental fact. The problem has to do with the generalizations that can be made from findings, not with their validity. The greater the size and diversity of the study population, the more secure one is in generalizing. Unfortunately, no population for a randomized trial, regardless of how it was selected, can ever match one's own population as seen in ordinary practice settings. Inferences are necessary in which one assumes that patients with characteristics similar to those studied will yield results similar to those seen in the study. In fact, it is often unreasonable to assume otherwise, unless there are sound reasons for doing so.

Generalizations to other types of study patients (e.g., to older patients or to patients who are more diseased than those studied) must be made on a judgmental, nonstatistical basis. The same is true for generalizations to related forms of treatment. Generalizations of this type are important, particularly in drug trials designed to focus on selected members of a larger family of drugs, such as in the UGDP, with tolbutamide as a member of the family of sulfonylurea compounds tested. There is no way of being certain as to whether or not the results associated with tolbutamide are also applicable to other members of that family of drugs without additional trials.

In the end, one's faith in the generalizations made depend in large measure on the study design and on the type and quality of data generated by that design. A poorly designed or executed trial that generates data of marginal quality, no matter how convincing the results may be, should not be used to make generalizations. Furthermore, one's faith in a set of results depends on the extent to which they are supported by results from previous trials. Unfortunately, the amount of information available in this regard is often limited because of the lack of previous trials. One cannot use observational data, especially when such data are collected in willy-nilly fashion and are subject to a variety of biases, to support or refute findings from designed trials. Trials, as noted by Fredrickson,[22] represent an ordeal, but they are indispensable if we are to assess the relative merits of the treatments we use.

References

1. Chalmers TC, Smith H Jr, Blackburn B, et al.: A method for assessing the quality of a randomized control trial. Controlled Clin Trials 2:31–49, 1981.

2. Freiman JA, Chalmers TC, Smith H Jr, et al.: The importance of beta, the type II error and sample size in the design and interpretation of the randomized control trial: Survey of 71 "negative" trials. New Engl J Med 299: 690–694, 1978.

3. Mosteller F, Gilbert JP, McPeek B: Reporting standards and research strategies for controlled trials. Controlled Clin Trials 1:37–58, 1980.

4. Meinert CL, Tonascia S: Clinical Trials: Design, Conduct, and Analysis. New York: Oxford University Press, 1986.

5. Kilo C, Miller JP, Williamson P: The Achilles heel of the University Group Diabetes Program. JAMA 243:450–457, 1980.

6. Canner PL: Monitoring treatment differences in long-term clinical trials. Biometrics 33:603–615, 1977.

7. Coronary Drug Project Research Group: Practical aspects of decision making in clinical trials: The Coronary Drug Project as a case study. Controlled Clin Trials 1:363–376, 1981.

8. University Group Diabetes Program Research Group: A study of the effects of hypoglycemic agents on vascular complications in patients with adult-onset diabetes: I. Design, methods and baseline characteristics. Diabetes 19(Suppl 2):747–783, 1970.

9. University Group Diabetes Program Research Group: A study of the effects of hypoglycemic agents on vascular complications in patients with adult-onset diabetes: II. Mortality results. Diabetes 19(Suppl 2):785–830, 1970.

10. Feinstein AR: Clinical biostatistics—VIII. An analytic appraisal of the University Group Diabetes Program (UGDP) study. Clin Pharmacol Ther 12:167–191, 1971.

11. Schor S: The University Group Diabetes Program: A statistician looks at the mortality results. JAMA 217:1671–1675, 1971.

12. Seltzer HS: A summary of criticisms of the findings and conclusions of the University Group Diabetes Program (UGDP). Diabetes 21:976–979, 1972.

13. Anturane Reinfarction Trial Research Group: Sulfinpyrazone in the prevention of cardiac death after myocardial infarction. New Engl J Med 298:289–295, 1978.

14. Anturane Reinfarction Trial Research Group: Sulfinpyrazone in the prevention of sudden death after myocardial infarction. New Engl J Med 302:250–256, 1980.

15. Temple R, Pledger GW: Special report: The FDA's critique of the Anturane Reinfarction Trial. New Engl J Med 303:1488–1492, 1980.

16. Meinert CL, Tonascia S, Higgins K: Content of reports on clinical trials: A critical review. Controlled Clin Trials 5:328–347, 1984.

17. Meinert CL: A critical eye: The science of reading research papers. Diabetes Spectrum 1:13–15, 1988.

18. National Cooperative Gallstone Study Group: Design and methodological considerations in the National Cooperative Gallstone Study: A multicenter clinical trial. Controlled Clin Trials 2:177–229, 1981.

19. National Cooperative Gallstone Study Group: Chenodiol (chenodeoxycholic acid) for dissolution of gallstones: The National Cooperative Gallstone Study: A controlled trial of efficacy and safety. Ann Intern Med 95:257–282, 1981.

20. Persantine—Aspirin Reinfarction Study Research Group: Persantine—Aspirin Reinfarction Study: Design, methods and baseline results. Circulation 62(Suppl II):II-1–II-42, 1980.

21. Persantine—Aspirin Reinfarction Study Research Group: Persantine and aspirin in coronary heart disease. Circulation 62:449–461, 1980.

22. Frederickson DS: The field trial: Some thoughts on the indispensable ordeal. Bull NY Acad Med 44:985–993, 1968.

Selected Readings

Bailar JC III, Mosteller F (eds.): Medical Uses of Statistics. Waltham, MA NEJM Books, 1986.

Breddin KH, Klimt CR (eds.): Second International Symposium on Long-Term Clinical Trials. Controlled Clin Trials 1:281–442, 1981.

Chalmers TC, Amacher P (eds.): Proceedings of a Conference on Recent History of Randomized Clinical Trials. Controlled Clin Trials 3:163–309, 1982.

Fletcher RH, Fletcher SW: Clinical epidemiology: A new discipline for an old art (editorial). Ann Intern Med 99:401–403, 1983.

Fletcher RH, Fletcher SW, Wagner EH: Clinical Epidemiology: The Essentials. Baltimore: Williams & Wilkins, 1982.

Friedman LM, Furberg CD, DeMets DL: Fundamentals of Clinical Trials. Boston: John Wright, PSG, 1985.

Hulley SB, Cummings SR, with major contributions by Browner WS, Newman TB, Hearst N: Designing Clinical Research: An Epidemiologic Approach. Baltimore: Williams & Wilkins, 1988.

Meinert CL: Clinical Trials Dictionary: Terminology and Usage Recommendations. Baltimore: The Johns Hopkins Center for Clinical Trials, 1996.

Piantadosi S: Clinical Trials: A Methodologic Perspective. New York: Wiley, 1997.

Roth HP, Gordon RH, Jr (eds.): Proceedings of the National Conference on Clinical Trials Methodology. Clin Pharmacol Ther 25:629–766, 1979.

Sackett DL, Haynes RB, Tugwell P: Clinical Epidemiology: A Basic Science for Clinical Medicine. Boston: Little, Brown, 1985.

Shapiro SH, Louis TA (eds.): Clinical Trials: Issues and Approaches. New York: Marcel Dekker, 1983.

Yusuf S, Wittes J, Probstfield J, et al.: Analysis and interpretation of treatment effects in subgroups of patients in randomized clinical trials. JAMA 266:93–98, 1991.

Appendices

APPENDIX I

World Health Organization Diabetes Programs

Hilary King

The World Health Organization (WHO) is the foremost intergovernmental agency in the health field and is a specialized agency of the United Nations. The highest governing body of the Organization consists of the Governments of 191 Member States, which convene in Geneva each May at the World Health Assembly. The functions of WHO include the provision of international leadership in public health, and of advice to member Governments on appropriate policies and strategies for health promotion and disease prevention and control.

The objective of WHO is the attainment by all peoples of the highest possible level of health, which is defined as "complete physical, mental and spiritual well-being, and not just the absence of disease or infirmity." For the past two decades, WHOs approach to achieving "health for all" has been through the concept of Primary Health Care. The most important components of this approach are universal accessibility of health services, community involvement, intersectoral action, and provision of appropriate and cost-effective technology. Recently, WHO launched an initiative for the renewal of the Health for All policy, to enable it to meet the challenges of the twenty-first century. The policy, together with a global health charter, will be submitted to the World Health Assembly in May 1998.[1]

WHO operates at three levels: globally, regionally, and nationally. Global activities are coordinated by WHO Headquarters in Geneva. Headquarters programs provide technical expertise and direction, set norms and standards in the health field, and coordinate global and interregional activities. There are six WHO Regions and Regional Offices: for the African Region, Brazzaville; for The American Region, Washington, DC; for the Eastern Mediterranean Region, Alexandria; for the European Region, Copenhagen; for the Southeast Asian Region, New Delhi; and for the Western Pacific Region, Manila. These offices are responsible for regional programs and for assistance with national program development. Nationally, the WHO Country Offices liaise directly with the national authorities to determine priorities and initiate health programs and activities.

The Diabetes Program at WHO Headquarters

The WHO Headquarters diabetes program operates under five principal areas of work:

The Normative Function

WHO Expert Committees in 1964[2] and 1979[3] and WHO Study Groups in 1985[4] and 1992[5] have each produced Technical Reports with recommendations on diagnosis, classification, treatment, management, and research needs for diabetes, which have received widespread international approval. The diagnostic criteria for abnormal glucose tolerance recommended in these reports have become the international standard. The classification and diagnostic criteria were recently reviewed at a WHO Consultation in 1996 (report in press) and were subject to some modification in light of new knowledge.

Epidemiology and Surveillance

The WHO diabetes program collates and disseminates global statistics on diabetes epidemiology. The first such publication of prevalence, estimates for 75 communities in 32 countries, appeared in 1993.[6] In 1997 numerical estimates and projections for the frequency of adult diabetes in all WHO Member States appeared in the World Health Report and a detailed report appeared in an International Journal in 1998.[18] In addition, the Program regularly advises on the planning and conduct of diabetes and noncommunicable risk factor surveys. Recent examples include Bolivia, Ghana, Qatar, Oman, Pakistan, and Uzbekistan. WHO has supported two international investigations in diabetes epidemiology, the WHO Multinational Study of Vascular Disease in Diabetes and the WHO Multinational Project for Childhood Diabetes (DIAMOND).

Training and Education

The Program assists with planning, fundraising, and conduct of epidemiology and public health training courses at the global and the regional level. Global courses have been held in Cambridge, United Kingdom, on seven occasions since 1981. Many leading diabetes epidemiologists have been participants of Cambridge courses and some have subsequently organized their own training courses at the regional level. Recent regional courses have been conducted in Cameroon, Colombia, Cyprus, Hawaii and South Africa. Currently, there is interest in developing training materials for dissemination via the Internet.

Development of National Programs

Following the Resolution on Prevention and Control of Diabetes Mellitus which was adopted by the World Health Assembly in 1989[7] as well as regional initiatives described below, many governments have developed their own national diabetes programs, with the assistance of WHO Headquarters and Regional Offices. WHO Headquarters arranged the preparation of guidelines for national diabetes program development.[8] National diabetes programs usually include the following key elements: an initial situational analysis, the definition of minimum standards of care, elaboration of preventive strategies, provision of essential drugs and supplies, training and health manpower development, establishment of a patient tracking and surveillance system for more effective health-care delivery, and a means of monitoring and evaluating the program. In 1994 the first global meeting on national diabetes programs was held in Geneva.[9]

A global Information Service

The Program receives numerous requests for information on all aspects of diabetes from national authorities, the private sector, individual health-care providers, students and people affected by diabetes and their families. Since 1995, the Program has released an annual newsletter called *World Diabetes*, which has proven a popular means of keeping in touch with its many friends and colleagues around the world.

The WHO Regional Diabetes Programs

The St. Vincent Declaration

The first WHO Region to adopt a supranational diabetes program was that of Europe, with the now well-known St. Vincent Declaration Action Program[10] coordinated jointly by WHO Europe and the International Diabetes Federation (IDF) European Region. The meeting which gave birth to the St. Vincent Declaration was held in the small town of St. Vincent, near Aosta in northern Italy in 1989—the same year as the adoption of the World Health Assembly resolution on diabetes. The Declaration set general goals and also specific targets for reducing morbidity and mortality due to diabetes. Guidelines for the prevention of specific complications were prepared.[11] This initiative has resulted in the establishment of national task forces and in diabetes program implementation an almost all countries of the Region. A key element of the project was the development of a basic data sheet, by which participating countries and institutions can monitor improvements in quality of diabetes care. See Appendix XI.

Eastern Mediterranean Program for Diabetes

Recognizing the growing problem of diabetes in populations of the Region, the WHO Regional Office for the Eastern Mediterranean instituted a regional diabetes program in 1991. Several regional meetings and consultations have taken place and these have resulted in the preparation of regionally appropriate guidelines for diabetes prevention and control[12] for standards of diabetes care and clinical practice guidelines[13] and for diabetes education.[14] Assistance has been given to epidemiological research and almost 20 Member States of the Region have begun planning or implementation of national diabetes programs.

Guidelines for the Management of Diabetes in Africa

The formation of a Pan-African Diabetes Study Group, with the support from IDF and WHO Regional Offices, has resulted in the appearance in 1996 of a consensus document on the treatment of noninsulin-dependent diabetes in Africa.[15] The objectives of the guidelines are the provision of information to promote early detection and effective management of diabetes, the achievement of lifestyle modification for prevention and control, the development of criteria for prevention, and treatment of diabetic complications and the integration of diabetes health care into noncommunicable disease programs within existing national health-care systems.

Diabetes Declaration of the Americas

In view of the emerging public health impact of diabetes, the Pan-American Health Organization (PAHO), which coordinates the work of WHO in the Region, recognized diabetes as a priority area for its newly formed Noncommunicable Disease Program in 1995. In due course, this led to official relations being established between PAHO and the IDF. At a meeting in Puerto Rico in 1996 a Declaration on Diabetes in the Americas was released. The Declaration was subsequently endorsed at the 1996 meeting of the PAHO Directing Council, confirming the official perception of diabetes as a condition of regional public health importance.[16] The Declaration is intended to set in motion similar processes as did the St. Vincent Declaration in Europe. An assessment of the state of readiness of national authorities is being conducted and minimum essential national targets have been distributed to all countries. An administrative structure is being developed and task forces will address major issues such as communications, education, policies, and procedures.

Other WHO Regional Initiatives

A meeting at the WHO Regional Office for South East Asia in New Delhi has led to the development of an initiative for the integrated prevention and control of noncommunicable diseases, with the focus on cancer, cardiovascular diseases, and diabetes. Demonstration projects will be established in several countries of the region. The WHO Regional Office for the Western Pacific is developing a regional profile on cardiovascular diseases and diabetes with the assistance of a WHO collaborating center in Australia.

Partnerships for Health

The WHO Collaborating Center Network

To assist it in its various tasks and program activities, the WHO diabetes program has developed a network of over 30 collaborating centers in the field of diabetes. They are well-recognized centers of excellence and they can do much to enhance the work of WHO. In the past, most centers have been situated in Europe and North America. Recently, there has been a determined attempt to create official links with diabetes centers in developing countries, with designations occurring in Africa, the Eastern Mediterranean, and South America.

Collaborating centers can assist WHO in many ways. Most are actively involved in training and dissemination of information, in addition to their usual clinical activities. Staff of the centers may act as WHO consultants on specific projects. Two recent WHO meetings on diabetes were organized by WHO collaborating centers, which also raised the necessary funds.

WHO and the International Diabetes Federation

The IDF is a nongovernmental organization (NGO), which currently represents individual member associations in 121 countries. The mission of IDF is to work with these associations to enhance the health of people with diabetes. IDF was formed in 1950, 2 years after

WHO, and it held its first congress in 1952. IDF entered into official relations with WHO in 1957. See Appendix II.

The WHO diabetes program and IDF have developed a strong partnership. The two organizations are complementary because WHO advises at the level of government, whereas IDF works more at the "grass roots." In terms of national program development, a joint approach may be highly effective, as has been demonstrated by the St. Vincent Declaration and Declaration of the Americas initiatives.

World Diabetes Day is another example of this partnership. World Diabetes Day is observed on 14 November each year (the birth date of Frederick Banting, who discovered insulin in 1921). The Day is a public awareness campaign that was initiated by the IDF in 1991, and which has been co-sponsored by WHO from the outset. Each year, a special theme is selected. World Diabetes Day offers the IDF the opportunity to distribute publicity and information to its member associations, which encourages them to organize events at the national and local level. WHO usually releases a press release through the United Nations media network and this results in attention in the international press and radio.

Recognizing the scope of joint activities, a WHO/IDF Working Group was established in 1995. This reviews progress on joint activities and plans for future projects and events.

WHO and the Private Sector

Traditionally, WHO programs were not encouraged to obtain resources from commercial enterprises. However, with the erosion of resources available for health promotion and disease prevention, a new attitude has emerged, whereby the private sector is seen as an ally of the international agencies. The WHO diabetes program is in the vanguard of this trend, which is not limited to the transfer of resources, but also involves active collaboration in projects. Currently, the large majority of program activities at Headquarters level are supported from external sources.

The World Health Report 1997: Conquering Suffering, Enriching Humanity

Each year, the World Health Organization issues its World Health Report, to coincide with the World Health Assembly. In 1997, for the first time, the report was focused on the growing threat to public health posed by the noncommunicable diseases, particularly cancers, cardiovascular diseases, chronic respiratory diseases, and diabetes.[17]

In the introduction it was noted that:

> Worldwide, life expectancy has increased dramatically during the last decades of the 20th century. But in celebrating our extra years, we must recognize that increased longevity without quality of life is an empty prize, i.e., **health expectancy** is more important than **life expectancy**

Unlike many infectious diseases, the majority of chronic diseases are preventable but cannot yet be cured. The emphasis must therefore be on preventing their onset, delaying their development in later life, reducing the suffering that they cause, and providing the supportive social environment to care for those disabled by them.

The World Health Report 1997 paid much attention to diabetes. It warned that diabetes was one of the most daunting challenges posed today by chronic diseases, by virtue of its frequency and the cost and suffering imposed by its complications. It included a description of diabetes in New Zealand, where the minority Maori and Pacific Islands communities were much more severely affected than were the majority population who are of European origin. This illustrates the fact that had become increasingly evident from epidemiological studies, that diabetes was no longer a disease of the affluent. The report concluded that *developing countries will bear the brunt of the diabetes epidemic in the 21st century.*

The World Health Report 1997 highlighted the recently completed WHO study to determine the worldwide frequency of diabetes. The results of this project indicated that approximately 135 million adults suffered from diabetes in 1995 and that this number will likely rise to 300 million by the year 2025, as a result of population ageing and urbanization. Seventy-five percent of these will reside in developing countries. The estimates and projections for each of the WHO regions is shown (Fig. I–1). The Report includes prevalence of diabetes as one of its chosen **basic health indicators** for its Member States, the first noncommunicable disease to appear in this context.

Traditionally, WHO and other international health agencies have accorded priority to basic public health (sanitation, safe water, vaccination, etc.) and to the major infectious diseases. The World Health Report 1997 provides a landmark and a turning point for those who have been advocating for greater attention to be accorded to diabetes and other chronic noncommunicable diseases. In 1998, a new administration took over the leadership of WHO. Substantial structural and administrative reforms have been introduced. In the process, noncommunicable diseases have been officially recognized as a priority area for the organization in the 21st century.

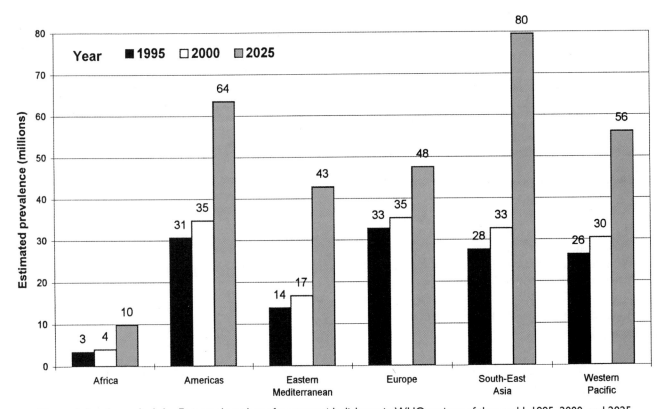

Figure I–1. Appendix I–1—Estimated number of persons with diabetes in WHO regions of the world, 1995, 2000, and 2025.

References

1. World Health Organization: Health for All in the 21st century. Newsletter, Summer 1987. Geneva: 1997.

2. World Health Organization: Diabetes mellitus. Report of a WHO Expert Committee. Technical Report Series no. 310. Geneva: 1965.

3. World Health Organization: Expert Committee on Diabetes Mellitus: Second Report. Technical Report Series no. 646. Geneva: World Health Organization, 1980.

4. World Health Organization: Diabetes mellitus. Report of a WHO Study Group. Technical Report Series no. 727. Geneva: 1985.

5. World Health Organization: Prevention of diabetes mellitus. Report of a WHO Study Group. Technical Report Series no. 844. Geneva: 1994.

6. King H, Rewers M, WHO Ad Hoc Diabetes Reporting Group: Global estimates for the prevalence of diabetes and impaired glucose tolerance in adults. Diabetes Care, 16:157–177, 1993.

7. World Health Organization: Prevention and control of diabetes mellitus. *In* Handbook of Resolutions. Vol. III, 2nd ed. (1985–1989). Geneva: 1990, p. 71 (WHA42.36).

8. Reiber G, King H: Guidelines for the development of a national programme for diabetes mellitus (WHO/DBO/DM/91.1). Geneva: World Health Organization, 1991.

9. King H, Gruber W, Lander T (eds): Implementing national diabetes programmes. Report of a WHO meeting (WHO/DBO/DM/95.2). Geneva: World Health Organization, 1995.

10. Diabetes Research and Care in Europe: the St. Vincent Declaration Action Programme (EUR/ICP/CLR 055/3). Copenhagen: WHO Regional Office for Europe, 1992.

11. Krans HMJ, Porta M, Keen H, Staehr Johansen K (eds): Diabetes care and research in Europe: The St. Vincent Declaration action programme. Implementation document. Giornale Italiano di Diabetologia 15:1, 1995.

12. Diabetes prevention and control. A call for action (WHO-EM/DIA/3/E/G). Alexandria, WHO Regional Office for the Eastern Mediterranean, 1993.

13. World Health Organization: Management of diabetes mellitus. Standards of care and clinical practice guidelines (WHO-EM/DIA/6/E/G). Alexandria: WHO Regional Office for the Eastern Mediterranean, 1994.

14. World Health Organization: Health education for people with diabetes (WHO-EM/DIA/7-E/G). Alexandria: WHO Regional Office for the Eastern Mediterranean, 1996.

15. Mbanya J-C, Bonnici F, Nagati K (eds): Guidelines for the management of non insulin dependent diabetes mellitus (NIDDM) in Africa. Athens: Novo Nordisk A/S, 1996.

16. Special Report: Diabetes—a Declaration for the Americas. Bulle Pan Am Health Organ 30:261–265, 1996.

17. World Health Organization: World Health Report 1997. Conquering suffering, enriching humanity. Geneva: 1997.

18. King H, Aubert RE, Herman WH: Global burden of diabetes, 1995–2025. Diabetes Care 21:1414–1431, 1998.

APPENDIX II

The International Diabetes Federation: Its Role, Objectives, Achievements and Perspectives

Jak Jervell

As of 1999, the International Diabetes Federation (IDF) is a federation of 161 member associations in 129 countries. Through its extended membership, the IDF directly represents an estimated 1.2 million individuals, more than 90% are people with diabetes and people close to them, less than 10% are health-care professionals. These numbers have grown rapidly in recent years, a trend that is expected to continue until all countries of the world have an IDF Member Association. The IDF also has individual members, including more than 300 life members. Many leading diabetes industry corporations are supporting are members.

IDF Leadership

Since the start of the IDF in 1950 until 1991, IDF presidents have all been medical professionals, usually professors of medicine. At the 14th IDF congress in Washington, DC, Wendell Mayes, Jr. became the first nonmedical president. He is the father of a son with diabetes, and has worked for a long time for diabetes through the American Diabetes Association and IDF. His managerial skills and personal qualities have demonstrated to all of us the value of joint leadership between nonmedical and medical experts in the IDF.

The IDF elects its president 3 years in advance. I was elected president-elect in Washington in 1991, and became president after Wendell in Kobe in 1994. Maria de Alva from Mexico was elected president-elect in Kobe in 1994, and became president after me in 1997. At the same IDF congress KGMM Alberti from the United Kingdom was elected president-elect, and will become president at the congress in Mexico City in November 2000. By electing Maria de Alva, the IDF council made two important statements. They elected the first person with diabetes and the first woman to be IDF President. She has had IDDM since childhood. Having diabetes and being a woman is of course no qualification for presidency. Maria, however, has demonstrated leadership qualities. In her own country she cofounded and is still active in the Mexican Diabetes

Federation. In the IDF, she was the chairperson of a Task Force on development of guidelines for member associations. Her work there resulted in the publication: "Together we are stronger. How to build Successful Diabetes Associations." This booklet will be the basis for much of the work in this triennium. The federation has several task Forces: on Regional Development, (chaired by Sterling Tucker, US), on Member Association Development (Bjørnar Allgot, Norway), on Insulin (Jean-Claude Mbanya, Cameroon and Earl Bell, South Africa), on Diabetes Health Economics (Rhys Williams, UK), on Appropriate Technology (KGMM Alberti, UK), Clinical Practice Guidelines (Philip Home, UK), Congress Development (Massimo Massi-Benedetti, Italy) Revenue Generation (Don Chisholm, Australia) and Finance and By-laws (Henry Rivera, US).

The IDF Mission

"The mission of the International Diabetes Federation is to work with our member associations to enhance the lives of people with diabetes."

IDF shall also be the voice of its member associations and people with diabetes in the international community. Many decisions that affect the lives of people with diabetes, their health-care providers, and the diabetes community are made in the World Health Organization (WHO), the World Bank, UNICEF, the European Union, and in multinational companies. The IDF is the only truly global advocate for people with diabetes. The World Health Assembly Resolution adopted on 19 May, 1989, regarding the prevention and control of diabetes was an important step. It was a direct consequence of efforts by the IDF, particularly by its president at the time, Professor Joseph Hoet. The Federation has since addressed the world's health ministers directly at the World Health Assembly in 1993, and the Executive Board of WHO in January 1994. The IDF has with the co-sponsorship of the WHO, also initiated an annual World Diabetes Day that has been successful in focusing public attention on diabetes worldwide. The strong support of WHO and its Director-General Hiroshi Nakajima, MD, is of great benefit to people with diabetes everywhere.

The Resolution was followed by the St. Vincent Declaration in Europe in October 1989. Close collaboration between WHO and the IDF in Europe has been established, and has led to major advances in diabetes care in many European countries. In the Eastern Mediterranean and Middle East-Region a similar collaboration has been started. In the summer of 1996 a Declaration of the Americas on Diabetes was adopted in San Jose, followed by it adoption also by the Executive Committee of PAHO (Pan-American Health Organization). Much has been achieved in developing guidelines suitable for national planning and diabetes management in the region. The collaboration between WHO and IDF, now formalized in a permanent working group, has given us a unique opportunity to influence national health-care programs, directly through our national member associations, and through WHO recommendations.

The Epidemic of NIDDM

There are at least 100 million people in the world with diabetes, and their number is rising. Most of them have noninsulin-dependent diabetes mellitus (NIDDM). The estimate has more than tripled during the last 7 years, as more epidemiological data have come in. Noteworthy is the fact that most countries with more than 10% diabetes in the adult population are either developing countries or underprivileged populations in developed countries.

We can expect a marked change in the age structure of the world population in the years to come. This change is a positive consequence of economic development, improved nutrition and better health care, leading to a marked decrease in mortality from infectious diseases, especially in children. However, when an increase in age comes together with a rise in the incidence of NIDDM in adults, the consequence is NIDDM epidemic. Another factor contributing to the marked rise in diabetes prevalence in the developing countries is rapid urbanization.

A third factor, which is receiving increased attention, is the possibility that a rapid change of lifestyle is especially damaging. This so-called Barker hypothesis; that intrauterine and early childhood malnutrition/undernutrition gives an increased risk for the so called noncommunicable diseases, including diabetes, in later life is a fascinating one. The diseases or conditions often described as part of the metabolic syndrome; NIDDM, hypertension, lipid disturbances and arteriosclerotic diseases, are in fact the ones included in this hypothesis. If the hypothesis is correct, the high prevalence of NIDDM in the adult populations in many developing countries is not due to genetics plus changing lifestyles

alone, but also a consequence of the rapidity of the change, from early undernutrition to later overnutrition within one lifetime.

The change in the disease spectrum in developing countries has been called the epidemiological transition, from communicable diseases to the chronic noncommunicable diseases. This epidemiological transition requires changes to be made: in health-care priorities; in the way we organize our cities and lives; in education, to prevent the consequences of changing lifestyles; and in research. IDF is eminently suited to vanguard these changes. Through our collaboration with WHO and other UN agencies, we have direct access to governments around the world, an access that has been used repeatedly during the last triennium. We shall continue our efforts to increase the awareness the rising diabetes prevalence, its impact and implications, and thus raise adequate resources for prevention, control, and research.

The Problems of People with IDDM

We do not know the true incidence of childhood diabetes in most places of the world because many die undiagnosed. Where good epidemiological studies have been done in developing countries, like in Karthoum, the incidence is as high as it is in the non-Scandinavian European countries, that is; about 10 per 100,000 children per year. And the number of children in developing countries is great.

Insulin does not reach everybody who needs it. There is, however, no lack of insulin in the world. Until recently insulin was made from pancreases of cattle and pigs. This resource is limited, and to counter the threat of insulin scarcity, genetic engineering was used. Today most insulin is made by micro-organisms, and the production can easily be increased to cover any needs.

There are great differences in the utilization of insulin in the world, with a much higher use in industrialized countries, as illustrated by Table II-1.

TABLE II–I   World Consumption of Insulin

	Insulin used (mill. units/year)	Nos. Treated (15000 units/year)	Population (in millions)
World	150 000	10 millions	5 500
Developing countries	45 000	3 millions	4 600
Industrialized countries	105 000	7 millions	880

In 1993 more than 2/3 of all insulin sold was used in countries with less than 1/5th of the world population. Table II-2 illustrates the great differences in utilization of insulin in different regions and countries around the world.

TABLE II–2 Insulin Utilization, Units/Mill. Inhabitants per Year

Whole world	27
Developing countries	10
Industrialized countries	120
Sub-Saharan Africa	4
Japan	30
North Africa	32
Egypt	44
Norway	153
USA	225

What are the reasons for these differences? When the sale of insulin is very low in a country or region e.g. sub-Saharan Africa, it must mean that either the incidence is very low and/or the survival time of persons with insulin-dependent diabetes are short. Some die undiagnosed and others die soon because insulin is not available or affordable. The prognoses may, however, also be poor because education and support is not given to the person with diabetes and her family. In recent studies in Khartoum in Sudan quite a high incidence, prevalence and mortality of childhood diabetes was found, to indicate that childhood diabetes is not uncommon in all parts of sub-Saharan Africa. There are other indications that the prognosis in IDDM in many developing countries is much poorer than in industrialized countries. Indeed, in 1988 Samad Shera wrote in the journal of the Diabetic Association of Pakistan, "Diabetes Digest":

"While the West is reaping the fruits of modern research, we are sadly decades behind. Particularly in the rural areas where the majority of our people live, a good number of young patients die undiagnosed because of virtually non-existent health care delivery systems and very poor diagnostic facilities. Those fortunate patients who survive, survive perilously due to lack of supply and proper storing facilities of life saving drugs like insulin, high economic cost of diabetic care, low and poor living conditions with all its attendant miseries. Thus many of our diabetic children die prematurely due to acute complications to which they are particularly susceptible. Over longer periods of time (months and years), lack of control in children, coupled with inadequate diet, give rise to the intermediate problems of growth failure and delayed development".

In a recent article from Africa it was calculated that the annual direct cost of diabetes care in 1989-90 was US $287 for a patient requiring insulin and $103 for a patient not requiring insulin. It was concluded that diabetes places a severe strain on the limited resources of developing countries. If African patients with diabetes have to pay for their treatment most will be unable to do so and will die. Another article from the same group in 1994 indicates that cost is the major factor in limiting availability-cost either for impoverished governments or impoverished patients. They point out, however, that this problem is but one of many problems facing sub-Saharan countries, most of which are in the midst of severe social and economic regression. Making some reasonable assumptions, they calculate that the total cost of care for children with diabetes in sub-Saharan Africa would be about US $25 million per year. There are, however, some developing countries which have managed to deal with the problem. One outstanding example is Egypt, which, although not as poor as the sub-Saharan countries, has a low national income per inhabitant and a high use of insulin. The Egyptian government has for a long time subsidized the price of insulin.

A high use of insulin may be due to a very high prevalence of insulin-dependent diabetes. Insulin is also often used for people with type 2 diabetes to achieve optimal glucose regulation. The extent to which this is done, varies according to clinical practice. In many developing countries insulin is not used in type 2 diabetes because of financial restraints, prejudice against injections etc. In the USA the very high insulin use is probably due to much insulin being used by people with type 2 diabetes, as the prevalence of type 1 does not seem to be exceptionally high. In Japan type 1 diabetes is uncommon, and by far the most insulin is used by people with type 2 diabetes. In Norway and other Scandinavian countries where the incidence of insulin-dependent diabetes is high, much of the insulin is probably used by people with IDDM.

In the rich part of the world, the treatment of IDDM will always be included in any written or unwritten priority list. Not so, however, in a poor country where many important public and private needs compete for the same very limited resources, and where a system for setting priorities, the infrastructure and public statistics are not web developed. If, however, a country decides it cannot afford to treat all people with insulin-dependent diabetes, this decision should at least be based on proper analyses of the situation and a setting of priorities.

The problems for a person with IDDM in a poor country is not only the problem of obtaining insulin and proper diabetes care, but often also the drain his disease causes on family resources. No one knows how often this leads to underutilization of insulin as a kind of slow suicide by neglect.

For the medical community in a poor country the situation is difficult. The gap between what can be achieved by good medical care in IDDM and what is actually being done, makes for some very complex situations, where a mixture of guilt and helplessness may make a rational approach difficult. The situation is often aggravated by overwork and a difficult personnel situation. It is sometimes necessary to remember that not all people using insulin are dependent on daily injections to prevent death, most NIDDM patients on insulin need it for better blood glucose control and not for short term survival.

The insulin manufacturers are also in a difficult situation. They are often blamed for not donating insulin or selling it very cheaply. Insulin, however is complicated to produce, whether it is from animal pancreases or by gene technology. The process is difficult to automate completely, and many safety measures have to be included. Insulin is also difficult to transport, does not stand heat and cold very well and has a limited shelf life. It can therefore never become really cheap. It is also difficult to sell insulin at a much cheaper price in some countries than in others because of the problems of reimportation and difficulties in getting the governments in the industrialized world to accept that insulin is sold at a cheaper price in other countries. The major insulin producers do, however, make considerable contributions in times of difficulties, whether they are due to natural or man-made causes.

To the IDF and other international organizations dealing with diabetes, the underutilization of insulin will no doubt remain a major concern for many years. The problem must always, however, be viewed against the backdrop of the total world situation of extremely uneven distribution of resources, education, infrastructure and management. The underutilization of insulin is an ethical problem, of course. However, it is much more a practical problem to be solved by proper analyses, wise decisions, planning and actions taken in each country. If this home work is done, help from the international community will probably also be easier to obtain.

Several international agencies have developed programs and are supplying insulin, either collected as such or bought from collected money, and given to medical centers in special need. An IDF task force on insulin has developed guidelines for such donations, to avoid misuse and ensure safe and appropriate delivery. If at all possible, such donations should be used to facilitate the making of a national plan to ensure insulin availability and proper care to people with insulin-dependent diabetes mellitus. Standardization of insulin strengths and color codes will also make insulin donations safer, and is being advocated strongly by the IDF in collaboration with the World Health Association and industry.

The IDF task force has, on the invitation from the national diabetes association, had a team on visit to Jamaica, one of the countries reporting that insulin is not always available, to discuss the situation with all involved parties. A report has been made with an analysis of the situation and suggestions for solving the problem. Some of the proposals of the team have already been implemented, and a dialogue between the parties involved with the situation has been started. The implementation and its effects will be evaluated. It is hoped to make similar visits to other countries with similar problems.

The underutilization of insulin in the world can only be helped by activities of many good men and women, by good planning and management, by giving IDDM management a higher priority then it has today in many poor countries, and by continuous efforts to raise the general awareness of the situation.

Appropriate Health Technology

"Methods, procedures, techniques and equipment that are scientifically valid, adapted to local needs, acceptable to those who use them and to those for whom they are used, and that can be maintained and utilized with resources the community and country can afford."

Today, many strengths of insulin are produced (U20, 40, 80, and 100) with many different color codes and other symbols. By 2000 most industrialized countries will have changed to U100. The IDF has been working and shall continue to work for only one strength of insulin (U100) before year 2000, and common color codes of all insulin. In this task we are working together with WHO, insulin manufacturers, and our member associations. More important, the federation and all its member associations are also working to ensure that unnecessary tariffs, taxes and costly distribution systems, which make insulin unnecessarily expensive, are abolished. Similarly, the producers of insulin should continue to provide insulin of adequate quality at prices appropriate to the resources available. The International Diabetes Federation should work for a permanent and sustainable solution to the insulin delivery, education, and monitoring problem.

Education and Public Awareness

Public awareness and understanding of diabetes is low. In the United States, diabetes is the third biggest cause of death by disease. But a 1991 survey found that only 6% of US citizens were aware of this. A survey in the United Kingdom found that nearly half of the population were unable to name any symptom of diabetes. Against this background it is not surprising that so few have been examined for diabetes and that many remain undiagnosed.

Poor understanding also breeds prejudice. In some countries people have been dismissed from their jobs as their diabetes was thought to be contagious. Some women with diabetes are subject to social rejection or deemed unsuitable as marriage partners. A survey in France found that diabetes was perceived as a punishment for past dietary excess. Worse still, diabetes as a condition was deemed most comparable with sexually transmitted diseases and alcoholism. Discrimination in the workplace and with matters such as health or life insurance is common. This is another reason why diabetes remains largely hidden from the public eye. Many people will not admit to having the condition, simply through fear of prejudice.

Education is the cornerstone of diabetes management at all levels. This involves the person with diabetes understanding their condition and being able to balance diet, exercise, and drug intake on a continual, daily basis. The US Center for Disease Control estimates that with proper education 50–80% of diabetic complications are preventable. Education could also prevent over 70% of diabetic ketoacidosis. Appropriate footcare can reduce amputations by 50%. Yet diabetes education often remains at a poor level. Only 1 in 10 people with diabetes in the United States have ever had any formal training in self-care and despite the fact that diabetes is the leading cause of blindness in the middle-aged, only 1 in 30 people has an annual eye examination. In parts of France over 50% of those with diabetes have not had an eye test for over 5 years.

Education of those with diabetes also has a very significant impact on health-care costs, to the state and to the patient. Pioneering teaching programs in Germany, Romania, Argentina, and Russia have recently reported significant reductions of mortality, acute complications, hospitalization, and sick day leaves. Cost–benefit analysis in selected programs in Russia indicate the possibility of "astronomical financial savings, along with dramatic improvements of diabetes care if made available to the whole country."

The IDF Bulletin is published four times per year in three languages, English, French and Spanish. It has "people who decide about diabetes" as its main target group. We want to fill a gap by informing health authorities, opinion leaders, and health professionals about diabetes issues and the impact of diabetes on public health and expenditure.

IDF Congresses

The IDF congresses are organized triennially, in 1991 in Washington DC, in 1994 in Kobe, in 1997 in Helsinki, in 2000 in Mexico City and in 2003 in Paris. It is one of the major scientific congresses of the world, including tracks on education, clinical diabetology, quality assurance and development, health economics, diabetes organizational work, and health-care delivery.

The IDF Action Plan

It is against this background that the IDF Board of Management defines ways in which the IDF could work to improve the global situation of people with diabetes. Keeping in mind its function as a federation of diabetes associations, and its role as the global advocate for people with diabetes, the IDF is focusing on four areas:

- the rapid global increase in the number of people with NIDDM, its prevention and management, especially in the developing world;

- the major difficulties facing people with IDDM, including the availability and cost of insulin;

- education—as important as insulin, other drugs and proper diet for people with diabetes; and

- the urgent need to increase awareness and knowledge of diabetes of decision makers and the general public.

In some cases, the IDF has formed special Task Forces to tackle specific global problems, such as availability and cost of insulin, and appropriate technology. In other cases, the IDF will rely on its new permanent Consultative Sections to address important issues, such as diabetes education and childhood and adolescent diabetes. In all cases, the IDF will work together with, and for the benefit of, its member associations, with the goal of helping them in their own development. Only through helping its member associations can the IDF really reach out and help individual people with diabetes and their health-care providers. This commitment to member associations will especially be demonstrated through the work of the Task Force on Member Association Development.

The IDF has been growing rapidly, in terms of association membership and the scope of its activities. In the coming triennium the focus will be particularly on developing its regional organizations to become stronger and more vibrant helpers of the member associations and stronger partners with the regional WHO organizations.

The present triennium 1997–2000 will be a full one for the International Diabetes Federation. Its new leadership, under the presidency of Maria de Alva, will remember the root of our existence and focus on our core constituents, IDF member diabetes associations. Simultaneously, we will continue to address diabetes issues on a global level as necessary by fostering relations with international bodies such as WHO, the World Bank and UNICEF, and with the multinational diabetes related industry. In short, the IDF will work for our members from all corners of the world, acting as the global advocate for people with diabetes.

Publications from the International Diabetes Federation can be obtained from its Executive Office: International Diabetes Federation, 1 rue Defacqz, B-1000 Brussels, Belgium. Tel.: + 32 2 538 5511; Fax: + 32 2 538 5114; Home page: http://www.idf.org/; E-mail: idf@idf.org.

APPENDIX III

American Diabetes Association

John H. Graham IV

The American Diabetes Association (ADA) has served since 1940 as an organized forum for America's efforts to fight diabetes. As is found with many successful institutions, the vision of ADA's founders is still evident in the current association of 1999. The ADA's mission is to prevent and cure diabetes and to improve the lives of people affected by diabetes. Throughout its 59-year history, the ADA has represented health professionals and the general public (patients and community leaders), fostered excellence in medical care, exchanged scientific information, issued authoritative opinions, raised public awareness, funded diabetes research, supported patient information activities, provided an umbrella for all organized diabetes efforts, and served as a model of excellence for others.

First, the ADA represents the efforts of all who have an interest in diabetes. The ADA's professional section and councils represent the interests of about 17,000 physicians, scientists, nurses, dietitians, podiatrists, pharmacists, social workers, and others who work as health professionals in diabetes. At the same time, people affected by diabetes and community leaders represent the interests of more than 16 million Americans, diagnosed and undiagnosed, impacted by this devastating and deadly disease.

Second, the ADA can be found at work in communities throughout America. In fact, it was representatives from communities that preceded and guided the establishment of ADA in 1940. This effort has now spread to over 600 communities in America. Our goal is to expand to over 2000 communities by the year 2000.

Such a broadly representative association has been the source of great strength in times of crisis. For example, the ADA's volunteers organized emergency insulin delivery to Puerto Rico during World War II, overcame calls to ban all artificial sweeteners from the United States market in 1977, advocated passage of vital legislation in 1974 to set up federal support for diabetes research and education, and in 1997 advocated

for the passage of legislation that enabled 3 million Medicare recipients to receive diabetes health management and education, medical nutritional therapy, durable goods, and other pharmaceuticals necessary to manage diabetes.

Third, the ADA continues to emphasize its original primary purpose: to improve the quality of care for all people with diabetes in America. The ADA was founded in 1940 by the efforts of Drs. Cecil Striker, Herman Mosenthal, and a small group of others, responding to the continued medical needs of their patients. The earliest programs included scientific meetings and papers, a journal (*The Proceedings of the American Diabetes Association*, vol. 1–10, 1941–1950) and support for governmental policies to improve the quality of care.

Especially from 1921 onward, early attention was focused on the discovery and manufacture of insulin to sustain life itself for the person with diabetes. This key discovery is credited to Drs. Banting and Best in Toronto in 1921. Both were named Honorary Presidents of ADA in 1941, and prestigious awards for scientific achievements are presented in their names annually at the ADA meeting. For other awards that are presented at the annual meeting see Tables III–1 through III–21.

Fourth, by 1940 it was apparent that a great deal more information about diabetes was needed. The ADA's founders included internists and surgeons, both of whom saw the generally poor quality of health of many people with diabetes under their care. Complications leading to blindness, kidney disease, painful and disabling neuropathy, and macrovascular disease leading to heart attacks, strokes, and lower limb amputation had become major concerns and remain so to this day. Furthermore, a 1997 study showed the direct and indirect costs of diabetes to be over $100 billion per year despite improvements in mortality and morbidity statistics during recent years.

The ADA was established as a forum for exchanging scientific information about diabetes and the numerous associated conditions. Major advances have been reported through the ADA's scientific meetings, postgraduate courses, symposia, and journals in the last 50 years. In 1994 at ADA's annual scientific meeting, the results of the landmark Diabetes Control and Complications Trial were announced. The results were clear. Controlling diabetes to near-normal levels had a positive impact on the onset and severity of diabetes complications.

Fifth, through nationwide coordinated efforts, the ADA has been able to reach out to primary care and other health providers. During the early years, the ADA promoted membership recruitment efforts broadly to the American Medical Association and the American College of Physicians. More recently, the ADA has launched publications and intensive symposia for such groups. The ADA's original journals were merged to form *Diabetes*, the world's premier diabetes research journal. *Diabetes Care* was launched to provide reports generally associated with clinical care and research. *Clinical Diabetes* is distributed to 60,000–65,000 primary-care physicians. The reception for *Clinical Diabetes* was so strong that the ADA received multimillion-dollar support in 1984 for continuing medical education (CME) programs. Since then, the ADA has received numerous grants to conduct CME programs on topics from cardiovascular disease to medical nutrition therapy for a wide range of primary-care providers. In 1988, ADA responded to another expressed need for the translation of research advances into practice by publication of *Diabetes Spectrum*.

Sixth, ADA has been the voice of authority in the diabetes field throughout its 59-year history. The ADA's founding in 1940 came at a difficult time for America, and ADA leaders were immediately called on by the government to advise about proper health policies, dietary and insulin needs, and prevention of medical quackery. Subsequently, ADA was called on to express expert scientific and medical opinion regarding various medical studies, sweeteners, employment discrimination, licensure, research, standards of care, and numerous other topics.

Seventh, the ADA has led efforts to increase public awareness about diabetes in America. National Diabetes Week was launched in 1948 with the primary purpose of detecting the hundreds of thousands of Americans then thought to have undetected diabetes. Since then, similar efforts have continued each year. During American Diabetes Month, November, in communities throughout America, the association strives to reach people with diabetes about the importance of eye and foot exams. During March, in communities throughout America, the American Diabetes Alert seeks to find those individuals who have diabetes and do not know it. In fact, in recent statistics announced by the government, diabetes has made great strides. We used to say there are 16 million Americans with diabetes and half do not know it. We are now able to say that there are 16 million Americans with diabetes and 6 million do not know it. We are beginning to see progress in the war against diabetes.

Eighth, the ADA has raised and spent well over $150 million for diabetes research awards and grants. The ADA's research program began in 1955 and has maintained its primary purpose of encouraging top candidates to begin a career in diabetes research. Notable scientists throughout America received their first funding from the ADA. This aspect of the ADA's work was a primary reason the ADA undertook a major restructuring in 1970 to convert from a purely professional society to a voluntary health agency to increase the potential for research contributions. In 1995, the association launched the American Diabetes Association Research Foundation to bring increased focus to research and more importantly provide a vehicle for major gifts to research. In 4 years, over $8 million has been raised through major gifts for diabetes research.

Ninth, the ADA is the leader in organizing and disseminating diabetes information in America. The ADA publishes *Diabetes Forecast*, a leading patient magazine in America. The ADA's community organizations conduct camp programs for diabetic youngsters in nearly every state, organize thousands of support group meetings each year, and supply patient information materials in English and Spanish through hospitals and health-care providers. With the advent of the Internet, the ADA's on-line activities have dramatically enabled the association to respond to people with diabetes electronically. For those seeking more traditional means, the ADA continues its Diabetes Information and Action Line (D.I.A.L.) for the purpose of addressing people's concerns with diabetes. In addition, the ADA operates two recognition programs. The first is to recognize those providers who meet the standards of a quality diabetes education program. The second recognizes those providers who meet the ADA's standards of care. The ADA was particularly excited about our partnership with National Committee for Quality Assurance (NCQA) in assuring that people with diabetes can receive quality care.

Tenth, the purpose of ADA's founding was to coordinate diabetes efforts in America. To bring more focus to that effort, in 1997 the American Diabetes Association Central Council and Board of Directors adopted a recommendation entitled Future Directions. Future Directions focuses the association's efforts on research, information, advocacy, and income development through community organization. Communities are where people live, work, play, volunteer, and donate. The Future Direction's initiative is designed to centralize the association in doing those things that are best done centrally such as technology, finance, and administration, and decentralizing those activities that are best done in communities such as reaching people with our message, recruiting more volunteers and raising dollars.

In communities, ADA volunteers and staff work with community leaders to deliver a wide range of program services. In this model, the ADA moved from 50 state affiliate associations separately incorporated to a regional structure under a single corporation. The association believes that this will enable us to better focus our energies and resources on those targets having the most impact on people with diabetes.

The ADA's Board of Directors is representative of all of these efforts and provides nationwide leadership to the work of the association. The ADA is the forum through which members of other diabetes groups in America coordinate their efforts on a broader scale. In addition, the ADA maintains relationships with numerous other not-for-profit organizations, professional and scientific societies, and other diabetes organizations. All during its 59-year history, the ADA has been a dynamic organization reflecting the zeal of its volunteer leadership and members. In 1940, the ADA began with 26 founders and 2 contributions totaling $1500. Four hundred members joined ADA in its first year. By 1999, the ADA has grown to an organization with a nationwide budget of over $190 million annually. Millions of people donate and hundreds of thousands provide volunteer time and energy to the association. As the ADA looks to the future, more and more every day, diabetes is viewed as a serious and costly disease. By focusing on our agenda of research, information and advocacy, made possible through an aggressive income development program, the association can focus its resources in communities where people live and work, and, thereby, continue to make an every day difference for people with diabetes.

TABLE III–I Banting Medal for Scientific Achievement

Name	Year	Name	Year
Elliott P. Joslin, M.D.	1941	Earl W. Sutherland, M.D.	1969
William Muhlberg, M.D.	1942	Paul E. Lacy, M.D.	1970
Fred W. Hipwell, M.D.	1943	George F. Cahill, Jr., M.D.	1971
Leonard G. Rowntree, M.D.	1944	Dorothy C. Hodgkin, Ph.D.	1972
Joseph H. Barach, M.D.	1946	Arnold Lazarow, MD, Ph.D.	1973
Bernardo A. Houssay, M.D.	1946	Albert Renold, M.D.	1974
H. C. Hagedorn, M.D.	1946	Roger H. Unger, M.D.	1975
R. D. Lawrence, M.D.	1946	Donald F. Steiner, M.D.	1976
Eugene Opie, M.D.	1946	David M. Kipnis, M.D.	1977
University of Toronto	1946	Stefan S. Fajans, M.D.	1978
G. H. A. Clowes, Ph.D.	1947	Charles R. Park	1979
Rollin T. Woodyatt, M.D.	1948	Norbert Freinkel, M.D.	1980
Herbert M. Evans, M.D.	1949	Lelio Orci, M.D.	1981
F. G. Young, D.Sc.	1950	Jesse Roth, M.D.	1982
C.N.H. Long, M.D.	1951	Arthur H. Rubenstein, M.D.	1983
R.R. Bensley, M.D.	1952	Daniel W. Foster, M.D.	1984
Shields Warren, M.D.	1953	Bjorn Nerup, M.D.	1985
Sir Henry H. Dale	1954	Albert I. Winegrad, M.D.	1986
Carl F. Cori, M.D.	1955	Joseph Larner, MD, Ph.D.	1987
William C. Stadie, M.D.	1956	Gerald M. Reaven, M.D.	1988
DeWitt Stetten, Jr., M.D., Ph.D.	1957	Ora Rosen, M.D.	1989
Jerome W. Conn, M.D.	1958	Daniel Porte, Jr., M.D.	1990
George W. Thorn, M.D.	1959	Mladen Vranic, M.D.	1991
Priscilla White, M.D.	1960	Gian Franco Bottazzo, M.D.	1992
Rachmiel Levine, M.D.	1961	C. Ronald Kahn, M.D.	1993
A. Baird Hastings, Ph.D.	1962	Philip E. Cryer, M.D.	1994
Bernardo A. Houssay, M.D.	1963	Franz M. Matschinsky, M.D.	1995
Solomon A. Berson, M.D.	1965	Peter H. Bennett, MB, Ch.B.	1996
Robert H. Williams, M.D.	1966	Alan D. Cherrington, Ph.D.	1997
Alexander Marble, M.D.	1967	Jerrold M. Olefsky, M.D.	1998
Arthur R. Colwell, M.D.	1968		

TABLE III–2   Outstanding Scientific Achievement (Sponsored by Eli Lilly and Company)

Name	Year	Name	Year
Solomon A. Berson, M.D.	1957	J. Denis McGarry, Ph.D.	1978
James B. Field, M.D.	1958	Leonard S. Jefferson, Ph.D.	1979
Marvin D. Siperstein, M.D., Ph.D.	1959	Jerrold M. Olefsky, M.D.	1980
Albert E. Renold, M.D.	1960	C. Ronald Kahn, M.D.	1981
Rosalyn S. Yalow, Ph.D.	1961	Michael P. Czech, Ph.D.	1982
Harry N. Antoniades, Ph.D.	1962	Howard S. Tager, Ph.D.	1983
James M. B. Bloodworth, Jr., M.D.	1963	Alan D. Cherrington, Ph.D.	1984
Roger H. Unger, M.D.	1964	Steven J. Jacobs, M.D.	1985
George F. Cahill, Jr., M.D.	1965	George S. Eisenbarth, M.D., Ph.D.	1986
Norbert Freinkel, M.D.	1966	Ralph A. DeFronzo, M.D.	1987
David M. Kipnis, M.D.	1967	John E. Gerich, M.D.	1988
Robert G. Spiro, M.D.	1968	Richard N. Bergman, Ph.D.	1989
Donald F. Steiner, M.D.	1969	Graeme I. Bell, Ph.D.	1990
Oscar B. Crofford, M.D.	1970	Jeffrey S. Flier, M.D.	1991
Daniel Porte, Jr., M.D.	1971	Simeon Taylor, MD, Ph.D.	1992
John H. Exton, Ph.D.	1972	Michael A. Brownlee, M.D.	1993
Arthur H. Rubenstein, M.D.	1973	Kenneth S. Polonsky, M.D.	1994
Jesse Roth, M.D.	1974	Barbara B. Kahn, M.D.	1995
Pedro Cuatrecasas, M.D.	1975	Jeffrey E. Pessin, Ph.D.	1996
Philip Felig, M.D.	1976	Gerald I. Shulman, M.D., Ph.D.	1997
Peter H. Bennett, M.D.	1977	Michael M. Myeckler, Ph.D.	1998

TABLE III–3   Outstanding Clinician in Diabetes (Sponsored by Pfizer's U.S. Pharmaceuticals Group, Pfizer Inc.)

Name	Year	Name	Year
.Edgar A. Haunz, M.D.	1975	O. Peter Schumacher, M.D., Ph.D.	1987
David Hurwitz, M.D.	1976	Allan L. Drash, M.D.	1988
Henry E. Oppenheimer, M.D.	1977	Fred W. Whitehouse, M.D.	1989
Priscilla White, M.D.	1978	James R. Gavin, III, M.D., Ph.D.	1990
Marvin E. Levin, M.D.	1979	Christopher D. Saudek, M.D.	1991
Harold Rifkin, M.D.	1980	Saul M. Genuth, M.D.	1992
James M. Moss, M.D.	1981	Alice N. Bessman, M.D.	1993
George P. Heffner, M.D.	1982	Lester Baker, M.D.	1994
Harvey C. Knowles, Jr., M.D.	1983	Lois Jovanovic-Peterson, M.D.	1995
Alan L. Graber, M.D.	1984	F. Xavier Pi-Sunyer, M.D.	1996
Burritt L. Haag, M.D.	1985	Bruce R. Zimmerman, M.D.	1997
Holbroke S. Seltzer, M.D.	1986	Julio V. Santiago, M.D. (posthumously)	1998

TABLE III–4   Kelly West Award

Name	Year	Name	Year
Peter H. Bennett, M.D.	1986	Trevor J. Orchard, M.D.	1993
Elizabeth L. Barrett-Connor, M.D.	1987	Ronald Klein, M.D., M.P.P.	1994
Ronald E. LaPorte, Ph.D.	1988	William C. Knowler, M.D., Dr.Ph.	1995
Harry Keen, M.D.	1989	Richard F. Hamman, M.D., Dr.Ph.	1996
Michael Stern, M.D.	1990	Steven M. Haffner, M.D., M.P.H.	1997
Paul Zimmet, M.D., Ph.D.	1991	Janko Tuomilehto, M.D., M.P.H., Ph.D.	1998
Maureen I. Harris, Ph.D., M.P.H.	1992		

TABLE III–5 Outstanding Physician Educator in Diabetes (Sponsored by Pharmacia, Uppsala, Sweden and Upjohn, Inc.)

Name	Year	Name	Year
Alexander Marble, M.D.	1975	Ronald A. Arky, M.D.	1987
Leona V. Miller, M.D.	1976	Daniel W. Foster, M.D.	1988
Philip W. Felts, M.D.	1977	Oscar B. Crofford, M.D.	1989
Frederick C. Goetz, M.D.	1978	Mayer B. Davidson, M.D.	1990
John K. Davidson, M.D. Ph.D.	1979	Marvin E. Levin, M.D.	1991
Leo P. Krall, M.D.	1980	John A. Colwell, M.D., Ph.D.	1992
John W. Runyan, M.D.	1981	John H. Karam, M.D.	1993
Ann Lawrence, M.D., Ph.D.	1982	Fred Whitehouse	1994
Donnell D. Etzwiler, M.D.	1983	Luther B. Travis, M.D.	1995
H. St. George Tucker, Jr., M.D.	1984	Edward S. Horton, M.D.	1996
Charles R. Shuman, M.D.	1985	Mark Molitch, M.D.	1997
J. Stuart Soeldner, M.D.	1986	Arthur Krosnick, M.D., F.A.C.P., C.D.E.	1998

TABLE III–6 Outstanding Educator in Diabetes (Sponsored by Bayer Corporation)

Name	Year	Name	Year
Rita M. Nemchik, R.N., M.S.	1977	R. Keith Campbell, R.Ph.	1989
Barbara M. Prater, Ph.D., R.D.	1978	Margaret A. Powers, R.D., M.S.	1990
Diana Guthrie, R.N., Ph.D.	1979	Judith Wylie-Rosett, R.D., E.D.	1991
Carelyn P. Fylling, R.N., M.S.	1980	Helen R. Bowlin, R.N., B.S., C.D.E.	1992
Barbara Christman Adair, R.N., M.S.N.	1981	Barbara J. Maschak-Carey, R.N.C.S.,	1993
Myrtis A. McSweeney, R.N.	1982	M.S.N., C.D.E.	
Maria Alogna, R.N., M.P.H.	1983	Jean Betschart, M.N., R.N., C.D.E.	1994
Margaret C. Yarborough, R.Ph.	1984	Linda B. Haas, M.N., R.N., C.D.E.	1995
Marion Franz, R.D., M.S.	1985	Ruth Farkas-Hirsch, M.S., R.N., C.D.E.	1996
Deborah A. Hinnen, R.N., M.N.	1986	Richard R. Rubin, Ph.D., C.D.E.	1997
Madelyn L. Wheeler, M.D., R.D.	1987	Anne S. Daly, M.S., R.D., C.D.E.	1998
Phyllis R. Crapo, R.D.	1988		

TABLE III–7 Albert Renold, M.D., Award

Name	Year	Name	Year
Peter H. Forsham, M.D.	1992	George F. Cahill, Jr., M.D.	1996
Jesse Roth, M.D.	1993	R. Paul Robertson, M.D.	1997
Harold E. Lebovitz, M.D.	1994	C. Ronald Kerhn, M.D.	1998
Daniel Porte Jr., M.D.	1995		

TABLE III–8 Outstanding Contribution to Camping and Diabetes (Sponsored by Becton Dickinson Consumer Products)

Name	Year	Name	Year
Donnell D. Etzwiler, M.D.	1979	Campbell P. Howard, M.D.	1889
Vivian Murray, R.D.	1980	Frank K. Thorp, M.D., Ph.D.	1990
Samuel Eichold, M.D.	1981	Doris A. Graves, M.D.	1991
Ronald Youngquist, M.D.	1982	Richard A. Guthrie, M.D.	1992
Kathleen Krauser, R.N.	1983	Marvin L. Rallison, M.D.	1993
Jerome R. Ryan, M.D.	1984	Jane K. Kadohiro, R.N., M.P.H., C.D.E.	1994
Robert K. Endres, M.D.	1985	John W. Stephens, M.D.	1995
Paul Madden	1986	Thomas A. Lera, Jr., M.D.	1996
Luther Travis, M.D.	1987	Lynda K. Fisher, M.D.	1997
Martha Leigh Spencer, M.D.	1988	Neil H. White, M.D., C.D.E.	1998

TABLE III–9   Outstanding Contribution to Diabetes in Youth (Sponsored by Boehringer Mannheim Corporation)

Name	Year	Name	Year
Aaron Fox Foundations	1973	Luther Travis, M.D.	1980
Harlan Hanson*	1973	Paul B. Madden, M.Ed.	1981
Joyce Kortman*	1973	Charlene Bandurski*	1982
Fred Wolinsky*	1973	Frank Robles, Ph.D.	1983
Melvyn Coldman*	1974	Linda Siminerio, R.N.	1984
Robert Jackson, M.D.	1974	Kathleen Wishner, M.D.	1985
Patricia McAlister*	1974	Nettie Richter*	1986
Priscilla White, M.D.	1975	Robert Endres, M.D.	1987
Caroline Sanders*	1975	Marilyn Moore	1988
Barbara Cavanaugh*	1976	Dorothy Becker, M.B.B.Ch.	1989
Mary Connolly*	1976	Don P. Wilson, M.D.	1990
Donnell Etzwiler, M.D.	1976	Fredda Ginsberg-Fellner, M.D.	1991
Abraham Silver, M.D.	1976	Stuart Brink, M.D.	1992
Matthew Steiner, M.D.	1976	Broatch Haig, R.D.	1993
Sheila Garvey, R.N.	1977	Francine R. Kaufman, M.D.	1994
Mary Olney, M.D.	1977	Georgeanna J. Klingensmith, M.D.	1995
Howard Traisman, M.D.	1977	William L. Clarke, M.D.	1996
Ronald Youngquist*	1978	Campbell P. Howard, M.D., C.D.E.	1997
Samuel Wentworth, M.D.	1979	Irene N. Sills, M.D.	1998

TABLE III–10   Outstanding Affiliate Service

Name	Year	Name	Year
Alice P. Hoover	1956	Harvey and Karen Carafiol	1977
C. Paul and Addie Lou Tiley	1957	Sydelle Feinman	1978
Louise Hayes Williams	1958	Jane Zarish	1979
Anna Smrha	1959	Nettie Richter	1980
Edith Jenkins	1960	Gilbert Marks	1981
Carolyn J. Spiegel	1961	Todd and Connie Leigh	1982
Mrs. Alan J. Arthur	1962	G. F. (Joe) DeCoursin	1983
Wilma Van Der Beek	1963	Sandra Lewis	1984
Pauline Steigerwald	1964	David Grier	1985
Helen Turner Whitney	1965	Timothy McGuckin	1986
Frances Vroom	1966	Harriet Silverberg	1987
Peter S. Kaufman	1967	Clydella Hentschel	1988
Lloyd C. Pray, Ph.D.	1968	Terry Golden, M.D.	1989
Mrs. Robert E. (Dorothy) Childs	1969	Anneliese Krauter	1990
Mrs. Henry A. Friedman	1970	David J. Jampole	1991
Lowell Echard	1971	Gloria Hirsch	1992
Jon W. Hall	1972	Jane Camporeale	1993
Dina Merrill	1973	Thomas P. Straus	1994
Mrs. Vernon B. (Dorothy) Child	1973	David I. Miller, M.D.	1995
Ruth Lawson	1974	Louis B. Chaykin, M.D.	1996
Beverly Holman	1975	Marvin D. Bordy, M.D.	1997
Samuel M. Shrilberg	1975	John N. Clore, M.D.	1998
Gordon P. Sprague	1976		

TABLE III–11   Youth Leadership (Sponsored by Equal Sweetener)

Name	Year	Name	Year
Kara Vereault	1985	Sara Murray	1992
Tom Casey	1986	Tandy L. McGee	1993
Susanna Maiuri	1987	Rhonda Joyce Pollard	1994
John Nawrocki	1988	Chantal Sampogna	1995
Joby Jobson	1989	Jeff Lahti	1996
Alison Schultz	1990	Chris Coombs	1997
Brian Steele	1991	N/A	1998

TABLE III–12   Outstanding Fund-Raising Service

Name	Year	Name	Year
Bruce Furness	1989	Carlene Watkins-Weinberger	1994
Arnold Soskin	1990	Gerald Bernstein, M.D.	1995
Donna Jean Hill, CFRE	1991	Darlene L. Cain	1996
Gerald F. Jones, Jr.	1992	Patricia Barnstable Brown	1997
Sylvia Luskey	1993	Gloria Hirsch	1998

TABLE III–13   Wendell Mayes, Jr. Medal

Name	Year	Name	Year
Wendell Mayes, Jr.	1986	Tom Parks	1993
Benjamin Greenspoon	1987	Wade Wilson	1994
Dorothea Sims	1988	Henry Rivera	1995
Lee Iacocca	1989	Todd E. Leigh	1996
William F. Talbert	1990	Ross V. Hickey, Jr.	1997
Maria L. de Alva	1991	Sterling Tucker	1998
Lee Ducat	1992		

TABLE III–14   Charles H. Best Medal for Distinguished Service in the Cause of Diabetes

Name	Year	Name	Year
Senator Gale W. McGee	1974	Senator Lowell Weicker	1987
Senator Richard Schweiker	1974	Neil Pettinga, Ph.D.	1987
Ray A. Kroc	1975	Richard Verville	1988
Oscar B. Crofford, M.D.	1976	Joan Foran	1988
Representative Louis Stokes	1977	Lions Clubs International	1989
Wayne Newton	1978	Wayne Parker	1990
President Gerald R. Ford	1979	Robert S. Bolan	1990
Jim (Catfish) Hunter	1980	Premiere Committee, Los Angeles	1990
David M. Kipnis, M.D.	1981	Eva R. Saxl	1991
Daniel T. Gillespie Family	1982	Frank Vinicor, M.D.	1991
J. William Flynt, M.D.	1983	Congressman Gerry Sikorski	1991
President Ronald Reagan	11/3/83	Rachmiel Levine, M.D.	1992
James M. Fowler, D.D.S.	1984	Holiday Sales Program	1993
Everett J. Grindstaff	1984	Diabetes Control and Complications Trial (DCCT) Study Group	1994
Keatha K. Krueger, Ph.D.	1985		
Nina Berlin	1985	Charles and Verda Kopke	1995
Jean F. Curran	1985	Order of the Amaranth, Inc.	1996
Dorothea F. Sims	1985	Michael Rossi	1997
Lester B. Salans, M.D.	1985	Diabetes Care & Education Practice Group of The American Dietetic Assocation	1997
Lee Iacocca	1985		
Honorable Gov. Robert Graham	1985		
John K. Davidson, M.D., Ph.D.	1986	Honorable Newt Gingrich	1998

TABLE III–15   Addison B. Scoville, Jr. Award for Outstanding Volunteer Service

Name	Year	Name	Year
Ernest M. Frost, Ed.D.	1975	Frederick C. Goetz, M.D.	1991
Wendell Mayes, Jr.	1977	Charles H. Kopke	1992
Alvin Z. Levine	1981	Deborah Hinnen, R.N., C.D.E.	1993
Robert L. Kroc, Ph.D.	1984	Denise Dodero	1994
Annette Shapiro	1986	Sydelle Feinman	1995
Oscar B. Crofford, M.D.	1987	Michael J. DeMarea, Jr.	1996
Virginia Hanson-Ullom	1988	David L. Shaw	1997
Sandra Segal Polin, M.P.A.	1989	Sara Nelson	1998
Jaime A. Davidson, M.D.	1990		

TABLE III–16   C. Everett Koop Medal for Health Promotion and Awareness

Name	Year	Name	Year
C. Everett Koop, M.D.	1990	Hillary Rodham Clinton	1994
Ted Turner	1991	Ronald Kotulak	1995
Governor Michael N. Castle	1992	The Honorable Jake Garn	1996
Governor Lowell P. Weicker	1993	N/A	1998

TABLE III–17   Harold Rifkin Award for Distinguished International Service in the Cause of Diabetes

Name	Year	Name	Year
Harold Rifkin, M.D.	1991	Meng H. Tan, M.D.	1996
Harry Keen, M.D.	1992	KGMM Alberti, F.R.C.P., Ph.D.	1997
Leo P. Krall, M.D.	1993	Errol Morrison, M.D.	1998
Wendell Mayes, Jr.	1994		
Hilary King, M.Sc., M.D., M.F.P.H.M., D.Sc.	1995		

TABLE III–18   Public Policy Leadership Award

Name	Year	Name	Year
Assemblyman Robert K. Sweeney and Senator Nicholas A. Spano	1995	Arlene B. Mayerson of Disability Rights Education & Defense Fund, Inc.	1997
Representative Elizabeth Furse	1996		
		Honorable George R. Nethercuth, Jr.	1998

TABLE III–19   Charles H. Best Medal for Service

Name	Year	Name	Year
Gail Velde	1974	William A. Mamrack	1989
Wendell Mayes, Jr.	1978	Sterling Tucker	1990
Myles H. Tanenbaum	1979	Arnold Bereson	1991
Benjamin Greenspoon	1981	Todd E. Leigh	1992
Harlan L. Hanson	1983	Ross V. Hickey, Jr.	1993
Gordon Stulberg	1984	Michael A. Greene	1994
Joseph H. Davis	1985	Douglas E. Lund	1995
Henry Rivera	1986	David H. McClure	1996
Sam A. Gallo	1987	Alan Altschuler	1997
S. Douglas Dodd	1988	Stephen S. Satalino	1998

TABLE III–20 Banting Medal for Service

Name	Year	Name	Year
Donnell D. Etzwiler, M.D.	1977	John A. Colwell, M.D., Ph.D.	1988
Norbert Freinkel, M.D.	1978	Charles M. Clark, Jr., M.D.	1989
Fred W. Whitehouse, M.D.	1979	Sherman M. Holvey, M.D.	1990
Ronald A. Arky, M.D.	1980	Edward S. Horton, M.D.	1991
Donald I. Bell, M.D.	1981	Jay S. Skyler, M.D.	1992
Oscar B. Crofford, M.D.	1982	F. Xavier Pi-Sunyer, M.D.	1993
Irving L. Spratt, M.D.	1983	James R. Gavin III, M.D., Ph.D.	1994
Allan L. Drash, M.D.	1984	Kathleen L. Wishner, Ph.D., M.D.	1995
Karl E. Sussman, M.D.	1985	Frank Vinicor, M.D., M.P.H.	1996
Harold Rifkin, M.D.	1986	Philip E. Cryer, M.D.	1997
Daniel Porte, Jr., M.D.	1987	Mayer B. Davidson, M.D.	1998

TABLE III–21 Rachmiel Levine, M.D. Award for Service

Name	Year	Name	Year
Patricia A. Lawrence, R.N., M.A.	1979	Madelyn L. Wheeler, M.S., R.D., C.D.E.	1992
Barbara Prater, R.D., Ph.D.	1981	Patricia D. Stenger, R.N., C.D.E.	1994
Florence R. Ruhland, R.N., M.Ed.	1983	Linda M. Siminerio, R.N., M.S., C.D.E.	1995
Patricia A. Schultz, R.N., M.S.	1986	Davida F. Kruger, M.S.N., R.N., C., C.D.E.	1996
Linda S. Hurwitz, R.N., M.S.	1988	Belinda P. Childs, R.N., M.N., C.D.E.	1997
Alan D. Cherrington, Ph.D.	1989	Christine A. Beebe, M.S., R.D., C.D.E.,	
Mary Louise Maras, R.D., C.D.E.	1990	L.D.	1998
Charlene Freeman, R.N., C.D.E.	1991		

APPENDIX IV

Camps for Children with Diabetes Mellitus

Marvin L. Rallison

It is not easy being a child with diabetes. Management of diabetes demands often confusing changes in the lifestyle of the diabetic child. How, what, and when a child may eat or play must be monitored and modified. Many children imagine they are alone in the world with diabetes, and wonder why they alone must poke their fingers to test for sugar in the blood and eat from a meal plan instead of just what they want, whenever they wish; and taking shots simply "sucks" when no one else has to.

It is even more of a challenge for a teenager with diabetes. Adolescence is characterized by growing independence, testing of parental authority, and coping with social and peer relationships. Increased physical growth, sexual development, and emotional tensions already demand continual adjustments in this period of life. Diabetes simply complicates the whole process. Physical and emotional changes of adolescence profoundly affect the metabolic control of diabetes and medical and emotional demands of diabetes make adjustment to adolescence more difficult.[1]

Children with diabetes may manipulate their diabetes care as a way of expressing their need for independence. They may react to what they perceive as unfair restrictions of their lifestyle by willful disregard of their diabetic diet, failure to take insulin, or deliberate attempts to precipitate diabetic acidosis. In the management of insulin-dependent diabetes, by far the most difficult variable to control and the least well understood is the patient's behavior and adjustment to life's situations.[2] See Chapter 47.

Goals of Camps for Children/Adolescents with Diabetes

Camps for diabetic children and adolescents have been established to help the child and his/her parents learn how to live with diabetes, how to keep it under control, and to help the child understand the need to care for diabetes while living a full and active life. The goals of camps for diabetic children include camping experiences, appropriate medical supervision, educational experiences, and comaraderie with other young diabetics. Emphasis vaies from camp to camp; some provide extensive camping skills, others emphasize social skills and friendship, and others emphasize learning how to better care for diabetes. Activities are geared to helping the diabetic child learn about his/her strengths and weaknesses. Diabetes camps provide a safe environment for fun-filled activites that promote a sense of accomplishment of living with diabetes and that enhance self-esteem and acceptance of a modified lifestyle at home[3]

Camps for diabetic children had their beginnings shortly after the discovery of insulin. In 1925 a summer camp was established near Detroit by Dr. Leonard Wendt, and shortly thereafter camps were started in Connecticut (NYDA). Cleveland (HoMitaKoda) and New England (Joslin/boys & Clara Barton/girls).[4] In 1995 there were over 60 summer camps listed with the American Diabetes Association (ADA) (accredited by the Am Camp Assoc), providing access for youth with diabetes to camps in nearly every state in the USA (Table IV–1), and many countries throughout the world, including Canada, Mexico, South America, Europe and Australia. Most ADA sponsored camps provide summer camping experience, but some also have winter camps, day camps, weekend retreats, and family camps.

Most camps are sponsored by a local ADA affiliate, though financing may come from fees and donations, sales of products or educational materials, or from civic organizations. Most camps operate under a camp committee, on which there is participation of parents, children, medical personnel, and camp staff. The direction of camp may be by a professional camp director with volunteer help or may be drawn from the camp committee or ADA affiliate, especially for short-term camps.

TABLE IV-1 ADA-Sponsored Summer Camps for Children with Diabetes—1995

State	Camp	Sessions	Fee	Capacity
Alabama	Cmp Seale Harris	1 wk × 3	$25	—
Arizona	Cmp AZDA	1 wk	$315	190
Arkansas	Cmp Yorkstown Bay	1 wk	$250	90
	Cmp Aldersgate	1 wk	$250	40
California	Cmp Chinook	2 wk × 4	$550	426
	Bearskin Meadows Cmp			
	Cmp de Los Ninos			
Colorado	Children's Diab Cmp	1 wk × 2	$275	150
Florida	Cmp Children/Youth	1 wk × 3	$400	310
Georgia	Cmp LiWiDia	1 wk × 2	$325	300
	Day Camp	4 dy × 1	$50	50
Hawaii	Diabetes Youth Cmp	1 wk		
Idaho	Cmp Hodia/Teen Cmp	1 wk × 2	$225	250
Illinois	Cmp Gran-ADA	1 wk	$260	100
	Triangle D Cmp	1 wk × 2	$250	200
Indiana	Cmp John Warvel	1 wk × 2	$180	400
Iowa	Cmp Herkto Hollow	1 wk × 1	$220	305
		4 dy × 2	$110	
Kansas	Cmp Discovery	1 wk × 3	$200	240
Kentucky	Cmp Hendon at KYSOC	1 wk	$225	110
Louisiana	LA Lions Cmp for Youth	1 wk × 2	$35	220
Maine	Cmp Kee-To-Kin (family)	1 wk	($250/300)	8
Maryland	Cmp Glyndon	1 wk × 4	$700	468
Massachussetts	Clara Barton Cmp (girls)	1 wk × 4	$950	362
		2 wk × 2		
	ElliotJoslin Cmp (boys)	1 wk × 4	$1150	380
		2 wk × 2		
Michigan	Midicha	1 wk × 2	$290	400
Minnesota	CmpNeedlepoint/Daypoint	1 wk × 2	$175	410
		4 dy × 1	$60	
Missouri	Cmp EDI	1 wk × 2	$550	146
	Cmp Shawnee	1 wk × 2	$150	270
	Cmp Red-Bird	4 dy × 1	$75	50
	Cmp Wyman	1 wk × 2	$550	146
Montana	Cmp DiaMont	1 wk × 1	$175	78
Nevada	Cmp Nevada	1 wk × 1	$300	75
New Hampshire	Cmp Carefree	2 wk × 1	$825	140
New Jersey	CmpNeJeDa	1 wk × 3		
New York	Cmp Sunshine	1 wk × 2	$395	190
North Carolina	Cmp Carolina Trails	1 wk × 1	$350	180
	Triangle Day Camp	5 dy		
North Dakota	Cmp Sioux	1 wk × 2	$0	90
Ohio	Cmp Korelitz	1 wk × 1	$220	100
	Cmp Tokumto	5 dy × 1	$50	20
Oklahoma	Cmp Ne Oca Da	1 wk × 1	$45	60
	Cmp O'Leary/Kno-Keto	1 wk × 1	$425	125
	Cmp Tom-a-Hawk	1 wk × 1	$50	20
Oregon	Gales Creek Cmp	1 wk × 2		
Pennsylvania	Diab Cmp at Crestfield	1 wk × 2	$300	200
	Cmp Setebaid	1 wk × 1	$300	84
South Carolina	Cmp Adam Fisher	1 wk × 1	$285	400
South Dakota	Cmp Gilbert	1 wk × 1		110
Tennessee	Cmp Sugar Falls	4 dy × 3		82

(continued)

TABLE IV–I   *(continued)* ADA-Sponsored Summer Camps for Children with Diabetes—1995

State	Camp	Sessions	Fee	Capacity
Texas	Cmp New Horizons	5 dy × 1		150
	Cmp Rainbow	5 dy × 1		85
	Cmp Sandcastle			
	Cmp Bluebonnet	5 dy × 1		100
	Cmp Independence	5 dy × 1		100
Utah	Cmp Utada	1 wk × 5	$190	500
	(winter/family)	3 dy × 5	$90	60/30
Washington	Cmp Sealth	1 wk × 2		unlimited
	Cmp Orkila	1 wk × 1	$420	unlimited
	Cmp Dudley	3 dy × 1	$95	unlimited
Wisconsin	Cmp Helen Brachman	1 wk × 2	$265	200
Wyoming	Cmp Hope			

(For dates, ages, and other information, contact the state affiliate of ADA or the ADA National Service Center, 1660 Duke Street, Alexandria VA 22314; telephone (703) 549–1500, ext. 2408.)

Camp sessions vary from 1 to 4 weeks or utilize long weekends (retreats, family camps); most provide 1 or 2 weeks. Some are open to all ages (usually 9–15 years), others are stratified according to age; some have separate sessions for boys and girls, but most are coeducational. For adolescent diabetics out-of-camp activities such as white-water rafting or wilderness backpacking may be provided. Day camps, family camps, and weekend retreats attempt to provide bridges between home and camp.[3]

Why Children Go to Diabetes Camps

When we inquired of children and their parents at Camp UTADA as to why diabetic children go to summer camp,[1] not too surprising was the agreement of children and parents that the most important reason for going to camp was to see and meet other young people with diabetes; parents rated it as being a more important reason than the children. For the children, the next most important reason was to learn how to eat properly; and the third reason was to have fun! For parents learning about giving insulin was second and dietary instruction third.

Of the learning experiences offered at camp, the children were equally interested in learning about insulin reactions (hypoglycemia), insulin injections, and diets. The parents thought meal planning was most important, insulin reactions and glucose monitoring slightly less so. Basically, for children camps are a social experience, a place to have fun and learn how to eat, take insulin, and treat insulin reactions. For their parents, there is hope that the child will learn some important new skills and interest in better management of their diabetes.

Medical Supervision and Educational Offering at Camps

Medical supervision and education are given considerable emphasis at camps for diabetic youth and guidelines for provision of adequate medical supervision are provided by the American Camping Association, which accredits most of the ADA-sponsored Camps. Some camps involve campers to a greater or lesser degree in the management and changes made at camp, while others provide meals, insulin regimens, and activities that are balanced by supervisors (camp counselors). We do not look upon diabetics as handicapped, but only in need of a little more-than-usual medical supervision to avoid frequent hypoglycemia. Medical problems seen in dispensaries of diabetes camps are usually the same as those seen in other camps: bumps, cuts, scrapes, rashes, upset stomachs, homesickness, etc., but about half the visits to the nurse are for treatment of low blood sugar reactions.[3]

Our medical supervision extends from Medical Director, who supervises the medical, dietetic, and educational programs at camp through unit doctors, nurses, dietitians, social workers, pharmacists, and cabin counselors to the child in each cabin, all of whom are involved in dynamic supervision and learning in management of diabetes at camp. We routinely hold "medical rounds" each evening with campers/counselors to discuss what we have learned from the day and to anticipate changes that might be helpful for the coming day.

The educational value of camps can be superlative. Some of the education for living with diabetes takes place in semiformal presentations, but more effective lessons are learned through the mingling of the child with peers. Guest speakers or cabin "workshops" can present topics such as advanced meal planning, exercise rules, sick-day guidelines, prevention of hypoglycemia, targets for blood glucose control, etc. in a nonjudgemental and pleasant manner, utilizing puppet shows, games, songs, or skits. Role playing together with peer pressure from doing things together is highly effective. The more the individual camper is involved in medical decisions and in educational experiences at camp, the more apt is the experience to be beneficial to camper and family and subsequently to health-care providers who supervise management of diabetes the rest of the year. Teenagers often respond best to successful young adult diabetics, at camp as counselors, staff or guest speakers, as a role model or hero, showing that young diabetics can prepare for college or a job, fall in love, get married and have children, and all while taking care of their diabetes.[3]

An added benefit from camp can be realized if within each cabin "family" of diabetics we can insert a student of medicine, pharmacy, nursing, dietetics, or social work so they can observe at first hand the day-to-day caprices of management of diabetes and the impact various devices have on the lifestyle of the young diabetic. Opportunities for research into what makes a young diabetic do what he does and finding better ways of managing diabetes at camp and at home infuses an academic flavor into the camping activities.[3]

Camping Programs at Camps for Diabetics

The programs at camps for diabetics should not differ much from programs available to nondiabetics. Camping skills, such as crafts, archery, games, obstacle courses, volley ball, base ball, hiking, nature strolls or demonstrations, etc. should be part of every camp curriculum, as should swimming, canoeing, or other water front activitites, if feasible. Diabetic children can take day hikes, prepare food for picnics, play games, engage in vigorous play etc. as long as adequate preplanning takes place to assure appropriate food for the occasion and appropriate changes in insulin administration. We often recommend a reduction in camp insulin by 10–20%, expecting activity at camp to be more vigorous than that at home.

Fireside programs help young diabetics to be comfortable exhibiting their skills in singing, acting, or playing musical instruments. We sing songs at campfire containing lessons about care of diabetes, encourage skits presenting the humorous lessons to be learned from camping experiences, all the while emphasizing friendships, how they are formed, fostered, and preserved. It is for comaradarie that most diabetics come

to camp and meeting other young people who also have to test their blood sugar, eat sensibly, and anticipate their special needs for a hike, swim, or lazy day on the beach is what makes camp special.

Day camps, family camps, or weekend retreats,involving family as well as the diabetic child, offer a special educational opportunity because they involve a parent (or grandparent) or all of the family and show how the diabetic fits into the family and demonstrates the dynamics of family activity. Sharing among families to find out what works best is a profitable family educational experience. This is particularly true of families with a very young diabetic child.

Special activities for teenagers are also extremely important in helping them to explore their feelings about life and the demands of diabetes. Camps can organize out-of-camp activities such as bicycle touring, white-water rafting, wilderness backpacking, spelunking, or special interest outings in which it can be demonstrated that even with vigorous activity, good control of diabetes can be maintained and a healthful, vigorous life can be enjoyed. Specific topics that can be discussed in small groups at the opportune moment include how to prepare for and find a job; career planning; college study; driving hazards; obtaining health insurance; avoiding peer pressure to smoke, drink, use drugs, or to become sexually active; dating, preparing for marriage; building a family, etc.

What Do We Accomplish at Camps for Diabetics?

Most parents and providers of health care feel that the educational and social experiences at camp are extremely valuable; admitting that some bad as well as good habits can be learned from peers at camp. Whether metabolic control acutually improves has been more difficult to document, but anecdotal evidence is uniform in attesting that camps promote healthy attitudes about diabetes management and foster self-esteem in the process.[3]

One of our diabetic counselors summed up her experiences of a week at camp UTADA in an essay entitled "What REALLY goes on at those diabetes camps?"

Just being surrounded by groves of aspen, fir and pine with a nearby fresh water stream, complete with swampy banks and willows and wildflowers... was partial therapy for the urban diabetic. Healthful food and plenty of it was provided for active diabetics, accompanied by diabetic banter of "Do your parents nag you about food?" Friendships come easily because of the common diabetic bond; no one feels left out.

Blood sugar testing and insulin injection times are a burden, made lighter because everyone participates... and it is exciting to help someone to their first ever shot, or most perfect blood sugar testing technique. How increased activity at camp shows up in blood sugar profiles is always a learning experience and figuring how to make appropriate changes is like a treasure hunt. Of all the camping activities, the horseback rides seemed to be the most popular, even when the horses could not be encouraged to more than a sedate stroll till they were headed back to the corral... then the group would come clattering back to the corral with a rosy flush of triumph on their cheeks.

Campfire programs contained perennial favorites such as songs about peanut butter, insulin shots, testing and a dead bird (camp mascot) and olios such as "Shooting of Dan Mcgrew" or "Casey at the Bat" and always taps and a moment of tranquility. And at the dance at the end of camp a hug from a naughty camper who finally admitted he would miss his counselor and hoped he could come back again. This friendship is what makes a week at camp so different from other weeks of the year.

P.S. Marshall, What REALLY goes on at those diabetes camps. Essay about Camp. Personal Communication, 1972.

And from a letter, written by a parent of a newly diagnosed diabetic, a similar message:

The joy that my son finds at camp is a miraculous, healing thing. I gave camp UTADA a boy fighting and avoiding his care... an incredibly negative attitude. He came home in charge of himself. He is doing his own thing, noting his needs and actually wanting to 'beat diabetes.' What is the magic of Camp? I think it is first of all the common ground. My son was with other kids with whom he could relate. The counselors have credibility, and can encourage right behavior. There is empathy, but not pity. A mother's instinct is to protect, but at camp kids are encouraged to get back into life in an insistent, yet loving way. Yes, there is a magic at Camp Utada; a magic found no where else for kids like my son... thank you.

References

1. Prater BM: Why diabetic children go to summer camp. J Am Dietetic Assoc 55:584–87, 1969.
2. Hinkle LE: The influence of the patient's behavior and his reaction to his life situations upon the course of diabetes. Diabetes 5:406, 1956.
3. Brink SJ: Diabetes camping and youth support programs. *In* Lifschitz F (ed): Pediatric Endocrinology, 3rd ed. New York: Marcel Deffer Inc., 1996, pp. 671–676.
4. Travis LB, Allen WR: Camps and similar programs. *In* Travis LB, et al. (eds): Diabetes Mellitus in Children and Adolescents. Philadelphia: W.B. Saunders, 1987, pp. 226–232.

APPENDIX V

European Association for the Study of Diabetes

Viktor Jörgens

The European Association for the Study of Diabetes (EASD) was founded in 1965 in Montecatini, Italy. The official language of the Association is English. The aims of the Association are to encourage and support research in the field of diabetes, rapidly diffuse acquired knowledge, and to facilitate its application. The Association is governed by a Council of 15 members (one third of whom retire each year), who are elected by the General Assembly, which is held at the time of the Annual Meeting. The President and two Vice-Presidents are elected from among the members of the Council.

The international membership of the Association embraces scientists, physicians, and laboratory workers interested in diabetes and related subjects. Any individual or corporation meeting such criteria, and on approval of the Council, may be a member of the Association as follows:

1. An Active Member is an individual holding a medical degree or a scientific worker with an academic degree, required to pay an annual membership fee, entitled to vote at General Assemblies, and eligible for election to the Council and to the Executive Committee.

2. A Junior Member is an undergraduate student or postgraduate science student, required to pay an annual membership fee, which does not include subscription to the journal *Diabetologia*, and entitled to vote at General Assemblies.

3. An Associate Member is an individual or corporation interested in diabetes or related subjects, required to pay an annual membership fee, but not entitled to vote or hold office.

4. A Supporting Member (divided into Gold and Silver Memberships) is an individual or corporation giving substantial material aid to the fight against diabetes, required to pay an annual membership fee, but not entitled to vote or hold office.

Paid-up Active Members of the Association receive the journal *Diabetologia*, the Official Announcement for the Annual Meeting, including the Abstract and Registration forms, as well as a triennial Membership Directory and information on prize nominations and application deadlines each year.

Currently, the Active Membership fee is DM 195 for members above 34 years of age and DM 130 for members younger than 35 years; Junior Membership amounts to DM 70 per year. The annual fees can also be paid in Pound Sterling. Membership includes subscription to the monthly journal *Diabetologia* and the abstract volume of the Association's Annual Meeting. Information on Annual Meetings, abstract and registration form are included in the January issue of *Diabetologia*. All Paid-up Members of the Association receive the Provisional Program of the abstracts and lectures to be presented at the Annual Meeting and in addition, a copy of the triennial membership Directory and information regarding prize nominations and application deadline each year.

The Active Membership of the Association currently numbers more than 5500 medical doctors and scientists from over 70 countries throughout the world. The Association also bestows Honorary Membership on any individual whose medical or scientific contribution to diabetes research is outstanding; the first Honorary Member of the Association was Charles Best. John K Davidson, the editor of this book, was elected Honorary Member of the European Association for the Study of Diabetes in 1998 honouring his outstanding contributions to clinical research in diabetes.

The Association has its official publication, the journal Diabetologia (Volume 1–42, 1965–1999) which publishes articles monthly on clinical and experimental diabetes and metabolism. In addition, there are rapid communications and review articles on selected topics of current interest by leading experts in the field. Manuscripts (original and 3 copies) by *regular mail* to: W. Waldhäusl, MD, Editor-in-Chief Diabetologia,

P.O.Box 27, A-1097 Wien, Austria, and by *registered or courier mail* to: W. Waldhäusl, MD, Editor-in-Chief Diabetologia Editorial Office, Lazarettgasse 14, A-1090 Wien, Austria, Fax: 00431404002728, e-mail: diabetologia@akh-wien.ac.at. Active members are entitled to a discount on subscriptions to several other diabetes research journals.

The Annual Meetings of the Association are held each year in September in European cities. Active members are entitled to attend the meetings at a considerably reduced registration fee. Abstracts to the Annual Meetings are invited from members as well as from nommembers. All abstracts are strictly anonymously reviewed by a Program Committee, chaired by the Honorary Secretary. Not only are the scores of the different subcommittees given anonymously, in addition, the Program Committee members do not know the name of the author and their places of employment when decisions on the final Program are made. The EASD was one of the first international Associations introducing anonymous review of abstracts, which seems to be the most democratic and fair procedure of handling the matter.

The high quality of scientific research presented is attested to by the increasing participation at the Annual Meetings, which in 1998 attracted nearly 10000 scientists and clinicians from around the world to the 34th Annual Meeting in Barcelona, Spain. To assist the participation of young members, the Association has established a Travel Fund from which over 100 awards are made available annually for the Annual Meeting. In addition, a number of Stayment Grants is made each year to assist the participation of colleagues coming from financially poor countries. The Meeting took place in Barcelona, Spain in 1998; the Annual Meeting of the EASD will be held in Brussels, Belgium in 1999, in Jerusalem, Israel in 2000, in Birmingham, United Kingdom in 2001 and in Budapest, Hungary in 2002. In 2003 the International Diabetes Federation will hold its meeting in Paris, France; the EASD Meeting in 2004 will take place in Munich, Germany and in Athens, Greece in 2005.

In 1995 for the first time a transatlantic scientific workshop was organized by the President of the Association, Prof KGMM Alberti. It included speakers from both sides of the Atlantic. A special volume of *Diabetologia* summarized this special event, which continued in 1996, 1997 and 1998.

The Association awards three major prizes annually: the Castelli Pedroli Prize, sponsored by the family of the late Maria Carla Castelli Pedroli, is awarded to a member whose published work in the previous 5 years has concerned the histopathology, pathogenesis, prevention, and treatment of the complications of diabetes mellitus; the recipient delivers the Camillo Golgi Lecture at the Annual Meeting. The Claude Bernard Medal is awarded to recognize an individual's innovative leadership and outstanding contribution to the advancement of knowledge in the field of diabetes mellitus and related metabolic diseases; the recipient delivers the Claude Bernard Lecture at the Annual Meeting. The Minkowski Prize is awarded to an individual member under the age of 40 years, whose distinction is manifested by publications that contribute to the advancement of knowledge concerning diabetes mellitus; the recipient delivers the Minkowski Lecture at the Annual Meeting.

Professor Albert Ernst Renold (1923–1988) was the founding Secretary of the Association from 1965–1970, and later served as President from 1974–1977. He played a major role in advancing diabetes research in Europe and throughout the world until his untimely death. To commemorate the considerable debt owed to Albert Renold for his inspirational leadership, the EASD has instituted the Albert Renold Fellowship designed to encourage young investigators (under the age of 40 years) who are members of the Association to visit another laboratory or laboratories to gain experience in new techniques and methodology, to receive postdoctoral training, or to carry out collaborative research. During the past years other research fellowships have been introduced: the EASD/Eli Lilly Research Fellowship in Diabetes and Metabolism; the EASD/Glaxo Wellcome Burden of Diabetes Research Fellowship; the EASD/Amylin - Paul Langerhans Research Fellowship for Research on the Physiology and Pathophysiology of the Beta-Cell; the EASD/Sankyo Insulin Resistance Project Award and the EASD Travel Fellowships for Young Scientists.

Annually the Association holds an EASD Scientists Training Course to attract new talent to diabetes research in new centers throughout the world. Nominations for all of the above are invited from the membership.

The Association has fifteen Study Groups: Artificial Insulin Delivery Systems (AIDSPIT), Metabolism and Insulin Action, Diabetic Pregnancy Study Group (DPGS), Diabetic Foot Study Group, Diabetes Education Study Group (DESG), Diabetes and Nutrition Study Group (DNSG), Diabetes Neuropathy Study Group (NEURODIAB), Diabetes Optimization through Information Technology Study Group (DOIT), European Diabetes Epidemiology Study Group (EDESG), EADS Islet Study Group, EASD Eye Complication Study Group (EASDEC), European Diabetes Nephropathy Study Group (EDNSG), Hypertension in Diabetes Study Group (HID), Lipoprotein Study Group, Psychosocial Aspects of Diabetes (PSAD). The Post Graduate Education Subcommittee (PGESC) is active in sponsoring workshops and courses for clinicians and educators. They also promote Study-Group Symposia as an official part of the program of the Annual Meeting.

Former Presidents of the Association include: J.P. Hoet, F.G. Young, K. Lundbaek, A.E. Renold, Sir P. Randle, W. Gepts, D. Andreani, P. Freychet, P. Lefèbvre, K.G.M.M. Alberti, and M. Berger. The Executive Director from 1965–1988 was Dr. (hc) J.G.L. Jackson (London). Current officers include: President: Prof. J. Nerup, Gentofte (retires 2001), Vice Presidents: P.A. Halban, Geneva (retires 1999), G.H. Tompkin, Dublin (retires 2000), immediate Past-President: M. Berger, Düsseldorf (1995-1998), Honorary Secretary: H. Porta, Torino (retires 2001), Honorary Treasurer: R.J. Heine, Amsterdam (retires 1999). The executive director is Dr. V. Jörgens, Düsseldorf.

All correspondence should be addressed to the EASD secretariat, Merowingerstrs. 29, D-40223 Düsseldorf, Germany. Tel: +49-211-316768, Fax +49-211-3190987, E-mail: easd@uni-dusseldorf.de; homepage: http: //www.easd.org.

The Juvenile Diabetes Foundation International—The Diabetes Research Foundation: Insulin is Not a Cure

The Juvenile Diabetes Foundation International

Brian Beauchamp

Insulin, which was discovered in 1922, makes it possible for people with diabetes to live longer. *But insulin is not a cure.* Even with treatment, all forms of diabetes can cause devastating complications that affect virtually every organ system in the body.

The Juvenile Diabetes Foundation International (JDFI) was founded in 1970 by a small group of parents whose children had diabetes. Over the years, that nucleus of families has grown to encompass tens of thousands of volunteers working in over 100 chapters and affiliates across the United States and around the world. But JDFI's mission remains the same: *to find a cure for diabetes and its complications through the support of research.* In fact, the JDFI gives more money to diabetes research than any other nonprofit, nongovernmental health agency in the world.

What is Diabetes?

Diabetes is a chronic, metabolic disorder. It impairs the body's ability to manufacture or use insulin, a hormone necessary to transport sugar (glucose) from the food we eat into the cells for energy and growth. There are three major forms of diabetes:

Type 1 Diabetes Mellitus (Insulin-Dependent, IDDM, or Juvenile Diabetes)

Type 1 diabetes can occur at any age but usually occurs before age 30. In this form of diabetes, the insulin-producing β cells of the pancreas are destroyed by an autoimmune response and can no longer produce insulin. The lack of endogenous insulin makes type 1 diabetes particularly difficult to control. Because it affects the young, complications such as blindness and kidney failure can occur at an early age. Treatment requires a strict regimen that includes a carefully calculated diet, home blood glucose testing up to eight times a day, and as many as six daily insulin injections.

Type 2 Diabetes Mellitus (Noninsulin-Dependent, NIDDM, or Adult-Onset Diabetes)

Type 2 diabetes typically occurs after age 45, but it can appear at an earlier age. In this form of diabetes, the pancreas still makes insulin, but either the amount of insulin produced is insufficient or the body cannot effectively utilize the insulin it makes. Treatment includes diet control, exercise, home blood glucose testing, and in some cases, oral medication. Approximately 40% of the people with type 2 diabetes require some insulin to manage their diabetes.

Gestational Diabetes

Gestational Diabetes develops during some pregnancies. Careful monitoring of blood sugar and sometimes insulin are required. This type of diabetes usually disappears when the pregnancy is over. Women who have gestational diabetes are at an increased risk for developing type 2 diabetes later in life.

The Human and Economic Costs of Diabetes

Diabetes affects all ethnic, racial, and socioeconomic groups. Worldwide, it is estimated that as many as 130 million people have diabetes. Furthermore, the incidence of this disease is increasing at an alarming rate. The World Health Organization predicts that by the year 2025 there will be 300 million individuals with diabetes in the world.

In the United States, 16 million people have diabetes. The US government reports the following morbidity statistics: Diabetes is the primary cause of new adult blindness, the number one cause of nontraumatic amputation, and responsible for nearly 30% of all new cases of kidney failure. Individuals with diabetes bear a two-to-four times greater risk of heart disease and stroke than those who do not have diabetes. A leading cause of premature death, this disease can shorten life expectancy by as much as one third. Every 3 min, diabetes claims the life of another child or adult.

Diabetes drains financial resources as well. The spiraling costs of this disease consume one out of every seven US health-care dollars and one out of four Medicare dollars. The lifetime cost of diabetes care for a person diagnosed at age three, calculated in today's dollar value, totals about $600,000.

Diabetes Research Funding

Since its inception, the JDFI has given over $260 million to diabetes research. In fiscal 1996–1997, JDFI awarded over $31 million to research projects in 15 countries on four continents. As JDFI membership continues to grow, annual research allocations are projected to increase even more. It is estimated that every dollar for medical research saves approximately eight dollars in health-care expenditures.

JDFI is committed to eradicating diabetes and its complications worldwide. The Foundation focuses its research funding in three general areas that will advance knowledge about all types of diabetes: (1) achieving normal blood glucose and metabolism; (2) preventing the onset of diabetes and its recurrence following transplantation; and (3) finding ways to prevent complications and treatments to improve the quality of life for those who live with diabetes.

All grant applications are reviewed by an international team of researchers and scientists who sit on JDFI's Medical Science Review Committee and by the volunteers appointed to JDFI's Lay Review Committee. This two-tiered review process ensures that all research JDFI funds is scientifically meritorious and mission-directed. Funding recommendations are presented to the international board of directors for final approval.

In 1990, the JDFI initiated the Only Remedy is a Cure Campaign. This $200 million campaign is dramatically accelerating the pace of diabetes research by establishing interdisciplinary research program projects in institutions all over the world to foster collaboration among preeminent diabetes researchers and scientists in other cutting-edge disciplines such as microbiology, immunology, genetics, and transplantation.

In addition, JDFI is pioneering unique partnerships with public and private entities, leveraging its dollars while changing the very nature of scientific research. Currently, the JDFI is collaborating with four of the US National Institutes of Health, the US Department of Veterans Affairs, and the Medical Research Councils of Canada and Australia.

For more information about the Juvenile Diabetes Foundation International, call: 1-800-JDF-CURE or 1-212-479-9500, write: Juvenile Diabetes Foundation International, 120 Wall Street, 19th Floor, New York, N.Y. 10005 or visit the Juvenile Diabetes Foundation International Web Site at *http://www.jdfcure.com*.

APPENDIX VII

Forms for the Diabetes Mellitus Problem-Oriented Record

John K. Davidson

The following forms may be used for collecting and assessing a defined diabetes mellitus data base and for constructing a complete problem list. The forms are divided into 10 sections as follows:

1. *Patient identification and demographic data*

2. *History (subjective).* Forty-three components (1–43) with subsets. Sections (1) and (2) are usually completed by a nurse or physician's assistant, but may be completed by the patient or a family member with physician input.

3. *Physical examination (objective).* Twenty-two components (44–65) with subsets.

4. *ECG (objective).* One component (66) with subsets. Section 4 is usually interpreted by a physician or a computer.

5. *Diet evaluation and prescription (subjective, objective, and plan).* Seven components (67–73) with subsets. Section 5 is usually completed by a registered dietitian (RD), but may be completed by a nurse, a physician's assistant, or a physician.

6. *Podiatry evaluation, education, and prescription (subjective, objective, and plan).* Seven components (74–80) with subsets.
Section 6 is completed by a podiatrist.

7. *Laboratory (objective).* Nine components (81–88) with subsets. Section 7 is completed by laboratory technicians.

8. *Diabetes mellitus problem status and subsets.* Type of diabetes mellitus (IDDM, NIDDM, or GDM), complications (acute, chronic), initial plans [tests, consultations, therapy (short-term fast, diet, exercise, insulin, other)].
Section 8 is completed by a physician.

9. *Complete problem list.* This section lists all identified problems at their contemporary levels of resolution (prepared by a physician).

10. *Checklist for patient education and responses, prescription(s), testing equipment, supplies, assigned primary-care professionals, and planned follow-up.*

Diabetes Mellitus Data Base

Birthdate _____/_____/_____ mo/day/yr   Age: _____ yr
Address _____
City _____ State _____ Zip _____
Telephone (_____) _____
Mode of transportation _____
Contact person _____
Relationship _____
Address _____
City _____ State _____ Zip _____
Telephone (_____) _____   Today's date____/____/____ mo/day/yr

Instructions: Circle Y for yes, NO for no, AB for abnormal, and NM for normal. For all Y or AB answers, circle the letters of the subitems under each item. When indicated, write UNK for unknown, or NA for not applicable in the blank or between Y and NO, or AB and NM.

Sex   Marital status   Employment status

   F—female   U—unmarried   H—homemaker _____

   M—male   M—married   E—employed _____

Race   S—separated   U—unemployed _____

   C—caucasian   D—divorced   D—disabled _____

   B—black   W—widowed   R—retired _____

   O—other   S—student _____

Access to previous patient records: Y   NO   UNK

Previous diagnosis: D—diabetes,   S—diabetes suspect,   N—no diabetes,   O—other _____

Date of diagnosis _____/_____ (mo/yr)   NA

History of diagnosis (include when, where, by whom, follow-up, blood, and urine glucoses):

_____

_____

_____

_____

How referred _____

History

                    Medications

Y   NO   1. *Current* medications (prescriptions and over-the-counter)–give dosages:

                     _____   _____

                     _____   _____

                     _____   _____

                     _____   _____

                    Substance abuse

Y   NO   2. Substance abuse

                     SM—smoker ____ number of cigarettes/cigars AL—alcohol use:

                     per: D—day, W—week, M—month   Q—quit drinking   D—drinking now

                     Q—quit smoking,   S—smoking now   ___ no of bottles beer: D—day, W—wk, M—mo

                     _____ number cigarette packs/years _____ ___ no of quarts wine: D—day, W—wk, M—mo

                     O—other substance abuse _____ ___ no of pints liquor: D—day, W—wk, M—mo

                     _____ ___ timespan use: W—wk, M—mo, Y—yr

                    Surgical procedures

Y   NO   3. Surgical procedures   Year   Where done and sequelae

                     _____   _____   _____

                     _____   _____   _____

                     _____   _____   _____

                     _____   _____   _____

                    Amputations

Y   NO   4. Amputations (include dates, where done, why, right or left)

                     AK—above the knee _____   S—Syme's _____

                     BK—below the knee _____   T—toes _____

                     TM—transmetatarsal _____   O—other _____

                     PR—prosthesis _____

                    Previous hospitalizations

Y   NO   5. Previous hospitalizations (nonsurgical, nonmetabolic imbalance)

                     _____

                     _____

                     _____

                     _____

Past tests/procedures (within last 5 years, indicate if abnormal or normal)

Y   NO   6. Previous x-rays mo/yr, where done:
C—chest _____   O—other _____

Y   NO   7. Previous ECG _____

Y   NO   8. Other _____

Weight (write NA in the blanks if not applicable, or UNK if unknown)

9. Maximum weight and age: _____ lb _____ yr (Nongestational): _____ lb
10. Weight at 20 years of age _____ lb
11. Weight at diabetes mellitus diagnosis _____ lb
12. Weight at insulin discontinuance _____ lb
13. Weight at oral agent discontinuance _____ lb

Initial symptoms

Y   NO   14. Initial symptoms (before diagnosis of diabetes mellitus)

WG—weight gain _____	S—skin infections _____
WL—weight loss _____	L—leg cramps/pain _____
PU—polyuria _____	P—pruritus _____
PD—polydipsia _____	I—impotence _____
PH—polyphagia _____	D—dizziness _____
BF—burning feet _____	T—tiredness _____
BI—bladder infection _____	V—vaginal infections _____
VD—visual difficulties _____	O—other _____

Insulin use

Y   NO   15. Insulin use at any time

a. _____/_____ mo/yr started: type, dose, units _____

b. _____/_____ mo/yr stopped: type, dose, units _____

c. _____/_____/_____ mo/day/yr last taken; *if still using*, type, dose, units _____

d. _____ number of W—wk,   M—mo,   Y—yr total insulin use _____

e. Type use (give dose units, when taken, past and present use)

NO—none _____	N—NPH _____
B—beef _____	L—lente _____
P—pork _____	S—sulfated _____
H—human (rDNA) _____	Sl—semilente _____
H(SS)—Human semisynthetic _____	U—ultralente _____
R—regular _____	PR—proinsulin _____
LI—Lispro _____	O—other _____

f. Maximum total dose, type, units, dose, why_____

Oral agent use

Y   NO   16. Oral agent use

a. _____/_____ mo/yr started _____

b. _____/_____ mo/yr stopped _____

c. _____/_____/_____ mo/day/yr last taken; if still using, type, and dose _____

d. Number of W—wk,   M—mo,   Y—yr total oral agent use _____

e. Agents used (past or present, when taken, past and present use) (UNK—unknown):

C—chlorpropamide/Diabinese _____	GB—glyburide (glibenclamide)/Dia Beta
T—tolbutamide/Orinase _____	(Micronase) _____
TZ—tolazamide/Tolinase _____	GZ—glipizide/Glucatrol _____
A—acetohexamide/Dymelor _____	P—phenformin/DBI-TD, DBI _____
M—metformin _____	AC—acarbose _____
ME—meridia _____	R—redux _____
FP—fenphen _____	F—fenfluramine _____
O—other _____	

Home-monitored glucosuria, ketonuria, and blood sugar

Y   NO   17.   Is patient testing?

         a.   Urine sugar? _____ urine acetone? _____ blood sugar? _____

         b.   Type of tests: urine _____   blood _____

         c.   Time of day: urine _____   blood _____

         d.   % positive tests: urine sugar _____   ketones _____

         e.   Range blood sugar levels (mg/dL) _____

            Comments _____

Metabolic imbalance

Y   NO   18.   Metabolic imbalance (include when, where, sequelae, laboratory values)

         DKA—diabetic ketoacidosis _____

         HHS—hyperglycemic hyperosmolar state _____

         H—hypoglycemia _____

         O—other _____

Family history of diabetes

Y UNK NO   19.   Family history of diabetes (if unknown, circle UNK between Y and NO)

         M—mother _____

         F—father _____

         B—brother   total no.: _____ no. with DM _____ no. with IDDM _____ no. with NIDDM _____

         S—sister   total no.: _____ no. with DM _____ no. with IDDM _____ no. with NIDDM _____

         G—grandparents _____

         C—children   total no.: _____ no. with DM _____ no. with IDDM _____ no. with NIDDM _____

Family history of other significant illness

Y   NO   20.   Family history: cardiac, high blood pressure, malignancies, obesity, ages at death, and causes

         M—mother _____

         F—father _____

         B—brother _____

         S—sister _____

         G—grandparents _____

         C—children _____

         O—other _____

Review of Systems/Past Illnesses

Y   NO   21.   Patient's chief complaint today? _____

General

Y   NO   22.   General

         WC—weight change _____   F—fever/chills _____

         M—malaise _____   MG—malignancies _____

         A—anemia _____   O—other _____

Integument

Y   NO   23.   Integument

         R—rashes _____   N—nails _____

         O—other _____

HENT (head, ears, nose, throat)

Y   NO   24.   HENT

         H—headaches _____   S—sinus drainage _____

         A—allergy _____   D—dentures _____

         T—thyroid _____   O—other _____

Visual

Y   NO   25.   Visual

         L—laser therapy _____   G—glasses _____

         B—legal blindness _____   GL—glaucoma _____

         D—decreased acuity _____   E—last eye examination _____

         O—other _____

Respiratory

Y   NO   26.   Respiratory
              D—dyspnea _____   C—cough _____
              H—hemoptysis _____   P—pain/discomfort _____
              T—tuberculosis _____   O—other _____

Cardiovascular

Y   NO   27.   Cardiovascular
              P—pain _____   M—myocardial infarction _____
              S—SOB _____   H—heart _____
              OR—orthopnea _____   ST—stroke _____
              C—claudication _____   O—other _____

Gastrointestinal

Y   NO   28.   Gastrointestinal
              I—indigestion _____   M—melena _____
              DS—difficulty swallowing _____   D—diarrhea _____
              P—pain _____   C—constipation _____
              NV—nausea _____   L—laxative abuse _____
              E—enema abuse _____   PC—pancreatitis _____
              LV—liver _____   O—other _____

Renal/genitourinary

Y   NO   29.   Renal-genitourinary
              D—dysuria _____   H—hesitancy _____
              F—flank pain _____   O—other _____
             30.   Number of urinations per day _____
             31.   Number of urinations per night _____

Reproductive

Y   NO   32.   Reproductive
              S—sexual difficulties _____
              genital infections (Syphilis,Gonorrhea, AIDS, Etc.) _____
              I—impotence _____   O—other _____

Y   NO   33.   Contraception (past and present, indicate dates)
              BCP—birth control pills _____
              S—birth control shots _____   O—other _____

Obstetrics/gynecology (female only, write NA in the blank if not applicable)
             34.   Age at menarche (yr) _____
             35.   Age at menopause (yr) _____
             36.   Total number pregnancies (zero if never preg.) _____
              L—livebirths _____   M—miscarriages/stillborns _____
              A—abortions _____   E—ectopic/tubals _____
             37.   Total number livebirths/stillborns birth weight ≥ 8.75 lb (zero if none) _____/_____

Y   NO   38.   Toxemia/preeclampsia ever _____

Y   NO   39.   OB/GYN
              M—menstrual irregularities _____
              P—postmenopausal bleeding _____
              V—vaginal discharge/itching/odor _____
              O—other _____

Neuromusculoskeletal

Y   NO   40.   Neuromusculoskeletal
              P--paresthesias _____   AR—arthritis _____
              W—weakness _____   PN—pain _____
              S—seizures _____   HI—head injuries _____
              F—fractures _____   O—other _____

Immunology

Y   NO   41.   Sensitivities/allergies

P—penicillin _____   I—insulin _____

F—food _____   IS—insect stings _____

O—other _____

Emotional/socioeconomic assessment

Y   NO   42.   Past psychiatric problems/hospitalizations _____

_____

_____

Y   NO   43.   Current emotional/socioeconomic problems _____

_____

_____

History-taker signature _____   ID number _____

Physical Examination

General status

AB   NM   44.   General status

a.   Frame: S—small,   MS—medium small,   M—medium,   ML—medium large,   L—large

b.   _____ present height (in) _____

c.   _____ present weight (lb) _____

d.   ideal body weight (Hamwi formula) _____

e.   temperature (Fahrenheit) _____

AB   NM   45.   General appearance _____

_____

Integument

AB   NM   46.   Integument

N—necrobiosis _____   H—hair distribution _____

A—lipoatrophy _____   L—lipohypertrophy _____

U—urticaria _____   S—scars _____

O—other _____

Eyes

AB   NM   47.   Eyes

a.   Acuity _____ right corrected

b.   Acuity _____ left corrected

C—cataracts _____   R—rubeosis irides _____

P—pupils _____   O—other _____

Fundoscopic

AB   NM   48.   Fundi

PPDR   M—microaneurysm,   H—hemorrhage,   X—exudate,   E—edema,   O—other ____

PDR: N—neovascularization,   O—other _____

V—vitreous hemorrhage _____

H—hypertensive retinal changes _____

O—other _____

HENTN

AB   NM   49.   HENTN

H—head _____   E—ears _____

N—nose _____   T—throat _____

TH—thyroid _____   C—carotid bruit _____

V—venous distention _____   O—other _____

Dental

AB   NM   50.   Dental

P—pyorrhea _____   C—caries _____

M—missing teeth _____   O—other _____

Lymph nodes

AB   NM   51. Lymph nodes
C—cervical _____   I—inguinal _____
A—axillary _____   O—other, _____

Thorax

AB   NM   52. B—breasts _____   L—lungs _____
O—other _____

Cardiovascular

AB   NM   53. Cardiovascular
A—apex impulse _____   S—sounds _____
M—murmurs _____   G—gallops _____
O—other _____

Blood pressure

54. Supine blood pressure   R—right _____ L—left _____
55. Sitting blood pressure   R—right _____ L—left _____
56. Standing blood pressure   R—right _____ L—left _____
57. Other blood pressure   R—right _____ L—left _____

Abdomen

AB   NM   58. Abdomen
L—liver _____   SP—spleen _____
A—ascites _____   OB—obese _____
M—masses _____   T—tenderness _____
R—rebound _____   S—sounds _____
O—other _____

Rectal

AB   NM   59. Rectal
H—hemorrhoids _____   O—other _____
a. Hemoccult: N—negative,   P—positive,   ND—not done and why _____

Genitalia

AB NA NM   60. Genitalia (female)
U—uterus _____   A—adnexa _____
C—cervix _____   E—external genitalia _____
V—vagina _____   O—other _____
a. Pap done: Y—yes,   N—no and why not   _____

AB NA NM   61. Genitalia (male)
E—external genitalia _____   P—prostate _____
O—other _____

Neuromusculoskeletal

AB   NM   62. Neuromusculoskeletal
C—cranial nerves _____   M—muscles _____
J—joints _____   O—other _____

AB   NM   63. Sensory
V—vibratory: R—right _____   L—left _____
L—light touch: R—right _____   L—left _____

AB   NM   64. Pulses (0 to 3+ and circle bruits)

	Fem.	Pop.	PT	DP	Other
R—right	a. _____	b. _____	c. _____	d. _____	e. _____
L—left	f. _____	g. _____	h. _____	i. _____	j. _____

AB   NM 65. DTR's: Motor reinforcement: Y—yes,   N—no
                 0—absent,   1—hypoactive,   2—active,   3—hyperactive,   4—clonus
                          Knee   Ankle   Plantar   Other
                 R—right   a. _____   b. _____   c. _____   d. _____
                 L—left   e. _____   f. _____   g. _____   h. _____

                 ECG
AN   NM 66. ECG
                 L–left ventricular hypertrophy RB–right bundle branch block (RBBB) N–normal sinus rhythm
                 P–previous infarction   LB–left bundle branch block (LBBB)   A–atrial fibrillation
                 O—other _____
                     a. _____ rate (beats per minute)
                     b. _____ PR,   _____ PRS,   _____ QT
                     c. Interpretation _____
                        _____
                        _____

                     Physician signature _____   ID number _____

Diet Evaluation Data

                 Diet History
Y   NO 67. Factors relating to diet
                     a. _____ number of members in household and who _____
                        _____
                     b. _____ meal preparers
                     c. Source of money for food: F—Food Stamps,   O—other _____
                     d. Meals away from home _____
                     e. Food intolerances/dislikes _____

Y   NO 68. Current diet
                     a. D—diabetic,   R—reduction,   N—nonprescribed,   O—other _____
                     b. Approximate caloric intake per day _____
                     c. Modifications (circle the numbers)

                        1. low sodium   2. high potassium   3. low potassium
                        4. low fat   5. low protein   6. Other _____

                     d. Compliance with prescribed diet
                        E—excellent,   G—good,   F—fair,   P—poor,   NA—not applicable
                     e. Nutritional supplements _____
                     f. Activity level _____
                     g. Patient education   —   grade completed (circle one or more)
                        A—reads words,   N—reads numbers,   P—poor vision,   U—unable to read or write
                     h. Current diet pattern, indicate food-preparation-amount:

Breakfast	Lunch	Supper	Snack

Recommended diet therapy

Y   NO   69.   Recommended diet

F—fast   __0__ (number calories) _____ number D—day, W—wk, M—mo

AF—after fast   _____ (number calories) _____ number D—day, W—wk, M—mo

L—long-term reduction   _____ (number calories) _____ number D—day, W—wk, M—mo

M—maintenance diet   _____ (number calories) _____ number D—day, W—wk, M—mo

G—weight gain diet   _____ (number calories) _____ number D—day, W—wk, M—mo

a.   _____ g CHO   _____ g protein   _____ g fat For which diet? _____

b.   Modifications (circle the numbers)

      1. low sodium   2. high potassium   3. low potassium

      4. low fat   5. low protein   6. Other _____

Y   NO   70.   Distribution of meals by fraction _____

Y   NO   71.   Diet pattern by exchange group currently prescribed

Group	B	MS	L	AS	S	HS
Milk						
Vegetable						
Fruit						
Bread						
Meat						
Fat						

Y   NO   72.   Patient education instructions

a.   Patient understanding of exchanges, diet, meal selection

     E—excellent,   G—good,   F—fair,   P—poor

b.   Patient motivation to adhere to diet

     E—excellent,   G—good,   F—fair,   P—poor

Y   NO   73.   Dietitian comments _____

_____

     RD signature _____ ID number _____

Podiatry (Lower Extremity) Data

Circulatory

AB   NM   74. Pulses: (0 to 3+ and circle bruits)

	Fem.	Pop.	PT	DP	Other
R—right	a. _____	b. _____	c. _____	d. _____	e. _____
L—left	f. _____	g. _____	h. _____	i. _____	j. _____

AB   NM   75. Circulatory

    V—varicosities _____   S—venous stasis _____

    T—thrombophlebitis _____   O—other _____

Sensory

AB   NM   76. L—light touch _____   V—vibratory _____

    J—joint position _____   O—other _____

Motor

AB   NM   77. Motor

    T—tone _____   M—muscle atrophy _____

    TR—tremor _____   H—hemiparesis _____

    O—other _____

Deep tendon reflexes

AB   NM   78. DTR's: Motor reinforcement: Y—yes,   N—no

    0—absent,   1—hypoactive,   2—active,   3—hyperactive,   4—clonus

	Knee	Ankle	Plantar	Other
R—right	a.. _____	b. _____	c. _____	d. _____
L—left	e. _____	f. _____	g. _____	h. _____

Musculoskeletal

AB   NM   79. Musculoskeletal

    P—pain _____   E—edema _____

    H—heat _____   R—rubor _____

    S—stiffness _____   D—deformity _____

    M—muscles _____   HT—hammer toes _____

    O—other _____

Dermatologic

AB   NM   80. Dermatologic

    H—hair changes _____   N—hypertrophic nail changes _____

    U—ulcers_____   S—sweating_____

    C—color changes _____   I—infections _____

    T—tumor_____   CL—callus _____

    CR—corns _____   O—other_____

Lower extremity status and therapy

Lower extremity status:

    NC—no complications

    L—lower extremity complications

        1. Arteriopathy

        2. Peripheral neuropathy

        3. Musculoskeletal

        4. DTR

        5. Dermatologic

Procedures performed

    D—debriding _____

    N—nail trim _____

    O—other_____

Patient instruction and care

    R—regular extremity hygiene and care _____

    S—special care _____

Consultations _____

_____

_____

Follow-up

    P—podiatry_____

    D—diabetes clinic, PRN podiatry _____

    O—other_____

Podiatrist signature _____   ID number _____

    Other signature _____   ID number _____

Laboratory Data

Plasma glucoses
81. Plasma glucoses
    a. Fasting and time_____ mg/dL, _____ Comments _____
    b. Second and time_____ mg/dL, _____ Comments _____
    c. Third and time _____ mg/dL, _____ Comments _____
    d. Other and time _____ mg/dL, _____ Comments _____

Glucosuria
82. Glucosuria (2 drop Clinitest method): 0, 1/4, 1/2, 1, 2, 3, 5%
    a. Fasting collection(%) _____ urinevolume _____ (g) glucose _____
    b. Second collection (%) _____
    c. Third collection (%) _____
    d. Other collection (%) _____

Ketonuria
83. Ketonuria: 0 = neg,   20 mg/dL = small,   40 mg/dL = moderate,   100 mg/dL = large
    a. Fasting collection (mg/dL) _____
    b. Second collection (mg/dL) _____
    c. Third collection (mg/dL) _____
    d. Other collection (mg/dL) _____

Proteinuria
84. Proteinuria dipstick
    a. Fasting collection _____ +
    b. Second collection _____ +
    c. Third collection _____ +
    d. Other collection _____ +

85. Glucosuria (grams urinary glucose in 24 hr)
    a. Fasting collection (%) _____
    b. Second collection (%) _____
    c. Third collection (%) _____
    d. Other collection (%) _____

Microscopic
86. Microscopic
    a. WBC: _____ hpf Comments _____
    b. RBC: _____ hpf Comments _____
    c. Other _____
       _____
       _____

Specific gravity
87. Specific gravity
    a. Fasting collection _____
    b. Second collection _____
    c. Third collection _____

Y   NO   88. C—CBC, S—SMA—6, M—SMA—12, L—lipid profile (total cholesterol, and VLDL, LDL, and
             HDL cholesterols), P—serum C—peptide, F—fructosamine, QUA—quantitative urine albu-
             min (normal <20 mg/24 hr, microalbuminuria 40–200 mg/24 hr, clinically proteinuric >300
             mg/24 hr), V—centrifuged urine sediment, H-HbA$_{1C}$ method , O—other _____
             Comments _____
             _____

Miscellaneous
Laboratory technician signature _____ ID number _____
Performed by _____ _____/_____/_____ (mo/day/yr)

Problem List

Instructions: Indicate the problem numbers, followed by the problem statement. Place an asterisk (*) after the problem for active problems (those for which you have included tests, consultations, and/or medications on the PROBLEM STATUS sheet).

no(s). _____ —diabetes status (see section labeled Diabetes Mellitus Problem Status

no(s). _____ —lower extremity status (see section labeled Podiatry Lower Extremity Status

no(s). _____
Problem statement _____
_____
_____
_____

no(s). _____
Problem statement _____
_____
_____
_____

no(s). _____
Problem statement _____
_____
_____
_____

no(s). _____
Problem statement _____
_____
_____
_____

no(s). _____
Problem statement _____
_____
_____
_____

no(s). _____
Problem statement _____
_____
_____
_____

no(s). _____
Problem statement _____
_____
_____
_____

no(s). _____
Problem statement _____
_____
_____
_____

Patient Education, Evaluation, and Therapy Checklist

Instructions: Review the checklist with the patient assigned to you before the patient leaves the initial visit.

Y   NO   Patient has received insulin this morning _____

_____

_____

Instructed:	Patient has received instructions in:	Patient response:

Y   NO   1. Urine testing
       a. Glucose _____
       b. Acetone _____

Y   NO   2. Home blood glucose monitoring
       a. Testing strip (type) _____
       b. Meter (type) _____

Y   NO   3. Understanding diabetes
       a. Symptoms and treatment _____
       b. Acidosis _____

Y   NO   4. Insulin administration
       a. Hypoglycemia _____
       b. Administration technique _____
       c. Disposable syringes and needles _____
       d. Insulin storage _____
       e. Rotate sites _____

Y   NO   5. General skin care, personal hygiene, bathing, dental care _____

Y   NO   6. Lower extremity hygiene and care _____

Y   NO   7. Dietary instruction _____

Y   NO   8. Goals for return visit _____

Y   NO   9. Other _____ _____

Patient has received prescriptions and/or equipment

Y   NO   1. Insulin, disposable syringes and needles

Y   NO   2. Clinitest, Acetest, test tube, dropper

       3. Blood testing strip and type _____
       Meter and type _____

Y   NO   4. ID card

Y   NO   5. Measuring cup, ruler, and spoon

Y   NO   6. Copy of *Diabetes Guidebook: Diet Section*

Y   NO   7. Lubrication cream

Y   NO   8. Prescriptions for other medications

_____ , _____

_____ , _____

Y   NO   Laboratory slips for other tests, procedures, x-rays

_____ , _____

_____ , _____

Y   NO   Other _____

Patient to return to diabetes clinic _____ (date and/or time span)

Patient to return to podiatry _____ (date and/or time span)

Patient's primary care clinic _____

Patient's assigned diabetes clinic nurse _____

Patient's assigned diabetes clinic physician _____

Patient's assigned diabetes clinic dietitian _____

The physician is to be promptly informed by the nurse of the results of consultations, laboratory tests, and procedures in person, by telephone, or by written memorandum.

Additional comments _____

_____

Nurse signature _____ ID number _____

Other signature _____ ID number _____

Problem Status (diabetes assessment, tests, consultations, medications for all active problems)

Criteria to support diagnosis of DM
      U—random urine glucose (>25 mg/dL)   _____ mg/dL ____/____ mo/yr
      P—random plasma glucose (>200 mg/dL)   _____ mg/dL ____/____ mo/yr
      M—2-hr postmeal (100 g carbohydrate) glucose (>175 mg/dL) _____ mg/dL ____/____ mo/yr
      F—fasting plasma glucose (>140 mg/dL)   _____ mg/dL ____/____ mo/yr
      G—glucose tolerance test (GTT)   _____ mg/dL ____/____ mo/yr
          (sum of fasting + 1 + 2 + 3 hr > 800 mg/dL)
      HN—high normal GTT (sum of F plus 1, 2, 3 hr post-100 g glucose load = 601–800 mg/dL)

Diabetes status
      N—no diabetes (sum GTT ≤ 600 mg/dL)
      HNGTT—sum GTT 601–800 mg/dL
      DM—diabetes mellitus (nongestational)
      1. IDDM (insulin-dependent) (type 1)
      2. NIDDM (non-insulin-dependent) (type 2)
      GDM—gestational diabetes mellitus

These criteria differ from those recently recommended (1997) by the American Diabetes Association. The ADA now accepts a fasting plasma glucose≥ than 126 mg/dL (7 mmol/l) × 2 or a two hour post 75-g glucose load plasma glucose > 140 mg/dL (7.8 mmol/l) × 2 as diagnostic of diabetes. The editor of this book believes that those levels are *too low*.

See Chapters 11 and 12 for further discussion concerning screening for and diagnosis of diabetes mellitus.

Indicate any complications
      MS—Acute complications (metabolic states)
        1.   DKA
        2   Hyperglycemic hyperosmolar state
        3.   Hypoglycemia
      MI—Chronic complications (microangiopathy)
        1.   Retinopathy
        2.   Nephropathy
      MA—Chronic complications (macroangiopathy)
        1.   Coronary artery disease
        2.   Peripheral vascular disease
        3.   Cerebral vascular disease
      N—Chronic complication (neuropathy)
        1.   Peripheral
        2.   Autonomic: C—cardiovascular,   GI—gastrointestinal,   GU—genitourinary
        3.   Cranial

Tests _____   Reason for _____

_____   _____

Consultations _____   Reason for _____

_____   _____

Therapy
    _____ number days fasting, diabetes clinic visit at intervals of _____ days   Present wt. _____ lb
    _____ number calories for weight loss (to IBW) for _____ weeks   Ideal body wt. _____ lb
    _____ number calories for weight gain (to IBW) for _____ weeks   Excess wt. _____ lb
    _____ number calories for maintenance of IBW   Estimated rate of
                                               weight loss _____ lb/wk

Patient goal: patient to achieve IBW of _____ lb by _____/_____ (mo/yr)

Exercise _____
Medication status _____

_____

_____

Other therapy _____
Physician signature _____   ID number _____
Other signature _____   ID number _____

APPENDIX VIII

Follow-up Visit(s) and Audit Forms

John K. Davidson

VIIIa. Diabetes Unit Walk-in Clinic Visit and Triage Form

Date _____

Patient Identification _____

Time In _____

Race _____ Sex _____   Method of Arrival _____

Subjective _____

   1. Referred Consultation   4. Blood Sugar Check ( )
      A. New Patient ( )   5. Dietary Consult ( )
      B. Established Patient ( )   6. Prescription Refill ( )
   2. B/P Check ( )   7. Other _____
   3. Foot Care ( )

Objective   Wt./IBW _____/_____ lbs. BP _____ Temp _____ Pulse _____ Resp. _____

_____

_____   Allergies

_____

_____

_____

_____

Assessment _____   Medications

_____

_____

_____

_____

_____

Plan _____

_____

_____   Lab Results

_____   FBG _____   PG _____   h.p.c. _____

_____ CO_2 _____   BUN _____   Cr _____

_____ K^+ _____   Na _____   Cl _____

_____   Urine ketones _____

   Other _____

Patient Education   Hyperglycemia _____   Hypoglycemia _____   Insulin Administration _____

Foot Care _____   Diet _____   Home Blood Glucose Monitoring _____   Urine Testing _____

Other _____

Patient Response   Able to verbalize understanding ( )   Unable to verbalize understanding ( )

               Able to return demonstration ( )   Unable to return demonstration ( )

Comments _____

Return Appointment _____   Discharge Time _____

Signature _____ R.N., N.P., P.A., R.D., D.P.M. No. _____

_____ M.D. No. _____

VIIIb.   Diabetes Clinic Follow-up Sheet

Patient Identification _____

Previous Rx: Diet: _____ Insulin: _____ OA: _____ Method of Arrival: _____

Date: _____ Time: _____

SUBJECTIVE _____

_____

_____

OBJECTIVE   ALLERGIES

WT/IBW _____/_____ lbs. Temp _____ Resp. Rate _____ _____

BP: Sit _____ Stand _____ Pulse: Sit _____ Stand _____ _____

PULSES   _____

Dorsalis Pedis R _____ L _____ Posterior Tibial R _____ L _____ _____

_____ MEDICATIONS

_____ _____

_____ _____

_____ _____

_____ _____

_____ _____

_____ _____

_____ _____

ASSESSMENT   LAB RESULTS

_____ FPG _____ PG _____ Hr _____

_____ Na _____ Cl _____ Cr _____

_____ K+ _____ CO_2 _____ BUN _____

_____ $HbAl_c$ _____ C-pep _____

_____ Date _____

_____ Urine S&A _____

PLAN   Blood Ac _____

_____ Cholest _____ TG: _____

_____ Date _____

_____ Other _____

_____

_____

_____

DIETITIAN

_____

_____

_____

_____

_____

_____

_____ R.N., N.P., PA. _____ R.D. _____ DPM No. _____

_____ M.D.No. _____

Return Appointment _____

Discharge Time _____

VIIIc. Diabetes Clinic Patient Education Instruction Form

Patient Identification _____

	Y	N	Reviewed but unable to perform

DIET
1. Has a copy of diet
2. Explains diet
3. States IBW
4. States recommendations regarding fluid intake

INSULIN
1. States times for injection
2. States type and dose of insulin
3. Demonstrates drawing up insulin
4. Demonstrates mixing insulin
5. Has literature on taking insulin

ORAL AGENTS
1. Type and Dose

HYPOGLYCEMIA
1. States symptoms of hypoglycemia
2. States what to do if hypoglycemia occurs

HGM
1. States goal (i.e. 80–150) of SMBG
2. States times and frequency of tests
3. Demonstrates UGM/BGM

FOOTCARE
1. Explains what to look for in daily foot checks
2. Demonstrates how to cut nails
3. Explains rationale for lubricating feet daily

EXERCISE
1. States recommendations

COMPLICATIONS
1. States when to call Nurse (i.e., foot changes, hypoglycemia, DKA, hyperglycemia or ill) or go to emergency room
2. Demonstrates ulcer/lesion care
3. Can state long-term complications of diabetes

OTHER MEDICATION
1. Explains reason for
2. States how and when to take
3. States side effects to look for

Signature _____

VIIId. Diabetes Clinic ICD-9-CM Diagnosis Codes

Date:

_____

CLINIC CODE

Diabetes Clinic
ICD-9-CH Diagnosis
Codes (Leave
attached to front of
Accounting Record)

PHYSICIAN: CHECK PROPER DIAGNOSIS CODE:
SPECIFY MORE DATA IN BLANK SPACES WHERE INDICATED BY*

Diabetes Mellitus
__ 250.00 No complica-
tions
__ 250.10 Ketoacidosis
__ 250.10 Acidosis—No
Coma
__ 250.10 Ketosis—No
Coma

**Diabetes Mellitus with
Complications**
__ 250.80 Bone Change
__ 250.90 Heart Disease
__ 250.50 Ophthalmic
Manifestation
__ 250.70 Peripheral
Circulation
Disorder
__ 250.60 Neurological
Manifestation
__ 250.40 Renal
Manifestation

Hypoglycemia
__ 251.2 Not Due to
Medication
__ 251.0 Due to Insulin
__ 251.0 Due to
Sulfonylurea
__ 251.0 Due to Other
Medication

OTHER DIAGNOSIS (not S/P or procedure) _____
SITE: _____
TYPE: _____
PHYSICIAN SIGNATURE   PHYSICIAN NUMBER

VIIIe. Diabetes Clinic Outpatient Accounting Record

Date:

_____ _____
Clinic Code

OUTPATIENT ACCOUNTING RECORD
MISCELLANEOUS VISITS

DIABETES CLINIC

AMBULATORY
CARE
_____
TIME OF VISIT
AM
PM

COPAYMENT

1 ☐ BLOOD GLUCOSE TESTING   3 ☐ PODIATRY   5 ☐ DIETARY CONSULTS

2 ☐ PRESCRIPTION REFILL   4 ☐ BLOOD PRESSURE CHECK

Diagnosis Or Approved Abbreviation   Physician Name   Physician No.

VIIIf.   Audit of Decompensated Diabetes Mellitus

Name _____ Hospital no. _____ Medicare? _____ Medicaid? _____

Birth date _____ Age _____ Sex _____ Race _____ Primary care clinic _____

Admission date _____ Discharge date _____ Ward _____

Was diabetes primary cause of admission? _____ Cause of admission if other than diabetes _____

Was diabetes undiagnosed prior to this admission? _____

Admission   PG _____ HCO_3 _____ Na _____ K _____ Cl _____ pH _____ BUN_____

         Ht. _____/_____ (ft/in)   Wt _____ lb   IBW _____ lb $\pm$ _____ IBW

Calculated serum osmolality _____ Calculated serum anion gap _____

Therapy prior to admission: Insulin (type, units) _____ Diet (cal) _____

Hospital therapy (first 24 hours):   Insulin (total units) _____ Fluid (liters) _____

                                              K^+ (mEq) _____ Na^+ (mEq) _____

Therapy on discharge: Insulin _____ Diet _____

DKA _____ Severe ($CO_2 < 10$) _____ Moderate (CO_2 10–20) _____ Mild ($CO_2 > 20$) _____

Hyperglycemic hyperosmolar state? _____ (osmolality > 350)

Uncontrolled hyperglycemia? _____ PG on discharge _____

Precipitating cause of decompensated diabetes? _____

Compliance with therapy before admission _____ Good _____ Fair _____ Poor

Date of initial diabetes clinic (DC) visit? _____ Date of last DC visit? _____

Date of next scheduled DC visit? _____ DC nurse _____

State of consciousness _____ Normal _____ Cloudy _____ Stupor _____ Coma

Side effects of therapy _____ Hypoglycemia (< 50 mg/dL) _____ Hypokalemia (< 3 mEq/L) _____

    Other _____

Complications _____ Malnutrition _____ Renal shutdown _____ Lactic acidosis _____ Pancreatitis

_____ Cardiac arrhythmias _____ Immunologic insulin resistance _____ Urinary tract infection (UTI)

_____ Aspiration pneumonia _____ Myocardial infarction (MI), stroke, thrombosis, embolus, etc.

_____ Vascular occlusion   Comments _____

_____ DRG No. _____

Date of death _____ Cause of death _____ ICD-9-CM Code No: _____

Cost of hospitalization _____

VIIIg.   Audit of Amputations and Other Surgical Services

Name _____ Hospital no. _____ Medicare? _____ Medicaid? _____

Birth date _____ Age _____ Sex _____ Race _____

Admission date _____ Amputation date _____ Discharge date _____

Admission diagnosis _____ Operative procedure _____

Service (vascular, orthopedic, other) _____ Death date _____ Cause _____

                                             DRG No. _____

                                             ICD-9-CM Code No: _____

Diabetes mellitus? _____   Nondiabetic? _____   Indeterminate? _____

Year diagnosed _____ Normal fasting PG? _____ PG not measured? _____

FPG > 140 mg/dL _____ Sum fasting and 1-, 2-, 3-hr post-100-g   Trauma? _____

GTT sum >   glucose load

   800 mg/dL _____   <600 mg/dL _____   _____

                        601–800 mg/dL _____   _____

Abnormal GTT? _____ Normal GTT? _____   _____

Last diabetes clinic visit? _____ Last podiatry visit? _____

Level of control (mean PG for 1 year prehospitalization) _____

   Good (<140 mg/dL) _____   Fair (141–175 mg/dL) _____

   Poor (175–210 mg/dL) _____   Very poor (>210 mg/dL) _____

APPENDIX IX

Index to Diagnoses, Drug-Related Adverse Reactions, and Procedures Associated with Diabetes Mellitus

John K. Davidson

IXa. *Disease categories* (ICD-9-CM)

IXb. *Drug-related adverse effects*

IXc. *Procedures* (ICD-9-CM)

The classification of diseases and procedures under leadership of the World Health Organization and other major health groups has developed significantly in recent years due to the rapid changes in medical practice and its financing. It has become essential that physicians get acquainted with contemporary coding of diseases and procedures. Those involved in the care of patients with diabetes mellitus have a particular need for such a knowledge of coding practices because of the complexity of the disease itself and its multiplicity of complications, concomitant problems, and treatment procedures. The *International Classification of Diseases, Ninth Revision, Clinical Modification (ICD-9-CM)* is the standard reference publication in this area and the source of information provided in this appendix.[1]

Coding for diabetes mellitus and diabetes-related disease categories is shown in Appendix IXa; for diabetes drug-related adverse reactions in Appendix IXb; and for procedures frequently carried out for diabetes and its complications in Appendix IXc. These *ICD-9-CM* categories are used in assigning hospitalized patients to diagnosis-related groups (DRGs), which in turn play an important role in the calculation of prospective payments to hospitals by Medicare, Medicaid, and other third-party payors (see Appendix X).

The concept of extending the *International Classification of Diseases* for use in hospital indexing was originally developed in response to a need for a more efficient basis for storage and retrieval of diagnostic data. Much of the early testing of the coding system in hospitals and medical centers in the United States was done in the 1950s. Development continued into the following decade, and by 1969, an international conference for the revision of the *International Classification of Diseases* could note that the eighth revision of *ICD* had been constructed with hospital indexing in mind, adding that the revised classification would be suitable for hospital use in some countries. A group of consultants then recommended that further detail be provided for coding of hospital and morbidity data, and through the cooperative efforts of the American Hospital Association, the United States Public Health Service, and other organizations, the *Eighth Revision, International Classification of Diseases, Adapted for Use in the United States* (PHS publication no. 1693) appeared in 1968. Commonly known as *ICDA-8*, this work began to serve as the basis for coding diagnostic data for official morbidity and mortality statistics in the United States. After *ICD-9* had been published, a steering committee was convened in 1977 by the National Center for Health Statistics to provide advice and counsel on the development of a clinical modification of that publication. Organizations represented on the Steering Committee were the American Association of Health Data Systems, American Hospital Association, American Medical Record Association, Association for Health Records, Council on Clinical Classifications (sponsored by American Academy of Pediatrics, American College of Obstetricians and Gynecologists, American College of Physicians, American College of Surgeons, American Psychiatric Association, and Commission on Professional and Hospital Activities), Health Care Financing Administration of the Department of Health and Human Services, and World Health Organization Center for Classification of Diseases in North America (sponsored by the National Center for Health Statistics and the Department of Health and Human Services).

Thus *ICD-9-CM* is a clinical modification of the World Health Organization's *International Classification of Diseases, Ninth Revision (ICD-9)*. The second edition of *ICD-9-CM* appeared in September 1980. According to Lester Breslow, chairman of the National Committee on Vital and Health Statistics:

the book had already proven useful in standardizing disease classification throughout the United States, and it stands as a significant achievement of the many clinicians, statisticians, epidemiologists, and nosologists who contributed to its development. The *ICD-9-CM* serves both to aid the clinical management of patients and to guide the formation of health care policy and priorities in the United States.[1]

The Ninth Revision of the *International Classification of Diseases (ICD-9)* is still being used in 1998, although discussions have taken place since 1985 concerning its possible replacement by ICD-10.[2–5]

References

1. International Classification of Diseases, Ninth revision, Vols. 1, 2, and 3, Ed. 2. Clinical Modification (ICD-9-CM). Department of Health and Human Services (DHHS) Publication no. [Public Health Service (PHS)] 80-1260. Department of Health and Human Services, Public Health Service–Health Care Financing Administration, 1980.

2. Bramer GR: International Statistical Classification of Diseases and Health Related Problems–Tenth Revision. World Health Stat Q 41:32–36, 1988.

3. Williams R, King H: ICD coding; what's in a number? Diabetic Med 6:385–386, 1989.

4. WHO: Diabetes Mellitus. Report of a WHO Study Group. Technical Report Series 727. Geneva: World Health Organization, 1985.

5. Jones MK, Schmidt KM, Aaron WS: St. Anthony's ICD-9-CM Code Book, vols. 1, 2, 3. Reston, VA: St. Anthony Publishing, Inc., 1996.

IXa. Disease Categories (ICD-9-CM) (See Appendix IX)

250 Diabetes mellitus
     Excludes
         Hyperglycemia NOS (790.6)
         Neonatal diabetes mellitus (775.1)
         Nonclinical diabetes (790.2)
         Diabetes mellitus complicating pregnancy, childbirth or the puerperium (648.0)
     Use the following fifth-digit subclassification with category 250:
         0 Adult-onset (non-insulin-dependent diabetes mellitus) or unspecified as to type
         1 Juvenile type (insulin-dependent diabetes mellitus)

250.0 Diabetes mellitus without mention of complication or manifestation classifiable to 250.1 through 250.9
       Diabetes (mellitus) NOS (see *Abbreviations*)
       Sugar

250.1 Diabetes with ketoacidosis
       Diabetic
           Acidosis ⎫
                    ⎬ without mention of coma
           Ketosis ⎭
           Acetonemia

250.2 Diabetes with hyperosmolar coma
       Hyperosmolar (nonketotic) coma

250.3 Diabetes with other coma
       Diabetic coma (with ketoacidosis)
       Hyperglycemic

250.4 Diabetes with renal manifestations
       Use additional code, if desired, to identify manifestation, such as:
       Diabetic
           Nephropathy NOS (583.81)

           Nephrosis (581.81)
           Hypertension-nephrosis syndrome (581.81)
           Intercapillary glomerulosclerosis (581.81)
           Kimmelstiel-Wilson disease or syndrome (581.81)

250.5 Diabetes with ophthalmic manifestations
       Use additional code, if desired, to identify manifestation, such as:
       Diabetic
           Cataract (366.41)
           Retinopathy (background 362.01/proliferative (362.02)
           Iritis (364.42)
           Retinal microaneurysms (362.01)
           Retinitis (362.01)
           Retinal hemorrhage (362.01)

250.6 Diabetes with neurologic manifestations
       Use additional code, if desired, to identify manifestation, such as
       Diabetic
           Amyotrophy (358.1)
           Mononeuropathy (354.0 to 355.9)
           Neurogenic Arthropathy (713.5)
           Peripheral autonomic neuropathy (337.1)
           Polyneuropathy (357.2)
           Dorsal sclerosis (340)
           Neuralgia (357.2)
           Neuritis (357.2)
           Neuropathy (357.2)

250.7 Diabetes with peripheral circulatory disorders
       Use additional code, if desired, to identify manifestation, such as
       Diabetic
           Gengrene (785.4)
           Peripheral angiopathy (443.81)

250.8 Diabetes with other specified manifestations
Use additional code, if desired, to identify manifestation, such as
  Diabetic bone changes (731.8)
  Secondary glycogenosis (259.8)
  Lancereaux's (diabetes mellitus with marked emaciation) (261)
  Lipoidosis (272.7)
  Ulcer (skin) (707.9)
  Ulcer (lower extremity) (707.1)
Excludes: intercurrent infections in diabetic patients
  Ulcer [specified site NEC (see *Abbreviations*)] (707.8)
  Xanthoma (272.2)

250.9 Diabetes with unspecified complication
  Uncontrolled NEC

251 Other disorders of pancreatic internal secretion

251.0 Hypoglycemic coma
  Iatrogenic hyperinsulinism
  Insulin coma
Use additional E code, if desired, to identify cause, if drug-induced (see Appendix VIIIb)

251.1 Other hyperinsulinism
  Hyperinsulinism
    NOS
    Ectopic
    Functional
  Hyperplasia of pancreatic islet B cells NOS
Excludes
  Hypoglycemia in infant of diabetic mother (775.0)
  Neonatal hypoglycemia (775.6)

251.2 Hypoglycemia, unspecified
  Hypoglycemia
    NOS
    Reactive
    Spontaneous
Excludes: leucine-induced (270.3)

251.3 Postsurgical hypoinsulinemia
  Hypoinsulinemia following complete or partial pancreatectomy
  Postpancreatectomy hyperglycemia

251.4 Abnormality of secretion of glucagon
  Hyperplasia of pancreatic islet A cells with glucagon excess

251.5 Abnormality of secretion of gastrin
  Hyperplasia of pancreatic A cells with gastrin excess
  Zollinger-Ellison syndrome

251.8 Other specified disorders of pancreatic internal secretion
  Steroid induced
    Correct substance, properly administered

251.9 Unspecified disorder of pancreatic internal secretion

  Islet cell hyperplasia NOS

258.1 Other combinations of endocrine dysfunction
  Schmidt's syndrome
  Dwarfism-obesity syndrome

271.4 Renal glycosuria
  Renal diabetes (true)

272.0 Pure hypercholesterolemia
  Familial hypercholesterolemia
  Fredrickson type IIa hyperlipoproteinemia
  Hyperbetalipoproteinemia
  Hyperlipidemia, group A
  Low-density-lipoid type (LDL) hyperlipoproteinemia

272.1 Pure hyperglyceridemia
  Endogenous hyperglyceridemia
  Fredrickson type IV hyperlipoproteinemia
  Hyperlipidemia, group B
  Hyperprebetalipoproteinemia
  Hypertriglyceridemia, essential
  Very-low-density-lipoid type (VLDL) hyperlipoproteinemia

272.2 Mixed hyperlipidemia
  Broad- or floating-beta-lipoproteinemia
  Fredrickson type IIb or III hyperlipoproteinemia
  Hypercholesterolemia with endogenous hyperglyceridemia
  Hyperbetalipoproteinemia with prebetalipoproteinemia
  Tubo-eruptive xanthoma
  Xanthoma tuberosum

272.3 Hyperchylomicronemia
  Bürger-Grütz syndrome
  Fredrickson type I or V hyperlipoproteinemia
  Hyperlipidemia, group D
  Mixed hyperglyceridemia

272.4 Other and unspecified hyperlipidemia
  Alpha-lipoproteinemia
  Combined hyperlipidemia
  Hyperlipidemia NOS
  Hyperlipoproteinemia NOS

272.5 Lipoprotein deficiencies
  Abetalipoproteinemia
  Bassen-Kornzweig syndrome
  High-density lipoid deficiency
  Hypoalphalipoproteinemia
  Hypobetalipoproteinemia (familial)

272.6 Lipodystrophy
  Barraquer-Simons disease
  Progressive lipodystrophy
Use additional E code, if desired, to identify cause, if iatrogenic (see Appendix VIIIb)
Excludes: intestinal lipodystrophy (040.2)

275.0 Disorders of iron metabolism
  Bronzed (bronze) diabetes
  Hemochromatosis

Pigmentary cirrhosis (of liver)
Excludes
    Anemia
        Iron deficiency (280.0 to 289.0)
        Sideroblastic (285.0)

275.3   Disorders of phosphate metabolism
        Phosphate

276.2   Acidosis
        Acidosis
            NOS
            Lactic
            Metabolic
            Respiratory
    Excludes: diabetic acidosis (250.1)

276.5   Volume depletion
        Dehydration
        Depletion of volume plasma or extracellular fluid
        Hypovolemia
    Excludes
        Hypovolemic shock
            Postoperative (998.0)
            Traumatic (958.4)

276.6   Fluid overload
        Fluid retention
    Excludes
        Ascites (789.5)
        Localized edema (782.3)

276.7   Hyperpotassemia
        Hyperkalemia
        Potassium (K)
            Excess
            Intoxication
            Overload

276.8   Hypopotassemia
        Hypokalemia
        Potassium (K) deficiency

276.9   Electrolyte and fluid disorders not elsewhere classified
        Electrolyte imbalance
        Hyperchloremia
        Hypochloremia

278.0   Obesity
    Excludes
        Adiposogenital dystrophy (253.8)
        Obesity of endocrine origin NOS (259.9)

648   Other current conditions in the mother classifiable elsewhere, but complicating pregnancy, childbirth, or the puerperium
    Includes: the listed conditions when complicating the pregnant state, aggravated by the pregnancy or when a main reason for obstetric care
    Excludes: those conditions in the mother known or suspected to have affected the fetus (655.0 to 665.9)

648.0   Diabetes mellitus
[0–4]   Conditions classifiable to 250
648.8   Abnormal glucose tolerance
[0–4]   Conditions classifiable to 790.2 complicating pregnancy, childbirth, or the puerperium
        Gestational
        Latent (chemical)

775.0   Syndrome of "infant of a diabetic mother"
        Maternal diabetes mellitus affecting fetus or newborn (with hypoglycemia)

775.1   Neonatal diabetes mellitus
        Diabetes mellitus syndrome in newborn infant

790.2   Abnormal glucose tolerance test
    Excludes
        That complicating pregnancy, childbirth, or the puerperium (648.8)
        Asymptomatic
        Chemical
        Latent (chemical)
        Nonclinical
        Stress
        Subclinical
        Subliminal

962   Poisoning by hormones and synthetic substitutes
        Excludes: oxytocic hormones (975.0)

962.0   Adrenal cortical steroids
        Steroid-induced diabetes
            Overdose or wrong substance given or taken

Abbreviations: NEC, not elsewhere classifiable (to be used only when the coder lacks the information necessary to code the term to a more specific category); NOS, not otherwise specified (equivalent of unspecified).

IXb. Drug-Related Adverse Effects

Table IXb–1 contains a classification of the drugs (different types of insulin, sulfonylureas, biguanides, acarbose, glucagon) that are used in the treatment of hyperglycemia in patients with diabetes mellitus. The table is keyed to the poisoning classification code (851 to 980) listed in *ICD-9-CM*, 1997. The table also contains a listing of external causes of adverse effects. An adverse effect is a pathological manifestation due to ingestion or exposure (e.g., hypoglycemia, allergy, dermatitis, hypersensitivity reaction, and so on.)

In addition to being identified by an appropriate poisoning code number (962.3 in *ICD-9-CM*, 1997), an adverse effect should also be identified by its appropriate external cause code number (see definitions below). The table headings pertaining to external causes are:

Accidental poisoning (E858)—accidental overdose of drug, wrong substance given or taken, drug taken

TABLE IXb-1   Table of Drugs Used to Treat Diabetes Mellitus with Diagnostic Categories of Poisoning and External Causes of Adverse Effects. (Adapted from *ICD-9-CM*, e Code Sections, and the American Hospital Drug Formulary, 1997, Washington, DC)

Drug	Poisoning by Overdose or Wrong Drug ICD-9-CM Code No.	External Causes (E Code)				
		Accidental Poisoning by Hormones and Synthetic Substitutes	Complications and Misadventures in Therapeutic Procedures	Suicide and Self-inflicted Poisoning	Homicidal Assault	Poisoning Undetermined Whether Accidentally or Purposely Inflicted
Insulin (all types)	962.3	E 858	E932.3	E950.4	E962.0	E980.4
Acetohexamide	962.3	E 858	E932.3	E950.4	E962.0	E980.4
Chlorpropamide	962.3	E 858	E932.3	E950.4	E962.0	E980.4
Tolazamide	962.3	E 858	E932.3	E950.4	E962.0	E980.4
Tolbutamide	962.3	E 858	E932.3	E950.4	E962.0	E980.4
Glyburide	962.3	E 858	E932.3	E950.4	E962.0	E980.4
Glipizide	962.3	E 858	E932.3	E950.4	E962.0	E980.4
Other Sulfonylurea	962.3	E 858	E932.3	E950.4	E962.0	E980.4
Phenformin	962.3	E 858	E932.3	E950.4	E962.0	E980.4
Other Biguanide	962.3	E 858	E932.3	E950.4	E962.0	E980.4
Acarbose	962.3	E 858	E932.3	E950.4	E962.0	E980.4
Glucagon	962.3	E 858	E932.3	E950.4	E962.0	E980.4
Other	962.3	E 858	E932.3	E950.4	E962.0	E980.4

inadvertently, and accidents in usage in medical and surgical procedures.

Therapeutic use (E932.3)—a correct substance properly administered in therapeutic or prophylactic dosage as the external cause of adverse effects.

Suicide attempts (E950.4)—instances in which self-inflicted injuries or poisonings are involved.

Assault (962.0)—injury or poisoning inflicted by another person with the intent to injure or kill.

Undetermined (E980.4)—to be used when the intent of the poisoning or injury cannot be determined whether it was intentional or accidental.

Reference: ICD-9-CM. E code sections, and The American Hospital Drug Formulary, 1997, Washigton, DC.

*The author expresses his gratitude to Philip Nant, R.Ph. of the Drug Information Center, Department of Pharmaceutical Services, Emory University Hospital, Atlanta, GA 30322 for supplying the information cited above.

IXc.   Procedures (ICD-9-CM)

Procedure classifications had not been a part of the *International Classification of Diseases* until the publications of *ICD-9* (see Appendix IX). The *ICD-9* Classification of Procedures in Medicine was published separately from the disease classification in a series of supplementary documents called fascicles. Each fascicle contains a classification of modes of therapy, surgery, radiology,

laboratory, and diagnostic procedures. The decision to publish each fascicle as a unique document was made in order to permit its revision on a separate schedule from the disease classification. Primary input to Fascicle V, "Surgical Procedures," came from the United States whose adaptations of *ICD* had contained a procedure classification since 1962.

The *ICD-9-CM* Procedure Classification is a modification of WHO's Fascicle V, "Surgical Procedures." The codes were expanded from three to four digits in *ICD-9-CM*, with approximately 90% of the rubrics referring to surgical procedures and the remaining 10% accounting for other diagnostic and therapeutic procedures. Rubrics in the range of 01 to 86 refer to surgical procedures, and rubrics 87 to 99 pertain to nonsurgical procedures. The structure of the classification is based on anatomy, not on surgical specialty.

The following listings are taken from *ICD-9-CM*, Vol. 3, and include many of the procedures encountered in treating individuals who have diabetes mellitus and its complications:

12	Operations on iris, ciliary body, sclera, and anterior chamber Excludes: operations on cornea (11.0 to 11.99)
12.9	Other operations on iris, ciliary body, and anterior chamber 12.97 Other operations on iris 12.98 Other operations on ciliary body 12.99 Other operations on anterior chamber

13 Operations on lens
13.1 Intracapsular extraction of lens
 Code also any synchronous insertion of pseudophakos (13.71)
   13.11 Intracapsular extraction of lens by temporal inferior route
   13.19 Other intracapsular extraction of lens
    Cataract extraction NOS
    Cryoextraction of lens
    Erysiphake extraction of cataract
    Extraction of lens NOS
13.2 Extracapsular extraction of lens by linear extraction technique
13.3 Extracapsular extraction of lens by simple aspiration (and irrigation) technique
    Irrigation of traumatic cataract
13.4 Extracapsular extraction of lens by fragmentation and aspiration technique
   13.41 Phacoemulsification and aspiration of cataract
   13.42 Mechanical phacofragmentation and aspiration of cataract by posterior route
    Code also any synchronous vitrectomy (14.74)
   13.43 Mechanical phacofragmentation and other aspiration of cataract
13.5 Other extracapsular extraction of lens
 Code also any synchronous insertion of pseudophakos (13.71)
   13.51 Extracapsular extraction of lens by temporal inferior route
   13.59 Other extracapsular extraction of lens
13.6 Other cataract extraction
 Code also any synchronous insertion of pseudophakos (13.71)
   13.61 Discission of primary membranous cataract
   13.62 Excision of primary membranous cataract
   13.63 Mechanical fragmentation of primary membranous cataract
   13.64 Discission of secondary membrane (after cataract)
   13.65 Excision of secondary membrane (after cataract)
    Capsulectomy
   13.66 Mechanical fragmentation of secondary membrane (after cataract)
   13.69 Other cataract extraction
13.7 Insertion of prosthetic lens (pseudophakos)
   13.70 Insertion of pseudophakos, not otherwise specified
   13.71 Insertion of intraocular lens of prosthesis at time of cataract extractions, one-stage
    Code also synchronous extraction of cataract (13.11 to 13.69)

   13.72 Secondary insertion of intraocular lens prosthesis
13.8 Removal of implanted lens
 Removal of pseudophakos
13.9 Other operations on lens
14 Operations on retina, choroid, vitreous, and posterior chamber
14.1 Diagnostic procedures on retina, choroid, vitreous, and posterior chamber
   14.11 Diagnostic aspiration of vitreous
   14.19 Other diagnostic procedures on retina, choroid, vitreous, and posterior chamber
14.2 Destruction of lesion of retina and choroid
 Includes: destruction of chorioretinopathy or isolated chorioretinal lesion
 Excludes: that for repair of retina (14.31 to 14.59)
   14.21 Destruction of chorioretinal lesion by diathermy
   14.22 Destruction of chorioretinal lesion by cryotherapy
   14.23 Destruction of chorioretinal lesion by xenon arc photocoagulation
   14.24 Destruction of chorioretinal lesion by laser photocoagulation
   14.25 Destruction of chorioretinal lesion by photocoagulation of unspecified type
   14.26 Destruction of chorioretinal lesion by radiation therapy
   14.27 Destruction of chorioretinal lesion by implantation of radiation source
   14.29 Other destruction of chorioretinal lesion. Destruction of lesion of retinal choroid NOS
14.3 Repair of retinal tear
 Includes: repair of retinal defect
 Excludes: repair of retinal detachment (14.41 to 14.59)
   14.31 Repair of retinal tear by diathermy
   14.32 Repair of retinal tear by cryotherapy
   14.33 Repair of retinal tear by xenon arc photocoagulation
   14.34 Repair of retinal tear by laser photocoagulation
   14.35 Repair of retinal tear by photocoagulation of unspecified type
   14.39 Other repair of retinal tear
14.4 Repair of retinal detachment with scleral buckling and implant
   14.41 Scleral buckling with implant
   14.49 Other scleral buckling
    Scleral buckling with
     Air tamponade
     Resection of sclera
     Vitrectomy
14.5 Other repair of retinal detachment
 Includes: that with drainage

14.51 Repair of retinal detachment with diathermy

14.52 Repair of retinal detachment with cryotherapy

14.53 Repair of retinal detachment with xenon arc photocoagulation

14.54 Repair of retinal detachment with laser photocoagulation

14.55 Repair of retinal detachment with photo-coagulation of unspecified type

14.59 Other

14.7 Operations on vitreous

14.71 Removal of vitreous, anterior approach
Open sky technique
Removal of vitreous anterior approach (with replacement)

14.72 Other removal of vitreous
Aspiration of vitreous by posterior sclerotomy

14.73 Mechanical vitrectomy by anterior approach

14.74 Other mechanical vitrectomy

14.75 Injection of vitreous substitute
Excludes: that associated with removal (14.71 to 14.72)

14.79 Other operations on vitreous

14.9 Other operations on retina, choroid, and posterior chamber

36 Operations on vessels of heart
Includes
Sternotomy
Median
Transverse } as operative approach
Thoracotomy
Code also cardiopulmonary bypass (extracorporeal circulation) (heart–lung machine) (39.61)

36.0 Removal of coronary artery obstruction
Coronary (artery)
Endarterectomy
Thromboendarterectomy } That with Angioplasty Graft patch
Direct relief of coronary artery obstruction

36.1 Bypass anastomosis for heart revascularization
Code also cardiopulmonary bypass (extracorporeal circulation) (heart–lung machine) (39.61)

36.10 Aortocoronary bypass for heart revascularization, not otherwise specified
Direct revascularization
Cardiac
Coronary
Heart muscle
Myocardial } With catheter stent, prosthesis, or vein graft
Heart revascularization NOS

36.11 Aortocoronary bypass of one coronary artery

36.12 Aortocoronary bypass of two coronary arteries

36.13 Aortocoronary bypass of three coronary arteries

36.14 Aortocoronary bypass of four coronary arteries

36.15 Single internal mammary-coronary artery bypass
Anastomosis (single)
Mammary artery to coronary artery
Thoracic artery to coronary artery

36.16 Double internal mammary-coronary artery bypass
Anastomosis, double:
Mammary artery to coronary artery
Thoracic artery to coronary artery

36.19 Other bypass anastomosis for heart revascularization

36.2 Heart revascularization by arterial implant
Implantation of
Aortic branches (ascending aortic branches) into heart muscle
Blood vessels into myocardium
Internal mammary artery (internal thoracic artery) into
Heart muscle
Myocardium
Ventricle
Ventricular wall
Indirect heart revascularization NOS

36.3 Other heart revascularization
Abrasion of epicardium
Cardio-omentopexy
Intrapericardial poudrage
Myocardial graft
Mediastinal fat
Omentum
Pectoral muscles

36.9 Other operations on vessels of heart
Code also cardiopulmonary bypass (extracorporeal circulation) (heart–lung machine) (39.61)

36.91 Repair of aneurysm of coronary vessel

36.99 Other operations on vessels of heart
Exploration
Incision
Ligation } of coronary artery
Repair of arteriovenous fistula

38 Incision, excision, and occlusion of vessels
Code also cardiopulmonary bypass (extracorporeal circulation) (heart–lung machine) (39.61)
Excludes: that of coronary vessels (36.0 to 36.99)

The following fourth-digit subclassification is for use with appropriate categories in section 38:

0 Unspecified site
1 Intracranial vessels
Cerebral (anterior) (middle)
Circle of Willis

Posterior communicating artery

2 Other vessels of head and neck
Carotid artery (common) (external) (internal)
Jugular vein (external) (internal)

3 Upper limb vessles
Axillary
Brachial
Radial
Ulnar

4 Aorta

5 Upper thoracic vessels
Innominate
Pulmonary
Artery
Vein
Subclavian
Vena cava, superior

6 Abdominal arteries
Celiac
Gastric
Hepatic
Iliac
Mesenteric
Renal
Splenic
Umbilical
Excludes: abdominal aorta (4)

7 Abdominal veins
Iliac
Portal
Renal
Splenic
Vena cava (inferior)

8 Lower limb arteries
Femoral
Common
Superficial
Popliteal
Tibial

9 Lower limb veins
Femoral
Popliteal
Saphenous
Tibial

38.0 Incision of vessel
[0 to 9]
Embolectomy
Thrombectomy
Excludes: puncture or catheterization of any
Artery (38.91, 38.98)
Vein (38.92 to 38.94, 38.99)

38.1 Endarterectomy
[0 to 6, 8]
Endarterectomy with
Embolectomy
Patch graft

Temporary bypass during procedure
Thrombectomy

38.2 Diagnostic procedures on blood vessels
38.21 Biopsy of blood vessels
38.29 Other diagnostic procedures on blood vessels
Excludes
Blood vessel thermography (88.86)
Circulatory monitoring (89.61 to 89.69)
Contrast
Angiocardiography (88.50 to 88.58)
Arteriography (88.40 to 88.49)
Phlebography (88.60 to 88.67)
Impedance phlebography (88.68)
Peripheral vascular ultrasonography (88.77)
Plethysmogram (89.58)

38.3 Resection of vessel with anastomosis
[0 to 9]
Angiectomy
Excision of
Aneurysm (arteriovenous) } With anastomosis
Blood vessel (lesion)

38.4 Resection of vessel with replacement
[0 to 9]
Angiectomy
Excision of
Aneurysm (arteriovenous) } With replacement
Blood vessel (lesion)

38.9 Puncture of vessel
Excludes: that for circulatory monitoring (89.61 to 89.69)
38.91 Arterial catheterization
38.93 Other venous catheterization
Excludes: that for cardiac catheterization (37.21 to 37.23)
38.94 Venous cutdown
38.98 Other puncture of artery
Excludes: that for:
Coronary arteriography (88.55 to 88.57)
Arteriography (88.40 to 88.49)
38.99 Other puncture of vein
Excludes: that for:
Angiography (88.60 to 88.69)
Extracorporeal circulation (39.61, 50.92)
Injection or infusion of
Sclerosing solution (39.92)
Therapeutic or prophylactic substance (99.11 to 99.29)
Perfusion (39.96 to 39.97)
Phlebography (88.60 to 88.69)
Transfusion (99.01 to 99.09)

39 Other operations on vessels
Excludes: those on coronary vessels (36.0 to 36.99)

39.0 Systemic to pulmonary artery shunt
Descending aorta-pulmonary artery ⎫
Left to right ⎬ Anastomosis (graft)
Subclavian-pulmonary ⎭
Code also cardiopulmonary bypass (extracorporeal circulation) (heart–lung machine) (39.61)

39.1 Intra-abdominal venous shunt
Anastomosis
Mesocaval
Portacaval
Portal vein to inferior vena cava
Splenic and renal veins
Excludes: peritoneovenous shunt (54.94)

39.2 Other shunt or vascular bypass
39.21 Caval–pulmonary artery anastomosis
Code also cardiopulmonary bypass (39.61)
39.22 Aorta–subclavian–carotid bypass
Bypass (arterial)
Aorta to carotid and brachial
Aorta to subclavian and carotid
Carotid to subclavian
39.23 Other intrathoracic vascular shunt or bypass
Intrathoracic (arterial) bypass graft NOS
Excludes: coronary artery bypass (36.10 to 36.19)
39.24 Aorta–renal bypass
39.25 Aorta–iliac–femoral bypass
Bypass
Aortofemoral
Aortoiliac
Aortoiliac to popliteal
Aortopopliteal
Iliofemoral (iliac–femoral)
39.27 Arteriovenostomy for renal dialysis
Anastomosis for renal dialysis
Formation of (peripheral) arteriovenous fistula for renal [kidney] dialysis
Code also any renal dialysis (39.95)
39.39 Other (peripheral) vascular shunt or bypass
Bypass (graft)
Axillary–brachial
Axillary–femoral (axillofemoral) (superficial)
Brachial
Femoral–femoral
Femoroperoneal
Femoropopliteal (arteries)
Femorotibial (anterior) (posterior)
Popliteal
Vascular NOS
Excludes: peritoneovenous shunt (54.94)

39.4 Revision of vascular procedure
39.41 Control of hemorrhage following vascular surgery
Excludes: that for control of hemorrhage (postoperative)
Anus (49.95)
Bladder (57.93)
Nose (21.00 to 21.09)
Prostate (60.94)
Tonsil (28.7)
39.42 Revision of arteriovenous shunt for renal dialysis
Conversion of renal dialysis
End-to-end anastomosis to end-to-side
End-to-side anastomosis to end-to-end
Vessel-to-vessel cannula to arteriovenous shunt
Removal of old arteriovenous shunt and creation of new shunt
Excludes: replacement of vessel-to-vessel cannula (39.94)
39.43 Removal of arteriovenous shunt for renal dialysis
Excludes: that with replacement (revision) of shunt (39.42)
39.49 Other revision of vascular procedure
Declotting (graft)
Revision of
Anastomosis of blood vessel
Vascular procedure (previous)

39.6 Procedures auxiliary to open heart surgery
39.61 Extracorporeal circulation
Artificial heart and lung
Pump oxygenator
Excludes
Extracorporeal hepatic assistance (50.92)
Hemodialysis (39.95)
39.62 Hypothermia (systemic) incidental to open heart surgery
39.63 Cardioplegia
Arrest
Anoxic
Circulatory
39.64 Intraoperative cardiac pacemaker
Temporary pacemaker used during and immediately following cardiac surgery

39.9 Other operations on vessels
39.93 Insertion of vessel-to-vessel cannula
Formation of
Arteriovenous ⎫
Fistula ⎬ by external cannula
Shunt ⎭
Code also any renal dialysis (39.95)
39.94 Replacement of vessel-to-vessel cannula
Revision of vessel-to-vessel cannula

39.95 Hemodialysis
Artificial kidney
Renal dialysis
Excludes: peritoneal dialysis (54.98)

52.8 Transplant of pancreas
52.80 Pancreatic transplant, not otherwise specified
52.81 Reimplantation of pancreatic tissue
52.82 Homotransplant of pancreas
52.83 Heterotransplant of pancreas

55 Operations on kidney
55.53 Removal of transplanted or rejected kidney
55.54 Bilateral nephrectomy
Excludes: complete nephrectomy NOS (55.51)

55.6 Transplant of kidney
55.61 Renal autotransplantation
55.69 Other kidney transplantation

84 Other procedures on musculoskeletal system

84.1 Amputation of lower limb
Excludes: revision of amputation stump (84.3)
84.10 Lower limb amputation, not otherwise specified
Closed flap amputation ⎫
Kineplastic amputation ⎪
Open or guillotine ⎬ Of lower
amputation ⎪ limb NOS
Revision of current ⎪
traumatic amputation ⎭

84.11 Amputation of toe
Amputation through metatarsophalangeal joint
Disarticulation of toe
Excludes: ligation of supernumerary toe (86.26)

84.12 Amputation through foot
Amputation of forefoot
Amputation through midde of foot
Chopart's amputation
Midtarsal amputation
Transmetatarsal amputation

84.13 Disarticulation of ankle

84.14 Amputation of ankle through malleoli of tibia and fibula

84.15 Other amputation below knee
Amputation of leg through tibia and fibula NOS

84.16 Disarticulation of knee
Batch, Spitler, and McFaddin amputation
Mazet amputation
S.P. Roger's amputation

84.17 Amputation above knee
Amputation of leg through femur
Amputation of thigh

Conversion of below-knee amputation into above-knee amputation
Supracondylar above-knee amputation

84.18 Disarticulation of hip

84.3 Revision of amputation stump
Reamputation ⎫
Secondary closure ⎬ Of stump
Trimming ⎭
Excludes: revision of current traumatic amputation (revision by further amputation of current injury) (84.00 to 84.19, 84.91)

84.4 Implantation or fitting of prosthetic limb device
84.40 Implantation or fitting of prosthetic limb device, not otherwise specified
84.45 Fitting of prosthesis above knee
84.46 Fitting of prosthesis below knee
84.47 Fitting of prosthesis of leg, not otherwise specified
84.48 Implantation of prosthetic device of leg

88 Other diagnostic radiology and related techniques

88.4 Arteriography using contrast material
Includes
Angiography of arteries
Arterial puncture for injection of contrast material
Radiography of arteries (by fluoroscopy)
Retrograde arteriography
Note: The fourth-digit subclassification identified the site to be viewed, not the site of injection
Excludes:
Arteriography using
Radioisotopes of radionuclides (92.01 to 92.19)
Ultrasound (88.71 to 88.79)
Fluorescein angiography of eye (95.12)
88.40 Arteriography using contrast material, unspecified site
88.41 Arteriography of cerebral arteries
Angiography of
Basilar artery
Carotid (internal)
Posterior cerebral circulation
Vertebral artery
88.45 Arteriography of renal arteries
88.46 Arteriography of placenta
Placentogram using contrast material
88.47 Arteriography of other intra-abdominal arteries
88.48 Arteriography of femoral and other lower extremity arteries
88.49 Arteriography of other unspecified sites

88.5 Angiocardiography using contrast material
Includes

Arterial puncture and insertion of arterial catheter for injection of contrast material
Cineangiocardiography
Selective angiocardiography
Code also synchronous cardiac catheterization (37.21 to 37.23)
88.53 Angiocardiography of left heart structures
Angiocardiography of
Aortic valve
Left atrium
Left ventricle (outflow tract)
Excludes: that combined with right heart angiocardiography (88.54)
88.54 Combined right and left heart angiocardiography
88.55 Coronary arteriography using a single catheter
Coronary arteriography by Sones technique
Direct selective coronary arteriography using a single catheter
88.56 Coronary arteriography using two catheters
Coronary arteriography by
Judkins technique
Ricketts and Abrams technique
Direct selective coronary arteriography using two catheters
88.57 Other and unspecified coronary arteriography
Coronary arteriography NOS
88.58 Negative-contrast cardiac roentgenography
Cardiac roentgenography with injection of carbon dioxide
88.6 Phlebography
Includes
Angiography of veins
Radiography of veins (by fluoroscopy)
Retrograde phlebography
Venipuncture for injection of contrast material
Venography using contrast material
Note: The fourth-digit subclassification (88.60 to 88.7) identifies the site to be viewed, not the site of injection
Excludes: angiography using
Radioisotopes or radionuclides (92.01 to 92.19)
Ultrasound (88.71 to 88.79)
Fluorescein angiography of eye (95.12)
88.7 Diagnostic ultrasound
Includes
Echography
Ultrasonic angiography
Ultrasonography

88.71 Diagnostic ultrasound of head and neck
Determination of midline shift of brain
Echoencephalography
Excludes: eye (95.13)
88.72 Diagnostic ultrasound of heart
Echocardiography
88.73 Diagnostic ultrasound of other sites of thorax
Aortic arch ⎫
Breast   ⎬ Ultrasonography
Lung   ⎭
88.74 Diagnostic ultrasound of digestive system
88.75 Diagnostic ultrasound of urinary system
88.76 Diagnostic ultrasound of abdomen and retroperitoneum
88.77 Diagnostic ultrasound of peripheral vascular system
Deep vein thrombosis ultrasonic scanning
88.78 Diagnostic ultrasound of gravid uterus
Intrauterine cephalometry
Echo
Ultrasonic
Placental localization by ultrasound
88.79 Other diagnostic ultrasound
Ultrasonography of
Multiple sites
Nongravid uterus
Total body
88.8 Thermography
88.81 Cerebral thermography
88.82 Ocular thermography
88.83 Bone thermography
Osteoarticular thermography
88.84 Muscle thermography
88.85 Breast thermography
88.86 Blood vessel thermography
Deep vein thermography
89   Interview, evaluation, consultation, and examination
89.0   Diagnostic interview, consultation, and evaluation
Excludes: psychiatric diagnostic interview (94.11 to 94.19)
89.01 Interview and evaluation, described as brief
Abbreviated history and evaluation
89.02 Interview and evaluation, described as limited
Interval history and evaluation
89.03 Interview and evaluation, described as comprehensive
History and evaluation of new problem
89.04 Other interview and evaluation
89.05 Diagnostic interview and evaluation, not otherwise specified

89.06 Consultation, described as limited
Consultation on a single organ system
89.07 Consultation, described as comprehensive
89.08 Other consultation
89.09 Consultation, not otherwise specified

89.1 Anatomic and physiologic measurements and manual examinations—nervous system and sense organs
Excludes
Ear examination (95.41 to 95.49)
Eye examination (95.01 to 95.26)
The listed procedures when done as part of a general physical examination (89.7)
89.13 Neurologic examination
89.14 Electroencephalogram
89.15 Other nonoperative neurologic function tests

89.2 Anatomic and physiologic measurements and manual examinations—genitourinary system
Excludes: the listed procedures when done as part of a general physical examination (89.7)
89.21 Urinary manometry
Manometry through
Indwelling ureteral catheter
Nephrostomy
Pyelostomy
Ureterostomy
89.22 Cystometrogram
89.23 Urethral sphincter electromyogram
89.24 Uroflowmetry (UFR)
89.25 Urethral pressure profile (UPP)
89.26 Gynecologic examination
Pelvic examination
89.29 Other nonoperative genitourinary system measurements
Bioassay or urine
Renal clearance
Urine chemistry

89.3 Other anatomic and physiologic measurements and manual examinations
Excludes: the listed procedures when done as part of a general physical examination (89.7)
89.31 Dental examination
Oral mucosal survey
Periodontal survey
89.32 Esophageal manometry
89.36 Manual examination of the breast
89.37 Vital capacity determination
89.38 Other nonoperative respiratory measurements
89.39 Other nonoperative measurements and examinations
Basal metabolic rate (BMR)
Gastric
Analysis
Function NEC

Excludes
Body measurements (93.07)
Cardiac tests (89.41 to 89.69)
Fundus photography (95.11)
Limb length measurement (93.06)

89.4 Cardiac stress tests and pacemaker checks
89.41 Cardiovascular stress test using treadmill
89.43 Cardiovascular stress test using bicycle ergometer
89.44 Other cardiovascular stress test

89.5 Other cardiac function tests
Excludes: fetal ECG (75.32)
89.51 Rhythm electrocardiogram
Rhythm ECG (with one to three leads)
89.52 Electrocardiogram
ECG NOS
ECG (with 12 or more leads)
89.54 Electrographic monitoring
Excludes: electrographic monitoring during surgery—omit code
89.55 Phonocardiogram with ECG lead
89.56 Carotid pulse tracing with ECG lead
89.57 Apexcardiogram (with ECG lead)
89.58 Plethysmogram
89.59 Other nonoperative cardiovascular measurements

89.6 Circulatory monitoring
Excludes: electrocardiographic monitoring during surgery—omit code
89.61 Systemic arterial pressure monitoring
89.62 Central venous pressure monitoring
89.63 Pulmonary artery wedge monitoring
Pulmonary capillary wedge (PCW) monitoring
Swan-Ganz catheterization
89.65 Measurements of systemic arterial blood gases
89.66 Measurement of mixed venous blood gases

89.7 General physical examination
89.8 Autopsy
90 Microscopic examination—I
The following fourth digit subclassification is for use with categories in section 90 to identify type of examination:
1 Bacterial smear
2 Culture
3 Culture and sensitivity
4 Parasitology
5 Toxicology
6 Cell block and Papanicolaou smear
9 Other microscopic examination
90.0 Microscopic examination of specimen from nervous system and of spinal fluid
90.1 Microscopic examination of specimen from endocrine gland, not elsewhere classified

90.2 Microscopic examination of specimen from eye

91 Microscopic examination—II

The following fourth digit subclassification is for use with categories in section 91 to identify type of examination:

1 Bacterial smear
2 Culture
3 Culture and sensitivity
4 Parasitology
5 Toxicology
6 Cell block and Papanicolaou smear
9 Other microscopic examination

91.0 Microscopic examination of specimen from liver, biliary tract, and pancreas

91.6 Microscopic examination of specimen from skin and other integument

Microscopic examination of
Hair
Nails
Skin
Excludes
Mucous membrane—code to organ site
That of operative wound (91.70 to 91.79)

91.7 Microscopic examination of specimen from operative wound

92 Nuclear medicine

92.0 Radioisotope scan and function study

92.01 Thyroid scan and radioisotope function studies
Iodine-131 uptake
Protein-bound iodine
Radioiodine uptake

92.02 Liver scan and radioisotope function study
Renal clearance study

92.03 Renal scan and radioisotope function study

92.04 Gastrointestinal scan and radioisotope function study
Radiocobalt B$_{12}$ Schilling test
Radioiodinated triolein study

92.05 Cardiovascular and hemopoietic scan and radioisotope function study
Bone marrow ⎫
Cardiac output ⎪ Scan or
Circulation time ⎬ function study
Spleen ⎭

92.09 Other radioisotope function studies

94 Procedures related to the psyche

94.3 Individual psychotherapy

94.34 Individual therapy for psychosocial dysfunction
Excludes: that performed in group setting (94.41)

94.38 Supportive verbal psychotherapy

94.39 Other individual psychotherapy
Biofeedback

94.4 Other psychotherapy and counseling

94.41 Group therapy for psychosexual dysfunction

94.42 Family therapy

94.5 Referral for psychological rehabilitation

94.51 Referral for psychotherapy

94.52 Referral for psychiatric aftercare
Excludes that in:
Halfway house
Outpatient (clinic) facility

94.55 Referral for vocational rehabilitation

94.59 Referral for other psychological rehabilitation

95 Ophthalmologic and otologic diagnosis and treatment

95.0 General and subjective eye examination

95.01 Limited examination
Eye examination with prescription of spectacles

95.02 Comprehensive eye examination
Eye examination covering all aspects of the visual system

95.03 Extended ophthalmologic workup
Examination (for)
Glaucoma
Neuro-ophthalmology
Retinal disease

95.04 Eye examination under anesthesia
Code also type of examination

95.05 Visual field study

95.06 Color vision study

95.07 Dark adaptation study

95.09 Eye examination, not otherwise specified
Vision check NOS

95.1 Examinations of form and structure of eye

95.11 Fundus photography

95.12 Fluorescein angiography or angioscopy of eye

95.2 Objective functional test of eye

95.21 Electroretinogram (ERG)

95.22 Electro-oculogram (EOG)

95.23 Visual evoked potential (VEP)

95.24 Electronystagmogram (ENG)

95.25 Electromyogram of eye (EMG)

95.26 Tonography, provocative tests, and other glaucoma testing

95.3 Special vision services

95.31 Fitting and dispensing of spectacles

95.32 Prescription, fitting, and dispensing of contact lens

95.33 Dispensing of other low vision aids

95.34 Ocular prosthetics

95.36 Ophthalmologic counseling and instruction
Counseling in
Adaptation to visual loss

Use of low vision aids

96　Nonoperative intubation and irrigation

96.0　Nonoperative intubation of gastrointestinal and respiratory tracts

　96.01　Insertion of nasopharyngeal airway

　96.02　Insertion of oropharyngeal airway

　96.03　Insertion of esophageal obturator airway

　96.04　Insertion of endotracheal tube

　96.05　Other intubation of respiratory tract

　96.06　Insertion of Sengstaken tube

Esophageal tamponade

　96.07　Insertion of other (naso-)gastric tube

Intubation for decompression

　96.08　Insertion of (naso-)intestinal tube

Miller-Abbott tube (for decompression)

　96.09　Insertion of rectal tube

Replacement of rectal tube

Abbreviations: See footnote following Appendix IXa.

APPENDIX X

Diagnosis-Related Groups and the Prospective Payment System for Hospitals

John K. Davidson

The 1965 Social Security Amendments (Public Law 89-7) established the Medicare program under Title XVIII and the Medicaid program under Title XIX. Medicare was divided into Part A (the Hospital Insurance Program) and Part B (which provided for voluntary supplementary insurance) to cover the cost of most physicians' services. In both Part A and Part B of Medicare, the beneficiary was required to pay a portion (20% or more) of the hospital and physician charges.

Costs for health care under the Medicare program have risen rapidly, from $1.1 billion in 1966 to $84.2 billion in 1982, of which $32.9 billion was spent for inpatient hospital care under Part A. Public Law 98-21 mandated a Prospective Payment System (PPS) for hospitals in 1983.

The law places physicians in a position where they must understand cost of hospital care, and they must become active participants in controlling those costs.

The cornerstone of the PPS is the diagnosis-related grouping system developed in the 1970s as a mechanism for utilization review. Diagnostic-related groups (DRGs) are derived from taking all possible diagnoses identified in the *ICD-9-CM* system (see Appendix IX), classifying them into 23 major diagnostic categories (MDCs) based on organ systems, and further breaking them into 467 distinct groupings, each of which is said to be "medically meaningful."

The following five pieces of information are necessary to assign a patient to a DRG: (1) the principal diagnosis and up to four complications or comorbidities, (2) treatment procedures performed, (3) age, (4) sex, (5) discharge status.

This information is submitted by the hospital to the fiscal intermediary, who has the responsibility for determining the DRG and calculating the appropriate payment.

Although the reimbursement formulas are quite complex, payment in general is the product of two factors: (1) the DRG weight, and (2) the dollar rate. The DRG weight is an index number that represents the relative hospital resources which are used, on average, for furnishing inpatient services. Weights apply equally to all hospitals in the system (5,200 hospitals as of September 1984). The other portion of the payment formula, the *dollar rate*, is now determined for all hospitals by the federal government. *Another factor* that contributes to the payment made to the hospital is the *regional wage index*. In 1989 in New York City it was 1.3183, whereas in Atlanta it was 0.9293.

To ensure the quality of care under the PPS, it was necessary for hospitals to enter into a contract with a peer review organization (PRO) by October 1, 1984. Hospitals that did not contract with a PRO are no longer eligible for payment from the Medicare program. The PROs are mandated to review the appropriateness of admissions, assignment of DRGs, and the quality of care.

In order to facilitate an understanding of the effects of DRGs on those who care for patients with diabetes mellitus, Figure X–1 and Table X–1 are presented in this appendix.

Two examples of payments from January 1 to September 30, 1990 to a major disproportionate share teaching hospital are shown in Table X–2. One example is from the medical partition for diabetic ketoacidosis (DKA), the other is from the surgical partition for an individual with diabetes mellitus (DM) and a lower extremity amputation.[1,2]

Examples:

For *294*: Relative weight was .8003 in 1985 and .7594 in 1996, LOS was 7.7 in 1985, and 5.7 in 1996.

For *295*: Relative weight was .7380 in 1985 and was .7159 in 1996, LOS was 5.6 in 1985 and 4.3 in 1996.[3]

It is important to assign and report correct codes to ensure appropriate reimbursement, based on the annual edition, issued by the U.S. Department of Health and Human Services each Oct. 1 and valid for 1 year (5th ed., Oct. 1, 1996–Sept. 30, 1997).[4,5]

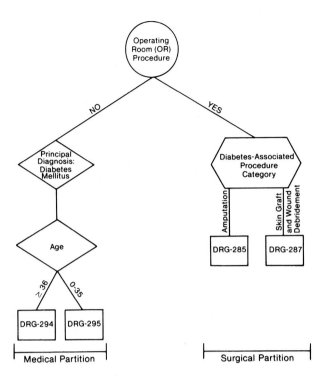

Figure X–1. Major diagnostic category 10: endocrine, nutritional, and metabolic diseases and disorders. In this figure a patient with diabetes mellitus is categorized under MDC 10: Endocrine, Nutritional, and Metabolic Diseases and Disorders. The first step is to ascertain if an operating room (OR) procedure was performed. If not, the program will branch to the medical portion of the decision tree depicted on the left of the diagram. The principal diagnosis is then noted with consideration for age, sex, or complicating factors. (In this example of uncomplicated diabetes, only age is depicted.) If the patient is 36 years or older, the DRG is 294. If the patient is younger than 36, the DRG is 295. If surgery was performed, the program would have branched to the right portion of the diagram: the surgical partition. The same method of categorization is performed, but it is based on the principal surgical procedure performed, and then, considering age or other relevant factors, the appropriate DRG is assigned. (*Source:* Adapted from DRGs and the Prospective Payment System: A Guide for Physicians. Chicago: American Medical Association, 1983. With permission.)

TABLE X–1 Major Diagnostic Category 10: Endocrine, Nutritional, and Metabolic Diseases and Disorders

Diagnosis-Related Groups (DRGs)	Title	Weight	Mean Length of Stay (LOS)
285	Amputations for Endocrine, Nutritional, and Metabolic Disorders	2.8360	24.0
286	Adrenal and Pituitary Procedures	2.8051	16.1
287	Skin Grafts and Wound Debride for Endocrine, Nutritional, and Metabolic Disorders	2.7851	22.8
288	OR Procedures for Obesity	1.5532	10.0
289	Parathyroid Procedures	1.3593	8.3
290	Thyroid Procedures	0.8460	6.0
291	Thyroglossal Procedures	0.4858	2.9
292	Other Endocrine, Nutritional, and Metabolic OR Procedures Age > 69 and/or CC	2.0096	10.8
293	Other Endocrine, Nutritional, and Metabolic OR Procedures Age < 70 w/o CC	1.4796	8.0
294	Diabetes Age > 36	0.8003	7.7
295	Diabetes Age 0–35	0.7380	5.6
296	Nutritional and Misc. Metabolic Disorders Age > 69 and/or CC	0.8886	7.3
297	Nutritional and Misc. Metabolic Disorders Age 18–69 w/o CC	0.7841	6.0
298	Nutritional and Misc. Metabolic Disorders Age 0–17	0.7460	5.4
299	Inborn Effors of Metabolism	0.9309	6.8
300	Endocrine Disorders Age > 69 and/or CC	0.9630	7.8
301	Endocrine Disorders Age < 70 w/o CC	0.8058	6.4

Abbreviations: OR, operating room; CC, comorbidity and/or complications.

Note: Although information in this table was current in mid-1985, DRG weights and other factors affecting hospital reimbursement are subject to change. For latest information on DRGs and the PPS, consult the Federal Register and other government publications and directives.

[*Source:* Adapted from DRGs and the Prospective Payment System: A Guide for Physicians. Chicago: American Medical Association, 1983. With permission.]

TABLE X–2   Prospective Payment System (PPS) Payments (1/1/90–9/30/90)

		Medical Partition			
Age	Diagnosis	DRG	Cost Weight	Length of Stay (Days)	PPS Payment to Hospital
≥ 36	DKA	294	0.7509	5.9	$3,576
0–35	DKA	295	0.7252	4.4	$3,454

		Surgical Partition			
Diagnosis	Level	DRG	Cost Weight	Length of Stay (Days)	PPS Payment to Hospital
Prime: DM					
Secondary: Gangrene					
Procedure: Amputation:	Toe	114	1.6119	14	$ 7,677
	BK	113	2.4616	14	$ 11,725
	AK	113	2.4616	14	$ 11,725

References

1. DRGs and the Prospective Payment System: A Guide for Physicians. Chicago: American Medical Association, 1983.

2. DRGs Definitions Manual Health Systems International. New Haven, Connecticut, 5th rev.

3. Federal Register, v. 61, no. 170/Fri. Aug. 30, 1996, p. 46266.

4. Jones MK, Schmidt KM, Aaron WS: St. Anthony's ICD-9-CM Code Book, Vols. 1, 2, 3. Reston, VA: St. Anthony Publishing, Inc., 1996.

5. Lourenz EW, Jones MK: St. Anthony's DRG Guidebook 1997. Reston, VA: St. Anthony Publishing, Inc., 1997.

The Saint Vincent Declaration

(a précis)

*Following a Meeting Organized by WHO & IDF in Europe
10-12 October 1989*

Diabetes Care and Research in Europe

Jean-Philippe Assal

Targets:

1. Elaborate, initiate and evaluate comprehensive programmes for detection and control of diabetes and of its complications, with self-care and community support as major components.

2. Raise awareness in the population and among health care professionals of the present opportunities and the future needs for prevention of the complications of diabetes and of diabetes itself.

3. Organize training and teaching in diabetes management and care for people of all ages with diabetes, for their families, friends and working associates and for the health care team.

4. Ensure that care for children with diabetes is provided by individuals and teams specialized both in the management of diabetes and of children, and that families with a diabetic child get the necessary social, economic and emotional support.

5. Reinforce existing centres of excellence in diabetes care, education and research. Create new centres where the need and potential exist.

6. Promote independence, equity and self-sufficiency for all people with diabetes - children, adolescents, those in the working years of life and the elderly.

7. Remove hindrances to the fullest possible integration of the diabetic citizen into society.

8. Implement effective measures for the prevention of costly complications:

   8.1 reduce new blindness due to diabetes by one third or more;

   8.2 reduce the numbers of people entering end-stage diabetic renal failure by at least one third;

   8.3 reduce by one half the rate of limb amputations for diabetic gangrene;

   8.4 cut morbidity and mortality from coronary heart disease in the diabetic by vigorous programmes of risk factor reduction;

   8.5 achieve pregnancy outcome in the diabetic woman that approximates that of the non-diabetic woman.

9. Establish monitoring and control systems using state-of-the-art information technology for quality assurance of diabetes health care provision and for laboratory and technical procedures in diabetes diagnosis, treatment, and self-management.

10. Promote European and international collaboration in programmes of diabetes research and development through national and regional agencies and WHO and in active partnership with diabetes patients' organizations.

APPENDIX XI–B

The Saint Vincent Declaration

*Diabetes Care and Research in Europe Recommendations
of the Working Groups*

Jean-Philippe Assal

Working Group on:
Reducing Blindness in Diabetes:
the best strategies

- develop and use registers on diabetic retinopathy within health care systems
- make commonly accepted definitions for visual impairment and blindness
- use information technology for data collection and processing

Working Group on:
Reducing Amputations
in Diabetes: the best strategies

- create optimal strategies to reduce amputation and speed up implementation
- screen for patients at-risk
- organize structured follow-up
- create models for practical organization
- create programmes for education of patients and health care personnel

Working Group on:
Successful Initiatives:
how were they accomplished?

- well defined unified aims and goals
- creation of appropriate expectations, motivations and liabilities - for people with diabetes, health care professionals and government
- comprehensive, structured documentation and evaluation
- ensure organization and management

- ensure education and empowerment
- ensure sufficient resources

Working Group on:
Optimizing Outcomes
of Pregnancy in Diabetes:
how can it be done?

- screening of all pregnant women for GDM between gestational week 24 and 28
- widespread use of WHO/IDF guidelines for pregnancy management to improve outcomes
- basic information sheet for diabetes and pregnancy to monitor and compare outcomes
- use WHO criteria: Gestational IGT(G-IGT) as diabetes mellitus during pregnancy
- reclassification after delivery and regular yearly control to identify glucose intolerance and other pathologies (signs of multimetabolic syndrome X) and prevent complications
- pre-pregnancy counselling for all women of child-bearing age who have diabetes
- during pregnancy, women with pre-existing diabetes and pregnant women with gestational diabetes to be cared for by interdisciplinary teams in (regional) centres of excellence for diabetes and pregnancy.

Working Group on:
SVD in an International
Perspective: the worldwide
impact

- make multidisciplinary programmes covering diabetes types 1, 2, 3, 4

- ensure WHO/IDF partnership with diabetes organizations and industry

- develop administrative structure in parallel with Declaration

- create a task force to develop a national plan

- include in national plan measurement of outcomes, analysis of drug availability and affordability and especially in developing countries, a tender system

Working Group on: Mobilizing the Front Troops: primary health care comes marching in

- build up a network of key persons in primary health diabetes care

- disseminate specific primary health care knowledge and skills regarding: organizational aspects; team guidelines; risk assessment; data collection and its use

- ensure continuous quality of care development in primary care as regards diabetes

- ensure data collection for evaluation and comparison purposes

- ensure allocation of financial support for further development of working group activities

Working Group on: Empowerment of Patients: how should it be done?

- educate persons with diabetes, their carers and the general public

- try to make group consultations an accepted part of diabetes health care delivery

- support diabetes associations at local and national levels

- establish 'consumer centres' (to advise persons with diabetes)

- publish a diabetes newsletter where one does not exist

- try to monitor and evaluate the results of programmes on empowerment

Working Group on: Improving Quality of Diabetes Care: the role of the laboratory

- for glucose in blood and urine: laboratories must monitor the accuracy and precision of their analyses

- for HbA_{IC}: the standards of European quality assurance system should be introduced and their use should be mandatory for all diabetes care centres

- self-monitoring of microalbuminuria should be implemented if simple, reliable and inexpensive methods are available

Working Group on: Improving Quality of Diabetes Care: the role of the pharmacist in the St. Vincent team

- ensure that, in lay terms, verbal information given by the pharmacist to patients is similar to that of other members of the health care team

- ensure that, for the sake of consistency, written information given by the pharmacist to patients is prepared together with other members of the health care team

- the pharmacist's activity in diabetes care should focus on Type 2 diabetes

- the pharmacist should keep patients' medication profiles at the pharmacy and hand a therapeutic card to the patient, including prescribed and non-prescribed medicines

- the pharmacist should maintain the confidentiality of patient data

- pharmacists should maintain a good relationship with the patient associations and refer persons with diabetes to the associations

- governments should be made aware of the pharmacist's role in diabetes care and their efforts to improve quality of care in this field

Working Group on: Education in Diabetes: how to obtain the best results:

- give education as well as insulin

- use structured education programmes

- develop programmes for therapeutic education

Working Group on: Information Technology Tools for Quality Development in Diabetes Care

- ensure integration of different technologies
- ensure benefit for the people who collect data
- ensure translation of data into quality

Working Group on: Epidemiology made Practical: what are the main issues?

- establish epidemiological indicators and operational definitions of events and outcomes in the assessment of effectiveness in diabetes care
- provide methodological support in the design and performance of epidemiological studies related to diabetes care and research in Europe
- provide expertise on the collection and interpretation of data related to diabetes epidemiology to assist SVD action programme managers and health authorities
- organize training seminars in diabetes epidemiology and the promotion of the development of networks aiming for comparability and validity of data and results across nations and regions

Working Group on: Improving the Quality of Patient Associations

- associations should agree on how to define a 'good association'
- ensure monitoring and evaluation of selected aspects of association activities
- associations of 'excellence' should assist the 'less accomplished' in becoming better

Working Group on: Implementing National Diabetes Programmes: lessons learned

- task forces should be multidisciplinary and ensure wide endorsement
- targets should be modest and changes achievable

- resources for change should be allocated at the clinical level
- data on aspects of health economy should be collected

Working Group on: The Role of the Media: have they contributed to improved diabetes care?

- diabetes magazines and newspapers should be encouraged to print information on current issues related to diabetes mellitus and on items regarding education of persons with diabetes
- articles in magazines regarding healthy lifestyles for persons with diabetes should be presented in a comprehensive and attractive fashion in order to reach more people
- the media of television is considered the most effective tool for dissemination of information during public awareness campaigns

Working Group on: Information Technology: 1) Lessons Learned - Future Strategies, 2) Confidentiality and Ethics in the Data Age: differences between theory and practice?

- disseminate the legal contents of the European directives on data privacy and the European recommendation on medical databases as a common background for data exchange
- generate awareness of the importance of confidentiality and data security in daily practice
- make health care professionals more aware of their duties and persons with diabetes more informed of their rights to privacy by providing comprehensive information
- implement data protection systems on a routine basis using existing solutions, password or smartcard/cryptography or hashing techniques, and firewall to protect data access-on site or on the network
- future use of databases and registers should be based on regular access rather than on explicit restriction

- a European code of conduct for databases (epidemiological, clinical and quality of care) should be developed and implemented and harmonized with the initiative from the international epidemiology association

Working Group on: Improving the Quality of Diabetes Care: the role of the nurse in the St. Vincent team

- create a database for identification of 'best practice'

- ensure additional training of nurses both in general and specific fields

- ensure training of the nurse within the frame of the health care team

Working Group on: Diabetes in Children and Adolescents: how can quality of care be improved?

- political pressure towards free availability of insulin and strips for home glucose monitoring for all children and adolescents under 18 years of age

- improve and individualize management and insulin treatment

- translate and distribute *'Consensus Guidelines for Management of Diabetes in Children and Adolescents'* and the *'BIS for children and adolescents'*

- improve quality of care through active use and benchmarking of the BIS within and between countries

- further develop networks of health professionals engaged in the care of children and adolescents

Working Group on: What is the Role of Industry in Improving Quality of Diabetes Care?

- prioritization is critical

- utilize criteria matrix

- regular St. Vincent and industry interface

- clarification of ownership of data

Working Group on: Diabetic Nephropathy: how can delivery of care be improved?

- develop and evaluate systems for integrated care for persons with diabetes in general and for those with nephropathy in particular

- support immediate implementation of minimal guidelines for: screening all persons with diabetes for microalbuminuria/nephropathy annually; in cases of positive tests, aim for: $HbA_{IC} < 8\%$, blood pressure, $<140/90$; total cholesterol $\leq 5.3\,mmol/L$; smoking cessation through special programmes

- existing knowledge should be used rather than wait for new data

Working Group on: Wellbeing and Quality of Life for Persons with Diabetes

- develop disease specific items for chronic disorders

- develop diabetes-specific items

- develop procedures for data analysis and translation of scales into local languages

Working Group on: The Common Enemy: stroke and heart disease

- reduce the risk of myocardial infarction and stroke by 30-40% in persons with diabetes

- prevention of myocardial infarction and stroke in high risk groups through treatment of hypertension and high lipid levels and improved lifestyles

- set up research following a pre-established priorities list

Further Information

An evaluation of the targets of the Working Groups to be made at the end of the ten-year period 1989-1999. Since the setting up of these initial 23 Working Groups, further groups have been formed and have been subdivided by area of interest, i.e. Education and Empowerment; Quality Development; Children and Adolescents; Outcomes; Expanding the Diabetes Team Partnership; Implementation and future developments. For further information please contact: Ms Helle Rink, SVD Secretariat, World Health Organization, Regional Office for Europe, Scherfigsvej 8, 2100 Copenhagen, Denmark.

APPENDIX XI–C

WHO-Euro Working Group Report on
Therapeutic Patient Education

Continuing Education Programmes for Healthcare Providers in the Field of Prevention of Chronic Diseases

Jean-Philippe Assal

At the request of Dr. J. E. Asvall, Regional Director of WHO-Euro in Copenhagen, Denmark, a WHO Working Group meeting was held in Grimentz, Switzerland in 1997. This meeting was aimed at producing a document dealing with the training of health care providers in the field of therapeutic patient education and long-term follow-up for chronic diseases. Fifteen experts coming from ten European countries critically discussed, appraised and produced this document, setting out proposals for continuing education programmes for health care providers working in the field of prevention of chronic diseases, taking into account translation difficulties, varying healthcare systems, as well as cultural and political influences with the different European countries. Recommendations were made to various bodies such as the health and pharmaceutical industries, institutes where health care providers are trained, member states and at the level of WHO-Euro.

This document is supported by the World Health Organization's *European Health 21, Target 18: By the year 2010, all Member States should have ensured that health professionals and professionals in other sectors have acquired appropriate knowledge, attitudes and skills to protect and promote health,* and it is significant to note that the World Health Organization puts Therapeutic Patient Education as one of the priorities in its training programmes for better long-term follow-up of patients.

Therapeutic Patient Education has been defined by the World Health Organization as follows:
 Therapeutic Patient Education ...

- **should enable patients to acquire and maintain abilites that allow them to optimally manage their lives with their disease;**

- **is a continuous process, integrated in health care, it is patient centred;**

- **includes organized awareness, information, self-care leaning and psychosocial support regarding the disease, prescribed treatment, hospital and other health care settings, organizational information, and behaviour related to health and illness;**

- **is designed to help patients and their families understand the disease and the treatment, cooperate with health care providers, live healthily and maintain or improve their quality of life.**

Listed below is a sample of the training modules suggested in this WHO-Euro Working Group Report:

Module 1: Adapting the behaviour of professionals to the specific features of chronic diseases

Objectives At the end of this one week module, participants will be able to:

- differentiate acute illness and crises from chronic diseases

- indicate how to change from a disease-centred to a patient-centred educational approach

- apply the theoretical implications of those approaches

- manage patients by means of a bio-psycho-social approach to which an educational and managerial approach has to be added

- integrate this approach in a multiprofessional and interdisciplinary model

Module 2: Understanding the patient with chronic disease

Objectives At the end of this one week module, participants will be able to:

- identify the patient's methods of coping with the disease and the treatment

- recognize and adapt to the patient's health beliefs and beliefs about the disease and its treatment

- adopt appropriate measures and attitudes to help the patient cope with difficulties

- practice active listening to the patient

- distinguish between the concepts of chronic disease and disability

Module 3: Taking account of patients' means of coping with their disease

Objectives At the end of this one week module, participants will be able to:

- select from each course key concepts illustrating its therapeutic content

- use different educational methods to explain to a patient one key concept

- construct different problem-cases to be solved

- describe and evaluate the patient's gains (skills and behaviour) related to the patient's own experience

- moderate a group discussion (patients, families) about the management of treatment

- create an assessment tool for the evaluation of patient performance

Module 4: Communicating with the patient

Objectives At the end of this one week module, participants will be able to:

- select the attitudes that favour communication

- assess a patient's emotional state

- hold support talks with patients individually

- moderate a group discussion

- define different profiles of attitudes

Module 5: Instructing the patient about the management of the treatment

Objectives At the end of this one week module, participants will be able to:

- recognize and indicate the difficulties that healthcare providers encounter

- explain to, and instruct, a patient about a prescription

- evaluate the extent to which a patient understood an explanation and instructions about a prescription

- recognise and deal with the difficulties related to the patient's adherence to treatment

- plan the therapeutic follow-up for the short and medium terms

Module 6: Assisting a patient in coping with the illness and the treatment

Objectives At the end of this one week module, participants will be able to:

- describe how an adult patient learns

- identify the three learning domains - intellectual, psychomotor and interpersonal communication

- state patients' learning objectives

- recognize the effect of patients' health beliefs on their learning process

- adapt the teaching to the patient's coping process

Module 7: Developing therapeutic education for patients

Objectives At the end of this one week module, participants will be able to:

- write learning objectives (of healthcare provider) relevant to the needs of the patient

- use methods and organization facilitating the patient's learning process

- choose and use different educational tools according to their efficacy

- organize educational programmes on the basis of individual patients' needs and educational abilities

- conduct group education

Module 8: Evaluation of a learning process and the methods used

Objectives At the end of this one week module, participants will be able to:

- distinguish the different functions of evaluation
- construct ways and markers to evaluate a given course
- evaluate the educational quality of a therapeutic education programme
- evaluate the educational quality of a therapeutic education session
- evaluate the impact of a therapeutic education programme

Module 9: Long term care of patients

Objectives At the end of this one week module, participants will be able to:

- describe how the patient relates to the disease and the treatment
- describe and manage the patient's personal health beliefs and conceptions
- adopt educational approaches and attitudes appropriate to the patient's difficulties
- take into account and use the `mistakes' made by the patient
- use means of preventing relapse

Module 10: Assessing one's learning gains

Objectives At the end of this one week module, participants will be able to:

- identify, among the learning objectives selected at the start of the modules, those they have achieved partially or not at all
- determine why this happened (poor time-planning, inefficient learning methods, etc.)
- prepare a plan of home-work in order to learn what is still missing
- prepare a plan of action for putting into operation the newly acquired competencies

Further Information

This Report is now in publication. For further details please contact: Prof. Jean-Philippe Assal, Chief, Division of Therapeutic Education for Chronic Diseases, University Hospital, Annexe Thury, 1211 Geneva 14, Switzerland.

APPENDIX XII

Values in Common and System International (SI) Units

John K. Davidson

Système International (SI) units have largely replaced common units in medical and scientific literature. For example, the common units for glucose of 140 mg/dL are now expressed in SI units as 7.8 mM. Table XII–1 lists SI units and common units, and factors for the conversion of common units to SI units and for conversion of SI units to common units.

TABLE XII–I   Système International (SI) Units for Plasma, Serum, or Blood Concentrations

Measurement	Conventional Unit	Conversion Factor	SI Unit	Significant Digits	Suggested Minimum Increments
Acetoacetate	mg/dL	97.95	μmol/L	XXO	10 μmol/L
Acetone	mg/dL	172.2	μmol/L	XXO	10 μmol/L
Adrenocorticotropin	pg/mL	0.2202	pmol/L	XX	1 pmol/L
Aldosterone	ng/dL	27.74	pmol/L	XXO	10 pmol/L
Amino acids					
Alanine	mg/dL	112.2	μmol/L	XXX	5 μmol/L
α-Aminobutyric acid	mg/dL	96.97	μmol/L	XXX	5 μmol/L
Arginine	mg/dL	57.40	μmol/L	XXX	5 μmol/L
Asparagine	mg/dL	75.69	μmol/L	XXX	5 μmol/L
Aspartic acid	mg/dL	75.13	μmol/L		5 μmol/L
Citrulline	mg/dL	57.08	μmol/L	XXX	5 μmol/L
Cystine	mg/dL	41.61	μmol/L	XXX	5 μmol/L
Glutamic acid	mg/dL	67.97	μmol/L	XXX	5 μmol/L
Glutamine	mg/dL	68.42	μmol/L	XXX	5 μmol/L
Glycine	mg/dL	133.2	μmol/L	XXX	5 μmol/L
Histidine	mg/dL	64.45	μmol/L	XXX	5 μmol/L
Hydroxyproline	mg/dL	76.26	μmol/L	XXX	5 μmol/L
Isoleucine	mg/dL	76.24	μmol/L	XXX	5 μmol/L
Leucine	mg/dL	76.24	μmol/L	XXX	5 μmol/L
Lysine	mg/dL	68.40	μmol/L	XXX	5 μmol/L
Methionine	mg/dL	67.02	μmol/L	XXX	5 μmol/L
Ornithine	mg/dL	75.67	μmol/L	XXX	5 μmol/L
Phenylalanine	mg/dL	60.54	μmol/L	XXX	5 μmol/L
Proline	mg/dL	86.86	μmol/L	XXX	5 μmol/L
Serine	mg/dL	95.16	μmol/L	XXX	5 μmol/L
Taurine	mg/dL	79.91	μmol/L	XXX	5 μmol/L
Threonine	mg/dL	83.95	μmol/L	XXX	5 μmol/L
Tryptophan	mg/dL	48.97	μmol/L	XXX	5 μmol/L
Tyrosine	mg/dL	55.19	μmol/L	XXX	5 μmol/L
Valine	mg/dL	85.36	μmol/L	XXX	5 μmol/L
Amino acid nitrogen	mg/dL	0.7139	mmol/L	X.X	0.1 mmol/L
Amylase	U/L	1.0	U/L	XXO	10 U/L
Androstenedione	μg/L	3.492	nmol/L	XX.X	0.5 nmol/L
Calcitonin	pg/mL	1.0	ng/L	XXO	10 ng/L
Calcium	mg/dL	0.2495	mmol/L	X.XX	0.02 nmol/L

(continued)

TABLE XII–I   *(continued)*   Système International (SI) Units for Plasma, Serum, or Blood Concentrations

Measurement	Conventional Unit	Conversion Factor	SI Unit	Significant Digits	Suggested Minimum Increments
Calcium ion	meq/L	0.500	mmol/L	X.XX	0.01 mmol/L
Carbon dioxide content	meq/L	1.00	nmol/L	XX	1 mmol/L
Cholesterol	mg/dL	0.02586	mmol/L	X.XX	0.05 mmol/L
Citrate (as citric acid)	mg/dL	52.05	μmol/L	XXX	5 μmol/L
Cortisol	μg/dL	27.59	nmol/L	XXO	10 nmol/L
C-peptide	ng/mL	0.331	nmol/L	XXX	0.01 nmol/L
Creatinine	mg/dL	88.40	μmol/L	XXO	10 μmol/L
Creatinine clearance	ml/min	0.01667	ml/s	X.XX	0.02 mL/s
cyclic AMP	μg/L	3.038	nmol/L	XXX	1 nmol/L
cyclic GMP	μg/L	2.897	nmol/L	XX.X	0.1 nmol/L
Dehydroepiandrosterone	μg/L	3.467	nmol/L	XX.X	0.2 nmol/L
Dehydroepiandrosterone sulfate	ng/mL	0.002714	μmol/L	XX.X	0.1 μmol/L
11-Deoxycortisol	μg/dL	28.86	nmol/L	XXO	10 nmol/L
Epinephrine	pg/mL	5.458	pmol/L	XXO	10 pmol/L
Estradiol	pg/mL	3.671	pmol/L	XXX	1 pmol/L
Estrone	pg/mL	3.699	pmol/L	XXX	5 pmol/L
Fatty acids, nonesterified	mg/dL	0.01	g/L	X.XX	0.01 g/L
Follicle-stimulating hormone	mIU/mL	1.00	IU/L	XX	1 IU/L
Fructose	mg/dL	0.05551	mmol/L	X.XX	0.1 mmol/L
Galactose	mg/dL	0.05551	mmol/L	X.XX	0.1 mmol/L
Gases					
P_{O_2}	mmHg	0.1333	kPa	XX.X	0.1 kPa
P_{CO_2}	mmHg	0.1333	kPa	X.X	0.1 kPa
Gastrin	pg/mL	1.0	ng/L	XXO	10 ng/L
Gastroinhibitory polypeptide	pg/mL	0.201	pmol/L	XXO	10 pmol/L
Glucagon	pg/mL	1.0	ng/L	XXO	10 ng/L
Glucose	mg/dL	0.05551	mmol/L	XX.X	0.1 mmol/L
Glycerol, free	mg/dL	0.1086	mmol/L	X.XX	0.01 mmol/L
Growth hormone	ng/mL	1.0	μg/L	XX.X	0.5 μg/L
β-Hydroxybutyrate	mg/dL	96.05	μmol/L	XXO	10 μmol/L
(as β-hydroxybutyric acid)					
17α-Hydroxyprogesterone	μg/L	3.026	nmol/L	XX.X	0.5 nmol/L
Insulin	μU/mL	6.0	pmol/L	XXX	5 pmol/L
Lactate (as lactic acid)	mEq/L	1.0	mmol/L	X.X	0.1 mmol/L
Lipase	U/L	1.0	U/L	XXX	1 U/L
Lipoproteins				X.XX	
LDL (as cholesterol)	mg/dL	0.02586	mmol/L	X.XX	0.05 mmol/L
HDL (as cholesterol)	mg/dL	0.02586	mmol/L	XXX	0.05 mmol/L
Luteinizing hormone	mIU/mL	1.0	IU/L	X.XX	1 IU/L
Norepinephrine	pg/mL	0.005911	nmol/L	XXX	0.01 nmol/L
Osmolality	mOsm/kg	1.0	mmol/kg	XX	1 mmol/kg
Pancreatic polypeptide	pg/mL	0.239	pmol/L	X.XX	1 pmol/L
Phosphate (as inorganic phosphorus)	meq/dL	0.3229	mmol/L	X.XX	0.05 mmol/L
Phospholipid phosphorus	mg/dL	0.3229	mmol/L	XX	0.05 mmol/L
Progesterone	ng/mL	3.180	nmol/L	XX	2nmol/L
Prolactin	ng/mL	1.0	μg/L	XX	1μg/L
Protein, total	g/dL	10.0	g/L	XX	1g/L
Pyruvate (as pyruvic acid)	mg/dL	113.6	μmol/L	XXX	1μmol/L
Renin	ng·mL^{-1}·h^{-1}	0.2778	ng·L^{-1}·s^{-1}	X.XX	0.02 ng·L^{-1}·s^{-1}
Serotonin	μg/dL	0.05675	μmol/L	X.XX	0.05 μmol/L
Somatostatin	pg/mL	0.611	pmol/L	XX	1pmol/L
Testosterone	ng/mL	3.467	nmol/L	XX.X	0.5 nmol/L
Thyroid-stimulating hormone	μU/dL	1.0	mU/L	X.X	0.1 mU/L
Thyroxine	μg/dL	12.87	nmol/L	XXX	1nmol/L
Triiodothyronine	ng/dL	0.01536	nmol/L	X.X	0.1 nmol/L
Urea nitrogen	mg/dL	0.3570	mmol/L	X.X	0.5 nmol/L
Vasoactive intestinal polypeptide	pg/mL	0.331	pmol/L	X.X	1 pmol/L

Largely from Young DS: Ann Intern Med 106:114–129, 1987. For insulin see Vølund A, Brange J, Drejer K, Jensen I, Markussen J, Ribel V, Sørensen AR, Schlichtkrull J: In vitro and in vivo potency of insulin analogues designed for clinical use. Diabet Med 8:839–847, 1991. (*Source*: Diabetes 47:306, 1998. With permission.)

Index

Page numbers in *italics* indicate figures. Page numbers followed by "t" indicate tables.